TEXTBOOK OF RADIOTHERAPY

GILBERT H. FLETCHER, M.D. *Radiotherapist, Professor of Radiotherapy Head of Department of Radiotherapy, The University of Texas M. D. Anderson Hospital and Tumor Institute, Houston, Texas*

TEXTBOOK OF RADIOTHERAPY

427 Illustrations

SECOND EDITION

LEA & FEBIGER   PHILADELPHIA

Library of Congress Cataloging in Publication Data

Fletcher, Gilbert Hungerford, 1911–
    Textbook of Radiotherapy.
  1. Radiotherapy. I. Title. [DNLM: 1. Radiotherapy.
WN 100 F612t 1973]
RM847.F53 1973   615'.842   73-6569
ISBN 0-8121-0438-2

Reprinted, 1975

ISBN 0-8121-0438-2

Library of Congress Catalog Card Number 73-6569

Published in Great Britain by Henry Kimpton Publishers, London

PRINTED IN THE UNITED STATES OF AMERICA

Preface

The basic pattern of the second edition has not been changed, being inspired by Paterson's first edition of *Treatment of Malignant Diseases by Radiotherapy*, with its subtitle, *A Practice of Radiotherapy*. Quoting Paterson, "The presentation of a definite outlook is of more value than the discussion of different principles and practices. It does not mean to imply that it is the only way, or the best, or the most correct method but may leave the reader with something concrete."

The clinical background pertinent to the justification and understanding of the techniques has been considerably expanded. Radiotherapy is a fast evolving speciality and since the first edition significant changes have happened in many areas. The results of treatment in the head and neck, breast and gynecological cancers treated at the M. D. Anderson Hospital have been exhaustively studied. This information is essential for the understanding of the particular techniques used.

The chapter on radiological physics is limited to practical points of treatment planning not discussed in the classical books of radiological physics.

Houston, Texas

As in the first edition, the major part of the textbook is based on the practices in existence at the M. D. Anderson Hospital. The radiotherapists at other institutions asked to participate in the first edition have been asked again to contribute, following the same pattern of presentation.

Although the main core of the treatment can be done with ^{60}Co units (similar to 4 to 6 Mev beams), the increasing availability of high energy photon beams and electron beams justifies the need to expand on their specific uses.

Radiotherapy operates more and more in a closely associated surgical context and to a chemotherapy context in some cancers. Specialists in various fields have been asked to expand on their initial chapters of the first edition.

We wish to acknowledge the editing of Miss Joan McCay and the secretarial help of Mrs. Barbara Foremsky and Mrs. Judy Lugrin. My family and the office force, headed by Mrs. Helen Atterbury, have borne the manifestations of a temperament worn thinner by the second edition than the first one.

GILBERT H. FLETCHER, M.D.

Contributing and Collaborating Authors

PETER R. ALMOND, B.S.C., M.A., Ph.D., Physicist and Professor of Biophysics, Chief Section of Radiation Physics, The University of Texas M. D. Anderson Hospital and Tumor Institute at Houston, Houston, Texas.

MALCOLM A. BAGSHAW, M.D., Professor of Radiology, Stanford University School of Medicine, Director, Division of Radiotherapy, Stanford Medical Center, Palo Alto, California.

FERNANDO G. BLOEDORN, M.D., Chairman and Professor, Radiotherapist-in-Chief, Department of Therapeutic Radiology, Tufts University School of Medicine, New England Medical Center Hospitals, Boston, Massachusetts.

JEAN BOUCHARD, M.D., Professor of Radiology and Chairman of Department, Faculty of Medicine, McGill University; Radiologist-in-Chief, Department of Therapeutic Radiology, Royal Victoria Hospital, Montreal, Canada.

GEORGE R. BROWN, M.D., Associate Radiotherapist and Associate Professor of Radiotherapy, The University of Texas M. D. Anderson Hospital and Tumor Institute at Houston, Houston, Texas.

ROBERT M. BYERS, M.D., Assistant Surgeon (Head and Neck Service), Assistant Professor of Surgery, The University of Texas M. D. Anderson Hospital and Tumor Institute at Houston, Houston, Texas.

JOSEPH R. CASTRO, M.D., Chief, Department of Radiation Therapy, Zellerbach Saroni Tumor Institute of Mt. Zion Hospital and Medical Center; Clinical Professor of Radiology (Radiation Oncology), University of California at San Francisco, San Francisco, California.

THOMAS E. DALY, D.D.S., Assistant Clinical Dental Surgeon, The University of Texas M. D. Anderson Hospital and Tumor Institute at Houston; Assistant Professor, The University of Texas Dental Branch at Houston, Houston, Texas.

LUIS DELCLOS, M.D., Radiotherapist and Professor of Radiotherapy, The University of Texas M. D. Anderson Hospital and Tumor Institute at Houston, Houston, Texas.

FREDERICK L. FAW, M.S., Physicist, Radiation Branch, National Cancer Institute, Bethesda, Maryland.

CARLOS H. FERNANDEZ, M.D., Assistant Radiotherapist and Instructor in Radiotherapy, The University of Texas M. D. Anderson Hospital and Tumor Institute at Houston, Houston, Texas.

LILLIAN M. FULLER, M.D., Radiotherapist and Associate Professor of Radiotherapy, The University of Texas M. D. Anderson Hospital and Tumor Institute at Houston, Houston, Texas.

DWIGHT W. GLENN, M.S., Physicist, Radiation Branch, National Cancer Institute, Bethesda, Maryland.

HELMUTH GOEPFERT, M.D., Research Project

Investigator, Head and Neck Surgery, The University of Texas M. D. Anderson Hospital and Tumor Institute at Houston, Houston, Texas, and Resident, Department of Otolaryngology, Baylor College of Medicine, Houston, Texas.

OSCAR M. GUILLAMONDEGUI, M.D., Assistant Surgeon (Head and Neck Service), Assistant Professor of Surgery, The University of Texas M. D. Anderson Hospital and Tumor Institute at Houston, Houston, Texas.

ULRICH K. HENSCHKE, M.D., Ph.D., Professor and Chairman, Department of Radiotherapy, College of Medicine, Howard University, Washington, D. C.

BASIL S. HILARIS, M.D., Associate Attending Radiation Therapist, Memorial Hospital, New York, New York.

PHILIP T. HUDGINS, M.D., Chief of Radiotherapy, Methodist Hospital; Clinical Associate Professor, Department of Radiology, Baylor College of Medicine, Houston, Texas.

RICHARD H. JESSE, M.D., Surgeon and Professor of Surgery, Chief, Section of Head and Neck Surgery, The University of Texas M. D. Anderson Hospital and Tumor Institute at Houston, Houston, Texas.

RALPH E. JOHNSON, M.D., Chief of the Radiation Branch, National Cancer Institute, Bethesda, Maryland

C. H. JONES, Ph.D., Senior Hospital Physicist, Physics Department, The Institute of Cancer Research, Royal Cancer Hospital, London, England.

MANUEL LEDERMAN, M.D., D.M.R.E., F.F.R., Deputy Director, Radiotherapy Department, Royal Marsden Hospital; Consultant Radiotherapist to Chelsea Hospital for Women, Moors Field Eye Hospital, and Royal National Throat, Nose and Ear Hospital, London, England.

ROBERT D. LINDBERG, M.D., Radiotherapist and Professor of Radiotherapy, The University of Texas M. D. Anderson Hospital and Tumor Institute at Houston, Houston, Texas.

LOWELL S. MILLER, M.D., Radiotherapist and Associate Professor of Radiotherapy, The University of Texas M. D. Anderson Hospital and Tumor Institute at Houston, Houston, Texas.

RODNEY R. MILLION, M.D., Chief of Radiotherapy, University of Florida Teaching Hospital; Professor, University of Florida, Gainesville, Florida.

ELEANOR D. MONTAGUE, M.D., Radiotherapist and Professor of Radiotherapy, The University of Texas M. D. Anderson Hospital and Tumor Institute at Houston, Houston, Texas.

R. F. MOULD, M.Sc., Ph.D., M.Inst.P., Principal Physicist, Westminster Hospital, London, SW1.

MURIEL C. PELHAM, B.S., Director of Dietetic Services, The University of Texas M. D. Anderson Hospital and Tumor Institute at Houston, Houston, Texas.

CARLOS A. PEREZ, M.D., Radiotherapist, Division of Radiation Therapy, Mallinckrodt Institute; Associate Professor of Radiotherapy, Washington University School of Medicine, St. Louis, Missouri.

BLANCHE POLUNSKY, B.S., Assistant Director of Dietetic Services, The University of Texas M. D. Anderson Hospital and Tumor Institute at Houston, Houston, Texas.

FELIX N. RUTLEDGE, M.D., Gynecologist, Professor of Gynecology, Head, Department of Gynecology, The University of Texas M. D. Anderson Hospital and Tumor Institute at Houston, Houston, Texas.

VINCENT A. SAMPIERE, Instructor in Physics, The University of Texas M. D. Anderson Hospital and Tumor Institute at Houston, Houston, Texas.

MELVIN L. SAMUELS, M.D., Internist, Associate Professor of Medicine, Chief, Section of General Medicine and Oncology, The University of Texas M. D. Anderson Hospital and Tumor Institute at Houston, Houston, Texas.

ROBERT J. SHALEK, Ph.D., Physicist, Professor of Biophysics, Chief, Section of Medical Physics, Head, Department of Physics, The University of Texas M. D. Anderson

Hospital and Tumor Institute at Houston, Houston, Texas.

JULIAN P. SMITH, M.D., Associate Gynecologist and Associate Professor of Gynecology, The University of Texas M. D. Anderson Hospital and Tumor Institute at Houston, Houston, Texas.

H. B. STALLARD, M.B.E., T.D., M.A., M.D., LL.D., F.R.C.S., Surgeon in Charge, Eye Department, St. Bartholomew's Hospital; Consultant Surgeon, Moorsfield Eye Hospital; Late Major, R.A.M.C., T.A., London, England.

HERMAN D. SUIT, M.D., D.Phil., Radiotherapist, Chief of Department of Radiation Medicine, Massachusetts General Hospital; Professor of Radiation Therapy, Harvard Medical School, Boston, Massachusetts.

WATARU W. SUTOW, M.D., Pediatrician, Professor of Pediatrics, Acting Head, Department of Pediatrics, The University of Texas M. D. Anderson Hospital and Tumor Institute at Houston, Houston, Texas.

ROBERT W. SWAIN, B.S., Physicist, Radiation Branch, National Cancer Institute, Bethesda, Maryland.

NORAH DUV. TAPLEY, M.D., Radiotherapist and Professor of Radiotherapy, The University of Texas M. D. Anderson Hospital and Tumor Institute at Houston, Houston, Texas.

CARL F. VON ESSEN, M.D., Professor of Radiology and Oncology, The University of California, San Diego; Chief, Radiation Therapy Division, University Hospital of San Diego County, San Diego, California.

CHARLES VOTAVA, JR., M.D., Associate Radiotherapist, Radiation Center, Latter-day Saints Hospital, Salt Lake City, Utah.

KENT C. WESTBROOK, M.D., Assistant Professor of Surgery, University of Arkansas Medical Center, Little Rock, Arkansas.

J. TAYLOR WHARTON, M.D., Assistant Gynecologist and Assistant Professor of Gynecology, The University of Texas M. D. Anderson Hospital and Tumor Institute at Houston, Houston, Texas.

IVOR GLYN WILLIAMS, M.B., F.R.C.S. (Eng.), F.F.R., D.M.R.E., Director of Radiotherapy Department, St. Bartholomew's Hospital; Consultant Radiotherapist, The Hospital for Sick Children, London, England.

Contents

1. General Considerations

2. Basic Principles of Radiotherapy

3. Head and Neck (Excluding Central Nervous System and Orbit)

13.

14.

15.

1. General Considerations

Radiation Measurement and Dosimetric Practices

VINCENT A. SAMPIERE, PETER R. ALMOND, and ROBERT J. SHALEK

It is the purpose of this section to present the methods of dose measurement and dose calculation in radiation therapy employed at The University of Texas at Houston M. D. Anderson Hospital and Tumor Institute. Those practical aspects of dosimetry which are required to implement the clinical methods described in this book will be emphasized. Since the methods utilized in interstitial and intracavitary radium treatment have been published recently[24,25] the discussions relating to these subjects will be limited and most of the section will be devoted to external beam techniques.

Basic Dose Determination

Measurement of Radiation Dose from Various Therapy Machines

The radiation doses delivered by various therapy machines are measured at regular intervals with a suitably calibrated ionization chamber described below.

In addition to a weekly calibration with a convenient instrument, it is advisable to employ a second independent method which can be utilized once or twice a year. For this purpose ferrous-sulfate chemical dosimetry is excellent since the yield of ferric ions is known and thus no further reference to radiation standards is required; however, the high total doses needed (4,000 to 8,000 rads) usually require long exposures.[23]

Calibration Jigs. X-ray and gamma-beam units have jigs constructed to ensure that chambers are held in identical relationship to the source each time a calibration is done. The jig is designed so that with the widest field, there is no chance of the primary beam hitting the jig itself.

Timer Errors. It is particularly important to determine the relationship of the exposure time to the time set on the timer. The difference arises from "end-errors" at the beginning and at the end of exposures. These end-errors produce the same time error regardless of the total length of exposure. While this error is usually insignificant compared to the time required for a clinical treatment, it may be appreciable in the small time required for the exposure of a 25-R or 100-R chamber. The timer error may be determined in a graphical manner by setting a number of different small times on the clock and taking readings with a dosimeter. Results are plotted and extrapolated to zero dose (Fig. 1-1). The slope is proportional to the exposure rate and the intercept on the horizontal axis is the time to be added to or subtracted from the time set on the timer. The graphical method depends upon the

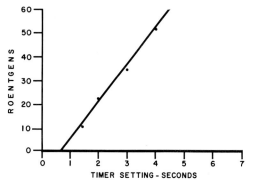

FIG. 1-1. Method of deriving timer errors. Timer errors arise from differences in true exposure time and that recorded by the timer. A plot of radiation dose versus timer setting extrapolated to zero dose indicates the amount of time to be added to or subtracted from the time set on the timer to give the true exposure time. In the instance shown the intercept, 0.7 seconds, should be subtracted from the time set on the timer in order to obtain the time of irradiation.

result in measured output variations of up to 15 per cent.

In the initial calibration of a radiation therapy unit, it is usual to measure the variation of exposure for the full range of treatment fields. It is convenient to express the change in output with change in field area as a ratio to the standard calibration field area (Fig. 1-2). The exposure rate for any field is then calculated by multiplying the exposure rate for the standard field by the appropriate ratio.

linearity of the measuring instrument. Another numerical method which is independent of instrument linearity calculates the timer error, α, by exposing the instrument to a single exposure yielding a reading M_1, in time t_1, and also to several (n) shorter exposures accumulating a total reading M_2 in a total time t_2. The two times should be equal or approximately so. Since the exposure rates in the two cases are equal, then

$$\frac{M_1}{t_1 + \alpha} = \frac{M_1}{t_2 + n\alpha}$$

and

$$\alpha = \frac{M_2 t_1 - M_1 t_2}{M_1 n - M_2}.$$

If α is positive it is added to the timer time; if α is negative it is subtracted from the timer time.

Field-Size Dependence. The radiation exposure in air varies with field size, trimmer position, and type of collimating system.

Scattering from collimating parts will be different for various field settings; this can

Kilovoltage X-ray Machines. The kilovoltage x-ray machines are calibrated on a weekly basis. The weekly calibration is compared with the current exposure rate in use. If a change of output has occurred between calibrations it is usually possible to make an estimate of the dose that the patient received with an uncertainty that is small compared with the total dose during the course of treatment. If there is more than a 2 per cent change, a repeat calibration is made. If the difference persists, new exposure rates are assigned to the machine. When the change is substantial, a daily calibration routine is initiated to observe any further fluctuations in the machine's performance.

^{60}CO. The cobalt units are calibrated monthly and the readings compared with the decay curve. If the readings and the decay curves differ by more than 2 per cent, an investigation is made to determine the cause. The most likely cause is a change in timer error caused by the shutter mechanism moving at a new speed. Otherwise the promulgated output of the machine is not altered except for the first day of each month in accordance with radioactive decay.

With the ^{60}Co irradiators, the exposure is measured in air for a 10 × 10 cm field with the center of the ionization chamber of the secondary standard at the point of measurement. The secondary standard is either a Baldwin-Farmer instrument or a Victoreen 100-R thimble chamber. The chamber is

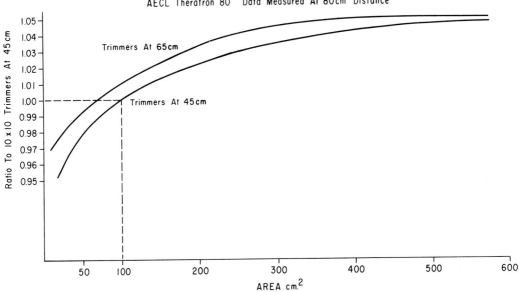

FIELD SIZE DEPENDENCE CURVE
AECL Theratron 80   Data Measured At 80cm Distance

FIG. 1-2. The relative exposure rate for two trimmer positions and various collimator settings. Measurements are at 80 cm distance for a particular *AECL* Theratron 80. The standard field size in this example is 10 × 10 cm with the trimmers at 45 cm.

fitted with the appropriate buildup cap (4 mm Lucite). The machines are calibrated in terms of exposure for a 10 × 10 field at 80.5 cm. The output is given by the following equation:

$$X_{air} = R \times N$$

X_{air} is the exposure in roentgens at the center of the chamber in the absence of the chamber, since the effects of its walls are included in the calibration factor; R is the chamber reading corrected for temperature and pressure (16) with the timer error taken into account; N is the exposure calibration factor for ^{60}Co gamma rays assigned to the chamber by the National Bureau of Standards with the stem correction taken into account. The given dose for any field size is then given by

$$D_{med} = R \times N \times A \times f_{med} \times \text{B.S.F.} \times \text{F.D.}$$

where D_{med} is the dose in rads in the medium; A is a factor which allows for the gamma-ray attenuation from the surface to 0.5 cm depth in tissue, $A = 0.985$; f_{med} is the rads per roentgen conversion for the medium ($f = 0.957$ rads/R for muscle); B.S.F. is the backscatter factor for the field size being used; and F.D. is the field size dependence measured in air (normalized to a 10 × 10 field). The dose at depth is then obtained by multiplying by the percentage depth dose for the appropriate field size and S.S.D.

Megavoltage X-ray. The dose delivered by the Allis-Chalmers Betatron is monitored by a transmission ionization chamber and a current integrator rather than by a timer, since the output fluctuates. Experience over the last ten years has shown this type of monitor to vary less than ±2 per cent under normal working conditions. Its accuracy is checked at least once a week with a 100-R Victoreen chamber in a cylindrical Lucite Buildup block with walls 4 cm thick, similar to that described in the literature.[27] It is important that the same field size be employed in each calibration since the stem effect for some 100-R Victoreen chambers may contribute up to 5 per cent of the observed reading, although for new chambers the stem effect is generally reduced to about 1 per cent. Correction factors for 22 Mev x-rays cannot be obtained at this time from the National Bureau of Standards. Chamber correction factors have been derived, however, from comparison of chambers with a local absorbed dose calorimeter and from comparison of the chambers with ferrous sulfate chemical dosimeters. The latter type of comparison is made once or twice a year. The correction factors used are in close agreement with those recommended by the Hospital Physicists Association[12] and by ICRU in Report 14.[15]

Electron Beam. The electron beam from the Siemens Betatron is monitored by a sealed ionization chamber placed in the edge of the beam. The output of the machine is measured with a Baldwin-Farmer ionization chamber. The chamber is placed in a Lucite phantom $15 \times 15 \times 10$ cm at a depth of 0.85 cm. The polystyrene phantom recommended by the American Association of Physicists in Medicine[2] may also be used. Calibration factors for the Baldwin-Farmer instrument for 6–18 Mev electrons have been derived by comparison with ferrous sulfate measurements in the same block. The correction factors derived are in close agreement with those reported in the literature.[1] The correction factors have also been checked with a local absorbed dose calorimeter. Because the measured output varies with respect to the monitor with time, the electron beam output is calibrated twice a week. Calibrations for special arrangements such as lead masks are carried out with the use of LiF thermoluminescent dosimeters (*TLD*).

In Vivo Dosimetry. In vivo measurements for verification of an individual treatment plan may be accomplished by the use of thermoluminescent dosimeters if the area of interest is accessible. The placement of such dosimeters via a nasogastric (Levin) tube is an example. Access to oral areas has been achieved by placing *TLD* in dental stents. The *TLD* is available in a variety of forms and configurations.

Usually, the dose to a given point delivered by a full treatment cycle is desired. To achieve a dose proportional to the total from a cycle, a selected fraction of the given dose to each field is treated on the same day with the dosimeter in place.

A carefully carried out measurement of this type may achieve ± 3 per cent over-all precision. The *TLD* is used in a relative sense, with a number of the dosimeters irradiated to a known dose. The dosimeters must either belong to a "batch" with known homogeneous response or have a known response relation to each other determined from prior irradiations.

Geometrical Parameters of the Beam

Source to Skin Distance (SSD). The source to skin distance (also known as *TSD* and *FSD* for target and focal skin distance respectively) refers to the distance usually along the central ray from the source of radiation to that part of the patient's skin that the beam enters.

Verification of the Inverse Square Law. With telecurie therapy machines, the apparent position of the source is sometimes closer to the patient than the physical position of the source. This effect is caused by small angle scattering in the head near the source and is thus highly dependent upon the machine design.

In the initial calibration of a unit, the effective source position can be determined experimentally by measuring the output at different distances with a constant collimator setting. The plot of the reciprocal of the square root of the dose rate, D.R., versus the distance yields a straight line. The intercept on the horizontal axis indicates the effective position of the source (Fig. 1-3). This distance can be used in inverse square calcula-

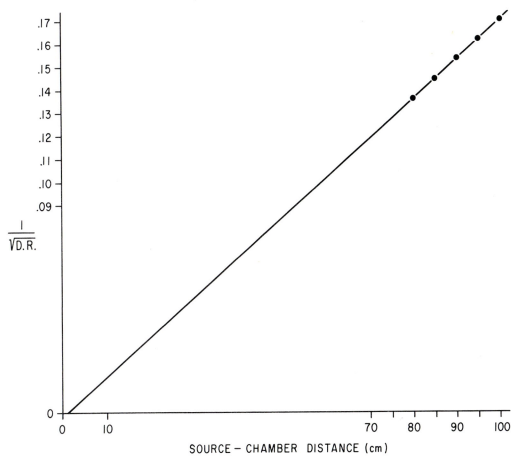

FIG. 1-3. The effective position of the source for a ^{60}Cobalt unit. The reciprocal of the exposure rate in air versus distance from the source is a linear relationship since,

$$D.R. = \frac{k}{d^2} \text{ and } d = \frac{\sqrt{k}}{\sqrt{D.R.}}$$

where D.R. is the exposure rate, d is the nominal distance from the source to the point of measurement and k is a proportionality constant.

tions relating distance and exposure rate for the same collimator setting.

Field Size Specification. ^{60}Co units of different manufacture with varying source diameters and collimation systems produce isodose patterns which can be different for the same field size specification, especially in the penumbra region. It is usual to define the radiation field with a particular percentage

isodose line of the radiation field. The actual percentage which is coincident with the light beam edge, and the width of the penumbra are important characteristics of each unit, therefore, when comparing treatment techniques between units, care should be given to the possible differences in these beam characteristics.

It is important to have isodose curves of good quality so that relationship of light beam and radiation beam is understood. If secondary blocking or penumbra trimmers are used in treatment, it is important to know their effect on the radiation beam (Fig. 1-4).

Modern ^{60}Co units with penumbra trimmers project a light field edge at the position where in air, the exposure rate is 50 per cent of that at the center of the field. In a phantom, the light field intersects between the 50 to 70 per cent isodose line along each edge of the field at the level of maximum dose. This specification of field size pertains to most of the clinical discussions in this book. However, the field size definition for published depth dose tables is to the 50 per cent

isodose in air and should be recognized in making comparisons.

Measurement of Field Size. Accurate measurement of field size in external beam therapy is necessary since exposure, backscatter factors, and depth dose percentages vary according to field area. The following aids are listed:

1) Field size: This is measured at the stated source-skin distance.

2) Sloping surface: The field is measured perpendicular to the central ray. The perpendicular measurement of field size is often difficult because of sloping skin surfaces; in

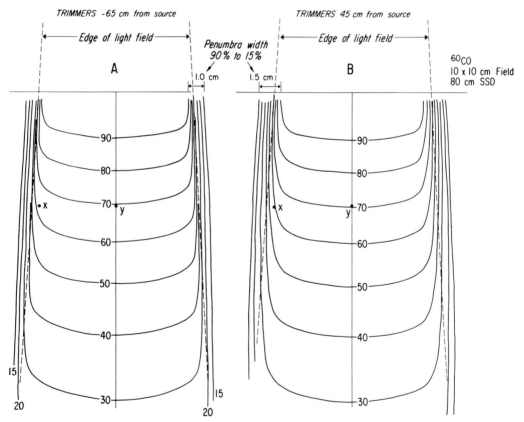

FIG. 1-4. Effect of the trimmer distance on the penumbra width of an AECL Theratron 80 is shown in **A** and **B**. A decrease in the separation between the 90 per cent and 15 per cent penumbra occurs with the trimmers at 65 cm from the source relative to the trimmers at 45 cm from the source.

The trimmer position is also relevant to the peripheral dose at a depth. Point X shown above is the perpendicular projection from the edge of the light field to a 7 cm depth. In **A** (trimmers at 65 cm), X is 10 per cent less than the central axis dose Y at the same depth and in **B** (trimmers at 45 cm) X is 16 per cent less than the central axis dose Y.

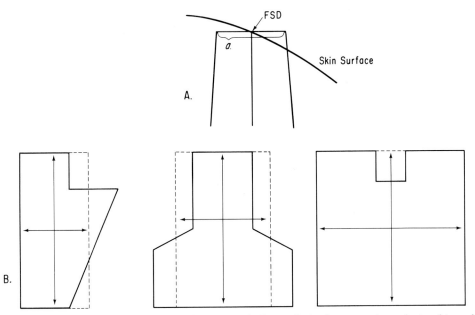

FIG. 1-5. Measurement of field sizes in unusual situations. **A.** For a radiation beam entering a sloping skin surface, the area of the beam is measured perpendicularly to the beam; one dimension of the field is a. **B.** The field areas taken to approximate a few irregularly shaped fields are shown.

such cases, measurement of one half of the field from central axis to edge may be doubled (Fig. 1-5A).

3) Irregularly shaped fields: It is helpful to approximate a rectangle which could be made from the irregular field drawn on the patient. To determine the area, the average width and length of the approximate rectangle are estimated as in Figure 1-5B.

The variation in dose across the field, particularly in areas of unusual shapes, can be calculated using the Clarkson method[4] where the scatter and primary radiation is calculated independently. An example of this variation is shown in Figure 1-6.

4) Elongation: A table of equivalent squares is used to determine the effective area of all rectangular fields.[6]

Alignment of Light Localizers. When light localizers are used to define a collimated radiation beam, it is necessary to routinely check the alignment of the light beam with the radiation beam. A misalignment of the light beam and the x-ray and gamma-ray

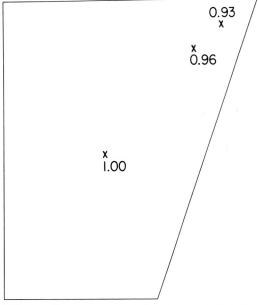

FIG. 1-6. The per cent depth dose to a constant depth was calculated to 3 selected points within an irregular-shaped cobalt field using the Clarkson method. The resultant percentages are shown as a ratio to the central axis dose and illustrate the reduction in dose due to the decreased scatter radiation.

beam may result from misadjustment of the light and mirrors or from location of the source off the axis of rotation of the light localizer. If the light source does not rotate with the light localizer, adjustment of the light to the radiation beam is usually straightforward, utilizing metal markers outlining the light field on a film. If the light beam and penetrating beam are aligned in one position of the light localizer, they will be aligned in all positions of the localizer. If the light source rotates with the light localizer, a more complex procedure, as demonstrated in Figure 1-7, is required.

Radiation Parameters of the Beam

Half-Value Layer (HVL). The *HVL* is the thickness of a specified material required to attenuate a radiation beam to half its original intensity under geometrical conditions in which little scatter from the absorbers reaches the detector. A small-beam size just large enough to insure full irradiation of the detector and a long distance from the absorbers to the detector (such as twice the distance from the source to the collimator) limits the scatter received into the detector.

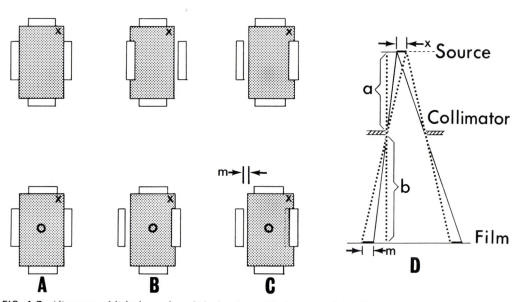

FIG. 1-7. Alignment of light beam from light localizer. Misalignment of the light beam to the radiation beam may result if the source of radiation is not on the axis of rotation of the light localizer or if the lights and mirrors are improperly adjusted. In types of light localizers in which the light system rotates, it is necessary to distinguish between these causes and to remedy the former before the latter. To test the alignment, a film is taken with strips of lead or other metal marking the edges of the field on a cardboard cassette. A corner of the film is marked. One exposure is taken with the localizer located at an arbitrarily selected 0 degree position (upper) and another exposure with the localizer rotated 180 degrees (lower with marked center). If the radiation beam and the light are in proper alignment, the resultant film is as shown in **A.** If the mirrors are out of adjustment, the result is as in **B.** If the radiation source is off the axis of rotation of the light localizer, the resultant film is as in **C.** The direction and the amount of movement of the source to place it on the axis of rotation is determined as in **D** from similar triangles: $x = m\dfrac{a}{b}$, where m is the discrepancy between the light and x-ray beam as in **C,** x is the required movement of the x-ray target, and a and b are the distances from the collimator to the target and the film. Adjustment of the lights and mirrors is accomplished by moving the light pattern to the radiation pattern.

Minimum scatter reaches the detector if the absorbers are placed at the collimator. Typical values are between 1 to 5 mm of aluminum in superficial x-ray machines, from 1 to 3 mm copper in kilovoltage machines and up to 15 mm of lead in megavoltage machines.

Backscatter Factors. The backscatter factors are defined as the ratio of the absorbed dose at a reference point in a phantom to the absorbed dose which would be measured at the same point in free air within a volume of the phantom material just large enough to provide maximum electronic buildup at the point of measurement. For up to 400 Kv radiation, the reference point is to be taken at the intersection of the central ray with the surface, while for radiation above 400 Kv, the reference point is to be taken at the position of the peak dose. Backscatter factors are functions of beam quality (*HVL*) and field size.[6,21]

Depth-Dose and Isodose Curves. The plot of dose along the central axis into tissue from the point of beam entry is called the central axis depth dose curve. The data are generally given as a ratio (expressed as a percentage) of the absorbed dose at a given depth to the absorbed dose at a fixed reference point on the central axis. For radiation up to 400 Kv the reference point is the surface. For radiation above 400 Kv, the reference point is at the position of the maximum absorbed dose, i.e., given dose. The central axis depth dose curve will vary with *SSD, HVL,* and field size. Lines of equal absorbed dose within a patient are referred to as isodose curves. They are usually expressed as percentages and are normalized to the same reference points as for the central axis depth-dose curves.

Production of Isodose Curves

Isodose curves for 60 cobalt can be obtained using automatic isosignal plotters which utilized a small ionization chamber in a water phantom. In our experience, film dosimetry at this energy can be misleading since the film response to the scattered radiation is greater than to the primary radiation.

Isodose curves for betatron x-rays and electron beams (6 to 18 Mev) have been determined using film. Kodak Translite or DuPont Adlux film has been found most suitable for the electron beam, and Kodak Type M industrial film found most suitable for the betatron x-ray beams. These film emulsions have a linear response with radiation dose to a density of at least 2.5. Translite and Adlux develop a suitable density with a maximum dose of about 200 rads while the Type M requires a dose of about 30 rads. Isodensity patterns on the films are read with the isosignal plotter or may be traced with a manually operated densitometer. It is advisable to determine the central axis depth dose by other methods to normalize the film isodose curves. For high energy x-rays, an ionization chamber is suitable for determining the central axis depth dose curve, but for high energy electrons care should be taken in using ionization chambers because of the change in response due to the polarization effect[17] and the displacement effect. Therefore, solid dosimeters such as the ferrous sulfate dosimeter and thermoluminescent dosimeter which have no polarization effect are more useful for electron beam dose distribution measurements.

Calculation of Treatment Time

Given Dose. The Given Dose is the absorbed dose at the point of maximum for the entering beam. Therapy prescriptions at this institution, with a few exceptions, are written in terms of tumor dose with the given dose calculated to deliver the prescribed tumor dose.

Time Calculator. The time required to determine the selected given dose to the patient may be calculated using an adopted circular slide rule.[3] The rule is constructed for individual radiation machines; markings upon the rule accommodate the dose variation to the patient with allowance for *SSD*, field size, and backscatter factor. One disc of the rule is fixed according to the radiation calibration of the machine. The index for the *SSD* is rotated to the proper field size; the time for a given radiation dose is read directly from another set of adjacent scales.

Error Detection. All therapy charts are checked weekly for calculative errors. This routine provides a quality control by an independent check on calculations affecting the treatment of each patient. This checking enables the therapist to make corrections for errors, if needed, during the course of radiation therapy.

The following items are checked: effective area for calculation, machine time calculation, central axis depth dose, total given dose versus dose prescription, addition of accumulated given dose, and weekly and final tumor doses. The occasional large error that has been discovered and corrected by this precaution more than justifies the effort and expense involved.

General Treatment Planning

A description of the radiation distribution in three dimensions throughout the volume of interest within the body with full allowance for tissue inhomogenities is feasible, but is more than is calculated at present for individual patients. Usually, a radiation distribution is calculated in a single plane that includes the central ray of one or more radiation fields entering the body. For stylized treatments, it is sufficient in many cases to precalculate the radiation distribution for a range of typical patient sizes and to refer to an atlas or table of dose distributions.

Patient Contours. For planning individual therapy, it is necessary to have at least one cross-sectional view of the patient in a plane which passes through the tumor. The antero-

posterior dimension in the abdominal region will change with the postion of the patient. If the patient is to be treated in more than one position, the dimensions of interest are measured with calipers in both positions and are averaged for use in depth dose calculations.

Two suitable methods for making the contour are the molding of plaster of paris bandage and the bending of lead wire about the patient in treatment position. If plaster of paris bandage is used, the contour can be obtained by folding the bandage or splints into strips approximately ½ inch wide and 8 layers thick. After moistening and squeezing between two fingers and the strips can be molded about the patient covering ½ of his total circumference, anatomical landmarks and field information can be indicated on the plaster bandage with a colored indelible pencil. After setting, the contour is removed and the second half of the contour can then be made.

If lead wire or solder is used, diameters of approximately ⅛ inch for body sections and ¹⁄₁₆ inch for head and neck sections should be used. The wire is bent about the patient in the treatment position and any anatomical landmarks or field information can be transferred to the wire with a wax pencil.

The two halves of the contours of either technique should be oriented about perpendicular axes on paper which has the average *AP*, *PA* and lateral diameters marked. The contour may be traced from the inside shape of the plaster or wire.

Combination of Isodose Curves. In multiport radiation beam treatment, dose in the tumor area is usually obtained by combining isodose curves. Figure 1-8, shows how two opposing fields are combined by inspection. First, the two individual isodose curves are placed in their treatment position on the contour of the patient. The intersection of two isodose curves is then found, for example: the 70 per cent isodose curve from one

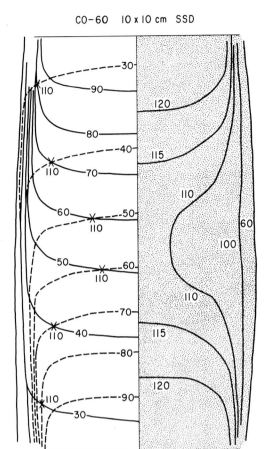

CO-60   10 x 10 cm SSD

FIG. 1-8. Method of combining by inspection. The left side of the central axis shows the individual isodose curve orientation on a patient contour. The intersection of the two curves showing a combined percentage of 100 is indicated. Other values would be similarly found and the resultant complete combination is shown on the right side of the central axis.

field intersects the 40 per cent isodose curve from the opposite field, which when added, gives 110 per cent. Additional intersections of two curves which add up to 110 per cent are found throughout the plane of tissues encompassed by the two fields. As one percentage curve is completed, another is developed until a complete distribution is drawn. With experience, it is possible to predict the approximate shape of the combined isodose curves distribution for any combination of

fields; with this ability, the direct compounding of isodose curves becomes very rapid. Where more than two fields are to be compounded, it is easiest to combine only two fields at one time, and the final combination is then the summation of the combined pairs.

Point-by-Point Calculations. Where many fields are involved and the dose must be determined for a few selected points within a patient's contour, it is sometimes quicker to sum the contribution from the various fields to the selected points of interest rather than attempt to combine the isodose curves into a full radiation distribution.

Computer Methods. Several computer programs are available for external beam therapy. The principle of calculation used in all of these programs is similar to manual computations in that dose distributions for single beams are compounded for individual patients. However, with a computer, the doses are summed for a large number of points on a grid, which allows plotting of isodose curves. Corrections are made for sloping skin surface.

A modification of the program written by Mauderli and Fitzgerald[19] is used on a large general-purpose digital computer to calculate dose distributions for rotation and fixed-field therapy. This method allows single beam distributions to be calculated from decrement line data, as well as digitized from existing isodose curves.

Another program in routine use has been developed for a small special-purpose digital computer, the Programmed Console,[11] to calculate fixed field dose distributions. It is particularly useful for treatment planning in instances where optimization of field placement or angulation is desired since parameters, such as position of the fields, can be changed easily and there is an immediate display of the isodose distribution on a cathode-ray tube. Hard copy of graphic data can then be drawn by an incremental plotter. An example of an isodose distribution for three fields calculated by the Programmed Console is shown in Figure 1-9.

Rotational Calculations. In rotation therapy, the dose to the axis of rotation can be quickly calculated by the use of tissue-air ratios found in BJR Supplement No. 10, described in Handbook 87, *Clinical Dosimetry.* For a complete isodose distribution, several manual methods of calculation are available; but in recent years, the manual methods have been replaced by digitalized computer methods at this institution, as indicated above.

Irregular Skin Surfaces. Isodose curves are usually measured in a water phantom with the beam entering perpendicularly. However, the surface of the patient where the beam enters is usually angled and curved. At megavoltage energies, it is possible to compensate for the irregular surface by a calculative procedure. The center of the field is usually, but not necessarily, considered at the nominal source-skin distance (Fig. 1-10A). Corrections are applied to the isodose curve to allow for the changing *SSD* relative to the nominal distance (Fig. 1-10B,C,D). A second approximate method is shown in Figure 1-11, using a $\frac{2}{3}$ shift method.[14]

Corrections for Lung Tissue. Lung corrections are made in calculations for patients in which the radiation beam traverses the lung in reaching the treated volume. A density of 0.35 gm/cm^3 is assumed for lung tissue.

From a demagnified transverse tomogram, the lung area is compressed by calculation to a unit density equivalence resulting in a smaller effective contour from which calculations for treatment are made. The procedure is as indicated in Figure 1-12. A second approximate method[14] is to increase the per cent depth dose from a ^{60}Co beam by 20 per cent after passing through 5–8 cm of lung tissue.

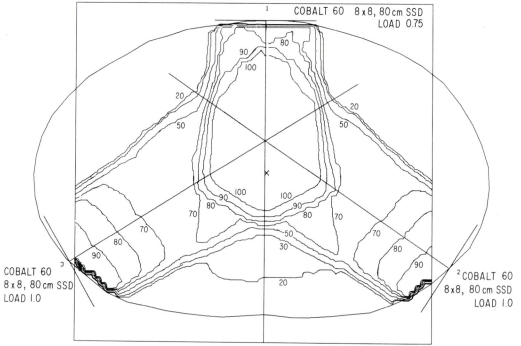

FIG. 1-9. An example of an isodose distribution as plotted by the program console. The computer has incorporated corrections for surface obliquity.

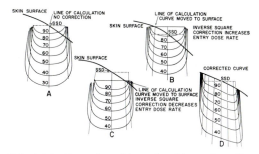

FIG. 1-10. Correction of irregular skin surface. Correction for varying *SSD* in different parts of the field may be corrected by calculation as shown in **A, B, C,** and **D**. Various rays from the source are chosen as lines of calculation. Upon each ray, the dose rate is corrected inversely as the square of the distance greater or less than the *SSD*. Thus in **B** on the ray of calculation, the skin is closer to the source; the dose rate at the surface is then:

Dose rate$_\text{surface}$

$$= \text{Dose rate}_\text{SSD} \times \left(\frac{SSD}{SSD - d}\right)^2$$

where *d* is the distance between the surface and the *SSD* along the direction of the radiation. If the skin is at a greater distance than the nominal *SSD* on the ray of calculation, *d* is added to the *SSD* in the denominator. The isodose curve is moved along the ray so that the isodose curve entry line intercepts the skin surface at the ray; the dose at a depth is the product of the inverse square correction and the dose indicated by the curve as in **D**. This method is an approximation which is useful only for source-skin distances close to the nominal distance.

Specialized Dosimetric Techniques

Wedge Filter—Megavoltage. Wedge-shaped filters constructed of lead or brass may be interposed in a radiation beam to cause the isodose curves to assume a planned assymetry. The resulting radiation distributions are of particular usefulness in instances where two beams enter the surface at angles of 60 to 90 degrees to each other; a large volume of tissue can be irradiated to a uniform dose by the proper relationship of wedged fields. (A wedge is usually defined by the angle

formed between the resultant 50 per cent isodose curve and a line perpendicular to the central axis.) The most frequently used wedges are 45 degrees and 60 degrees. The curves are expressed in percentages of the given dose, i.e., dose that would be given if the wedge were not present. It is usual to place the wedge at least 15 cm from the patient to reduce the number of secondary electrons arriving at the skin.

Design of Wedge Filters and Calculation of Curves. Wedge filters of any shape can be designed for megavoltage equipment by calculating the absorption necessary to distort the open-field isodose curve to the desired slope. The angulation produced in the iso-

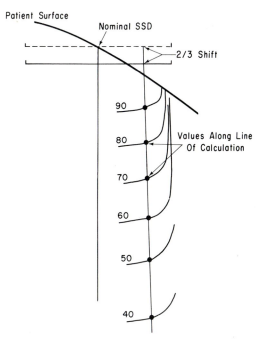

FIG. 1-11. The isodose curve shift method for ^{60}Co. Another approximation method to correct for the sloping skin effect is accomplished by shifting the isodose curve $^2\!/_3$ of the distance between the nominal *SSD* and the skin surface on a line of calculation as shown in **E**. No inverse square correction is made. Along each line of calculation the corrected position of the isodose curves is indicated by the position the curves assume when shifted the $^2\!/_3$ distance.

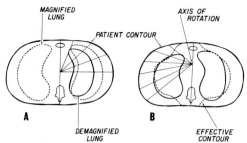

FIG. 1-12. Correction for the distortion of the radiation pattern of beams traversing lung. A transverse tomogram through the center of the treatment fields is used to determine the cross-sectional geometry of the patient's lungs. The lungs are corrected for the magnification of the film by drawing rays at regular intervals originating from the center of the tomogram (Fig. 1-12A). The distance from the center of the lungs is reduced by magnification of the film and the lungs are located within the contour drawn of the patient. In the figure, the outline of the patient is that determined from the contour taken at the level of treatment. In deriving the effective contour, rays are drawn at regular angular intervals from the center of rotation or the intersection of the central rays of the fixed radiation fields. The distance from the center to the reduced unit density contour is obtained by adding the thickness of tissue to the lung thickness multiplied by 0.35. The points on the various rays are corrected, yielding the reduced contour as shown on **B**.

dose curve will vary with depth, thus a 45-degree wedge will have that angle at a selected depth but not at other depths. The procedure for the calculation of wedges is given in Figure 1-13.

Treatment Planning with Wedges. The contour of the patient, in a plane which passes through the tumor, is obtained by the methods described; usually the plane is perpendicular to the long axis of the patient. All localization of anatomy pertinent to planning, such as the tumor, spinal cord, lens, etc., can be drawn within this contour.

The choice of wedge angle depends upon which wedge arrangement produces a radiation distribution that most closely approxi-

mates the tumor shape and avoids over-irradiation of critical regions. The choice of the relationship between the entry beams is usually such as to cause the isodose curves of one field to be parallel with those of the other. Two 45-degree wedges (Fig. 1-14A) will produce a boxlike volume of uniformly irradiated tissue when set at approximately 90 degrees to each other while two 60-degree wedges when set at approximately 60 degrees to one another (Fig. 1-14B) will produce a more triangularly shaped volume of uniformly irradiated tissue.

Inverse square corrections described before are made on each curve to allow for sloping or irregular skin surfaces. The curves then are combined to show the resultant radiation distribution.

Cardboard Cutouts for Wedged Pair

Treatment. A problem which is always present in dosimetry is the transfer of the treatment plan to the patient and a daily assurance of the accuracy of the radiation treatment. A practical, simple procedure is the use of a cardboard cutout.

After the final treatment plan is decided, the necessary skin marks such as edges of fields, source-skin distance and anatomical landmarks can be transferred from the patient's treatment plan, using secretary's carbon paper, to a cardboard cutout which is cut to fit the patient's contour as shown in Figure 1-15. Final verification films with the treatment machine are taken to assure that the treatment field includes the volume to be treated. A pocket level is fastened to the cutout in a position parallel to a predetermined horizontal line on the treatment plan. The cardboard cutout can then be used to transfer these field-defining borders and source-skin distance marks to the patient; the cutout is used on a daily basis for positioning the patient.

Upon completion of treatment, the cardboard cutout becomes a permanent part of the patient's record and can be used for fu-

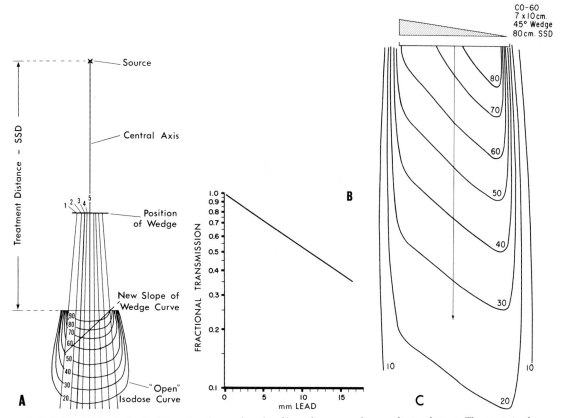

FIG. 1-13. Method of calculating the shape of wedge filters for megavoltage radiation beams. The steps in the calculation are as follows:

1) The source, the wedge, the skin surface, and the open-field isodose curve are located in their relative positions, full scale, as shown in **A.** The wedge is usually located at the end of the cone or at the face of the light localizer.

2) A line of the desired slope is drawn from a point on the edge of the 50 per cent curve (or other curve) which is still in the full beam.

3) From the source or target, diverging straight lines are drawn which pass through the wedge and the isodose curve. These lines, called increment lines, should be spaced approximately 1 cm apart at the surface of the isodose curve.

4) A given increment line will pass through the new slope at some point of dose level higher than the 50 per cent isodose curve. The thickness of lead (or other material) required to reduce the transmission of the open-field beam on the increment line to the intensity chosen for the sloping line is obtained from reference to the absorption curve **(B)** which is the absorption curve obtained with a small radiation field. For example, if increment lines at the position of the new slope passes through the unwedged curve at the 60 per cent level, the reduction in intensity is calculated as follows: $^{50}/_{60} = 0.83$ transmission through wedge. From **B** it is seen that 3 mm of lead will reduce the transmission to 83 per cent. The thickness of lead on increment line 2 is to be 3 mm.

5) The thickness of lead for other increment lines is calculated in a similar manner, thus defining the wedge. The wedge-filtered field is shown in **C.** The resultant isodose curve is expressed as a percentage of the dose to the open unwedged field.

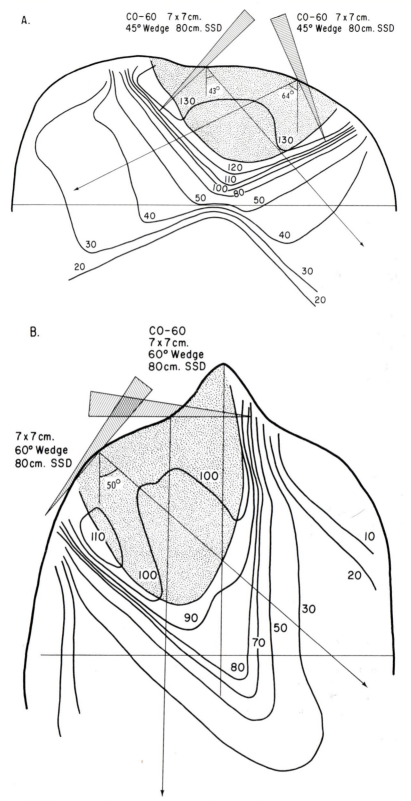

FIG. 1-14. Dose distribution resulting from treatment with two 45° wedges is shown in A. Dose distribution resulting from treatment with two 60° wedges is shown in B.

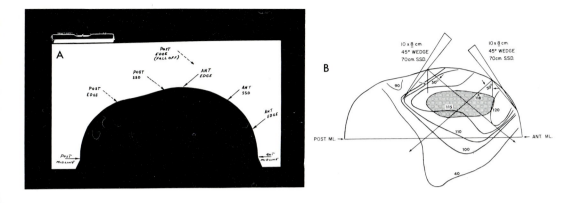

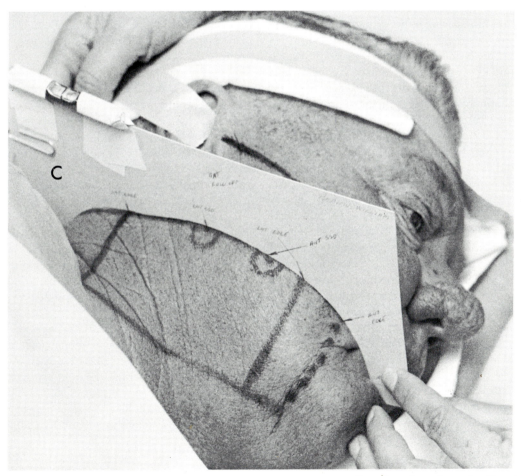

FIG. 1-15. Beam alignment utilizing a cardboard cutout. **A.** Cardboard cutout. **B.** Isodose plan with a wedge-filtered field for which a cardboard cutout was utilized for beam alignment. **C.** Alignment of a patient with a cardboard cutout.

ture reference to the position of the treatment fields.

Tissue Compensating Filters. In treating anatomical locations such as soft palate, epiglottis or tongue, which have metastatic disease in the neck, a common field arrangement is opposing lateral fields. The diameters through the superior and inferior levels of this type of treatment field can be significantly different, resulting in undesirable variations in the radiation distribution between the two levels (Fig. 1-16A).

The use of tissue compensating filters can eliminate this problem while still preserving the skin-sparing effect of high energy beams (Fig. 1-16B).

The technique used at this institution is similar to that published by Hall and Oliver[10] and includes the selection of the nominal *SSD* point near the shortest *SSD* of the treatment field.

A matrix column of rods is attached to the machine while in treatment position; each rod is then brought into contact with the patient's surface (Fig. 1-16C) within the field. Measurement of each rod relative to the rod at the *SSD* location will indicate the air gap and bolus necessary to achieve a uniform dose. A compensating filter is built using aluminum rods with a $\frac{3}{8}''$ square cross section (Fig. 1-16D). Each compensating rod is positioned on a square which has a bolus thickness requirement determined in the above step. The aluminum compensator-tissue ratio is 0.325; i.e., 0.325 cm of aluminum compensates for 1 cm of tissue.

Breast Technique. When treating the intact breast or chest wall on the ^{60}Co unit by means of two tangential fields, a special

auxillary collimator blocks one-half the field, reducing penumbra on that side as shown in Figure 1-17. In this manner, the volume of lung tissue receiving radiation is reduced. A portion of the treatment is given with bolus to insure that the surface receives an adequate radiation dose.

Two volume distributions are calculated, one with bolus and one without bolus, on a contour taken through the center of the breast. The lower edges of both fields are marked on the contour and their separation is compared with the measured breast bridge separation. A line connecting both of these marks forms the base line used for orienting the angulation of the treatment field. The central axis of the lateral tangential field is always parallel to this baseline. The central axis of the medial tangential field is either parallel to or angulates 10 degrees downward from the central axis of the lateral field, depending on whether or not the internal mammary chain is included in the tangential treatment. Inverse square corrections to the entering beam are made on the distribution without bolus.

Hodgkin's Disease—Mantle Field Calculations. With the mantle field technique, the following points are routinely calculated: lower, mid- and upper mediastinum axillae and neck, all at mid-diameter depths; in addition the supraclavicular is calculated to a 0.5 cm depth.

In fields of extremely irregular shape, such as the mantle, point calculations such as those mentioned above can be made to any depth and position within the field using the Clarkson method.[4]

This technique divides the radiation contribution to a particular point into two sepa-

FIG. 1-16. The effect of tissue compensating filters. A illustrates the dose nonuniformity occurring in two planes shown in the insert. This effect is due principally to the changing SSD at the contour levels. B illustrates the improvement of dose uniformity in the same contour levels by the insertion of a tissue-compensating filter in each field. C illustrates the method of determining the *SSD* of various points within the treatment field. Columns of rods moved to the surface of the patient indicate the thickness of compensation necessary at each rod position to produce the effect of a flat skin surface. D shows a completed tissue compensator ready for insertion into the treatment field.

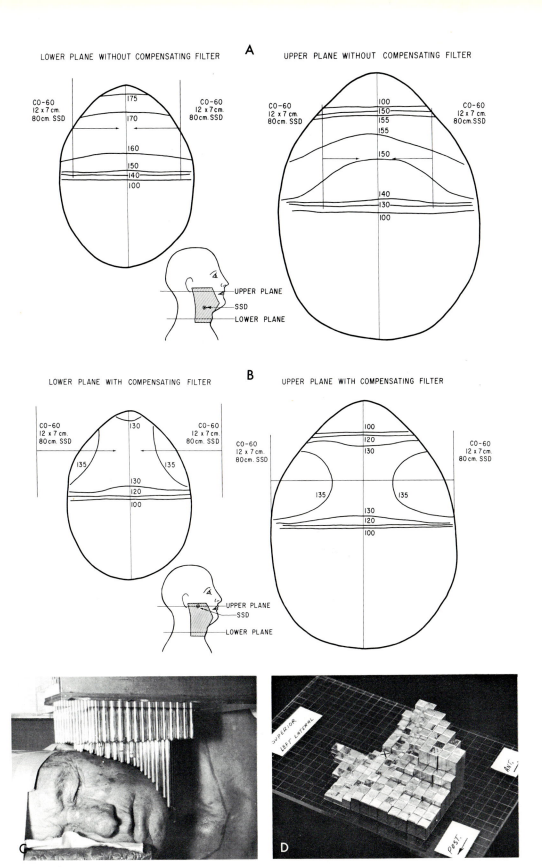

LOWER PLANE WITHOUT COMPENSATING FILTER   A   UPPER PLANE WITHOUT COMPENSATING FILTER

CO-60
12 x 7 cm.
80cm. SSD

CO-60
12 x 7 cm.
80cm. SSD

UPPER PLANE
SSD
LOWER PLANE

LOWER PLANE WITH COMPENSATING FILTER   B   UPPER PLANE WITH COMPENSATING FILTER

CO-60
12 x 7 cm.
80cm. SSD

CO-60
12 x 7 cm.
80cm. SSD

UPPER PLANE
SSD
LOWER PLANE

C   D

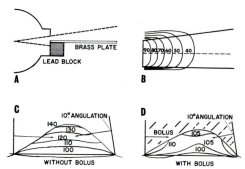

FIG. 1-17. Treatment of the intact breast or chest wall with tangential radiation fields from a ^{60}Co irradiator. **A.** Auxilliary collimator for reduction of penumbra on one side of the field. The collimator is composed of a lead block and a brass plate which serves to reduce penumbra and to act as an *SSD* indicator. **B.** The isodose curve is shown that results from the use of the auxilliary collimator. **C.** The distribution of radiation in a typical treatment is shown without bolus. **D.** The radiation distribution with bolus is shown.

The bolus portion of treatment helps deliver a more uniform radiation distribution throughout the intact breast and also increases the surface dose for chest wall irradiation following simple mastectomy by ensuring electronic buildup at the skin surface.

rate parts: primary and scatter radiation. The scatter contribution to a point within the field is calculated using special scatter function rulers constructed from standard depth dose tables.[6]

The original publication considered the primary radiation to be constant across the entire field for any given depth. Modifications of the basic technique, including corrections for off-axis effect on the primary radiation, have recently been introduced.

Lung Blocks. Lung blocks for the mantle field are made for the individual patient and are cut with a band saw from 5 cm lead stock. The shape of the block is obtained by projecting a shadow from the blocking tray to the lung block outline drawn on a radiograph taken of the patient in treatment position. This is done on a simulator in which the

geometry duplicates the treatment situation. Completed lung blocks are arranged on the blocking tray and a verification film with the patient in treatment position is made prior to treatment.

Lung Technique. Treatment is delivered through two opposing fields (anterior and posterior) with given dose loadings of 2:1 for anterior lesions, 3:2 for midline lesions, or 1:1 for posterior lesions. An outline of the treatment field is drawn with a wax pencil on a sheet of plastic positioned over the patient. Diameter and surface distance measurements are made at *SSD* and calculative points. Normally the points of calculation are the mid-mediastinum, spinal cord at the level of the upper mediastinum, and the center of any boost field that might be used.

Calculations are based on data from an isodose curve of appropriate dimension or the Clarkson method depending on the shape of the field drawn on the patient. Appropriate inverse square corrections are made depending on the surface distance above the points of calculation.

Strip-Field Technique. The strip-field technique permits the treatment of a large volume of the abdomen to a larger dose than would be possible by conventional techniques.[5] The method is adapted here for use with a cobalt unit with adjustable diaphragms. Field widths of 10, 7.5, and 5 cm are obtained with the regular adjustable diaphragm; the 2.5 cm width field, however, is achieved using additional lead blocks. Radiation fields of increasing widths, starting with 2.5 cm, are treated to equal given doses on various days (Fig. 1-18A). (Examples of calculation of dosage and daily prescription can be found in the ovarian tumor chapter in this book.) The curve in Figure 1-18C shows the average percentage of given dose at mid-thickness of a patient together with the maximum and minimum dose seen at the center of a patient. Doses of 6 per cent or less of the full beam are counted as zero in compounding the over-all depth dose distribution of the combined strip fields. These maxima and minima occur only if the anterior and posterior fields are placed exactly in apposition. In practice, it is very unlikely that this amount of variation will be seen. The depth dose data for this technique should be calculated for each type of therapy machine as differences in the shape of the isodose curves between machines will yield differ- ences in the cummulative per cent depth dose.

Accessories. For some types of treatment, it is advantageous to employ extra beam blocking to shield structures or to shape the edge of the field more precisely to the volume under treatment. For these purposes, the half value layer measured with a small field (and therefore the "narrow beam" absorp-

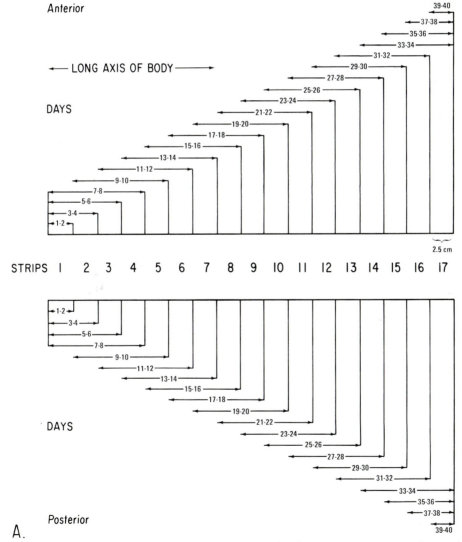

FIG. 1-18. Diagrams and graph relating to the strip technique. **A.** The treatment sequence to the anterior and posterior surfaces is shown. Half the prescribed given dose is delivered each day to the anterior and posterior strips.

ISODOSE DISTRIBUTION AT THE COMPLETION OF TREATMENT TO BOTH SIDES

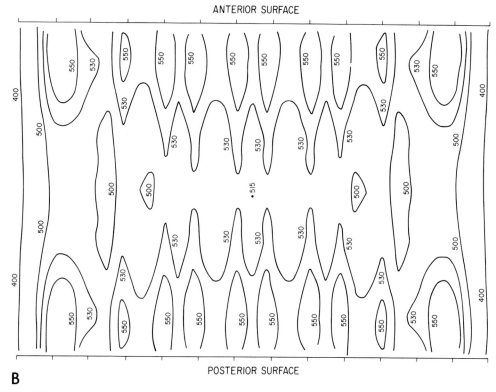

B

FIG. 1-18B. An example of the combined isodose distribution upon completion of treatment in the sagittal plane that includes the longitudinal axis of the body. The total given dose to each strip is 100 per cent. This distribution is computer generated for an Eldorado 8 Cobalt unit, *SSD* 80 cm, trimmers at 65 cm from the source (except for the 2.5 cm field).

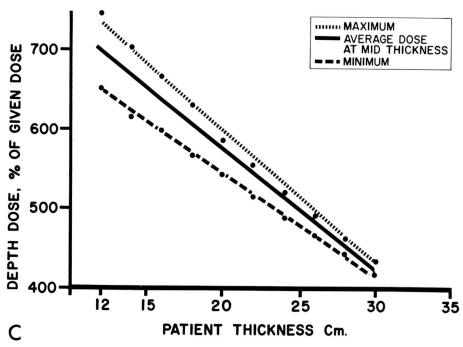

C

FIG. 1-18C. The dose to the longitudinal mid-line expressed as a per cent of given dose to one field versus the anteroposterior patient thickness. This graph is valid for an Eldorado 8 Cobalt unit, *SSD* 80, with trimmers at 65 cm from the source (except for the 2.5 cm field).

tion) is used. The thickness of lead required for various attenuations for different radiations is shown in Table 1-1. If transparent plastic is employed to hold such blocking, the absorption of the x- and gamma-rays in the plastic should be allowed for or the plastic should be thin enough to neglect the absorption. A 4 mm thick Lucite blocking tray (3 per cent absorption) that attaches to the collimator is suitable for most treatment fields. A thicker, 9 mm, Lucite tray (5.5 per cent absorption) is necessary for larger blocking trays. This type of tray is needed in large field therapy such as mantle fields where a great amount of weight has to be supported over a large area. It is important to have a secure mounting (usually to or on the treatment table) for the safety of the patient. A caution to be considered in the use of trays is the possibility of secondary electrons in the forward direction. If the tray is at least 15 cm from the skin, the dose contributed by these electrons to the skin is negligible. An investigation with lithium fluoride powder, using a 10 × 10 cm ^{60}Cobalt field, has indicated that a plastic tray located at 15 cm from the skin caused 43 per cent of full electronic build-up compared to 55 per cent at 10 cm, 75 per cent at 5 cm, and 36 per cent at 20 cm. The percentage of electron contamination increases with larger field sizes.

Separation between Adjacent Fields. The ideal separation between two adjacent fields is dependent upon the size of the penumbra

Table 1-1. *Millimeters of Lead Required for Various Attenuations*

	Reduction to		
	50%	5%	1%
250 Kvp x-ray	0.3	1.7	2.5
300 Kvp x-ray	0.6	2.7	4.2
Gamma, ^{137}Cs	5.4[9]	23	36
Gamma, ^{60}Co	10.4[9]	45	69
22 Mevp x-ray	13	56	86

DIAGRAM ILLUSTRATING THE REQUIRED FIELD SEPARATION TO YIELD DOSE UNIFORMITY BETWEEN ADJACENT FIELDS

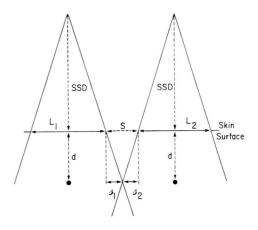

$$\mathcal{S}_1 = 1/2\ L_1 \left(\frac{d}{SSD}\right)$$
$$\mathcal{S}_2 = 1/2\ L_2 \left(\frac{d}{SSD}\right)$$
$$S = \mathcal{S}_1 + \mathcal{S}_2$$

(L_1) and (L_2) : Field Lengths
(d) : Depth of Dose Specification
(SSD) : Source-Skin Dist.
($\mathcal{S}_1$) and ($\mathcal{S}_2$) : Field "Half-Separations"
S : Field Separation

FIG. 1-19. Diagram illustrating the required field separation at the surface to achieve dose uniformity between adjacent fields. The light defining the edge of field coincides with the exposure rate which is 50 per cent of that at the central ray.

and the divergence of the two fields being used.

An article by Glen and co-workers[9] for a particular unit describes the separation needed between two adjacent fields to achieve uniform depth dose to a particular depth in the junction area relative to the same depth at the central axis of the two treatment fields.

When the light field defines 50 per cent of the maximum of the penetrating beam, the crossing of the light edges at the depth of interest will approximately insure dose uniformity in the junction regions (Fig. 1-19).

When the junction area is critical or when more than a single depth is needed, the combining of isodose curves which have a high degree of accuracy in the penumbra region is recommended for separation analysis (Fig. 1-20).

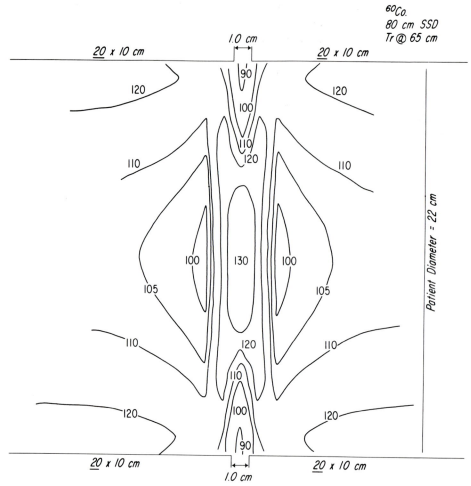

FIG. 1-20. Separation between adjacent fields. The isodose distribution for two pairs of opposing fields with a 1 cm separation between the field edges and a 22 cm diameter patient. The complexity of isodose distribution in the adjacent area and the resultant need to analyze the entire distribution rather than a particular point is illustrated.

Lead Shields. In superficial and electron beam therapy, it is often necessary to have a beam defining aperture near or in contact with the patient, especially when delicate structures such as the lens of the eye are close to the lesion being treated. In order to make a lead shield of a patient's face that fits, in a reproducible manner, for many treatments, it is convenient to make a positive reproduction of the face—preferably in dental stone. The lead shield can then be formed upon the dental stone from lead of a thickness sufficient to reduce the dose to about 5 per cent of its original value.

Fetus Protection. Protective shielding of the fetus is routinely provided for pregnant patients undergoing radiation therapy.

Five sheets of lead each measuring $30 \times 30 \times .7$ cm are positioned on a rigid support over the abdomen of the patient. For mediastinal and mantle type fields, the superior edge of the lead should be positioned close to the inferior edge of the treatment field. Most of the radiation which can be shielded originates as scatter from the primary and secondary collimating systems; there is also leakage from the unit housing.

A critical factor in the effectiveness of the shielding is the distance from the bottom edge of the treatment field to the fetus. Shielding is less effective when this distance is short because of the increased scatter contribution from within the patient. If the distance is 15 cm or greater, the use of shielding can reduce the dose to the fetus by a factor of $\frac{1}{2}$ to $\frac{1}{4}$ the dose the fetus would receive without shielding (Fig. 1-21).

Intracavitary and Interstitial Radiation

Intracavitary and interstitial radiation provide a high radiation dose in or near the tumor where radiation is desired and a rapidly diminishing radiation dose rate to regions outside the tumor. A disadvantage of interstitial and intracavitary radiation, which has undoubtedly limited its popularity, is the radiation which the physician, nursing and other personnel receive in the procedure. To a large extent, the radiation hazard to personnel has been reduced by the use of afterloading techniques which permit implantation with unloaded applicators and the subsequent application of radioactive sources after the patient has arrived at the ward.[26]

Interstitial Radiation Therapy. In external beam therapy, it is usual for the radiation dose distribution to be described by isodose curves in a plane intersecting the beam or beams. However, in interstitial radium therapy the calculation by manual methods by

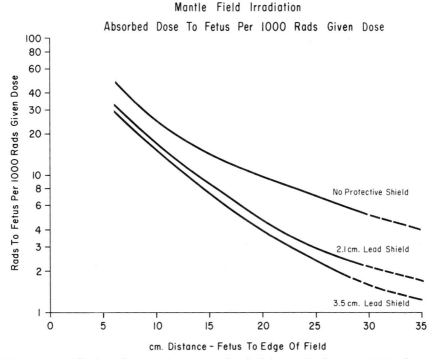

FIG. 1-21. Experimentally derived curves showing the absorbed dose to the fetus per 1,000 rads given dose by ^{60}Cobalt to a mantle-shaped field. The dose to the fetus is relative to the distance of the closest field edge and to the absence or addition of protective lead sheets suspended above the abdomen of the patient.

isodose curves resulting from multiple radioactive sources is a very laborious process which is not feasible as a method for routine treatment. Instead, tabular systems from which a single dose rate would be calculated from the geometry of the implant and the radioactivity in the sources were devised in the early 1930's. The physics of linear radioactive sources and groups of sources has been reviewed[24], and the calculation of doses delivered clinically utilizing the Paterson–Parker system has been given a detailed account.[22] In the view of the authors, there is no need here to elaborate further upon the radium systems except to make a single exhortation as strongly as possible: *It is imperative that a radiotherapist use one radium system to the exclusion of others.*

It seems likely that calculations of full isodose distribution by computer methods will become more widespread. It is possible for radiotherapists to utilize computers hundreds or thousands of miles away for the calculation of individual treatments; however, with the proliferation of computers it is likely that the distances between the user and the computer will grow smaller.

The computer methods for linear sources and seeds have been described.[18,25] The precise details of the format of input data to the computer can be obtained together with the program from the authors of the references. An example of a computer calculation is shown in Figure 1-22.

One major point to be considered in the transfer of clinical experience from the Paterson–Parker system to computer methods is the relationship of the single stated dose in roentgens derived from the Paterson–Parker tables and the dose distribution in rads delineated by the computer. To derive absorbed dose in rad from the roentgens calculated from the Paterson–Parker tables, four correction factors are required:

1) Γ factor: The Paterson–Parker tables were prepared using 8.4 roentgens per hour as the dose rate in air from a point source

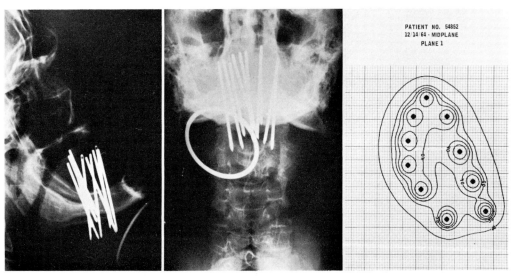

FIG. 1-22. An interstitial radium implant in the floor of the mouth. The implant is composed of ten Indian-club needles, 1.8 mg radium each, 4.5 cm active length, 0.65 mm platinum filtration. The anteroposterior and lateral radiographs together with isodose curves in a plane bisecting the needles are shown. A 1 mm grid is in the background. The numbers on the curves refer to rads/hr. The curves were drawn and labelled by an incremental plotter as directed by the output of the computer.

of radium filtered by 0.5 mm platinum. More recent measurements indicate that this dose rate is 8.25 roentgens per hour. Thus, the dose rate derived from Paterson–Parker tables is reduced by the ratio of 8.25 over 8.4.

2) Oblique filtration: In the preparation of the Paterson–Parker tables, the attenuation of dose due to oblique filtration was not allowed for completely. For this reason, the dose from a typical implant is approximately 2 to 4 per cent less than that calculated by the Paterson–Parker tables.

3) Tissue Absorption: Since the Paterson–Parker tables give exposure in air, no allowance was made for tissue absorption. In the computer calculations, dose rates are decreased 1 per cent per centimeter up to 4 cm distance from the source to allow for tissue absorption.[20]

4) Absorbed Dose: The exposure dose in roentgens is multiplied by 0.957[13,14] to obtain the absorbed dose in muscle expressed in rad.

When all these correction factors are considered, the conversion factor from Paterson–Parker roentgens to rad in muscle varies from 0.987 to 0.910 for planar and volume implants of usual size. It is recommended that a single conversion factor of 0.90 rad per "roentgen" (as calculated by Paterson–Parker tables) be applied to obtain the absorbed dose in rad for planar and volume implants.[24]

Uterine Cervix. The most extensive and successful use of radium has been in treatment for carcinoma of the uterine cervix. The computation of three-dimensional dose distributions to the corpus, paracervical areas, and parametria is too tedious and time consuming to be done manually on a routine basis. A method which provides considerable information from calculations in one plane has been utilized for a decade[7,8] and is demonstrated in Figure 1-23. Recently a computer method has become available[25] which

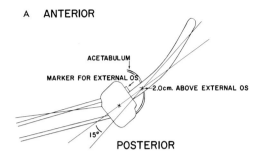

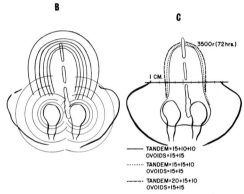

FIG. 1-23. Manual calculation of the dose distribution in treatment of carcinoma of the cervix. From anteroposterior and lateral radiographs a single isodose curve and the doses extending laterally to the pelvic wall in a plane related to the radium geometry can be calculated in a reasonable time. The plane is defined by the centers of the colpostat sources and a point 2 cm. above the external *os* (usually the upper end of the lowest intrauterine source). As shown in **A**, the angle of the intrauterine tandem to the calculation plane is derived from the lateral radiograph; a library of isodose projections of various tandems upon the calculation plane have been developed for angles at 15-degree intervals. The appropriate curve for the tandem together with the isodose curves for the colpostat sources is overlaid upon the anteroposterior radiograph as shown in **B**. The final compounding of the curves is shown in **C**. The curves have been enlarged by the factor 1.21 to allow for the average magnification of the radiograph. (**B** and **C**, Courtesy: Fletcher, *Carcinoma of the Uterine Cervix, Endometrium and Ovary*, Chicago, Year Book Medical Publishers, Inc., p. 69, 1962.)

permits the rapid calculations of families of
isodose curves in arbitrary planes through
and around the radium system (Fig. 1-24
and 1-25).

BIBLIOGRAPHY

1. Almond, P. R.: The use of ionization chambers for the absorbed dose calibration of high
   energy electron beam therapy units, *Int. J.
   Appl. Rad.*, 21, 1, 1970.
2. American Association of Physicists in Medicine: Protocol for the dosimetry of high energy electrons, *Phys. Med. Biol.*, 11, 505, 1969.
3. Braun, E. J., Van Roosenbeek, E., and Shalek,
   R. J.: A dose-time calculator for roentgen-
   and gamma-ray beams, *Am. J. Roentgen.*, 84,
   770, 1960.
4. Clarkson, J. R.: A note on depth doses in
   fields of irregular shape, *Brit. J. Radiol.*, 14,
   265, 1941.
5. Delclos, L., Braun, E. J., Herrera, R. J., Sampiere, V. A., and Van Roosenbeek, E.: Whole
   abdominal irradiation by cobalt-60 moving
   strip technique, *Radiology*, 81, 632, 1963.
6. Depth dose tables for use in radiotherapy,
   Brit. J. Radiol., Supplement 10, 1961.
7. Fletcher, G. H., Wall, J. A., Bloedorn, F. G.,
   Shalek, R. J., and Wootton, P.: Direct measurements and isodose calculations in a radium therapy of carcinoma of the cervix,
   Radiology, 61, 885, 1953.
8. Fletcher, G. H., Stovall, M., and Sampiere, V.:
   In *Carcinoma of the Uterine Cervix, Endometrium
   and Ovary*, Chicago, Year Book Medical Publishers, Inc., p. 69, 1962.
9. Glenn, D. W., Faw, F. L., Kagan, A. R., Johnson, R. E.: Field separation in multiple portal
   radiation therapy, *Am. J. Roentgenol.*, 102, 199,
   1968.
10. Hall, E. J. and Oliver, R.: The use of standard
    isodose distributions with high energy radia-
    tion beams—the accuracy of a compensator
    technique in correcting for body contours,
    Brit. J. Radiol., 34, 43, 1961.
11. Holmes, W. F.: External beam treatment
    planning with the programmed console,
    Radiology, 94, 391, 1970.
12. Hospital Physicists' Association: A code of
    practice for the dosimetry of 2 and 8 MV
    x-ray and cesium-137 and cobalt-60 γ ray
    beams, *Phys. Med. Biol.*, 9, 457, 1964.

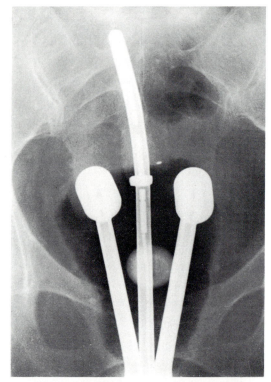

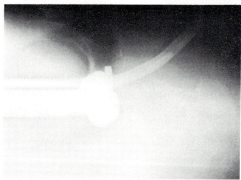

FIG. 1-24. Computer methods in cervix calculation.
The same computer program used for the
calculation of the isodose distributions
around interstitial implantations (Fig. 1-22)
is suitable for the calculation of isodose
curves around gynecological intracavitary
radiation. The planes of calculation may be
chosen arbitrarily. The anteroposterior and
the lateral radiographs of an implantation
with Fletcher-type afterloading applications
are shown in **A** and **B**. In the radiograph,
the sources are inactive; thus four sources
appear but only three were used in treatment in the uterine tandem. The isodose
curves developed by the computer are
shown in Fig. 1-25.

INSERTION 2   15+15+10   20+20
PLANE 2   LAT THROWOFF

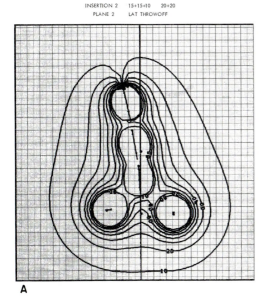

A

INSERTION 2   15+15+10   20+20   PLANE 1   SAGITTAL PLANE

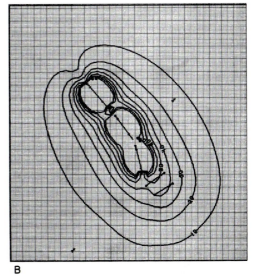

B

INSERTION 2   15+15+10   20+20   PLANE 3   PELVIC BRIM

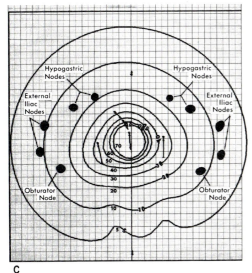

C

FIG. 1-25. Computer methods in cervix calculations. In **A,** the plane shown is the same as shown for the manual calculation of another case in Fig. 1-23; this plane is defined by the centers of the colpostat sources and a point 2 cm above the external *os*. In **B,** the isodose distribution in the "sagittal plane" is shown; the plane is not a true sagittal plane but one that includes the intrauterine tandem and proceeds from anterior to posterior. In **C,** the radiation distribution in the plane called the pelvic brim is shown. This plane is chosen on the lateral film by the physician and is defined by the superoposterior surface of the symphysis pubis and the junction of the first and second sacral vertebrae. The approximate location of various lymph nodes in the pelvis is shown. The curves were drawn and labelled by an incremental plotter as directed by the output of the computer.

13. ICRU Radioactivity: Report 10c of the International Commission on Radiological Units and Measurements. National Bureau of Standards (U. S.) Handbook 86, 1963a.

14. ICRU Clinical Dosimetry: Report 10d of the International Commission on Radiological Units and Measurements. National Bureau of Standards (U. S.) Handbook 87, 1963b.

15. ICRU Report 14: Radiation dosimetry: x-rays and gamma rays with maximum photon energies between 0.6 and 50 MeV (ICRU Publications, Washington), 1969.

16. Johns, H. E. and Cunningham, J. R.: *The Physics of Radiology,* Springfield, Charles C Thomas, p. 241, 1969.

17. Laughlin, J. S.: Electron beams of *Radiation Dosimetry Volume III,* Attix and Tochlin, New York, Academic Press Inc., p. 91, 1960.

18. Laughlin, J. S., Siler, W. M., Holodny, E. I., and Ritter, F. W.: A dose description system

for interstitial radiation therapy, *Am. J. Roentgen.*, 89, 470, 1963.

19. Mauderli, C. R., Fitzgerald, L. T.: A computer program for rotational treatment planning, *Am. J. Roentgen.*, 94, 880, 1965.

20. Meisberger, L. L., Keller, R., and Shalek, R. J.: The effective attenuation in water of the gamma rays of gold-198, iridium-192, cesium-137, radium-226, and cobalt-60, *Radiology* 90, 953, 1968.

21. Review of supplement No. 10, Depth dose tables for use in radiotherapy, *Brit. J. Radiol.*, 41, 932, 1968.

22. Shalek, R. J. and Stovall, M.: In *Radiation Therapy in the Management of Cancers of the Oral Cavity or Oropharynx,* Springfield, Charles C Thomas, p. 295, 1962.

23. Shalek, R. J. and Smith, C. E.: Chemical dosimetry for the measurement of high-energy photons and electrons, *Annals New York Academy of Sciences,* 161, 44, 1969.

24. Shalek, R. J. and Stovall, M.: In *Radiation Dosimetry,* F. H. Attix, W. C. Roesch, and E. Tochilin, eds., New York, Academic Press, Inc., p. 743, 1969.

25. Stovall, M. and Shalek, R. J.: The M. D. Anderson method for computation of isodose curves around interstitial and intracavitary radiation sources. III. Roentgenograms for input data in the relation of isodose calculations to the Paterson–Parker system, *Am. J. Roentgen.*, 102, 677, 1968.

26. Suit, H. D., Moore, E. B., Fletcher, G. H., and Worsnop, B. R.: Modification of Fletcher ovoid system for afterloading, using standard-sized radium tubes (milligram and microgram), *Radiology,* 81, 126, 1963.

27. U. S. National Bureau of Standards: Protection Against Betatron Synchrotron Radiation up to 100 Million Electron Volts (U. S. National Bureau of Standards Handbook No. 55), Washington, D. C.

Special Gamma-Ray Techniques

LUIS DELCLOS

Head and Neck

Surface and Intracavitary Applicators

Most of the squamous cell carcinomas in the head and neck area are treated at this institution by either a radium implant or by external beam (photons and/or electrons) as outlined in other sections of this book. There are situations where a surface or intracavitary applicator is the treatment of choice.

Surface applicators, or molds, can only be used when the tumor is very superficial, either in the skin or mucous membranes, or if the tumor lies between 2 surfaces close enough to allow a satisfactory dose distribution between applicators placed on each side.

The rapid fall-off is an advantage as it spares the underlying structures. Applicators can be made so that the patient carries them for a few hours a day, removing them for meals and at bedtime.

The applicators are made of Lucite. Radium or a radioactive isotope such as cobalt, iridium, cesium, etc., may be used. The sources are distributed and the dose calculated according to the Paterson–Parker rules for planar molds.[10,12]

The area, or volume to which an adequate dose must be given is delineated to determine the required distance from the radioactive sources to the surface. Distances greater than 3 cm are impractical because of the space problem or the large amount of radioactive material needed.

Use of radioactive substances other than radium, such as cesium or iridium may be an advantage from the point of view of protection of the surrounding tissues.

Surface applicators will be the treatment of choice in the following situations:

1) Squamous and basal cell carcinoma extending along a convex surface such as the scalp or the forehead. These are generally relatively superficial lesions, sometimes extensive, with a thin layer of subcutaneous tissue only between the tumor and the underlying bone.

2) The tip of the nose (Fig. 1-26).

3) Squamous cell carcinoma of the mucosa of the hard palate (Fig. 1-27) and, lower and upper gum which cannot be reached with an intraoral cone.

4) Occasional superficial lesions of the floor of the mouth.

5) Lip: Although most of the lesions of the lips can be treated by external irradiation, with a lead shield behind, or by means of a radium implant, it should be mentioned that a "double mold" could be used because of the excellent cosmetic results (Fig. 1-28).

6) Lesions of the ear: The use of gamma-ray will minimize the risk of subsequent cartilage necrosis (Fig. 1-29).

7) Superficial tumors of the edge of the

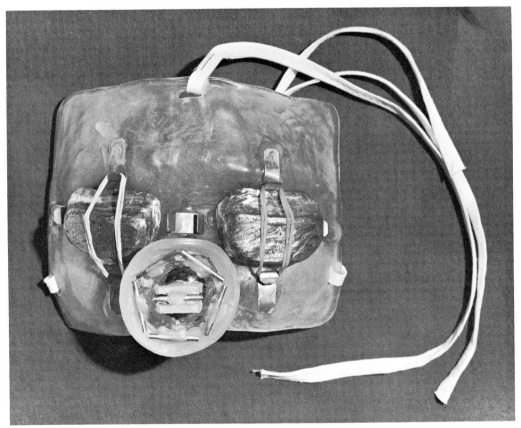

FIG. 1-26. Curved single circle for the treatment of postsurgery residual basal cell carcinoma on the tip of the nose of this 59-year-old patient. A surface dose of 6,300 rads (4,320 rads at 0.5 cm) has been administered in 9 doses, the patient wearing the applicator for 2 hours 2 minutes daily in 8 treatment days. The eyes were protected with lead reducing the irradiation to the lens below 200 rads; 5 × 20 mg and 1 × 5 mg radium tubes were used. Similar applicators can be loaded with iridium, cesium, or cobalt if available.

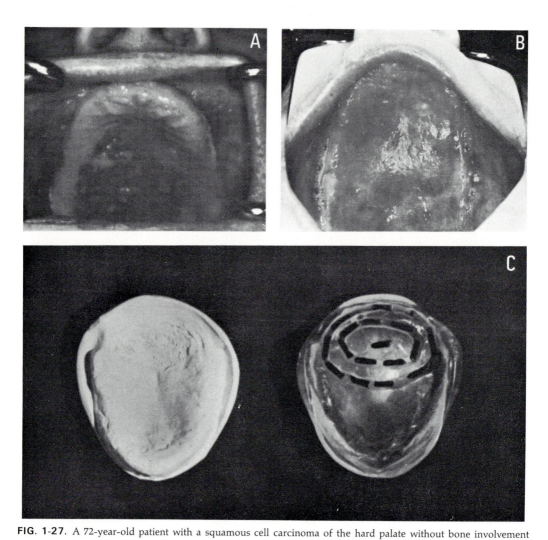

FIG. 1-27. A 72-year-old patient with a squamous cell carcinoma of the hard palate without bone involvement in a leukoplakic oral cavity **A.** This lesion was a second primary as will be explained later. Because of the location it could not be covered by an intraoral cone (neither x-ray nor electrons) or implanted (the mucosa was too thin making even the use of radon or gold seeds difficult). With external irradiation we would have irradiated a large volume of tissue. It was selected to use an intraoral surface applicator (radium) which was worn 8 days for 5 hours a day (February 1966). A dose of 8,000 rads was delivered to the surface and 5,867 rads to a depth of 3 mm. **B.** Palate 1 year later completely healed. There was no evidence of disease in the primary site at the time of the patient's death in November 1970.

In 1963 the patient had a "commando" with partial glossectomy for a carcinoma of the tongue (first primary) followed by post-operative irradiation with megavoltage (^{60}Co). In June 1970, $3\frac{1}{2}$ years after treatment of the palate and 7 years after treatment of the tongue she developed a third primary in the left lower gum extending to the floor of the mouth with metastases in the left neck. Local excision, partial glossectomy and skin graft were performed. This area healed well and in November 1970 she was taken to the operating room for a radical neck dissection, however, she died from heart failure during the anesthetic. **C.** Shows a Lucite applicator of the type used with the above-mentioned patient but carrying gold seeds. Cesium, cobalt, or iridium can also be used. (Courtesy: Delclos, *J. Prosth. Dent.,* 15, 157, 1965.)

nostril or nasal vestibule, including the anterior part of the septum, can be irradiated effectively by means of a central linear source (Fig. 1-30). A large dose can be delivered to the tumor-bearing surface without excessive irradiation of a larger volume of normal tissue.

8) Antrum: For incomplete surgical removal of a tumor or recurrent lesion, the whole surface of the cavity may be treated using an intracavitary applicator (Fig. 1-31). The shape of the cavity is irregular and therefore, the position and number of radioactive sources are adjusted so that there is adequate dose to the surface where tumor is present. This calls for individualization as the cavities vary so much in size and shape. Measurement at different points over the surface and adjustments of the radioactive sources may have to be made during the treatment.

Chest Wall

Surface Molds

The availability of electron beams has reduced the need for large surface applicators; however, when these beams are not available and it is desirable to irradiate a large thin layer of skin with a minimum of penetration, as frequently occurs with patients after a radical mastectomy, a surface mold can be used.

The radium or sealed radioactive isotope (iridium, cobalt, cesium, tantalum, etc.) is mounted on the "mold" according to the Paterson–Parker rules for rectangles (Fig. 1-32).[12] The distance between the radium and the skin depends upon the depth below the surface that we wish to irradiate adequately; the shorter the distance the thinner the slab of tissue that will receive a se-

---

Calculation of the Radium Applicator for the Hard Palate

Area (ellipse): $\pi/4 \times 5.0 \times 3.9 =$

15.3cm^2 @ 0.7 cm:

405 mghr/1000 r elongation:

$$\frac{5.0}{3.9} = \frac{1.3}{1} = 2\%$$

Correction for elong: $405 \times 1.02 = 413$ mghr/1000 r
\# cells available: 26×3 mg cells $\therefore$

$26 \times 3.18 = 82.7$ mg.

Distribution Rules (use rules for circle):

effective circular diameter: $\pi/4\ d^2 = 15.3$ cm^2 $\therefore$

$d = 4.4$ cm.

$$\frac{\text{Diameter}}{\text{distance}} = \frac{4.4}{.7} = 6.3$$

$\therefore$ we must use 2 concentric circles with a center spot.
80% outer circle = $.80 \times 82.7 = 66.2$ mg $\simeq$ 20 cells
3% center spot = $.03 \times 82.7 = 2.5$ mg $\simeq$ 1 cell
Remainder in inner = $82.7 - 66.2 - 2.5 = 14$ mg $\simeq$ 5 cells

Dose rate @ surface (0.7 cm): $\dfrac{82.7}{413} \times 1000 =$

200 r/hr.

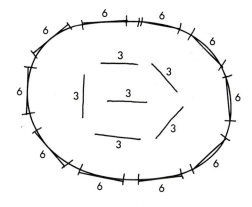

Dose rate @ 3 mm below surface: $552 \times 1.02 = 563$ mghr/1000 r

$$\frac{82.7}{563} \times 1000 = 147 \text{ r/hr.}$$

Aim: 8000 r in 8 days @ surface

Total Hrs.: $\dfrac{8000}{200} = 40$ hrs $= 5$ hr/day $\times$ 8 days

Dose @ 3 mm below surface: $40 \times 147 - 5876$ r/40 hrs.

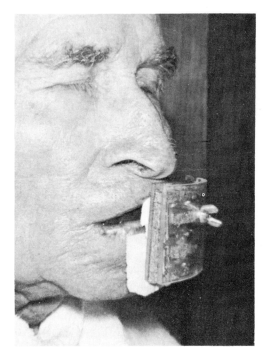

	$h = 1.5$ cm		
Height = 3 cm			
Distance from Ra	2.5 cm	2.0 cm	1.5 cm
Length of plane	2.9 cm	3.2 cm	3.5 cm
Effective area	8.7 cm^2	9.6 cm^2	10.5 cm^2
mg-hr./1,000 rads	1,344	1,011	748
rads/hr.	76.4	101.6	137.3

Inner Mold

Area = $4.0 \times 3.0 = 12$ cm^2 $h = 0.5$ cm

Distance from Ra	0.5 cm	1.0 cm	1.5 cm
mg hr./1,000 rads	290	533	789
rads/hr.	153.4	83.5	56.4

The mold was applied in this fashion for nine hours over a two-day period. This delivered the following dosages:

Outer	Skin	Center of lip	Mucosa
9 hrs. ×	137.3	101.6	76.4
	1,236 rads	914 rads	688 rads
Inner			
9 hrs. ×	56.4	83.5	153.4
	508 rads	752 rads	1,381 rads
Total	1,744 rads	1,666 rads	2,069 rads

It was then decided to lengthen the planes of the outer mold to allow more adequate margin around the tumor (to approximately 1.5 cm).

The inner mold remained unchanged. The following factors were obtained:

Outer Mold   Height = 3 cm $h = 1.5$ cm

Distance from Ra	2.5 cm	2.0 cm	1.5 cm
Length of plane	3.8 cm	4.2 cm	4.6 cm
Effective area	11.4 cm^2	12.6 cm^2	13.8 cm^2
mg-hr./1,000 rads	1,432	1,121	843
rads/hr.	71.7	91.6	121.8

Solving by simultaneous equations:

	Skin	Mucosa
Total dosage required	5,500 rads	6,300 rads
From first 9 hours	1,744	2,069
Needed	3,756	4,231

x = hrs. inner mold y = hrs. outer mold

$$153.4x + 71.7y = 4,231$$
$$56.4x + 121.8y = 3,756$$
$$260.8x + 121.8y = 7,193$$
$$56.4x + 121.8y = 3,756$$
$$204.4x = 3,427$$
$$x = 16.8 \text{ hrs. (inner mold)}$$
$$2577 + 71.7y = 4,231$$
$$71.7y = 1,654$$
$$y = 23.1 \text{ hrs. (outer mold)}$$

To be delivered in 5 days

$$\frac{16.8}{5} = 3.4 \text{ hrs. each day (inner mold)}$$

$$\frac{23.1}{5} = 4.6 \text{ hrs. each day (outer mold)}$$

Total dosage in eight days

Skin: 5,500 rads
Center of lip: 5,185 rads
Mucosa: 6,300 rads

SQUAMUS CARCINOMA Gr. II LOWER LIP
RADIUM MOLD – 2 PLANE " SANDWICH "

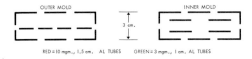

RED = 10 mgm., 1.5 cm. AL TUBES   GREEN = 3 mgm., 1 cm. AL TUBES

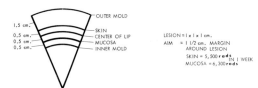

LESION = 1 x 1 x 1 cm.
AIM = 1 1/2 cm. MARGIN
AROUND LESION
SKIN = 5,500 rads IN 1 WEEK
MUCOSA = 6,300 rads

FIG. 1-28. Patient with a squamous cell carcinoma of the lower lip wearing a "double mold". The tumor is "sandwiched" between the two applicators.

The treatment was performed in November 1961. The patient died from intercurrent disease in 1969 with no evidence of disease in the lips. The cosmetic result was excellent.

Total Radium:

Outer Mold =

10 × 10 mg × 0.9 filt. corr. =   90   mg
4 × 3 mg × 1.06 filt. corr. =   12.7 mg
                                102.7 mg

Inner Mold =

14 × 3 mg × 1.06 filt. corr. = 44.5 mg

The mold was planned with the following factors:

Outer Mold   Length of planes

Outer mold   = 4.5 cm
Skin   = 3.5 cm
Center of lip = 3.2 cm
Mucosa   = 2.9 cm
Inner mold   = 4.0 cm

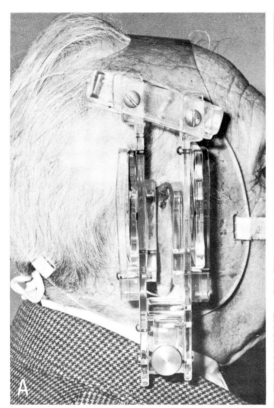
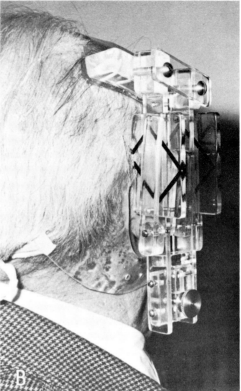
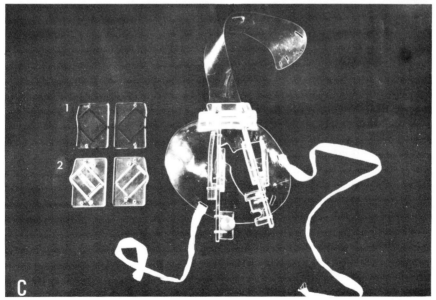

FIG. 1-29. Double (sandwich) applicator for the ear. Because of the underlying cartilage, this lesion is best treated using a gamma applicator. To reduce the exposure of the personnel involved, the applicator was constructed so that the daily fitting and removal of the apparatus could be done with "dummies." Once the applicator was properly placed the radium carrier was inserted in a few seconds. **A** and **B.** Applicator in position. **C.** Applicator with (1) dummy carrier for fitting and (2) radium carrier. (Courtesy: Delclos, and Cordovilla, *Radiologia*, In press.)

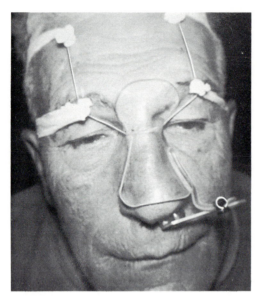

FIG. 1-30. Patient with a squamous cell carcinoma of the vestibule of the nose wearing a Lucite applicator containing a single linear source. An impression of the nostril is taken and a single radium tube is placed parallel to the area we plan to irradiate. Attempts are made to keep the normal mucosa at a greater distance so that it receives a smaller dose; this is not difficult because with such short treating distances the "inverse square law" plays an important part.

In October 1961, 8,100 rads were given at 0.5 cm depth in 19.25 hours. The applicator was worn 5 days for 3 hours and 51 minutes daily. In January 1972, no evidence of disease or complication.

with adhesive tape. Some of these molds can be remotely afterloaded eliminating the hazards of strong radiation.[9]

The irradiated area should be larger than the obvious nodules; experience shows that if irradiation is limited to the immediate vicinity of the skin nodules, further recurrences beyond the edge of the irradiated area is the rule.

Implants

These will cover a similar area to the mold, but it is the choice for the case with thicker flaps.

Radium needles can be used, but to minimize exposure of the operating room and nursing personnel we recommend the use of some sort of afterloading system. There are innumerable reports describing techniques

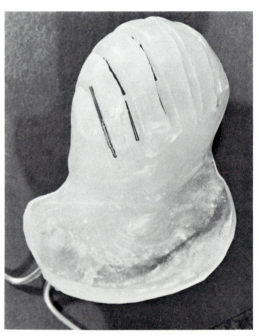

FIG. 1-31. Intracavitary applicator to irradiate residual tumor in the defect resulting from antrectomy for a squamous cell carcinoma of the maxillary antrum. (Made in the Section of Orthodontics, The University of Texas Dental Branch, under the direction of J. B. Drane, D.D.S.)

lected minimum dose. The maximum practicable distance is about 3 cm, as greater distances will require too much radium. A dose of 4,500 to 5,500 rads can be given in 6 to 10 days.

The radioactive material is mounted on a suitable material of the correct thickness ("distance"); among the different materials available, self-adhesive "Elastofelt" is the most popular; it is light, flexible, and can be accurately fitted with a minimum of secondary radiation. The "mold" should be reinforced by a few layers of plaster of Paris bandage to prevent springing of the curved surface of the thorax. It is secured in position

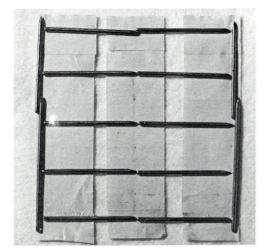

FIG. 1-32. Elastofelt surface applicator "loaded" with radium needles which have been distributed according to Paterson-Parker rules. This is the treatment of choice for skin and subcutaneous nodules in a previously untreated thin chest wall. (Courtesy: Delclos, *Tumors of the Skin,* Chicago, Year Book Medical Publishers, Inc., p. 294, 1963.)

proved to be very valuable when a less rigid system is desired and for lesions too large to be encompassed by the commercially available radium needles with a maximum

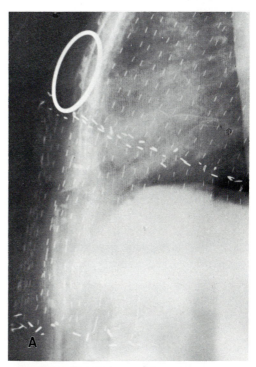

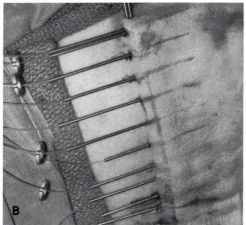

FIG. 1-33. **A.** X-ray films showing a chest wall implant done with ^{192}Ir seeds in nylon ribbons. **B.** The ribbons are afterloaded into stainless steel needles implanted into the skin flaps and arranged according to Paterson-Parker rules for implants of large areas. This technique has been developed by Henschke.

and instrumentation for the use of afterloading in interstitial therapy using radium (as early as 1910 by Abbe)[17] or any other suitable solid isotope.[4,5,6,7,8,11,13,14,15,16] Iridium wires or plastic ribbons carrying iridium seeds, which can be afterloaded into needles previously arranged according to the Paterson–Parker rules for large areas[12], seems to be a good choice (Fig. 1-33). This technique is a further development by Henschke[6,7] of the flexible carrier method, which was first used by Haines in 1937.[5]

Miscellaneous Gamma-Ray Implants

There are situations, for instance lesions of the lateral border of the tongue, buccal mucosa (Fig. 1-34) or the anal margin (Fig. 1-35) where, because of the extent of the disease or the route of growth, it may be desirable to employ longer and more flexible radioactive sources than radium needles. [192]Ir seeds in nylon ribbons have

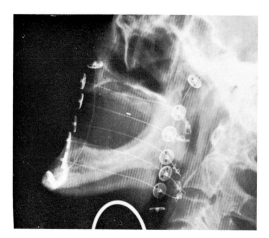

FIG. 1-34. X-ray film showing a single plane implant of a poorly differentiated squamous cell carcinoma of the buccal mucosa covering an area 6.5 × 6.5 cm. A minimum tumor dose of 2,500 rads was delivered in 50 hours at a distance of 0.5 cm to each side of the implant following the administration of 5,000 rads in 5 weeks (9–12 Mev electrons, 8 × 8 cm field). The x-ray film was taken with inactive stainless steel wires within the teflon tubings, later replaced by ^{192}Ir wires.

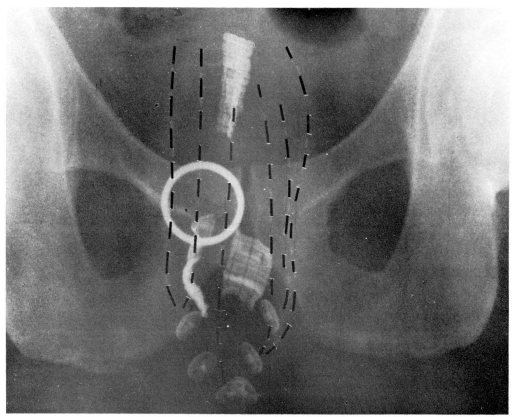

FIG. 1-35. Forty-five year-old white male seen at Syracuse Memorial Hospital. Biopsy of squamous cell carcinoma. The lesion was too large for a radium implant; ^{192}Ir seeds in nylon ribbons were ordered. May 26, 1964—Single plane curved implant done. No evidence of disease in May 1970. Good function.

active length of 4.5 or 5 cm. An afterloading technique is described by Henschke in the following section.

BIBLIOGRAPHY

1. Delclos, L.: In *Tumors of the Skin,* Chicago Year Book Medical Publishers, Inc., p. 294, 1963.
2. Delclos, L.: Radiotherapy for head and neck cancer; Teamwork: Problems common to physician and dentist, *J. Prosth. Dent.,* 15, 157, 1965.
3. Delclos, L. and J. J. L. Cordovilla: An afterloading ear applicator to carry radium or substitute, *Radiologia,* In press.
4. Fishman, R., and Citrin, L. I.: A new radium implant technique to reduce operating room exposure and increase accuracy of placement, *Amer. J. Roentgen.,* 75, 495, 1956.
5. Haines, I.: A new method in the use of radon gold seeds, *Amer. J. Surg.,* 38, 235, 1937.
6. Henschke, U. K.: In *Therapeutic use of Artificial Radioisotopes,* P. F. Hahn, ed., New York, John Wiley and Sons, Inc., p. 375, 1956.
7. Henschke, U. K.: In *International Conference on the Peaceful Uses of Atomic Energy,* Vol. 10, New York, United Nations Publications, p. 48, 1956.
8. Henschke, U. K., James, A. G., and Myers, W. G.: Radiogold seeds for cancer therapy, *Nucleonics,* 11, 46, 1953.
9. Joslin, C. A. F., Liversage, W. E., and Ramsey, N. W.: High dose-rate treatment moulds by afterloading techniques, *Brit. J. Radiol.,* 42, 108, 1969.
10. Meredith, W. J.: *Radium Dosage: The Manchester System,* Edinburgh, E. and S. Livingstone Ltd., 1947.
11. Mowatt, K. S. and Stevens, K. A.: Afterloading—A contribution to the protection problem, *J. Fac. Radiologists,* 8, 28, 1956.
12. Paterson, R.: *Treatment of Malignant Disease by Radiotherapy,* 2nd., Baltimore, The Williams & Wilkins Company, 1963.
13. Pierquin, B., Chassagne, D., and Gasiorowski, M.: Technique et dosimetrique de curie puncture par fils d'or 198. *J. de radiol. et d'electrol.,* 40, 690, 1959.
14. Pierquin, B., *Precis De Curiethérapie,* Masson et Cie, Editeurs, Paris, 1964.
15. Suit, H. D., Shalek, R. J., Moore, E. B., and Andrews, J. R.: Afterloading technique with rigid needles in interstitial radiation therapy, *Radiology,* 76, 431, 1961.
16. Wolever, T. H., and Brooks, Q. T.: A new method of implantation of the base of the tongue, *Radiology,* 74, 102, 1960.
17. *Arch. Roentgen Ray.,* 15, 74, 1910 (Short paragraph describing Dr. Abbe's method of afterloading).

Afterloading for Interstitial Gamma-Ray Implantation

ULRICH K. HENSCHKE AND BASIL S. HILARIS

"Afterloading" is a technique for interstitial and intracavitary radiation therapy, which we have advocated since 1953. Its advantages, mainly lower radiation exposure and greater accuracy, are now generally recognized. Afterloading techniques should be used today in every institution in which many patients are treated with interstitial and intracavitary radiation therapy.

Afterloading for interstitial implants requires a separate discussion of "removable implants" and "permanent implants," since different afterloading techniques must be used.

Afterloading for Removable Implants

"Removable implants" are implants in which the radioactive sources are completely removed after the desired dose has been delivered; the classic example is a radium needle implant.

The principal advantage of a removable implant is the better control of the distribution of the radioactive sources and of the dose. Both can be adjusted within wide limits after the implantation by removing radioactive sources at different times. In contrast, with a permanent implant, neither the distribution nor the dose can be readily changed after the initial insertion.

For afterloading of removable interstitial implants, we have developed a special "nylon ribbon" into which any number of small (3 mm long and 0.5 mm diameter) radioactive "seeds" can be loaded. They can be spaced at any distance, thus permitting heavy end loading.

Stainless steel encased iridium seeds of these dimensions (either activated to ^{192}Ir or inactive for activation in other reactors) and sets of nylon ribbons, custom loaded with these ^{192}Ir seeds, are available from the Department of Radiotherapy of Howard University, Washington, D. C. 20001. ^{192}Ir sources in form of platinum-cladded wires, which the user can cut to the desired active length, are also available from the Centre d'Études Nuclear de Sacley, Jif-Sur-Yvette, France.

Figure 1-36 illustrates the use of these nylon ribbons with ^{192}Ir seeds for afterloading of needles. As the first step (Fig. 1-36A), empty, hollow needles are implanted. The needles are made from standard 17-gauge "hypodermic" stainless steel tubing and are closed and beveled on one end. They can be

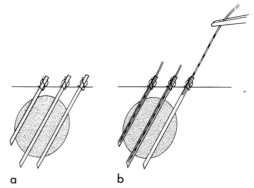

FIG. 1-36. Afterloading of a removable implant. **A.** Insertion of empty hollow needles. Used mainly in tumors which are accessible from only one side. For greater accuracy, plastic stabilizers can be used to hold the needles in position. **B.** Afterloading of needles with ^{192}Ir seeds in nylon ribbons. Each nylon ribbon comes with 12 seeds spaced 1 cm apart, but any number of seeds can be cut off to obtain the desired active length.

adapted in the operating room to any length simply by breaking them off on the open end after notching with a file. The needles are held in position by a surgical suture which is tied around a ball on the needle. The ball is made of plastic or metal and is held on the needle with a set screw.

As the second step (Fig. 1-36B) the inserted needles are afterloaded with the ^{192}Ir seeds in nylon ribbons. The active length of these nylon ribbons is adjusted by cutting off the seeds which are not desired, and the remaining nylon ribbon is inserted with a long clamp.

Afterloading of needles can be used wherever radium needles have been used in the past. This technique is of special value if the tumor is accessible from one side only. Excellent distribution can be achieved and maintained if "stabilizers" are used for the needles. Stabilizers are simply metal or plastic pieces of one-quarter to one-half inch thickness, into which holes for the needles are drilled in the desired direction. Figure 1-37 shows a stabilized needle afterloading implant for a carcinoma of the female urethra.

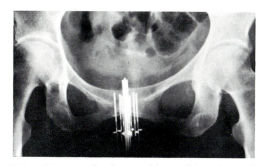

FIG. 1-37. Example of removable needle implant with stabilizer. C.G./74-year old housewife with a squamous cell carcinoma of the urethra. Six needles were spaced at 1 cm distance around the urethra and held in place by a plastic template, which was attached to a metal catheter in the urethra. Patient living and well without functional defects 8 years after implant.

Figure 1-38 illustrates the use of the nylon ribbons with ^{192}Ir seeds for afterloading of plastic tubes. These are preferable to needles in neck and breast tumors and in other tumors which are accessible from two sides. Nylon tubing of the same outer and inner diameter as the 17-gauge needles has proved most satisfactory in our experience. To secure the nylon tubes to the skin, one can use the same aluminum or plastic balls with set screws which are employed with the needles (Fig. 1-38A). One can also use a special stainless steel button with a central tube, which when slightly squeezed holds the nylon tube in place. To insert these nylon tubes a 17-gauge stainless steel needle is inserted first. We prefer to use needles of at least 20 cm length, since the direction of the needle in the tissue can be judged more easily with the longer needles. Usually we insert all needles first and then the nylon tubes. The nylon tubes have been pulled to

a thinner diameter at one end and this end is threaded through the needle first. Alternatively, one can connect the nylon tube and the stainless steel needle by an inner stylet, which provides the necessary rigidity to push the nylon tube into position.

As the second step (Fig. 1-38B), the plastic tubes are afterloaded with the ^{192}Ir seeds in nylon ribbons. Since the plastic tubes are open on both sides, all the inactive ends of the nylon ribbons can be pulled through the plastic tubes first while the ends with the ^{192}Ir seeds remain in the lead container. The active ends are then pulled into place one by one after the superfluous seeds have been cut off. The nylon ribbon is then secured within the outer nylon tubes by tightening the set screw of the ball on one side. Figure 1-39 illustrates the use of the technique.

Table 1-2 lists the radioisotopes which have been used for afterloading of removable implants, arranged according to their half lifes. None of these is ideal in every respect; but ^{192}Ir, which we introduced into Curietherapy in 1953, has emerged as the isotope of choice for afterloading of interstitial implants.

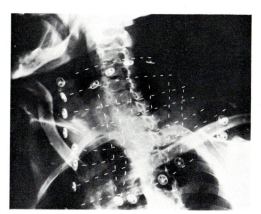

FIG. 1-39. Example of a removable plastic tube implant. S.W./55-year old designer with a large $10 \times 6 \times 5 \, cm^3$ carcinoma, which had recurred after surgery and cobalt teletherapy. A two-plane afterloading implant was done with 179 ^{192}Ir seeds in 14 nylon ribbons. Patient living and well 10 years after implant.

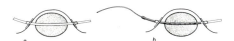

FIG. 1-38. Afterloading of a removable plastic tube implant. **A.** Insertion of empty plastic tubes. Used mainly in tumors which are accessible from two sides. **B.** Afterloading of plastic tubes with ^{192}Ir seeds in nylon ribbons.

Table 1-2. *Radioisotopes for Removable Implants*

Radioisotope	Half Life	Half Value Layer
^{226}Ra	1600 years	$\frac{1}{2}$ inch lead
^{137}Cs	27 years	$\frac{1}{4}$ inch lead
^{60}Co	5.3 years	$\frac{1}{2}$ inch lead
^{182}Ta	118 days	$\frac{1}{2}$ inch lead
^{192}Ir	75 days	$\frac{1}{10}$ inch lead
^{198}Au	2.7 days	$\frac{1}{10}$ inch lead

^{226}Ra has such a long life that no dose adjustments are necessary. However, radium presents the greatest hazard in case of capsule breakage, and its high gamma energy makes shielding difficult. Another disadvantage for afterloading is the large diameter of the radium needles, which requires needles and plastic tubes of at least 2 mm outer diameter.

^{137}Cs has a relatively long half life; only yearly dose adjustments are required. ^{137}Cs is safer than radium and its lower gamma energy eases the shielding problem considerably. Unfortunately ^{137}Cs, like radium, cannot be produced in very small sizes. Consequently, the diameter of needles and tubes for afterloading has to be substantially larger than for the following radioisotopes.

^{60}Co can be produced in very small diameters and is safer than either radium or cesium, especially if a suitable cobalt alloy wire is used instead of pure cobalt wire. Encapsulation is still mandatory to avoid contamination, but the diameter can be held to such small dimensions that the needles and the plastic tubes for afterloading can be of the same or even smaller size than the commonly used radium needles. ^{60}Co shares with radium the disadvantage of a high gamma energy, which makes shielding difficult. Another disadvantage of ^{60}Co is the need for monthly dose adjustments. ^{182}Ta is commercially available in form of platinum-shielded ^{182}Ta wire, which can be cut to any desired length. Compared with ^{192}Ir, tantalum is difficult to shield because of its high gamma energy, and for this reason ^{192}Ir is generally preferable.

Of all isotopes listed in Table 1-2, ^{192}Ir has by far the highest cross section. It therefore can be produced in the smallest sizes or alternatively at the lowest cost. Shielding is facilitated by its relatively low gamma energy. Its relatively short half life is a disadvantage. However, since ^{192}Ir is so inexpensive to produce, one may discard the sources after each use. If this is done, the short half life may at times be a blessing in disguise, for instance, if a source is accidentally lost in a patient. In such a case, it would not be mandatory to remove it since a single ^{192}Ir source can be tolerated in the tissue without major complications.

^{198}Au has such a short half life that ordinarily one would not consider it for removable implants, especially since it has no advantages over ^{192}Ir. However, if an institution used gold extensively for permanent implants and carries out removable implants only occasionally, one might consider the use of gold seeds for the latter as well.

Afterloading for Permanent Implants

An important advantage of a permanent implant is that no hospitalization is required since the sources can be inserted under local anesthesia and since no complications ensue in the immediate postinsertion period. This is of special value in the palliative management of many patients with advanced but accessible cancer for whom hospitalization would impose an additional economic and emotional burden. A permanent implant is usually a more simple procedure than is the removable implant and can be carried out more quickly, especially in tumors in the abdominal and thoracic cavities. A permanent implant in these locations is also a safer procedure, since the chances of infection, of dislodging or losing the sources are much less than with a removable implant.

To understand the importance of afterloading for permanent implants, one must appreciate the fact that in many locations good implants are possible only if one can carefully palpate the position of the tips of the needles and adjust them precisely. With the usual implanters, which are already loaded with one or several seeds, excessive exposure to the fingertips of the operator occurs. In touching the tip of a needle containing a seed, the fingertip is only 1 mm away from the seed. This gives in one second the same exposure to the fingertip as one would receive in three hours at a distance of 10 cm from the seed. This simple calculation readily explains why damage to the fingertips is found so often in physicians who have tried to do careful permanent implants. It also underscores the essential point in carrying out permanent implants; that is, to maintain a distance of at least 10 cm from the radioactive seeds at all times.

Figure 1-40 illustrates the afterloading technique which we have developed for permanent implants. It permits more accurate control of the distribution than is possible with the usual introducers and guns. As the first step (Fig. 1-40A), unloaded hollow needles, each 15 cm long, are inserted in and around the tumor. If feasible, the tumor should be so exposed that one hand can be placed under it. By measuring the length of the needles outside the tumor, the shape and size of the implanted volume can be determined. The number of sources required to give the desired dose is then calculated. Next,

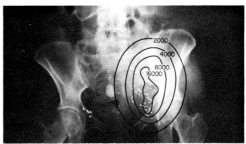

FIG. 1-41. Example of permanent afterloading implant. C.Q./64-year old housewife with a large 7 × 5 × 4 cm³ pelvic wall recurrence from a bladder carcinoma, which had not responded to cobalt teletherapy and was unresectable. Marked pain and swelling of the left leg for several months. Nonfunctioning left kidney. Ninety radon seeds each 0.75 cm were permanently implanted through 17 needles and the uterus was sutured over the implant. The computer calculated isodose curves illustrate the high doses which can be safely given with an interstitial implant. Excellent regression of the tumor was demonstrated at another exploration 6 months later. She died 2 years later however, with recurrent disease.

an instrument with a depth gauge is attached to each needle in turn (Fig. 1-40B). Through it the required number of radioisotope sources are introduced one by one into the tissue and deposited at the desired depth. Figure 1-41 gives an example of the technique.

This technique is a refinement of an insertion procedure first described by us in 1953[1,2] and has been used at the Memorial Center for most larger implants since 1957.[3] It has greatly extended the scope of permanent implantation by increasing accuracy in distribution and dose and by eliminating radiation exposure during the critical phase of the insertion of the needles.

Table 1-3 lists the radioisotopes for permanent implants which have been used in clinical practice.

^{222}Rn seeds are still used most often for permanent implants. They are much safer than radium capsules or needles, but have the same undesirable high gamma energy as radium, which makes protection difficult.

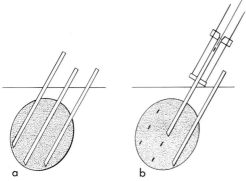

FIG. 1-40. Afterloading for permanent implants. **A.** Insertion of empty hollow needles. **B.** Afterloading of the needles with radioactive seeds, which are spaced with the help of the depth gauge on the instrument.

Table 1-3. *Radioisotopes for Permanent Implants*

Radioisotope	Half Life	Half Value Layer
^{222}Rn	3.84 days	$\frac{1}{2}$ inch lead
^{198}Au	2.7 days	$\frac{1}{10}$ inch lead
^{192}Ir	74.5 days	$\frac{1}{10}$ inch lead
^{131}Cs	9.8 days	$<\frac{1}{1000}$ inch lead
^{125}I	60 days	$<\frac{1}{1000}$ inch lead

^{198}Au seeds have the important advantage of easier protection but the shorter half life of the ^{198}Au seeds (2.7 versus 3.85 days for radon seeds) is a definite disadvantage: Gold seeds deliver the total dose in a much shorter time than do the radon seeds and this must be considered less favorable from the radiobiological point of view. In addition, the shorter half life is a practical disadvantage since due to the faster decay, gold seeds have a suitable strength for a shorter time than radon seeds.

^{192}Ir is a fascinating isotope for permanent implantation and has been used by us in 350 patients from 1956 to 1960. With its long half life of 74.5 days, ^{192}Ir provides continuous effective irradiation over several months, which, on the basis of a number of radiobiological studies, appears as a most promising way to increase the selective damage to the cancer cell. Unfortunately, permanent ^{192}Ir implants have the drawback that the implanted patient remains radioactive for a long time and thus radiation safety precautions are often necessary for months.

^{131}Cs was our original choice of a radioisotope with low energy for permanent implants, and we still feel that its half life of about 10 days would be most suitable. However, we carried out only one implant with ^{131}Cs seeds in 1965, because the cost of ^{131}Cs seeds is in the order of $50.00 per seed.

^{125}I seeds cost only about one-tenth as much, and we have used them therefore in all subsequent permanent implants with low energy seeds. Up to July 1970, we had carried out 254 permanent implants with ^{125}I seeds. The greatly improved radiation protection with these ^{125}I seeds is reflected in the reduction of the film badge readings to negligible levels. Our clinical results have been satisfactory, comparing favorably with the results obtained with the high energy isotopes (radon, gold and iridium).

ACKNOWLEDGMENT

This work was supported in part by PHS Grant EC 00113 from the Bureau of Radiological Health, Rockville, Maryland.

BIBLIOGRAPHY

1. Henschke, U. K., James, A. G., and Myers, W. G.: Radiogold seeds for cancer therapy, *Nucleonics,* 11, 46, 1953.
2. Henschke, U. K.: In *Radioisotopes in Medicine,* G. A. Andrews, M. Brucer, and E. B. Anderson, eds., Oak Ridge, Tennessee, Oak Ridge Institute of Nuclear Studies, Inc., United States Atomic Energy Commission, p. 711, 1953.
3. Henschke, U. K., Hilaris, B. S., and Mahan, G. D.: Afterloading in interstitial and intracavitary radiation therapy, *Amer. J. Roentgen.,* 90, 386, 1963.
4. Hilaris, B. S., Henschke, U. K., and Holt, J. G.: Clinical experience with long half life and low energy encapsulated radioactive sources in cancer radiation therapy. *Radiology,* 91, 1163, 1968.
5. Hilaris, B. S.: Techniques of interstitial and intracavitary radiation. *Cancer,* 22, 745, 1968.

Electron Beam

NORAH duV. TAPLEY

Basic Physics

The characteristics of the electron beam are:

1) Rapid dose build-up. The 100 per cent dose is reached at one cm depth and the dose approaches 90 per cent or higher within the first millimeter of tissue, which explains the modest skin sparing of the electron beam. The ratio of surface dose to dose at depth of maximum build-up increases as the electron energy increases. Various methods of dose determination give surface doses of 85 per cent for 7 Mev, 87 per cent for 9 Mev, 89 per cent for 11 Mev, 97 per cent for 15 Mev, and 98 per cent for 18 Mev.[1]

2) Sharp dose fall-off. A high dose level is maintained to a depth determined by the energy of the beam with the dose falling off sharply beyond this depth. At 7 Mev, the 80 per cent dose level decreases abruptly beyond 1.9 cm; at 18 Mev, an 80 per cent or higher dose level is maintained to 4.8 cm and drops to 12 per cent at 8 cm (Fig. 1-42).

3) Constriction of isodose curve at depth. There is significant tapering of the 80 per cent isodose curve (Fig. 1-43) at energies above 9 Mev. The decreased area included by the 80 per cent curve at depth relative to the surface area of the field cannot be avoided even with optimal cone design and is worse for small fields at the higher ener-

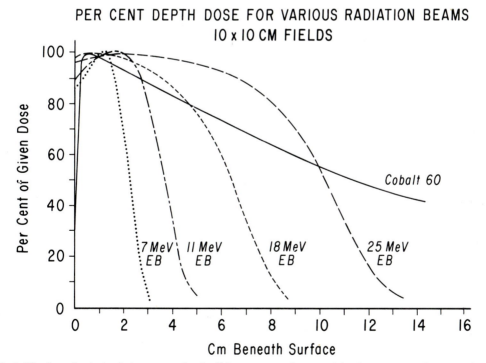

**PER CENT DEPTH DOSE FOR VARIOUS RADIATION BEAMS
10 x 10 CM FIELDS**

FIG. 1-42. Central axis depth dose curves for the ^{60}Co gamma ray beam and for the 7, 11, 18 and 25 Mev electron beams. With electrons the build-up is rapid, approaching 100 per cent near the surface; the fall-off in dose is sharp beyond the 80 per cent point for 7, 11, and 18 Mev electrons.

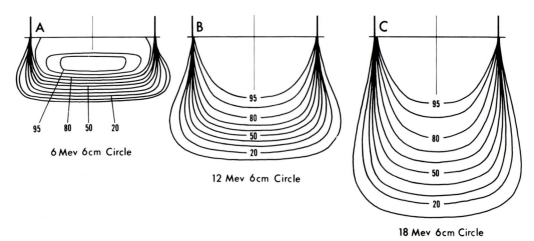

FIG. 1-43. Electron beam isodose curves measured in a water phantom.

Field size—6 cm circle.

1) 6 Mev The 80 per cent curve is at 1.9 cm. There is little radiation beyond 2 cm.

2) 12 Mev The 80 per cent curve is at 3.6 cm.

3) 18 Mev The 80 per cent curve is at 4.7 cm. The decrease in percentage depth dose is less rapid than at 6 Mev, but little radiation extends beyond 8 cm. Note that the 80 per cent isodose line is not flat at the geometric edge of the field. A generous field must be used. (Courtesy: Tapley and Fletcher: *Radiologic. Clin. N. Amer., 7,* 301, 1969.)

gies. At 18 Mev, there is 0.75 cm constriction at all margins of the effective portion of the beam, i.e., the 80 per cent curve, which is located at 4.8 cm depth. A field which at the surface is defined as a 6 cm circle will have an effective diameter of 4.5 cm across the 80 per cent isodose curve. The margins of the field at the 80 per cent depth receive doses ranging from 70 to 50 per cent.

4) Air spaces. The energy lost by electrons in traversing air is approximately 4 per cent per centimeter of air. *In situ* measurements[3] have shown a marked increase in percentage depth dose for both 9 and 18 Mev electron irradiation across lung tissue when compared with water phantom values for the same depth. The highest depth doses were measured *in vivo* with the thinnest chest wall.

With chest walls less than 1.6 cm thick, the radiation dose delivered to the underlying lung tissue is large when electrons of higher than 6 Mev energy are used to treat the chest wall after radical mastectomy. The incidence of pulmonary fibrosis is decreased by using 6 Mev electrons. *In vivo* dosimetry suggests

that 9 Mev electrons may be used if the chest wall measures from 1.5 to 2.5 cm, with approximately ±10 per cent dose variation within the substance of the chest wall. The dose will rapidly decrease and will reach a low level in the underlying pulmonary tissue.

5) Bone. The range of the electrons within different materials depends primarily on the electron densities of those materials. The density of compact bone, as in the mandible adjacent to the tonsillar area, is taken to be 1.85 gms/cm³. Considering the ratio of the electron density of bone to that of muscle, 1 cm of bone should produce approximately the same attenuation as 1.65 cm of muscle.

With lithium fluoride dosimeters in patients undergoing treatment for lesions in the tonsillar area[2], the average percentage decrease in dose compared with the water phantom value was approximately 10 per cent. However, the actual percentage decrease varies widely, depending on the thickness of the ramus of the mandible (measured by transverse tomography), and especially on the depth of the dosimeter. The corrected dose may be computed by the simple formula: Depth $+0.65$ (cm bone) $=$ Effective Depth (E.D.). No correction for bone absorption need be applied in the average patient for 12 and 15 Mev electron irradiation when the sternum (predominantly spongy bone) is interposed in the beam.

Normal Tissue Reactions

Skin

Large areas of skin tolerate high given doses with 6 and 9 Mev electrons; a moist reaction, when it occurs, is patchy and superficial and will heal quickly. With given doses of 5,000 to 6,000 rads in 4 or 5 weeks to large fields on the chest wall and the lateral neck, including the supraclavicular region, moist reactions are rare. Most patients receiving treatment to the chest wall with the 6 or 9 Mev electron beam (given dose of 5,500 rads in 4 weeks) to areas measuring 200 to 350 sq. cm have had a dry skin reaction. Over half of the patients receiving given doses of 6,500 rads in 5 weeks to 7,500 rads in 6 weeks to fields measuring less than 80 sq. cm developed heavy dry peeling.

When 12, 15, and 18 Mev electrons are used, a dry skin reaction is usually seen if the given doses do not exceed 5,500 rads in $4\frac{1}{2}$ weeks to 7,000 rads in 6 weeks. Severe late skin changes rarely occur with dose levels under 7,000 rads in 6 or 7 weeks. With given doses of 6,600 rads in 5 weeks to 8,100 rads in $6\frac{1}{2}$ weeks, almost 50 per cent of patients will develop moist skin reactions, limited in extent and patchy rather than confluent. Healing time is usually 7 to 14 days; it is rarely more than 28 days. With doses above 6,500 rads in 5 weeks, a significant number of patients have developed telangiectasias and patchy depigmentation.

Mucous Membranes

The acute mucous membrane reactions seen with the electron beam are similar to those produced by the photon beam for the same doses but are sharply localized to the treated side. No reaction is seen in the contralateral mucous membrane. Limiting the high dose to one side of the oral cavity insures less discomfort for the patient, improved nutrition during the course of therapy, and decreased interference with salivary gland function.

When the electron beam is combined with the 18 to 22 Mev photon beam in the treatment of more deeply located lesions or those requiring high tumor doses, the mucosal reaction on the entrance side will be a patchy or confluent exudate whereas the opposite side will show erythema only.

Muscle and Connective Tissue

For the first $3\frac{1}{2}$ years, the 6 to 18 Mev electron beam was either the single modality of treatment or provided additional dosage to a limited volume following comprehensive ^{60}Co treatment. The technique most often used was a single appositional portal. It was recognized that the homogeneously high dose through the treated tissue volume might lead to excessive injury of the skin and subcutaneous tissues. Analysis of the results in the first series of patients showed an unacceptable degree of late radiation sequelae in the normal tissues of some patients.

The incidence of subcutaneous fibrosis in patients treated with the electron beam alone or when combined with the other irradiation, either megavoltage photon beam or interstitial radium is compared in Table 1-4. Fewer patients develop fibrosis when the electron beam is combined with other radiation in treatment for floor of mouth and tonsillar area lesions where there is a large treatment volume. No difference is seen in the treatment of lesions of the hypopharynx and supraglottic larynx where the treatment volume is smaller.

In order to lessen the high dose to the skin and subcutaneous tissues and to avoid underdosing, which might result from shadow-

Table 1-4. *Incidence of Subcutaneous Fibrosis After Electron Beam Therapy: Primary Lesions of Upper Respiratory and Digestive Passages May 1963–Dec. 1966*

Anatomical Sites	No. Pts. Treated	Fibrosis		
		E.B. Alone	E.B. Combined with External Photon Beam or Interstitial Gamma Ray	E.B. Boost
Buccal mucosa & Gingiva	33	12% ($3/25$)	14% ($1/7$)	0% ($0/1$)
Floor of mouth	45	22% ($4/18$)	8% ($2/26$)	0% ($0/1$)
Tonsillar area	91	18% ($2/11$)	3% ($1/31$)	14% ($7/49$)
Hypopharynx & Supraglottic	32	0% ($0/12$)	12% ($1/8$)	8% ($1/12$)

ing by bone, the electron beam is frequently combined with 18 or 22 Mev photons or with interstitial therapy in suitable situations. With the former technique, the intense mucosal reactions with confluent exudate is confined to the homolateral side and the reaction on the contralateral side is limited to erythema without mucosal studding. Moderate to severe dryness and loss of taste sense, commonly occurring with parallel opposing portals, are rare.

Basic Concepts

Laboratory studies[5] comparing the electron beam with megavoltage photon irradiation have shown a relative biological effectiveness (*RBE*) close to 1.0. The working concept has been to evolve patterns of use of 6 to 18 Mev electrons, utilizing special treatment techniques, fitted to clinical situations where satisfactory management had not been achieved with the photon beam.

The characteristics of the electron beam are of distinct advantage in treating malignant lesions at a limited depth. A sterilizing dose of radiation can be delivered to the tumor while the total volume of tissue included in the high dose range is sharply limited. The electron beam is well suited for intraoral and transvaginal therapy.

The principal areas of application suitable for the 6 to 18 Mev electron beam are:

1) Skin and lip cancers.
2) Chest wall and neck
   a) elective after surgery or
   b) for recurrent disease.
3) Primary lesions of the head and neck, located at 2 to 6 cm depth
   a) total treatment with electron beam alone or in combination with the photon beam using equal given doses or with interstitial therapy or
   b) boost treatment to the primary.
4) Boost to nodes.

The selection of treatment technique, the combination of electrons and photons, and the ratio of given doses of each beam depends upon the maximum depth of the lesion to be treated. A variation of combination treatment is that of additional or "boost" therapy using reduced portals, in order to raise to a high level the total tumor dose to the initial gross disease.

In the clinical applications of the electron beam, treatment aims and therapeutic principles are based upon the basic parameters of radiation therapy that have been established for megavoltage photon irradiation. The alterations in the accepted time-dose relationships have been minimal. Treatment techniques have been modified only as dic-

tated by the special characteristics of the electron beam.

The minimum tumor dose is not significantly altered with a megavoltage photon beam if a 1 or 2 cm error in the estimated depth of the tumor is made, but with the electron beam the maximum depth of the lesion must not exceed the depth of the 80 per cent isodose curve, taken as the minimum tumor dose (Fig. 1-44). When 18 or 22 Mev photons are combined with the 18 Mev electron beam in a 1:1 ratio of given doses, the location of the minimum 80 per cent tumor dose is not as critical because the

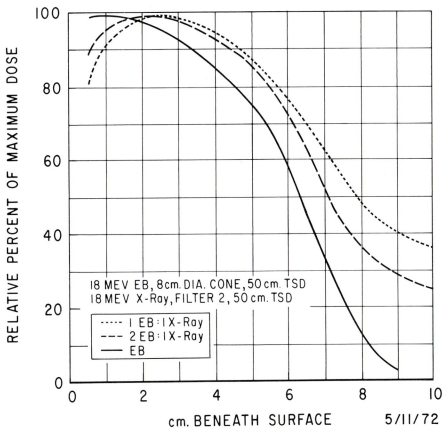

Percent Depth Doses with Combined Electron and Photon Beams

18 MEV EB, 8cm. DIA. CONE, 50cm. TSD
18 MEV X-Ray, FILTER 2, 50cm. TSD

..... 1 EB:1 X-Ray
--- 2 EB:1 X-Ray
— EB

cm. BENEATH SURFACE   5/11/72

FIG. 1-44. Combined 18 Mev electron and photon beam depth dose curves. With a 1:1 ratio of electron and photon given doses, the calculated 80 per cent dose level is located more than 1 cm deeper than with 18 Mev electrons alone.

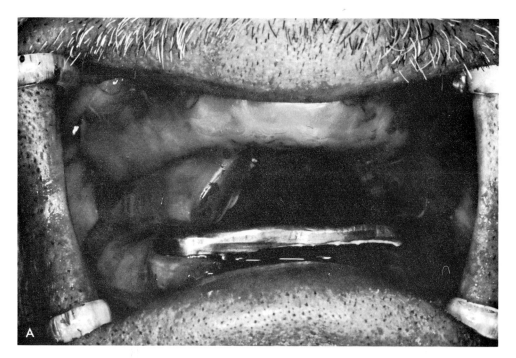

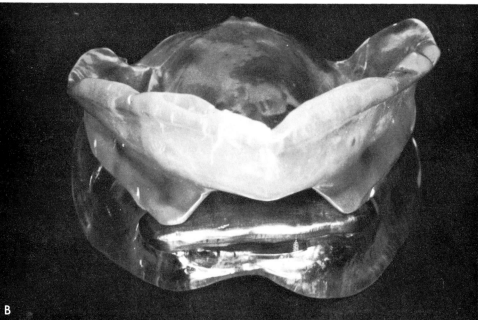

FIG. 1-45. A. Carcinoma of the anterior gingiva and floor of mouth, invading the root of the tongue. An intraoral stent is in position in the mouth to flatten the tongue and to protect the hard palate. B. Lucite upper and lower plates with a lead block inserted between to protect the palate. With a submental portal using the 18 Mev electron beam, 2 to 4 mm of lead is adequate to protect the mucous membrane because of partial absorption of the beam by the submental tissues and the tongue. (Courtesy: Tapley and Fletcher: *Radiologic Clin. N. Amer.*, 7, 301, 1969.)

decrease in percentage depth dose beyond this point is not as precipitous.

With the sharp fall-off in dose, the structures deep to the treatment target receive relative protection. Nine millimeters of lead will absorb close to 95 per cent of 18 Mev electrons; 6 Mev electrons require only 2 millimeters of lead. Added distance alone offered by intervening tissues significantly decreases the dose to deeper structures. For this reason, in treating lesions of the oral cavity, intraoral stents are made for the individual patients and provide protection either by containing lead or by increasing the distance according to the thickness of tissue-equivalent Lucite of which they are made. These stents (Fig. 1-45A and B) provide protection for the teeth, gingiva, tongue, and floor of mouth.

A differential in depth dose may be achieved by Lucite blocking of a portion of the field, as in treatment of the neck when it is desired to treat one area to a depth of 2 cm and an adjacent area to a depth of 3 cm. With the 12 Mev electron beam, the addition of 1 cm of Lucite will provide a dose distribution comparable to the 9 Mev electron beam in the area covered by the Lucite. This technique is used only when a portion of the treatment is to be given with the electron beam since all skin sparing is lost by the interposition of tissue-equivalent material.

The constriction of the useful portion of the beam, particularly at high energies and with small fields (Fig. 1-43), requires extra care in centering the lesion with reference to the beam (Figs. 1-46A, B and C). It must be remembered that the area covered by the 80 per cent curve of the 18 Mev electron beam will be decreased by 0.5 to 0.75 cm at all margins of the field, requiring a proportionately larger portal to ensure coverage of the entire lesion and a satisfactory surrounding margin.

A control rate of 81 per cent for T_1–T_3 tonsillar area lesions treated with the electron beam alone or combined with the megavoltage photon beam is comparable to the local control rate in patients having received photon beam treatment. The advantage of the combined technique is provided by the decrease in the number and severity of radiation sequelae in the normal tissues. Surgical resection of recurrences following electron beam therapy has been possible without undue delay in healing and has provided a significant salvage rate. The electron beam "boost" dose, through a small, appositional field, can be increased over the dose that can be given with a glancing ^{60}Co field, since the treatment volume is decreased in two dimensions, by shrinking the size of the field and by limiting the depth of the high dose by using a lower Mev. In the elective treatment of potentially involved adjacent lymphatic drainage areas, the given dose with the 9 or 12 Mev electron beams is 5,000 to 5,500 rads in 4 to $4\frac{1}{2}$ weeks.

Clinical Applications

Skin Lesions

The 6 Mev electron beam is used for the treatment of superficial lesions of the skin, including the eyelids. The estimated 80 per cent surface dose rapidly builds up to 100 per cent which eliminates the need for bolus material. The homogeneous dose distribution and the rapid decrease in depth dose permits the delivery of a high dose to a limited depth. The beam energy is selected according to the estimated depth of the lesion. Nine or 12 Mev electrons are used if there is infiltration of underlying structures.

Carcinomas of the eyelids are treated with 6 Mev electrons. The field is defined by a cut-out in a fitted lead mask (Fig. 1-47), used to shield orbital structures. With a given dose of 5,500 rads in $4\frac{1}{2}$ weeks or 6,000 rads in 5 weeks, excellent cosmetic and functional results were seen at one to 5 years after treatment in 55 patients with carcinomas of the eyelids, including the medial canthus.

Superficial skin lesions are treated with 6 Mev electrons; the given doses are 5,000

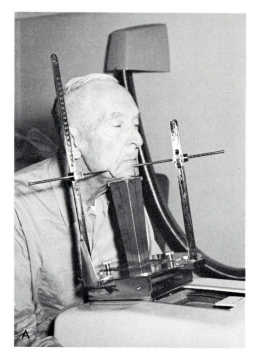

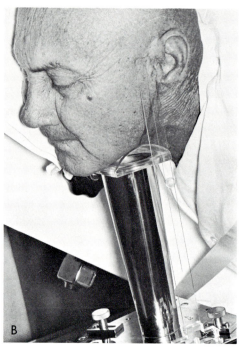

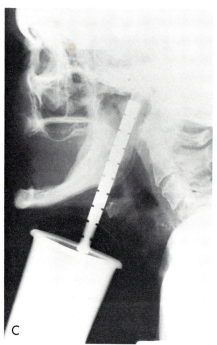

the marks on the patient's face. These assist in positioning the patient daily.

B. This 69-year-old patient had 2 exophytic lesions of the laryngeal surface of the epiglottis; squamous cell carcinoma, grade II, staged T_2N_0. Treatment was given with parallel opposing 6 cm fields with the 22 Mev photon beam, 5,500 rads tumor dose in 5 weeks. A 5 cm submental field with 18 Mev electrons was used to add 1,000 rads tumor dose. The patient showed no evidence of disease $8\frac{1}{2}$ years after treatment. The submental compression cone is shown in treatment position. A Lucite strip to define the central axis of the beam is aligned with a mark on the skin. The skin mark, placed during fluoroscopy, was aligned with the epiglottis.

C. Film taken on the simulator showing the compression cone of the submental portal and the distance from the cone surface to the base of the tongue. The indentations at each centimeter of the measuring device show that the distance to the dorsum of the tongue is approximately 4.5 cm. With the 18 Mev electron beam, the dose to the area of the tumor will be no less than 80 per cent of the given dose. (Courtesy: Tapley and Fletcher: *Radiologic Clin. N, Amer.*, 7, 301, 1969.)

FIG. 1-46. A. Anterior floor of mouth carcinoma. Treatment position for submental electron beam portal. The metal pointers are aligned with the central axis of the beam and with

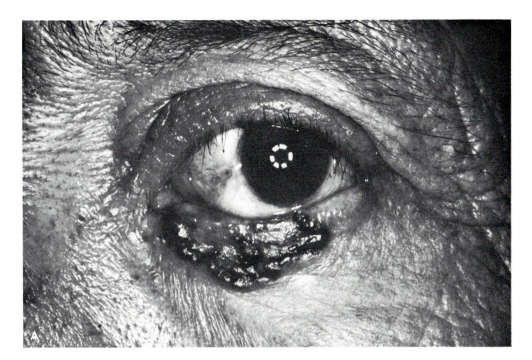

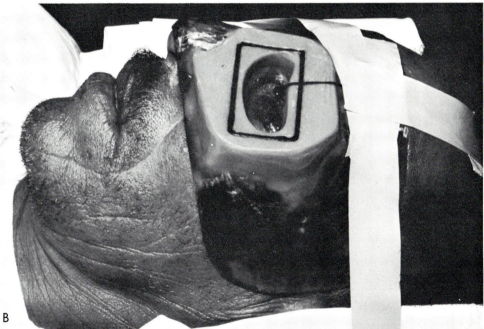

FIG. 1-47. This 53-year-old male was seen in April 1968 with a 6-month history of a lesion of the left lower eyelid which gradually increased in size and became slightly ulcerated. The lesion was pigmented, thick and nodular and measured 2.5 cm. It did not involve the lid conjunctiva. On biopsy it was a basal cell carcinoma.

A lead mask was made and the entire lower lid was treated with the 6 Mev electron beam. The total given dose was 5,500 rads in 37 elapsed days. In follow-up $3\frac{1}{2}$ years after completing treatment the eyelid was in good condition with no evidence of recurrence or of ectropion. There was no tearing and no conjunctivitis.

A. Lesion of lower eyelid extending laterally from the medial canthus. **B.** The patient is shown in treatment position. The cut-out in the lead mask defines the field. The treatment portal is fitted to the wax seating. A lead eye shield is inserted under the eyelids. The upper lid is retracted out of the treatment field. (B Courtesy: Tapley and Fletcher: *Radiologic Clin. N. Amer.,* 7, 301, 1969.)

rads in 3 weeks to 6,500 rads in 5 weeks. For large infiltrative skin lesions, the Mev is selected for the estimated depth of the lesion and the dose is 7,500 rads in 6 weeks to 8,500 rads in 7½ weeks. A decreased field and lower Mev are used after 5,000 to 6,000 rads are given.

Cancers of the lip, previously untreated or recurrent after excision, are treated with 6 to 12 Mev electrons. With a wide margin included around the lesion, the given dose is 5,000 rads in 4 weeks, followed by an additional 2,000 to 2,500 rads delivered by a radium needle implant. If interstitial radium is not used, 1,500 to 2,000 rads are added at reduced energy and with a smaller portal. The underlying structures are protected by a stent containing lead. The skin and mucosal reactions are brisk but healing is rapid. The late results are very satisfactory both cosmetically and functionally. The skin and lip are soft and atrophy is minimal.

Parotid Gland Tumors

The technique used in the treatment of parotid gland tumors is described in Chapter 3—Malignant Tumors in Salivary Glands.

Floor of Mouth and Undersurface of Tongue

Lesions of the floor of the mouth and the undersurface of the tongue are treated with the electron beam if they are not considered suitable for primary interstitial gamma-ray therapy. A superficial carcinoma of the anterior floor of the mouth, if it can be adequately encompassed by an intraoral cone, receives a given dose of 6,000 rads in 4 weeks with 6 or 9 Mev electrons. More advanced lesions receive 4,000 rads in 4 weeks or 5,000 rads in 5 weeks with the external photon beam, supplemented respectively by 3,000 to 3,500 rads or 2,500 to 3,000 rads with a radium needle implant. In lesions extending onto the gum (Fig. 1-48A), 1,000 to 2,500 rads may be added through an intraoral cone, if the cone covers it well (Fig. 1-48B and C), for a total of 6,500 rads in 5½ to 6 weeks. Infiltrative lesions of the floor of the mouth, which are fixed to the periosteum of the mandible or which extend onto the gingiva, are treated with the 18 Mev electron beam through a submental field (Fig. 1-46A) combined with parallel opposed 18 Mev photon beam fields. The total tumor dose is 6,500 rads in 6 weeks

FIG. 1-48. This 75-year-old male was seen in November 1968, with an exophytic squamous cell carcinoma of the anterior floor of mouth and gingiva, with a pressure defect of the mandible on x-ray examination, staged T_3N_0. The plan of treatment was to begin therapy with an intraoral cone using the 12 Mev electron beam to give 1,900 rads in 7 treatments followed by parallel opposed 22 Mev photon fields to 5,000 rads at the midline and a submental field (Figure 1-46A) with 18 Mev electrons to provide an additional 1,250 rads given dose. The calculated tumor doses were 7,500 rads in 7½ weeks provided by:

    Intraoral cone—12 Mev electrons—1,500 rads
    Parallel opposed fields—22 Mev photons—5,000 rads
    Submental field—18 Mev electrons—1,000 rads

The patient had a small recurrence on the gingiva 9 months after radiation therapy was completed. This was resected without removing the mandible. At 2 years a right radical neck dissection was done for metastatic preglandular nodes. The patient had a stroke and expired 4 years after radiation treatment.

    A. Exophytic lesion of the anterior floor of mouth and gingiva prior to treatment. **B.** Patient in treatment position. The intraoral cone, 4 cm in diameter, is maintained in position by an intraoral stent. **C.** Lesion photographed through intraoral stent after receiving 1,900 rads given dose with the 12 Mev electron beam. Exudate covers the lesion. The tongue is held back by a Lucite bar across the upper third of the stent. (B, C Courtesy: Tapley and Fletcher: *Radiologic Clin. N. Amer.*, 7, 301, 1969.)

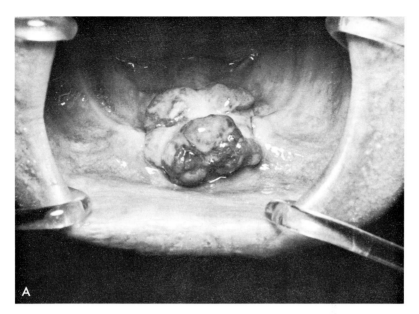

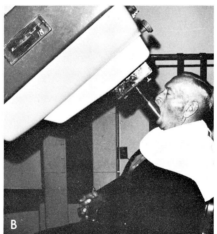

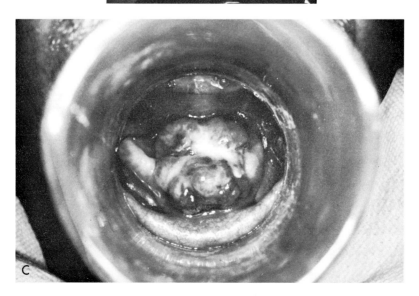

or 7,000 rads in 7 weeks provided equally by the two modalities.

Small carcinomas of the undersurface of the tongue close to the tip are treated with an 18 Mev submental electron beam field followed by interstitial radium. The tongue is maintained in position (flattened into the floor of the mouth) by an intraoral stent (Figs. 1-45A and B). This is to ensure that the lesion remains within the high dose range of the 18 Mev electron beam. The tumor dose, taken as the 80 per cent dose, is 4,000 rads in 4 weeks or 5,000 rads in 5 weeks. A radium needle implant provides an additional tumor dose of 3,000 to 3,500 rads if 4,000 rads have been given with the electron beam or 2,500 to 3,000 rads if 5,000 rads have been given.

Gingiva and Gingivobuccal Sulci

Small, superficial lesions of the gingiva are treated with the electron beam alone, either through an intraoral cone exclusively or a cone combined with an external appositional electron beam portal. The tumor dose is 6,000 rads in 5 weeks or 6,500 rads in 6 weeks. Larger lesions of the gingiva and lesions of the buccal-gingival sulci usually require a combination of electron and megavoltage photon beams in a 2:1 ratio of electron to photon given doses, the total tumor dose ranging from 6,000 rads in 5 weeks to 6,500 rads in 6 weeks or 7,000 rads in 7 weeks, depending upon the size and extension of the lesion. An intraoral stent which contains lead is always used with the electron beam to protect the tongue and the mucous membranes of the opposite oral cavity.

Buccal Mucosa

Although it is tempting to use the electron beam alone to treat carcinomas of the buccal mucosa, previous experience demonstrated an undesirable degree and duration of acute reactions as well as later sequelae of severe skin changes and fibrosis with trismus. The current technique for buccal mucosa lesions combines the electron beam with interstitial radium. The tongue is protected by an intraoral stent containing lead.

If the lesion extends posteriorly toward the pterygoid space, and especially if the patient presents with trismus, a lateral field with 18 or 22 Mev photons is used to build up the depth dose of the 18 Mev electron beam and to spare the skin and subcutaneous tissues. The treatment may be given in a 1:1 ratio of electrons to photons, or an added tumor dose of 1,500 to 2,000 rads may be given with the photon beam after 5,000 rads tumor dose in 5 weeks has been given with the electron beam.

Retromolar Trigone-Anterior Faucial Pillar

There is a percentage of bone exposure and mandibular necrosis in lesions of the faucial arch treated with ^{60}Co, either with single homolateral portals or wedge-paired filters, with a control rate for T_1 and T_2 lesions of approximately 90 per cent.[4] Pronounced dryness of the mouth and throat with persistent impairment in the sense of taste are frequent when parallel opposing portals are used.

Limited lesions of the retromolar trigone are well lateralized and do not present the problem of shadowing by bone even if they extend into the posterior sulcus of the buccal mucosa. If an intraoral cone can be used to provide part of the treatment (1,000 to 1,500 rads tumor dose), these lesions may be treated with a single lateral 18 Mev electron beam field. The total tumor dose is 6,000 rads in 5½ weeks or 6,500 rads in 6 weeks depending upon the size of the portal.

Carcinomas of the anterior tonsillar pillar (T_1-T_3, N_0-N_1), with minimal extension into the soft palate or tongue, receive combined treatment in a 1:1 or 1:2 ratio with the electron beam and 18 or 22 Mev photon irradiation because a greater depth dose is necessary and because interposed bone will further decrease the depth dose. With equal given doses using the 18 Mev electron and photon beams, the 80 per cent tumor dose is located at a depth of approximately 6 cm (Fig. 1-44) unless shifted toward the surface by heavy cortical bone in the mandible. Corrections are made for mandible thickness, if necessary, when calculating the tumor dose with the electron beam. The combined tumor dose is 6,000 rads in 5 weeks for limited lesions and 6,500 rads in 6 or 6½ weeks or 7,000 rads in 7 weeks for more extensive lesions. When possible, the final 1,000 to 1,500 rads tumor dose is given through a reduced field. The subdigastric node area is included in the treatment field of the primary lesion. The mucositis is sharply limited to the affected side with essentially no mucosal reaction on the opposite side (Fig. 1-49). Acute radiation morbidity is decreased and late dryness is negligible.

In more advanced lesions or when neck nodes are involved, after 5,000 rads or 6,000 rads with parallel opposed portals with ⁶⁰Co, the electron beam alone or in a 1:1 ratio with the 18 Mev photon beam may be used for additional irradiation. This "boost" to the

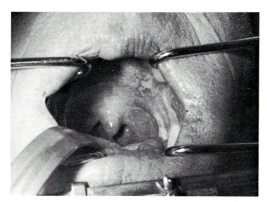

FIG. 1-49. This patient had squamous cell carcinoma of the anterior tonsillar pillar. Treatment was given with combined 18 Mev electron and photon beams in a 1:1 ratio of given doses. At a tumor dose of 6,000 rads in 6 weeks, the mucositis is sharply localized to the left oral cavity. (Courtesy: Tapley and Fletcher: *Radiologic Clin. N. Amer.,* 7, 301, 1969.)

primary provides 7,000 rads total tumor dose to a limited volume.

Tonsillar Fossa and Glossopalatine Sulcus

In lesions arising in the tonsillar fossa, after the primary lesion and the upper neck nodes have received a tumor dose of 5,000 to 6,000 rads with opposed ⁶⁰Co portals, the electron beam may be used alone, but usually is combined with the 18 Mev photon beam in equal doses, to add a tumor dose of 2,000 or 1,000 rads to the primary lesion through a reduced field, to a total dose of 7,000 rads. If lymph node metastases are present in the neck and radical neck dissection is not feasible, an electron beam boost of 1,000 to 1,500 rads is given to the nodes.

Base of Tongue

Base of tongue tumors, frequently located near the midline or extending across it and with a high incidence of bilateral cervical node metastases, require through and through treatment with parallel opposed portals. After treatment with ⁶⁰Co or the photon beam to a tumor dose of 5,500 to 6,000 rads, a submental field (Fig. 1-46B and C) is used to add 2,000 to 2,500 rads tumor dose to the primary lesion to achieve a total tumor dose of 7,500 rads in 7½ weeks or 8,000 rads in 8 or 8½ weeks. The beam passes through untreated skin, avoiding the already irradiated mandible. The dose received by the base of the tongue is 80 to 90 per cent of the electron beam given dose.

Submental boosts should not be used to treat the base of the tongue when the maximum depth of the tumor from the submental skin exceeds 5 cm with a resulting unacceptably low depth dose with the 18 Mev electron beam. If the tumor in the base of the tongue involves the dorsum of the tongue, the boost is given through a reduced lateral photon beam field because the distance from the submental skin will exceed 5 cm.

Supraglottic Larynx and Hypopharynx

In tumors of the unilateral supraglottic structures, the 15 Mev electron beam provides sparing of the opposite laryngeal structures. After 5,000 rads with ^{60}Co, 1,500 to 2,000 rads tumor dose is given through an appositional electron beam portal (Fig. 1-50).

The total dose is 6,500 rads in 6½ weeks or 7,000 rads in 7 weeks. The mucosal reaction is confined to the high dose area.

With extensive lesions of the suprahyoid epiglottis parallel opposing ^{60}Co portals are used to deliver 5,000 to 6,000 rads tumor dose. A submental field (centered lower than for the base of the tongue) is then used with 15 or 18 Mev electrons to add 2,000 rads

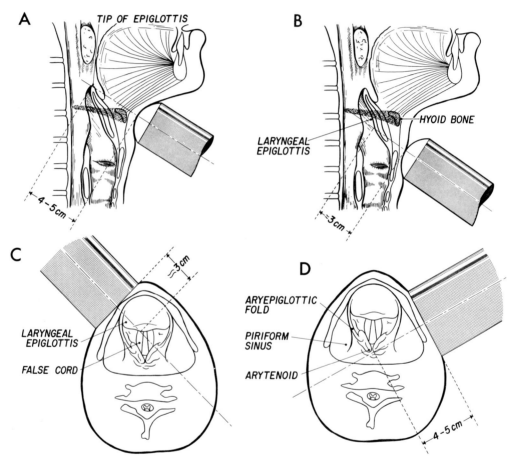

FIG. 1-50. Portal applications for hypopharynx and larynx lesions. **A.** Lingual epiglottis—submental compression cone. The distance from skin surface to tip of epiglottis is 3 to 3.5 cm ensuring a minimum 80 per cent tumor dose with 18 Mev electrons. A similar port application, with increased upward angulation is used for base of tongue lesions. **B.** Laryngeal epiglottis—submental cone with cephalad angulation decreased. The lower margin of the field is at the thyroid notch, the upper margin at the hyoid bone. **C.** Angle (base) of epiglottis and false cord—portal *appositional* to slope of neck with central axis of beam perpendicular to and isodose curves parallel to the vocal cord. The anterior edge of the beam is at the midline. Since the distance from skin surface to true cord is 3 to 3.5 cm, 15 Mev electrons can be used. **D.** Pyriform sinus and arytenoid—appositional portal with anterior margin of beam moved approximately 1.0 cm posterior from midline of neck. The field size is increased to 6 × 6 or 6 × 8 cm.

tumor dose if 5,000 rads tumor dose in 5 weeks has been given, and 1,000 rads tumor dose if 6,000 rads in 6 weeks have been given.

Lateral pharyngeal wall and pyriform sinus lesions can be treated with the 12 to 15 Mev electron beam alone if there is no extension to the posterior pharyngeal wall or into adjacent laryngeal structures. The tumor dose is 6,500 rads in $6\frac{1}{2}$ weeks or 7,000 rads in 7 weeks. Skin reactions have not been severe. Laryngeal edema is no problem because of sparing of the opposite side of the larynx. With more extensive lesions or with thick overlying tissues, 5,000 rads in 5 weeks are given with ^{60}Co followed by the 15 or 18 Mev electron beam to provide a total tumor dose of 7,000 rads in 7 weeks.

Cervical Lymph Nodes

The physical characteristics of the electron beam permit ideal irradiation of the cervical lymphatics in a multiplicity of clinical situations.

The most common clinical situations are:

1) Irradiation of one entire neck as the sole modality of elective treatment.

2) Irradiation of one entire neck after radical neck dissection

    a) as elective treatment or

    b) for recurrent disease.

3) Irradiation of the spinal accessory chain of nodes.

4) Irradiation of extensions of surgical scars not easily included in the treatment field when postoperative treatment is given with the photon beam.

5) Additional local dosage ("boost" therapy) after photon irradiation of residual masses or areas of high risk of infestation.

Elective treatment to the whole neck, with or without later neck dissection, is given with the electron beam when there is a high risk of lymphatic infestation which is limited to one side. Treatment may be given to the neck in conjunction with treatment of the primary lesion or the site of the primary lesion, if excision has been done. For example, after removal of a malignant tumor of the parotid gland, if there is known or suspected residual disease and if the tumor is of high grade malignancy, the parotid area is irradiated with combined photon and electron beams and the entire ipsilateral neck is treated with the 9 or 12 Mev electron beam (Fig. 1-51).

With a clinically negative neck, the given dose is 5,000 rads in 4 weeks or 5,500 rads in $4\frac{1}{2}$ weeks; this provides a dose to the lymphatics in the range of 4,500 to 5,000 rads. Similar treatment may be provided for an oral cavity lesion with a clinically suspicious node, followed by a radical neck dissection.

In the operated neck, the treatment field must include all extensions of the surgical scar. If the anterior limb of the neck incision extends directly across the thyroid cartilage, it is necessary for the larynx to remain in the field without shielding until at least 4,500 rads have been given. If possible, 6 Mev is used which will limit the dose to the ipsilateral laryngeal structures.

Indications for treatment of the whole neck after radical neck dissection are:

1) Multiple positive nodes in the surgical specimen.

2) Total replacement of a node by tumor or rupture of a cystic node.

3) Tumor found in connective tissue.

4) Tumor found in the perineural lymphatics.

Healing must be complete before irradiation is started, usually 14 to 21 days after surgery. The field is defined with a lead cutout (Fig. 1-52). If the flaps are very thin, the entire neck may be treated at 6 Mev; with thicker flaps 9 Mev is necessary. When there are large, partially fixed or fixed nodes which have been removed from the upper neck or if the involved nodes were attached to the periosteum of the mandible, the neck field is divided with the upper neck being treated at 9 to 15 Mev and the lower neck being treated at 6 Mev (Fig. 1-53). The larynx is included in the lower portion of the field and

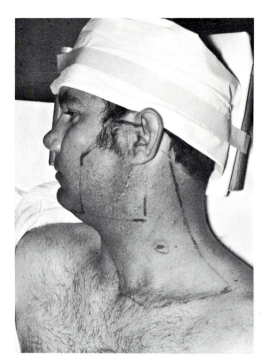

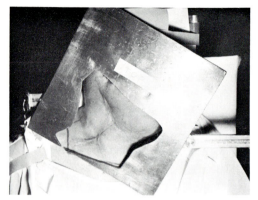

FIG. 1-52. Whole neck treatment with 9 Mev electron beam after radical neck dissection. Unless the dissection scar extends across the anterior neck, the larynx is usually shielded with a small lead block after 4,000 to 4,500 rads given dose. The field is defined with a lead cut-out (0.5–1.0 cm thick) which is placed as close to the patient as possible. If the distance from the cut-out to the patient does not exceed 5 cm, the edges of the radiation field are relatively sharply defined. (Courtesy: Tapley and Fletcher: *Radiologic Clin. N. Amer.*, 7, 301, 1969.)

FIG. 1-51. This 37-year-old male was referred for radiation therapy in February 1972 after a total parotidectomy for high grade mucoepidermoid carcinoma of the left parotid gland. Sacrifice of the 7th nerve was necessary because the tumor was wrapped around it. Because of nerve involvement and the relatively undifferentiated tumor, radiation therapy was recommended for the parotid bed area and for the entire ipsilateral neck.

The parotid area was treated with a single left lateral 10 × 8 cm portal using 18 Mev electron and photon beams in a 1:1 ratio of given doses. In 5½ weeks, the large field received 5,000 rads at 5 cm depth and an additional 500 rads with the photon beam through a small field limited to the base of the skull. The entire neck was treated with 11 Mev electrons to a given dose of 5,000 rads in 4 weeks. The neck field was defined with a lead cut-out. The patient developed mild hoarseness and had marked throat soreness when the given dose to the neck had reached 3,750 rads in 3 weeks. There was minimal ipsilateral laryngeal edema and exudate along the lateral pharyngeal wall. Because of the thickness of the neck soft tissues since there had not been a neck dissection, 11 Mev electrons were considered necessary. The resulting depth dose

is irradiated with the lower Mev. The given dose is 5,000 rads in 4 weeks or 6,000 rads in 5 weeks except in patients with extensive fixed disease who require a boost field to the area. An additional 1,000 to 1,500 rads may be given through a sharply reduced field.

Treatment may be given with the electron beam for recurrent disease. The given dose will be higher, usually 6,000 rads in 5 weeks to the whole involved neck and, through a reduced field, an additional 1,000 to 1,500 rads to the site of recurrence. With a planned

produced intense mucosal reactions. The electron energy was decreased to 9 Mev for the remainder of the treatment and the severity of the mucosal reaction subsided.

The patient is shown in treatment position with the treatment fields defined for the parotid bed area and for the entire neck. The surgical scar can be seen in the preauricular area and extends from the subdigastric area upward behind the ear. (Courtesy: Tapley and Fletcher: *Amer. J. Roentgen.*, In press.)

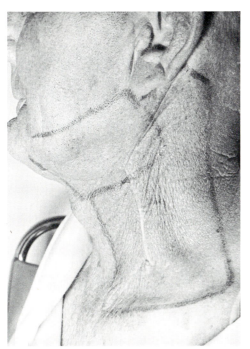

FIG. 1-53. This 64-year-old male was first seen at M. D. Anderson Hospital in June 1966, with a history of having had a radium needle implant in July 1965, for carcinoma of the lower lip. In March 1966, the lip lesion recurred. On examination the patient had a mass overlying the left mental foramen as well as the recurrence on the lip. The recurrent lip lesion was resected and a left radical neck dissection done. The pathology report described squamous cell carcinoma, Grade II. In the neck, 6 of 51 nodes contained tumor deposits and tumor was found in connective tissue.

The patient received postoperative irradiation to the entire neck with the electron beam. The upper portion of the field overlying the mandible (measuring 6 × 10 cm) was treated to a given dose of 6,500 rads in 5½ weeks with 15 Mev electrons. The remainder of the neck, including the mastoid tip was treated with 9 Mev electrons to 6,000 rads given dose in 5 weeks.

The patient showed no evidence of disease in June 1971. The irradiated tissues are in good condition, soft and pliable on palpation, 5 years after treatment was completed. (Courtesy: Tapley and Fletcher: *Amer. J. Roentgen.*, In press.)

high dose, it is essential to shield the larynx when 4,500 rads have been given. If the recurrent disease is in the vicinity of the laryngeal structures, a Lucite block 1 or 2 cm thick can be placed over the larynx to decrease the depth dose.

With electron beam irradiation to the whole neck, the acute reaction is a brisk erythema followed by dry desquamation. When the given dose is more than 5,500 rads in 4½ weeks, patches of moist desquamation usually are seen in the high dose areas, but healing occurs in 7 to 10 days. Moderate pharyngeal mucositis usually occurs, producing some discomfort on swallowing. The reaction in the larynx is almost always minimal and edema of the laryngeal structures is limited to the ipsilateral side. In the unoperated neck, fibrosis does not develop and skin changes are minimal (Fig. 1-54). In the operated neck, there may be minimal to moderate subcutaneous fibrosis. Telangectasias may occur but are infrequent unless the given dose has exceeded 6,000 rads.

Seventy-five patients have received electron beam treatment to one entire neck and 6 patients to both necks from May 1963 through December 1969. Treatment has been given electively after radical neck dissection has been performed for extensive neck disease or for recurrent disease in the neck occurring 2 to 26 months after radical neck dissection. Freedom from recurrence of disease has been achieved most often in those patients without gross disease who have been treated electively. Table 1-5 shows that 11 of 31 patients receiving elective irradiation after neck dissection are alive with no evidence of disease up to 8 years after treatment and that 9 patients died from intercurrent disease or distant metastases but were free of disease above the clavicle. Of 16 patients receiving treatment for recurrent neck disease, only 1 patient has remained alive free of local or generalized disease.

Irradiation of the spinal accessory chain nodes is indicated in a variety of situations. If the primary lesion is treated with parallel

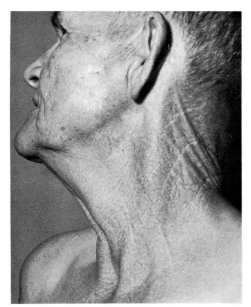

FIG. 1-54. This 61-year-old male, seen in 1966, had a history of skin cancers of the face treated by excision and radium several years previously. He developed a mass in the left upper neck which extended into the superficial lobe of the parotid. A partial parotidectomy was performed but no attempt was made to resect the entire tumor. The tumor was reported to be poorly differentiated squamous carcinoma with extensive invasion of the perineural lymphatics. When the patient was seen for radiotherapy, there was a firm mass anterior to the ear and induration in the upper neck.

Treatment was given to the parotid area with combined 18 Mev photon and electron beams. In 6 weeks the dose was 6,000 rads at 5 cm depth. The entire neck was treated with the 9 Mev electron beam, giving 6,000 rads in 5 weeks. In November 1971, 68 months later, the patient was well and the irradiated tissues were in excellent condition.

The patient is shown $6\frac{1}{2}$ years later with essentially normal appearing tissues except for some scarring at the site of radium treatment for a previous skin cancer in the left cheek. (Courtesy: Tapley and Fletcher: *Amer. J. Roentgen.*, In press.)

opposing fields with a 1:1 loading, the fields are extended back over the chains until the midline tumor dose reaches 4,500 rads. To exclude the spinal cord from further irradiation, the primary fields are moved forward and the 6 or 9 Mev electron beam then treats the posterior strips to at least 5,000 rads at 1 cm depth (Fig. 3-17). When parallel opposing fields with a 2:1 loading are being used to treat the primary lesion, a posterior strip on the contralateral side may be treated by the 9 Mev electron beam and by the exit dose of the ipsilateral field which extends back over the spinal cord (Fig. 3-55).

Boost treatment through a reduced field may be given after the area of the primary and both necks have received 5,000 rads with ^{60}Co. The electron beam is used at varying energies to increase the dose to involved nodes in the neck (Fig. 2-48B and 3-16) or to areas of high risk of infestation (Fig. 3-18B) without increasing the dose significantly to the deeper structures such as the pharynx, larynx, or spinal cord. The additional dosage may be 1,000 to 2,500 rads given dose in 4 to 10 treatments through a field limited to the area of residual adenopathy or induration. The electron beam is also used to treat a field-within-a-field if a lymph node continues to enlarge under treatment (Fig. 2-48A). The field is limited to the palpable mass, giving 250 rads twice a week using 9 or 12 Mev to a total dose of 1,500 to 2,000 rads. The concomitant additional treatment replaces the boost usually given at the end of treatment.

BREAST CANCER

The techniques and applications of the electron beam in the treatment of breast cancer are described in Chapter 6—Management of Localized Breast Cancer.

Table 1-5. *Results of Electron Beam Treatment: Cervical Lymphatics*
May 1963–Dec. 1969
Reviewed April 1972

	Elective Treatment After Radical Neck Dissection	Treatment for Recurrence After Radical Neck Dissection
Total Patients	31	16
Alive and No Recurrence of Neck Disease	11	2*
Dead and Free of Disease Above the Clavicle	9 (4 died from *DM***) (5 died from Intercurrent Disease)	6 (3 died from *DM***)
Dead with Recurrence of Neck Disease	11 (5 outside field 6 within field) (6 died with *DM***)	8 (4 within field 4 within + outside field) (4 died with *DM***)

*1 patient developed a recurrence within the field which was removed by cryosurgery, with no further recurrence.
** *DM*—distant metastasis.

BIBLIOGRAPHY

1. Almond, P. R., Wright, A. E., and Lontz, J. F., II: The use of lithium fluoride thermoluminescent dosimeters to measure the dose distribution of a 15 Mev electron beam, *Physics in Medicine and Biology*, 12, 389, 1967.
2. Almond, P. R., Wright, A. E., and Boone, M. L. M.: High energy electron dose perturbations in regions of tissue heterogeneity. Part II: Physics models of tissue heterogeneities, *Radiology*, 88, 1146, 1967.
3. Boone, M. L. M., Crosby, E. H., and Shalek, R. J.: Skin reactions and tissue heterogeneity in electron beam therapy. Part II: *In vivo* dosimetry, *Radiology*, 84, 817, 1965.
4. Grant, B. P., and Fletcher, G. H.: Analysis of complications following megavoltage therapy for squamous cell carcinomas of the tonsillar area, *Amer. J. Roentgen.*, 96, 28, 1966. ✏
5. Sinclair, W. K., and Kohn, H. I.: The relative biological effectiveness of high-energy photons and electrons, *Radiology*, 82, 800, 1964.
6. Tapley, N. duV., and Fletcher, G. H.: Radiation therapy with electron beam: Current techniques, *Radiologic Clin. N. Amer.*, 7, 301, 1969.
7. Tapley, N. duV., and Fletcher, G. H.: Applications of the electron beam in the management of the lymphatics of the neck in head and neck cancers, *Amer. J. Roentgen.*, In press.

Parallel Opposing Portals Technique

In Collaboration with
NORAH duV. TAPLEY

A treatment technique comprises a variety of physical parameters, including the effective energy of the beam, the number of portals directed to the treatment volume, whether one or all fields are treated each day, and time-dose-fractionation factors. For example, with the technique of parallel opposing portals, when using ^{60}Co and treating only one field per day, the dose to the lateral tissues will be higher than the dose to the central area whereas with a 22 Mev photon beam, there is reversal of this dose distribution (Fig. 1-55).

The factors affecting the distribution of the biological dose throughout the treatment volume are: 1) width of field separation, 2) equal or differential loading, and 3) the lateral tissue high dose (edge effect) created by

treating only one field per day. When calculating the given doses needed to achieve a particular tumor dose, there is a tendency to be concerned exclusively with the dose at the midline or at a single point in the bulk of the tumor and to overlook the dose delivered to normal structures within the treatment volume. Figures 1-56 and 1-57 show the volume distribution for various portal arrangements and beam energies.

With ^{60}Co or 3 to 6 Mev, in particular with a single homolateral portal, the subcutaneous tissues and structures near the surface are heavily irradiated. The single homolateral field technique with the ^{60}Co unit in treating tonsillar area lesions produced the highest incidence and severity of osteonecrosis (18 per cent necessitating surgery)[1] and should

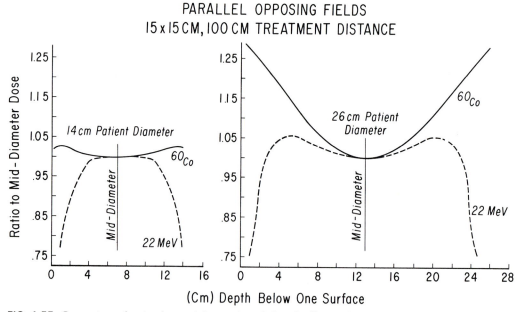

FIG. 1-55. Comparison of ratio of central dose to lateral dose for ^{60}Co and 22 Mev at 100 cm *TSD* with various widths of separation.

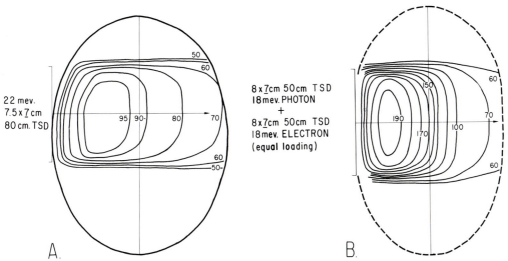

FIG. 1-56. A. Single homolateral portal with 22 Mev beam—gradient approximately 10 to 15 per cent across treatment volume. **B.** Equal loading with 18 Mev electron and photon beams. The lateral soft tissues and the primary tumor at a depth of 5 to 6 cm receive equally high doses. The opposite side of the pharynx and the contralateral parotid gland receive nondamaging doses.

not be used. With a 22 Mev beam and a single homolateral portal, the skin reaction is minimal on the entrance side and is moderate on the opposite side; the dose to the contralateral oropharynx is diminished by 10 to 15 per cent, producing a less severe mucositis (Fig. 1-56A). An even more favorable ratio of homolateral dose to opposite dose is achieved with combined 18 Mev electron and photon beams with the dose to the opposite oropharynx being in the range of 50 per cent of the dose in the tumor at 5 or 6 cm depth (Fig. 1-56B).

PATTERNS WITH PARALLEL OPPOSING TECHNIQUES

Radiation energies in the 3 to 6 Mev range remain effective with the parallel opposed portals technique when an equally high dose is needed to treat both the lymph glands near the skin surface and the more deeply located primary tumor, as in carcinomas of the tonsillar fossa or base of the tongue. With the disease centrally located, a 1:1 loading with ^{60}Co provides homogeneous high dosage

with no sparing of the lateral tissues (Fig. 1-57A). In treating disease located unilaterally in nodes just under the skin surface and with the primary lesion at a depth of 3 to 5 cm, a satisfactory dose distribution is achieved with ^{60}Co or 3 Mev equivalent energy using a 2:1 loading (Fig. 1-57B and 1-57C).

With field separations of more than 14 cm, a favorable midline dose-lateral dose ratio can be achieved only with energies in the 18 to 30 Mev range (Fig. 1-55). The higher energies are of advantage for centrally located lesions of the head and neck such as those of the soft palate and posterior pharyngeal walls when large areas of the neck do not require irradiation (Fig. 1-57D). High tumor doses can be delivered with minimal skin changes and a low risk of subcutaneous fibrosis. Surgical excision of relatively common failures in lesions of the posterior pharyngeal walls can be done with fewer complications. For tumors that are located in the thorax, abdomen and pelvis, a 25 or 35 Mev beam is advantageous with parallel opposing portals and is effective with lateral portals.

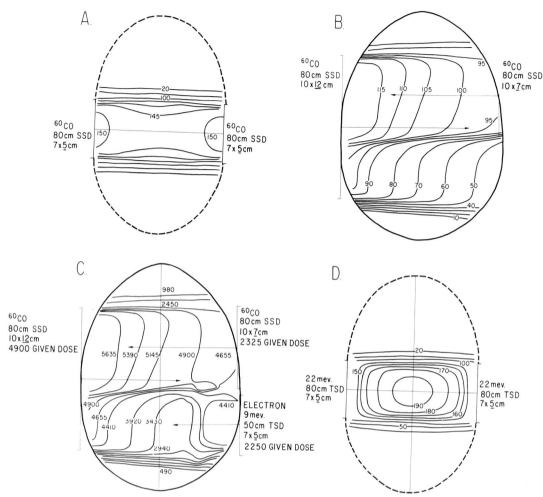

FIG. 1-57. A. Parallel opposing portals with ^{60}Co beams. The central dose is slightly lower than the dose to the lateral subcutaneous tissues. **B.** Treatment plan for patients with lateralized lesions and homolateral neck nodes. The contralateral portal covers only the primary lesion and excludes the spinal cord. **C.** Same pattern as "B" with the addition of a 9 Mev electron beam field to cover the contralateral spinal accessory chain. This technique is used for patients with tonsillar fossa lesions where there is risk of involvement of the opposite spinal accessory chain of nodes. **D.** Parallel opposing portals with 22 Mev beams. The central dose is higher than the dose to the lateral tissues.

VARIATIONS IN TISSUE THICKNESS WITHIN TREATED VOLUME

In the treatment of lesions of the oral cavity, oropharynx and hypopharynx, there may be considerable variation in the thickness of tissues in the path of the opposing beams. The differences in tissue doses may not be significant enough to adjust with compensa-

tors (Fig. 1-58). If the larynx is included, the difference in thickness becomes significant and the dose delivered to the larynx will be as much as 10 per cent higher than the tumor dose calculated at the midline from the *SSD* point (Fig. 1-59). Patients who have had extensive surgical procedures may have considerable variation in the thickness of the different structures included in the large vol-

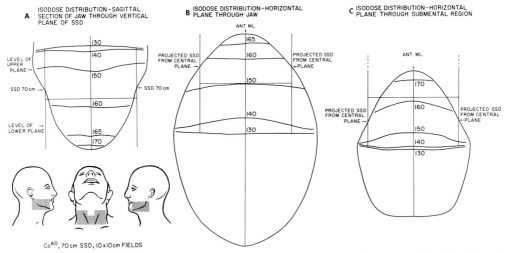

FIG. 1-58. Dose distributions with ^{60}Co in a patient treated for squamous cell carcinoma involving the entire tongue. The total treatment included the combination of intra-arterial 5-Fluorouracil for the first 10 days with external irradiation through 2 parallel opposing portals. The tumor dose was 6,000 rads in 6 weeks. The larynx is excluded from the parallel opposed fields and is blocked in the anterior neck field. The various isodose distributions show that the differences in thickness throughout the treatment volume do not produce sufficient variation in dosage to justify the use of compensators.

ume which must be treated to encompass the entire surgical area. Compensators are then necessary. For the last week of treatment of oral cavity and oropharynx lesions with parallel opposed portals, fall-off of the beam should be avoided in the submental area; this is a form of compensating technique.

At 4,500 rads tumor dose (5,000 rads if the dose rate is 850 rads per week), the posterior margins of the lateral portals are moved forward to remove the spinal cord from the treatment beams. Additional dosage to the posterior ipsilateral and contralateral spinal accessory chains or to the posterior portion of a large node then is best given with the 6 or 9 Mev beam (Fig. 1-57C).

DIFFERENTIAL LOADING

When the 2:1 loading technique is used for asymmetrical lesions, tumor dose calculations must be made at the midline, in the center of the lesion and 1 cm deep to the skin on the side involved. The maximum tumor dose is taken at the depth selected as the center of the lesion, usually 3.5 to 4.5 cm and not "at the midline" to avoid excessive dosage laterally (Figs. 1-60 and 1-61). To further avoid excessive dose to the subcutaneous tissues, the 22 Mev photon beam is often used for the last 1,500 to 2,000 rads tumor dose, being given to the primary lesion through reduced portals.

EDGE EFFECT (LATERAL TISSUE DAMAGE)

For a detailed discussion of the biological factors to be considered in the treatment of one field per day versus all fields each day, see the section on Clinical Parameters, Chapter 2. Wilson and Hall[2], in their discussion of the effect on the lateral soft tissues of the high doses which are delivered when treating one field per day, have designated this "the edge effect". This descriptive term must not be confused with the penumbra or low dose area at the edges of a treatment beam.

To achieve biological homogeneity of dose throughout the treated volume, when using

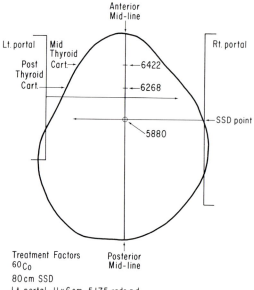

Anterior
Mid-line

Lt. portal | Mid Thyroid Cart.→

Rt. portal

Post Thyroid Cart.

←6422

←6268

←SSD point

5880

Treatment Factors
⁶⁰Co
80 cm SSD
Lt. portal - 11 x 6 cm, 5175 rads g.d.
Rt. portal - 11 x 9 cm, 2725 rads g.d

Posterior
Mid-line

FIG. 1-59. This 74-year-old male had squamous cell carcinoma, grade II, of the infrahyoid epiglottis extending to the right aryepiglottic folds. There was fixation of the right hemilarynx and a fixed 6 × 7 cm mass in the right subdigastric area. The tongue deviated to the right, indicating paralysis of the hypoglossal nerve. The plan of treatment was to use ⁶⁰Co parallel opposing fields with a 2:1 loading in favor of the right side and to deliver 850 rads tumor dose per week up to 7,500 rads in 8½ weeks to the midline at the level of the angle of the jaw. The right field extended posteriorly to cover the large node whereas the left field extended only to the vertebral body. The 9 Mev electron beam was used to treat the contralateral spinal accessory chain of nodes.

The following given doses were delivered:

5,175 rads ⁶⁰Co to large ipsilateral (right) field

2,725 rads ⁶⁰Co to smaller contralateral (left) field

6,000 rads ⁶⁰Co to the right lower anterior neck

5,000 rads ⁶⁰Co to the left lower anterior neck

1,500 rads 9 Mev electron beam to right posterior neck

3,000 rads 9 Mev electron beam to left posterior neck

The left posterior neck was treated on the days that the left opposed portal was

3 to 6 Mev beams both fields should be treated each day. This avoids the severe fibrosis which results from the biological damage to the lateral normal tissues which is greater with alternate day treatment.

Although the treatment to enlarged nodes is biologically more effective when a large dose is given every other day, there is no advantage to the centrally located primary tumor—it receives an equally effective dose each day. With central tumors (*e.g.,* base of tongue, posterior pharyngeal wall, nasopharynx) even if clinically positive nodes are present, each field is treated every day. With laterally located tumors (*e.g.,* tonsillar area) and node(s), using 3 to 6 Mev and 2:1 loading, treatment is given to the homolateral field on successive days and to the contralateral field on the third day. This increases

treated. The right posterior spinal accessory chain of nodes was treated with the electron beam after the right portal was moved forward to exclude the spinal cord.

The tumor dose of 850 rads had been delivered posteriorly where the neck thickness was greater than at the level of the larynx. At 6 weeks and 2 days the dose to the larynx was 6,422 rads whereas the midline dose at the maximum neck thickness was 5,880 rads. The patient developed marked arytenoid edema and mucositis due to the higher laryngeal dose, the rapid dose rate, and the large treatment volume. If the dose schedule had been based on 850 rads per day to the laryngeal structures, the dose to the large right neck node would have been lower than the dose actually given but could have been augmented by a concomitant field-within-a-field.

The figure shows a diagram of a contour of the neck and alignment of the treatment portals. The asymmetry on the right is caused by the large neck mass. The larger right portal extends posteriorly over the spinal accessory chain of nodes. Calculations of the dose distribution throughout the area of the tumor showed a 9 per cent difference between the midline dose at the SSD point and the dose more anterior in the larynx. This higher dose caused arytenoid edema, most marked on the right.

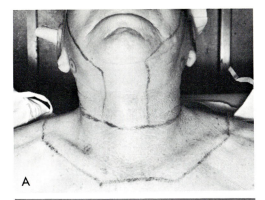

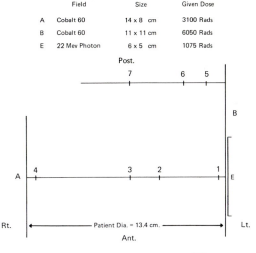

	Field	Size	Given Dose
A	Cobalt 60	14 x 8 cm	3100 Rads
B	Cobalt 60	11 x 11 cm	6050 Rads
E	22 Mev Photon	6 x 5 cm	1075 Rads

Post.

7   6   5

B

A   4   3   2   1   E

Rt. ◄———— Patient Dia. = 13.4 cm. ————► Lt.

Ant.

Lt.

Point	Distance From Field B Surface	Total Accumulated Dose
1	0.5 cm	8015 Rads
2	4.0 cm	7880 Rads
3	6.7 cm (Mid.–Diameter)	7430 Rads
4	12.9 cm	6595 Rads
5	1.0 cm	5870 Rads
6	2.0 cm	5535 Rads
7	6.7 cm (Mid.–Diameter)	4115 Rads

A

B

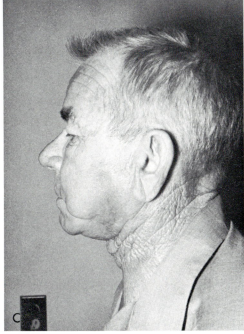

C

FIG. 1-60. This 63-year-old male had a massive squamous cell carcinoma (staged T_4N_3A) arising in the left tonsillar fossa. The lesion extended into the lateral border of the tongue, down to the base of the tongue and valleculae, up along the soft palate, and posteriorly into the pharyngeal wall. There were large matted left neck nodes measuring more than 6 cm. The plan of treatment was to use ^{60}Co parallel opposing portals with a 2:1 loading in favor of the left side to deliver 7,500 rads tumor dose at a rate of 850 rads per week. Only the left posterior cervical nodes were to be included in the ^{60}Co field. The right accessory chain would be treated with the electron beam and the lower neck with an anterior ^{60}Co field.

From February 5 to April 8, 1969, the primary lesion received 6,500 rads tumor dose with parallel opposing ^{60}Co portals and 1,000 rads tumor dose boost with the 22 Mev photon beam. The total dose to the midline was 7,500 rads in 9 weeks. The left neck received 6,000 rads given dose in 6 weeks with ^{60}Co; the right neck received 5,200 rads given dose.

In November 1970 the patient was seen after removal of 3 molar teeth. There were erythema, heat, and induration over the left mandible and fibrosis of the left upper neck with trismus. The patient was placed on antibiotics and by January 1971 the erythema had disappeared. On examination of the tonsillar fossa there was no evidence of disease. There was a 1 cm ulceration on the left posterior mandible at the site of the previous extractions. Examination of the neck showed induration on the left with subcutaneous fibrosis. A hemimandibulectomy was done in March 1971 because of painful radionecrosis. In January 1972, 35 months after radiation treatment, the patient was doing well with no evidence of disease. The fibrosis is asymptomatic.

A. Anterior view of the parallel opposed treatment portals which cover the tonsillar area and upper necks. The larynx is excluded from these fields. **B.** Distribution of doses. With a 2:1 loading the dose in the left neck at 0.5 cm depth is 8,015 rads, 22 per cent higher than the dose of 6,595 rads in the right neck at 0.5 cm depth. This is a desirable dose distribution with the enlarged left upper neck nodes. **C.** The patient in November 1970 showing fibrosis in the left upper neck prior to hemimandibulectomy.

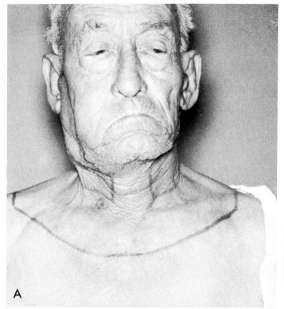

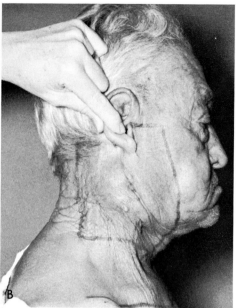

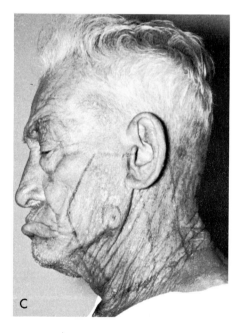

FIG. 1-61. This 68-year-old male, with a 6-month history of a right neck mass, had a squamous cell carcinoma of the right tonsillar fossa, Stage T_4N_3A. The lesion extended to the midline of the soft palate and almost to the midline of the base of the tongue. The entire right lateral and posterior pharyngeal walls were involved down to the level of approximately C6. The tumor almost completely filled the pyriform sinus and its most inferior aspect could not be visualized well by indirect laryngoscopy. There was an area of erythroplasia on the left side of the soft palate which extended into the left tonsillar fossa. The right subdigastric mass meas-ured 10 cm in length, 8 cm in width, and was 4 to 5 cm thick. The left neck was negative.

The plan of treatment was to use parallel opposing ^{60}Co fields to deliver 850 rads tumor dose per week to a total of 5,500 rads and then to re-evaluate for further treatment. The lower necks were to receive 5,000 rads given dose including the supraclavicular regions without blocking the midline because the large fixed nodes extended inferiorly.

From 12-29-70 through 2-24-71, treatment was given with a combination of ^{60}Co 22 Mev x-rays and 9 Mev electrons. The total midline tumor dose was 6,000 rads followed by a boost of 1,000 rads with the 22 Mev photon beam. The left spinal accessory chain received 2,700 rads with the 9 Mev electron beam. The posterior portion of the right neck node mass received 1,200 rads boost with the 9 Mev electron beam.

At discharge there was no visible tumor in the oropharynx. There was a residual fixed mass in the right mid-neck and in April 1971 a modified right neck dissection was done. There was no tumor in the specimen. In July 1971, the patient presented with a 3 × 3 cm ulcerated lesion of the *left* anterior tongue border and a skin nodule on the left side of the chin. Pulmonary metastases were present. As a palliative procedure, a partial glossectomy was done in August 1971. The patient died with metastatic disease in October 1971.

A, B, C. Treatment portals. Parallel opposed portals with right lateral portal extending posteriorly to cover large neck mass. The left lateral portal excludes the spinal cord and the dose to the spinal accessory chain nodes is boosted with a 9 Mev electron beam strip.

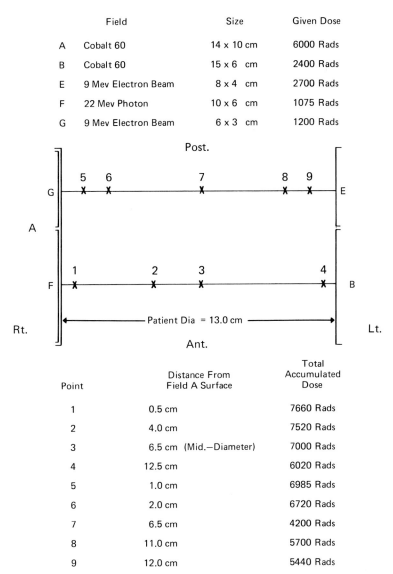

Field		Size	Given Dose
A	Cobalt 60	14 x 10 cm	6000 Rads
B	Cobalt 60	15 x 6 cm	2400 Rads
E	9 Mev Electron Beam	8 x 4 cm	2700 Rads
F	22 Mev Photon	10 x 6 cm	1075 Rads
G	9 Mev Electron Beam	6 x 3 cm	1200 Rads

Point	Distance From Field A Surface	Total Accumulated Dose
1	0.5 cm	7660 Rads
2	4.0 cm	7520 Rads
3	6.5 cm (Mid.—Diameter)	7000 Rads
4	12.5 cm	6020 Rads
5	1.0 cm	6985 Rads
6	2.0 cm	6720 Rads
7	6.5 cm	4200 Rads
8	11.0 cm	5700 Rads
9	12.0 cm	5440 Rads

FIG. 1-61D. Distribution of doses. The midline dose in the tumor area is 7,000 rads whereas the dose to the spinal cord is 4,200 rads. The dose in the right posterior node mass at 1 cm depth is 6,985 rads whereas the dose at 1 cm depth on the left is 5,440 rads. With a 2:1 loading, the dose differential ranges from 7,660 rads in the right subcutaneous tissues to 6,020 rads in the left subcutaneous tissues at the level of the primary tumor.

the biological effectiveness to the nodes without altering the daily dose to the primary lesion.

It is not necessary to treat every field every day with the 18 to 25 Mev beams because, as seen in Table 1-6, the lateral tissue dose is not greatly increased over the midline dose unless the separation is more than 30 cm. The edge effect, associated with the 3 to 6 Mev beams, is magnified by treating 4 days (or worse, 3 days) a week instead of 5 days a week because the individual fractions are larger. Even in head and neck lesions with a maximum separation of 14 to

Table 1-6. *Lateral Soft Tissue Doses*

	^{60}Co 15 × 15 cm 100 cm SSD			22 MeV 15 × 15 cm 100 cm *TSD*		
Diameter Cms	Maximum Dose (0.5 cm)	Midline Dose	Lateral (Exit) Dose at 1 cm	Maximum Dose (4.0 cm)	Midline Dose	Lateral (Exit) Dose at 1 cm
14	274	200	138	215	200	158
16	291	200	129	223	200	152
18	310	200	121	233	200	147
20	330	200	114	242	200	141
22	351	200	105	251	200	136
24	375	200	98	262	200	131
26	398	200	92	272	200	126
28	425	200	87	284	200	122
30	452	200	82	294	200	118

With ^{60}Co for the same dose at the midline, the maximum dose at 0.5 cm increases and the dose to the opposite lateral tissues decreases as the transverse diameter increases. With the 22 MeV photon beam a much more favorable ratio is maintained between the midline dose and the maximum dose at 4 cm.

15 cm, treatment should be given to every field each day.

TREATMENT OF NODES

In the treatment of carcinomas of the head and neck, large metastatic nodes may be present in the spinal accessory chain or may protrude posteriorly beyond the margin of the sternocleidomastoid muscle. In a 2:1 loading these large nodes may be covered by the ipsilateral field only in order to decrease the dose to the spinal cord. The dose they receive will be low, particularly when the weekly tumor dose to the primary lesion is calculated at 850 rads. A boost must be given with a separate "field-within-a-field" over the nodes, delivering 250 rads twice a week. A posterior glancing field delivering 5 × 300 rads is used for very large protruding nodes

and precludes the need for additional treatment when the fields are moved forward off the spinal cord at 4,500 rads tumor dose (Fig. 1-62).

If irradiation of the spinal accessory chain of nodes is indicated, both parallel opposed fields may extend back over the spinal accessory chain to a midline tumor dose of 4,500 rads. The 6 to 9 Mev electron beam is then used over the posterior strips to bring the posterior dose at 1 cm to 5,000 rads in the clinically negative chain or to 6,000 rads in the clinically positive chain (Figs. 1-61 and 1-62).

DOSIMETRY FORM

In order to facilitate calculation of the rather complex dosimetry of the parallel opposing portals and to depict the dose dis-

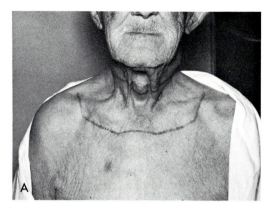

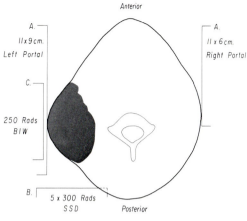

Anterior

A.
II x 9 cm.
Left Portal

A.
II x 6 cm.
Right Portal

C.

250 Rads
BIW

B.
5 x 300 Rads
SSD

Posterior

A. Right & Left ^{60}Co Portal

B. Left Posterior ^{60}Co Portal

C. Field Within-a-Field
6 Mev Electron Beam

FIG. 1-62. This 83-year-old male had squamous cell carcinoma of the uvula, staged T_1N_3A. The patient had first noted a mass in the left neck in September 1971 which was biopsied in December and a lesion of the uvula was found. On admission in January 1972, there was a 1.5 cm exophytic lesion of the uvula which extended slightly onto the left posterior tonsillar pillar and a fixed 6 × 6 cm mass in the left subdigastric area, extending posteriorly.

The plan of treatment was to begin therapy with an intraoral cone using 140 Kv x-rays, giving 1,500 rads air dose in 5 fractions. At the same time, the left neck mass was to receive 1,500 rads given dose in 5 fractions with a posterior glancing ^{60}Co field. Treatment would then continue with parallel opposing ^{60}Co fields, equally loaded, to 5,500 rads midline at 850 rads tumor dose per week, excluding the spinal cord at 4,500 rads. The lower necks would receive 5,000 rads given dose through a single anterior portal. After 1½ weeks treatment, in order to increase the dose to the neck mass and to free it so that a modified neck dissection could be done after completion of treatment, the treatment plan was changed to a 2:1 loading in favor of the left side. The right portal was moved forward to exclude the spinal cord. A 7 Mev electron beam strip was added to the right posterior neck.

After 4½ weeks of treatment the neck mass measured 3 × 3 cm and was mobile and discrete. By the 7th week, the node was smaller and a moist reaction had developed in the left neck. The uvula tumor was no longer visible. At this point, because of the age of the patient and the good response in the neck node, the surgeon decided not to do a modified neck dissection. The patient was, therefore, given 2 weeks' rest and treatment to the node was continued with the 9 Mev electron beam, giving an additional 1,500 rads in 6 fractions.

A. The large left neck mass can be seen bulging laterally just above the line of the junction of the upper and lower neck fields. **B.** The diagram shows a contour of the neck at the level of the enlarged nodes and the placement of the treatment portals as initially planned in this patient. The posterior glancing field covers the node mass; the fall-off over the skin enhances the skin reaction.

tribution, a tabular form has been developed as shown in Figure 1-63. This form should be part of the treatment chart and the doses at each point listed on the form should be calculated. The form also can be used for treatment planning, thus providing an analy-sis of the dose distribution in the nodal area and the primary tumor. It can be rapidly seen whether a 1:1 loading or a 2:1 loading is to be preferred, and when additional treatment to the spinal accessory chain nodes is needed.

DOSE DETERMINATION FORM FOR
PARALLEL OPPOSED PORTAL TECHNIQUE

	PRIMARY Weekly Rate: Loading:			NODES Subdigastric Nodes in Primary Field			Posterior Nodes In Primary Field		Lower Neck	
Total TD (indicate depth in cm.)	Max.	Min.	Midline	R	L		R	L	R	L
From R						From R				
From L						From L				
From Others: (Specify)						Postero-Anterior				
Total						Anterior Posterior				
B O O S T From R						Total				
From L						Miscellaneous Boosts:				
From Others (Specify)										
Total						Space for contour or drawings				
No. of Fractions										
No. of Days										
NSD										
Spinal Cord Dose										

FIG. 1-63. Form for determining doses both to the primary treatment volumes and to all areas of the neck. It is important to calculate the doses delivered to the posterior nodes by the primary treatment fields so that the additional dosage given to the posterior strips will not be excessive.

BIBLIOGRAPHY

1. Grant, B. P., and Fletcher, G. H.: Analysis of complications following megavoltage therapy for squamous cell carcinomas of the tonsillar area, *Amer. J. Roentgen.*, 96, 28, 1966.

2. Wilson, C. S., and Hall, E. J.: On the advisability of treating all fields at each radiotherapy session, *Radiology*, 98, 419, 1971.

2. Basic Principles of Radiotherapy

Radiation Biology: A Basis for Radiotherapy

HERMAN D. SUIT

In cellular and tissue radiation biology, significant advances have been made over the past 15 years; these provide the basis for a beginning understanding of the response of normal and malignant tissues to irradiation. The aspects of radiation biology which are most relevant to clinical radiotherapy are the quantitative evaluation of the cell lethal response to irradiation, repair of radiation damage by the cell, and the effect of irradiation to alter kinetics of proliferation of cells of tumor and normal tissues. This section will review pertinent findings in cellular radiation biology which are related to these aspects of the radiation response. Then, the implications of extrapolating those findings on individual cells to the response of normal and malignant tissues will be compared with the experimentally observed responses of irradiated tissues. No attempt is made to cover all of the relevant or interesting aspects of the subject but only selected points of special concern. The reader is referred to several excellent books and symposia on this subject.[2,9,22,49]

Cellular Radiobiology

Relationship Between Cell Lethal Response and Radiation Dose

The large body of data derived from *in vitro* studies of the relationship between cell lethal response and radiation dose represent confirmation and extension of the now classic (1956) report of Puck and Marcus.[46] Earlier they had developed methods for the culture of individual mammalian cells and showed that those cells could proliferate and produce a clone when plated on special media. Importantly, they used this capacity of the cell to produce a clone as a measure of its viability. That is, in their studies a cell was counted as viable only after it had demonstrated its reproductive integrity by proliferating to produce progeny of more than 50 cells by the ninth day of culture (Fig. 2-1). Cells might be capable of performing various and complex metabolic functions but would be scored as "nonviable" unless they had demonstrated an ability to sustain proliferation.

As the definition of cell death is the loss of proliferative capacity, the loss of cell viability need not be closely related in time with cell lysis. In fact, several studies[46,75] have shown that nonviable cells may survive in a metabolic sense for prolonged periods and may even pass through one or more divisions before lysis. This has been strikingly demonstrated by cine-photography observations on mammalian cells irradiated *in vitro*.[75] Indeed, pedigrees of progeny produced from a single irradiated cell may show as many as 8 to 9 divisions along certain branches of

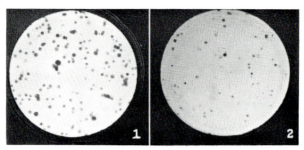

FIG. 2-1. Appearance of clones developing from normal and irradiated HeLa cells.

1) Colonies developing on a plate seeded with 200 S_3 HeLa cells and incubated nine days in growth medium.

2) Colonies developing on a plate identical with that of 1 in every respect except that the plate was irradiated with 300 r before incubation. (Courtesy: Puck, *J. Exp. Med., 103,* 653, 1956.)

the pedigree before all the cells of the abortive colony undergo lysis. After moderate radiation doses, most "nonviable" cells lysed during an attempted cell division. At higher doses, lysis of cells occurred during interphase. Consequently, the time after irradiation that the radiation killed cells or their abortive progeny undergo lysis would be a function of radiation dose and duration of the intermitotic period. Thus, the proportion of cells that had lysed at a specified time after a certain radiation dose would be expected to be larger for irradiation of a rapidly dividing cell population than of a slowly dividing one.

Following development of their beautiful technique for culture *in vitro* of individual mammalian cells, Puck and Marcus[46] proceeded to perform the first measurements of mammalian cell radiosensitivity. Their investigations were based on a HeLa cells line which had been derived from a human uterine carcinoma. The experimental technique can be visualized by inspection of Figure 2-1. Their experimental method of procedure was: 1) to count the number of colonies that developed on a plate that had been seeded by a known quantity of cells and not subsequently irradiated, 2) to compute the plating efficiency or the ratio of number of colonies observed/number of cells plated, 3) to count the number of colonies that developed on a plate that had been seeded by a known quantity of cells and then irradiated, 4) to

compute from numbers 2 and 3 the fraction of cells surviving the irradiation, and 5) to repeat this study for a range of radiation doses. Their experimental results are shown in Figure 2-2. The equation included in the Figure 2-2 was proposed as a description of the relationship between radiation dose (D) and fraction of cells that survived irradiation (S).

From these data, the loss of cell viability following irradiation was found to be a complex exponential function of dose. We will first consider the practical meaning of this statement and then discuss the equation shown in Figure 2-2.

The statement that the response is an exponential function of dose means that a specified radiation dose kills a constant fraction of irradiated cells. This means that the fraction of cells killed is independent of the number of cells irradiated, while the absolute number of cells killed by a specified dose varies with the number of cells irradiated. Sample calculations to illustrate this process are given in Table 2-1. For these computations, 380 rads is specified as the dose which kills 90 per cent of the irradiated cells. Thus, 380 rads given to a population of 10^{10} cells would kill 9×10^9 cells. However, if 10 viable cells were irradiated, the same dose of 380 rads would be expected to kill only 9 cells. Accordingly, the first 380 rads to a cell population would be much more damaging

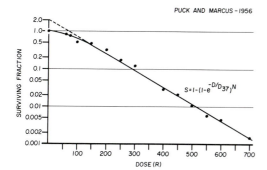

FIG. 2-2. Proportion of HeLa cells surviving as a function of radiation dose. Cell viability assayed by the cell's ability to form colonies when plated out on special culture media (a method similar to assay of survival of bacterial cells). (Courtesy: Puck, *J. Exp. Med.,103,* 653, 1956.)

in terms of the number of cells killed than the second or subsequent dose increments. It is apparent that, in concept, this process is similar to decay of a radioactive isotope (a constant fraction of the isotope disintegrates per unit of time) or to absorption of x-rays in matter (radiation dose is reduced by a constant fraction per unit of absorbing material).

If the calculated numbers of surviving cells and corresponding radiation doses (as given in Table 2-1), were plotted on loglinear paper, the curve connecting the points would be a straight line originating at a survival fraction of 1.0 for zero dose. However, the curves which best fit the various reported experimental data are not simple straight lines. Rather they are similar to the one of Puck and Marcus shown in Figure 2-2, which is characterized by a "shoulder" in the low dose region.

A survival curve of this shape is often referred to as a "multitarget" survival curve. The multitarget-single hit response law was developed to describe the survival curve when these conditions obtained: (1) all cells in the population contain N targets; (2) targets are of uniform size; (3) a target is inactivated by a single hit; and (4) cell death occurs only when N targets have been hit,

i.e., cells which retain at least one undamaged target survive. The equation describing this curve is:

$$S = 1 - (1 - e^{-D/D_{37}})^N$$

S = Surviving fraction

D = Radiation dose

D_{37} = Dose increment that reduces the survival fraction by a factor of 0.37 in the straight line portion of the curve. D^{37} is sometimes designated D_0 or the mean lethal dose. In formal multitarget terms it is the dose which would, on the average, inactivate one target.

e = Base of natural logarithmus
 = 2.71828

N = The ordinate intercept of the back extrapolation of the straight line portion of the curve to zero dose. This is usually called the extrapolation number. N would also correspond to the target number in a pure multitarget system.

A derivation of the equation for the multitarget survival curve is presented in Appendix 1. The e or base of the nature logarithmus is present because of the integral calculus required in the derivation of the equation. The origin of the number 37 is apparent by considering the following: In the simple situation where $N = 1$, $S = e^{-D/D_{37}}$, and when $D = D_{37}$, $S = e^{-1} = 0.37$.

This multitarget survival curve is shown in Figure 2-3. In Figure 2-3A the curve is drawn on a long-linear grid and in this form two important features of this curve are clearly shown: in the shoulder region, dose is relatively ineffective (width of the shoulder for a given D_{37} determines the value of N); the curve is a straight line after the shoulder, and the slope is $1/D_{37}$. By using units of D/D_{37} on the horizontal axis instead of radiation dose in rads the curve is shown in a general form. From such a curve, survival fractions (S values) may be computed for cells of various radiosensitivities (D_{37} values).

Table 2-1. *Number of Cells Killed with each 380 rad Radiation Dose Increment for Model Cell Population**

Accumulated Dose in Rads†	Radiation Dose in Increments of 380 rads	Number of Viable Cells Irradiated	Number of Cells Killed	Number of Cells Surviving
380	380 × 1	10,000,000,000	9,000,000,000	1,000,000,000
760	380 × 2	1,000,000,000	900,000,000	100,000,000
1140	380 × 3	100,000,000	90,000,000	10,000,000
1520	380 × 4	10,000,000	9,000,000	1,000,000
1900	380 × 5	1,000,000	900,000	100,000
2280	380 × 6	100,000	90,000	10,000
2660	380 × 7	10,000	9,000	1,000
3040	380 × 8	1,000	900	100
3420	380 × 9	100	90	10
3800	380 × 10	10	9	1

*Initial population size = 10^{10} viable cells; 90 per cent of cells irradiated are killed by 380 rads; 10 per cent of cells irradiated survive 380 rads.
†The total dose given at each level, *i.e.*, 1 × 380 or 10 × 380, were given as a single treatment. This is, no time elapsed between dose increments.

As a point of interest, the same curve is plotted on linear coordinates in Figure 2-3B. Because of the greater convenience of handling a straight line, the log-linear plot is usually the form in which this relationship is used.

One additional term is introduced here: Dq. This is a convenient description of

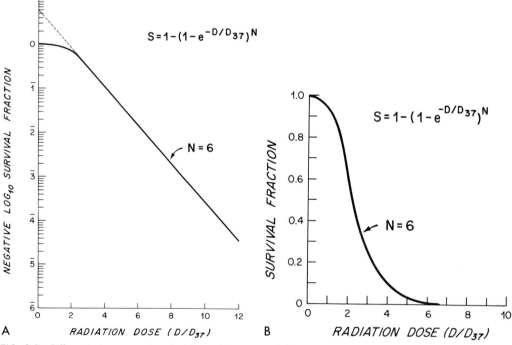

FIG. 2-3. Cell survival curve as described by multitarget-single hit response model. **A.** Plot of curve on log-linear grid. In this example, target number is set at 6. **B.** Plot of same curve on a linear grid.

shoulder width of the survival curve where the survival curve cannot be determined at low doses. Specifically, Dq is $D_{37} \times LnN$ and this corresponds to the dose at which a back extrapolation of the straight line portion of the survival curve indicates 100 per cent survival. This is illustrated in Figure 2-4: a Dq for single dose irradiation and two dose irradiation. In the latter instance, a first dose (D1) reduces survival fraction to 0.1 then variable second doses are given so that a survival curve is generated for the 10 per cent of cells which survived D1. In this example Dq is the difference between the dose at which the second survival curve back extrapolates to a survival fraction of 0.1 and D1.

If a particular end-point of an *in vivo* system being studied required as a minimum dose one which yielded a survival fraction of ≤ 0.1, and the number of colony forming units were unknown then N could not be

determined directly. However, by determining a survival curve for single dose irradiation and a survival curve for split dose irradiation (first dose yielding a survival fraction of ≈ 0.1) the Dq could be computed and therefore N estimated. Such an approach has definite limitations because the distribution of radiosensitivities (D_{37}, N) of the cells surviving at the time of the second dose may not be the same as the first dose, (*i.e.* slopes of the two survival curves may not be exactly the same). Despite these restrictions, Dq is useful in estimating the shoulder width for irradiation of cells *in vivo*.

The multitarget-single hit survival curve has zero slope in the very low dose region, because hits must be accumulated in order that any one cell receives hits at all N targets. That is, at very low doses, there would be no killing. In fact, experimental data show cell killing at very low doses. This finding indicates that some radiation is absorbed in events which produce nonrepairable damage. Apparently some cells are killed by single hit-single target events ($N = 1$) while other cells are killed according to more complex mechanisms, *e.g.* multitarget. In Figure 2-5 are shown cell survival curves for the situation where 0.0, 0.1, 0.2, or 0.3 of the dose produces single hit-single target killing. Obviously this factor does not affect survival for large single doses but would be important for small doses or for radiation given continuously at a low dose rate. Equation for the multitarget-single hit response law may be rewritten to allow for the proportion of dose (ω) which achieves single hit-single target killing:

$$S = e^{-\omega D/D_0}[1 - (1 - e^{-(1-\omega)D/D_0)N}].$$

For purposes of simplicity, in the sequel ω will be set at 0.0 and not considered unless specifically mentioned.

Although the data from most *in vitro* studies on mammalian cells have been fitted satisfactorily by a multitarget type of curve for values of S down to levels of 10^{-4} to 10^{-5}, the radiotherapist is interested in knowing

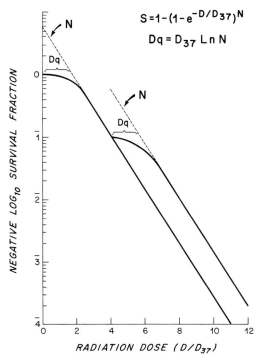

$$S = 1 - (1 - e^{-D/D_{37}})^N$$

$$Dq = D_{37} \, Ln \, N$$

FIG. 2-4. Plot of cell survival curve for single dose and split dose irradiation (D^1 yields survival fraction of 0.1) to demonstrate Dq.

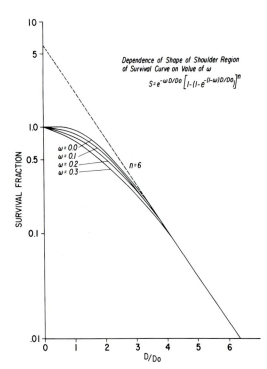

Dependence of Shape of Shoulder Region of Survival Curve on Value of ω

$$S = e^{-\omega D/D_0}\left[1-(1-e^{-(1-\omega)D/D_0})\right]^n$$

$\omega = 0.0$
$\omega = 0.1$
$\omega = 0.2$
$\omega = 0.3$

$n = 6$

FIG. 2-5. Plot of cell survival curve for multitarget model which illustrates the effect of ω on the shoulder region of the curve where ω is the proportion of the energy absorbed in production of single hit or nonrepairable events. (Courtesy: Suit, Withers, Brown and Thomson: (In preparation).)

the fit of the data to the curve at small values of S, *e.g.*, 10^{-9} and particularly for radiation given as a number of daily treatments. Hewitt and Wilson[34] have developed an elegant *in vivo* technique for obtaining survival fraction data on cells of certain transplantable tumors. They determined the number of cells, obtained from irradiated tumors, required to yield a 50 per cent tumor transplant take rate as a function of radiation dose. Their tumor transplantation results were expressed in terms of survival fractions. These were fitted satisfactorily by a multitarget curve. For one murine leukemia cell line, they obtained good fit of data to the curve for values of S down to $\approx 10^{-7}$ following single radiation doses.[33] Survival fraction data on the bacteria Serratia marcescens fitted acceptably a multitarget curve

($N = 1.3$) for values of S down to $<10^{-9}$ (Dewey)[15]. However, it is necessary to point out that there are experimental results from mammalian cells which have not been satisfactorily described by the multitarget survival curve. Rather, those data were better described by the more complicated multihit response law. The multihit response law was developed for the situation where the cell has one or more targets or sensitive sites each of which must be hit N times before the cell is killed. The slope of the cell survival curve for the multihit response differs from that of the multitarget in that there is no straight line portion, but the curve continues to bend down slightly with increasing dose. At very large doses the curve approaches a straight line whose slope is the same as for the curve with $N = 1$.

The true dose response law is probably much more complex than either the multitarget or multihit response law, *viz.*, the number of targets per cell and the number of hits required to inactivate each target may be variable. Discussion of these various models is beyond the scope of this section and the interested reader is referred to Zimmer.[86] Because the "multitarget" response law does fit so much of the available data and is relatively simple, it will be used in this section as a convenient means of describing experimental data.

Experimentally Determined Values for D_{37} and N

A wide variety of mammalian cell lines of both normal and malignant origin have been employed in determinations of D_{37} and N values by both *in vitro* and *in vivo* techniques. For aerobic cells the values for the parameters D_{37} and N have been $D_{37} \approx 165$ rads*

---

*In accordance with the fact that most clinical radiotherapy is now based on megavoltage techniques values for D_{37} are given in terms of ^{60}Co rads, unless specified otherwise. That is, results from studies based on 50 to 250 Kv x-rays are multiplied by the RBE correction factor of $\dfrac{1.00}{0.85}$ or 1.17.[52]

(110 to 240 rads) and $N \approx 2$ to 10 (1.5 to 20). Radiosensitivity of cells is the same for cells irradiated as suspension of individual cells or as intact tissue; that is, the cell contact experienced by cells comprising tissue does not affect their sensitivity. This has been shown for bone marrow and for several tumors.

The D_{37} increases directly with cell radio-resistance, *i.e.,* higher D_{37} indicates a more radioresistant or less radiosensitive cell. Figure 2-6 illustrates the effect of variation of N on the survival curve. If a heterogeneous cell population comprised of two cell lines characterized by a common D_{37} but differing N values and are irradiated by a single dose which reduces S to a level ≤ 0.1, the ratio of the S's for two cell lines would be the ratio of their N values. In the example shown, the

ratio is 5. However, for smaller doses or larger survival fractions this ratio decreases with decreasing dose. Thus the relative effect of differences in N values on survival fraction is dose dependent over dose range yielding $S \geq 0.1$.

Radiation Sensitivity and Cell Replication Cycle

The localization and extent of damage to the molecular structure(s) of the cell that causes cell death is largely unknown. Present evidence strongly indicates that unrepaired radiation-induced changes in the genetic material or deoxyribonucleic acid (*DNA*) are the dominant causes of cell death. The reader is referred to the review by Terasima[71] of this aspect of cellular radiobiology.

Because of the high probability that *DNA* is the critical structure in the cell, with respect to cell killing by radiation, we will now consider radiosensitivity in relation to *DNA* synthesis by the cell.

As a result of the research of Howard and Pelc[36] we know that the cell replication cycle may be described with respect to two major events in the cycle: synthesis of sufficient *DNA* to produce an additional set of chromosomes and the mitotic process itself. This replication cycle is represented by four stages: S or *DNA* synthesis period; M or mitotic period; a G_1, or first gap period, between M and S; and a G_2 or second gap period, between S and M (Fig. 2-7). The duration of the S, G_2, and M periods have shown slight variation among the different cell lines studied, and the total time for the three periods has been ≈ 10 to 15 hours. By contrast, G_1 may vary from extremely short times (<1 hour) to quite long periods. Indeed, cells of some tissues such as liver parenchyma, apparently stay in a long and variable G_1 and enter S only when additional cells are needed, *e.g.* after partial hepatectomy. Such long G_1 stages are designated by some as G_0.

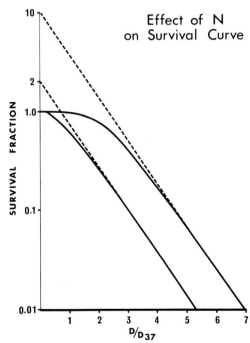

FIG. 2-6. Effect of N on survival fraction. In this example, the N values are 2 and 10, *i.e.,* differing by a factor of 5. S or survival fractions at any specified dose level differ by a factor of 5, provided $S \leq 0.1$. At larger values of S (>0.1) the ratio of survival fractions would be less than 5 and the ratio approaches 1 at extremely small doses.

Investigations in a number of laboratories have shown that cell radiosensitivity in terms

Stages of Cell Replication Cycle

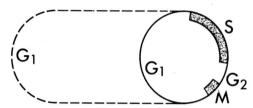

FIG. 2-7. Stages of cell replication cycle.

S = period of *DNA synthesis*

G_2 = time between completion of S and mitosis

M = mitosis

G_1 = period between end of M and start of S

The figure is drawn to indicate that S, G_2, and M periods are relatively constant, while G_1 may be quite variable.

of D_{37} and N varies as the cell progresses through the cell replication cycle.[54] This is described as the "age response function" of the particular cell line. See Figure 2-8 for an illustration of effect of cell age on cell survival. There are several general points which

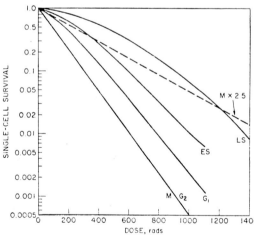

FIG. 2-8. Single cell survival data for various stages of the cell cycle of Chinese hamster cells, V_{79} line. (The broken line is a hypothetical curve for anoxic mitotic cells, assuming a dose-modifying factor of 2.5). (Courtesy: Sinclair: In *Time and Dose Relationships in Radiation Biology as Applied to Radiotherapy*, Brookhaven National Laboratory report 50203 (C-57), 1969, p. 98.)

may be made: 1) age response function shows some variation between various cell lines, 2) changes in sensitivity are largely due to variation in N rather than D_{37}, 3) maximum sensitivity occurs in M and G_2 phases; cells at the G_{1-s} interface being only slightly less-sensitive; and cells in late S being most resistant; and 4) the differential in survival between cells at different phases of the cell cycle increases with radiation dose *e.g.* not readily detectable at doses of 200 rads to 300 rads, but may be greater than a factor of 10 at doses of 800 to 1,200 rads. Figure 2-8 illustrates survival curves for Chinese Hamster cells irradiated at M, G_2, G_1, early S and late S. Thus, a population of actively dividing cells would be composed of subpopulations which were heterogeneous with respect to radiation sensitivity. Accordingly, the distribution of cells around the cell cycle would not be the same immediately after irradiation as it were before treatment. There would be a higher proportion of resistant cells in the survivors *i.e.* an induced partial synchrony. The surviving cells would continue to progress through the cell cycle with the result being that the effectiveness of a second or a subsequent dose would be affected by this partial synchrony. Implication of this for fractionated irradiation of tissue will be considered in a later section.

EFFECT ON CELL SURVIVAL CURVE OF CELL POPULATIONS HETEROGENEOUS WITH RESPECT TO RADIOSENSITIVITY

In general, the slope of the cell survival curve will indicate the D_{37} of the most resistant subgroup in the irradiated population provided the minimum survival fraction studied is small as compared with the fraction of the total population made up by the resistant subpopulation. The N value indicated by a survival curve based on a mixed population will depend on: the number and relative abundance of the several subpopulations, and the D_{37} and N of each subpopulation. Theoretical curves presented in Figure 2-9 illustrate that the survival curve for a

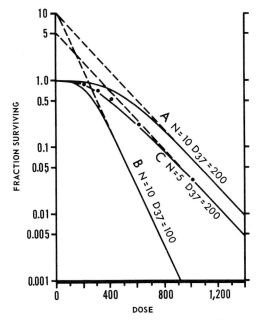

FIG. 2-9. Theoretical survival curve (C) for cell population made up of equal numbers of cells of two subpopulations differing in radiosensitivity.

A—D_{37} = 200 rads; N = 10
B—D_{37} = 100 rads; N = 10

Curve C has an apparent N of 5 and D_{37} of 200 rads and they differ from curve C by a maximum of 9 per cent. (Courtesy: Dewey, *Nature, 194,* 660, 1962.)

homogeneous cell population (uniform D_{37} and N) may be distinguished only with the greatest difficulty from that obtained from irradiation of a number of subpopulations, each with different D_{37} and N values.[16] These considerations are highly relevant to interpretation of the survival curves derived from asynchronously dividing cell populations where there is a distribution of D_{37} and N values.

RADIOSENSITIVITY AND CHROMOSOME NUMBER AND MORPHOLOGY

The great bulk of radiobiological data has been interpreted as indicating that the molecular changes produced by radiation that are effective in producing a cell lethal response are those in nuclear *DNA*.[71] Consequently, a reasonable expectation has been that radiosensitivity would be affected by chromosome number and morphology. Studies of hypodiploid and hypotetraploid lines of Ehrlich ascites carcinoma cells[51] and of a murine leukemia cell line[5] showed that D_{37} was the same for both ploidy numbers while N for the tetraploid line was considerably larger than for the diploid line.

Till[76] reported no significant variation of D_{37} or N among five sublines of the L cell, with modal chromosome numbers varying from 59 to 109. Finally N is $\approx$ one for G_2 and M cells which have just completed *DNA* synthesis and have two full sets of chromosomes. Chromosomal morphology or configurations might affect sensitivity. Notation is made of the fact that morphology of the chromosome is different in G_1, S, and G_2 cells. In summary, in mammalian cells, a correlationship between radiosensitivity and chromosome number of morphology has not been established.

Modification of Cellular Radiosensitivity

MOLECULAR OXYGEN

The most thoroughly authenticated modifier of cellular radiation sensitivity is molecular oxygen. In every reported study of mammalian cells where the cell lethal response has been the endpoint, radiation sensitivity was found to be strongly dependent on the oxygen tension in the cell at the instant of irradiation. The ratio D_{37} anoxic cells/D_{37} aerobic cells is 2.3 to 3.0.[27] However, N was independent of oxygen tension[21,51] or was reduced for hypoxic cells.[38,47]

The D_{37} increases very rapidly with small changes in oxygen tension in the range of severe to moderate hypoxia, as shown by the work of Dewey[15], based on the bacteria *Serratia marcescens* (Fig. 2-10). The dependence of radiosensitivity on oxygen tension is in the

2. Basic Principles of Radiotherapy

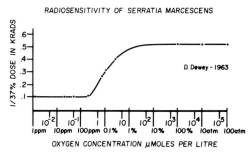

FIG. 2-10. Radiosensitivity of the bacteria *Serratia marcescens* as a function of the oxygen tension in the cell at the time of irradiation. (Courtesy: Dewey, *Radiat. Res., 19,* 64, 1963.)

range of 300 to 10,000 ppm ($\approx$.2 to 10 mm Hg). Rather similar but less extensive data have been obtained for mammalian cells.

A detailed explanation in biophysical and chemical terms for the mechanism of this oxygen effect has not been developed. Molecular oxygen is known to be highly reactive with many organic radicals, serving as an electron donor. Ionizing radiation induces radical formation by removing an electron. Molecular oxygen would be expected to react with these radiation-induced radicals in biologically important molecules, to produce nonrepairable biochemical changes, *e.g.* peroxides, etc. In the absence of oxygen, the damaged site in the molecule would have a higher probability of being repaired by simple electron capture process. For a fuller discussion of this aspect of oxygen effect, see reference.[29]

PYRIMIDINE AND PURINE ANALOGS

As stated earlier, radiation damages to the *DNA* molecules are considered to be the most important ones in the cell killing action of radiation. Cellular radiosensitivity has been increased by allowing the cell to incorporate into its *DNA* molecules certain of the analogs of the four base constituents of *DNA:* thymine, cystosine, adenine, and guanine. The degree of sensitization has been

found to be a function of the extent that the analog replaced the natural base. Five-bromodeoxyuridine (5-BUdR), a well-studied thymidine analog, is a potent sensitizer of mammalian cells; cells cultured in the presence of this compound may show a decrease in D_{37} by a factor up to 2 to 3.[17,38,41] At this magnitude of sensitization the extent of thymine replacement produced definite toxic effects on the cells. In addition to decreasing D_{37}, the N is also diminished, but not to 1.0 except at definitely toxic dose levels. Only those cells that had passed through an S period (*DNA* synthesis) during exposure to the analog would be sensitized. That is, cells which remained in G_1 period during the time that the analog was in culture would not be sensitized.

Of special relevance to attempts to use such agents to modify radiosensitivity of tumor cells has been the finding that—at least for 5-BUdR—the sensitizing effect is independent of the oxygen tension at the time of irradiation.[38] Accordingly, the D_{37} for a normal cell irradiated under hypoxic conditions would be some four to nine times that for a similar cell whose *DNA* contained 5-BUdR and was irradiated under aerobic conditions.

RADIATION PROTECTION: SH COMPOUNDS

A large number of compounds possessing active sulfhydryl groups have been proven highly effective as radiation protective agents. The SH group could be effective by repairing the radiation-induced radicals in the *DNA* molecule by the donation of an H atom to the site of the radical and thereby restore the *DNA* molecule to an active form. These agents are effective in protection of aerobic and anoxic cells.[15] To date, these agents have had no role in modification of response of human tissue to radiations as all agents tested in man have been found to be quite toxic at systemic dose levels which are not protective at the cellular level.

Repair of Radiation Injury by Mammalian Cells

"SUB-LETHAL" DAMAGE REPAIR

Cells which survive a first radiation dose (D_1) repair the radiation damage rapidly and within 2 to 6 hours they have been restored almost to their pretreatment status, as assessed by response to a second dose (D_2). This was first pointed out by Elkind and Sutton[18] and has been confirmed in many other laboratories in studies of mammalian cells *in vitro* and *in vivo*. In their experiments Elkind and Sutton administered radiation as either a single dose ($v = 1$) or as two doses ($v = 2$) separated by a variable time (ti). The proportion of cells surviving graded doses was measured for single and split dose irradiations. Results from a typical experiment are shown in Figure 2-11. They found that 1,120 rads given as a single dose yielded $S = 0.001$. In contrast, if treatment were given as an initial dose of 505 rads and then after 18 hours of incubation under standard conditions the remaining 615 rads were given, S had increased from 0.001 to 0.005. That is, there were five times as many survivors after the two dose as after the single dose irradiation. This increase in survivors is due to the repair of radiation damage during the time interval between D_1 and D_2. As illustrated in Figure 2-11 the shape of the cell survival curve (B) based on the cells which survived an initial treatment of 505 rads, 18 hours earlier, was essentially the same as that obtained for previously unirradiated cells (A). There had been essentially a full return of the shoulder region of the curve, or N, during the 18 hour period. Apparently the cells which survived the D_1 of 505 rads were restored to approximately the pretreatment status by the time of D_2. Thus S following 1,120 rads given as a split dose was larger by a factor of 5.1, than S following 1,120 rads given as a single dose. This difference was the same as N of 5.2 for the control cells.

Important to the radiation therapist who

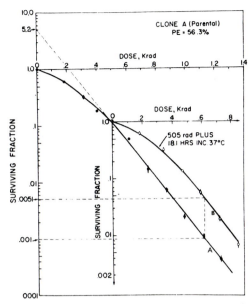

FIG. 2-11. Repair of sub-lethal cellular injury by hamster cells between irradiation doses when irradiated *in vitro*. See text. (Courtesy: Elkind, *Radiat. Res.*, *13*, 556, 1960.)

employs multiple small doses in clinical treatments, this repair of radiation damage has been shown to occur after each of several successive radiation doses.

Figure 2-12 is a plot of the fraction of cells surviving 1,499 rads given in two doses with t_i of 0 to 14 hours.[20] S increased rapidly for 2 hours but then decreased between 2 and 6 hours. This was followed by a subsequent increase in S to a value $\simeq$ that obtained at the 2-hour point. Then S remained at a steady level until cell proliferation commenced. This variation in the apparent recovery as a function of time following irradiation is a reflection of two processes. First, a very large number of damaged sites in the surviving cells are rapidly repaired. This produces the prompt return of the shoulder on the survival curve. There is no subsequent loss of this repair. The second process, which probably explains the variations in S after the 2-hour point, is the progression of surviving cells to positions in the cell replication cycle of differing radiosensitivity. The first dose of radiation kills predominately the most sensitive cells; immediately following the first dose, most of the surviving cells would be in relatively resistant stages. Later, they move into the more sensitive stages, and a dose at that time would be relatively more effective. Thus, the shape of a curve of the type presented in Figure 2-12 would be a function of the repair of damaged sites in the individual cells, the variations in D_{37} and N in the different stages in the cell cycle (determining the survival fraction in each stage), and the rate of movement of the surviving cells through the cell cycle. An additional factor is the size of the first and the second dose. For the recovery curve to show a maximum effect both the first and second doses must yield survival fractions of $\leq.1$ or beyond the shoulder.[85]

Extensive studies on repair of radiation damage in mammalian cells have been performed. Despite this work the biochemical processes involved cannot be specified. Several rather general statements can be made. The form of damage which is assessed by the split dose experiment can proceed at an essentially full rate in the face of chemical blockage of *DNA* and protein synthesis. Apparently, blockage of *RNA* synthetic activity will suppress repair activity. Hypo-

thermia in the range 18–24°C effects only a slight reduction in repair. Further cells which are exposed to severe hypoxia (≤ 10 ppm) for long periods cannot repair[8,30,35]; oxygen must be present during the time interval between D_1 and D_2 for maximal recovery.[8,35]

"POTENTIALLY LETHAL DAMAGE" REPAIR

Whitmore et al.[82] proposed the term potentially lethal to describe damage which is lethal under normal conditions but which may be repaired sufficiently to permit survival if the cells are exposed to appropriate post-treatment conditions. For example, he found survival of LP_{59} cells to be increased if the cells were exposed to 5°C for a brief period following treatment. Presumably, the reduced temperature favored reconstitution of damaged sites over progression of the biochemical reactions to produce damage which could not be repaired. There are various other procedures which permit repair of the potentially lethal damage. Probably there is no physical or chemical difference in "sub-lethal" and "potentially lethal" damage but one is studied by split or multidose irradiation while the other is studied by varying the post-irradiation conditions.

NON-REPAIRABLE AND NON-LETHAL DAMAGE

Data from studies on cells surviving large radiation doses show clearly that the initial and rapid repair process is not effective in fully restoring the cell to its preirradiation condition. Cells that constitute the surviving fraction, *i.e.* those cells retaining a capacity for sustained proliferation, may show biological properties that differ markedly from that of the unirradiated cell line. In a systematic study based on V79-1 hamster cell line cultured *in vitro*, Sinclair[53] found that many of the cells surviving doses of 1,500 r produced "small colonies" and their cells were characterized by increased radiosensitivity, (decrease in D_{37} but no change in N) de-

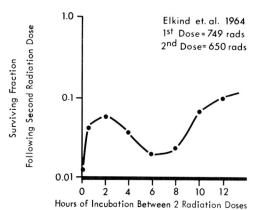

FIG. 2-12. The survival fraction of Chinese hamster cell line V79-379-A when irradiated *in vitro* by 1,499 rads given in two doses separated by varying periods of incubation at 37°C. (Courtesy: Elkind, *Nature, 202,* 1190, 1964.)

creased plating efficiency, change in median cell volume, gross chromosome abnormalities, lengthened intermitotic time, and increase in the probability of daughter cell death. Thus, those viable cells demonstrated a number of radiation-induced heritable changes, *i.e.* their radiation damage had not been completely repaired. It is of special interest that these altered cell properties were maintained in some of the cell lines cultured continuously for many months. He suggested that at higher radiation doses these "sub-lethal" changes might accumulate and become lethal.

That the repair of damage produced by doses of 100 to 200 rads is incomplete and that this damage persisted in viable colonies for many generations was strikingly demonstrated by the cinephotography study of LP_{59} cells already mentioned.[75] In some cell pedigrees there was a markedly elevated frequency of cell pyknosis and lysis in the first 5 to 6 generations after irradiation even though a viable colony was eventually established. This is a class of radiation damage which persists for very long times and causes death of cells in generations remote from the "irradiated and surviving" cell.

Tissue Radiobiology

The various concepts already discussed under cellular radiobiology are directly applicable to tissue or organ radiobiology. Response of a tissue or a group of tissues to irradiation is of course more complex than the response of an individual cell. This is so as the observed changes in an irradiated tissue(s) reflect the total or integrated reaction of the various tissue elements (*viz.* epidermal, dermal, vascular, etc.) and each of these is in turn the resultant of responses of the constituent cells of the particular tissue. In addition to the effects on cells comprising different tissues there may be physiological changes induced in the tissue of interest which would modify the reaction. For example, after an initial treatment the surviving

cells may go into a phase of accelerated proliferation which would markedly affect response to fractionated irradiation. If there is gross damage to a vessel, then cells adjacent to the vessel may die (infarct) or if there is a reduced blood flow the cell may become hypoxic and hence relatively radioresistant.

The dominant factors in determining the character of the observed response of tissue (or group of tissues) is the proportion of cells inactivated (killed) by the radiation, the distribution of cell lysis times, *i.e.* times between irradiation and lysis or dissolution of the cell, the capability of the surviving cells in each tissue to proliferate and to reconstitute the tissue, and the capability of the reconstituted tissues to reform the original tissue complex, *e.g.* organ. Reaction of tissue to irradiation might be minimal (undetectable) if the tissue were comprised of non-dividing (or almost non-dividing) cells as lysis occurs principally at the time of attempted division. In contrast, if the cells were dividing rapidly there would be observed a rapid series of changes. In accordance with this, the expected and the observed changes in brain and in the jejunum are markedly different.

Tumor Biology

At this point brief consideration will be given to selected aspects of tumor biology. Tumors *per se* are comprised of tumor cells and stromal elements. The tumor cells are in several categories: viable and actively proliferating; viable but not in active cell cycle (in a prolonged G_1 phase) but with the capacity for proliferation; nonviable but histologically intact; and nonviable and pyknotic. Supporting the tumor is normal tissue stroma which consists of blood and lymph vascular system, connective tissue and nerve tissue.

The proportion of tumor tissue which is comprised of histologically intact tumor cell elements can vary from ≈ 5 to 10 per cent up to almost 100 per cent. This will depend on the particular tumor and upon the size of tumor. Study by the Chalky technique of the mouse mammary carcinoma employed in our laboratory, indicated that ≈ 60 per cent of the tumor is made up of intact tumor cells (studied at a tumor diameter of 8 mm). That is, 40 per cent of the tumor volume represents gross necrosis and stromal elements.[50] The percentage of tumor which is intact tumor tissue would be much higher at tumor sizes of 1 to 2 mm diameter and some extent lower for tumors of 12 and 16 mm diameter. At all tumor sizes there are pyknotic tumor cells scattered throughout the areas of apparently intact tumor tissue.

For certain tumors there is a definite architectural pattern which is determined by the distribution of areas of necrosis. This is a reflection of the distribution of vessels and specifically the distance between vessels. Figure 2-13, a photomicrograph of the mouse mammary carcinoma used in our laboratory, shows tumor cells arranged radially around a central vascular core. This tumor appears to exist in cords and that these cords are delimited by the surrounding necrotic tissue. Radii of these cords are $\approx 90\,\mu$ and this corresponds to ≈ 10 cell layers. The corded structure is not observed until the tumor is ≈ 10 to 12 mm in diameter and there is necrosis; necrotic areas are not present in small tumors. Interesting work in tumor biology has been performed in developing models of tumor morphology at different stages of tumor growth, calculation of distributions of various metabolites (pO_2, glucose, CO_2, lactic acid), and measurements of proliferative activity of tumor cells in various regions of the tumor.

The best available analysis suggests that oxygen is the critical metabolite and that necrosis appears at distances from the capillary which corresponds to the diffusion dis-

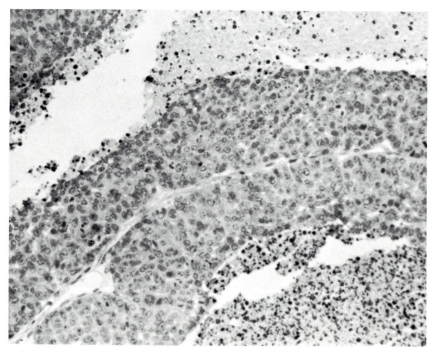

FIG. 2-13. Photo micrograph of a C_3H mouse mammary carcinoma. Note that the tumor is growing as a cord of cells with a central vascular axis and that this cord of intact tumor is surrounded by necrotic tissue. There would be expected to be a rather steep oxygen tension gradient across the cord radius, oxygen tension being maximal near the central vascular structure. Photomicrograph by Helen B. Stone.

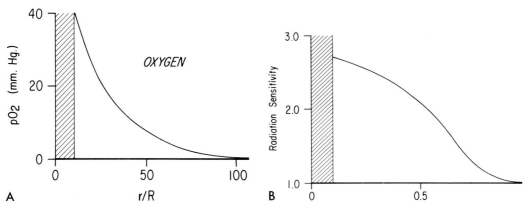

FIG. 2-14. **A.** Plot of the calculated pO_2 as a function of distance from capillary in terms of diffusion distance of oxygen (at diffusion distance $pO_2 = 0$). **B.** Radiation sensitivity of cells as a function of distance from capillary in terms of diffusion distance. (Courtesy: Tannock: *J. Nat. Cancer Inst.,* (In Press).)

tance of oxygen, *i.e.* necrosis or cell death is observed at the distance required for the pO_2 to fall to ≈ 0.[70] Accordingly there would be a decrease in pO_2 and radiosensitivity along the radius from capillary to the necrotic region. The predicted changes in pO_2 and radiation sensitivity as a function of distance from capillary are illustrated graphically in Figure 2-14 (calculations made by Tannock). Further, the rate of cell proliferation decreases with a decrease in pO_2.[4] Accordingly there would be expected broad distributions of cellular radiosensitivity and proliferative activity within the tumor tissue, *i.e.* there is not simply one compartment of aerobic, radiosensitive and actively dividing cells and a second compartment of hypoxic, radioresistant, and non-proliferating cells. Much of the writing on the role of hypoxic cells in determining response of tumor tissue to irradiation has been based on use of a simple model which features aerobic cells (minimum D_{37}) and hypoxic or anoxic cells (maximum D_{37}). This has been justified upon the need for simplification. In this section such a simplified approach will be used. The above paragraph is included to emphasize that the biological reality is much more complex than our calculations indicate.

Kinetics of cell proliferation in many tumors of laboratory animals and of man have

been studied. Mention will be made here of the study by Tannock of the C_3H mammary carcinoma used in our laboratory.[69] The basic technique is to inject one dose of tritiated thymidine (³HTdR) intraperitoneally and to sacrifice the animal at various times later and prepare autoradiographs of the tumor. Thymidine is one of the pyrimidine bases of the *DNA* molecule and it is incorporated exclusively into the *DNA* being synthesized at the time of injection. Cells in *S* period at injection or their progeny will therefore be labeled or show grains over their nucleus in the autoradiograph. If the animal were sacrificed at 30 minutes after injection of ³HTdR then all labeled cells would have been *S* phase. No *M* or G_1 cells would be labeled. If the animal were sacrificed at 4 hours, nearly all cells in mitosis would be labeled; *i.e.* all cells in *M* at 4 hours after injection would be cells which had been in *S* at time 0 but had progressed through G_2 and into *M* during the 4 hours. By 12 hours only a small proportion of *M* cells should show grain counts: cells in *M* phase at 12 hours would have been in G_1 phase when the injection was made. Therefore, by plotting the per cent of labeled mitotic figures against time, a curve of the type shown in Figure 2-15 can be constructed. From such a curve the mean duration of G_2, *S*, total cell

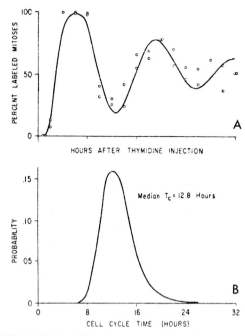

FIG. 2-15. A. Labeled mitoses results and computed curve for carcinoma cells of the C$_3$H mammary tumor; 100 mitoses per point were scored with use of a grain-count threshold of 5 grains/cell. **B.** Computed distribution of cell cycle times for C$_3$H mammary carcinoma cells. (Courtesy: Tannock: In *Time and Dose Relationships in Radiation Biology as Applied to Radiotherapy*, Brookhaven National Laboratory Report 50203, (C-57), 1969, p. 218.)

upon pO$_2$, the findings in Table 2-2 are particularly interesting: mitotic index and labeling index decreased markedly with distance from the capillary. Actually in the cell layer next to the necrotic region essentially no mitotic figures or labeled cells were found.

Another parameter of tumor cell proliferation is the *GF* or growth fraction. A tumor cell population may be classified as *P* cells (actively proliferating or in active cycle) and *Q* cells (non-proliferating or quiescent cells). The growth fraction corresponds to the fractional increase in *P* cells during one mean cycle time. For example, consider a tumor which contains 10^6 *P* cells, but after one mean cell cycle time there are 1.4 × 10^6 *P* cells instead of the expected 2 × 10^6 if all progeny of *P* cells were in fact *P* cells. The growth fraction would, in this instance, be 0.4. This means that 0.6 × 10^6 cells or 60 per cent of the increase in cell number are *Q* cells. These *Q* cells may remain in the tumor for a long time but would not divide. By standard autoradiographic studies following injection of tritiated thymidine, data may be developed from which the growth fraction can be calculated. The proportion of cells which are labeled in autoradiographs prepared from tissue collected at 30 to 60 minutes after injection is defined as the labeling index or *LI*. This would be determined by the ratio T_s/T_c (T_s is the length of the *s* phase, T_c is the length of the cell cycle) if all cells were in cycle. If, however, the experimentally determined *LI* were less than the observed T_s/T_c then only a fraction (*GF*) of the total

cycle may be estimated. For this tumor the cell time was calculated to be 12.8 hours with $S = 7.2$ hours, $G_1 = 3$ hours, and $G_2 = 3$ hours. With respect to the earlier statement that cell proliferative activity was dependent

Table 2-2. *Proliferation Activity of Cells of a C3H Mouse Mammary Carcinoma as a Function of Position in Tumor Cord*

	Central Region	Intermediate Region	Peripheral Region
Mitotic Index % (Mean + S.D.)	4.3 ± 0.4	2.5 ± 0.3	0.6 ± 0.2
Labeling Index % (Mean ± S.D.)	50.0 ± 2.5	29.6 ± 4.8	10.3 ± 3.4

Adapted from: Tannock, In *Time and Dose Relationships in Radiation Biology as Applied to Radiotherapy*, Brookhaven National Laboratory Report 50203 (C-57), 1969, p. 215.

cell population is actively proliferating. In this instance, the growth fraction may be derived from simple cell kinetic data as follows:

$$GF = LI \times \frac{Tc}{Ts} \times \frac{1}{\lambda}, \text{ where } \lambda \text{ is a constant.}$$

For the mouse mammary carcinoma under discussion the growth fraction was calculated to be 0.5.

Tumor cell number often increases more slowly than is indicated by the proliferative activity as determined by standard assays of cell proliferation, *e.g.* mitotic index, labeling index, etc. This slow growth in cell number is due not only to the fact that the growth fraction is less than 1.0, but also that there is a very large proportion of the cells lost during each cell cycle time. This loss of progeny has been referred to by Steele as the "cell loss factor" and is designated ϕ.[57,58] Cell loss may be due to cell death at attempted division, exfoliation into the blood or lymph vascular spaces, shedding of cells to the surface or into interior body cavities, etc.

Because of this cell loss, the observed population doubling time, Td is greater than that expected on the basis of mean cell cycle time and growth fraction. The term potential doubling time (T) is used to designate the population doubling time if there were no cell loss; $T = \lambda \frac{ts}{LI}$. If cell loss is the only factor making Td longer than T, then $\phi = 1 - \frac{T}{Td}$. If ϕ were 0.6, Td would be 2.5 times T (ratio of $T/Td = 0.4$). For mammary carcinoma ϕ was calculated to be 0.6.

This factor is especially important in that for many of the human carcinomas which have been studied ϕ was usually >0.5 and as high as 0.9. The observed growth of tumor is therefore often much slower than predicted from the measured cell cycle time due to a growth fraction less than 1 and a high cell loss factor. Volume doubling time of human tumors are often in the range of

months to years but the mean cell cycle time is in the range of 24 to 96 hours. This emphasizes that slow growth does not *per se* indicate a low proliferative activity by the cells.

Radiation Therapy of Laboratory Animal Tumors

Dose Response Curves for Animal Tumors

Responses of certain laboratory animal tumors to x-irradiation will be considered with reference to the review of cellular radiation biology presented in the above section. Do the constituent cells of a solid tumor respond to irradiation on an individual cellular basis, or are there factors inherent in the relationship between the cells of a tumor and/or between the cells and the organism of which they are a part that modify that response? Can the response of a solid tumor to a specified dose of radiation be predicted by considering the tumor as a population of a finite number of cells whose individual cellular radiosensitivities are defined by the multitarget relationship in terms of D_{37} and N. If this relationship does obtain for cells constituting tumor tissues *in vivo* and a single surviving cell were to proliferate to produce a local recurrence, then the probability of a tumor lethal response to a single radiation dose could be predicted by knowing only the number of viable tumor cells and their distribution of radiosensitivities, in terms of D_{37} and N values. Accordingly, one should find that the shape of the dose response curve is predictable and that there is an orderly relationship between tumor cell number and the TCD_{50} (the dose which would be expected on the average to yield control of half the irradiated tumors).

The end-point of tumor response which is of greatest interest to the clinical radiation therapist is tumor control or tumor destruction. Investigations employing laboratory animal tumor systems are attractive because it is feasible to generate complete dose response curves using this end-point. These curves may be obtained for radiation administered under different conditions, various schedules of dose fractionation, and combination of radiation with chemotherapeutic agents, surgery, immunotherapeutic procedures. A dose response curve for a C_3H mouse mammary carcinoma is shown in Figures 2-16 and 2-17. For this assay, 250 Kv x-radiation was administered as a single dose under clamp induced hypoxia. The tumors were 8 mm in diameter. In Figure 2-16 the data are plotted on linear grid and the resultant curve is of the S shape type. Plotted on a probability-log grid in Figure 2-17, the dose response curve is a straight line. From such a curve the TCD_{50} may be read directly. The

TCD_{50} is preferred to any other tumor control probably because it may be estimated with the greatest accuracy for a given number of animals in an experiment.

EXPERIMENTAL PROCEDURE FOR ESTIMATION OF THE TUMOR CONTROL DOSE 50 OR TCD_{50}

To perform a TCD_{50} assay of C_3H mouse mammary carcinoma, recipient mice are assigned by a random number procedure to one of several radiation dose levels at the time of tumor transplantation. The growing tumors are measured 3 times per week and as they approach the volume at which they are to be irradiated they are measured on a daily basis. In the assay illustrated in Figure 2-16 and Figure 2-17, radiation was given on

TUMOR CONTROL DOSE RESPONSE CURVE

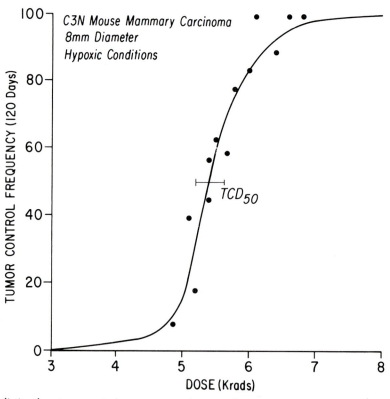

FIG. 2-16. Radiation dose-tumor control response curve for 8 mm diameter mammary carcinoma of the C_3H mouse treatment by single radiation doses and under conditions of clamp induced hypoxia.

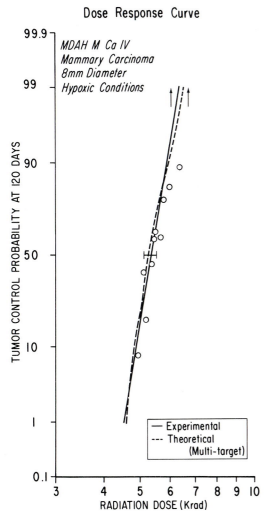

FIG. 2-17. Dose response curve for 8 mm diameter mammary carcinoma irradiated clamp hypoxia by single radiation doses. The dotted line is the curve which would be predicted by the multitarget-single hit response law if conventional values for D_{37} and N are assumed.

the day the diameter reached 8 mm. Thus, range of tumor volume at time of treatment is minimal. Animals are examined weekly for presence of tumor at the treated site during the first 120 days after irradiation. The proportion of mice which have local control of tumor at each dose level at 120 days following irradiation is tabulated, then a regression line is fitted through these local control re-

sults and the TCD_{50} calculated. Almost all local recurrences are scored by day 100–120. The TCD_{50} for this tumor system at 300 days is only ≈ 5 per cent higher than it is at 120 days.

SHAPE OF RADIATION DOSE-TUMOR CONTROL RESPONSE CURVE

Figure 2-17 shows a theoretical dose response curve for a model tumor with these properties: a fixed number (M) of cells, cell response is described by multitarget-single hit response law, D_{37} and N are constant for all cells, and tumor recurs if one cell survives irradiation.* Also included in this figure are the experimental data points and the regression line fitted through those points for an 8 mm diameter mouse mammary carcinoma irradiated under clamp hypoxia conditions. Although there are uncertainties in the values taken for M, D_{37}, and N, the slopes of the theoretical and experimental curve are not distinguishable over the range TCD_1 to TCD_{99}. These curves show the maximal steepness of a response curve. Less steep curves would be expected where the individual tumors in the tumor population being studied were variable in cell number, distribution of cell sensitivities, or if there were variation in host reaction to its tumor.

TCD_{50} and Tumor Volume for Single Dose Irradiation

The effect of tumor volume on the likelihood of successful treatment by radiation therapy has long been of interest to the clinician. According to the tumor model de-

*Referring to equation 2-4 of Appendix 2. $TCD_p \approx D_{37}$ $[1nM + 1nN - 1n(-1np)]$. $P =$ probability of killing all of M cells, i.e. $TCD_{10} \approx D_{37}$ $[1nM + 1nN - 1n(-1n0.1)]$. Inspection of this equation shows that TCD_p varies directly with the expression of $D_{37}[-1n(-1np)]$. The theoretical curve was computed using the following assumptions: $M = 2.5 \times 10^8$ (number of clonogenic cells); $N = 6$. Therefore, for the experimentally determined TCD_{50} of 5,400 rads, the D_{37} would be 270 rads. Then TCD_p values were computed for p varying from 0.01 to 0.99.

scribed above the dependence of TCD_{50} on tumor cell number (M) would be approximated by this equation: $TCD_{50} \approx D_{37}$ $[1nM + 1nN - 1n(-1n\ 0.5)]$. This applies only to response to single dose irradiation. A graphic representation of this equation is given in Figure 2-18. The slope is dependent on D_{37} while the intercept is determined by N. For this model, TCD_{50} increases by $2.3 \times D_{37}$ for each 10 fold increase in cell number. Accordingly, the TCD_{50} would increase by 2.3×400 or 920 rads if the number of hypoxic cells were greater by a factor of 10.

The correlation between TCD_{50} and tumor volume (and presumably cell number) has been examined in 16 dose response studies, based on tumors varying in volume at the time of treatment from 0.16 to 1,000 mm³;

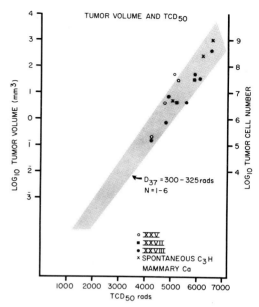

FIG. 2-19. TCD_{50} values determined from 16 response curve studies. (Volume range: 0.16 to 1,000 mm³.) (Courtesy: Suit, In *Cellular Radiation Biology*, Baltimore, Williams & Wilkins Company, p. 514, 1965.)

these include spontaneous tumors, autotransplants, and isotransplants of mammary carcinoma of the C₃H mouse. Studies are shown in Figure 2-19. TCD_{50} increased by 690–750 rads for each 10 fold increase in tumor volume.

As illustrated in Figure 2-19, the 16 experimentally determined TCD_{50} values fell within a band which would be defined by curves where $D_{37} = 300$ rads, $N = 1$ and for $D_{37} = 325$ rads, $N = 6$.

Recently, cell survival curves have been developed for two mouse mammary carcinomas: D_{37} was estimated to be 300–360 rads.[11,50] These values are in the central portion of the range of radiosensitivities for hypoxic mammalian cells of 250 to 589 rads as listed in Table 2-3.

Tumor Regression and Probability of Local Control

Is there a correlation between the rate at which a tumor regresses following irradiation

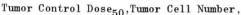

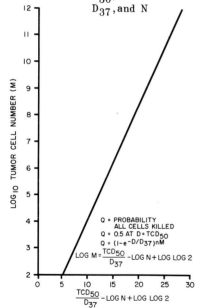

FIG. 2-18. Predicted relationship between D_{37}, N, TCD_{50}, and M or tumor cell number, provided the multitarget response described relationship between cell killing and radiation dose and a single surviving cell would produce an observed recurrence. (Courtesy: Suit, In *Cellular Radiation Biology*, Baltimore, Williams & Wilkins Company, p. 514, 1965.)

Table 2-3. *"Oxygen Effect Factor"* for Several Mammalian Cell Lines

Cell Line	Viability Assay	D_{37} Aerobic	D_{37} Anoxic	Oxygen Effect Factor	References
Murine Leukemia	*in vivo*	65	365	2.3	Hewitt and Wilson[34]
Murine Bone Marrow	*in vivo*	95	250	2.6	Till[76]
Human Liver Cell	*in vitro*	140*	310*	2.3	Dewey[15]
Ehrlich Ascites Cells	*in vivo*	134*	415*	3.1	Silini and Hornsey[51]
L-P 59 Cell	*in vitro*	148*	412*	2.8	Humphrey, Dewey, and Cork[38]
V 79-1	*in vitro*	187	589	3.1	Elkind[21]

*These experiments were performed with 200 to 250 Kv x-rays. In accordance with the policy used in this section the D_{37} values as listed are in terms of Co^{60} rads; the experimentally determined values were multiplied by the RBE correction factor of $\frac{1.00}{0.85}$.

and the probability that the tumor will be controlled permanently by the treatment? To investigate this question, growth curves of 142 spontaneous mammary carcinomas of the C_3H mouse were prepared for the periods of growth prior to irradiation, regression of tumor following treatment, and the regrowth of tumor.[60]

Individual tumor growth curves for two tumors that received 6,600 rads (local control rate of 73 per cent) are shown in Figure 2-20. In one instance as shown in Figure 2-20 (upper curve) there was a rapid regression of tumor and then complete absence of palpable tumor until after day 100 when local recurrence was noted. This contrasts with the course followed by the tumor growth curve in Figure 2-20 (lower curve) where there was a very slow regression over a period of 320 days. On histological examination at the 320-day point, the small persistent nodule contained no recognizable malignant cells.

Figure 2-21 shows the proportion of tumor volume remaining at 21 days for the entire series of tumors following single radiation doses which yielded local tumor control rates varying from 0.3 per cent (4,125 rads) to 99.7

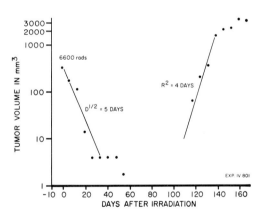

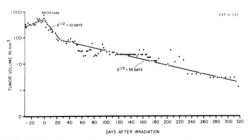

FIG. 2-20. Regression curves for spontaneous mammary carcinomas in two individual C_3H mice following single radiation doses of 6,600 rads (this dose yields a local control rate of 73 per cent). (Courtesy: Suit, *Radiology, 84,* 1100, 1965.)

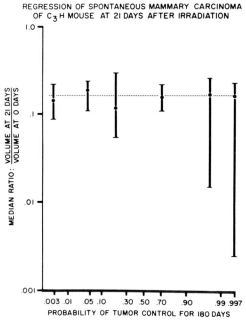

REGRESSION OF SPONTANEOUS MAMMARY CARCINOMA
OF C₃H MOUSE AT 21 DAYS AFTER IRRADIATION

FIG. 2-21. Regression of the spontaneous mammary carcinoma of the C_3H mouse at 21 days following single doses of radiation given under conditions of local tissue anoxia. Probability of local control of tumor for 180 days extended over the range of 0.003 to 0.997. The points represent median values of the ratio of tumor volume at 21 days after treatment to the volume at the time of treatment. Brackets enclose the 95 per cent confidence intervals around the median values. Distribution free confidence interval for the median from Table XVII, Lienert[40]. (Courtesy: Suit, *Radiology*, 84, 1100, 1965.)

An explanation for these findings may be that for permanent local control of tumor, radiation dose must be sufficient to injure lethally all tumor cells. Therefore, even radiation doses which are quite ineffective in terms of achieving sterilization of tumor, *e.g.* TCD_1, would be expected to damage lethally almost all tumor cells, say $\gg 99.99$ per cent. Certainly over short periods of observation, gross measurements of tumor size would not enable one to discriminate between survival fractions of 10^{-4} and 10^{-7}, *i.e.* a low and a high probability of tumor control.

According to this reasoning, in observing a tumor following large dose irradiation, the experimentor measures the diameters of a mass of nonviable tumor cells and only describes the rate of removal of lysed tumor cells and tumor stroma.

SIGNIFICANCE OF MORPHOLOGICALLY "INTACT" TUMOR CELLS PERSISTING IN IRRADIATED TUMOR

The demonstration of morphologically intact and normally staining tumor cells in tissue after irradiation treatment is often considered prima-facie evidence for persistence of viable tumor cells which, if undisturbed, would proliferate and produce recurrent growth.

Following irradiation of the spontaneous mammary carcinomas in the C_3H mouse, there is often a persistent nodularity or thickening at the site of the primary tumor for many months following the original treatment although this is not followed by local recurrence. The residual nodularity of the primary tumor was studied histologically in 21 nodules at 48 to 110 days following radiation doses varying from 5,760 to 9,400 rads, *i.e.*, a local control rate of 20 to 99.7 per cent. In each instance, these residual nodules showed morphologically intact and normally staining tumor cells. These nodules would be considered by the standard surgical pathological criteria as containing "viable" tumor cells. In a few instances, tumor nodules ex-

per cent (9,400 rads). Even over this range of dose there was no correlation between tumor regression following treatment and the likelihood of tumor control for 180 days. Thus, these data from the spontaneous mammary carcinoma of the C_3H mouse indicate no relationship between observed tumor regression and probability of local control of tumor over the range of dose used.

Thomlinson and Craddock[74] studied the effect of single dose irradiation (3,000–6,000 rads) on the growth curve of a benzypyrene induced fibrosarcoma in rats. For this tumor also, the slope of the post-treatment regression curve was independent of dose.

amined at greater than 110 days also showed "viable" tumor cells by these criteria.

Were these persistent cells viable but failed to proliferate and produce a recurrence as a result of the severe radiation-induced changes in the tissues of the tumor bed? As a test of the viability of these intact cells, transplantation studies were performed. A series of the spontaneous mammary carcinomas were irradiated with doses that yielded local control rates of <1 per cent, 20 per cent, and 95 per cent. At approximately 28 days following irradiation, the nodules were removed and divided into several portions. One portion was submitted for histological study and the others were transplanted into young adult isologous animals. The histological slides prepared from these nodules were interpreted by the surgical pathologist as showing persistent "viable" tumor cells. However, successful transplantation of tumor occurred only from the nodules that received a dose that yielded local control at a rate of <1 or 20 per cent.[59] The local control rate of tumor corresponded closely to the observed tumor transplant take rate although the histological changes observed in the nodules were not dose dependent (at this time following irradiation and for the dose levels used). These results were consistent with the data on tumor regression rate following irradiation. Therefore, in at least this animal tumor system, neither rate of tumor regression nor persistence of histologically intact cells in irradiated tissue indicated the probability of regrowth of tumor. The only proof that tumor cells remaining in irradiated tissue are viable is the demonstrated ability of these cells to proliferate, *i.e.* to produce a recurrence.

TCD$_{50}$ as Modified by Immunological Reaction Between Host and Tumor

Experimental evidence shows that nearly all tumors of experimental animals induced by carcinogenic chemical compounds, oncogenic viruses and plastics carry weak but specific antigens. Isologous animals can be partially immunized against the isotransplantation of these tumors. Many human tumors have been shown to possess specific antigens and that the patient (host) reacts to those antigens makes it pertinent to consider the significance of an immunological reaction by the host against the tumor on the response of tumor to local irradiation.

The number of cells required to transplant induced tumors of experimental animals can be sharply modified by altering the immunological status of the host or by prior exposure to the tumor, *i.e.* immunization, whole body irradiation, etc.[25,45] Cohen[12] reported that the TCD_{50} for a mammary carcinoma was 7,900 R when transplanted in C$_3$H mice, which had been made immunologically incompetent by prior whole-body irradiation as compared with 5,700 R for tissues growing in normal mice.

In a similar study[64], the TCD_{50} for a methylcholanthrene induced fibrosarcoma was determined for tumor which had been transplanted into normal, previously immunized (3 injections of 2×10^7 radiation killed cells), or immunologically depressed recipients (400 rads whole body irradiation at 24 hours before transplantation). The TCD_{50} values were: 3,500 rads, 2,700 rads, and 4,300 rads respectively as listed in Table 2-4. For this tumor system, the immunological status of the host *at the time* of transplantation was a powerful factor in the response of tumor to local x-irradiation. In contrast, the TCD_{50} was not affected by standard immunization procedures or by whole body irradiation *after* the tumor had been irradiated locally. Much additional research is necessary in this area to establish the efficacy of various immunotherapy procedures when combined with radiation therapy of established tumors in experimental animals. This is especially so as it has now been demonstrated that certain procedures can stimulate production of enhancing antibodies: apparently these are produced by the host during tumor growth and do affect the effectiveness of the host immune reaction (block the action of sensi-

Table 2-4. *TCD$_{50}$ values for a C3H/He Fibrosarcoma (Tumor was 8 mm in diameter at treatment. Radiation was administered under conditions of local hypoxia)*

Condition of Mouse at Time of Transplantation	TCD$_{50}$ (rads)	95% Confidence
Normal	3,480	(3,280–3,700)
Actively Immunized	2,740	(2,270–3,310)
Immune Depressed*	4,510	(4,080–4,550)

*400 rads whole body irradiation given 24 hours before transplantation. (Courtesy: Suit and Kastelan: *Cancer,* 26,232, 1970.)

tized lymphoid cells to inactivate the tumor cell).

Radiation Dose Fractionation and Tissue Response

The effect of dividing a total radiation dose into a number of equal fractions on the dose which is required to yield a specified response in tissue will be determined by a complex interaction of at least 4 factors. These may be referred to as the 4 R's of fractionation. These are 1) repair of radiation damage; 2) redistribution of cell age (sensitivities); 3) repopulation; 4) reoxygenation or improvement in the oxygen tension in the irradiated tissue during fractionated irradiation. There are almost certainly other factors but these are important determinants of responses which reflect cell killing. The discussion of the effect of dose fractionation will be directed to these 4 factors with respect to tumor tissue and then to normal tissue.

REPAIR OF RADIATION DAMAGE

Elkind[19] has reported that the response of cells growing *in vitro* to five successive radiation doses of 505 rads separated by 22 hour periods was essentially equal to that which would be predicted if there had been full recovery (return of shoulder region) between each irradiation. His experimental results are reproduced in Figure 2-22. Those data nicely demonstrate the fact that the dose which

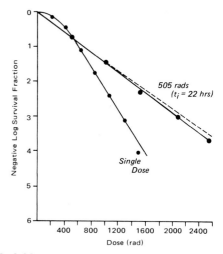

FIG. 2-22. Response of Chinese hamster cells to irradiation *in vitro* by single dose or multiple doses of 505 rads with 22 hours between doses (t_i). Solid curves are best fits through the experimental data. The dashed line indicates the survival curve had there been complete "recovery" during each of the 22 hour periods. (Courtesy: Elkind and Sutton: *Radiat. Res., 13,* 556, 1960.)

yields a specified survival fraction is increased if dose is given in multiple fractions instead of a single fraction. For example, a single dose of 1,425 rads resulted in a survival fraction of 2×10^{-4}; however, when the radiation was given in 5 equal fractions (22 hours between fractions) a total dose of 2,425 rads was required to reduce survival to the same level.

As the extrapolation number is a good indicator of the capacity for repair of radiation damage, it is useful to consider the dependence of the fractionation effect on the extrapolation number. Figure 2-23 demonstrates the manner in which the TCD_{50} would be expected to depend upon fractionation number (ν) when tumor cells are characterized by N values of 1, 2, 4, 6, and 10. For these calculations a model tumor comprised of 10^6 cells is employed; cells are uniformly sensitive and do not proliferate between fractions ($q = 1.00$)*.

As expected TCD_{50} is markedly dependent upon N for fractionated irradiation. Of course, TCD_{50} is independent of ν in the special case of $N = 1$. When $N = 2$, TCD_{50} increases regularly with ν, at least up to $\nu = 100$. For the N values of 4–10 (range of N found for most cells studied *in vivo* except for lymphoid, germinal, and bone marrow cells) TCD_{50} is sensitive to N value for ν in the range of 1–30 but approaches a common maximum value at $\nu = 60$ to 100. This re-

*For this model ω is set at 0.3, *i.e.* 0.3 of the dose produces damage which inactivates cells according to the single hit-single target model.

sults from the low dose per fraction: cells are killed only by the single target-single hit mechanism because insufficient radiation damage is accumulated at any one treatment for inactivation by the multitarget-single hit process.

The dependence of TCD_{50} upon ν has been determined experimentally for a mouse mammary carcinoma irradiated at 8 mm diameter; data are shown in Figure 2-24. Each treatment was administered under clamp-hypoxia so that differences in tumor tissue pO_2 during the course of fractionated irradiation would not affect the experimentally observed values. For this tumor the TCD_{50} increased as ν was raised from 1 to 2 to 5 to 10. In these assays, time between fractions (t_i) was 24 hours. These data points could be fitted by a curve similar to those shown in Figure 2-23 where N was intermediate between 6 and 10. The slope of the curve fitting these data points would be influenced by a changing distribution of cell ages (cell radiosensitivities) during the course of treatment as well as proliferation during t_i. There

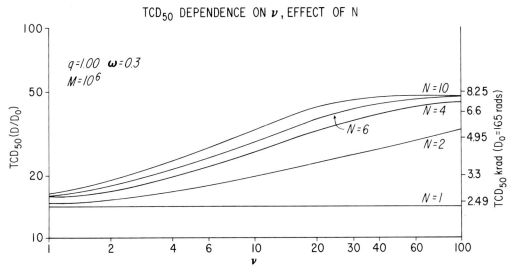

FIG. 2-23. Theoretical relationship between TCD_{50} and fractionation number (ν) over a range for ν of 1 to 100 for a tumor of 10^6 viable cells. The curves have been drawn for tumor cell populations characterized by N values of 1, 2, 4, 6, and 10. In all instances, the stipulations are made that: 1) there is no proliferation of viable cells during the course of treatment ($q = 1.0$) and 2) that $\omega = 0.3$. (Courtesy: Suit, Withers, Brown and Thomson: (In preparation).)

FIG. 2-24. Experimentally determined TCD_{50} values for an 8 mm diameter mammary carcinoma growing as transplants in the C_3H mouse. Radiation was administered in 1, 2, 5, or 10 equal dose fractions; there were 24 hours between each treatment session. All treatments were given under condition of local tissue hypoxic (clamp technique). Slope of the regression line through the data points is 0.27. (Courtesy: Suit and Howes: (In preparation).)

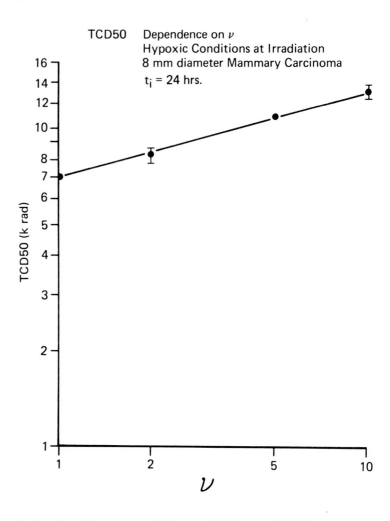

is no good method for allowing for the effect of altered distribution of cell ages and is therefore not attempted. Theoretical study by Young and Fowler[85] indicated that although redistribution of cell ages may make a significant effect on response to 2 or a small number of fractions it is not likely to be a big factor for more fractionated irradiation.

CELL PROLIFERATION BETWEEN TREATMENTS

At some point as intertreatment intervals are lengthened, proliferation of tumor cells would be expected to affect significantly the response of tissue to fractionated irradiation. The effect of cell proliferation on TCD_{50} of

a model tumor is illustrated in Figure 2-25: a family curves relating TCD_{50} and ν for different values of q. Here, q is defined as the fractional increase in viable cell number during each intertreatment interval. For example if q were 1.2, then during each time period between irradiations, the number of viable cells would be increased by 20 per cent. The range of q values used in this figure were selected on the basis of the values judged most likely to apply to clinical setting. As shown, the effect of q becomes progressively more prominent as ν is increased: greater total time available for cell proliferation (no allowance was made for the radiation induced mitotic block). Unless q is large, *viz.* greater than 1.10, cell proliferation would not

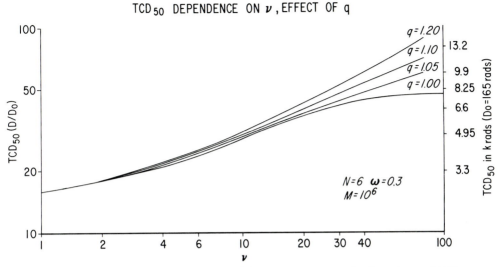

FIG. 2-25. The predicted effect of cell proliferation between treatments on the dependence of TCD_{50} on ν. A family of curves for q values of 1.00 to 1.20; q is the fractional increase in viable cell number during the intertreatment interval. For these calculations the tumor model is given as 10^6 viable cells; N value for all cells is set at 6; and W is specified to be 0.3. No allowance for changing distribution of cell sensitivities has been attempted. (Courtesy: Suit, Withers, Brown and Thomson: (In preparation).)

be a prominent factor in tumor response to fractionated irradiation for fractionation numbers up to 10-15. However, for the usually employed fractionation numbers in clinical radiation therapy of 30–40 a q value of 1.05–1.10 would be significant. Experimental data relevant to these considerations are presented in Figures 2-26 and 2-27. Again, all treatments were given under clamp-hypoxia so that the TCD_{50} would be primarily dependent upon the total number of viable cells in the tumor and be uninfluenced by changes in tumor oxygen tension. In Figure 2-26 are presented TCD_{50} results versus time between doses for $\nu = 2$, 5, and 10. TCD_{50} was found to increase more rapidly with prolongation of t_i for $\nu = 10$ than for $\nu = 2$. This was not unexpected because of these factors: 1) the dose per fraction decreased with larger number of fractions viz. 1,300 rads ($\nu = 10$), 2,200 rads ($\nu = 5$), and 3,500 rads ($\nu = 2$); 2) the mitotic delay or the block in cell progression would decrease as dose per fraction diminished; 3) the total time over which treatment was given increased with fractionation number for a stated intertreat-

ment interval, *viz.* where t_i was 1 day the total treatment times were 1 day ($\nu = 2$), 4 days ($\nu = 5$), and 9 days ($\nu = 10$). Data from experiments where intertreatment times of 8 or 12 hours were employed (2–3 treatments per day) yielded TCD_{50} values the same as where t_i was 24 hours. That is TCD_{50} for $\nu = 10$ was the same for treatment given as 1, 2 or 3 sessions per day. These findings indicate that for single doses of at least 1,300 rads, no effective cell proliferation occurs for intertreatment periods of 1 day or less. However, the prompt increase in TCD_{50} as time between irradiation is raised to 48 hours and then to 72 hours indicates active cell replication between irradiations. Figure 2-27 presents the data given in Figure 2-26 so as to demonstrate the effect of overall time of treatment on the TCD_{50}. For assays using $\nu = 5$, TCD_{50} for $t_i = 3$ or $t_i = 5$ days was significantly higher than for $t_i = 1$ day. This indicates that tumor cell proliferation was occurring during these long intertreatment intervals. It is interesting that this proliferation activity was occurring at the same time that the gross tumor was decreasing in size.

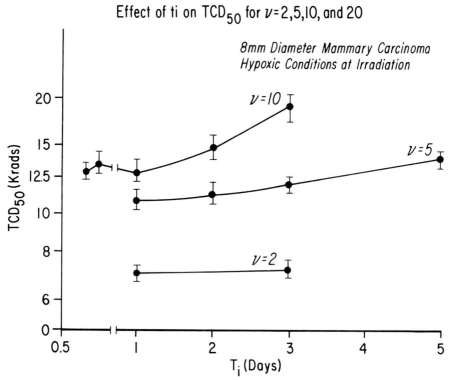

FIG. 2-26. Effect of time between dose fractions on the TCD_{50} for a C_3H mouse mammary carcinoma irradiated under hypoxic conditions (clamp induced). Total number of dose fractions 2, 5, and 10. (Courtesy: Suit and Howes: (In preparation).)

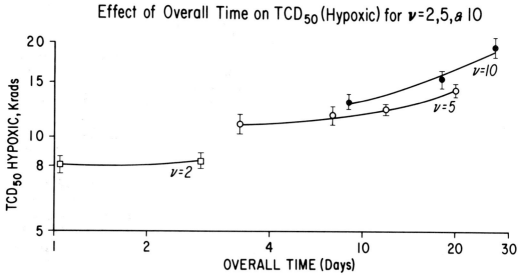

FIG. 2-27. Experimentally determined effect of total time of treatment on TCD_{50} for an 8 mm diameter C_3H mouse mammary carcinoma irradiated in 2, 5, or 10 equal doses. All irradiations administered under conditions of local hypoxia (clamp technique). (Courtesy: Suit and Howes: (In Preparation).)

In some experimental tumor systems evidence has been developed which shows that following a single large radiation dose, surviving cells enter a period of increased proliferative activity. For example, Hermens[31,32] found that between 0 and 4 days after a single dose of 2,000 rads delivered to a R-1 rhabdomyosarcoma there was only a slow increase in number of viable cells. However, between day 4 and 10 there was a more rapid increase in viable cell number; this was accompanied by a decrease in mean cell cycle time, see Figure 2-28. Van Peperzeel has also observed a shortening of mean cell cycle time during a phase of rapid regrowth following a single dose of 210 rads to a transplanted mouse mammary carcinoma.[79] This intense proliferative response to radiation injury may not be a general phenomenon as indicated by Denekemp's study of 4 tumors.[14] Following single doses of 1,000 to 1,500 rads there was no detected change in cell cycle time. Additional laboratory work on this phenomenon is in progress. In particular, the clinician would like to know for the *individual* patient if there is effective cell proliferation during the course of treatment: over weekend, between treatments (especially if only 2 or 3 treatments are given per week) or during the split in split course therapy. For certain tumors (*e.g.* certain lymphomas and sarcomas) which are characterized by rapid growth there might well be a net increase in the number of viable cells during 24 hour time periods between doses of 150 to 200 rads. This is an area of research which might yield results of practical clinical value.

REOXYGENATION

As stated earlier, the molecular oxygen tension in mammalian cells at the time of irradiation can modify the cellular D_{37} by a factor of two to three. Thomlinson and Gray[73] proposed that adjacent to the necrotic areas observed in solid tumors, there are viable cells which are severely hypoxic and hence, radioresistant. Such cells would be expected to affect strongly the efficacy of radiation therapy. The influence of the presence of a very small fraction of anoxic cells in an otherwise aerobic tumor cell population on the tumor control dose response curve can be appreciated by the following considerations: the TCD_{50} for a tumor of 10^6 viable and aerobic cells treated by 30 equal doses ($D_{37} = 165$ rads, $N = 4$, $\omega = 0.3$, $q = 1.0$) would be 5,960 rads; however, if 1 per cent of the cells were hypoxic (10^4 cells) the TCD_{50} would be 10,800 rads ($D_{37} = 400$ rads, $N = 4$, $\omega = 0.3$, $q = 1.0$). Therefore, it is of interest to examine tumors of experimental animals for the presence of hypoxic cells and to evaluate the effectiveness of various methods of reducing the effect of hypoxic cells on the response of tumor tissue to irradiation.

Goldacre and Selven[26] have shown that in the spontaneous and transplanted murine mammary carcinoma there are usually large areas where there is no demonstrable blood

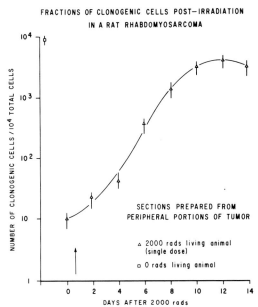

FRACTIONS OF CLONOGENIC CELLS POST—IRRADIATION IN A RAT RHABDOMYOSARCOMA

SECTIONS PREPARED FROM PERIPHERAL PORTIONS OF TUMOR

△ 2000 rads living animal (single dose)

□ 0 rads living animal

NUMBER OF CLONOGENIC CELLS / 10^4 TOTAL CELLS

DAYS AFTER 2000 rads

FIG. 2-28. A plot of the relative number of clonogenic tumor cells in the peripheral regions of a rat rhabdomyosarcoma of the rat following a single dose of 2,000 rads. (Adapted from: Hermens: Unpublished data, 1971.)

flow by plasma staining techniques. From these apparently necrotic areas, cells were obtained which were viable as proven by their ability to produce tumor growth when transplanted.

Powers and Tolmach[44] demonstrated the presence of two cell populations in their murine lymphosarcoma: about 99 per cent of the cells had a D_{37} corresponding to that for the same cells irradiated *in vitro* under oxygenated conditions while about 1 per cent of the cells had a radiosensitivity corresponding to that which would be predicted for anoxic cells (Fig. 2-29). Severely hypoxic cells are present in virtually all tumors of experimental animals which have been studied.

The remaining important factor to consider in the discussion of dose fractionation

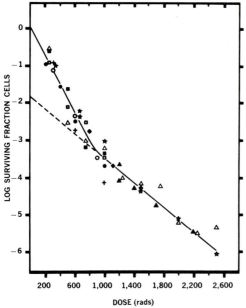

FIG. 2-29. Survival of 6C$_3$HED mouse lymphosarcoma cells irradiated *in vivo*. Each symbol refers to a separate experiment. Each point involved determination of the number of cells required to produce tumors in 50 per cent of 30 mice, using the endpoint dilution method of Hewitt. This number of unirradiated cells was generally in the range of two to five cells. (Courtesy: Powers, *Nature, 197,* 710, 1963.)

and response of tumor tissue is the process of "reoxygenation".[72] By this is meant that the number of hypoxic cells in the tumor decreases more rapidly than would be expected on the basis of radiation killing of hypoxic cells. The most feasible interpretation is that many of the hypoxic cells become aerobic as a result of the radiation induced changes which are produced in the tumor during the course of fractionated irradiation, *e.g.* reduced distances between capillaries, reduced intratumoral pressure, diminished oxygen utilization due to killing of aerobic cells adjacent to capillaries resulting in more oxygen being available for the previously hypoxic cells. Figure 2-30 is a schematic representation prepared by Thomlinson[72] of changes in proportion of viable cells which might occur during tumor growth and following a single radiation dose. The basic concept is that immediately following irradiation the proportion of hypoxic cells among the total *surviving* cells would be much higher than prior to treatment. Changes in this proportion with time would depend upon the changes in distribution of oxygen tension within the tumor.

There are data from several laboratories which indicate that there is some improvement in oxygenation of tumor tissues after a single dose or during multidose therapy. One of the most comprehensive of these studies is that by Howes[37] who made estimates of proportion of cells in a 5–6 mm diameter mammary carcinoma (C$_3$H mouse) as a function of time following a single dose of 1,500 rads, Figure 2-31. In the unirradiated tumor $\approx$12 per cent of the cells were estimated to be hypoxic. According to the data analysis of Howes there was evidence of improved-oxygenation by 6 hours and the calculated proportion of cells which was hypoxia had decreased to $\approx$0.1 per cent by 72 hours. This had not returned to control levels by 168 hours. The reader should appreciate that these figures represent only rough approximations, as no means are available to distinguish changes in tumor sensitivity due

FIG. 2-30. Diagram of changes in the proportion of anoxic clonogenic cells in a tumor. **A.** When a tumor is very small there are likely to be no anoxic cells: in some tumors they probably never occur. **B.** If any anoxic cells are produced they appear as the tumor grows. **C.** The proportion becomes limited to a level characteristic of the type of neoplasm, dependent on its growth rate, degree of differentiation and site. **D.** If a dose of radiation be given, R_1, the proportion of anoxic clonogenic cells amongst the survivors of radiation injury rises, perhaps to 100 per cent. **E.** The proportion remains high until the effect of irradiation begins to develop. **F.** As injury leads to cell death the anoxic proportion falls because of (a) increased availability of oxygen to hypoxic cells following reduced consumption by damaged cells, and (b) improved circulation following shrinkage of the tumor. **G.** Surviving cells regrow the tumor at a rate dependent on the postirradiation environment. **H.** The mean proportion of anoxic clonogenic cells reaches a minimum at a time dependent on the type of tumor and its growth rate; this time is optimal for a second dose, R_2. **I.** The characteristic level is restored. **J.** Late radiation ischemia is not likely to alter the anoxic proportion greatly unless it were previously zero. (Courtesy: Thomlinson: *Frontiers of Rad. Ther. & Oncology,* 3, 109, 1968.)

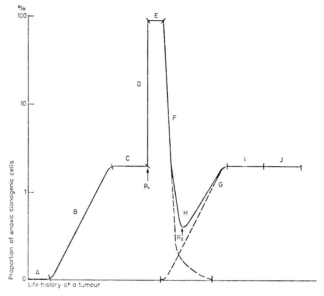

to improved oxygenation from those consequent of a more favorable distribution of cell ages. However, the data of Howes and similar data of others represents good evidence that oxygenation of several murine tumors improved during the first few days post-treatment.

Another set of data pertinent to this point is that presented by Suit and Maeda[63] showing that the ratio $\dfrac{TCD_{50}\ \text{hypoxia}}{TCD_{50}\ \text{air}}$ for the 8 mm diameter mouse mammary carcinoma was ≈ 1.05 for single dose irradiation but was ≈ 1.4 for $\nu = 10$ with 24 hours between fractions. This finding is also consistent with the idea that there is improved oxygenation as fractionated irradiation progresses. Further support for this is given in Figure 2-32 which shows TCD_{50} values from recent experiments where radiation was given under air conditions: $\nu = 2, 5,$ or 10 and for various intertreatment time periods.

For any given ν value, TCD_{50} values were independent of total times of treatment tested up to 18 days and that TCD_{50} was the same for $\nu = 2$ and $\nu = 5$. These results indicate not only that reoxygenation compensated for the cell proliferation which occurred during the intertreatment interval but also that "reoxygenation" partially overcame the effect of repair of radiation damage. Contrast this with the presentation in Figure 2-27 where effects of changes in oxygen tension were excluded by irradiation use clamp technique: TCD_{50} increased with fractionation number and with time between fractions.

Irradiation Under Conditions of Normal and Increased Tissue Oxygen Tension

There has been an intense interest by physicians on the use of hyperbaric oxygen or

FIG. 2-31. Estimate of the proportion of hypoxia cells in a mammary carcinoma growing as a transplant in the anterior chest of a C_3H mouse as a function of time after a single dose of 1,500 rads. (Adapted from: Howes: *Brit. J. Radiol.*, 42, 441, 1969.)

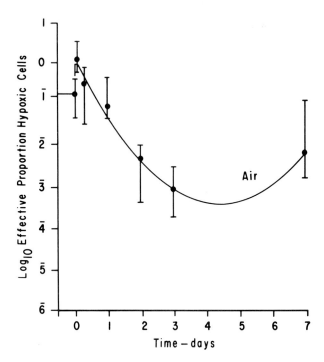

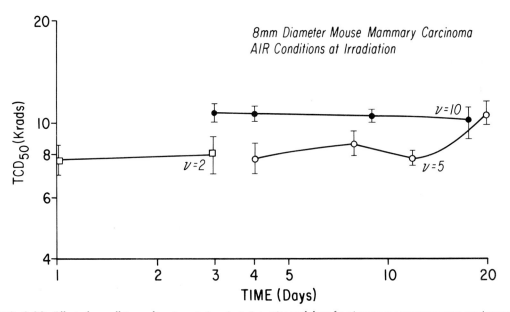

FIG. 2-32. Effect of overall time of treatment given in 2, 5, or 10 equal dose fractions to mouse mammary carcinoma treated under "air" or normal conditions. (Courtesy: Suit and Howes: (In preparation).)

high LET radiations in clinical radiation therapy to reduce the likelihood of treatment failures because of the hypoxic cells. See Chapter 15 for a review of clinical work with these approaches. Here results of laboratory studies of hyperbaric oxygen and radiation therapy will be considered. In the next section a limited review of radiation therapy utilizing high LET beam will be given.

EFFECT OF TUMOR VOLUME

Radiation dose-tumor control response curves are presented in Figure 2-33 for early generation isotransplants of a C_3H mouse mammary carcinoma treated by single radiation doses at two volumes: 250 mm^3 and 0.6 mm^3. The tumors were irradiated either under clamp hypoxia, normal condi-

tions (air breathing animal) or the animal in an environment of high pressure oxygen (44 psi) for 15 minutes before and then during the irradiation. As shown there was a marked effect of tumor volume on the relative position of the "air" curve to the $O_2$44 psi and the "anoxia" curve. In the large tumors there were grossly demonstrable areas of necrosis. For these tumors the "air" and "anoxia" curves were almost equal, but under "$O_2$44 psi" conditions the tumors were significantly more sensi-

tive: $\dfrac{TCD_{50} \text{ anoxia}}{TCD_{50} \ O_2 44 \text{ psi}} \approx 1.5$. Respiration of

oxygen at 30 psi was less effective and the corresponding ratio was ≈ 1.2. In the

smaller tumors the ratio $\dfrac{TCD_{50} \text{ anoxia}}{TCD_{50} \ O_2 44 \text{ psi}}$

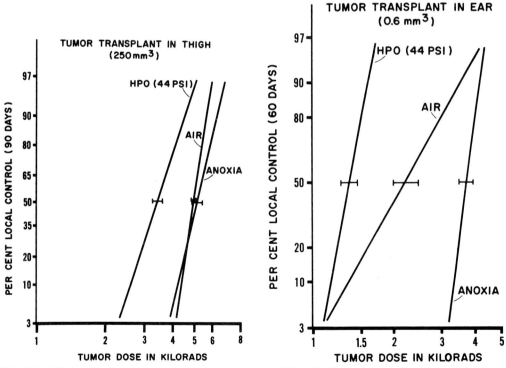

FIG. 2-33. Effect of high pressure oxygen tension on the TCD_{50} for large (250 mm^3) and small (0.6 mm^3) isotransplants of the C_3H mouse mammary carcinoma. Treatments were given as single doses under conditions of local tissue anoxia, normal blood flow and the animal breathing air, or high pressure oxygen, *i.e.*, the animal breathing 100 per cent O_2 at 44 psi for 15 minutes prior to and then during local irradiation. (Courtesy: Suit, *Amer. J. Roentgen., 96*, 177, 1966.)

was 2.8, *i.e.* essentially a maximal effect. A point of interest in Figure 2-33 (lower curve) is that for the small tumor the slope of the dose response curve for air conditions was relatively flat. This indicates that there was a prominent variation amongst tumors in the proportion of tumor cells which were hypoxic, *viz.*, in some tumors nearly all cells were aerobic while in others there were variable proportions of hypoxic cells.

In summary these data have shown that for this tumor, tumor volume is an important determinant of the effectiveness of hyperbaric oxygen as a radiation sensitizer of tumor tissue.

Van den Brenk[78] and Thomlinson[72] have studied response of other tumors to single radiation doses and observed an even more prominent effectiveness of hyperbaric oxygen than described for the mammary tumor.

EFFECT OF DOSE FRACTIONATION

Now we may consider the relative effectiveness of hyperbaric oxygen to improve results of radiation given in a series of equal doses when treatment is administered either under hypoxia, air or $O_2$30 psi conditions. Using the C_3H/He mouse, $O_2$44 psi could not be studied because of the severe toxicity of repeated exposure to oxygen at this high pressure. Accordingly, our experiments using fractionated irradiation have been based on $O_2$30 psi which is well tolerated for prolonged and multiple exposures. Figure 2-34 shows that the TCD_{50} is essentially independent of fractionation number or total time over which treatment is administered for irradiation under $O_2$30 psi conditions. This indicates that the effectiveness of hyperbaric oxygen adequately compensates for the net effect of cell proliferation and of repair of radiation damage over the range of ν and t_i values investigated. Since the dose to elicit a particular response of mouse skin increases rapidly dose fractionation and prolongation of total treatment time the "clinical" effectiveness of hyperbaric oxygen and irradiation of these mouse tumors improves with fractionation and protraction of treatment.

In all experimental animal tumor systems studied, response of tumor tissue to frac-

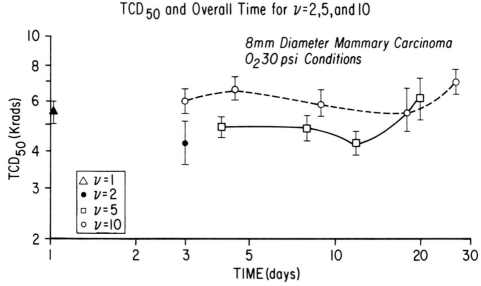

FIG. 2-34. Effect of overall time of treatment of 8 mm diameter mouse mammary carcinomas for $\nu = 1, 2, 5,$ and 10 when radiation is administered under $O_2$30 psi conditions. (Courtesy: Suit and Howes: (In preparation).)

tionation irradiation is augmented if given under hyperbaric oxygen conditions. Further, data from our system demonstrates that $O_2$30 psi is much more effective than breathing pure oxygen or 95 per cent oxygen and 5 per cent CO_2 at normal pressure. Also for $O_2$30 psi conditions in this tumor system, a maximal sensitizing effect is achieved by respiration of $O_2$30 psi for 5 minutes; there is no advantage of breathing oxygen for 15 minutes.

High LET Radiation Therapy

PHYSICAL CONSIDERATIONS

Radiobiological studies at the cellular and tissue level have established that there are wide variations in the efficiency with which energy absorbed from the various particulate and electromagnetic radiations produce effects in biological material. This variation in efficiency is a result of the differing spatial distributions of energy loss as the particle or photon traverses the cell (Fig. 2-35). Linear energy transfer or *LET* may be expressed as Kev of energy lost by the particle per micron of path length (Kev/μ). For high energy pho-

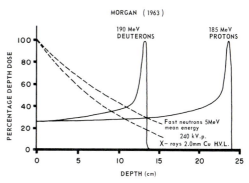

MORGAN (1963)

FIG. 2-36. A plot of absorbed dose as a function of depth or particle path length for 190 Mev deuterons and 185 Mev protons. Both particles have a charge of 1+ but differ in mass by a factor of $\approx$2. The very sharp and limited increase in dose at end of track length is the "Bragg Peak". Dotted lines refer to depth dose curve for 240 Kvp x-rays and for a neutron beam whose mean energy is $\approx$5 Mev. (Courtesy: Morgan, R. L., In *Cancer Progress*, R. W. Raven, ed., London, Butterworth & Company, Ltd., p. 176, 1963.)

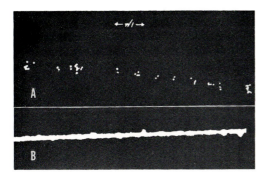

FIG. 2-35. **A.** Cloud chamber tract of a fast electron illustrates that ionization occurs in clusters. Successive clusters are separated by approximately 1μ. **B.** Cloud chamber tract of a proton ejected by a neutron; note the high density of ion pairs. (Courtesy: Bacq and Alexander, *Fundamentals of Radiobiology*, 2nd. ed., New York, Pergamon Press, Inc., p. 1, 1961.)

tons, *e.g.* ^{60}Co gamma-rays, the *LET* is at a minimum value of $\approx$0.3 Kev/μ but for charged particles of certain energies the *LET* is much higher, *e.g.*, 189 Kev/μ for certain fission fragments. The *LET* of charged particles is proportional to the square of the charge and is an inverse function of the kinetic energy (velocity) of the particle. Accordingly, at the terminal portion of the track length, there is a rapid increase in *LET* and hence, absorbed dose. This local increase in *LET* or dose is referred to as the "Bragg Peak", and is illustrated in Figure 2-36. The depth at which the Bragg Peak appears for a given particle is proportional to energy, but the width and height of the peak are related only to the charge on the particle and the composition of the absorbing material.

The neutron is a particle with no charge and whose mass is approximately that of the proton. Although neutrons have no charge, they are high *LET* radiations. This results from the neutron-atomic nucleus reaction which produces a proton whose energy depends on the neutron energy and the atomic number of the reacting atom. Therefore, the *LET* and hence biological effectiveness of neutrons will be the result of the *LET* of the products of neutron-atomic nuclei reactions and not due to direct effects of the neutrons. In tissue, fast neutrons lose energy primarily by reaction with hydrogen atoms to produce recoil protons. These recoil protons produce the high *LET* effects of neutron irradiation. See Figure 2-35 to compare the relative ion density produced by an electron and recoil proton. Because of this high probability of a neutron-hydrogen atom reaction, the absorbed dose in tissues high in hydrogen, *e.g.* fat, would be higher than those low in hydrogen, *e.g.* bone.

Cellular Radiobiological Aspects

Data from an extensive series of experiments based on *in vitro* studies of a line of Chinese hamster cells[55] are listed in Table 2-5. These data show the dependence of D_{37} and N value on the *LET* of the radiation beam. For these cells D_{37} decreases by a factor of 1.7 (170/100) as *LET* increases from 3 (250 Kv x-rays) to 189 (carbon ions). However, N values decreased by a factor of about 3.5 over the same range of *LET*. Now we may consider the term Relative Biological Effectiveness or *RBE*; this is the ratio of the dose for a test radiation to dose of control radiation to produce a specified effect. Usually the control or reference radiations are 250 kvp x-rays. The dose ratio to yield $S = 10^{-1}$ and

$S = 10^{-8}$ for 250 Kv x-rays ($D_{37} = 170$ rads, $N = 5$) and 106 Mev carbon ions ($D_{37} = 100$ rads and $N = 1.6$) would be 2.4 and 1.7 respectively. For small single doses, the differential effectiveness of two radiations is strongly dependent on the relative N values. At large individual doses, *RBE* is largely a function of differences in D_{37} values.

It also follows that if *RBE* were used to describe the ratio of absorbed doses to produce a specified effect, then *RBE* would clearly be a function of the dose fractionation schedule. N exerts a powerful influence on the dependence of the TCD_{50} on dose fractionation; refer to Figure 2-23. Accordingly, *RBE* must be specified for each fractionation schedule employed in the study, *i.e.*, an *RBE* determined by a single dose study (large single doses) would not be expected to apply to a multidose radiation treatment featuring small individual doses.

Another factor that significantly modifies the *RBE* is the oxygen tension in the biological material at the instant of irradiation. As described earlier, the "oxygen effect" factor is ≈ 2.0 to 3.0 for 250 Kv x-rays or ^{60}Co gamma rays (D_{37} anoxic cells/D_{37} aerobic cells). In sharp contrast the effectiveness of high *LET* radiations, is much less dependent on oxygen tension. Alper[1] has reviewed oxygen enhancement ratios determined in 15 experiments using neutrons (*LET* varying from 20 to 40 Kev/μ) and x-rays. The ratio of oxygen effect (x-rays) to oxygen effect (neutrons) was 1.3 to 2.8 with an average of ≈ 1.7. A review of *OER* for fast neutrons of

Table 2-5. D_{37} *and N Values for a Chinese Hamster Cell Line as Influenced by LET*

Radiation	LET Kev/μ	D_{37} (rads)	N
250 Kv x-ray therapy	2.0	170	5.0
Helium	19.1	165	2.6
Lithium	72.7	143	1.9
Boron ion	126.5	107	1.3
Carbon ion	189.0	100	1.6

widely varying energies have indicated that the *OER* is relatively independent of neutron energy over the range of 6 to 30 Mev.[6] If the *RBE* for two radiations, *i.e.*, x-rays and neutrons, were 2.0 when studied at aerobic conditions, the *RBE* could be expected to be ≈ 3.4 if irradiations were performed under anoxic conditions. In summary, the observed *RBE* would be determined not only by the *LET* of the two radiations being compared, but also by the size of the individual dose, and the oxygen tension at each irradiation.

LABORATORY ANIMAL STUDIES

Despite sizeable *RBE* values, no therapeutic benefit could be expected to result from the use of high *LET* instead of low *LET* radiations unless there were a favorable differential of *RBE* values for cells of the critical normal tissue and the tumor cells. There are two situations where this might obtain. Firstly, such a differential could exist provided a radiobiologically significant fraction of the tumor cells are hypoxic (reoxygenation is not complete) because effectiveness of high *LET* radiations is only weakly dependent upon pO_2, *viz* $OER = 1.1-1.7$ while for low *LET* radiations the *OER* is 2.5–3.0. Secondly, N is usually smaller for high than for low *LET* irradiation and therefore a favorable differential might develop if the reduction of log N were greater for tumor than for the critical normal cells. This would also result in a greater *RBE* for tumor cells than for the normal cells, and have a more effective treatment. The ratio of *RBE* tumor tissue/*RBE* normal tissue has been designated Therapeutic Gain Factor (Bewley and Hornsey[7]). A clinically promising situation exists if the gain factor is $\geq 1.10-1.15$.

There are scant data indicating the relative effectiveness of high *LET* radiations in treatment of experimental animal tumors. Early studies of Gray and Reed[28] showed that 2.8 Mev neutrons were clearly more effective than radium gamma rays in control of experimental animal tumors. Field and Jones and

Thomlinson[23,24] employed the Hammersmith cyclotron to compare the "clinical effectiveness" of fast neutron and x-rays in treatment of a fibrosarcoma in rats. They found that for radiation administered in 1, 2, or 5 fractions, the fast neutrons produced a greater damage to tumor for a given damage to skin than did the x-rays. However, the work of van Putten et al.[80] with an experimental osteosarcoma indicated that the therapeutic gain in using fast neutrons instead of x-rays in treatment of this tumor would be quite small.

In summary, data from laboratory studies using animal tumor systems known to contain hypoxic cells demonstrate that fast neutrons are more effective than x-rays as radiation therapy beams. The gain factor would vary from tumor to tumor and might be quite small for some tumors.

Radiobiologic Basis for Combining Radiation Therapy and Surgery

Is there a rational basis for the use of less than radical doses when radiation therapy is combined with surgery? If so, what dose levels would likely be of benefit? The aim of radiation therapy would be to damage lethally those "viable" tumor cells which would not be removed in the surgical specimen or which would be spilled into the wound. Cells from either source could proliferate and produce a recurrence. Here a "viable" cell is a cell that has the capacity of sustained proliferation; however, this capacity is not necessarily exercised unless the cell is in a favorable environment.

NUMBER OF CELLS REQUIRED TO PRODUCE A RECURRENCE

Apparently fewer "viable" cells are required to produce a recurrence when the cells constitute established tumor tissue than when they are spilled or dispersed into tissues as individual cells. This is almost certainly true in the instances of the C_3H mouse mammary carcinoma. To transplant this tumor into isologous animals using individual cells in suspension, most researchers have found that an inoculum containing $\geq 10^4$ "viable" cells is required. This contrasts to results obtained when these same cells constituted tumor tissue irradiated *in situ* as a solid tumor. Apparently a single surviving tumor cell would proliferate and produce a tumor regrowth.[61] Cohen and Cohen[13] found that the TCD_{50} for their mouse mammary carcinoma was 5,780 R for radiation administered in a tumor *in situ* but was only 2,850 R for irradiation of tumor fragments irradiated *in vitro* prior to implantation. These results from mammary carcinoma tissue do not necessarily apply to other tumor types. Studies in several laboratories have shown that some murine lymphomas may be transplanted by 5 cells individually suspended in the inoculum.

A relevant clinical experiment has shown that very large numbers of dispersed human cancer cells ($\geq 10^5$) are required to produce the disease when autotransplanted* into the subcutaneous tissue of the thigh.[56] Accordingly, the radiation dose required to prevent tumor transplantation from tumor cells spilled into the operative wound would be expected to be very much less than the dose which inactivate small foci of established tumor growing beyond the surgical margins.

TREATMENT OF SMALL FOCI OF ORGANIZED CARCINOMA TISSUE LYING BEYOND SURGICAL MARGINS

The relationship between TCD_{50} given in 30 equal exposures and the number of viable tumor cells is presented graphically in Figure 2-37. According to this model, a tumor of 10^4 aerobic cells would have a TCD_{50} of 30×165 or 4,950 rads (if given in 20 fractions the dose would be 4,400 rads).

---

*Autotransplantation of tumor results when tumor is removed from one site and transplanted to another site in the same animal. A metastasis may be considered as an autotransplant.

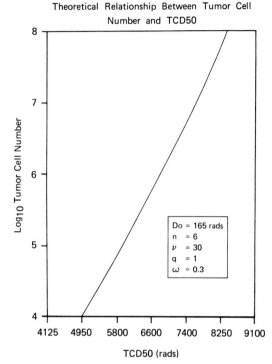

FIG. 2-37. Relationship between TCD_{50} and tumor cell number for model tumors with the indicated values for the pertinent parameters.

These calculations emphasize that readily tolerated doses can be highly effective in treatment of small extensions of tumor composed entirely of aerobic cells. These same considerations obtain when planning treatment of "subclinical" or nonpalpable disease. This is discussed more fully in the next section on "Clinical Parameters". Treatment of small foci of organized tissues should be equally effective as either preoperative or postoperative irradiation.

TREATMENT OF CELLS SPILLED INTO THE OPERATIVE FIELD

If $\approx 10^5$ viable tumor cells were spilled into the operative wound during surgical manipulation of the specimen and $\geq 10^3$ such cells establish one autotransplant, the radiation dose to prevent transplantation would be 2,000–2,300 rads if given in 10 equal doses. Thus, prevention of recurrences due to contamination of the wound with tumor cells would be a simple task.

LABORATORY ANIMAL EXPERIMENTS

Data from studies based on laboratory animal tumor systems have shown that radiation therapy given before excision is effective in reducing the incidence of local recurrence. Inch and McCredie[39] employed early generation isotransplants of the C_3H mouse mammary carcinoma, growing in the subcutaneous tissue of the back. They reported that 2,000 rads* minimum tumor dose given 24 hours preoperatively reduced local recurrence rate at 100 days from 43 to 34 per cent. Similar studies on a variety of other tumors have been described by Powers.[43] In a spectrum of tumors studied by him, some instances of definite increase in local control rate was achieved by doses of 1,000 to 2,000 rads, but in other tumor systems the recurrence rate was only slightly modified by presurgical doses of 3,000 to 4,000 rads.

PREOPERATIVE IRRADIATION AND INCIDENCE OF DISTANT METASTASES

Another useful aspect of preoperative irradiation may be speculated. Clinical and laboratory animal tumor studies[10,48] have shown that during manipulation of tumors, many tumor cells appear in the blood. Presumably, these cells would increase the probability of subsequent appearance of metastatic disease. If the yield of metastases were low in relation to the number of cells appearing in the blood stream, *e.g.* one metastasis on the average for $\geq 10^3$ cells released into the blood (a relationship similar to that for development of tumor from cells spilled into operative wounds), then a small dose of radiation therapy given preoperatively would be expected to reduce drastically the proba-

bility of metastases developing from cells released into the systemic circulation at surgery.

According to this reasoning, the radiation should be administered not only prior to excision but also prior to manipulation and biopsy.

TUMOR BED EFFECT

Following radiation therapy, changes induced in the normal tissues might be expected to affect the survival time of viable tumor cells spilled into the operative wound at subsequent surgery and thereby modify the minimum number of cells that would be able to establish a focus of tumor growth. Such a "tumor bed effect" has been discussed by Summer et al.[67] They found that radiation doses of the order of 1,500 to 3,000 r, given as single doses to normal tissue prior to an inoculation of large numbers of mouse mammary carcinoma cells, delayed the appearance of a palpable tumor and increased survival time of the animal. We have found that prior treatment of the tissues of a mouse leg to 3,500 rads or 5,000 rads does not affect the number of cells required to transplant the tumor but prolonged the time between inoculation of tumor cells and appearance of tumor.[77]

Radiobiological Basis of "Shrinking Field Technique"

Early clinical practice of radiotherapy as developed by the French school of Coutard, Regaud, and Baclesse emphasized the need to reduce field size as treatment progressed so as to permit the highest possible dose to the central tumor mass with an acceptable level of normal tissue damage.

There is now a sound radiobiological basis for that practice. Clinically, best results can be expected when radiation dose distribution is planned in accordance with probable distribution of tumor cells. Figure 2-38 illustrates the treatment plan for a model tumor.

---

*This would correspond to 2,340 rads ^{60}Co radiation if a *RBE* factor of 0.85 were used.

For most tumors, there are extensions of disease away from the main mass of tumor so that the number of tumor cells per unit volume of tissue decreases very rapidly with distance from the central lesion. There is, of course, a reciprocal increase in volume of involved tissue. According to the tumor cell distribution assumed in Figure 2-38 a TCD_{90} could be expected to result from a treatment where the peripheral portions of the treated tissue received 75 per cent of the dose given to the central region. The dose of 371×20 could not be tolerated if it were given to the largest field used and if only areas B or C were treated, marginal recurrences would be expected. Actual use of such a technique must be based on sound clinical knowledge of the patterns of spread of the particular type of tumor under treatment.

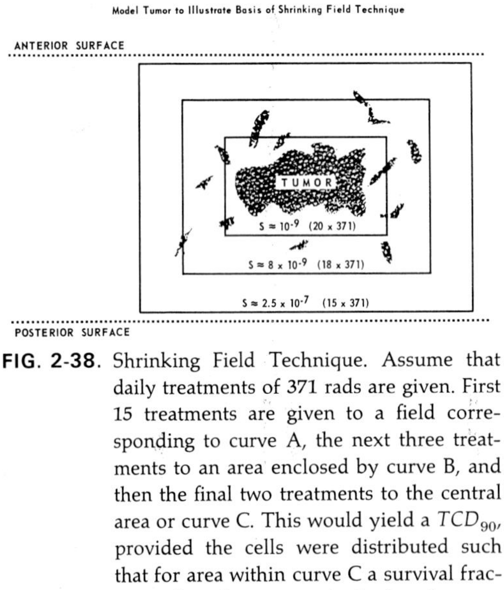

Model Tumor to Illustrate Basis of Shrinking Field Technique

ANTERIOR SURFACE

$S \approx 10^{-9}$ (20 x 371)

$S \approx 8 \times 10^{-9}$ (18 x 371)

$S \approx 2.5 \times 10^{-7}$ (15 x 371)

POSTERIOR SURFACE

FIG. 2-38. Shrinking Field Technique. Assume that daily treatments of 371 rads are given. First 15 treatments are given to a field corresponding to curve A, the next three treatments to an area enclosed by curve B, and then the final two treatments to the central area or curve C. This would yield a TCD_{90}, provided the cells were distributed such that for area within curve C a survival fraction of 10^{-9} was required, that for area enclosed by B-C a survival fraction of 8×10^{-9} was required, and that for area enclosed by A (B and C) a survival fraction of 2.5×10^{-7} was required. It is important to realize that the number of tumor cells/mm³ of tissue might be very low in the peripheral portions of the treatment fields but the total number of cells could be substantial because of the large volumes of tissue involved.

General Comments Regarding Dose Fractionation

The discussion and data presented thus far on the subject of dose fractionation have been directed primarily at the response of tumor tissue. Clearly though, the effect of radiation on normal tissue which surrounds the tumor is as important as the effect on the tumor in determining the "clinical success" of the treatment. In an attempt to optimize treatment either in mouse or man, full attention must be given to the biology and radiobiology of the tumor tissue and the normal tissue(s) which is dose limiting. As the response of tumor tissue has been treated in some detail only a summary statement can be included on response of normal tissue.

Response of Normal Tissues to Local Irradiation

Data now exist from a large number of ingenious and complex experiments on normal tissues of the mouse and rat from which estimates of the values for the parameters of radiation sensitivity of the constituent cells have been derived. These studies have featured single and multidose irradiation. Normal tissues studied are: bone, marrow, skin, gut (stomach, jejunum, and colon), hair follicles, cartilage, lung, testis, lymphoid cells, and the connective-vascular tissue which produce callus at fracture site.[84] The experimental procedures and details of results will not be presented here. Estimates of D_{37} for the normal cells have not been different from the D_{37} values for the various tumor cells studied with the exception that the cells of bone marrow, lymphoid tissue, and gonadal tissue are more sensitive (D_{37} in the range of ≈ 50–100 rads) as compared with D_{37} of ≈ 150 rads for cells of other systems. For most of the normal tissues investigated, the experimental techniques employed did not yield data from which a direct estimate of N value could be derived. Indirectly, this has been achieved by determining the radiation dose which elicits a specifically defined response for radiation administered in two fractions ($\nu = 2$) and in a single dose ($\nu = 1$). Provided the size of the first and the second dose were sufficient to yield a survival fraction which was beyond the shoulder region of the survival curve then the increase in dose required when two fractions were employed instead of a single dose can be accepted as an approximation of the dose equivalent of the extrapolation number. Data from this type of experiment for the various tissues mentioned have been reviewed by Withers.[84] There is little or no difference in repair activity between cells of normal tissue and tumor tissue; if there is a real but small difference it favors normal tissue.

Advantage to Patient in Treatment of All Fields on Each Treatment Day

In planning radiation therapy it is essential that the clinician think in terms of isoeffect curves and distributions of biological damage and not only in terms of isodose curves and patterns of distribution of physical dose. The point being that an iso-effect distribution may be quite different from an isodose distribution when multiple field techniques are employed and there is a failure to treat all fields on each treatment day. That is, distributions of dose in rads need not correspond to distribution of damage to tissue. This problem of the relative damage produced by one or multiple fields per day has been discussed by Wilson and Hall[83] in terms of cell survival curves and NSD. The point is most readily understood by consideration of a simple cell survival curve. Examine Figure 2-39 which is the experimental cell survival curve for asynchromously dividing Hela cells. Our example is as follows: treatment is being given by a simple parallel opposed pair of 15 × 15 cm fields; separation is 20 cm, and per cent depth dose at 4 mm 10

HELA CELL SURVIVAL CURVE

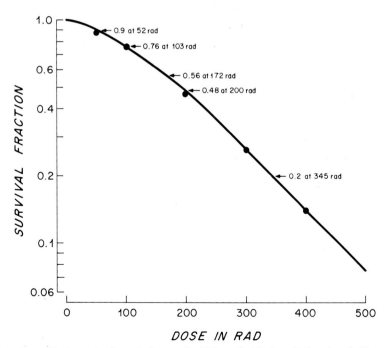

FIG. 2-39. Experimentally determined survival curve for HeLa cells (single radiation doses). The numbers shown are calculated survival fractions for doses of interest in the discussion of the relative effects of treating a patient with one or with two fields per day. (Courtesy: Wilson and Hall: *Radiology,* 98, 419, 1971.)

and 20 cm are 100 per cent, 58 per cent and 30 per cent respectively. Therefore to give 200 rads to the central region the treatment could be a dose of 345 rads to one field (345 rads at 4 mm depth, 200 rads at 10 cm, and 103 rads exit dose) or 172 rads to the anterior and to the posterior field (224 rads at 4 mm depth, 200 rads at 10 cm). On Figure 2-39 are indicated the cell survival figures for 52, 103, 172, 200 and 345 rads; these are .90, .75, .56, .48, .20 respectively. Accordingly, if 400 rads were administered to the midpoint the dose at 4 mm depth would be 44 rads. Of clinical interest is the calculated survival fraction at 4 mm depth of 0.15 and 0.26 for treatment using 1 field and 2 fields per day respectively. For a course of 30 treatment sessions the survival fractions at 4 mm depth would be 4.4×10^{-13} and 1.68×10^{-9} respectively. See Table 2-6. These calculations demonstrate a marked advantage by using a 2 field per day technique: a vastly greater damage to superficial tissue when only 1 field is used per day.

If the survival curve for cells of human skin and connective tissue cells have broader shoulder regions than do Hela cells (as seems likely) then the differential effect on super-ficial tissues between one or multiple field per day treatment will be much greater than indicated in this example. This differential in favor of treating all fields each day would be expected to diminish as beam energy increased (depth dose improved). That is, the advantage in use of multiple fields per day would be less with 22 Mev x-ray beam than with ^{60}Co beams. It is relevant that most clinicians who worked with 250 Kv x-ray units treated all fields every day. They appreciated the fact that with the poorly pene-trating (lack of skin sparing effect) 250 Kv beams all fields had to be treated each day. The effect is less dramatic but still real with ^{60}Co treatments. From these calculations and clinical observations a safe rule in radiation therapy would be to treat all fields on each treatment day where radical dose levels are to be employed.

BIBLIOGRAPHY

1. Alper, T.: Comparison between the oxygen enhancement ratios for neutrons and x-rays, as observed with Escherichia coli B, *Brit. J. Radiol.*, 36, 97, 1963.

Table 2-6. *Survival Fraction* *

		1 field per day	2 fields per day
Two fractions (400 rad tumor dose)	Radiation Dose at 4 mm depth	448	448
	Cell Survival Fraction	0.15	0.26
Thirty Treatments (6,000 rad tumor dose)	Radiation Dose	6,720	6,720
	Cell Survival Fraction	4.4×10^{-13}	1.68×10^{-9}

*Survival fraction for tissue cells at 4 mm depth when 400 rads (2 fractions) or 6,000 rads (30 fractions) are given with parallel opposed 10 × 10 cm fields (20 cm separation; depth doses at 4 mm, 10 cm, and 20 cm are 100%, 58%, and 30% respectively). Treatments given by using 1 field or 2 fields per day. Survival fractions are calculated using the survival curve parameters from Figure 2-39 based on HeLa cells.

2. Andrews, J. R.: *The Radiobiology of Human Cancer Radiotherapy,* Philadelphia, W. B. Saunders Co., 1968.

3. Bacq, Z. M. and Alexander, P.: *Fundamentals of Radiobiology,* 2nd Ed., New York, Pergamon Press, Inc., 1961, p. 1.

4. Bedford, J.: Oxygen tension in cell proliferation, In *Time and Dose Relationships in Radiation Biology as Applied to Radiotherapy,* Brookhaven National Laboratory Report 50203 (C-57), 1969, pp. 225–227.

5. Berry, R. J.: Quantitative studies of relationships between tumor cell ploidy and dose response to ionizing radiation *in vivo.* Modification of radiation response in a previously irradiated tumor, *Radiat. Res.,* 18, 236, 1963.

6. Berry, R. J.: Hypoxic protection against fast neutrons of different energies—A review, *Eur. J. of Cancer,* 7, 153, 1971.

7. Bewley, D. K. and Hornsey, S.: In *Biological Effects of Proton and Neutron Irradiations,* Vol. II, I.A.E.A., Vienna, 1964, 173.

8. Bryant, P. E.: In *Time and Dose Relationships in Radiation Biology as Applied to Radiotherapy,* Brookhaven National Laboratory Report 50203 (C-57), 1969, p. 76.

9. Carmel NCI-AEC Conference, *Time and Dose Relationships in Radiation Biology as Applied to Radiotherapy,* Brookhaven National Laboratory Report 50203 (C-57), 1969.

10. Clifton, E. E. and Agnostino, D.: Cancer in the blood of simulated colon cancer resectable & unresectable: Effect of fibrinolysin and heparin on growth potential, *Surgery,* 50, 395, 1961.

11. Clifton, K. H., Briggs, R. C. and Stone, H. B.: Quantitative radiosensitivity studies of solid carcinomas *in vivo:* Methodology and effect of anoxia, *J. Nat. Cancer Inst.,* 36, 965, 1966.

12. Cohen, A. and Cohen, L.: Radiobiology of the C_3H mouse mammary carcinoma: The effect of body dose on the radiocurability of the tumour treated *in situ, Brit. J. Cancer,* 7, 452, 1953.

13. Cohen, A. and Cohen, L.: Radiobiology of the C_3H mouse mammary carcinoma: Comparative radiosensitivity of the tumour prior to implantation and of the established tumour *in situ, Brit. J. Cancer,* 7, 231, 1953.

14. Denekamp, J. and Thomlinson, R. H.: The cell proliferation kinetics of four experimental tumors after acute x-irradiation, *Cancer Res.,* 31, 1279, 1971.

15. Dewey, D. L.: The x-ray sensitivity of Serratia marcenscens, *Radiat. Res.,* 19, 64, 1963.

16. Dewey, W. C. and Cole, A.: Effects of heterogeneous populations on radiation survival curves, *Nature,* 194, 660, 1962.

17. Djordjevic, B. and Szybalski, W.: Genetics of human cell lines: III. Incorporation of 5-bromo and 5-iododeoxyuridine into deoxyribonucleic acid of human cells and its effect on radiation sensitivity, *J. Exp. Med.,* 112, 209, 1960.

18. Elkind, M. M. and Sutton, H.: X-ray damage and recovery in mammalian cells in culture, *Nature,* 184, 1293, 1959.

19. Elkind, M. M. and Sutton, H.: Radiation response of mammalian cells grown in culture, *Radiat. Res.,* 13, 556, 1960.

20. Elkind, M. M., Alescio, T., Swain, R. W., Moses, W. B. and Sutton, H.: Recovery of hypoxic mammalian cells from sublethal x-ray damage, *Nature,* 202, 1190, 1964.

21. Elkind, M. M., Swain, R. W., Alescio, T., Sutton, H. and Moses, W. B.: In *Cellular Radiation Biology,* Baltimore, Williams & Wilkins Company, 1965, p. 442.

22. Elkind, M. M. and Whitmore, G. F.: *The Radiobiology of Cultured Mammalian Cells,* New York, Gordon and Breach Science Publishers, Inc., 1967.

23. Field, S. B. and Jones T.: The relative effects of fast neutrons and x-rays on tumour and normal tissue in the rat, I. Single doses, *Brit. J. Radiol.,* 40, 834, 1967.

24. Field, S. B., Jones, T. and Thomlinson, R. N.: II, Fractionation: Recovery and reoxygenation, *Brit. J. Radiol.,* 41, 597, 1968.

25. Foley, E. J.: Antigenic properties of methylcholanthrene-induced tumors in mice of the strain of origin, *Cancer Res.,* 13, 835, 1953.

26. Goldacre, R. J. and Sylven, B.: On the access of bloodborne dyes to various tumour regions, *Brit. J. Cancer,* 16, 306, 1962.

27. Gray, L. H.: Radiobiologic basis of oxygen as a modifying factor in radiation therapy, *Amer. J. Roentgen,* 85, 805, 1961.

28. Gray, L. H. and Read, J.: Comparison of the lethal effect of neutrons and gamma-rays on mouse tumors by irradiation of grafted tumors *in vivo* and by irradiation of tumor fragments *in vitro, Brit. J. Radiol.,* 21, 5, 1948.

29. Gray, L. H. and Scott, O. C. A.: In *Oxygen in the Animal Organism,* London, Pergamon Press, 1964, p. 537.

30. Hall, E. J. and Cavanagh, J.: The effect of hypoxia on recovery of sublethal radiation damage in Vicia seedlings, *Brit. J. Rad.*, 42, 270, 1969.

31. Hermens, A.: Unpublished data, 1971.

32. Hermens, A. F. and Barendsen, G. W.: Changes of cell proliferation characteristic in rat rhabdomyosarcoma before and after irradiation, *Europ. J. Cancer*, 5, 173, 1969.

33. Hewitt, H. B.: In *Radiation Effects in Physics, Chemistry and Biology*, Amsterdam, North Holland Publishing Co., 1963, p. 234.

34. Hewitt, H. B. and Wilson, C. W.: A survival curve for mammalian leukemia cells irradiated *in vivo*, *Brit. J. Cancer*, 13, 69, 1959.

35. Howard, A.: The role of oxygen in the repair process. In *Time and Dose Relationships in Radiation Biology as Applied to Radiotherapy*, Brookhaven National Laboratory Report 50203 (C-57), 1969, p. 70–76.

36. Howard, A. and Pelc, S. R.: Synthesis of deoxyribonucleic acid in normal and irradiated cells and its relation to chromosome breakage, *Heredity* (Suppl.) 6, 261, 1952.

37. Howes, A.: An estimation of changes in the proportions and absolute numbers of hypoxic cells after irradiation of transplanted C_3H mouse mammary tumor, *Brit. J. Radiol.*, 42, 441, 1969.

38. Humphrey, R. M., Dewey, W. C. and Cork, A.: Effect of oxygen in mammalian cells sensitized to radiation by incorporation of 5-bromodeoxyuridine into the DNA, *Nature*, 198, 268, 1963.

39. Inch, W. R. and McCredie, J. A.: Effect of a small dose of x-irradiation on local recurrence of tumors in rats and mice, *Cancer*, 16, 595, 1963.

40. Lienert, G. A.: Verteilungsfreie methoden in der biostatistik verlag ariton hain, Meisenheim am Glan, Germang, Table 17, p. 359, 1962.

41. Moehler, W. C. and Elkind, M. M.: Radiation response of mammalian cells grown in culture III. Modification of x-ray survival of Chinese Hamster Cells by 5-Bromodeoxyuridine, *Exp. Cell Res.*, 30, 481, 1963.

42. Morgan, R. L.: In *Cancer Progress*, R. W. Raven, Editor, London, Butterworth & Co, Ltd, 1963, p. 176.

43. Powers, W. E.: Radiation biologic considerations and practical investigations in pre-operative radiation therapy, *J. Canad. A. Radiologists*, 16, 217, 1965.

44. Powers, W. E. and Tolmach, L. J.: A multicomponent x-ray survival curve for mouse lymphosarcoma cells irradiated *in vivo*, *Nature*, 197, 710, 1963.

45. Prehn, R. T. and Main, J. M.: Immunity of methylcholanthrene-induced sarcomas. *J. Nat. Cancer Inst.*, 18, 769, 1957.

46. Puck, T. T. and Marcus, P. I.: Action of x-rays on mammalian cells, *J. Exp. Med.*, 103, 653, 1956.

47. Revesz, L. and Littbrand, B.: Variation of the relative sensitivity of closely related neoplastic cell lines irradiated in culture in the presence or absence of oxygen, *Nature*, 203, 742, 1964.

48. Roberts, S. S.: In *Dissemination of Cancer, Prevention and Therapy*, New York, Appleton-Century-Crofts, Inc., 1961, p. 61.

49. Schwartz, E. E.: *Biological Basis for Radiotherapy*, Philadelphia, J. B. Lippincott Co., 1966.

50. Shirakura, I. and Suit, H. D.: Unpublished data.

51. Silini, G. and Hornsey, S.: Studies on cell survival of irradiated ehrlich ascites tumor. III. A comparison of the x-ray survival obtained with a diploid and tetraploid strain, *Int. J. Radiat. Biol.*, 5, 147, 1961.

52. Sinclair, W. K.: The relative biological effectiveness of 22 MeVp X-rays, Cobalt-60 gamma rays, and 200-Kvep X-rays, *Radiat. Res.*, 16, 394, 1962.

53. Sinclair, W. K.: X-ray induced hertable damage (small-colony formation) in cultured mammalian cells, *Radiat. Res.*, 21, 584, 1964.

54. Sinclair, W. K.: Dependence of radiosensitivities upon cell age. In *Time and Dose Relationships in Radiation Biology as Applied to Radiotherapy*, Brookhaven National Laboratory report 50203 (C-57), 1969, p. 97.

55. Skarsgard, L. D., Kihlman, B. A., Parker, L., Pujara, C. M. and Richardson, S.: Survival, chromosome abnormalities, and recovery in heavy-iron-and x-irradiated mammalian cells, *Radiat. Res.* (Suppl.) 7, 208, 1967.

56. Southam, C. M., Brunschwig, A., and Dizon, Q.: In *Biological Interactions in Normal and Neoplastic Growth*, Boston, Little Brown and Co., 1962, p. 723.

57. Steel, G. G.: Cell loss as a factor in the growth rate of human tumours, *Europ. J. Cancer*, 3, 381, 1967.

58. Steel, G. G., Adams, K. and Barrett, J. C.: Analysis of the cell population kinetics of transplanted tumours of widely-differing growth rate, *Brit. J. Cancer*, 20, 784, 1966.

59. Suit, H. D. and Gallager, H. S.: Intact tumor cells in irradiated tissue, *Arch. Path.*, 78, 648, 1964.

60. Suit, H. D., Lindberg, R. L. and Fletcher, G. H.: Prognostic significance of extent of tumor regression at completion of radiation therapy, *Radiology*, 84, 1100, 1965.

61. Suit, H. D., Shalek, R. J. and Wette, R.: In *Cellular Radiation Biology*, Baltimore, Williams & Wilkins Co., 1965, p. 514.

62. Suit, H. D. and Maeda, M.: Oxygen effect factor and tumor volume in the C_3H mouse mammary carcinoma, *Amer. J. Roentgen.*, 96, 177, 1966.

63. Suit, H. D. and Maeda, M.: Hyperbaric oxygen and radiobiology of a C_3H mouse mammary carcinoma, *J. Nat. Cancer Inst.*, 39, 639, 1967.

64. Suit, H. D. and Kastelan, A.: Immunological status of host and response of a methylcholanthrene-induced sarcoma local x-irradiation, *Cancer*, 26, 232, 1970.

65. Suit, H. D. and Howes, A. E.: The effect of intertreatment interval and fractionation numbers on response of a mouse mammary carcinoma, (In preparation).

66. Suit, H. D., Withers, H. R., Brown, B. W. and Thomson, J. M.: Consideration of dose per fraction and continuous irradiation in radiation therapy, (In preparation).

67. Summer, W. C., Clifton, K. H. and Vermund, H.: X-irradiation of the tumor bed, *Radiology*, 82, 691, 1964.

68. Tannock, Ian F.: Effects of PO_2 on cell proliferation kinetics. In *Time and Dose Relationships in Radiation Biology as Applied to Radiotherapy*, Brookhaven National Laboratory Report 50203 (C-57), 1969, p. 215.

69. Tannock, Ian F.: Population kinetics of carcinoma cells capillary endothelial cells and fibroblasts in a transplanted mouse mammary tumor, *Cancer Res.*, 30, 2470, 1970.

70. Tannock, Ian F.: Oxygen diffusion and distribution of cellular radiosensitivity in tumor, *J. Nat. Cancer Inst.* (In press).

71. Terasima, Toyozo: On the role of DNA in cell killing by radiation. In *Time and Dose Relationships in Radiation Biology as Applied to Radi-*

otherapy, Brookhaven National Laboratory Report 50203 (C-57), 1969, p. 82.

72. Thomlinson, R. H.: Changes in oxygenation in tumours in relation to irradiation, *Frontiers of Radiation Therapy and Oncology*, 3, 109, 1968.

73. Thomlinson, R. H. and Gray, L. H.: The histological structure of some human lung cancers and possible implications for radiotherapy, *Brit. J. Cancer*, 9, 539, 1955.

74. Thomlinson, R. H. and Craddock, E. A.: Response of experimental tumour to x-rays, *Brit. J. Cancer*, 21, 108, 1967.

75. Thompson, L. H. and Suit, H. D.: Proliferation kinetics of x-irradiated mouse L cells studied with time-lapse photography, II. *Int. J. Rad. Biol.*, 15, 347, 1969.

76. Till, J. E.: Radiosensitivity and chromosome numbers in strain L mouse cells in tissue culture, *Radiat. Res.*, 15, 400, 1961.

77. Urano, M. and Suit, H. D.: Experimental evaluation of tumour bed effect of C_3H mouse mammary carcinoma and for C_3H mouse fibrosarcoma, *Radiat. Res.*, 45, 41, 1970.

78. van den Brenk, H. A. S., Elliott, K., and Hutchings, H.: Effect of single and fractionated doses of x-rays on radiocurability of solid Ehrlich tumor and tissue reactions *in vivo* for different oxygen tension, *Brit. J. Cancer*, 16, 518, 1962.

79. van Peperzeel: *Patterns of Tumor Growth After Irradiation*, Drukkerij van Denderen, 1970.

80. van Putten, L. M., Lelieveld, P. and Broerse, J. J.: Response of a poorly reoxygenating mouse osteosarcoma to x-rays and fast neutrons, *Europ. J. Cancer*, 7, 153, 1971.

81. Vos, O., Budke, L. and Vergroesen, A. L.: Protection of tissue culture cells against ionizing radiation. I. The effect of biological amines, disulphide compounds and thiols., *Int. J. Radiat. Biol.*, 5, 543, 1961.

82. Whitmore, G. F. and Gulyas, S.: Studies on recovery processes in mouse L cells, *N.C.I. Monograph 24, Radiobiol. Radiotherapy*, 1967, p. 141–156.

83. Wilson, C. S. and Hall, E. J.: On the advisability of treating all fields at each radiotherapy session, *Radiology*, 98, 419, 1971.

84. Withers, H. R.: Capacity for repair in cells of normal and malignant tissues, In *Time and Dose Relationships in Radiation Biology as Ap-*

plied to Radiotherapy, Brookhaven National Laboratory Report 50203 (C-57), p. 54.

85. Young, J. M. and Fowler, J. F.: The effects of x-ray induced synchrony on two-dose cell survival experiments, *Cell Tissue Kinet.*, 2, 95, 1969.

86. Zimmer, K. G.: *Studies on Quantitative Radiation Biology*, New York, Hafner Publishing Co., Inc., 1961.

Appendix 1

Derivation of equation of multitarget survival curve:

$$S = 1 - (1 - e^{-D/D_{37}})^N$$

p = probability of cell death; this probability increases with increase of dose x

$1 - p$ = probability of a cell surviving = S

$\therefore dp = \beta(1 - p)\, dx$, i.e., dp = (a constant, β) (S) (increase of radiation dose)

$$\int_0^{'} \frac{dp}{1 - p} = \int_0^{\infty} \beta\, dx$$

$$-\ln(1 - p) = \beta x$$

$$1 - p = e^{-\beta x}$$

$p = 1 - e^{-\beta x}$, this is for the situation where cell death results from a single event occurring in a critical area of the cell.

x = radiation dose

β = a constant ($1/D_{37}$)

When $\beta x = 1$, $p = 1 - e^{-1} = 1 - 0.37$
$$= 0.63$$

$\therefore$ the radiation dose that equals $\frac{1}{\beta}$ is the dose that yields a hit in a target with a probability of $1 - 1/e$ or 0.63. For the single target, single hit model such a dose would yield a survival fraction of 0.37 and may be referred to as the D_{37}.

$p = (1 - e^{-\beta x})^N$ where cell death resulted only if N number of independent sites are inactivated in the cell (assuming equal probability in activation for each of N sites). Probability of cell death is the product of the probabilities of inactivating N sites.

$$\therefore S = 1 - (1 - e^{-\beta x})^N$$
$$= 1 - (1 - e^{-D/D_{37}})^N$$

A model for the cell lethal effect of irradiation could assume that each of N targets or sensitive sites in the cell had to be "hit" more than one time and that the number of hits per target and the probability of hitting specific targets (*i.e.*, variation in target size) could be variable.

Appendix 2

Derivation of Relationship Between Probability of a Tumor Lethal Response and the Number of Tumor Cells Present and Their Radiosensitivity

Equation 2-1:

$$S = 1 - (1 - e^{-D/D_{37}})^N$$

$$p = 1 - s$$

$$Qp = (1 - e^{-D/D_{37}})^N$$

= probability of killing a single cell, *i.e.*, $M = 1$

S = fraction of cells surviving

D = radiation dose

D_{37} = dose that reduces S by a factor of 0.37 in the straight line portion of the curve

e = base of natural systems of logarithms = 2.71828 . . . .

N = extrapolation number

p = fraction of cells killed

M = number of viable cells in the tumor

Equation 2-2:

$$Qp = (1 - e^{-D/D_{37}})^{N \cdot M}$$

Qp = probability of killing all of M cells, *i.e.*, product of probabilities of killing each of M cells

= 0.5 at TCD_{50}, i.e., that dose yielding no surviving cells in half the tumors

$$-1nQp = N \cdot M \cdot [-1n(1 - e^{-D/D_{37}})]$$
$$\approx N \cdot M \cdot e^{-D/D_{37}},$$

with $- 1n(1 - e^{-D/D_{37}}) \approx e^{-D/D_{37}}$,

where $D/D_{37}, \gg 1$

$$1n(-1nQp) \approx 1nN + 1nM - D/D_{37}$$

Equation 2-3:

$$TCD_p \approx D_{37}[1nN + 1nM - 1n(-1nQp)]$$
$$= \text{dose yielding a local control rate } p$$

Equation 2-4:

$$TCD_{50} \approx D_{37}[1nN + 1nM + 1n \, 1n2] \text{ when}$$
$$p = 0.5, \text{ i.e., a 50\% local control rate}$$

Clinical Parameters

Tumor Control Versus Dose

Original Concept of Cancerocidal Dose

The concept of an "all or none" cancerocidal dose has dominated radiotherapy since the discovery of radium and x-rays. The goal of the early antibacterial chemotherapy, the *therapia magna sterilisans,* was the origin of this concept. The radiation dose effective to sterilize cancer was taken as being 110 per cent of the skin erythema dose, based on the belief that a dose slightly higher than the one needed to kill the epithelium of the mother organ would eradicate tumors originating from that epithelium. However, as early as 1914, it was recognized that the total dose given in one exposure would not sterilize a tumor.[52] It was thought preferable to divide the dose into several exposures in order to irradiate the cells in a more sensitive stage, mitosis being considered the stage of greatest radiosensitivity.

The concept of intrinsic radiosensitivity originated with the belief that a particular type of cancer could not be eradicated unless a dose specific for that cancer was given. For example, Lenz[40] stated on adenocarcinoma of the breast: "The demonstration of persisting

cancer after tumor doses of about 4,500 roentgens corroborates our belief that such doses are too low to destroy cancer of the breast completely and will produce only temporary growth restraint". This concept was not consistent with Miescher's dose-response curve for skin cancer obtained in 1934[44] as well as the dose-response curve of Strandqvist published in 1942 (Fig. 2-40).[58] In 1947, a dose-response curve was published for carcinomas of the skin treated with a single dose.[30] It is apparent from the sig-

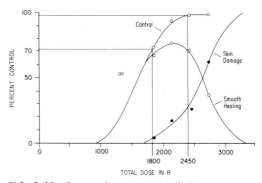

FIG. 2-40. Curve of tumor control (1 year recurrence-free), curve of skin complications (within 1 year), and curve of smooth healing calculated by Strandqvist using the iso-effect equivalent single doses. (Courtesy: Strandqvist: *Acta Radiol. Suppl.,* 55, 1, 1944.)

moid dose-response curve that an "all or none" cancerocidal dose does not exist. For a certain dose, a percentage of the tumors is controlled, which places tumor control, at least in part, on a probabilistic basis.

Most radiotherapists ignored the significance of the size of the tumor.[41] Paterson, in the first edition of his textbook[47] and in his study of optimal dosage[48] selected, using external beam, 5,000 roentgens in 3 weeks or 5,500 roentgens in 5 weeks as the optimal dose for squamous cell carcinomas, irrespective of the size of the lesion. Using interstitial radium therapy, larger tumors requiring larger implants were given a lesser dose because of diminished tolerance.[48] In a recent clinical trial[31], the dose was set between 3,500 to 4,500 rads given in 21 days 3 times a week, the smaller dose being used when larger volumes were irradiated. In contrast, Baclesse had the concept that the cancer at the site of origin was more radioresistant than that at the periphery. He designed the shrinking field technique which delivers higher doses to the central mass. Clinically uninvolved areas of the regional lymphatics were given significantly lower doses when treated electively.

Tumor Control by Irradiation

Tumor-control dose is a better term than is the term, cancerocidal dose, as any amount of irradiation is lethal to a percentage of the total cancer cell population. The curves of clonogenic ability and the oxygen effect have shown that the total number of cells and the percentage of cells in an anoxic state are paramount factors in determining the dose required to eradicate a cancer, *i.e.*, control of the disease is essentially a function of tumor size and tumor bed. A smaller dose should be required to eradicate small aggregates of cancer cells (microscopic or not clinically detectable) than the dose required to eradicate a palpable mass because a small aggregate has fewer cells and a lesser, if any, anoxic compartment. It should also be possible to establish a correlation between tumor size and tumor-control dose. In addition, if a reoxygenation effect actually occurs in cancers in man, it should be evidenced by higher control rates if, for the slow regressing infiltrating tumors, appropriately adjusted total doses are given in longer treatment times.

Control of Subclinical Disease

The emphasis in radiation therapy has been directed almost uniquely to the eradication of grossly detectable cancer with little attention being given to the amount of irradiation necessary to control occult deposits.

Table 2-7 shows increasing control rates with increasing dose levels.[20] The 90 per cent plus control point is firm for both squamous

Table 2-7. *Per Cent of Control of Subclinical Disease in Function of Dose**

Adenocarcinoma of the Breast		Squamous Cell Carcinoma of the Upper Respiratory and Digestive Tracts	
3,000–3,500 rads (89 patients)	60–70%	3,000–4,000 rads (50 patients)	60–70%
4,000 rads (121 patients)	80–90%	5,000 rads (356 patients)	>90%
5,000 rads (273 patients)	>90%	6,000 rads (65 patients)	>90%

*1,000 rads/week—5 days a week. (Courtesy: Fletcher, In *Biological and Clinical Basis of Radiosensitivity*, October, 1971, Publication pending.)

cell carcinomas of the upper respiratory and digestive tract, and for adenocarcinomas of the breast; the other control points are shown as ranges because of variations in dose. The doses are deliberately not normalized to rets in order to show the actual treatment schedules. This does not imply, however, that other treatment schedules, possibly more economical in number of fractions, would not achieve the same results.

Using Cohen's mathematical model[14], one can calculate that 4,000 rads given in 20 fractions in 4 weeks, control almost 90 per cent of aggregates containing 10^6 cells; that 3,200 rads given in 22 days (equivalent to 2,000 rads given in 5 consecutive days) control 40 per cent of 10^6 cell aggregates and 99 per cent of 10^5 cell aggregates. The slope of the dose-response curve is very steep up to the 90 per cent control point (Fig. 2-41).[32] These calculations agree with our clinical data. The steepness of the curve and the low doses

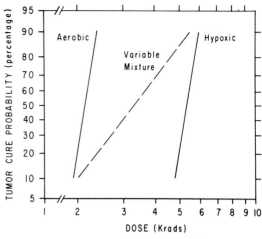

FIG. 2-42. Theoretical tumor-cure probability control curves based on the results of animal tumor studies for homogeneously aerobic or hypoxic tumors and for a series of tumors in which the proportion of hypoxic cells was variable. The shallow slope of this latter, variable mixture, curve reflects a wide range of probabilities for cure of individual tumors in a series in which hypoxia may vary from complete to non-existent. (Courtesy: Withers and Suit: In *Biological and Clinical Basis of Radiosensitivity*, Milton Friedman, Ed., Publication pending.)

employed suggest that the tumor cell aggregates in the undisturbed lymphatics are oxic.

Control of Gross Cancer

A dose-response curve can only be elicited when groups of homogeneous tumors are given a range of radiation doses. Theoretical tumor-probability control curves have been drawn with the expected slopes for series of homogeneously oxic or hypoxic tumors and for a series in which the oxygenation was variable from tumor to tumor (Fig. 2-42).[64]

Tumor rets ($T^{0.11}$ not included) should theoretically be used for dose-response curves of tumor; however, the curves keep the same relative slopes using normal tissue rets. Tumor rets should not be used to determine clinical treatments, but used only as an arbitrary device to put dose and time into one figure, allowing two-dimensional repre-

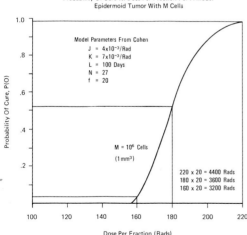

FIG. 2-41. Probability of cure versus dose per fraction for a model epidermoid tumor with M cells. For a 10^6 (1 mm³) cell aggregate the probability of cure drops from 99 per cent with 4,400 rads to 52 per cent with 3,600 rads and to less than 5 per cent with 3,200 rads (approximately equivalent to 2,000 rads in 5 consecutive days). (Courtesy: Herring and Compton: Report # EMI-216 from Enviro-Med. Inc., La Jolla, California, July 10, 1970.)

sentations. There are data in conflict with the *NSD* basis[18], which suggest that tumors can respond to irradiation by having their growth accelerated.[60]

PRIMARY LESIONS

Tumors of all sites cannot be grouped indiscriminately to obtain dose-response curves. A superficially extensive lesion on the faucial arch is not equivalent to a spheroidal lesion of the same maximum diameter in the tonsillar fossa. The incidence of failures by *T* stages differs in the different anatomical sites of the faucial arch and oropharynx.[27] Necrotic tumors, which are poorly vascularized have a higher failure rate than do the exophytic and even the infiltrative ones.[27] Differences in tumor cell composition and proportion of anoxic cells must account for these clinical facts.

At M. D. Anderson Hospital, it was not until the 1960's when results in patients treated since 1954 were analyzed, that specific dosage schedules were established for varying tumor sizes, though from 1954 on, larger tumors generally received higher doses. Table 2-8 shows a sharp rise in the control rates of T_2 and T_3 lesions of the supraglottic larynx whereas practically all T_1 le-

sions were controlled at all dose levels, and a percentage of T_4 lesions were controlled at all dose levels with no improvement in control rate with increasing dose.[53] A dose-response curve was elicited for cancers of the cervix treated with external irradiation alone except in the massive lesions where control rate does not improve above 1,750 rets (Table 2-8).[8] Higher doses are necessary to control larger masses of adenocarcinoma of the breast (Table 2-9).[7] A dose-response curve was not elicited for squamous cell carcinomas of the vocal cords.[34]

The steep rise in control rates for the

Table 2-9. *Adenocarcinoma of Breast Curie Foundation (1960–1966)*

*Correlation of Local Control in Function of Volume of Tumor and Dose**

	T_2†	T_3††
<7,000 rads	38% (8/21)	0% (0/25)
7,000–8,000 rads	66% (23/35)	32% (9/28)
8,000–9,000 rads	64% (16/25)	56% (24/43)

* 6,000 rads in 7 weeks then 2,000–3,000 rads boost in 2–3 weeks.
† T_2: 2–5 cm
†† T_3: >5 cm
(Courtesy: Calle, Personal Communication.)

Table 2-8. *Dose-Response Curves*

	Local Control Supraglottic Larynx Lesions			Control within the Irradiated Area in Cancers of the Cervix Treated with External Irradiation Only		
rets*	T_1	T_2-T_3	T_4	rets*	Stage I, II, IIIA	Stage IIIB, IV
1,701–1,800	4/5	1/6	5/9	≤1,575	0/2	0/30
1,801–1,900	4/5	10/15	5/8	1,750	3/8	9/20
1,901–2,000	8/8	18/23	2/6	≥1,950	12/14	11/34
2,001–2,100	1/1	7/8	2/3			

*1,000 rads per week with 5 treatment days. (Modified from: Fletcher, Time-Dose Relationships in Radiation Biology as Applied to Radiotherapy. BNL (C-57) Biology and Medicine TID-4500, Brookhaven National Laboratories, Upton, N. Y., p. 260, 1970.)

$T_2 - T_3$ lesions of the supraglottic larynx (Fig. 2-43) suggests that if a fraction of the cells critical to tumor survival (clonogenic cells) were initially anoxic, they become oxic soon enough during treatment so that the tumor population has a response curve similar to that which would occur if it were composed of homogeneously oxic tumors. Large tumors (T_4) are apt to have nonmalignant components because of inflammation, necrosis, and connective tissue reaction; their size may give a false estimate of the malignant cell content. Furthermore, in cellular composition, a T_4 lesion of the suprahyoid epiglottis differs from a T_4 lesion of the infrahyoid epiglottis with invasion into the pre-epiglottic space in that the latter usually is associated with infection. These T_4 lesions are heterogeneous with respect to both oxygenation and number of malignant clonogenic cells. This could explain the lack of systematic increase in local control rates with increasing doses. The flatness of dose-response curves in vocal cord cancers probably can be accounted for by the fact that in a significant percentage, the recurrences are actually new lesions and, that a built-in bias is present in this series of patients because those with the larger tumors systematically received higher doses.[34]

METASTATIC NODES

A control rate of 96 per cent was obtained in clinically positive axillary nodes of patients with cancer of the breast (Table 2-10). Assuming that 38 per cent of these patients with clinically positive nodes were histologically negative[15], at least 100 of the patients would have histologically positive nodes. With doses of 6,000 rads in 6 weeks to 7,000 rads in 7 weeks, the minimum control rate, therefore, would be 93 per cent.

From various analyses of the management of clinically positive neck nodes in patients with squamous cell carcinoma of the mucous membrane of the upper respiratory and digestive tract, it seems that 50 per cent of 2 to 3 cm nodes are controlled with 5,000 rads in 5 weeks and that 80 per cent are controlled with 7,000 rads in 7 weeks (Table 2-10).[46] A high percentage of nodes 3 to 5 cm in diameter is sterilized by 6,500 rads in $6\frac{1}{2}$ weeks to 7,000 rads in 7 weeks.[62]

CORRELATION OF DOSE VERSUS VOLUME

Table 2-11 correlates tumor volume versus dose for control of the cellular exophytic lesions of similar clinical variety in the supraglottic larynx and tonsillar fossa. Table 2-12 consolidates the data on subclinical disease and gross cancer showing clearly that in order to obtain equivalent control rates, higher doses are needed for larger tumors. The increased total doses have, on the main, been given in longer treatment times. Table

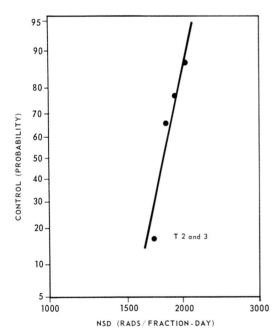

FIG. 2-43. Graph of probability of control versus NSD.

The ordinate scale has been obtained by logarithmically representing the probability from 5 to 50, and from 95 to 50 in reverse. This has the effect of linearly displaying the normal sigmoid-response curve. (Courtesy: Shukovsky: *Amer. J. Roentgen.*, 108, 27, 1970.)

Table 2-10. *Percentage of Control of Metastatic Nodes in Function of Dose, Primary Lesion Being Controlled*

Jan. 1955–Dec. 1967   Analysis Jan. 1972

Patients with late Stage III (UICC) adenocarcinoma of the breast. Clinically positive axillary nodes*	Metastatic squamous cell carcinoma to neck nodes
No. patients with no evidence of disease on the chest wall or retained breast— 161**	Primary controlled
	2–3 cm***
6,000 rads in 6 wks	5,000 rads
to	(Pre-op) 50% control†
7,000 rads in 7 wks	7,000 rads 80% control††
	(Irradiation only)
Axillary control 96% (154/161)	3–5 cm****
	6,500–7,000 rads 70% control†
	(Pre-op)

≈ 1,000 rads per week, 5 days a week.
* At least 62% expected to be histologically positive
** Fletcher, *Cancer,* 29, 545, 1972.
*** Northrop, Fletcher, Jesse, and Lindberg: *Cancer,* 29, 23, 1972.
**** Votava, Fletcher, Jesse, and Lindberg: *Radiology,* 105, 417, 1972.
† Specimen of neck dissection negative.
†† Ninety per cent of tonsillar nodes ≈ 3 cm in diameter permanently disappeared. Ninety per cent of nodes ≈ 3 cm in diameter, are histologically positive so that the probability of control of truly invaded nodes would be 80%.
(Courtesy: Fletcher, *Brit. J. Radiol.,* 46, 1, 1973.)

Table 2-11. *Dose-Tumor Volume Relationships for Squamous Cell Carcinomas of Supraglottic Larynx and Tonsillar Fossa*

Rets 1,000 rads/wk 5 days/wk	$T_1(L + T)^*$ (<2 cm)	$T_2(L + T)^*$ (2–<4 cm)	$T_3(L + T)^*$ (4–6 cm)	$T_4(T)^*$ Massive (>6 cm)
1,700–1,799 (1,750 ≈ 6,000 rads/6 wks)	5/6 1,700	6/11	3/5	1/1
1,800–1,899 (1,850 ≈ 6,500 rads/6½ wks)	11/12	12/16 1,800	6/13	0/3
1,900–1,999 (1,950 ≈ 7,000 rads/7 wks)	11/11	17/21	17/24 1,900	0/1
2,000–2,175 (2,100 ≈ 7,800 rads/8 wks)	2/2 2,100	12/13 2,100	8/8 2,100	3/3 2,000 / 2,175

* *T*: Tonsillar Fossa, *L*: Supraglottic Larynx, only exophytic lesions of the supraglottic larynx are treated with irradiation; the infiltrative T_3 lesions and T_4 lesions are generally treated by laryngectomy. (Courtesy: Fletcher, *Brit. J. Radiol.,* 46, 1, 1973.)

Table 2-12. *Dose-Tumor Volume Relationships* for Approximately Ninety Per Cent Control in Squamous Cell Carcinomas of the Upper Respiratory and Digestive Tracts*

Subclinical disease in lymphatics of the neck (All anatomical sites)	Gross Disease Supraglottic Larynx and Tonsillar Fossa			
	<2 cm	2–4 cm	4–6 cm	Massive (>6 cm)
≤ 1,575 rets	1,800 rets	1,900 rets	2,000 rets	2,100 rets
	6,090 rads/	6,800 rads/	7,310 rads/	7,890 rads/
(5,000 rads/5 wks)	30 tx/6 wks	35 tx/7 wks	37 tx/7½ wks	40 tx/8 wks

*The number of rads and weeks are for 1,000 rads per week which, on the main, have been the dose-time schedules used in the material analysed. Longer treatment times are used in the supraglottic larynx lesions than in those of the tonsillar fossa. (Courtesy: Fletcher, *Brit. J. Radiol.*, 46, 1, 1973.)

2-13 shows that these data fit with control rates obtained in other series.[55]

The increased amount of irradiation is less than 10 per cent of the total dose from T_2 to T_3 and T_3 to T_4 lesions (Table 2-12). The explanation for this small increment is that: 1) assuming that the tumor mass is composed only of malignant clonogenic cells, the increase in size, *e.g.* from 3 cm (10^9 cells) to 6 cm in diameter does not add quite a decade (10^1), 2) a specified dose of irradiation kills a constant fraction of irradiated cells (it takes the same dose to kill 90 per cent of cells in a cell population of 10^{10} and in a population of 10^2), and 3) as a few malignant clonogenic cells, perhaps one only are sufficient for regrowth of the tumor, a few hundred rads more tumor dose can be vital to the eradication of a tumor. These facts are against the intuitive concept that large increments of dose are needed for masses which are clinically evaluated as large or even massive. For

Table 2-13. *Squamous Cell Carcinoma of the Tonsillar Fossa*

Local Recurrence Rates

Stage	Shukovsky & Fletcher		Perez et al.*		Fayos & Lampe**	
			6,000–6,500 rads in 6–6½ wks.			
T_1	0%	0/14	0%	0/5	20%	2/10
T_2	14%	6/41	28%	4/14	15%	7/47
T_3	21%	11/53	40%	10/25	45%	14/31
T_4	38%	8/21	59%	10/17	64%	9/14
All T_3 + T_4 patients	25.5%	19/74	49.5%		43/87	
T_3 + T_4 patients treated with 6,000–6,500 rads in 6 to 6½ weeks	50%	8/16				
T_3 + T_4 patients treated with >6,500 rads in 6½ weeks	19%	11/58				

*Perez, Ackerman, Mill, Ogura, and Powers: *Amer. J. Roentgen.*, 114: 43–58, 1972.
**Fayos and Lampe: *Amer. J. Roentgen.*, 111, 85–91, 1971. (Courtesy: Shukovsky and Fletcher, *Radiology*, In press.)

well-vascularized tumors, like those of the tonsillar fossa, the overall treatment time may not be critical above 5 weeks.[55] For large breast tumors, the Baclesse technique of 100-days treatment[3] produced, at M. D. Anderson Hospital, a much higher percentage of controls than the technique of treating in 4 to 6 weeks.[1,29] This suggests that long protraction allows reoxygenation in those poorly vascularized cancers (Table 2-14).

Tumor Control Related to Growth Pattern

Some concepts, for examples that adenocarcinoma of the cervix is less radiosensitive than is squamous cell carcinoma, that adenocarcinoma of the breast is more radiosensitive in the nodes than in the breast, and that squamous cell carcinoma of the head and neck is more radiosensitive in the primary site than in metastatic nodes, need to be revised. Growth patterns vary not only with different histological types but are also dependent upon the mother organ, which produces tumors with different clinical characteristics. Malignant tumors of the salivary glands often grow slowly, reaching large volumes before the patients seek medical help. The difficulty of eradicating the large amount of cancer has been the basis for the radio-resistant reputation of the malignant salivary

Table 2-14. *Local Control in Patients with Advanced Breast Cancer Treated with Irradiation Only*

Jan. 1955–Dec. 1967

	< Whole breast involved*	Whole breast involved*
M.D.A.H., HOUSTON, TEXAS 9,000 rads/14 wks with 250 Kv ≈ 2,160 rets (10% RBE) 9,000 rads/11 wks with ^{60}Co ≈ 2,140 rets	Edema, ulceration, skin fixation < ½ breast satellite nodules in continuity with primary limited inflammatory features Pectoral fascia fixation 229 78% (5-yr. survival rate 30%)	Edema, ulceration, skin fixation > ½ breast peripheral satellite nodule, massive inflammatory Chest wall fixation 144 70% (5-yr. survival rate 10%)
PRESBYTERIAN HOSPITAL NEW YORK CITY, NEW YORK 4,000 rads/4 wks with 250 Kv ≈ 1,500 rets (10% RBE) 5,000 rads/4 wks with 22 Mev ≈ 1,700 rets Atkins: *Am. J. Roent.*, 1961, 85, 860	Lesions suitable for simple mastectomy 15% (3/20) (5-yr. survival rate 11%)	
MASSACHUSETTS GENERAL HOSPITAL BOSTON, MASSACHUSETTS 4,000–5,000 rads/35–40 days with 250 Kv ≈ 1,700 rets (10% RBE) 5,000–6,000 rads/4–5 wks with 2 Mev ≈ 1,900–2,000 rets Griscom & Wang: *Radiology*, 79, 18, 1962		Lesions similar to those of the MDAH patients 35% (3-yr. survival rate 5.5%)

*Any one or a combination of these features. (Courtesy: Fletcher, *Brit. J. Radiol.*, 46, 1, 1973.)

gland tumors. Adenocarcinoma of the cervix, usually of endocervical origin, grows locally and spreads to the myometrium, attaining a large volume. Control by irradiation is complicated by two factors: 1) the cellular mass is large, with a probably significant anoxic compartment, and 2) the tumor cells in the myometrium are further away from the radium sources than are the cells confined to the cervix. When squamous cell carcinoma originates in the endocervix and invades the myometrium to form a barrel-shaped lesion, the same situation exists and local failures are not uncommon.

Adenocarcinoma of the breast can grow to enormous dimensions while the infested nodes are generally smaller, the smallest being those in the supraclavicular area. The breast is largely a nonfunctional organ with a poor blood supply; the peripheral lymphatic areas are well vascularized. Hence, cancer in nodes is more easily controlled than is the primary tumor, the doses being 6,000 rads in 6 weeks to 7,000 rads in 7 weeks for the node and 9,000 to 10,000 rads in 11 to 12 weeks for the primary. The situation may be the reverse in squamous cell carcinoma of the head and neck, as the larger volume of cancer can be in the nodes. Less irradiation is needed for breast or prostate metastases to bone, since the metastases are diffuse and produce relatively small tumor masses, than for metastases from adenocarcinomas of the GI tract and kidney, which usually produce large masses before being symptomatic.

Intrinsic Radiosensitivity

The radiosensitivity of tumors of various histological types reflect, to some degree, the radiosensitivity of the tissue of origin. Tumors originating in the reproductive organs, such as the seminomas, are very radiosensitive. This is in accordance with the law of Bergonie and Tribondeau.[6] Experimental data obtained from clonogenic ability curves show that comparable doses render the same percentage of mammalian cells incapable of unlimited divisions. This does not agree with all clinical observations; for example, large masses of seminoma are eradicated by considerably lower doses than the doses used for large epithelial tumors. The lymphomas require less dose than do the epithelial tumors.

The radiosensitivity of squamous cell carcinomas versus that of the adenocarcinomas has long been argued. The concept that radiosensitivity depends upon the degree of differentiation has also been argued. Present clinical data show that all squamous cell carcinomas, adenocarcinomas of the breast and uterus, mucoepidermoid, malignant mixed, and adenoidcystic carcinomas of the salivary glands are equally radiosensitive, other factors being equal. The fact that the lymphoepitheliomas are controlled with doses lower than those needed for epithelial tumors may be because the tumor mass consists in part of the very radiosensitive lymphocytes.[9] Large masses of oat cell carcinoma of the lung are controlled with relatively low doses. The characteristic of these two tumors to grow fast may account for the increased apparent rate of volume reduction.[60]

The doses necessary to control the sarcomas (excluding the lymphomas) are not well defined. Subclinical aggregates of soft tissue sarcoma cells are controlled by doses only slightly higher than those needed to control subclinical aggregates of squamous cell carcinomas and adenocarcinomas of the breast and uterus.

Regression Rate and Tumor Dose Determination

In our center, prior to the early 1960's, the total radiation dose selected for the treatment of individual squamous cell carcinomas of the head and neck region was to a great extent, decided by the clinical status of the tumor after a minimum course of therapy. For example, if a T_3 squamous cell carcinoma of the tonsillar fossa was planned to receive a basic dose of 6,000 rads in 6 weeks and if disease had clinically disappeared by the fourth week of therapy, the lesion was considered to be "radiosensitive" and no further treatment was given. In contrast, if induration and nodularity persisted after the delivery of 6,000 rads, the lesion was classed as "radioresistant" and an additional 1,000 to 1,500 rads were given through reduced fields.

A study of the incidence of local recurrences, related to stage of disease and clinical evaluation of tumor activity at the completion of treatment, showed that local control in the T_3 and T_4 squamous cell carcinomas of the oropharynx was not clearly correlated with the rate of tumor regression.[59] The same observation was made for advanced cancers of the cervix treated only by external irradiation.[8] These observations are at variance with other studies where the chance of local control was correlated with rate of volume reduction.[60] Gross and microscopic changes in malignant tissues after irradiation depend on the rate of lysis of nonviable cells and removal of tissues, malignant or not, from the area. The highly cellular tumors with sparse stroma undergo rapid regression, for instance, the exophytic tumors of the tonsillar fossa area, supraglottic larynx and vocal cords clinically disappear, almost without exception, after 4,000 rads in 4 weeks. Viable tumor cells are still present microscopically after clinical disappearance of gross cancer.

The size of the mass of cancer, the tumor bed, and the tolerance of the supporting structures are the main factors in determining the total dose and over-all treatment time. The observed regression of tumor during therapy is related to the clinical variety of the tumor. Provided that an adequate tumor dose is given, increasing with tumor size, 5 to 7 weeks treatment gives the same rate of control in the squamous cell carcinomas of the tonsillar fossa.[55] For supraglottic larynx tumors, the treatment time must be 7 weeks because of lesser tolerance of the larynx. Infiltrating tumors, like the squamous cell carcinomas of the base of the tongue and large adenocarcinomas of the breast require long treatment times with a time adjusted total dose.

Normal Tissue Tolerance

Physical and Biological Dosage

Because treatment practices varied widely during the first half of the century, the available data concerning tolerance of normal tissues were limited and unreliable. The advent of megavoltage permitted simple techniques which, in the absence of differential bone absorption, yielded accurate dosimetry. Furthermore, in the last two decades, differences between centers in basic dosage determination have been reduced to less than 5 per cent.[56,57]

The belief that reactions varied widely from patient to patient was not substantiated in a study of mucosal reactions (Fig. 2-44). In 1957, when a second ^{60}Co unit was obtained, it was soon noted that mucous membrane reactions in patients treated with the new unit were more intense than in those treated with the first unit. Careful investigation of the calibration log book of the first unit showed that the time on and off had not been included in the reading of the 25 r chamber. With the first ^{60}Co unit, the doses were 5 per cent less at 70 cm *SSD* and 7 per cent less at 50 cm *SSD* than with the new unit. This difference in dosage determination was first recognized at the clinical level. The change from the roentgen to the rad was made at the M. D. Anderson Hospital in February 1959. With the various factors that were included (^{60}Co correction factor, stem factor, and the error in the initial dosage determination with the first ^{60}Co unit), the rad was 10 per cent stronger than the roentgen. However, it was decided to keep the same number of rads as had previously been given in roentgens in the treatment schedules. A number of laryngeal edemas occurred in vocal cords treated after February 1959.[24] In November 1961, a slightly different time-dose relationship was adopted (only a 2 per cent diminution in *NSD*), with subsequent disappearance of laryngeal edemas (Table 2-15). With the 22 Mev photon beam the

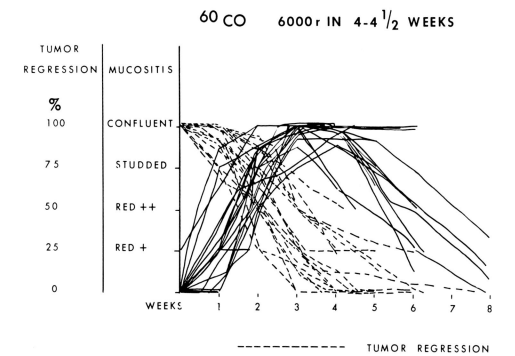

FIG. 2-44. Tumor regression and mucositis; 5,500 rads in 4 to $4\frac{1}{2}$ weeks with ^{60}Co.

Thirteen hundred and seventy-five rads per week to the soft palate produces a confluent mucositis which starts at the end of the second week of treatment, reaches its peak in the middle of the third week and, on the average, begins to regress at the fifth week. It is healed by the eight to the ninth week. The curves which show no down slope are those of patients who were unable to return weekly after the completion of treatment for charting reactions. (Courtesy: Fletcher, MacComb, and Shalek: *Radiation Therapy in the Management of the Oral Cavity and Oropharynx,* Springfield, Ill., Charles C Thomas, p. 51, 1962.)

change from the roentgen to the rad resulted in an increase of 7 per cent. When the same doses in rads were given to the whole pelvis for cancer of the uterine cervix, there was an increased incidence and severity of sigmoiditis.

With treatments changed to 3 days instead of 5 days a week in the irradiation of breast cancer, the same total dose was maintained in the effort to decrease the incidence of failures within the irradiated area, *i.e.,* breast, axilla, and supraclavicular nodes. It had been the practice to use bolus for part of the treatment in order to obtain a brisk erythema since breast cancer characteristically invades the superficial dermal lymphatics. Enhanced skin reactions were observed in patients randomized for treatment with the 3-day rather than the 5-day schedule but, with adjustment in the amount of bolus used, identical skin reactions were obtained with each schedule. Tumor control was increased but there was a concomitant rise in complication rate (Table 2-16).[45] Complications included woody fibrosis, frozen shoulders, multiple rib fractures, and chest wall necrosis. This exemplifies the Holthusen graphic representation of the narrow margin between tumor control and increased complications.[33] Although the control rate is clearly better with the 3-days a week schedule, the complications are prohibitive.

Table 2-15. Variations in Dose-Time Relationship
(All Patients Treated with ^{60}Co, 5 days/week)
Feb. 1959–Dec. 1967   Analysis June 1971

NSD	No of Patients	No of Recurrences	Average NSD of Recurrence	No of Complication (Edema or Nec.)	Average NSD of Complication
Feb. 1959–Nov. 1961					
5,500 rads/4 weeks ⟶ 1872	68 [49-T_1 / 19-T_2	14 [9-T_1 / 5-T_2	T_1 1978	6 [5-T_1 / 1-T_2 9%	2023
+ 500 rads/2 days ⟶ 1965			T_2 1977		
+ 1000 rads/5 days ⟶ 2045					1965
Nov. 1961–Dec. 1967					
6,000 rads/5½ weeks ⟶ 1828	236 [151-T_1 / 85-T_2	41 [16-T_1 / 25-T_2	T_1 1842	3 [1-T_1 / 2-T_2 1.5%	1950
+ 500 rads/2 days ⟶ 1936			T_2 1937		
+ 1000 rads/5 days ⟶ 1990					

(Courtesy: Horiot, Fletcher, Ballantyne, and Lindberg, *Radiology*, 103, 663, 1972.)

Table 2-16. *Failures and Severe Complications in Patients Treated with Protracted Irradiation Alone with* ^{60}Co

5 days per week: 88 Patients   3 days per week*: 57 Patients

Failures	5x/week	3x/week	Severe Complications	5x/week	3x/week
Breast, axilla, supraclavicular area separately or combined	27%	12%			
			Severe axillary fibrosis and frozen shoulder	2%	11.5%
			Chest wall necrosis and fibrosis; multiple rib fractures	3%	13%

* With 3 days versus 5 days per week, the increase in biological effectiveness is 7 to 10 per cent according to the NSD formula for the tissues of the shoulder and axilla (anterior supraclavicular and axillary portal (1 loading); posterior axillary portal (0.5 loading) 2 and 2 days per week, and 15 per cent for the breast and chest wall, the tangential portals being treated alternately (2.5 fractions versus 1.5 fractions)). (Courtesy: Montague, *Radiology,* 90, 962, 1968.)

The dose-response curve of complications is steep. If a treatment schedule is close to maximum tolerance, a 10 per cent increase in biological effectiveness may lead to disaster. Every change in the basic factors of radiotherapy requires a long follow-up period. The principal complication of megavoltage is fibrosis, which progresses steadily for years after treatment. A follow-up of at least 5 years and probably 10 years is necessary to derive the equivalence of different dose-time fraction schedules.

DOSE VOLUME RELATIONSHIP

It has been recognized since the early days of radiotherapy that radiation tolerance decreases as the area of skin or the volume of tissue irradiated increases. Tables based on clinical data have been formulated giving dose-time-area relationships for the various degrees of skin reactions.[17,47] Paterson had derived semiempirical data from an analysis of successes, failures, and necroses in oral cavity and oropharynx tumors, treated either by interstitial radium implants or external irradiation.[48] Jolles[37] and Cohen[10,11] have published tables and graphs correlating volume and dose, seemingly developed from surveys and extrapolations more than from actual clinical facts. VonEssen correlated time and area for skin cancers.[61] Despite this interest, the volume factor has not been ade-

quately studied in relation to the production of complications and only spotty data are available. Fig. 2-45 shows in the incidence of complications in the treatment of squamous cell carcinoma of the supraglottic larynx, the relationship of volume, which is a function of portal size, versus dose-time.

Radiation tolerance decreases quickly with increased volume and slightly different treatment geometries producing different volume distributions may be associated with more or fewer complications. Table 2-17 tabulates, by technique, the incidence and severity of bone complications in the radiation treatment of tumors in the tonsillar area, using equal tumor doses and treatment times.[28] With a single homolateral field or paired wedge filter fields, the dose to the mandible is higher than that used in the parallel opposing fields technique. Many apparently conflicting data in the literature could easily be reconciled if treatment factors were reviewed not only in terms of total dose, total treatment time, and fractions, but also the volume of specific tissues irradiated with different treatment techniques.

Time Factor

History

The time factor has been the one parameter in radiation therapy which probably has

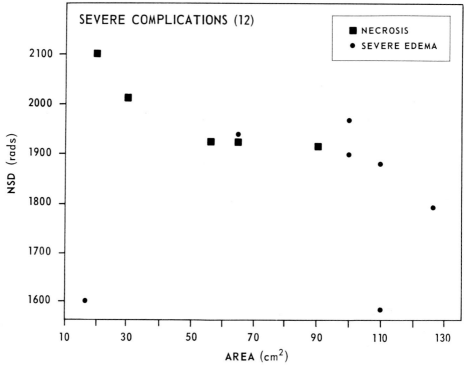

FIG. 2-45. Scattergram of complications in supraglottic squamous cell carcinoma. (Courtesy: Shukovsky: *Amer. J. Roentgen.*, 108, 27, 1970.)

received the most attention, striving, by manipulating it, to increase the ratio of tumor control versus normal tissue damage. There is a vast literature on the subject replete with conflicting data and little practical information.

In 1918, the first experiment on human skin was published which demonstrated that a specific physical dose of radiation would be less biologically effective if given in multiple fractions.[39] This was the origin of the concept of recovery between fractions. In 1927, Regaud and Ferroux reported that sterilization of the testicles could be achieved

Table 2-17. *Incidence of Bone Exposure and Osteonecrosis by Techniques of Irradiation of Tonsillar Area Tumors*

Technique	Number of patients	Number of patients with bone exposure	Number of patients with necroses requiring mandibulectomy
Single homo-lateral field	50	48.0% (24)	18.0% (9)
Parallel Opposing fields	78	30.8% (24)	5.1% (4)
Paired wedge filter field	22	45.5% (10)	13.6% (3)

Modified from: Grant and Fletcher, *Amer. J. Roentgen.*, 96, 28, 1966.

with less skin damage if fractionation was used.[50] This experiment provided some experimental data for the developing concept of the ratio of damage to normal tissue versus tumoricidal dose.

In the 1930's the effect of fractionation, primarily on skin reactions, was extensively studied. The best known studies are those of Reisner in 1933[51] and of MacComb and Quimby in 1936[43], establishing the concept of recovery with experimentally produced skin reactions. Through the 1930's various fractionation schemes were established in clinical centers in England, the Scandinavian countries, and in continental Europe primarily at the Curie Foundation. Doses and treatment times varied widely. For example, in the treatment of patients with cancer of the larynx, the tumor dose was 6,000 to 6,500 gamma roentgens in 12 to 14 days at the Radiumhemmet with teleradium units, whereas in England, using similar equip-

ment, the tumor dose was around 6,000 gamma roentgens in 6 weeks. At the Christie Hospital, Manchester[47], it was the practice with external beam therapy, to give 5,000 roentgens tumor dose in 3 weeks or 5,500 roentgens tumor dose in 5 weeks. At the Curie Foundation such doses could not be given and at the most were 4,500 to 5,000 roentgens in 6 weeks. Baclesse gave total tumor doses between 7,000 to 7,500 roentgens in 70 to 80 days.[2,3,4] These puzzling differences in the practices of radiotherapy in the 1940's and through part of the 1950's, resulted in the commonly made statement that, for mysterious reasons, what could be done at one center could not be done at another center.

The iso-effect curves of Strandqvist show no advantage to prolongation of the treatment times since all the curves are parallel (Fig. 2-46). However, it is obvious that if the iso-effect curves for normal tissues and

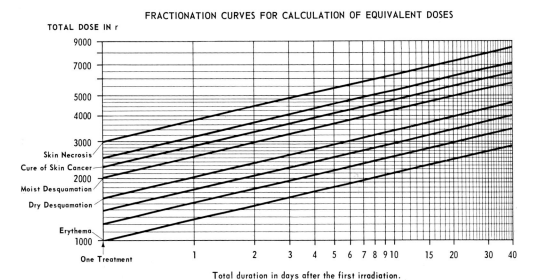

FRACTIONATION CURVES FOR CALCULATION OF EQUIVALENT DOSES

TOTAL DOSE IN r

Total duration in days after the first irradiation.

FIG. 2-46. Strandqvist curves on log paper. The slope of the curves, 0.22, is the same for the tumoricidal dose for squamous cell carcinoma and for various degrees of skin reactions.

A detailed review of the material used by Strandqvist shows that practically all of the 280 patients with basal cell and squamous cell carcinomas of the skin and lip in Strandqvist's study were treated within 14 days. Only 8 were treated between 14 and 21 days and one patient was treated for 45 days. In Strandqvist's monograph there is no experimental data to determine that the slope for skin reactions is the same as the slope for sterilization of skin cancer. However, Strandqvist showed that the data of Reisner and MacComb-Quimby fitted his slope for skin reactions. (Courtesy: Strandqvist: *Acta Radiol.* Suppl. 55, 1, 1944.)

tumor truly had the same slope, there would be no reason not to treat every lesion with a single dose of irradiation, but this is known to produce prohibitive complications in inner organs. Zuppinger[65], utilizing late skin changes, derived a different iso-effect curve for normal tissues, which showed an advantage of long treatment times. Cohen[10,11] estimated the slope for skin reaction to be 0.30 based both on the skin erythema data of Reisner and Quimby and on tables of skin tolerance of irradiated patients published by Ellis in 1942.[17] Later Cohen[12,13] suggested that the slope was 0.33 based on the skin damage of irradiated patients. It is of historical interest that both Quimby and Cohen in an early publication[10] considered the number of fractions unimportant, the determining factor being the total dose in the same over-all time.[10,43] Iso-effect curves became very popular and were drawn for various types of tumor.[12,26] Formulae for optimal dosage were developed which included *RBE*, volume, dose, and time.[10,11,37]

There were radiotherapists who thought that the same total dose delivered in the same over-all time offered greater tissue-sparing if given in more fractions. Although this was not universally accepted, it became a predominant concept which Baclesse carried to its maximum clinical effectiveness at the Curie Foundation, treating every field every day 6 days a week. Some radiotherapists even made it a practice to treat the same field twice a day. I, myself, with 250 Kv, gave 125 rads to each upper neck field every day instead of 250 roentgens on alternate days and had the impression that it produced less skin damage, which was, until megavoltage, the main obstacle to the delivery of adequate dosage. Therefore, it is not correct, as sometimes stated in recent years, that the practice of treating 5 days a week evolved because there are 5 working days in the week. The concept, right or wrong, that the same dose given in more fractions damages the normal tissues less, has been the basis underlying the practice of daily treatment.

Limitations of the NSD

It is beyond controversy that, for normal tissues, a dose of radiation is more effective when given in less over-all treatment time and when the number of fractions in which it is given is decreased. A formula to calculate varying fraction-dose-time schedule equivalents has been sought since the early days of radiotherapy. Unfortunately, the slopes for recovery of normal tissue and tumor tissue have not been definitively determined.

In the irradiation of vocal cord cancers, the elimination of edema and necrosis (Table 2-15) by dose-time alterations with only a 2 per cent diminution in *NSD* is evidence that tolerance expressed in *NSD* is not applicable in this situation. An explanation may be that the effect of the treatment time ($T^{0.11}$) is underestimated with low *LET* radiation, the exponent being possible 0.22.[16] It is also clear that the tolerance of connective tissues will have decreased *NSD* values with increasing irradiated volumes. According to Table 2-18, 1,900 rets are equivalent to 6,100 rads in 5 weeks, or 6,500 rads in 6 weeks, or 6,850 rads in 7 weeks. Previous experience in the irradiation of larynx tumors showed that a high percentage of patients would develop severe edema if supraglottic tumors were irradiated with 6,100 rads in 5 weeks through portals which could not be smaller than 35 cm² [24], whereas with 6,850 rads in 7 weeks only an occasional, selfhealing, edema will develop. Again, the explanation may be in the underestimation of the effect of the over-all treatment time. Furthermore, with reduction of field size from 5,000 to 6,000 rads and 6,000 rads to the total dose of 7,000 rads, the volume receiving the maximum dose is less than if 6,100 rads are given in 5 weeks without field reduction.

The *NSD* can be used as an arbitrary device to give a first approximation in selecting total dose, number of fractions, and over-all treatment time. For example, if one gives 850 rads per week instead of 1,000 rads per week,

Table 2-18. *Nominal Standard Dose Equivalents in Weeks*

Rets	5 Weeks ($N = 25; T = 35$)	6 Weeks ($N = 30; T = 42$)	7 Weeks ($N = 35; T = 49$)
1700	5450	5800	6100
1800	5750	6150	6500
1900	6100	6500	6850
2000	6400	6850	7200

$^{7000}/_7$ weeks $\simeq$ 1950 rets

$$NSD\text{—(nominal standard dose)} = \frac{D \text{ (total dose)}}{N^{0.24} T^{0.11}}$$

N—number of fractions
T—Time of therapy in days

the total dose must be increased. The increase is 10 per cent according to the *NSD*. Failures and complications with a new schedule must be carefully watched.

Fractionation Corrected Dosimetry

Specifying the number of treatment days per week is not enough since the computing of isodose curves is not correlated with the time factor unless all fields are treated every day.[63] This is illustrated in Figure 2-47 where one sees a substantial difference in rets in an apparently homogeneous volume distribution. The center of the tumor receives fewer rets than expected, a potential reason for failure. If the upper neck is treated every other day, the neck nodes will get a high dose one day and a low dose the next day, which is more effective than two equal doses.

Reoxygenation

Animal tumor system studies indicate that there is reoxygenation of surviving anoxic cells between dose fractions.[35] With small doses per fraction, most of the reoxygenated cells will be killed, allowing further reoxygenation of the anoxic survivors. When this process is repeated many times the significance of initially hypoxic cells is diminished and perhaps eliminated.

Are there clinical data which suggest that

there is reoxygenation during radiotherapy of human cancers? There should be a difference between the critical over-all treatment times for tumors which are highly cellular, regress rapidly, and clinically disappear by the third or fourth week of treatment and for those tumors in muscle or in connective tissue with a slow regression rate.

Exophytic tumors of the tonsillar fossa regress very rapidly; most disappear clinically by the third to fourth week of treatment. In 1954 in the early days of the megavoltage program, some oropharyngeal lesions of limited volume were treated with 6,000 rads in 4 to 5 weeks. The analysis shows no difference in control rates for tumors of the tonsillar fossa treated from 4 to 7 weeks.[55] In contradistinction, although the numbers are too small for a statistically valid comparison, there is a suggestion that tumors of the base of the tongue have a higher percentage of local failures when the treatment time is 4 to 5 weeks rather than $6\frac{1}{2}$ to 7 weeks.[27]

Tumors of the breast, generally a poorly vascularized organ, especially in older patients, reach a large size with considerable connective tissue reaction. Baclesse, who initiated protracted treatment (up to 100 days for cancer of the breast), reported a significant difference in local control in patients treated in less than 10 weeks and those treated in 10 to 16 weeks.[3]

At MDAH, Baclesse's protracted treatment schedule has been used for the inoperable

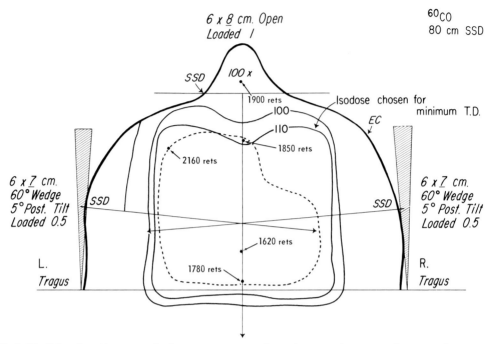

FIG. 2-47. Using the 110 per cent isodose curve a tumor dose of 6,000 rads at 850 rads per week was given. The volume distribution in rets is unhomogeneous. The biological dose is least in the center of the tumor which receives the same dose every day whereas it is high in the anterior aspect of the nostrils which receive a higher dose every other day.

breast cancers, *i.e.*, 100 days with 250 Kv and 11 weeks with ^{60}Co.[25] Table 2-14 compares local control rates in the MDAH series with those in series from other institutions treated in 4 to 6 weeks. A strikingly lower local control rate is found in the Presbyterian Hospital series.[1] These were patients suitable for simple mastectomy, *i.e.*, the majority of the lesions were less advanced than those of the MDAH patients. Furthermore, the longer survival times of the MDAH patient subjected them to an increased risk of a local recurrence. A similar difference is seen on comparing patients with very advanced lesions in the Massachusetts General Hospital series[29] and the MDAH series. Although the doses in rets in the other series are less than the doses used at MDAH, the local control rates are so strikingly lower that there is a suggestion that the long treatment time is a contributing factor in the higher control rates for the patients treated at MDAH.

Repopulation

Table 2-19 compares the cumulative recurrence rates in advanced T_3 and T_4 lesions of the upper respiratory and digestive tracts in patients treated with the split-course technique to a tumor dose of 7,000 rads in 10 weeks with a 3-week rest and in similar lesions treated with 850 rads per week to a total dose of 7,500 to 8,000 rads in 9 to $9\frac{1}{2}$ weeks. The over-all tolerance of the normal tissues is clinically thought to be the same in the two techniques. Although the numbers are small there is a suggestion that continuous treatment is superior to the split-course. The explanation may be repopulation of the clonogenic cells during the rest interval.

To obtain control of tumor masses, there is a minimum weekly dosage rate. Baclesse observed that with doses less than 700 roentgens per week practically no metastatic neck nodes were controlled.[5] With correction for

Table 2-19. Cumulative Recurrence Rates in T_3^* and T_4^* Squamous Cell Carcinoma of the Upper Respiratory and Digestive Tracts (Analysis January 1972)

	No. Pts.	Residual	6 mo	12 mo	24 mo	36 mo
Split course 3,000 rads/3 wks; 3 wks. rest; 4,000 rads/4 wks Total time 10 weeks.**	23 3/65 to 7/67	5	48% (11)	74.5% (17)	79% (18)	(all pts. dead)†
850 rads for 5 days/wk for 8 wks then 1,000–1,500 rads 1–1½ wks Total dose 7,500–8,000 rads in 9–9½ wks**	20 8/68 to 2/70	2	20% (4)	40% (8)	45% (9)	10††

* T_3 > 4 cm in diameter; T_4 massive
** 5 days a week treatment
† All patients dead, 4 from intercurrent disease, one from distant metastases
†† 3 patients died from intercurrent disease, one patient is alive at 28 months with neck disease only. Five patients are NED at 24 mos, 26 mos, 26 mos, 28 mos, 32 mos
(Courtesy: Fletcher, Brit. J. Radiol., 46, 1, 1973.)

RBE and rad, one can estimate that 800 rads per week is the minimum megavoltage dose. Not uncommonly, neck metastases will grow during treatment even when 1,000 rads are given per week. From the observation of a significant number of cases, a weekly tumor dose of 1,500 rads is necessary to control fast growing masses. To initiate regression, 250 rads are given twice weekly to an additional total dose of 1,500 to 2,000 rads through a small field covering only the palpable node(s) within the large treatment fields (Fig. 2-48).

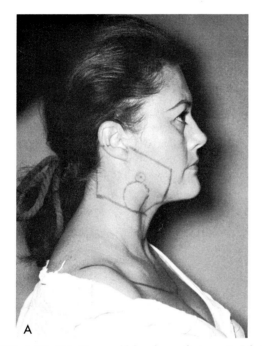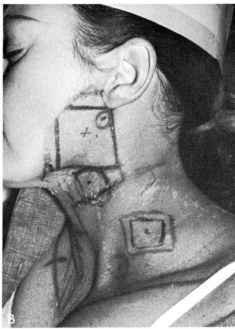

FIG. 2-48. This 43-year-old female was first seen in July 1970 with a 2 cm squamous cell carcinoma with spindle component of the base of the tongue and with bilateral neck nodes. In the right neck there was a subdigastric node measuring 2.5 × 3 cm and also a node in the jugular chain which measured 1 × 1.5 cm. There were two jugular nodes in the left neck, the largest measuring 2 × 2 cm at the level of the hyoid bone.

From July 20, 1970 to September 22, 1970 at a rate of 850 rads per week, 6,000 rads were given to the midline of the base of the tongue and upper necks with parallel opposing ^{60}Co fields. An additional 1,000 rads tumor dose was given to the primary lesion with a left lateral 18 Mev photon beam making a total of 7,000 rads in 8 weeks to the primary. At 4,500 rads tumor dose the fields were moved forward to exclude the spinal cord. The right lower neck received 5,500 rads given dose and the left lower neck received 6,000 rads given dose with an anterior ^{60}Co field. In the second treatment week, because the right subdigastric node was increasing in size, the 12 Mev electron beam was used to treat a 4 × 6 cm field-within-a-field, (A), 250 rads twice each week, to 2,000 rads given dose. When the ^{60}Co portals were moved off the spinal cord at 4,500 rads tumor dose, 9 Mev electron beam posterior strips were used to treat both spinal accessory chains to 5,500 rads at 1 cm depth. The 2 palpable jugular nodes in the left neck received 6 Mev electron beam boosts of 1,000 rads given dose through 3 cm circular and 3 × 4 cm fields (B).

At the completion of treatment, the disease in the base of the tongue and in the necks had disappeared. The patient showed no evidence of disease in April 1972.

A. In the upper right neck field a circle about 4 cm in diameter outlines the growing cervical node. An appositional 12 Mev electron beam field was used to treat it twice a week. **B.** This is the left neck in the last week of treatment. The upper field covering the angle of the mandible is the boost photon beam field for the primary. The circle in the midneck and the small rectangles in the lower neck are the boost 6 Mev electron beam fields for the cervical nodes.

Baclesse's Protracted Technique[2,3,4]

For advanced lesions of the head and neck and in debilitated or very old patients, the Baclesse technique with protraction over 60 to 70 days to avoid marked mucosal reactions is very useful. When giving 850 rads tumor dose per week, the total tumor dose must be increased by 10 per cent. Severe mucosal reactions do not develop, making the treatment less taxing for the patient. Additionally chemotherapy can be given in association with irradiation without excessive reactions.

Altered Fractionation Schemes Split-Course Technique

The treatment technique designated "split course" consists of two courses of treatment separated by a rest period, *i.e.,* 3,000 rads in 3 weeks, 3-week rest, and another 3,000 rads in 3 weeks. Most authors have reported a decrease in radiation reactions and some authors have reported increased survival rates. The rationale is to take advantage of the reoxygenation which has occurred when the treatment is restarted.

At MDAH, a small number of T_3 and T_4 lesions of the oropharynx were treated with 3,000 rads given in 3 weeks, a 3-week rest period, and another 3,000 rads in 3 weeks, followed by an extra 1,000 rads through reduced portals, the total dose being 7,000 rads in 10 weeks. With this technique very little palliation was obtained, even for a limited time (Table 2-19).[42]

THREE-DAYS-A-WEEK TREATMENT

With 3-days-a-week treatment, even if the total dose is decreased by 10 to 12 per cent to provide an equivalent dose, the edge effect of the large fractions must be taken into consideration and every field must be treated each treatment day. Fractions larger than 400 roentgens given with the 800 Kv unit at St. Bartholomew's Hospital in the late 1930's produced severe fibrosis.[36]

The only 3-days-a-week treatment situation which does not require treating every field each treatment day is that for very short-term palliation. This may be used for debilitated patients to avoid frequent trips to the hospital.

HIGH-DOSE, FEW-FRACTIONS TECHNIQUE

Such fractionation schemes as 1,250 rads *TD* given twice, 3 weeks apart, or 850 rads given twice within 48 hours (*NSD* equivalent of 3,000 rads in 3 weeks), a 3-week rest, and again twice 850 rads, have been tried for bronchogenic carcinoma. A scheme of 6 times 500 rads in 3 weeks was tried in locally advanced breast cancer. In both situations, growth restraint was very limited. The few patients with bronchogenic carcinoma who lived more than a few months had fatal complications. The patients with breast cancer who survived a year or more developed crippling fibrosis.

The schedule of a small number of high dose fractions should be reserved for very short-term palliation, such as growth restraint of fungating masses, in patients close to death from disseminated cancer.

External Beam Equipment

At the present time, the majority of skin cancers are excised, radiotherapy being preferred only for lesions in locations such as the eyelids and around the nose where excision may require complex and multiple surgical procedures. The number of such patients hardly justifies the installation of superficial kilovoltage equipment. Furthermore, the electron beam can be used if a 4 to 6 Mev linear accelerator is available. If one's practice includes a large number of patients with cancer of the cervix, a 300 Kv unit with variable voltage from 150 to 300 Kv is very useful for transvaginal irradiation to control bleeding.

Do energy levels above 20 Mev offer any advantages over 3 to 6? Figure 2-49 shows

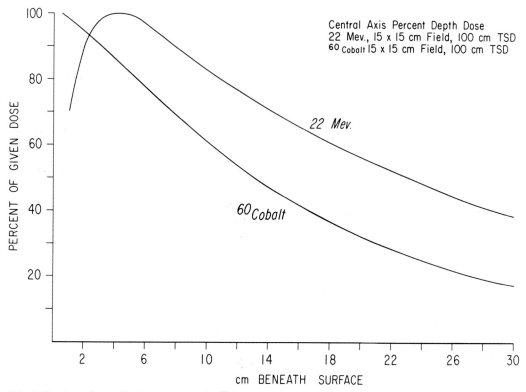

FIG. 2-49. Central axis depth dose curves for ^{60}Co and 22 Mev with 100 cm *TSD*.

the central axis depth doses for ^{60}Co (which is equivalent to 3 Mev) and a 22 Mev beam. The ratio of the central dose to the lateral dose for various thicknesses is favorable with the 22 Mev beam (Fig. 1-55). In addition to a favorable ratio, it is not necessary to treat every field every day with 22 Mev beam because, as seen in Table 1-6 the midline dose is not too different from the lateral tissue dose. If 3 to 6 Mev is used, it is imperative to treat every field every day because the biological damage to lateral normal tissues would be comparatively greater with alternate day treatment than the damage to the centrally located tumor. The edge effect is magnified by treating 4 days (or worse, 3 days) a week instead of 5 days a week because the individual fractions are larger.

For tumors that are located in the thorax, abdomen, and pelvis, a 25 Mev beam is advantageous with parallel opposing portals and is effective for lateral portals. It also has advantages for centrally located lesions of the head and neck such as those of the soft palate and posterior pharyngeal walls. High tumor doses can be delivered with better tolerance of the mucosa and with a minimum of skin changes and subcutaneous fibrosis. Besides adding to the patient's comfort, surgical excision of relatively common failures in lesions of the posterior pharyngeal walls can be done with fewer complications.

The electron beam energies of the greatest usefulness are from 6 to 9 Mev. Six Mev is adequate for treatment of the chest wall after radical mastectomy and 6 or 9 Mev are suitable for most situations in the neck.

Interstitial and Intracavitary Gamma-Ray Therapy

For interstitial gamma-ray therapy of oral cavity cancers and for intracavitary gamma-ray therapy of cancers of the cervix, vagina, and corpus, radium is still the most useful gamma-ray emitter. Forty years of clinical experience has been accumulated with specific dosage rates and volume distributions. With the very critical tolerance of normal tissue, new variables should not be lightly introduced in treatment for these highly curable lesions.

Clinical Relative Biological Effectiveness of Different Megavoltage Beams

The relative biological effectiveness (*RBE*) is the specific response of biological material to different wave lengths of ionizing radiation, other factors being equal. The relative *RBE* of 1 to 3 mm Cu *HVL* versus 1 to 25 Mev is approximately 0.85 to 0.9.[38] The tolerance and recovery of the supporting organs depends upon the amount of irradiation the surrounding structures receive. The treatment geometry with various megavoltage beams is not the same, since the physical characteristics of various photon and electron beam energy levels can be utilized to assure anatomical coverage with simple, reproducible patterns.

In the treatment of pelvic malignancies with 22 Mev photon, 1,000 rads per week through a 15 × 15 cm AP and PA portal (even better with the box technique) are well tolerated; with 3 to 6 Mev, 850 to 900 rads only are tolerated because the central dose is lower than the dose to the lateral tissues. With the electron beam, the tolerance is improved because of the rapid fall-off in dose. The irradiated volume is sharply reduced, and therefore, higher doses are possible.

Causes of Failure

The possible causes of further active disease in the vicinity of the primary cancer are multiple.

1) Geographical miss.

Part of the tumor was not included in the irradiated volume.

a) When the active disease becomes clinically manifest one can retrospectively, by studying the volume distribution related to the initial description of the disease, arrive at the conclusion that the beam actually missed a part of the cancer.

b) Unusual extensions; for instance, squamous cell carcinoma of the floor of the mouth may spread along the periosteum at such a distance, that one would not encompass it even with a generous target volume.

2) New primary.

Squamous cell carcinomas of the upper respiratory and digestive tracts have the tendency to be multicentric with a high percentage of the patients developing new cancers. When a cancer develops in the vicinity of the treated volume, it is always a question that it may be a recurrence or a new primary.

3) Technical errors.

a) Obvious "cold spots" (as in cancer of the uterine cervix when the vaginal colpostats are anterior to the tandem and a recurrence develops on the posterior lip which is in a "cold spot" area). Similarly some "cold spots" can be detected in interstitial implants of the oral cavity.

b) Systematic cause of underdosage detected after analysis of a series of patients correlating failures at a specific area leading to investigating some hidden flaw in the treatment technique. An example is the incidence of recurrences anteriorly on the buccal mucosa or on the gum in those patients with squamous cell carcinomas of the faucial pillar and retromolar trigone, who were treated with the 22 Mev photon beam alone or half 22 Mev photon beam and 18 Mev electron beam.[27] With the 22 Mev photon beam, the maximum build-up is at 4 cm depth so that inside of the cheek (at about 1.5 to 2 cm depth), the dose may be only 80 to 90 per cent. With the combination photon and electron beam, because of the constriction of the isodose curves of the electron beam, 15 to 20 per cent less dose can be given close to the geometrical edge of the field. A difference of 10 to 15 per cent less than the proposed dose is sufficient to produce a significant incidence of failures. This is important to recognize in the planning and the carrying out of the treatments. A few malignant clonogenic cells are sufficient for continued activity of the tumor.

4) No obvious cause.

The control of cancers is partly based on a random basis like the survival of cells in tissue culture. This is demonstrated by the sigmoid response curve of cancers treated with increasing doses, like the one obtained for skin cancers (Fig. 2-40).

Basic Principle of Radiotherapy

The basic principle of radiotherapy is to obtain maximum control of tumors with a minimum of complications. This was graphically illustrated by Holthusen in 1936[33] (Fig. 2-50), and was verified by Strandqvist on application to the treatment of skin cancer (Fig. 2-40). This concept, central to radiotherapy, is the choice between increasing the percentage of controls at the expense of complications, major or minor. For skin cancers doses can be given which produce a relatively low tumor control rate but result in normal skin, or those doses which provide almost 100 per cent tumor control but produce atrophy, telangiectases, and a percentage of necroses.[58] In the treatment of T_1 lesions of the vocal cord, one can obtain 90 per cent control with perfect voices, but if a control rate close to 100 per cent is sought, severe edema would result in a significant percentage of patients and possibly minor edema would develop in many patients. This would defeat the very purpose of choosing radiotherapy over partial laryngectomy, *i.e.*, the anticipation of a normal voice with irradiation.

Optimal control rates are not the same for all types of disease, organ location, and stage of disease. A control rate of 90 per cent for early lesions is satisfactory because the sigmoid curve begins to flatten out and an increased control rate is obtained at the expense of a disproportionate incidence of complications and sequelae. With advanced lesions, complications must be accepted to obtain even a modest control rate. Techniques which produce no complications and a significant incidence of failures should be rendered more radical. Conversely, with no failures but with significant complications, the technique must be made less radical.

The following illustration of this principle has been abstracted in some detail from an earlier publication.[54]

Retinal and Optic Nerve Complications in a High Dose Irradiation Technique of Ethmoid Sinus and Nasal Cavity Tumors

A group of patients received high doses of megavoltage radiation to the retina and optic nerve for treatment of ethmoid sinus and nasal cavity malignant neoplasms. These tumors involved the nasal cavity, ethmoids, medial orbital wall and/or the ethmoidomaxillary plate. The purpose of the treatment technique was to avoid irradiation of the sensitive parts of the eye, *i.e.*, lens and cornea, while covering the tumor adequately and delivering a very high dose to the main bulk of disease. The basic field arrangement was an anterior L-shaped portal transecting the ipsilateral globe with the patient looking superiorly and laterally to avoid corneal irradiation. With this technique, treatment was given half with ^{60}Co and half with 22 Mev x-rays.

Doses were calculated from isodose curves obtained from simulated localization films and patient contours. A minimum tumor dose of 6,000 rads was given at 6 to 8 cm depth in 6 weeks. The dose to the main bulk of the tumor was 7,000 to 7,500 rads in 6 weeks. Retinal and optic nerve doses were determined in retrospect by superimposing on these isodose curves appropriate diagrams from a cross-sectional anatomy atlas (Figs. 2-51 and 52A).

While sparing the most sensitive parts of

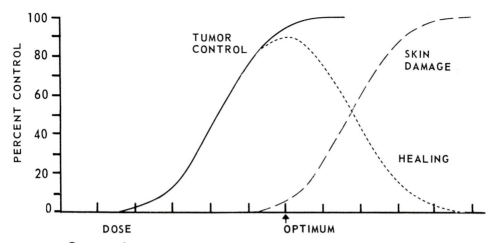

Curves of increasing percentage tumor control respectively with skin damage and healing after Holthusen.

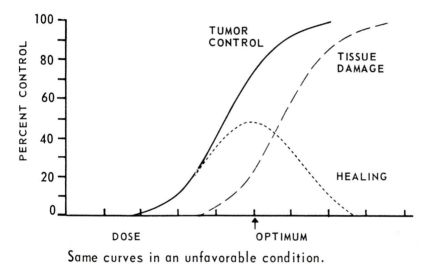

Same curves in an unfavorable condition.

FIG. 2-50. Tumor control curves versus complication curves. *Top:* Curves of increasing percentage of tumor control with skin damage and healing. *Bottom:* Same curves in an unfavorable condition. (Courtesy: Holthusen: *Strahlentherapie,* 57, 254, 1936.)

the eye, this technique delivered high doses to the retina and optic nerve which lie adjacent to the medial orbital wall when the patient is looking laterally. Because of the depth of the tumor the dose was chosen to include the entire ethmoid sinus, and sometimes the sphenoid sinus, the dose to the retina and/or optic nerve was 15 to 25 per cent greater than the minimum tumor dose.

The effectiveness of this technique in treating the entire primary tumor and the careful selection of cases is reflected by only one of the 30 patients having had disease recur behind the blocked part of the eye. This was achieved despite a 20 per cent (6 of 30) incidence of bony orbit destruction found on tomograms. The local control rate for the squamous cell carcinomas alone is 87 per cent (13 of 15).

This technique has preserved the lens, as

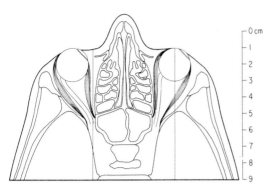

FIG. 2-51. Frontal section through globes, optic nerves, and paranasal sinuses. Vertical lines approximate limits of the field. (Modified from: Pernkopf: *Atlas of Topographical and Applied Human Anatomy,* Vol. I, Philadelphia, W. B. Saunders Co., p. 51, 1963.)

only 2 patients developed cataracts. However, 9 patients developed loss of vision. These 9 patients lost sight in 12 eyes because of 1) macular and retinal degeneration, 2) optic nerve atrophy, and 3) central retinal artery thrombosis.

There is a definite dose-time-effect relationship in those patients who lost their sight from retinal degeneration and optic nerve atrophy (Fig. 2-53). When Ellis' nominal standard dose is used, all of the doses are

above 2,000 rets. The one patient with preservation of vision above this level has had 2 lens prescription changes since irradiation 8 years ago. With this correction, he has useful vision, with the irradiated eye functioning as well as the contralateral eye.

No patient having received less than 2,000 rets has lost his sight from retinal degeneration or optic nerve atrophy. However, 2 patients of 7 had central retinal artery thrombosis. Neither patient had a history of diabetes or vascular disease.

The use of posterior lateral wedges eliminates the excessive dose to the retina and optic nerve (Fig. 2-52B). However, it may result in less effective tumor control because the main bulk of the neoplasm receives a smaller dose than in the technique described. If the control rate falls too low, the previous technique will be reinstituted.

Planning and Choice of Technique

It is a common statement that there are various ways to achieve the same results. That is not correct if one analyzes not only the "crude control" but all phases of the end

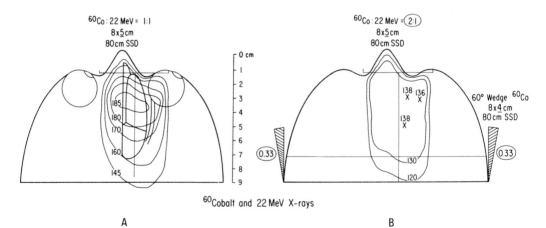

A   B

FIG. 2-52. A. Isodose distribution with half ^{60}Co and half 22 Mev x-rays. The globes and right optic nerve, nasal cavity, ethmoids, and sphenoid sinus have been sketched in for convenience. **B.** Recently instituted portal arrangement including lateral 60° wedge filters. (Courtesy: Shukovsky and Fletcher: *Radiology,* 104, 629, 1972.)

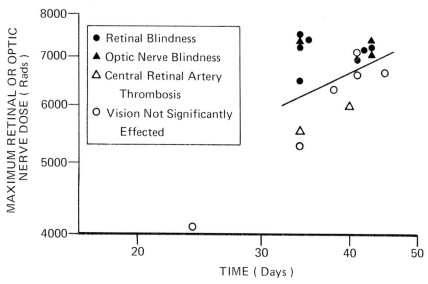

FIG. 2-53. Time-dose scattergram for loss of vision. (Courtesy: Shukovsky and Fletcher: *Radiology, 104, 629, 1972.*)

results, including complications and sequelae.

Modalities of treatment must be chosen which deliver adequate tumor doses with the least irradiation of surrounding structures. Techniques should be selected which buffer one another; techniques with additive drawbacks should not be combined. The ease by which lethal tumor doses can be delivered by megavoltage techniques should not lead to the abandonment of interstitial gamma-ray implants for oral cavity cancers and of intracavitary radium therapy for cancers of the uterine cervix. External beam therapy, which irradiates much larger volumes of tissue to high doses, results in a greater incidence of both minor and major complications and sequelae.

The utilization of various radiotherapeutic techniques should not be merely blind duplication from papers, textbooks or short observation periods in a radiotherapy center. The following basic features of a treatment plan must be thoroughly understood and tested. They are:

1) The basic dosage determination.
2) The beam characteristics.

3) The precise description of tumor dose(s).

4) The volume distribution and the anatomical structures included in this volume.

5) The dose-time fractionation schedule, *i.e.,* over-all time and total number of fractions for each portal.

Interaction of Surgery and Irradiation

Introduction

The combination of surgery and irradiation has been used since the early days of the century, either as preoperative or post-operative or separately for the primary lesion and the regional lymphatics. The evaluation of the effectiveness of combined therapy has been cyclically positive and negative.

The quantitative data now available on the doses of irradiation which produce percentages of control of subclinical disease has given a rational basis for the planning of strategies which fit the varied clinical situations presented by different organs and histologies.

The basis in all strategies is that moderate amounts of irradiation eradicate a high percentage of subclinical aggregates of cancer cells at the periphery of the central mass, along routes of spread and in the regional lymphatics.

Preoperative Irradiation

The purposes of preoperative irradiation are:

1) To eradicate subclinical disease which might have spread beyond the margins of the surgical resection.

2) To diminish the number of viable cells so that implants in the surgical area are less probable. Experimental tumor biology has shown that a large number of viable cells are required to establish an implant.

3) Theoretically, preoperative irradiation should diminish the incidence of distant metastases. Surgical manipulations increase the number of tumor cells circulating in the blood but no correlation has yet been shown between the number of circulating cancer cells in the blood of patients and the incidence of distant metastases.

Even relatively modest doses given preoperatively have a measure of effectiveness. This is particularly true for subclinical disease which does not contain anoxic cells.

Postoperative Radiotherapy

Although radical surgical procedures interfere with the blood supply to the region, the tissues are not anoxic and subclinical aggregates of cancer cells do not have markedly lowered radiosensitivity even if located in somewhat hypoxic tissues. Six thousand rads can be given to the area of a resected primary lesion if it is uncertain whether disease was left behind, in particular, in poorly vascularized tumor beds (bone, cartilage, fascial planes, nerve sheaths, etc.). Five thousand rads can be given to the regional lymphatics without producing sequelae. These doses are adequate to eradicate subclinical

disease remaining after the surgical procedure. Irradiation should be started within a few weeks after surgery, before the cells have grown into a gross recurrence.

Combination of Conservative Surgery with Irradiation

The inability of any type of superradical surgery to eradicate cancer when advanced past a certain stage, is due to the diffuse spread of the disease. More extensive dissection or thinning of flaps do not alter the outcome. This point is well illustrated in advanced cancers of the breast and pyriform sinus. A conservative procedure limited to removal of the main masses is a useful approach in many situations.

The sequence of irradiation and the surgical procedure varies depending upon the site of disease. For large neck nodes, 5,000 rads are usually given to the whole neck followed by a modified neck dissection. For large lesions of the uterine cervix a conservative extrafascial hysterectomy is done after irradiation. Removal of the mass in the breast by simple mastectomy and simple excision of palpable nodes in the axilla is done first, followed by irradiation. A simple mastectomy can be done without complications after 5,000 rads but tradition prevails to perform the surgical procedure first. Node dissections which are not truly "en bloc" dissections, such as the retroperitoneal lymphandenectomies, are best combined with 5,000 rads, either given postoperatively or 2,500 rads preoperatively and 2,500 rads postoperatively.

The usefulness of this approach will be dealt in details in the various chapters. A new method is the "shelling out" of the soft tissue sarcomas followed by irradiation of the operated field. Another area which should become prominent in local control rate is the management of the rectosigmoid adenocarcinomas; the incidence of pelvic recurrences should be diminished and colostomies could be eliminated with the renewed use of an anterior instead of an abdomino-peritoneal resection, followed by irradiation unless the tumor is quite early.

The Quality of Life

The goal of cancer treatment, be it surgical, radiotherapeutic or a combination of both, must be not only to eradicate the disease and keep the patient alive, but to maintain for the patient a desirable quality of life. Sequelae, even though they may not be fatal or crippling, may still diminish normal functions and create cosmetic blemishes incompatible with a normal life. For instance, pneumonitis resulting from high dose mediastinal irradiation for lymphoma produces minimal to moderate dyspnea, which does not leave the patient in a normal state. Mutilating surgical procedures may leave the patient an emotional cripple, with no desire to live. Furthermore, sequelae which initially are minor may become symptomatic later in life with limitation of the individual's activity.

Treatment must be based on the rules rather than the exceptions of tumor behavior and treatment should not be extraradical to avoid any possible untoward happenings. Contralateral neck metastases rarely develop in patients with lesions of the buccal mucosa; only an occasional patient dies from lack of control of contralateral metastases. It is, therefore, not justified to irradiate both sides of the neck with 5,000 rads in all patients. This cannot be done without irradiating the oral cavity and oropharynx mucosa with some resulting dryness.

Radicalism, both in dose and irradiated volume, must be balanced against the probability of lack of control of the primary lesion and/or the appearance of new disease and the chances of combating the disease if it does appear. The physician has the choice to lose one or two patients out of 100 or to produce some measure of complications or sequelae in all. This decision, as to importance of the quality of life, remains a matter of philosophy, varying with the environment, the patient, and the oncological team.

BIBLIOGRAPHY

1. Atkins, H. L., and Horrigan, W. D.: Treatment of locally advanced carcinoma of breast with roentgen therapy and simple mastectomy, *Amer. J. Roentgen.*, 85, 860, 1961.
2. Baclesse, F.: Carcinoma of the larynx, *Brit. J. Radiol.*, Supp. 3, 1949.
3. Baclesse, F.: L'etalement ou le "Fractionnement" dans la roentgentherapie seule des epitheliomas du pharynx et du larynx, de L'uterus et du vagin, du sein (Etude de 1.449 cas), *Acta Unio Internationalis Contra Cancrum*, 9, 32, 1953.
4. Baclesse, F.: Clinical experience with ultra-fractionated roentgen therapy. In *Progress in Radiation Therapy*, F. Buschke, ed., New York, Grune and Stratton, 1958.
5. Baclesse, F.: Radiotherapy of carcinoma metastatic to the cervical lymph nodes. In *Treatment of Cancer & Allied Diseases. The Head and Neck*, Vol. 3, 2nd ed. (New York, Paul B. Hoeber, Inc.), p. 641, 1959.
6. Bergonié, J., and Tribondeau, L.: Interpretation of some results of radiotherapy and an attempt at determining a logical technique of treatment, *Radiat. Res.*, 11, 587, 1959. Translation of original article in *C. R. Acad. des Sci.*, 143, 983, 1906.
7. Calle, R.: Personal communication, 1972.
8. Castro, J. R., Issa, P., and Fletcher, G. H.: Carcinoma of the cervix treated by external irradiation alone, *Radiology*, 95, 163, 1970.
9. Chen, Kuang, Y., and Fletcher, G. H.: Malignant tumors of the nasopharynx, *Radiology*, 99, 165, 1971.
10. Cohen, L.: Clinical radiation dosage (Part I), *Brit. J. Radiol.*, 22, 160, 1949.
11. Cohen, L.: Clinical radiation dosage (Part II), *Brit. J. Radiol.*, 22, 706, 1949.
12. Cohen, L., and Kerrich, J. E.: Estimation of biological dosage factors in clinical radiotherapy, *Brit. J. Cancer*, 5, 180, 1951.
13. Cohen, L.: Radiotherapy in breast cancer. 1. The dose-time relationship: Theoretical considerations, *Brit. J. Radiol.*, 25, 636, 1952.
14. Cohen, L.: Theoretical iso-survival formulae for fractionated radiation therapy, *Brit. J. Radiol.*, 41, 522, 1968.

15. Cutler, S. J., and Connelly, R. R.: Mammary cancer trends, *Cancer,* 23, 767, 1969.

16. Dutreix, J., Wambersie, A. and Bounik, C.: Cellular recovery in human skin reactions. Application to dose/number of fractions/overall time relationship in radiotherapy, In preparation.

17. Ellis, F.: Tolerance dosage in radiotherapy with 200 Kv x-rays, 15, 348, 1942.

18. Ellis, F.: Nominal standard dose and the ret, *Brit. J. Radiol.,* 44, 101, 1971.

19. Fletcher, G. H.: Time-dose relationships in radiation biology as applied to radiotherapy. BNL (C-57) Biology and Medicine TID-4500, Brookhaven National Laboratories, Upton, New York, p. 260, 1970.

20. Fletcher, G. H.: Dose response curve of subclinical aggregates of epithelial cells and its practical application in the management of human cancers, In *Biological and Clinical Basis of Radiosensitivity,* Milton Friedman, ed., A collection of papers presented at an International Conference at the Instituto Regina Elena, Rome, Italy, October 1971, Publication pending.

21. Fletcher, G. H.: Local results of irradiation in the primary management of localized breast cancer, *Cancer,* 29, 545, 1972.

22. Fletcher, G. H.: Clinical dose response curves of human malignant epithelial tumors, *Brit. J. Radiol.,* In press.

23. Fletcher, G. H., MacComb, W. S., and Shalek, R. J.: *Radiation Therapy in the Management of Cancer of the Oral Cavity and Oropharynx* (monograph), Springfield, Ill., Charles C Thomas, 1962.

24. Fletcher, G. H., and Klein, R.: Dose-time-volume relationship in radiation therapy of laryngeal tumors, *Radiology,* 82, 1032, 1964.

25. Fletcher, G. H., and Montague, E. D.: Radical irradiation of advanced breast cancer, *Amer. J. Roentgen.,* 93, 573, 1965.

26. Friedman, M., and Pearlman, A. W.: Time-dose studies in irradiation of mycosis fungiodes, *Radiology,* 66, 374, 1956.

27. Gelinas, Michel, and Fletcher, G. H.: Incidence and causes of local failure of irradiation in squamous cell carcinoma of the faucial arch, tonsillar fossa and base of tongue, *Radiology* (publication pending).

28. Grant, B. P., and Fletcher, G. H.: Analysis of complications following megavoltage therapy

for squamous cell carcinomas of the tonsillar area, *Amer. J. Roentgen.,* 96, 28, 1966.

29. Griscom, N. T., and Wang, C. C.: Radiation therapy of inoperable breast carcinoma, *Radiology,* 79, 18, 1962.

30. Hale, C. H., and Holmes, G. E.: Carcinoma of skin: Influence of dosage on the success of treatment, *Radiology,* 48, 563, 1947.

31. Henk, J. M., Kunkler, P. B., Shah, N. K., Smith, C. W., Sutherland, W. H., and Wassif, S. B.: Hyperbaric oxygen in radiotherapy of head and neck carcinoma, *Clin. Radiol.,* 21, 223, 1970.

32. Herring, D. F., and Compton, D. M. J.: The degree of precision required in the radiation dose delivered in cancer radiotherapy. Report #EMI-216 from Enviro-Med. Inc., La Jolla, California, July 10, 1970.

33. Holthusen H.: Erfahrungen über die verträglich keitsgrenze für Röntgenstrahlen und deren Nutzanwendung zur verhütung von schäden, *Strahlentherapie,* 57, 254, 1936.

34. Horiot, J-C, Fletcher, G. H., Ballantyne, A., and Lindberg, R. D.: Analysis of failures of early vocal cord cancers, *Radiology,* 103, 663, 1972.

35. Howes, A. E.: An estimation of changes in the proportions and absolute numbers of hypoxic cells after irradiation of transplanted C_3H mouse mammary tumours, *Brit. J. Radiol.,* 42, 441, 1969.

36. Innes, G.: Personal communication, 1962.

37. Jolles, B., and Mitchell, R. G.: Optimal skin tolerance dose levels, *Brit. J. Radiol.,* 20, 405, 1947.

38. Kohn, H. I.: In *Progress in Radiation Therapy,* New York, Grune & Stratton, p. 62, 1958.

39. Kronig, S., u. Friedrich, W.: Physikalische und biologische Grundlagen der Strahlentherapie, *Sonderband der Strahlentherapiem,* 1918.

40. Lenz, Maurice: Tumor dosage and results in roentgen therapy of cancer of the breast, *Amer. J. Roentgen.,* 56, 67, 1946.

41. Lenz, Maurice: Tissue dosage in roentgentherapy of mammary cancer, *Acta Radiol.,* 18, 583, 1947.

42. Lindberg, R. D., and Fletcher, G. H.: Clinical experiences with altered fractionation, *Revista Interamericana de Radiologia,* 7, 15, 1972.

43. MacComb, W. S. and Quimby, E. H.: The rate of recovery of human skin from the

effects of hard or soft roentgen rays or gamma rays, *Radiology*, 27, 196, 1936.

44. Miescher, G.: Erfolge der karzinombehandlung an der Dermatologischen Klinik Zurich. Einzeitige Höchstodsis und Fraktionierte Behandlung, *Strahlentherapie*, 49, 65, 1934.

45. Montague, E. D.: Experience with altered fractionation in radiation therapy of breast cancer, *Radiology*, 90, 962, 1968.

46. Northrop, M. F., Fletcher, G. H., Jesse, R. H., and Lindberg, R. D.: Evolution of neck disease in patients with primary squamous cell carcinoma of the oral tongue, floor of mouth, and palatine arch and clinically positive neck nodes neither fixed nor bilateral, *Cancer*, 29, 23, 1972.

47. Paterson, R.: *The Treatment of Malignant Disease by Radium and X-ray; Being a Practice of Radiotherapy*, Baltimore, Williams & Wilkins Company, 1949.

48. Paterson, R.: Studies in optimum dosage, *Brit. J. Radiol.*, 25, 505, 1952.

49. Pernkopf, E.: *Atlas of Topographical and Applied Human Anatomy*, Vol. I, Philadelphia, W. B. Saunders Co., p. 51, 1963.

50. Regaud, C., and Ferroux, R.: Discordance des effets de rayons X, d'und part dans le testicule, par le fractionnment de la dose, *Compt. rend Soc. de Biol.*, 97, 431, 1927.

51. Reisner, A.: Hauterythem und Röntgenstrahlung, *Ergben. d. med. Strahlenforschg.*, 6, 1, 1933.

52. Schwarz, G.: Heilung teifliegender Karzinome durch Röntgenbestrahlung von der Körperoberflache, *München. Med. Wchnschr.*, 61, 1733, 1914.

53. Shukovsky, L. J.: Dose-time volume relationships in squamous cell carcinoma of the supraglottic larynx, *Amer. J. Roentgen.*, 108, 27, 1970.

54. Shukovsky, L. J., and Fletcher, G. H.: Retinal and optic nerve complications in a high dose irradiation technique of ethmoid sinus and nasal cavity, *Radiology*, 104, 629, 1972.

55. Shukovsky, L. J., and Fletcher, G. H.: Time-dose and tumor-volume relationships in the irradiation of squamous cell carcinoma of the tonsillar fossa, *Radiology*, In press.

56. Sinclair, W. K.: The specification of radiation dose in publications, *Radiology*, 71, 575, 1958.

57. Sinclair, W. K., Laughlin, J. S., Rossi, H. H., Ter Pogossian, M., and Moos, W. S.: Intercomparison of x-ray exposure using Victoreen dose meters at various energies, particularly 22 Mevp, *Radiology*, 70, 736, 1958.

58. Strandqvist, M.: Studien über die Kumulative Wirkung der Röntgenstrahlen bei Fraktionierung, *Acta Radiol.* (Stockholm), Supplement 55, 1944.

59. Suit, H. D., Lindberg, R. D., and Fletcher, G. H.: Prognostic significance of extent of tumor regression at completion of radiation therapy, *Radiology*, 84, 1100, 1965.

60. vanPeperzeel, H. A.: Effects of single doses of radiation on lung metastases in man and experimental animals, *European J. Cancer*, Publication pending.

61. vonEssen, C. F.: Roentgen therapy of skin and lip carcinoma: Factors influencing success and failure, *Amer. J. Roentgen.*, 83, 556, 1960.

62. Votava, Charles, Jr., Fletcher, G. H., Jesse, R. H., and Lindberg, R. D.: Management of cervical nodes either fixed or bilateral from primary squamous cell carcinoma of the oral cavity and faucial arch, *Radiology*, 105, 417, 1972.

63. Wilson, Charles S., and Hall, Eric J.: On the advisability of treating all fields at each radiotherapy session, *Radiology*, 98, 419, 1971.

64. Withers, H. R., and Suit, H. D.: Is oxygen important in the radiocurability of human tumors? In *Biological and Clinical Basis of Radiosensitivity*, Milton Friedman, ed., A collection of papers presented at an International Conference at the Instituto Regina Elena, Rome, Italy, October 1971, *Publication pending*.

65. Zuppinger, A.: Spätveränderungen nach protrahiert-fraktionierter Röntgenbestrahlung im Bereich der oberen Luft und Speisewege, *Strahlentherapie*, 70, 361, 1941.

3. Head and Neck

Feeding Head and Neck Patients Undergoing Radiation Therapy

BLANCHE POLUNSKY and MURIEL PELHAM

Maintenance of good nutrition is necessary during the treatment of cancer patients. Feeding the cancer patient who is receiving radiation therapy in the head and neck area presents various problems. The dietitian, as a member of the team of therapists, can help guide the patient in adjusting his eating habits to those foods which he can tolerate and hence prevent weight loss and the resulting complications.

At the start of a 6 week course of treatment, the patient usually has little discomfort and follows his normal eating pattern. However, it is during this first week of treatment that the dietitian should have her first meeting with the patient. If possible, she should speak to the patient and to his family, since at this time, it may be difficult for the patient to absorb the advice given by the dietitian because the period is one of great adjustment for him. It is a period of severe mental stress and strain, discomfort and pain connected with the disease. It is better for the dietitian to meet the patient and his family in an area removed from the examining room; in a relaxed atmosphere, the patient will discuss his problems more freely. It is essential for the dietitian to establish rapport with the patient, in order to maintain his confidence in her assistance later as problems develop.

A routine should be instituted for each patient with follow-up meetings scheduled at least once a week unless further problems arise. The results of the weekly interviews should be charted on a simple form. His weight should be noted at the start of treatment and he should be weighed each week since the loss or gain in pounds is an indication of how well the patient is eating. A basic meal plan including the addition of supplementary feedings must be started at the beginning of therapy and this regimen with modifications should be followed during the total period of treatment. It is important for the diet to be relatively high in total calories and proteins, even if the distribution of other nutrients varies from the normal requirements temporarily during this time. A copy of the diet should be given to the patient for reference during the treatment period.

Depending upon the extent and the location of the treated area, the dietitian from experience, is aware of the reactions to foods which the patient will face. For example, patients who undergo radiation therapy in the areas of the vocal cord, the thyroid, or the ear, do not seem to have eating problems. Such patients have gained 4 to 8 pounds during the 6 weeks of treatment. However, the patients who are being treated because of tumors in the tonsillar region, the palate, the tongue, and especially in the nasopharynx area, experience the most severe reactions to their therapy and have the greatest loss of weight. Even with continued instruction, such patients may lose 3 to 15 pounds during their treatment period. Dietary instruction should be oriented to the psychological, as well as the physical, needs of the patient and should be given in a firm but encouraging manner. The concept of the dietitian having a special interest in his problems appeals to him and the patient generally reacts favorably to her suggestions. The dietitian must recognize his need to eat and act like other people, so that even though his food may be modified in texture and consistency, it is important to maintain his meal plan as close to normal as possible.

Generally, during the second and third week of treatment, he will experience some reactions to food. One of the first food reactions seems to be a burning sensation in the throat when the patient swallows citrus juices. The substitution of bland fruit nectars or apply juice may be suggested since these are better tolerated. He will also experience some loss of appetite, loss of sense of taste, and soreness of the mouth. The dietitian must encourage the patient and emphasize the importance of eating even though he is not hungry or it hurts him to swallow. She can teach him to substitute food aromas for the sense of taste needed to stimulate his appetite. Since extremes in food temperature increase the soreness in the mouth, it is better to have all foods served at room temperature. Highly seasoned foods should be eliminated during this period since the spices tend to irritate the membranes of the mouth.

As the weeks progress, the reactions become more severe. The patient encounters extreme difficulty in swallowing and will stop eating unless continually encouraged by the dietitian and his family. One complication of his treatment is a lack of saliva, thus foods tend to "stick" in his throat and give a sensation of nausea. Moistening the food with gravy or sauces will help the patient in swallowing. Medications also can be used

before meals to anesthetize the throat area so it is less painful to swallow. Again, the patient's diet should be modified to adjust texture, consistency and size portions depending upon the patient's needs. As the need arises, raw or coarse foods are eliminated, meats are ground, and the diet changed to a soft, semisoft, or liquid consistency. Food supplements should be included as an additional source of calories and protein, but the patient should be cautioned to use these feedings to supplement rather than supplant his three meals a day.

It is interesting to note that during a 3 year study period when the dietitian consulted with each patient undergoing radiotherapy treatment, there was a considerable decrease in the number of patients who needed to be tube fed or admitted to the hospital because of severe weight loss. This psychological need for the patient to discuss his problems with the dietitian must be emphasized.

In some instances, however, patients experience such excruciating pain when swallowing that the physician may decide that a tube feeding is more desirable. As a general rule, when a patient has lost 10 pounds by the third or fourth week of treatment, a nasogastric tube is inserted and the patient is fed with a formula. Again the dietitian must consider the psychological effect on this patient when she assists him. Food—real food—and odors and flavors of real food are important to people and that is why she should recommend using real foods in these tube feedings. Again the basic plan of three meals a day is followed. Any liquid foods which are readily definable, such as milk, coffee, or juice are served individually, in addition to the formula made of blended foods. The patient should have cream and sugar for his coffee and salt to season his food. The formula will vary in color in accordance with the foods used. Different juices, cereals, meats, and vegetables should be used for each meal to avoid the monotony of the same thing all the time.

The importance of getting the cancer patient to eat cannot be overemphasized. Each patient must be handled individually and the dietitian should work with him very closely to adapt his diet to his needs as his treatment progresses. Her understanding and encouragement during this critical time, helps maintain the nutritional well being of the patient and assists him throughout the treatment period.

When the patient is ready for discharge, the dietitian should instruct him about his future meal plans. Generally the patient will experience some problems for about two weeks after his last treatment but then he will gradually progress to the normal diet. If possible, the dietitian should plan to see the patient during his follow-up visits to the hospital to ensure that he is maintaining good nutritional progress.

Diet Modifications

Mechanical Diet

This is a modification in texture of the regular diet and is recommended for use when chewing or swallowing become difficult. The preparation methods and the foods allowed are in accordance with individual patient tolerance rather than therapeutic restriction. The meat is ground in order to facilitate chewing and foods should be moist for ease of swallowing; other modifications may be made according to individual patient's needs.

Suggested Meal Plan

BREAKFAST

Pear nectar, cooked farina, scrambled egg, toast, butter, jelly, milk, coffee or tea, cream, sugar.

DINNER

Cream soup, ground roast beef with gravy, mashed potatoes, buttered carrots, bread, butter, chocolate pudding, milk, coffee or tea, cream, sugar.

SUPPER

Ground chicken with cream gravy, buttered noodles, green peas, bread, butter, applesauce, milk, coffee or tea, cream, sugar.

Baby Soft Diet

This diet is indicated when the patient is having extreme difficulty in chewing or swallowing. It is a modification of the mechanical diet. The meats and vegetables are blended in order to be of a smooth consistency.

Suggested Meal Plan

BREAKFAST

Pear nectar, cooked farina, scrambled egg, milk, coffee or tea, cream, sugar.

DINNER

Strained cream soup, blended beef with gravy, thin mashed potatoes, blended carrots, chocolate pudding, milk, coffee or tea, cream, sugar.

SUPPER

Strained cream soup, blended chicken with cream gravy, buttered noodles, blended peas, baked custard, milk, coffee or tea, cream, sugar.

When only small servings of food are tolerated at mealtime, between-meal supplementary feedings should be added.

Supplementary Feedings

Some of the recipes for the supplementary feedings used in this hospital are as follows:

FORTIFIED MILK

One cup milk, ⅓ cup instant nonfat dry milk. Mix together.

HIGH PROTEIN EGGNOG

One cup milk, 2 eggs, ⅓ cup instant nonfat dry milk, 1 teaspoon sugar, ½ teaspoon vanilla. Beat egg well, add part of milk and instant nonfat dry milk, dissolve, add rest of milk, sugar, and vanilla.

HIGH PROTEIN MILKSHAKE

One cup milk, 1 scoop ice cream, ⅓ cup instant nonfat dry milk (for malt add 2 teaspoons malt). Flavor: 2 tablespoons chocolate syrup, or 1 teaspoon vanilla, or 2 tablespoons coffee. Dissolve instant nonfat dry milk; add flavoring and ice cream. Beat well.

SUSTAGEN OR GEVRAL

To one cup milk add 4 tablespoons Sustagen or 2 tablespoons Gevral. For flavor add 2 tablespoons chocolate syrup, or 1 teaspoon vanilla, or 2 tablespoons coffee, or ½ can strained baby banana.

Other commercial products are also available which can be used for supplementary feedings. Some readily acceptable products which provide a palatable and nourishing drink are Meritene, Nutrament, and Instant Breakfast.

Tube Feeding

Regular Tube Feeding

This diet is based on the baby soft diet. It is adequate in all essential nutrients as established by the National Research Council except niacin. It may be used in instances where the patient is unable to chew or swallow, but must be fed by tube. The composition of this regular tube feeding is as follows: 2,765 calories, 90 gm protein, 145 gm fat, 275 gm carbohydrate, total volume 3,600 cc.

Preparation of Formula

The ingredients (except eggs) should be heated until lukewarm. Everything including eggs, is then blended together in an electric blender, or by rotary beater, strained, and administered at body temperature. If the complete formula is not used at once, the remainder should be refrigerated, then heated to body temperature before serving. The glasses of formula should be stirred before pouring into the tube in order to suspend the solids which tend to settle to the bottom on standing.

Suggested Daily Meal Plan

BREAKFAST

One cup citrus juice (as orange, grapefruit, or tomato juice). Three glasses formula made of: ½ cup strained cooked refined cereal (as farina, cream of wheat, cream of rice), 1 raw egg, 1½ cups milk, ¼ cup corn syrup, 1 tablespoon oil. One cup coffee, ½ ounce cream, 2 teaspoons sugar.

LUNCH AND SUPPER

One cup juice. Three glasses formula made of: 1 jar (3½ ounces) strained baby meat, ½ cup strained cooked vegetable, 2 cups milk, 2 tablespoons oil. One cup coffee, ½ ounce cream, 2 teaspoons sugar.

Light Tube Feeding

This diet eliminates meat and vegetables from the formula. This tube feeding may be indicated when the patient is unable to tolerate these foods. It is adequate in all essential nutrients as established by the National Research Council except niacin and thiamine. The composition of this light tube feeding is as follows: 2,100 calories, 80 gm protein, 100 gm fat, 220 gm carbohydrate, total volume 3,300 cc.

Preparation of Formula

The ingredients (except eggs) should be heated until lukewarm. Everything, including eggs, is then blended together in an electric blender, or by rotary beater, strained, and administered at body temperature. If the complete formula is not used at once, the remainder should be refrigerated, then heated to body temperature just before serving. The glasses of formula should be stirred before pouring into the tube in order to suspend the solids, which tend to settle to the bottom on standing.

Suggested Daily Meal Plan

BREAKFAST

One-half cup citrus juice (orange, grapefruit, or tomato juice). Three glasses of formula made of: $\frac{1}{2}$ cup strained cooked refined cereal (as farina, cream of wheat, cream of rice), 1 raw egg, $1\frac{1}{2}$ cups milk, $\frac{1}{4}$ cup corn syrup, 1 tablespoon oil. One cup coffee, $\frac{1}{2}$ ounce cream, 2 teaspoons sugar.

LUNCH AND SUPPER

One-half cup juice. Three glasses formula made of: 2 cups milk, 2 raw eggs, 1 cup water. One cup coffee, $\frac{1}{2}$ ounce cream, 2 teaspoons sugar.

No Milk Tube Feeding

This feeding is based on the baby soft diet, but eliminates milk. This diet may be indicated when a patient is allergic or unable to tolerate milk, or when diarrhea develops. It is low in fat and below the recommended daily dietary allowance for calcium, niacin, and thiamine, as established by the National Research Council. The composition of this no milk tube feeding is as follows: 2,650 calories, 80 gm protein, 125 gm fat, 300 gm carbohydrate, total volume 3,600 cc.

Preparation of Formula

The ingredients (except eggs) should be heated until lukewarm. Everything, including eggs, is then blended together in an electric blender or by rotary beater, strained, and administered at body temperature. If the complete formula is not used at once, the remainder should be refrigerated, then heated to body temperature before serving. The glasses of formula should be stirred before pouring into the tube in order to suspend the solids, which tend to settle to the bottom on standing.

Suggested Daily Meal Plan

BREAKFAST

One cup citrus juice (orange, grapefruit, or tomato juice). Three glasses formula made of: 1 cup strained cooked refined cereal (farina, cream of wheat, cream of rice), 2 raw eggs, $1\frac{1}{2}$ cups water, $\frac{1}{4}$ cup corn syrup, 2 tablespoons oil. One cup coffee, 2 teaspoons sugar.

LUNCH AND SUPPER

One cup juice. Three glasses formula made of: 1 jar ($3\frac{1}{2}$ ounces) strained baby meat, $\frac{1}{2}$ cup strained cooked vegetable, 2 raw eggs, $1\frac{1}{2}$ cups juice, $\frac{1}{2}$ cup water, 2 tablespoons oil.

Dental Care in the Irradiated Patient

Basic Problems

Changes occur in irradiated bone and are of prime importance in the production of complications. Among these changes are:

1) The numbers of osteoblasts and osteoclasts are diminished.

2) Vessels of irradiated bone show a loss of tonus and a decreased diameter.

3) Normal metabolism of bone is impaired.

Consequently, there is increased susceptibility to infection and the processes of repair are extremely limited or nonexistent.

Subclinical or chronic states of infection can often be controlled by normal bone metabolism. In irradiated bone, these types of infections set up a progressive series of events which often leads to an acute infectious episode. Infection in irradiated bone gives rise to more destruction of bone because of the lysis action of the infected material itself. Leukocytes at the site of infection cause further breakdown by means of additional resorption.

Because of the effect of radiation on healing processes, it is difficult for continued healing to occur after radiation therapy has started. Reepithelialization is slow or impossible and because the body's defense mechanism is weakened the bone can become infected.

In 1966, a research project was initiated to find a correlation between the dental procedures performed prior to and after completion of radiotherapy and postirradiation complications, mainly bone necrosis and postirradiation decay of the teeth.

Of the patients, 60 per cent presented with all or some teeth remaining. The patients were put in one of four dental groups. The edentulous group and those whose teeth sta-

tus were classified as poor, fair, or good. Different procedures were done for patients in each group. Patients in the poor group had all remaining teeth extracted. Patients in the fair group had teeth which would be in the beam of radiation extracted. Patients in the good group had no extractions prior to the start of radiation therapy. It was found that the greatest amount of bone necrosis occurred in groups that had oral surgical intervention. The least amount of bone necrosis was found in the groups that had no oral surgery prior to the start of radiation therapy (Table 3-1).

Of the necroses in both the poor and the fair groups, 50 per cent occurred at the sites where extraction had been done prior to the start of radiation therapy.

It was believed that either a much longer healing time would be needed if teeth were to be extracted before irradiation or that a new set of policies for extraction should be initiated. At the present, new patients do not have elective extraction of teeth except when the tooth is in exceptionally poor condition and if it can be extracted atraumatically and adequately healed in a short time. Teeth that

Table 3-1. *Radiation Complications Study 1/66–12/70*

Group 1/1/66–12/31/70	Number of Patients	Number of Bone Necrosis
Group I Edentulous	124	12 (10%)
Group II Poor	46	10 (22%)
Group III Fair	81	32 (39.5%)
Group IV Good	53	10 (19%)

are expected to be a source of severe local irritation during and after treatment may be extracted.

The goals of teeth care if patients are to be treated with radiation are:

1) To decrease the incidence and severity of bone necrosis.

2) To reduce the incidence and severity of postirradiation decay of the teeth by the use of topically applied sodium fluoride.

3) To ultimately fit dentures after treatment reactions have subsided.

Preirradiation Care

Patients have a visual examination of all hard and soft tissues of the oral cavity, and all pertinent x-ray examinations. Dental findings recorded include: the condition of the mucosa and bone, teeth, gingival tissues, existing restorations, prostheses, complete charting of all dental findings. After complete evaluation of all dental findings, patients are presently placed in one of our four dental groups. Dental procedures are done according to groups.

Group I—Edentulous

1) Criteria for assignment to edentulous group.

a) The patient is edentulous upon clinical examination.

b) On radiographic examination, the patient may show root tips, cysts, or granulomas although no tooth fragments are visible.

2) Procedures performed for edentulous patients.

a) Surgical removal of any symptomatic cysts, infected retained root tips, or alveolar hyperplasia.

b) Complete hygiene instruction and precautionary instruction about trauma and premature use of a prosthesis.

Group II—Poor

1) Criteria for assignment to the dentally poor group.

a) Teeth are beyond repair by ordinary dental procedures.

b) Teeth that have decay which extends into or in close proximity of pulpal tissues throughout the mouth.

c) Generalized oral sepsis present.

d) Generalized periodontal problem.

e) May have chronic perapical abscesses or granulomas.

f) Previous dental restorations are of poor quality.

g) Marked mobility of the teeth.

h) X-ray examination reveals that at least one half of the bone supporting the roots of the teeth is missing.

2) Procedures performed for the dentally poor group.

a) Removal of *all* remaining teeth prior to irradiation with primary closure and adequate healing prior to start of radiation therapy.

b) Antibiotic coverage during healing stage.

c) Surgical preparation of the alveolar ridges to later support a prosthesis.

d) Complete hygiene instruction and precautionary instruction about premature use of a prosthesis and trauma.

Group III—Fair

1) Criteria for assignment to the dentally fair group.

a) Teeth are restorable by ordinary dental procedures.

b) Periodontal pockets are of less than 3 mm depth.

c) No oral sepsis present.

d) Carious lesions are not in close proximity to the pulp.

e) Mobility must be only slight or moderate if present.

f) X-ray examination shows at least one half of the bone still present around root surfaces of the teeth.

g) No more than 20 restorable carious lesions.

h) The condition of the existing restorations must not be of poor quality.

2) Procedures performed for the dentally fair group.

a) Removal of only those teeth that are completely nonsalvageable when adequate healing can be obtained in a short time.

b) Antibiotic coverage during the healing stage if teeth are extracted.

c) Dental prophylaxis of remaining teeth including brush training.

d) Restorations of remaining teeth as needed.

e) Construction of individual custom-made fluoride carriers.

Group IV—Good

1) Criteria for assignment to dentally good group.

a) The patient must not have a severe malocclusion.

b) Oral hygiene is good.

c) Few carious lesions are present.

d) The carious lesions that are present must not be in close proximity to the pulpal tissues and are correctable by conventional dental procedures.

e) Moderate mobility if present in an isolated area.

f) Existing dental restorations are of good quality.

g) The bone level upon radiographic examination is within normal limits for the patient's age group.

h) Dental prophylaxis is basically all that is needed to bring the periodontium into a good state of health.

2) Procedures for those of the dentally good group.

a) Periodontal evaluation and a dental prophylaxis including brush training.

b) Restorations in needed areas.

c) No extractions prior to radiation therapy.

d) Construction of individual custom-made fluoride carriers.

Patients in the dentally fair and dentally good groups are supplied with custom-made mouth guards of flexible plastic material when their use is indicated. The guards keep the patient from chewing or biting on the irradiated or edematous tissues. They are particularly useful when the lesion is located on the buccal mucosa, oral tongue, floor of mouth, or lip.

Preirradiation Extraction of Teeth

In cases where extraction of teeth is done prior to radiation therapy, gingival tissues must be approximated to eliminate socket openings and underlying bone is contoured so that primary closure is possible in extraction sites. All loose spicules and sharp projections of bone must be removed so that eventual puncture or erosion of bone through gingival tissues will not occur. Closure should be neither too loose nor too tight. Looseness of closure sites allows entrance of debris; closures that are too tight often tear the gingival tissues allowing bone exposure.

Sufficient time must be allowed, not only for the gingival tissues to heal but for adequate blood clot organization in the socket itself. It is from this original clot formation that all subsequent bone formation and healing will take place. Healing usually cannot be achieved in less than ten days and, in many cases three weeks or longer will be necessary depending upon the amount of trauma caused by removal of the teeth and contouring of the bone. In many cases where a traumatic procedure was performed, such as removal of impacted teeth or multiple difficult extractions, many weeks are necessary for healing because bone exposure and eventual bone necrosis develop without adequate healing of dental tissues.

One must be cautious in recommending extraction prior to therapy. Only teeth which are completely unsalvageable and which would require extraction shortly after treatment and those which, if left in place, would be the source of severe postirradiation complications (creation of soft tissue necrosis by friction) should be removed. If great difficulty in extraction of teeth is contemplated, or if it is thought that healing will be inadequate, or those cases where there is a problem of tumor growth, size, or contiguity to the teeth extracted, teeth should not be considered for elective removal.

Postirradiation Care

It is imperative to follow patients as closely as possible, at least every three months for the initial two years after therapy. Most complications occur within the first two years. If a patient is to develop postirradiation decay of the teeth, it often begins within one year from completion date of the radiation therapy.

Postirradiation Decay Factors

1) Radiation reduces normal salivary gland activity. It has been found that the majority of our patients presenting with radiation decay were treated with parallel opposed supervoltage portals coincident with irradiation of large volumes of salivary gland tissue.

2) The teeth are generally found to be involved with continuous plaque formation.

3) Fair to poor oral hygiene exists.

4) Patient's inability to understand or to perform home care correctly.

5) Teeth in the direct field of radiation are often found to have direct damage to the tooth structure itself. The major contributing factor appears in the amount of the saliva and in the reduction in the pH.

Radiation decay, usually found within the first year after radiation therapy, may progress for many years before total crown amputation of the teeth is seen. The process appears to quicken in mouths that have much root cementum exposed. Oral hygiene is an important factor in preventing progression of radiation decay and the amount of plaque formation or debris present is directly proportional to the advancement of the decay process.

PREVENTIVE MEASURES DEALING WITH IRRADIATION DECAY

In our study it was found that those patients who received fluoride, had adequate home care instruction, and good oral hygiene exhibited much less postirradiation decay of the teeth than those that did not have the benefit of cleaning, home care instruction, and fluoride (Table 3-2).

1) Cleaning: All patients are given dental prophalaxis whereby all debris, tartar, and stains are removed from the gingival crevices and all surfaces of the teeth. All tooth surfaces are polished to insure that no food debris can attach itself to the tooth.

2) Patient education: After the oral cavity is brought to a healthy state it is important that the patient be thoroughly educated and taught home care.

3) Construction of fluoride carriers (Fig. 3-1): These are individual custom-made mouth guards which are made for each patient. The patient is instructed in proper use of the guard and in local application of the fluoride solution to the gingiva and tooth surfaces.

4) Technique for fabrication of fluoride carriers: A technique for making the individual fluoride carriers used to help prevent postirradiation decay of the teeth is outlined. (Note: Ability to prevent decay is directly proportional to the patient's cooperation in the use of the fluoride and adequate home care.)

Impressions are made of the upper and lower arches with alginate impression material. These alginate impressions are then poured in dental stone. After they have set, the stone casts are separated from the impressions. The casts are trimmed in a horseshoe-shaped fashion. The lower cast has the lingual portion (where the floor of the mouth and the tongue section would be) trimmed away, forming a horseshoe. The upper cast has the palatal section trimmed out. This horseshoe appearance of the upper and lower arch facilitates molding of the material while making the individual guard.

Table 3-2. *Radiation Complications Study 1/66–12/70*

Group Randomized 1/1/66–12/31/70		Total No. Patients	Patients' Radiation Decay
Group III	Control	43	29 (67%)
Fair	Fluoride	38	13 (34%)
Group IV	Control	26	17 (65%)
Good	Fluoride	27	5 (18%)

Material used for making a mouth guard is "Sta-guard" plastic (Stalite, Inc., 4480 E. 11th Avenue, Hialeah, Florida 33013) used in conjunction with the vacutrol unit (Jelrus Technical Products Corp., New Hyde Park, New York) both of which are available through local dental supply houses. The Sta-guard material comes in boxes of 12

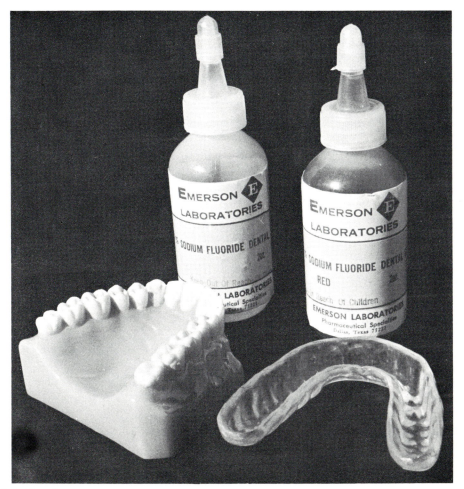

FIG. 3-1. Fluoride carrier.

sheets, $5\frac{1}{2} \times 5\frac{1}{2}$ inches square and approximately 3 mm in thickness. The material is placed in water at or above 180 degrees F until the material becomes very soft and flexible. The material is then placed upon the stone cast under the vacuum unit and compressed upon the stone cast. It is kept under vacuum for one minute; the pressure is released. While the material is still rather warm, it is further adapted using wet cellophane, into the interproximal areas of all the teeth. After this has been completed throughout both buccal and lingual sufaces, the cast and material, still together, are immersed in cold water to harden the material to its original state. After the material has cooled, cast is marked so that the proper length of the custom carrier can be determined for each arch. We like to include a margin of 3 to 4 mm excess beyond the gingival margin of the casts to allow for adequate fluoride coverage of all of the tooth surfaces. The Sta-guard material on the casts is marked with a felt-tip marking pencil. The material is removed from the stone cast and is trimmed with scissors at the marked line. After trimming with scissors there is a right angle in the junction line. The Sta-guard material is then smoothed on a lathe with the use of arbor bands. The Sta-guard individual mouth piece is again placed on the stone cast and is fire polished to remove any rough edges for better adaptation to the stone cast and is again smoothed with wet cellophane.

Fluoride Formula: The type of fluoride in use at this institution is a 1 per cent Sodium Fluoride Solution similar to that orginally used by the United States Public Health Service and by the Peace Corps. At the start of our program, the formula was prepared at M. D. Anderson Hospital. Presently we obtain our supply from Emerson Laboratories Inc., Dallas, Texas 75221. This change was necessary because of the large volume required. The type we are now using is made according to the following formula:

Sodium Fluoride	7.0	Gm
Sodium Phosphate, Tribasic	7.0	Gm
Sodium Carboxymethyl-cellulose ether sodium salt	19.6	Gm
Citric Acid	3.5	Gm
Saccharin Sodium	0.14	Gm
	or 140	mg

Add 1 cc of flavoring agents listed below:

This is mixed in a blender to a very viscous consistency. The flavoring agent consists of the following:

Lemon Oil, terpeneless	2.	cc
Orange Oil, terpeneless	2.	cc
Tween 20	4.	cc
Alcohol, Ethyl (95%)q.s. to	40.	cc

Caution: If a patient has a number of silicate cement fillings, it might be better to use a neutral gel, that is, one which does not contain citric acid. One may wish to use more or other flavoring agents.

In order to disclose plaque deposits clearly, we add 50 to 100 mg of Red #3 dye (Magnus, Mabee, and Reynard, Inc., 16 Desbrosses Street, New York, New York) to 100 cc of the Gel. Plaque and debris are clearly stained by this method. Two different solutions are prepared, one with the disclosing solution and one without. The patients are started on fluoride with the red disclosing solution. After they have demonstrated good oral hygiene and effective results from the use of this solution, they are switched to the clear solution with occasional use of the red solution to check oral hygiene and brushing techniques.

Being viscous, the material is put into a 2 to 3 oz squeeze bottle and is squeezed into the custom-made latex carrier. It is not necessary to fill the carrier completely, but only to *coat* it, since it is a custom-fitted appliance and any excess over that required for coating would simply spill out into the mouth. It unually takes, on a full upper arch where all teeth are present or a full lower, approximately 10 drops of fluoride gel. The fluoride is spread around by the use of a cotton tip applicator. The patients are instructed to brush their teeth first and have them completely clean, then wear the fluoride carrier with the solution in place for five minutes each day. Upon removal of the carrier they are told to empty the mouth and rinse. Any areas of plaque that have been disclosed by the disclosing solution should be brushed off. The patient is cautioned that if any excess does flow out into the mouth, it should be emptied into the basin. Even though it is of low toxicity, it is not wise for them to swallow any more than is necessary.

The patients are asked to use the topical fluoride for five minutes each day for an indefinite period of time. When the patient stops using the fluoride, the decay process once again resumes.

Close follow-up of these patients is mandatory. They must be seen quite often to be shown areas missed in brushing and the early areas of radiation decay requiring special attention. They must be constantly encouraged to use the fluoride.

MANAGEMENT OF RADIATION DECAY

There are several methods to manage failure to control radiation decay. Silver fillings or any other appropriate filling material can be used in conjunction with continued use of fluoride. After numerous gum line fillings have been done, the decay process appears to slow considerably because normal surfaces that would be attacked by the decay process are now filled. The material of choice is silver because it is easily patched and channeled for additional restorations. Sometimes, in the anterior mouth, synthetic porcelain fillings are used for aesthetic reasons. When treatment for the milder stages of radiation decay fails we often have the patient increase the time and frequency of applications to 10 or 15 minutes three times a day.

If the decay process is advanced, fluoride will only slightly halt progression. When the tooth is so badly decayed that a filling will no longer stay, these teeth are often merely smoothed so that there will be no sharp irritating edges. The mere existance of a decayed tooth in the arch is no reason for extraction. It may be in an irradiated area where an extraction could lead to further complications such as bone necrosis. Any acute or subacute infection as a result of pulp exposure resulting from the decay process can usually be adequately handled by use of antibiotics, root canal therapy, or both.

REMOVAL OF TEETH AFTER RADIATION THERAPY

Removal of teeth is indicated only after a failure of other methods of management such as filling, root canal therapy, antibiotics, analgesics, etc. When there is constant acute or subacute pain, infection or severe mobility, teeth often can be extracted with minimum trauma. The patient is placed on antibiotics for a period of several days before extraction of the root segment and kept on antibiotics for a period of 7 to 10 days after extraction. The patient must be taught the importance of good home care of the extraction site and be followed closely for any extraction sequelae.

Management of Necrosis

Different onset, clinical appearances, and prognosis are noted in osteoradionecrosis. In a patient who has had radium implant, for example, the adjacent aspect of the mandible receives an appreciable dose of irradiation yet the fall-off is such that there are areas of little or no damage. If bone exposure occurs, the chance of healing is better than in those patients receiving external irradiation alone or external irradiation combined with an implant because a large volume of bone is irradiated.

CONSERVATIVE TREATMENT FOR NECROSIS

The first management of bone necrosis should be conservative. No surgical intervention should be attempted unless there has been continuous failure using conservative procedures. Surgical intervention in irradiated bone may extend the necrotic site to include areas that clinically are not necrotic, because of the inability of bone to repair properly after radiation damage. Healing of bone exposure and bone necrosis is promoted if infection is brought under control. If gross infection is not present and the area of bone necrosis is not too great, the body will treat the bone fragments as foreign bodies and seek to sequestrate them. This process may take months or years. Conservative treatment such as zinc peroxide packs, topical 1 per cent neomycin solutions, systemic antibiotics, etc., are indicated for limited necrosis. Other conservative procedures include gentle removal of loose spicules of bone above the gingival crest to keep them from irritating surrounding tissues. Good oral hygiene is imperative. Food debris must be carefully flushed from the area to lower the total bacteria count. The patient must be cognizant of the importance of his total involvement in the care of the area if conservative procedures are to be beneficial.

RADICAL TREATMENT FOR NECROSIS

When conservative treatment fails and there is irretractible pain, recurrent severe infection and/or trismus, the patient is a candidate for more aggressive procedures to eliminate necrotic bone. This may be done by partial or total mandibular resection. Radical surgery for necrosis should, when possible, extend outside of the irradiated portion as the cut end of the bone may also become necrotic because of previous subclinical radiation damage. Often a partial resection, including *all* irradiated bone, is better than marginal resection, since the lat-

ter often requires an additional surgical procedure.

CONTROL OF POSTIRRADIATION TOOTH SENSITIVITY

It is not uncommon for patients to present with extremely sensitive teeth. Sensitivity and/or pain can do much to undermine the patient's nutritional status and/or psychological well-being. Use of fluoride to help prevent postirradiation decay can often eliminate postirradiation sensitivity. Patients started initially on fluoride rarely develop this sensitivity. In cases of extreme sensitivity, the custom-made mouthguard is worn with 1% sodium fluoride for periods of up to 10 minutes 2 or 3 times a day.

Management of Problems of Trismus

The muscles of mastication may have been irradiated and therefore may be severely fibrosed, often depending on whether the patient received treatment from both sides or was treated unilaterally. Patients are instructed to exercise so they will not lose inter-arch space. The patient opens his mouth as wide as he can twenty times, 3 times a day. The patient must stretch the muscles to the point where there is discomfort or no benefit will be achieved by this exercise program. Once trismus is evident, measurement of the opening is recorded and the patient is put on intensified home exercises to regain the lost space. When home exercises fail, various types of prosthetic appliances with springs and elastics must be fabricated to mechanically drive these ridges apart and attempt to stretch these muscles.

Oral Care for Pediatric Patients

Soft tissue sarcomas, especially rhabdomyosarcoma, are often encountered and the necessity for immediate initiation of therapy is obvious. The patients are made comfortable by dental cleaning and polishing, and the patients and their parents are told of the importance of long-range conservative treatment of these teeth. When the deciduous teeth and jaws are irradiated, often it is found that there will be lack of growth if the patient becomes a long-term survivor. Therefore, if there are various permanent tooth components that may not erupt, it is important to conserve the deciduous teeth that are present. We have found that fluoride works equally well for the pediatric patient as in the adult. Adequate home care must be given and an intensified preventive program established.

Construction of Dentures for the Postirradiated Patient

If the patient has been free of all major treatment sequelae many months after irradiation, one evaluates each patient individually to see if he is a candidate for denture construction. Some patients will never be ready for a prosthesis because of severe post-radiation complications, while others will be ready within a year to a year and a half after treatment. Treatment sequelae should be resolved before one constructs a prosthesis and then only with full knowledge that complications can follow because of use of the prosthesis.

Prostheses after radiation are similar in many ways to regular complete or partial dentures that nonirradiated patients wear. However, in the radiated patient extreme care is taken in fitting, adjustment of the occlusion, elimination of over-extension of the borders of the prosthesis, and premature contact of occlusion. All materials used for making impressions are nonirritating, no heated compound material or any irritating impression material is used. Both the fabrication and finish of the prosthesis is done atraumatically. Soft denture base material should be used cautiously. Presently hard denture base prostheses are preferred, but each patient must be evaluated individually.

Recent results have shown that most patients are able to wear complete or partial dentures after aggressive radiation therapy if care is taken in the construction of these prostheses. Dry mucous membranes are more subject to tear from friction than are moist normal mucous membranes, therefore adaptation on the under surfaces of the denture should be so constructed that the material is nonirritating. Adjustment should be done immediately when local irritation is present. The patient is most vulnerable to bone necrosis or soft tissue necrosis in the immediate postinsertion stages. The bone necrosis that results from insertion of a prosthesis can be managed as any other type of bone necrosis. With care, this bone necrosis can be kept to a minimum by correct construction and adequate adjustment of the prosthesis. Some patients will develop soft tissue necrosis after insertion of the prosthesis. Our special group of study patients has shown that all full or partial denture-caused soft tissue necrosis (15), have healed at this time by such conservative procedures as modification of the prosthesis or changing of the lining material; 81 patients received prostheses postirradiation (64 full dentures and 17 partial dentures), and only 5 patients developed bone necrosis. Four were healed by conservative treatment and one is still evident.

Interaction of Surgery and Irradiation
In Head and Neck Cancers

In Collaboration with

RICHARD H. JESSE, JR., and KENT C. WESTBROOK

The interaction of surgery and irradiation in the management of cancer is not limited to combining the two disciplines in the management of a particular type of cancer. Rather, it includes interaction between the surgeon and radiotherapist as team members to select the optimal therapy for each patient which may be surgery alone, irradiation alone, or a combination of both.[2,4,5] Definitive treatment should prevent subsequent development of clinical carcinoma from occult tumor deposits as well as eradicating gross disease. To achieve these purposes, the treatment team must be flexible, varying its approach according to the anatomical site of origin, local extension of the primary cancer, and the initial amount of neck disease. Additionally, the patient's age, general condition, habits, and desires must be considered.

The use of superradical surgery or superradical irradiation to have a few more patients free of cancer is not compatible with providing a comfortable quality of life. In planning each patient's therapy, the treatment team must balance the risk of recurrence and/or occurrence of new disease against discomfort and complications.

A flexible interaction of surgery and irradiation yields a maximum of patients free of disease, functionally and cosmetically acceptable with minimal morbidity. The surgeon and radiotherapist, as team members, must be aware of the role each will play from the initiation of therapy. If both surgery and irradiation are to be employed, the desirability of modifying each in a combined approach must be discussed.

Recurrence of cancer at the primary site after surgery is the result of microscopic disease present along fascial planes, nerve sheaths, periosteum, or bone which is beyond the limits of resection. The surgeon is often unaware of microscopic disease at the line of resection and needs the radiotherapist to eradicate residual cancer at the periphery of the primary site.

The radiotherapist, conversely, easily eradicates cancer at the periphery of the lesion where the amount of cancer is small and the cells are well oxygenated. However, he may fail in the center of large masses, either primary or metastatic, which contain hypoxic areas. A geographical miss occurs when the radiotherapy (external or interstitial) does not cover the cancer due to misjudgement regarding tumor extent or extension of microscopic disease along unexpected routes.

Because of the failure of either surgery or radiotherapy alone to control advanced disease, surgical procedures are frequently combined with preoperative or postoperative irradiation. The therapy sequence is determined primarily by the extent of the required surgery related to the difficulty of performing extensive surgical procedures after irradiation of 5,000 rads is given to the primary cancer and the entire neck.

Preoperative Irradiation

The purposes of preoperative irradiation are:

1) To eradicate subclinical disease beyond the margins of surgical resection.

2) To diminish tumor implantation by decreasing the number of viable cells in the operative field. A large number of viable cells is required to establish an implant as shown by experimental tumor biology.

3) To diminish the incidence of distant metastases by decreasing viability of cells entering the bloodstream at the time of surgery. Surgical manipulation increases the number of tumor cells in the bloodstream but no proven correlation exists between circulating cancer cells and the incidence of distant metastases.

In order to accomplish these goals, at least 5,000 rads should be given to the primary lesion and the entire neck. The treatment team must realize that this high dose of preoperative irradiation compromises healing ability and may increase complications unless appropriate measures are taken. Healing after radiotherapy varies with the radiation dose, the size of the portals, the extent of the surgical procedures, and the nutritional status of the patient. The nutritional factor is crucial. Difficult swallowing caused by the cancer itself or irradiation mucositis may cause malnutrition, negative nitrogen balance, and poor healing. When 5,000 rads are given in 5 weeks or 6,000 rads in 6 weeks, the surgeon must evaluate the patient carefully and delay surgery several weeks until there is positive nitrogen balance.

Normal healing will occur in patients whose entire neck is irradiated up to 6,000 rads in 6 weeks if only a unilateral radical neck dissection is performed. Simultaneous bilateral radical neck dissections should not be done in patients after high-dose irradiation through large portals. The blood supply, compromised by the irradiation, is further reduced by the large incision required for such a procedure. Wound separation may expose the carotids with catastrophic results. Bilateral radical neck dissections should be staged one month apart in heavily irradiated patients.

Resection of an area of heavily irradiated oropharyngeal mucosa results in a high incidence of nonhealing of the mucosal suture line unless special precautions are taken. Closure of large lateral oropharyngeal defects is best accomplished by using a forehead pedicle (Fig. 3-2). If the anticipated defect is large and poor healing is anticipated, the pedicle may be outlined and raised 7 to 10 days preoperatively. Large hypopharyngeal wall defects in the heavily irradiated patients should be closed with a thoracoacromial pedicle based on the internal mammary artery as described by Bakamjian[1] (Fig. 3-3). Split-thickness grafts or cervical pedicles from the irradiated area rarely result in a good covering for the carotid artery.

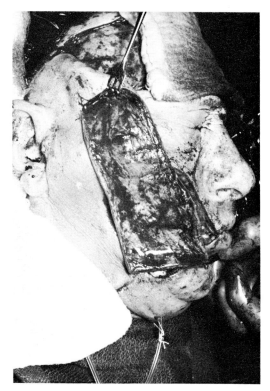

FIG. 3-2. A forehead pedicle is rotated to replace a large mucosal defect. (Courtesy: Fletcher, Lindberg, and Jesse, In *Surgical Oncology*, Hans Huber Publishers, Bern, Switzerland, 1970, p. 347.)

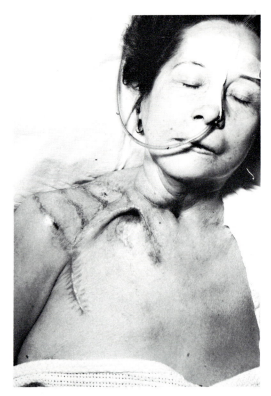

FIG. 3-3. Thoraco-acromial pedicle replaces the total circumference of the pharynx. (Courtesy: Fletcher, Lindberg, and Jesse, In *Surgical Oncology*, Hans Huber Publishers, Bern, Switzerland, 1970, p. 347.)

Almost any surgical procedure can be accomplished through this incision if it extends well into the contralateral side of the neck. Cervical flaps in the irradiated patient must retain the platysma muscle to insure an adequate blood supply. Patients in whom disease invades the platysma and skin should probably be treated by irradiation alone. If removal of both platysma and skin is necessary, a pedicle must be supplied from a non-irradiated area.

If an extensive procedure is planned, the radiotherapist should modify the irradiation portals to spare possible donor areas for skin flaps. Alteration of the portals, however, must not spare skin areas which have a reasonable chance of containing cancer.

When laryngectomy is necessary for an advanced laryngeal lesion usually enough pharyngeal mucosa is present for closure. However, in the heavily irradiated patient, the surgeon should leave a small controlled fistula by suturing the mucosa to the skin for 1 to 2 cm (Fig. 3-4). This prevents breakdown of the remaining suture line which, if it occurs, usually drains over the area of the carotid artery. The fistula is easily closed as an office procedure 3 to 4 weeks later.

Surgical procedures in heavily irradiated patients must be modified to insure healing. The neck incision in irradiated patients should always be bifurcate rather than trifurcate. Our most frequent incision is a high thyroid collar incision with a single vertical line curving up to the mastoid tip (Fig. 3-5).

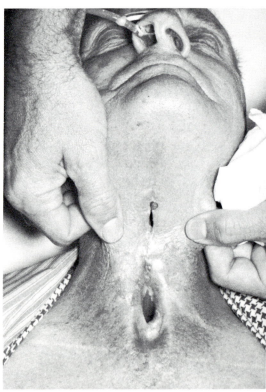

FIG. 3-4. A controlled pharyngeal fistula is created following laryngectomy in a heavily irradiated field. (Courtesy: Fletcher and Jesse, *Current Problems in Radiology*, Robert D. Moseley, Editor, Year Book Medical Publishers, Inc., Chicago, Ill. 1, 4, 1971.)

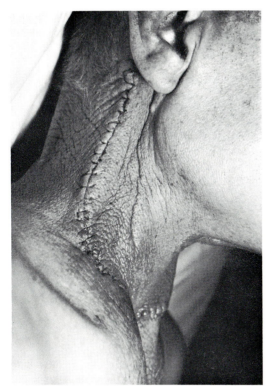

FIG. 3-5. This incision is employed for radical neck dissection in most patients and is mandatory in postirradiated patients. (Courtesy: Fletcher, Lindberg, and Jesse, In *Surgical Oncology,* Hans Huber Publishers, Bern, Switzerland, 1970, p. 347.)

Postoperative Irradiation

The purposes of postoperative irradiation are:

1) To treat known disease which was not resected.

2) To decrease recurrence in the surgically treated field by destroying foci of cells left.

3) To eradicate new disease in adjacent areas by sterilizing microscopic foci of cancer (contralateral neck, etc.).

The use of postsurgical irradiation requires modified surgical techniques in order to minimize morbidity. The oral, pharyngeal, and laryngeal mucosa often have multifocal areas of cancer some distance from the main tumor, and the contralateral neck may also contain metastatic deposits. The surgeon therefore must either remove only the gross cancer and rely on irradiation treatment of areas of microscopic disease, or perform a superradical procedure designed to remove all possible microscopic spread. The latter procedure involves the risks of both prolonged healing and delay in postoperative radiation therapy. The surgical procedure must not remove so much tissue that irradiation is technically impossible. For example, a laryngopharyngectomy with bilateral radical neck dissection leaves only the skin over the vertebral bodies containing the spinal cord (Fig. 3-79) and irradiation is impossible. The better choice would be to remove gross clinical disease in the neck by modified or partial neck dissection which leaves sufficient tissue for postoperative radiation therapy (Fig. 3-80).

The surgical procedure must provide rapid primary healing so irradiation will not be delayed. Immediate repair is essential so staged reconstruction is not used. Split-thickness grafts and undelayed pedicle flaps from the neck, forehead, or chest must be used to secure prompt healing. Most patients should begin radiotherapy within 3 weeks of their operation.

Postoperative radiotherapy is given to the opposite side of the neck as well as to the surgically disturbed area. This is necessary to prevent the appearance of new disease in high-risk patients. The contralateral neck may not be irradiated in well-lateralized lesions which carry a minimal risk of contralateral metastases, e.g., buccal mucosa cancer with a minimal number of cancer cells in the connective tissue of the surgical specimen.

Radical surgical procedures interfere somewhat with the blood supply to the center of the operative field. The tissues and subclinical cancer deposits in them are not anoxic and have only a slightly lowered radiosensitivity. The site of the resected primary and upper portion of the neck can be irradiated with 6,000 rads in 6 weeks without producing significant sequelae. The lower portion of the neck receives 5,000 rads in 5 weeks.

Management of Recurrences

Management of Surgical Recurrences and Probable Postoperative Residual

Most recurrences or new manifestations of malignant tumors of the head and neck appear within 6 months of surgery and essentially all appear within one year.[3] Early recurrences after surgery usually are widely spread with multiple manifestations either in the head and neck or at distant sites. A recurrence appearing after one year is more likely to be isolated. This may indicate a lesser biological potency of recurrence in that particular patient and, therefore gives a better prognosis. Active disease is present above the clavicle in 80 per cent of the patients who die because of their disease.

Table 3-3 is a tabulation of patients remaining free of cancer according to whether they had immediate irradiation for lack of surgical clearance or delayed irradiation for discernible recurrence. The group of patients with elective postoperative irradiation have a statistically significant higher *NED* rate. Treatment should not await recurrence in patients with a high risk of failure after a surgical procedure. Such patients should be

Table 3-3. *Disease Control.** *Immediate Postoperative Irradiation Versus Irradiation for Gross Recurrence*

	Immediate Postoperative Irradiation**	Irradiation for Gross Recurrences
Patients treated	19	147
Patients *NED*	8	16
Per cent *NED*	42%†	11%†

*Follow-up of 1 to 6 years
**Lack of clearance in surgical specimen
†$p < .001$
(Modified from: Fletcher and Evers, *Radiology,* 95, 185, 1970.)

Table 3-4. *Disease Control Above Clavicles. Localized Irradiation Versus Whole Neck Irradiation*

	Localized Irradiation	Whole Neck Irradiation
Patients Treated*	109	44
Patients *NED* above clavicles	29	18
Per cent *NED* above clavicles	26.5%†	41%†

*Patients were treated for lack of clearance in the surgical specimen or gross recurrence.
†$p < .05$ for the test with one-sided alternative.
(Modified from: Fletcher and Evers, *Radiology,* 95, 185, 1970.)

given postoperative irradiation to the primary site and entire neck as soon as the wound heals.

Postsurgical residual disease is usually disseminated with often microscopic deposits some distance from the initial obvious initial recurrence. Therefore, patients irradiated for the first postsurgical recurrence must be comprehensively treated to include the area of the primary and the whole neck (Table 3-4).

The following cases illustrate these points:

Case I: Male, age 45, was irradiated at another institution for a pyriform sinus tumor. It recurred and the patient had a laryngectomy and radical neck dissection at our institution in September 1964. On March 16, 1965, the patient developed pain from a retropharyngeal node which was proved positive by biopsy. Irradiation was given to the upper part of the neck, including the retropharyngeal area.

On October 5, 1965, another node was noted in the right supraclavicular area. Treatment was given to both supraclavicular areas with a boost to the palpable node. Further disease developed and the patient died within a year.

Case II: Female, age 54 was seen on April 29, 1964 with a squamous cell carcinoma of the buccal mucosa extending to the hard palate. Excision of the lesion was done but the patient developed a recurrence in the lower left gingivobuccal gutter on September 4, 1964. This was treated locally with a tumor dose of 6,150 rads in 30 days.

On April 16, 1965, a recurrence appeared in the left upper neck overlying the mastoid tip. The whole left side of the neck was treated, but eventually the patient died from disease on June 11, 1966.

Case III: Male, age 60, on December 20, 1967, because of a squamous cell carcinoma of the oral tongue, Grade II, had a combined resection of the primary with a right radical neck dissection and a left suprahyoid neck dissection. Tumor was close to the margin of resection. At the surgeon's request, only the upper neck, including the parapharyngeal lymphatics, was treated with 6,000 rads in 6 weeks from January 23, 1968 to March 4, 1968 with 2 parallel opposing portals. The lower margin of the field stopped at the thyroid notch. On May 30, 1968, a 3 cm node developed in the right supraclavicular area. A given dose of 5,000 rads was administered through an anterior portal with ^{60}Co and a supplement of 1,600 rads over the node was given with the electron beam. In July 1968, a third node appeared in the right parotid area plus nodes in both supraclavicular regions. The patient died from disease in September 1968.

Surgery for Radiation Recurrences

Failures after irradiation can be classified as residual cancer at the completion of treatment, early recurrence (before 6 months), or late recurrence (after 6 months).

RESIDUAL AND EARLY-RECURRING CANCER

Biopsy of clinically evident residual disease should not be done earlier than 8 to 10 weeks after completion of treatment. The presence of histologically intact tumor cells shortly after irradiation may be misleading. The management of biopsy-proved residual

or recurrent cancer 2 to 6 months after completion of radiation therapy is often very difficult. The timing of the surgery is most important because the patients often have not recovered from radical irradiation and are still in negative nitrogen balance.

Patients with residual cancer 6 weeks after radical irradiation (6,000 rads or more) should be operated upon as soon as nitrogen balance is restored. Since the risk of wound disruption and carotid artery rupture is high, the most conservative surgical procedure which removes the original primary lesion and original palpable nodes should be performed. It is not necessary to remove in the irradiated area large areas which were initially uninvolved as experience has shown that subclinical disease in those areas is well controlled by the irradiation therapy. Cancer appearing at the original site after an apparent radiation cure is often small if it is located in the center of the original cancer where radiation therapy was ineffective because of a great number of anoxic cells. This can be handled by a conservative surgical excision.

If, however, residual or recurrent disease develops at the periphery of the irradiated site, the recurrences are often multiple. They may be hidden under an intact mucosa and frequently extend some distance from the edge of the irradiated field. The surgical procedure necessary to eradicate this type of disease is often extensive. Any surgical procedure less than an extremely radical one is doomed to failure. Since it is difficult to determine the extent of the recurrence before operation, the surgeon often finds it difficult to plan adequate flaps for repair. The probability of controlling cancer in this type of patient is small.

LATE RECURRENCES

Usually the later the recurrence, the less extensive it is. Postirradiation recurrences occurring more than 12 months after therapy are easiest to control surgically. Such recurrences are apt to be single and less extensive than early recurrences. The surgical procedure can be somewhat less radical than that necessary for patients with early postirradiation recurrence. The patients with late recurrences have usually regained their weight and wound healing is reasonably good.

Complications of Head and Neck Irradiation

Major complications of soft tissue and bone necrosis, laryngeal edema, spinal cord myelitis, etc, are infrequent. Minor complications such as dryness of the mucosal membranes and fibrosis of muscles and connective tissues are fairly common and create moderate to considerable discomfort. Five thousand rads given in 5 weeks, 5 fractions per week, produce dryness of the mouth and/or throat, but no detectable tissue fibrosis. This dose to the lower portion of the neck through an anterior portal produces little if any discernible change in the neck. Sites of excised primaries in the oral cavity, pharynx, and larynx, or both subdigastric areas must not be irradiated with parallel opposing portals unless the patient has significant risk of developing recurrence. Such a technique delivers 5,000 rads to the mucosa of the oral cavity and of oropharynx and produces dryness.

Necrosis

With the aim of obtaining a high percentage of local cures by irradiation, the team must expect that a certain number of patients will develop necrosis. The surgeon must be ready to help relieve the pain associated with tissue necrosis.

The basic cause of radiation necrosis is the adverse effect of the radiation upon the blood supply to the local area. Contributing factors, however, are significant and include chemical irritants, mechanical irritants, systemic factors, and bacterial infection. Many of these patients are alcoholics and heavy users of tobacco. The continued irritation of alcohol

and tobacco contributes to mucosal breakdown. Poorly fitting dentures is a mechanical irritant and poor dental hygiene creates other problems.

An important systemic factor is the negative nitrogen balance present in many patients. Patients frequently lose their appetite because of the discomfort of the cancer, the irradiation effect on the taste, and excessive mouth dryness. Bacteria in a dry mouth cause carious teeth which are an avenue of infection into the bone.

The radiotherapist, surgeon, and dental members of the team must explain to the patient the consequences of neglect concerning the above factors. A program of preventive treatment must be planned and implemented. First, the patient must eat an adequate diet to maintain or gain weight during and after radiotherapy. The patient should be weighed weekly and a feeding tube inserted if the weight loss exceeds 5 pounds. Second, the patient must eliminate or decrease alcohol and tobacco consumption. Third, management of the remaining teeth should be carefully assessed with a dental consultant. Prior to radiation therapy, salvageable teeth are repaired and only those which cannot be adequately restored are removed. Fewer patients will develop necrosis if radiotherapy is delayed for 2 weeks following extraction of teeth in the irradiated field.

Posttherapy, a program of fluoride treatment, careful scaling, repair of caries and education of the patient to use good oral hygiene should be outlined. The crown of a decayed tooth is allowed to slough and the root tip is allowed to remain in the bone under intact mucosa unless a periapical abscess develops. If an abscess develops, the tooth or its root may be removed under antibiotic coverage if absolutely necessary.

If breakdown of the mucosa develops, recurrent tumor must be ruled out. Biopsy is mandatory for questionable areas. If the mucosal breakdown is due to necrosis, conservative therapy is instituted. Irrigations with salt and soda solution, one-half teaspoonful of each to one quart of lukewarm water, is helpful in ridding the necrotic crater of debris and bacteria. These irrigations are particularly important immediately after meals. One per cent Neomycin solution on a small gauze pack is placed on the necrotic area 4 times daily after the patient has irrigated and is held in place for at least one hour. If the physician and patient are persistent in these measures, 90 per cent of the necrotic areas will heal.

Soft tissue necrosis persisting after prolonged conservative therapy, can occasionally be excised and grafted. This is particularly true in those necrotic areas occurring after radium needle implant giving locally a high dose of irradiation. The problem of necrosis is more serious when bone is involved. Exposed bone will eventually sequestrate. The surgeon should usually wait until the sequestrum is loose and can be easily lifted out. Small particles of exposed bone in shallow ulcers can sometimes be removed surgically under antibiotic coverage, allowing the surrounding mucosa to grow over the defect and close it.

Exposed bone is painful, but patients vary greatly in their ability to withstand pain. In approximately 10 per cent of the patients who have exposed bone, in spite of all careful conservative therapy, osteonecrosis of the mandible persists and progresses with pain unbearable for the patient. When this occurs, the offending portion of bone should be removed. Repeated inflammation of the surrounding soft tissue, particularly if abscess formation occurs, may also necessitate bone removal.

Resection, when necessary, is usually accomplished intraorally through an incision made directly through the gum. In selected patients, particularly those whose radiation has been delivered interstitially with the external cortex of the bone receiving somewhat less than the maximal dose of irradiation, the bone can be saucerized and packed open.

This technique is particularly useful when necrosis approaches the anterior midline and when resection of the full thickness of the mandible would result in a serious disability. A procedure of this type can be expected to succeed only in patients who will cooperate fully, in regard to controlling both their smoking and drinking habits and in practicing meticulous oral hygiene.

The full thickness of the mandible is usually sacrificed in patients who received the majority of their irradiation with an external beam unit, who have necrosis of the full thickness of the mandible, and who have necrosis laterally or posteriorly in the oral cavity. An incision is made directly through the gum and a subperiosteal resection is done. The resulting mandibular bed is packed and no attempt is made to close the soft tissue defect. The resulting defect heals from the bottom and the packing is changed regularly until complete healing occurs.

BIBLIOGRAPHY

1. Bakamjian, V. Y.: A two-stage method of pharyngeal esophageal reconstruction with primary pectoral skin flap, *Plas. and Reconstr. Surg.*, 36, 173, 1965.
2. Fletcher, G. H., Lindberg, R. D., and Jesse, R. H.: The combination of radiation and surgery in oropharynx and laryngopharynx squamous cell carcinoma. In *Surgical Oncology*, F. Saegesser and J. Pettavel, Editors, Hans Huber Publishers, Bern, Switzerland, 347, 1970.
3. Fletcher, G. H., and Evers, W. T.: Radiotherapeutic management of surgical recurrences and postoperative residuals in tumors of the head and neck. *Radiology*, 95, 185, 1970.
4. Fletcher, G. H., and Jesse, R. H.: Interaction of surgery and irradiation in head and neck cancers, *Current Problems in Radiology*, Robert D. Moseley, Editor, Year Book Medical Publishers, Inc., Chicago, Illinois, 1, 4, 1971.
5. MacComb, W. S., and Fletcher, G. H.: *Cancer of the Head and Neck*, Baltimore, Maryland, Williams and Wilkins Company, 1967,

Neck Nodes

In Collaboration with

RICHARD H. JESSE, JR., ROBERT D. LINDBERG and KENT C. WESTBROOK

GUIDELINES FOR MANAGEMENT

With increased effectiveness of irradiation, surgery, or the combination of both in the management of the primary lesions of the head and neck, disease in neck nodes has become a major cause of treatment failure.

Until recently, neck treatment had not been individualized. Radical neck dissection, unilateral or bilateral, had not been questioned as the preferred treatment either electively for occult metastasis or therapeutically for clinically apparent metastasis. In the light of accumulated clinical data, the surgeon's ingrained concepts need reevaluation and a fresh approach combining radiation therapy with surgical procedures must be considered.[7]

No general policy can be formulated for treatment for cervical metastases. Treatment of an individual patient is determined by the anatomical site of origin of the cancer, initial staging of the primary lesion, and initial staging of cervical nodes.

Large primary lesions usually exhibit a high incidence of metastases. Biologically virulent tumors of the nasopharynx, tonsillar fossa, base of tongue, and pyriform sinus may present with extensive neck disease although having small primary lesion. The incidence of distant metastases correlates with the extent of initial neck involvement.[4]

The incidence of recurrent cancer in the neck of patients after radical neck dissection has been reported by Beahrs[2] as 26.5 per cent and by Strong[19] as 36.5 per cent. Strong's series is more revealing when the pathological status of the surgical specimen is considered. Fifty-four per cent of patients with positive nodes and 71 per cent of patients with positive nodes at multiple levels developed recurrent disease. This recurrence may be due to microscopic cancer in lymphatic channels which is not totally removed by the most carefully performed radical neck dissection. Preoperative irradiation of 2,000 rads tumor dose to the neck given in 96 hours (equivalent to 3,000 rads in 3 weeks) diminished somewhat the incidence of recurrent disease in the radically dissected neck in Strong's series.[19] In our own material, pre- or post-operative irradiation dramatically

Table 3-5. *Squamous Cell Carcinoma of Tonsillar Fossa, Base of Tongue, Supraglottic Larynx, and Hypopharynx—1948 through 1967—Failures in Ipsilateral Side of Neck (Primary Controlled when Neck Disease Becomes Manifest) Patients have Survived at Least 24 Months*

Treatment	N_0 Neck Treatment			N_1	N_2A	N_2B	N_3A	N_3B	Total
	None	Partial	Complete						
Radiation	—	13/85	1/50	8/52	6/22	7/27	8/21	11/35	54/292–18.5%
Surgery	16/29	8/23	2/28	5/47	1/13	7/30	5/12	7/17	51/199–25.6%
Combined	—	1/5	0/6	0/21	0/17	0/28	3/13	5/15	9/105– 8.6%

(Courtesy: Barkley, Fletcher, Jesse, and Lindberg, *Amer. J. Surg.*, 124, 462, 1972.)

diminished the incidence of recurrences (Table 3-5).[10,1] In most clinical situations, therefore, the surgeon needs the help of the radiotherapist to eradicate diffuse microscopic disease in the heavily infested neck.

Irradiation of the neck lymphatics may be given:

1) To eradicate existing clinically positive nodes.

2) To diminish the incidence of recurrence in the radically dissected neck (Table 3-5).

3) To eradicate occult metastases in initially uninvolved areas (Tables 3-5, 6, 7, 8).

Moderate irradiation (5,000 rads) alone, while effective for minimal metastasis, is not consistent in controlling large metastatic cervical masses. In one series[16], 56 per cent of clinically positive nodes were histologically negative following irradiation. There is no way to predict which nodes have regrowth potential if not removed. Conversely, high-dose irradiation (7,000 rads or more) may control advanced metastatic disease but produces a woody, painful neck. We prefer to combine moderate doses of irradiation (preoperatively or postoperatively) with either a radical or modified neck dissection.

Indications for surgical resection after preoperative irradiation for squamous cell carcinoma depend upon the number, the size, and the location of the initial nodes related to the radiation dose and the response to it. A single first level node, size 2–3 cm, receiving 7,000 rads or a single first level node under 2 cm receiving 6,000 rads usually does not require surgical excision. All other situations with clinically positive nodes require a modified or radical neck dissection including: 1) a node below the first level of lymphatic drainage, 2) multiple positive nodes at different levels, 3) a node initially greater than 3 cm, 4) a node receiving under 5,000 rads, and 5) a node which persists at the end of radiation therapy.

Postoperative radiotherapy (5,000 rads to entire neck) is used to control occult disease and is indicated if node(s) clinically are over 3 cm, invade connective tissue histologically,

or if multiple nodes are positive histologically in the surgical specimen.

Patients who develop new neck disease have a significantly higher incidence of distant metastases than those who are clinically free of disease above the clavicle as actively growing cancer is a source of further metastases (Fig. 3-6).[8,16] Therefore, elective irradiation, if it can be accomplished simply, is justified to prevent further neck disease which will require radical treatment.

In summary, metastatic neck disease is a major problem in patients with head and neck cancer. Surgery alone results in high recurrence rates and radical radiotherapy alone produces significant morbidity. The

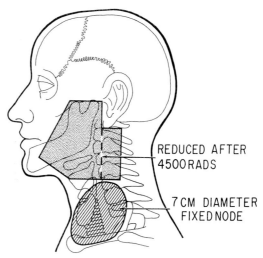

FIG. 3-6. Male, age 63, seen in September 1959 with T_2 squamous cell carcinoma of the left anterior faucial pillar. There were no palpable nodes in either side of the neck. A tumor dose of 6,000 rads was given in 34 days with a 2:1 loading in favor of the involved side.

Thirteen months after the initial treatment, the patient was seen in the follow-up clinic with a 7 cm node occupying the left lower neck. In addition, the patient had a left hilar mass which was probably a metastasis from the initial lesion, although it could conceivably have been a second primary. The node was treated with 10 × 600 rads given dose which produced considerable shrinking of the mass. The patient died eventually from disseminated cancer.

judicious use of a moderate dose radiotherapy and a modified surgical procedure decreases neck recurrences significantly with negligible morbidity. The therapeutic goal includes not only the treatment of known disease but also the prevention of future disease. Modified neck dissection, while contrary to established surgical concepts, is effective when combined with irradiation in controlling cancer while preserving function and cosmetic appearance.

Topographical Distribution

Analysis of the location of clinically positive cervical nodes at admission to our hospital was undertaken to determine the topographical distribution of nodal metastases. Each side of the neck is divided into 9 nodal regions (Fig. 3-7).

1) The *submental nodes* are located in the triangle bounded by the anterior bellies of the digastric muscles and the hyoid bone.

2) The *submaxillary nodes* lie along the lower border of the mandible in the submaxillary triangle and are divided into 3 groups—preglandular, prevascular, and retrovascular.

3) The *subdigastric nodes* are located below the posterior belly of the digastric muscle at the level of the greater cornu of the hyoid bone and include the upper jugular nodes as well as the tonsillar node.

4) The *midjugular nodes* are located at the bifurcation of the common carotid just below the hyoid bone.

5) The *low jugular nodes* are located along the lower third of the internal jugular vein.

6) *Upper posterior cervical nodes* lie at the upper end of the spinal accessory chain. The uppermost node is beneath the sternocleidomastoid muscle at the tip of the mastoid process.

7) *Midposterior cervical nodes* include those of the spinal accessory chain at the same level as the midjugular nodes.

8) *Low posterior cervical nodes* are located at the lower end of the spinal accessory chain.

9) *Supraclavicular nodes* including the anterior scalene group are located just above the clavicle in the transverse lymphatic chain which connects the jugular and spinal accessory chains.

The location of involved nodes is usually predictable for a given primary site. Initial metastasis from keratinizing squamous carcinoma is usually limited to the first node level for a specific site, but with advanced

NODAL REGIONS OF THE NECK

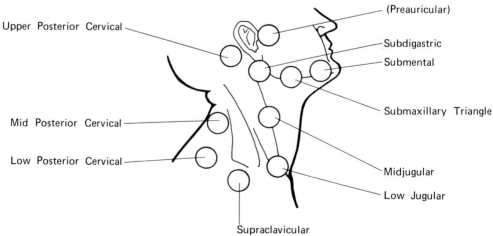

FIG. 3-7

disease spread to other levels is common. Metastatic cancer from anaplastic squamous carcinoma of lymphoepithelioma more frequently involves multiple levels of lymph nodes. Initial and later spread to the contralateral neck is usually into the corresponding first level.

The staging of cervical metastasis employed at M. D. Anderson Hospital is as follows:

N_0: No clinically positive node.

N_1: Single clinically positive node less than 3 cm in diameter, not fixed.

N_2A: Single clinically positive node greater than 3 cm in diameter, not fixed.

N_2B: Multiple ipsilateral clinically positive nodes, not fixed.

N_3A: Clinically positive unilateral fixed node(s).

N_3B: Clinically positive bilateral nodes, fixed or not fixed.

The distribution of clinically positive nodes and the N Stage on admission are shown for oral tongue and floor of mouth (Fig. 3-8); retromolar trigone/anterior faucial pillar, soft palate, and tonsillar fossa (Fig. 3-9); base of tongue and oropharyngeal walls (Fig. 3-10); and supraglottic larynx, hypopharynx, and nasopharynx (Fig. 3-11).[11]

Study of the distribution of clinically positive lymph nodes shows the following:

1) *Oral tongue.* The subdigastric nodes are most commonly involved, followed by the submaxillary triangle nodes and the midjugular nodes. The submental, low jugular, and posterior cervical nodes seldom are involved.

2) *Floor of mouth.* The nodes of the submaxillary triangle most commonly are involved: subdigastric nodes also are frequently involved. The submental nodes rarely are involved in spite of the anterior location of the tumors. The low jugular and posterior cervical nodes rarely are involved.

3) *Oropharynx.* The subdigastric nodes are most commonly involved for all anatomical sites. The submaxillary nodes occasionally are involved and submental nodes rarely.

a) Retromolar trigone-anterior faucial pillar. The most commonly affected node is the tonsillar node in the subdigastric group. Because of the anterior location of the retromolar trigone-anterior faucial pillar in the oropharynx, the incidence of metastasis in the submaxillary triangle is significant. The midjugular nodes are as often involved. The posterior cervical nodes rarely are involved.

b) Soft palate. Because it is a midline structure, the incidence of bilateral subdigastric nodes is high.

c) Tonsillar fossa. The tonsillar node of the subdigastric group is almost always the first to be involved. The incidence of involvement of mid- and low-jugular nodes is also significant. Metastasis to the posterior cervical nodes is common, both ipsi- and contralaterally.

d) Base of tongue. Since the base of tongue also is a midline structure, bilateral metastases are common. The midjugular nodes often are involved. A few patients present with positive posterior cervical nodes. The low jugular and supraclavicular nodes rarely are involved.

e) Oropharyngeal walls. The main spread is along the jugular chain bilaterally since the posterior pharyngeal wall is a midline structure. The upper jugular nodes in the subdigastric group most commonly are involved, followed by the midjugular nodes. The incidence of posterior cervical node involvement is high, whereas supraclavicular node involvement is rare.

4) *Supraglottic larynx.* The main spread is along the jugular chain, and upper jugular nodes are most commonly affected, followed closely by midjugular nodes. The incidence of bilateral metastases is significant. The posterior cervical nodes seldom are involved. The submental and submaxillary triangle nodes almost never are involved.

5) *Hypopharynx.* The majority of metastases are to the jugular chain—upper, mid, and lower, in decreasing order of frequency. Since most of these lesions arise in the pyriform sinus, the frequency of bilateral metas-

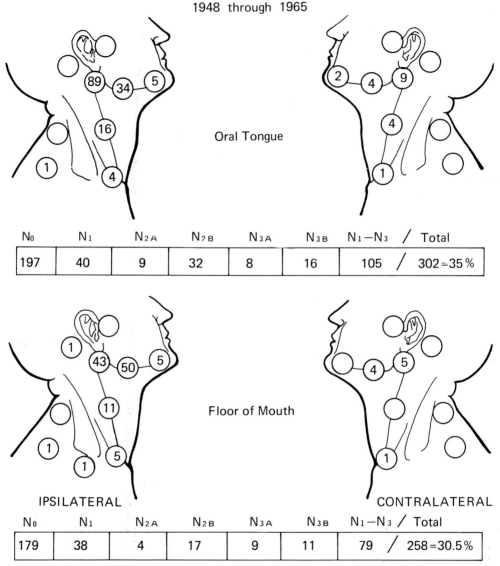

FIG. 3-8

Oral Tongue

N_0	N_1	N_{2A}	N_{2B}	N_{3A}	N_{3B}	N_1-N_3	/	Total
197	40	9	32	8	16	105	/	302 = 35%

Floor of Mouth

IPSILATERAL   CONTRALATERAL

N_0	N_1	N_{2A}	N_{2B}	N_{3A}	N_{3B}	N_1-N_3	/	Total
179	38	4	17	9	11	79	/	258 = 30.5%

tases is low. Ipsilateral posterior cervical nodes occasionally are involved. The submental and submaxillary triangle nodes almost never are involved.

6) *Nasopharynx.* Nasopharyngeal lesions have the greatest incidence of bilateral metastases and posterior cervical chain involvement of any type of head and neck cancer. The submental and submaxillary nodes al-

most never are involved. The incidence of supraclavicular metastasis is significant.

Elective Irradiation of Subclinical Disease

The presence of subclinical disease (disease present but not clinically detectable) in the cervical lymphatics has been well docu-

NODAL DISTRIBUTION ON ADMISSION
1948 through 1965

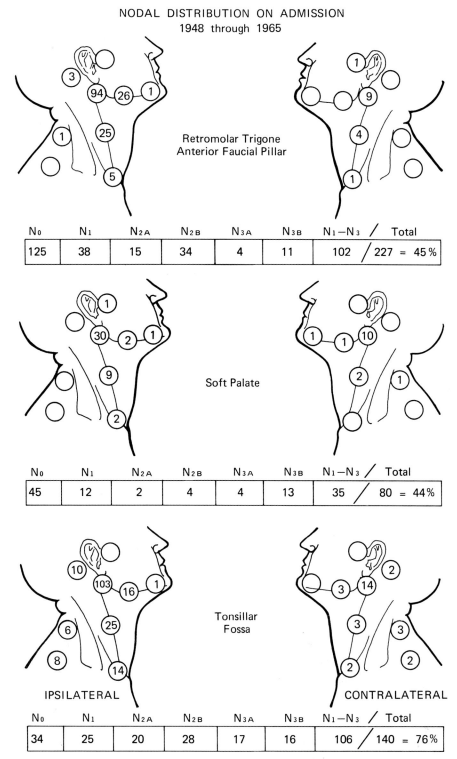

Retromolar Trigone
Anterior Faucial Pillar

N_0	N_1	N_{2A}	N_{2B}	N_{3A}	N_{3B}	N_1-N_3 / Total
125	38	15	34	4	11	102 / 227 = 45%

Soft Palate

N_0	N_1	N_{2A}	N_{2B}	N_{3A}	N_{3B}	N_1-N_3 / Total
45	12	2	4	4	13	35 / 80 = 44%

Tonsillar
Fossa

IPSILATERAL   CONTRALATERAL

N_0	N_1	N_{2A}	N_{2B}	N_{3A}	N_{3B}	N_1-N_3 / Total
34	25	20	28	17	16	106 / 140 = 76%

FIG. 3-9

NODAL DISTRIBUTION ON ADMISSION
1948 through 1965

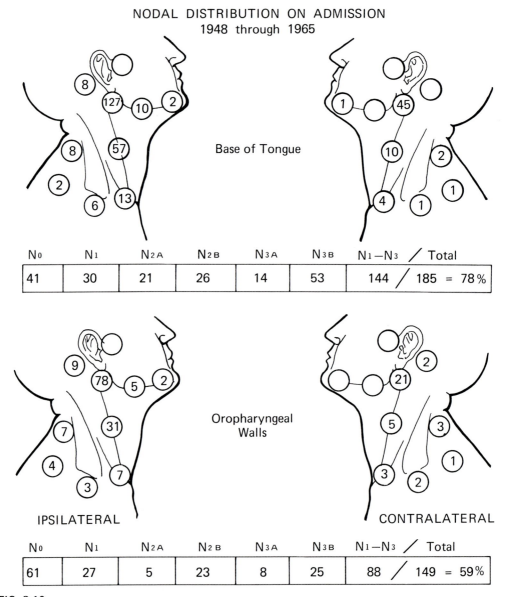

Base of Tongue

N0	N1	N2A	N2B	N3A	N3B	N1—N3	/	Total
41	30	21	26	14	53	144	/	185 = 78%

Oropharyngeal Walls

IPSILATERAL   CONTRALATERAL

N0	N1	N2A	N2B	N3A	N3B	N1—N3	/	Total
61	27	5	23	8	25	88	/	149 = 59%

FIG. 3-10

mented by elective radical neck dissections. The incidence of neck metastases in clinically negative necks in patients with squamous cell carcinoma of the mobile tongue has been reported to be from 40 to 60 per cent[9,13,17,18] and as high as 22 per cent in patients with early lesions.[14] A prolonged controversy over the advisability of elective neck dissection has resulted from this knowledge. Most patients with squamous cell carcinomas of the nasopharynx, faucial arch, tonsillar fossa, and base of tongue are treated by irradiation. Treatment is given to both sides of the neck. The upper neck is treated through parallel opposed portals to the upper border of thyroid cartilage and the lower neck with an anterior portal shielding the larynx. The dose to the upper neck nodes is never less than

NODAL DISTRIBUTION ON ADMISSION
1948 through 1965

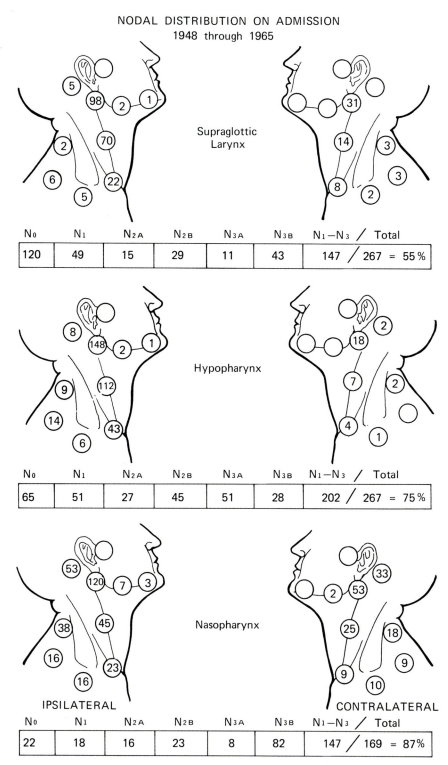

Supraglottic Larynx

N₀	N₁	N₂ₐ	N₂в	N₃ₐ	N₃в	N₁–N₃ / Total
120	49	15	29	11	43	147 / 267 = 55%

Hypopharynx

N₀	N₁	N₂ₐ	N₂в	N₃ₐ	N₃в	N₁–N₃ / Total
65	51	27	45	51	28	202 / 267 = 75%

Nasopharynx

IPSILATERAL   CONTRALATERAL

N₀	N₁	N₂ₐ	N₂в	N₃ₐ	N₃в	N₁–N₃ / Total
22	18	16	23	8	82	147 / 169 = 87%

FIG. 3-11

5,000 rads, often 6,000 rads. The given dose to the lower neck is 5,000 rads. The dose to the midjugular nodes may be as low as 4,500 rads. The nodes in the supraclavicular fossa and posterior cervical triangle, located immediately under the skin, receive 5,000 rads. Early in the megavoltage irradiation program all patients with base of tongue and tonsillar fossa lesions did not receive treatment to the lower neck. Patients with faucial arch lesions have been treated by more variable approaches. Some received irradiation to only the ipsilateral or bilateral subdigastric areas rather than to the entire neck. Table 3-6 compares the appearance of neck disease in the two groups of patients.[3,15] New neck disease appeared in 12 per cent of the patients whose neck was only partially irradiated. Less than 10 per cent of these patients were initially staged N_3 and therefore have a low risk of occult disease. In contradistinction, new disease appeared in only 1.7 per cent of the patients whose entire neck was irradiated, generally with a primary cancer of the nasopharynx, tonsil, and base of tongue. More than one-third of these were initially staged N_3 and therefore have a high

risk of occult disease. The lower incidence of new disease in this group (a higher risk group) attests to the value of elective radiotherapy.

Table 3-7 is a composite of results of various studies.[8,12,16] The appearance of new disease in the contralateral side of the neck in patients with lesions of the floor of the mouth, oral tongue, faucial arch, supraglottic larynx, and pyriform sinus who receive various amounts of external irradiation to the first level lymphatics with a significant contribution to the equivalent contralateral lymphatics. Only 3 per cent (6/187) developed new disease compared with 24 per cent (46/187) for patients treated with an ipsilateral radical neck dissection only.[16]

The diminution in contralateral disease, compared with the expected rate, is 60 to 70 per cent in patients receiving 3,000 to 4,000 rads in 3 to 4 weeks to the opposite submaxillary and subdigastric area. No patient with a faucial arch lesion developed contralateral neck disease when the opposite subdigastric nodes were given 5,000 rads in 5 weeks. Postoperative radiotherapy (6,000 rads to the opposite upper neck and 4,500 to 5,000 rads to the lower neck) eliminates more than 90 per cent of the contralateral metastases in patients with supraglottic or pyriform sinus lesions.

Table 3-8 shows that:

1) The number of patients initially with a clinically negative neck who develop subsequent disease in the neck is low compared with published reports. This is particularly impressive in patients with faucial arch lesions who have a high rate of clinically positive nodes on admission (Fig. 3-8) and therefore should have a high incidence of subclinical metastasis.

2) No increase in the incidence of new neck disease occurs as the staging of the primary increases. This unexpected finding is probably the result of a more systematic use of high-dose external irradiation to the upper neck in patients with large lesions.[8,12]

With a minimum of 5,000 rads to the high

Table 3-6. *Control of Subclinical Disease in Squamous Cell Carcinomas of the Nasopharynx, Tonsillar Fossa, Base of Tongue and Faucial Arch-Primary Lesion and Initial Neck Disease Controlled**

New Disease in Areas of Neck Initially Clinically Negative	
Partial Neck Irradiation	Whole Neck Irradiation
185 pts. (12 N_3)**	284 pts. (100 N_3)**
	4,500–5,000 rads/5 weeks to initially uninvolved areas
12.0% (22/185)	1.7% (5/284)

* All treatments 1,000 rads per week 5 days a week.
** Either fixed node(s) (N_3A) or bilateral clinically positive node(s) (N_3B) in the upper portion of the neck. (Courtesy: Berger, Fletcher, Lindberg, and Jesse, *Amer. J. Roentgen.*, 111, 66, 1971.)

Table 3-7. *Control of Subclinical Disease in Squamous Cell Carcinomas of the Floor of Mouth, Oral Tongue, Faucial Arch, Supraglottic Larynx, and Pyriform Sinus-Primary Lesion and Initial Neck Disease Controlled**

	New Disease in Opposite Side of the Neck Initially Clinically Negative					
	Without Irradiation				*With Irradiation*	
Floor of Mouth $(N_1$ & $N_2)$†	47.5%	(9/19)	10.5%	(3/28)	⎧3,000 rads/3 wks	⎧to opposite
Oral Tongue $(N_1$ & $N_2)$†	27.0%	(8/30)	9.0%	(2/22)	⎨ to ⎩4,000 rads/4 wks	⎨ subdigastric & submaxillary ⎩triangle nodes
Faucial Arch $(N_1$ & $N_2)$†	30.0%	(3/10)	0%	(0/72)	5,000 rads/5 wks	⎧to opposite ⎨ subdigastric ⎩nodes
Supraglottic Larynx and Pyriform Sinus†	20.0%	(26/128)	1.5%	(1/65)	⎧6,000 rads/6 wks upper neck ⎨5,000 rads/5 wks given dose to ⎩lower neck	
Total	24.0%	(46/187)	3.0%	(6/187)		

* All treatments 1,000 rads per week 5 days a week

† N_1: Single clinically positive node $\leq$ 3 cm

N_2: Single clinically positive node $>$ 3 cm not fixed or multiple clinically positive ipsilateral nodes. (Courtesy: Fletcher, In *Biological and Clinical Basis of Radiosensitivity*, Publication pending.)

and midjugular nodes, no patient with squamous cell carcinoma of the supraglottic larynx developed neck disease in a neck initially staged N_0 (Table 3-9).

Although irradiation with 5,000 rads in 5 weeks does not produce detectable fibrosis, it should be used only when there is significant probability of occult disease. Both subdigastric areas cannot be irradiated without including the mucosa of the oral cavity and

Table 3-8. *Percentage of Patients with Squamous Cell Carcinoma Initially N_0 Developing Neck Disease by T Staging*

	Oral Cavity				Faucial Arch		
Primary Stage	No Pts	Percentage of Pts Having Had Partial Neck Treatment*		Percentage of Pts Developing Neck Metastases		$\frac{2}{3}$ of the Patients Have Had Area I or Areas I and II Irradiated	Percentage of Pts Developing Neck Metastases
T_1	169	5%	(9/169)	23%	(39/169)	Usually angle node only, occasionally all subdigastric nodes irradiated.	16% (7/43)
T_2	200	24%	(48/200)	26%	(52/200)		18.5% (12/65)
T_3	110	52%	(57/110)	29%	(32/110)	All subdigastric nodes usually irradiated	10% (4/39)
T_4	42	69%	(29/42)	26%	(11/42)		16% (2/12)

* Irradiation limited to the subdigastric and submaxillary triangle nodes. (Courtesy: Fletcher and Jesse, *Current Problems in Radiology*, Robert D. Mosely, Ed., Year Book Medical Publishers, Inc., Chicago, Illinois, 1, 3, 1971.)

Table 3-9. *Evolution of Neck Disease in N₀* *Patients with Squamous Cell Carcinoma of the Supraglottic Larynx with Primary Controlled by Methods of Treatment. January 1948–December 1967, Minimum 2-Year Follow-Up*

Site	No. of Pts by Initial Treatment of Primary	No. of Pts Developing Neck Nodes
Suprahyoid Epiglottis	2 Surg.	0
	14 XRT†	0
	1 Preop.	0
Infrahyoid Epiglottis	20 Surg.	8
	6 XRT†	0
	1 Postop.	0
False Cords	16 Surg.	4
	12 XRT†	1**
Arytenoids	1 Surg.	1
	4 XRT†	0
Aryepiglottic Folds	4 Surg.	1
	8 XRT†	0
Total	43 Surg.	14
	44 XRT†	1
	1 Postop.	0
	1 Preop.	0

*Clinically negative neck.
**5 × 5 cm portal, a node developed above the treatment field in the high jugular area.
†XRT: irradiation

oropharynx. Irradiation doses of 5,000 rads produce some dryness. Irradiation of the lower neck may interfere with treatment of the supraclavicular areas for possible future primary carcinomas of the lung as well as of the head and neck area. Figure 3-12 outlines the lymphatic areas for planning the irradiation portals.

ORAL TONGUE, FLOOR OF MOUTH, AND FAUCIAL ARCH
N₀ **PATIENTS**
(TABLES 3-10 AND 11)

Elective treatment of the entire ipsilateral side of the neck (either by surgical resection or by radiotherapy) is not used routinely for

patients with a small unilateralized lesion (1 cm) who do not have clinically positive nodes. The ipsilateral submaxillary triangle and subdigastric nodes usually receive a

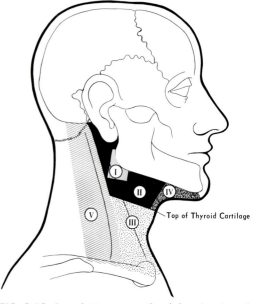

FIG. 3-12. Lymphatic areas outlined for planning of radiation portals:

Area I. Includes only the subdigastric (tonsillar, sentinel) node at the angle of the jaw.

Area II. Includes a field bounded posteriorly by a line bisecting the sternomastoid muscle, inferiorly by an imaginary line drawn at the upper border of the thyroid cartilage, and anteriorly by the anterior border of the submaxillary gland. Superiorly, it extends slightly over the lower border of the mandible.

Area III. That portion of the neck bounded anteriorly by the midline, posteriorly by a line bisecting the sternocleidomastoid muscle, superiorly by the upper border of the thyroid cartilage and inferiorly by the clavicle.

Area IV. Includes the submental area from the point of the chin superiorly to the upper border of the thyroid cartilage inferiorly and has a common boundary with Area II laterally.

Area V. The entire posterior triangle of the neck. (Courtesy: Jesse, Lindberg, Barkley, and Fletcher, *Amer. J. Surg.,* 120, 505, 1970.)

Table 3-10. *Policy of Treatment for Lesions of Oral Tongue and Floor of Mouth*

	N_0	N_1	N_2A	N_2B	N_3A	N_3B
T_1	Treat primary only	5,000 rads upper neck bilaterally plus radical neck dissection or 5,000 rads entire neck plus modified neck dissection	Primary Treated with Irradiation 5,000 rads to entire neck followed with radical or modified neck dissection(s)			
T_2	5,000 rads to ipsilateral upper neck and slightly less to contralateral upper neck		Primary Treated with Surgery For fixed nodes, 5,000 rads preoperatively to entire neck and primary lesion. For multiple nodes or cancer in connective tissue, 5,000 rads postoperatively to entire neck.			
T_3						
T_4						

Note: 1. Nodes at multiple levels require radical neck dissection.
     2. Status of irradiated primary considered at time of neck dissection.

therapeutic dose of irradiation in patients with all but the smallest primary lesions. As the size of the primary lesion increases, however, a more extensive surgical procedure or a larger radiation portal is required which often removes or covers the first level of lymph nodes. This dose of irradiation usually sterilizes the subclinical metastases in these nodes and the rate of development of clinical metastases does not increase, as expected, with increasing T stage (Table 3-8). Since the entire side of the neck is not treated, some patients will develop nodes outside the radiated field and subsequent therapy, usually radical neck dissection, controls the metastasis in 75 per cent of the patients who have the primary lesion controlled.[8,12] Both sub-

digastric areas are included in the radiation fields for faucial arch (soft palate, anterior tonsillar pillar, and retromolar trigone) lesions (Fig. 3-13), except for very early retromolar trigone or anterior tonsillar pillar lesions.

N_1 AND N_2 PATIENTS

Radical neck dissection is adequate in eliminating cancer in the neck if the cancer is limited to a single small node at the first level of metastasis. Radical neck dissection is less effective if the node is large, if connective tissue is infiltrated histologically, or if multiple nodes are histologically positive. Ipsilateral neck dissection cannot prevent the

Table 3-11. *Soft Palate, Anterior Faucial Pillar, and Retromolar Trigone*

	N_0	N_1	N_2A	N_2B	N_3A	N_3B
T_1	Treat primary and Area I	5,000 rads upper neck bilaterally plus radical or modified neck dissection if ipsilateral lower neck irradiated	5,000 rads to entire neck. Neck dissection(s) or combined resection if primary uncontrolled			
T_2	5,000 rads upper neck bilaterally					
T_3	5,000 rads to entire neck					
T_4						

Note: Angle node (Area I) receives high dose irradiation with treatment of primary and neck dissection is not necessary if this is the only positive node.

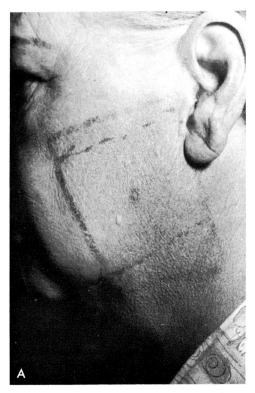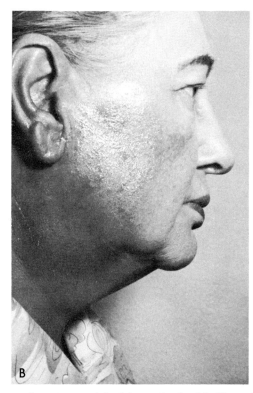

FIG. 3-13. Female, age 58, seen on 4-24-70 with squamous cell carcinoma of the left anterior faucial pillar and soft palate, staged T_3N_0.

Treatment was given with the 22 Mev photon beam, a single left lateral portal delivering a tumor dose of 6,500 rads in 6 weeks and 2 days. At 5,000 rads the portal was reduced as shown in A. The dose in the contralateral subdigastric node area, calculated at 85 per cent of the given dose, was 4,250 rads.

At completion of therapy, there was no visible tumor. There was marked mucous membrane reaction. There was a moderately dry reaction of the skin exposed to the treatment portal and a brisk erythema of the skin covering the opposite subdigastric area (B).

The patient is NED in July 1972. (Courtesy: Fletcher, and Jesse, In *Current Problems in Radiology*, Robert D. Moseley, Editor, Year Book Medical Publishers, Inc., Chicago, Illinois, 1, 3, 1971.)

appearance of nodes in the opposite neck. Subclinical disease in the opposite side is usually limited to the subdigastric area and radiation can prevent its clinical manifestation (Table 3-7).

In N_1 patients with floor of mouth or oral tongue primaries, the upper neck receives irradiation bilaterally with the primary treatment. The lower ipsilateral neck must be treated either with a radical neck dissection or irradiation (Fig. 3-14). If a small node (N_1) in the first lymph node level of the neck receives less than 6,000 rads, it is imperative

to do a neck dissection within 6 to 8 weeks. A full radical dissection is done if the lower neck has not been irradiated and a modified dissection is done if it has been irradiated. Small nodes (N_1) receiving over 5,000 rads may be watched beyond 6 to 8 weeks if control of the primary is in doubt (Fig. 3-14). For N_1 patients with faucial arch lesions, the node at the angle of the jaw receives a high-dose (6,000 rads plus) as irradiation treatment of the primary includes Area I. Such N_1 patients, with only this node positive, will probably not need surgery as the high-dose therapy will sterilize the node, provided the ipsilateral lower neck has been irradiated.

For N_2A patients, combined radiation and surgery are used for the neck if the primary lesion is to be treated with radiation therapy. If nodal disease is at the first level, the ipsilateral first level receives 5,000 rads in 5 weeks and the contralateral side receives slightly less in conjunction with treatment of the primary. The ipsilateral lower neck must either be treated with 5,000 rads or a full radical neck dissection performed within 4 to 6 weeks. If the lower neck is treated with irradiation, a partial neck dissection (limited to the original node bearing area) is adequate. Patients presenting with a neck node below the first level should receive a full neck dissection.

For patients with multiple positive nodes (N_2B), both full necks are given 5,000 rads tumor dose in 5 weeks along with treatment for the primary (Fig. 3-15). In 4 to 6 weeks, an ipsilateral radical neck dissection is done if the primary is controlled. A combined resection is done if the primary is active. In the N_2B clinical setting, a complete radical neck dissection is necessary as the disease is not limited to one area.

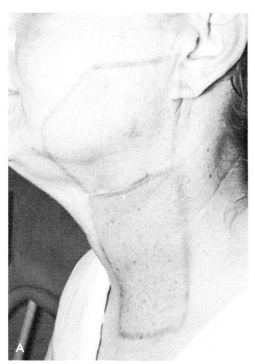 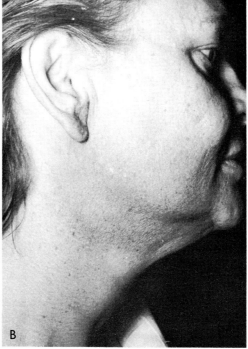

FIG. 3-14. A. Female, age 52, seen on 7-15-70 with a deeply infiltrative squamous cell carcinoma of the posterolateral border of the tongue classified late T_2. There was a 1-cm hard node (N_1) in the subdigastric area. Five thousand rads tumor dose were given in 5 weeks with the 22 Mev betatron covering areas I and II. Then, 2,500 rads were added to the primary with a radium implant. Five thousand rads given dose were delivered to the mid and low jugular node to permit delaying a radical neck dissection until the primary lesion was considered controlled. Eventually no radical neck dissection was performed as the single node disappeared under treatment and never regrew. **B.** Shows the erythema in the opposite subdigastric area, the dose calculated being 4,250 rads. The patient developed a soft tissue necrosis which healed. The patient is *NED* in March 1972. (Courtesy: Northrop, Fletcher, Jesse, and Lindberg, *Cancer,* 29, 23, 1972.)

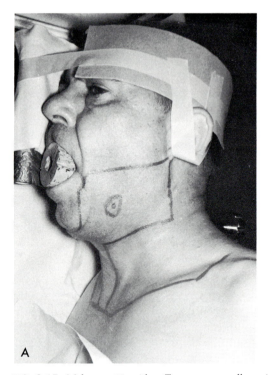 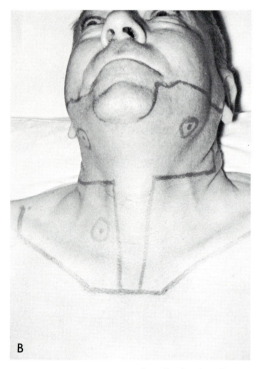

FIG. 3-15. Male, age 63, with a T_3 squamous cell carcinoma of the floor of the mouth and 2 hard nodes, one
1 cm in diameter in the submaxillary triangle and one 1.5 cm in diameter in the subdigastric area.
From 10-30-69 through 12-4-69, a midplane tumor dose of 5,000 rads was given with parallel opposing
^{60}Cobalt portals **(A)** The lower portion of the neck received 5,000 rads given dose through a single
anterior portal **(B)**. On 12-15-69 the patient had an interstitial radium needle implant to the primary
which delivered 2,940 rads in 98 hours.
On 2-16-70, the patient had a radical neck dissection; no tumor was found in the specimen. There
was slightly delayed healing. In April 1972, the patient had no evidence of disease. (Courtesy: Fletcher
and Jesse: *Current Problems in Radiology,* Robert D. Moseley, Editor, Year Book Medical Publishers, Inc.,
Chicago, Illinois, 1, 3, 1971.)

N_3 PATIENTS

A significant number of patients with advanced nodal disease may be salvaged by
radiation combined with surgical procedures.[20] Irradiation must include the entire
neck as these patients usually have extensive
subclinical disease.

N_3A patients (node fixed to skin, carotid
artery, or prevertebral muscle) should never
have primary radical neck dissection since
recurrence is frequent. Proper treatment
consists of 5,000 rads or more to the entire
neck preoperatively and 6,000 rads over the
node. This usually renders the neck mass
operable and permits either a radical or
modified neck dissection.

N_3B patients (bilaterally positive nodes)
are seen in two clinical settings. The first is
a midline carcinoma usually arising in the
soft palate (uvula) or the floor of the mouth.
These nodes are usually not fixed and each
side of the neck is treated separately according to its clinical stage as outlined above for
N_1 or N_2 neck. Should bilateral neck dissections be necessary following irradiation, the
procedures should be staged about 4 weeks
apart to decrease morbidity. Occasionally
bilateral nodes associated with a midline lesion are fixed on one side and their treatment
is exemplified by this case history:

Patient presented with a squamous cell
carcinoma of the soft palate and an 8 cm,
fixed, subdigastric node in the right side and

Table 3-12. *Tonsillar Fossa*

	N_0	N_1	N_2A	N_2B	N_3A	N_3B
T_1	5,000 rads to upper neck		6,000 rads upper neck bilaterally and 5,000 rads lower neck bilaterally.			
T_2			Neck dissection(s) or combined resection if primary uncontrolled			
T_3	5,000 rads to entire neck	Neck dissection for residual node				
T_4						

two 1 cm subdigastric nodes in the left side. Five thousand rads tumor dose were given to the primary tumor and the entire neck with photon beam irradiation. With the electron beam, an additional 1,000 rads were administered both to the palate with an intraoral cone and to the left subdigastric nodes through a small lateral portal. Six weeks later, the nodes in the left side had disappeared while a 3 cm induration remained in the right subdigastric area. A right radical neck dissection was performed with one subdigastric node positive of 29 nodes recovered. The nodes in the left neck were not removed as they were initially small, received 6,000 rads, and had disappeared. The patient died of a bronchogenic carcinoma 5 years later without recurrence in the head and neck area.

The second clinical setting with bilateral neck nodes (N_3B) occurs when the ipsilateral lymphatic channels are blocked by metastases forcing cells from a laterally located primary cancer. This forces cells to metastasize into the contralateral side of the neck. Frequently, there will be a fixed ipsilateral node(s) and a nonfixed contralateral node(s). The entire neck is irradiated to at least 5,000 rads in 5 weeks and neck dissections, either total or partial as indicated, are staged 4 to 8 weeks later.

OROPHARYNX (TABLES 3-12, 13 AND 14)

The parapharyngeal nodes of Rouviere are involved in approximately 30 per cent of patients with lesions of the tonsillar fossa and pharyngeal walls. These lymphatics should be included in the radiation fields since the nodes are difficult to remove surgically. The general treatment plan is to irradiate both sides of the neck in patients whose

Table 3-13. *Base of Tongue*

	N_0	N_1	N_2A	N_2B	N_3A	N_3B
T_1	Treat primary and upper neck		6,000 rads upper neck bilaterally and 5,000 rads lower neck bilaterally.			
T_2		6,000 rads upper neck bilaterally	Neck dissection(s) or combined resection if primary uncontrolled			
T_3		5,000 rads lower neck bilaterally				
T_4		Radical or modified neck dissection in 6 wks for residual node				

Note: 1. Nodes may be treated to 7,000 rads if located in Area I or II.

Table 3-14. *Oropharyngeal Walls*

	N_0	N_1	N_2A	N_2B	N_3A	N_3B
T_1	7,000 rads to primary through bilateral ports if posterior wall	7,000 rads to primary 5,000 rads to entire neck.	7,000 rads to primary 5,000 rads to entire neck Neck dissection(s) if primary controlled			
T_2						
T_3	2 : 1 loading if lateral wall	Neck dissection if primary controlled				
T_4						

primary is also irradiated. Exceptions are made for those patients with small primary cancers (≤ 1 cm) and no nodes on admission.

For well-differentiated squamous cell carcinoma, 5,000 rads are given to the entire neck. If the original node is less than 3 cm at the angle of the jaw and receives in excess of 7,000 rads, surgery may not be performed. If the nodes are large or multiple, a partial or radical neck dissection follows. The effectiveness of preoperative irradiation as opposed to radical neck dissection alone in preventing recurrence in the radically dissected neck is seen in Table 3-5. For fixed node(s), a simple dissection may be done

after irradiation (Fig. 3-16). If the tumor is anaplastic or lymphoepithelioma, greater dependence is placed upon radical irradiation and surgery is rarely performed.

SUPRAGLOTTIC LARYNX (TABLES 3-15 AND 16)

The neck management for cancer of the supraglottic larynx varies with the treatment of the primary disease. Since most lesions of the suprahyoid epiglottis are treated by radiation therapy, the upper neck necessarily receives irradiation. If the neck is N_0, a rather generous field including the subdigastric and

Table 3-15. *Exophytic Supraglottic Larynx Treated by Radiotherapy*

	N_0	N_1	N_2A	N_2B	N_3A	N_3B
T_1	7,000 rads to primary, 5,000 rads to high and mid-jugular nodes bilaterally	6,000 rads to upper neck bilaterally 5,000 rads to lower neck bilaterally Neck dissections(s) (modified or radical) for nodes larger than 3 cm or small nodes receiving under 6,000 rads.				
T_2						

Table 3-16. *Infiltrative Tumor of Infrahyoid Epiglottis, False Cords, Aryepiglottic Folds Primary Treated with Larygectomy*

	N_0	N_1	N_2A	N_2B	N_3A	N_3B
T_3	Wide field laryngectomy radical neck dissection or only postoperative irradiation to entire neck	Postoperative irradiation is routinely given fixed nodes (N_3A, some N_3B): preoperatively 5,000 rads to entire neck followed by laryngectomy and neck dissection(s) (modified or radical)				
T_4						

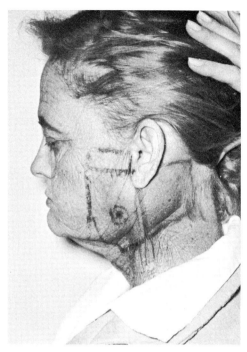

FIG. 3-16. This 57-year-old female was seen in February 1971 with squamous cell carcinoma, Grade III, of the left tonsillar fossa. With a large fixed node at the angle of the jaw, measuring 7 × 6 cm and several other smaller, questionable positive nodes along the jugular chain, the staging was T_2N_3A.

From February 9, 1971 to April 2, 1971, with parallel opposed ^{60}Co fields, the patient received a midline dose of 6,500 rads given at the rate of 850 rads tumor dose per week. The large left lateral portal received a given dose of 5,000 rads. The lower necks were treated with a split field, 5,000 rads given dose in 5 weeks to the right neck and 6,000 rads to the left neck. An additional 1,150 rads with the 22 Mev photon beam were given to the primary through a reduced field. The total tumor dose to the tonsillar fossa lesion (4 cm depth) was 7,500 rads in 8½ weeks. It had been decided in consultation with the head and neck surgeon that the subdigastric node would loosen enough for a partial neck dissection if minimum tumor dose of 6,000 rads was given to the whole node. The posterior aspect of the fixed node received an additional 1,750 rads with the 15 Mev electron beam. The right posterior neck received 2,475 rads given dose with the 6 Mev electron beam to bring the dose at 1 cm depth to 5,100 rads.

On May 3, 1971, the patient had resection of the residual tumor mass in the left neck, and a superficial parotidectomy. A modified left upper neck dissection was done. The mass extended along the internal jugular vein into the retropharyngeal space up to the base of the skull, and to the deep lobe of the parotid. The recovery was essentially unremarkable. The bulk of the mass was completely acellular, with a few scattered islands of recognizable neoplastic squamous cells. There was hyperplastic disorganization sufficient to suggest that the cells were no longer viable. The patient showed no evidence of disease in April 1972.

The patient is shown toward the end of the course of therapy with the boost electron beam field placed over the posterior aspect of the bulging upper neck node.

midjugular nodes are irradiated to 5,000 rads. The field is then reduced to give the necessary dose to the primary lesion. If nodes are clinically present, either unilaterally or bilaterally, the upper and middle portions of the neck receive 6,000 rads in 6 weeks bilaterally while the lower portion of the neck receives 5,000 rads in 5 weeks through an anterior portal. Surgery may not be performed if the nodes were originally less than 3 cm, received 7,000 rads and have disappeared. If the nodes were large, a unilateral or bilateral radical or modified neck dissection is done 4 to 6 weeks after completion of radiation therapy (Fig. 3-17).

The management of lesions of the remainder of the supraglottic larynx (*i.e.*, the infrahyoid epiglottis, false cords, and aryepiglottic folds) is individualized according to the size and nature of the primary lesion. Exophytic lesions are usually treated by irradiation and the neck is managed as described for the suprahyoid epiglottis. Large and infiltrative tumors are managed surgically.

If the neck is N_0, the surgical dissection includes bilateral removal of the upper and

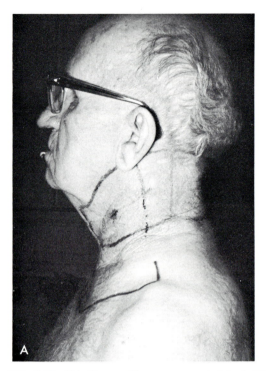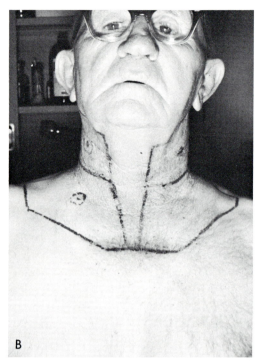

FIG. 3-17. This 70-year-old man was seen in March 1970 with a recent biopsy scar in the right subdigastric area surrounded by induration. There was a 2.5 cm node in the left midjugular area. The posterior aspect of the suprahyoid epiglottis was thickened and distorted and biopsy showed squamous cell carcinoma. The node histology was poorly differentiated squamous cell carcinoma. The patient's disease was staged T_1N_3B.

From 4-2-70 to 5-20-70 the primary lesion received 6,600 rads with parallel opposing ^{60}Co fields and the lower necks received 5,000 rads given dose. After 4,500 rads tumor dose the primary treatment portals were reduced to exclude the spinal cord. The 6 Mev electron beam was used to treat both posterior cervical node areas to bring the minimal tissue dose to 5,500 rads.

Approximately 6 weeks after completion of the irradiation, simultaneous modified bilateral neck dissections were done with excision of the scar in the right neck. The sternocleidomastoid and anterior jugular vein were not removed. Of 22 nodes recovered from the right neck, 5 showed necrotic tissue with peripheral fibrosis and focal cholesterol slits consistent with degenerative cancer. From 35 nodes recovered from the left modified neck dissection, one contained necrotic tissue with peripheral fibrosis and inflammation consistent with degenerative metastasis. No viable tumor was identified in any of these specimens. The patient was seen in March 1972 with no evidence of disease.

The patient is shown after the upper fields have been removed forward to exclude the spinal cord and posterior strip fields have been defined for electron beam treatment.

midjugular nodes (wide-field laryngectomy). The nodes are examined histologically at the time of surgery. If the nodes are negative, no further surgical treatment is given to the neck. If the nodes are positive, the surgeon must either do a radical neck dissection on the positive side or depend upon postoperative radiation therapy to sterilize occult deposits of cancer.

If the neck is clinically positive (N_1 and N_2), a radical neck dissection may be done on the positive side and upper and midjugular nodes are dissected on the contralateral side. Postoperative radiation therapy is administered to both sides of the neck and to the primary area. When there are fixed or bilateral neck nodes (N_3A, N_3B) associated with supraglottic cancers, 5,000 rads or more

Table 3-17. Nasopharynx

	N_0	N_1	N_2A	N_2B	N_3A	N_3B
T_1	7,000 rads to primary, 5,000 rads to entire neck, palpable nodes to 6,500 to 7,000 rads					
T_2	Surgery used only for recurrences					
T_3						
T_4						

are given preoperatively followed by partial or radical neck dissection(s) and laryngectomy.

Table 3-5 shows a reduction of recurrences in the radically dissected neck and Table 3-6 shows a striking diminution in the appearance of contralateral clinical metastasis in those patients having had postoperative irradiation.

NASOPHARYNX (TABLE 3-17)

The treatment policy for cancer of the nasopharynx is irradiation of the entire neck in conjunction with the primary regardless of node status. Radical neck dissection is employed only for recurrent neck disease since irradiation has proven effective in controlling the cancer in all but a few patients.[5]

Hypopharynx Including Pyriform Sinus (Table 3-18)

Laryngopharyngectomy is the initial treatment for the majority of patients with cancer of the hypopharynx. An ipsilateral radical neck dissection is performed if nodes are clinically positive. The contralateral jugular nodes are removed but, even if positive, a radical neck dissection is not performed on the contralateral side. The entire neck, the retropharyngeal nodes, and the primary site are irradiated postoperatively. The recurrence rate in the radically dissected neck is

Table 3-18. *Hypopharyngeal Walls and Pyriform Sinus*

	N_0	N_1	N_2A	N_2B	N_3A	N_3B
T_1	Irradiation to primary and entire neck plus retropharyngeal nodes followed by neck dissection if nodes > 2 cm					
T_2 early						
T_2 late			Laryngopharyngectomy, ipsilateral radical neck dissection and retropharyngeal node dissection, contralateral modified neck dissection. Postoperative irradiation to entire neck and retropharyngeal nodes.			
T_3	Wide field laryngopharyngectomy					
T_4	plus postoperative irradiation to entire neck and retropharyngeal nodes.					

much lower in patients receiving the combined treatment than in those treated with surgery alone (Table 3-5). Cancer appearing in the contralateral neck of patients electively irradiated is nonexistent in our series (Table 3-7).

For the relatively small number of patients with hypopharyngeal cancer and a clinically negative neck, elective irradiation is preferred over elective neck dissection. If the primary lesion is small, radiation therapy is used to preserve the larynx. The primary lesion receives 6,500 to 7,000 rads in $6\frac{1}{2}$ to 7 weeks while the entire neck and retropharyngeal nodes receive 5,000 rads.

Few patients present with a small primary lesion and clinically positive nodes. These patients receive 6,500 to 7,000 rads in $6\frac{1}{2}$ to 7 weeks to the entire primary lesion and 5,000 rads to the entire neck. A radical or modified neck dissection is performed 4 to 6 weeks later.

Treatment for Cancer in the Neck Appearing Secondarily

The guidelines used for the simultaneously treated neck apply to patients in whom neck disease appears later after the initial treatment. Radical neck dissection alone is usually adequate if the node is single, relatively small, and at the first level.

Pre- or postoperative irradiation or irradiation alone is frequently indicated if nodes appear within months of the initial treatment of the primary (Fig. 3-18). Patients with extensive metastasis in the ipsilateral neck subsequent to treatment of the primary have a high probability of contralateral neck involvement. Clinical appearance of contralateral disease can be prevented by irradiation and is preferable to elective or therapeutic radical neck dissection.

Preoperative irradiation is preferred when nodes are multiple, fixed, or bilateral. The entire upper neck receives a minimum of 5,000 rads through parallel opposing portals while the lower neck receives 5,000 rads given dose through an anterior portal. This dose produces a moderate dryness of the mouth and throat. It is, however, a small price to pay when contrasted to the high risk of further metastasis in undissected portions of the neck. Metastases which are fixed or particularly large may receive booster doses of irradiation. Surgical procedures adapted to the clinical situation follow.

First level nodal metastasis, which develops after the primary lesion has been controlled for one year, are almost invariably single and can be controlled by surgical resection only. If multiple nodes are positive, postoperative radiotherapy is employed. If the probability of disease in the contralateral

---

FIG. 3-18. This 52-year-old male was admitted in April 1970 with a 1.2 cm slightly raised and ulcerated area on the right side of the undersurface of the tongue with good oral mobility. The clinical staging was T_1N_0. The patient gave a history of numerous attacks of sialadenitis in the submaxillary glands.

In April 1970, the tongue lesion was widely excised and primary closure was done. Six months later sudden swelling developed over the left submaxillary gland which regressed with antibiotics and probing the submaxillary duct. One month later the gland again became enlarged and tender. After adequate treatment with antibiotics, the gland was removed. There was an acute and subacute chronic sialadenitis with a small focus of squamous carcinoma in a lymph node overlying the gland.

Because the metastasis had appeared in the contralateral side, there was significant risk of new disease in the ipsilateral neck and 5,500 rads were given to the upper necks through parallel opposing portals and 5,000 rads in 5 weeks were given to the lower necks (A). A boost of 1,000 rads was given to the area of the scar in the left submental region through an appositional 7 × 12 cm field with 9 Mev electrons (B). The patient shows no evidence of disease 2 years later.

The scar of dissection stops at the midline. The creases in the skin in the contralateral neck must not be mistaken as being continuation of the scar.

The patient is NED February 1972. (Courtesy: Fletcher, and Jesse, In *Current Problems in Radiology,* 1, 3, 1971.)

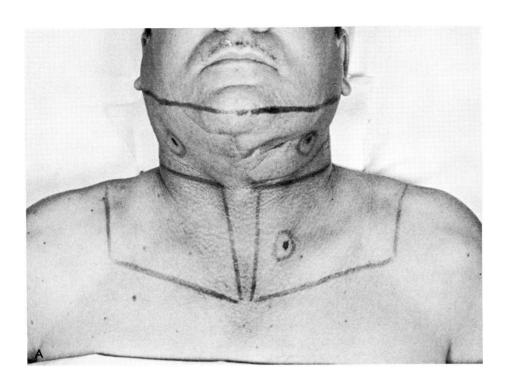

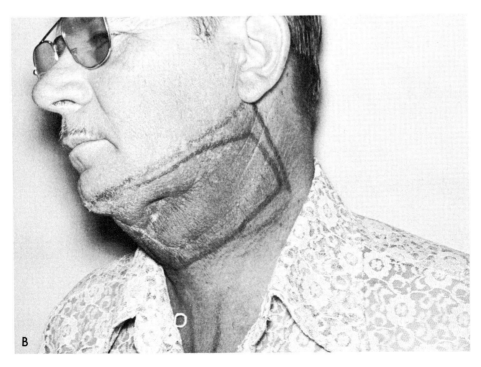

neck is low, one may gamble in not irradiating the contralateral neck in order to avoid dryness. In this situation, the electron beam is useful for irradiation of the dissected neck.

Unresectable Nodes

Interstitial implants can be added to external beam treatment if nodes do not become resectable after external irradiation. Total doses of 8,000 to 9,000 rads are an effective method of treatment.

Unresectable nodes, appearing after the initial treatment and not located over vital structures may be treated with 6,000 rads in 10 to 12 treatments. They often undergo permanent regression.

Lower Neck Irradiation

Irradiation to the lower neck is administered through an anterior split field (Fig. 3-19). If the lower neck is clinically negative, the split is complete down to the manubrium taking care not to shield the midjugular nodes. Treatment consists of 5,000 rads given dose in 5 weeks. If the lower neck is clinically positive, only the larynx is shielded, and an additional 1,000 to 2,000 rads are given through reduced portals.

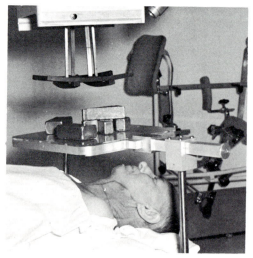

FIG. 3-19. Lower neck treatment position.

Employing the ^{60}Cobalt unit, the tumor dose to the lower jugular, supraclavicular, and posterior cervical triangle nodes is the same as the given dose since they are located immediately under the skin. The midjugular nodes are at the most 2 to 2.5 cm deep and the tumor dose to these nodes is about 90 per cent of the given dose.

Hypothyroidism rarely develops even though midline shielding covers only the isthmus of the thyroid and not the lobes. Since hypothyroidism is a remote possibility, the physician should observe the patient carefully for the symptoms and signs of this condition.

BIBLIOGRAPHY

1. Barkley, H. T. Jr., Fletcher, G. H., Jesse, R. H. Jr., and Lindberg, R. D.: Management of cervical lymph node metastasis: Primary lesions of the tonsillar fossa, base of tongue, supraglottic larynx and hypopharynx, *Amer. J. Surg.*, 124, 462, 1972.
2. Beahrs, O. H., and Barber, K. W.: The value of radical dissection of structures of the neck in the management of carcinomas of the lip, mouth, and larynx, *Arch. Surg.*, 85, 49, 1962.
3. Berger, D. S., Fletcher, G. H., Lindberg, R. D., and Jesse, R. H.: Elective irradiation of the neck lymphatics for squamous cell carcinoma of the nasopharynx and oropharynx, *Amer. J. Roentgen.*, 111, 66, 1971.
4. Berger, D. S., and Fletcher, G. H.: Distant metastases in patients with squamous cell carcinoma of the nasopharynx, tonsillar fossa, and base of tongue free of disease at the primary site and in the neck, *Radiology*, 100, 141, 1971.
5. Chen, K. Y., and Fletcher, G. H.: Malignant tumors of the nasopharynx, *Radiology*, 99, 165, 1971.
6. Fletcher, G. H.: Elective irradiation of subclinical disease in cancers of the head and neck, *Cancer*, 29, 1450, 1972.
7. Fletcher, G. H., and Jesse, R. H.: Interaction of surgery and irradiation in head and neck cancers, in *Current Problems in Radiology*, Robert D. Moseley, Editor, Year Book Medical Publishers, Inc., Chicago, Illinois, 1, 3, 1971.

8. Jesse, R. H., Barkley, H. T., Jr., Lindberg, R. D., and Fletcher, G. H.: Cancer of the oral cavity. Is elective neck dissection beneficial? *Am. J. Surg.,* 120, 505, 1970.

9. Kremen, A. J.: The case for elective (prophylactic) neck dissection, J. Conley, (Ed), In *Cancer of the Head and Neck,* Washington, D. C., Butterworth, Inc., p. 183, 1967.

10. Lindberg, R. D., and Jesse, R. H.: Treatment of cervical lymph node metastasis from primary lesions of the oropharynx, supraglottic larynx and hypopharynx, *Amer. J. Roentgen.,* 102, 132, 1968.

11. Lindberg, R. D.: Distribution of cervical lymph node metastases from squamous cell carcinoma of the upper respiratory and digestive tracts, *Cancer,* 29, 1446, 1972.

12. Lindberg, R. D., Barkley, H. T., Jr., Jesse, R. H., and Fletcher, G. H.: Evolution of the clinically negative neck in patients with squamous cell carcinoma of the faucial arch, *Amer. J. Roentgen.,* 111, 60, 1971.

13. Lyall, D., Schetlin, D. F.: Cancer of the tongue, *Ann. Surg.,* 134, 313, 1958.

14. Martin, H. E., Munster, H., and Sugarbaker, E. D.: Cancer of the tongue, *Arch. Surg.,* 41, 888, 1940.

15. Million, R. R., Fletcher, G. H., Jesse, R. H.: Evaluation of elective irradiation of the neck for squamous cell carcinoma of the nasopharynx, tonsillar fossa, and base of tongue, *Radiology,* 80, 973, 1963.

16. Northrop, M., Fletcher, G. H., Jesse, R. H., and Lindberg, R. D.: Evolution of neck disease in patients with primary squamous cell carcinoma of the oral tongue, floor of mouth, and palatine arch and clinically positive neck nodes neither fixed nor bilateral, *Cancer,* 29, 23, 1972.

17. Roux-Berger, J. L., Baud, M., and Courtial, J.: Cancer de la partie mobile de la langue. Le curage ganglionaire prophylactique est-il justifie? Statistique de la Foundation Curie, *Mem. Acad. chir.,* 75, 120, 1949.

18. Southwick, H. W., Slaughter, D. P., and Trevino, E. T.: Elective neck dissection for intraoral cancer, *Arch. Surg.,* 80, 905, 1960.

19. Strong, E. W.: Preoperative radiation and radical neck dissection. *Surg. Clin. N. Amer.,* 49, 271, 1969.

20. Votava, C., Fletcher, G. H., Jesse, R. H., and Lindberg, R. D.: Management of cervical nodes either fixed or bilateral from primary squamous cell carcinoma of the oral cavity and faucial arch, *Radiology,* 105, 417, 1972.

Skin and Lip

CARL F. VON ESSEN

Skin cancer, other than melanoma, is rarely a fatal disease. The majority of lesions grow slowly, and because over 90 per cent arise in exposed areas, they are usually detected in early stages of development. These tumors are often readily curable and therefore the selection of the optimum treatment modality should be considered with respect to the expected cosmetic effects, the relative comfort, time and cost of treatment to the patient, as well as upon the probability of cure.

Curability of the common epithelial skin tumors by competent surgery is not questioned by reasonable radiation therapists nor should the converse be challenged. The remaining factors, then, should direct the form of treatment in the large majority of cases.

Radiation therapy has a special role in the palliation of the widespread cutaneous manifestations of lymphomas and some multicentric diseases such as Kaposi's sarcoma. Some tumors are radioresistant or are located in sites that tolerate irradiation poorly. These include the melanomas, fibrosarcomas, and carcinomas arising in the scrotum, vulva, and portions of the extremities.

The use of ionizing radiation, by preference, supposes the expectation of a high probability of eradicating the lesion, preservation of the normal tissues with little or no blemish, and the achievement of all of this without trauma and with minimal time and cost for the patient. This will demand a good clinical knowledge of anatomical factors, radiobiology, and a judicious computation of all the physical factors in radiation therapy, including treatment volume, quality of irradiation, dosage, overall treatment time and fractionation.

Biological Principles

Anatomy of the Integument

An understanding of the origin of malignant neoplasms of the skin and of approaches to treatment is aided by knowledge of its basic structure. The epidermis varies in thickness from 60 microns (0.06 mm) in the eyelid and vulva to 1 mm in exposed sites such as the palms and soles. Epidermal cells which extend into the dermis (dense connective tissue) and occasionally into the looser subcutaneous connective tissue include those of the fat and sweat glands and the hair follicles. It is important to recall that the epidermis is avascular, all nutrition being supplied by a network of capillary loops extending into the papillae of the upper layer of the dermis. Furthermore, the superficial dermis contains only capillary vessels, all arterioles extending in a network in the subcutaneous tissue and lower dermis. The accessory glandular structures vary greatly in number throughout different body regions. They have an important role in the re-epithelialization of the epidermis after injury. Epithelial outgrowth is often noted from sites of hair follicles and sweat glands after superficial desquamation following thermal burns

or radiation therapy. It is noteworthy that the incidence of basal cell carcinomas has been correlated with the incidence of sebaceous glands.[18]

Because of the vital role that the dermis and subcutaneous tissue play in the nutrition of the integument, all therapeutic approaches should emphasize maximum protection of these structures consistent with therapeutic results. It is likely that late radiation sequelae such as necrosis or carcinogenesis relate to severe dermal and subcutaneous tissue injury rather than to more superficial cell damage which may be healed by re-epithelialization.[37]

The generation time of the basal germinative cell is in the order of 120 hours in "resting" epithelium. Following radiation this generation time is greatly shortened provided that adequate nutrition is available.[11] Cells lining the accessory glands, especially the hair follicles, follow a similar growth pattern.

The three important basic elements of the skin, the epithelial cell, the endothelial cells, and the fibroblast exert their prime effects in response to injury by incontinuity spread of sheets of cells or by migration of individual cells through vascular channels and intercellular spaces.

Neoplasms of the Integument

Histological study will often give clues to the biological behavior of the tumor. The gross characteristics of the neoplasm *i.e.,* degree of ulceration, sharpness of margins, underlying fixation, edema, inflammation, will also indicate the behavior patterns. The mode of spread will dictate the correct form of treatment; in general, if highly destructive, surgery and repair by grafts; if less destructive or beyond surgical control, radiotherapy.

BASAL CELL CARCINOMA

Although all neoplasms may adopt different behavior patterns that can be intercompared, the basal cell tumors appear to have several highly characteristic patterns. A convenient division can be made of six types; the ulcerative, adenocystic, morphea, terebrant, multiple superficial and the metastasizing forms.

Ulcerative Basal Cell Carcinoma (the rodent ulcer) is the most common variety seen in clinical practice. The site of predilection is the face, particularly the regions above the mouth, including the nose, nasolabial fold, eyelids, and cheek. The lesions begin as colorless papules, soon develop central umbilication after achieving a diameter of a few millimeters, and will ulcerate shortly thereafter, presumably because of outgrowth resulting in central necrosis. The margins are classically pearly, *i.e.,* translucent and pale, and enlarged capillaries can be seen entering the lesions. By palpation the lesions are moderately firm as compared to nonpigmented benign nevi. Marginal biopsies will show small to large nests of dark staining cells with artificial separation from the surrounding stroma. Nests of cells beyond the visible and palpable margin may be present and the characteristics of these nests, small and infiltrating, or large and well-defined, are of importance in establishing therapeutic margins. Progression of the tumor is associated with increasing ulceration, usually in a lateral dimension, but also in depth.

Adenocystic Basal Cell Carcinoma appears as a papule which will progress to quite large dimensions without ulceration. The tumor cells develop large cystic spaces. The neoplasm is poorly invasive. It is stated to be relatively radioresistant but this may be attributed to the large volume to area ratio of these tumors with consequently larger numbers of cells per unit area and to cystic spaces which may regress slowly.

Morphea (or serpiginous) Carcinoma develops and spreads as a flat, quite superficial, neoplasm with irregular, pearly borders which leave behind areas of shiny atrophic scarring. This is sometimes termed a healing process but sections of the scar will reveal nests of viable appearing tumor cells. Superficial progression appears to continue and deep ulceration is not a part of the behavior. However, because of the extensive central scarring by the neoplasm the therapeutic approach may warrant excision and repair by grafting.

Terebrant Carcinoma originates most commonly in the triangular region of the upper cheek under the eyelids extending to the nasolabial fold.[4] It may present as a small ulcerated tumor on inspection, but by palpation and histological examination there is an early extension into deeper structures and infiltrations in all dimensions by small nests of undifferentiated basal cells. This variety may invade the orbit, nose, and maxilla producing marked destruction. It is highly important that this variety is recognized and treated vigorously.

Multiple Superficial Tumors are relatively non-invasive and have a tendency for spontaneous healing. There is little role for radiotherapy of these lesions.

Metastasizing Basal Cell Carcinoma cannot be identified as such until evidence of metastasis develops. Generally it is found that metastasis occurs in far advanced ulcerated tumors or in those tumors that have received repeatedly unsuccessful treatment, surgical or radiological. The rare case will develop widespread hematogenous metastases.

SQUAMOUS CELL CARCINOMA

Histological variants have more often been described than morphological forms. The various grades extend from the well differentiated form, forming keratin pearls, and with distinct intercellular bridges to an anaplastic variety difficult to distinguish from reticulum cell sarcoma. The most common carcinoma of the skin, however, is the well differentiated form and the site of predilection is the mucosa of the lower lip with the ears, lower portion of the face and neck less commonly involved.

INVASIVE ACANTHOSIS

These neoplasms are often referred to as pseudocarcinomas.[27] They represent a family of similar types with the predominant lesion called keratoacanthoma (molluscum sebaceum). The histological features closely resemble those of well differentiated epidermoid carcinoma. The lesions are usually single, rapidly growing, and develop prominent central cores containing necrotic, sebaceous material. However, multiple lesions have been described. The keratoacanthomas, by definition, are self-healing, possibly on the basis of an inflammatory reaction secondary to keratin deposits. The therapeutic approach is conservative because of this tendency to heal. However, the possibility of malignancy warrants that the form of treatment should be directed towards complete eradication of the neoplasm. Waiting for spontaneous regression is hazardous from two standpoints; progression of the lesion will produce destruction of normal structures resulting in a poor cosmetic result even if spontaneous regression occurs; and the lesion may be or become a progressive epidermoid carcinoma.

MALIGNANT MELANOMA

The diagnosis of malignancy rests ultimately on histologic interpretation. However, the criteria are by no means universal. The separation of an early malignant melanoma from an active junctional nevus, a juvenile melanoma, extramammary Paget's disease of the vulva, and even pigmented basal cell carcinoma may be difficult. The lesion is often highly malignant by early treatment appears to be helpful in increasing the general cure rate. In this country the accepted

standard for treatment has been wide excision with incontinuity dissection of the draining regional lymphatic system. However, elsewhere, the use of high dosage superficial irradiation has been advocated.[20,25,28]

CUTANEOUS LYMPHOMAS

This group of neoplasms is exceptionally suited for control by certain radiation techniques. The malignant lymphoma cells are relatively radiosensitive and large areas of skin are often involved, contraindicating surgical removal, while the disease may be symptomatically limited to the skin, thus contraindicating systemic chemotherapy.

Lymphosarcoma may arise apparently from the skin *de novo* or as metastases from known primaries elsewhere in the body. The appearance may be that of discrete or confluent erythematous macular eruptions or, occasionally, a generalized erythroderma. The disease may remain limited to the skin for a considerable time but inevitably all cases will demonstrate progression to systemic involvement and eventual death.

Leukemia Cutis may present from any of the various forms of leukemia. The management is palliative and may depend a great extent upon the status of the primary disease.

Cutaneous infiltrates of Hodgkin's disease are occasionally seen and can be controlled by suitably designed radiation therapy. Very rarely it may develop as an apparent primary lesion in the skin.

MYCOSIS FUNGOIDES

Controversy and confusion have clouded both the criteria of diagnosis and the principles of management of this uncommon disease. It has been suggested that the diagnosis of mycosis fungoides should be restricted to that neoplastic process which remains limited to the skin throughout the life of the patient.[6] Similar neoplastic infiltrates that sooner or later appear in other organs and structures will usually be found to fall into the category of lymphosarcoma or reticulum cell sarcoma. The rate of progression of disease varies widely, not only between patients but also in various surface areas of individual patients. The initial stages, usually not diagnosed, appear to be parapsoriatic lesions which may gradually involve the whole body surface. At some stage the lesions become plaque-like, pruritic and range from discrete to confluent. If a sufficiently large percentage of the body surface is involved, the application of total cutaneous electron irradiation may prove to be of distinct palliative benefit. However, other stages may supervene; the infiltrates may increase in thickness and tumorous areas will develop with ulceration. The depth of these tumors will exceed the effective range of electrons and, therefore, they are best treated by localized x-irradiation of suitable energy. Because the disease is relatively chronic and the disease apparently cannot be prevented from recurring in treated sites, the dosage should be conservative and the areas treated should be carefully recorded.

However, this conservative concept is challenged by Fuks and Bagshaw[17] who report a group of patients surviving from 3 to 11 years after electron beam irradiation and who have remained free of disease. They believe it is justified to refer patients with early and relatively localized mycosis fungoides for total skin electron irradiation in the hope of achieving permanent disease control.

Some chemotherapeutic agents (methotrexate, vinblastine, vincristine) hold promise of temporary control and alternation of treatment modalities may serve to prolong relatively symptom-free life.

KAPOSI'S SARCOMA

This poorly understood disease is encountered most often in the lower extremities of males of Mediterranean, African and Near East origin. This progression is slow and death may occur from systemic disease but more often death is intercurrent. On the basis that disease may be unicentric some authors have proposed radical management, either by radiation[10] or chemotherapeutic perfusion. Evidence is still lacking that this approach significantly alters the natural course of disease. It is, therefore, the consensus that conservative management by localized x-irradiation to lesions as they arise is the treatment of choice.

BENIGN CONDITIONS OF THE SKIN

The scope of radiation therapy in the management of benign inflammatory, hyperplastic, and neoplastic conditions has diminished through the last 25 years with the development of steroids, antibiotics, chemotherapeutic agents, and improved surgery. Recent knowledge, however, of the hazards of systemic steroid medication, and of the transient effects of topical applications of steroids, has served to stimulate the continued use of ionizing radiation in a small group of benign conditions.

Dermatoses which respond to steroid medication are, in general, responsive also to ionizing radiations. The principles of action probably lie in the lymphocytolytic effects of both agents, the possible basis of "anti-inflammatory" effects. Radiation therapy may be justified in cases of localized drug resistant eruptions. Suitable treatment patterns (area, depth, dose) designed to minimize radiation to underlying and peripheral areas generally involve very low energy x-irradiation (10 to 80 Kv). The prime hazard is the possibility of excessive cumulative dosage if retreatment is sought by the patient from different radiotherapists without mention of previous treatment. With proper attention it appears that the risk of skin damage or subsequent changes is negligible.[15,30]

Similar considerations exist for infections of the skin and its appendages.

Hyperplastic Conditions, such as keloids developing in surgical or traumatic scars may be of cosmetic and symptomatic disability to the patient. The most effective management is surgical excision followed by a single dose of irradiation of the order of 800 to 1,000 rads limited to the scar and designed to reach the depth of the incision. Radiation is best carried out immediately following surgery.

Benign Neoplasms. A more conservative approach to the treatment of hemangiomas has developed since a better understanding of the natural history of these lesions was presented.[7] The lesions are self-limited and may eventually involute. There is, however, an indication to treat as early as possible the rapidly growing capillary hemangioma of infancy, particularly when it is situated at or near natural orifices. Untreated, the hemangioma may interfere with function (breathing, eating, defecation, sight, etc.). Such lesions invariably ulcerate, and following involution will leave extensive, possibly deforming, scarring. A modest dose of ionizing radiation may prevent many or all of these sequelae. On the other hand, a hemangioma with cavernous and capillary elements not exhibiting growth and not interfering with function is probably best untreated.

Therapeutic Principles

The Dose-Time-Area Concept

There is a relationship between the radiation dose required to achieve a given effect such as tumor regression, and the time required to administer that dose. This function can be expressed by:

$$D = kT^n$$

where D is the dose required for the given effect, T is the overall time, and n is an exponent less than one.

Strandqvist[29] employed this approach in deriving a function for curability of skin cancer and for normal tissue reactions. In his work the value (n) was identical (0.22) for both tumor curability and for skin reactions and it was expressed as a linear function on logarithmic scales of time and dose.

Analysis of other data by Cohen[8] suggested, however, that the slopes for skin reactions and for tumor curability differed and that the slope for tumor curability was less steep than that for skin reactions. These findings helped to explain the empirically discovered superiority of dose protraction in many clinical radiotherapy situations.

A corroboration was noted by this author[34] who also found in his clinical material that the slope for 99 per cent tumor curability to be considerably flatter than those of Strandqvist or Cohen (Fig. 3-20). A reason for the discrepancy between these findings may be that tumor size or irradiated tissue volume (essentially equivalent to area in the case of superficial skin malignancies) was not studied as a separate variable by Strandqvist. The larger lesions were gener-

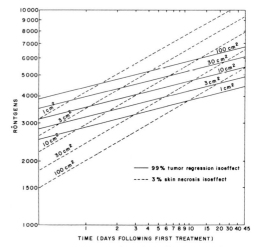

FIG. 3-20. Time-Dose plot of isoeffect curves for various areas of irradiated skin and tumor using the indices of 3 per cent skin necrosis and 99 per cent tumor curability respectively. The slope for skin tolerance is 0.27 and for tumor curability is 0.14. Transforming the time scale to $T = 1$ for the first treatment these values approximate 0.32 and 0.17 respectively. (Courtesy: von Essen, *Radiology,* 81, 881, 1963.)

ally irradiated over longer time intervals, presumably because of empirical experience that better results followed longer protraction of irradiation of large tumors. Thus the plot of tumors treated and recorded on X-Y coordinates of time and dose was not random but influenced by tumor size and consequently by irradiated area—the greater areas being irradiated over longer time spans. Because larger tumors are more radioresistant by virtue of increased cell numbers and possibly by increased hypoxia, the apparent time-dose iso-effect slope was steeper than would probably be the case if tumors of a given size were irradiated randomly over the usual time scale (1 day to about 6 weeks) used in radiation therapy.

Strandqvist's slope of 0.22 on the logarithmic Y-scales of dose in roentgens and X-scale of elapsed time in days with an initial point of 8 hours (0.35 days) can consequently be reconciled with the derivation of a slope of 0.14 for tumor regression if a mean value is obtained from a second slope derived for skin tolerance. This has been found to range from 0.26 to 0.33.[1,8,9,34] The data showing that larger tissue areas tolerate less irradiation have been presented by Jolles and Joyet and Hohl[21,22] among others. The means of the value 0.14 and of the range 0.26 to 0.33 is in the range of 0.20 to 0.24. This range of values overlaps the slope of 0.22 derived by Strandqvist. These relationships are depicted on a three-dimensional model shown in Figure 3-21 and on cross-sectional graphs (Fig. 3-22). The line of intersection of the two planes in fact approximates almost exactly the slope of the Strandqvist iso-effect line.

What is the radiobiological basis for these mathematically defined relationships? Ex-

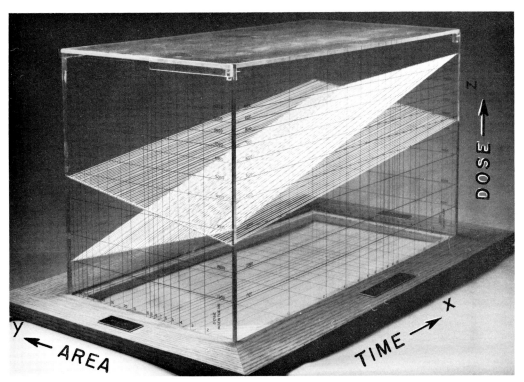

FIG. 3-21. A three-dimensional model portraying the graphic data of Figure 3-20 on logarithmic scales. The X-axis gives cumulative time in days, the Y-axis area in cm², and the Z-axis cumulative dosage in roentgens. The light plane is the 3 per cent skin necrosis isoeffect plane. The dark plane is the 99 per cent tumor cure isoeffect plane. (Courtesy: von Essen, *Radiology*, 81, 881, 1963.)

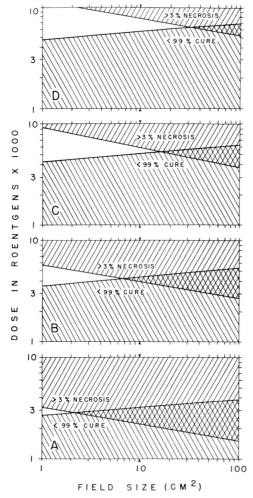

FIG. 3-22. Graphic cross-sections through the model shown in Figure 3-21 taken perpendicular to the time (X) axis. **A.** Single treatment (0.35 days), **B.** 5 days, **C.** 21 days, **D.** 45 days.

host-tumor relationship *in situ:* following any injury the host seeks to repair the injured site by means of cellular repopulation, by either in continuity proliferation or by seeding through the blood and lymphatic channels. If an overwhelming injury occurs such as that following a single large dose of irradiation, healing will follow in a certain time interval and will depend in its effectiveness upon the volume injured, as shown by DuNouy for surgical wounds.[13] A large volume exposed to sudden injury will result in an abrupt loss of cellular continuity mitigating against the ability of the repopulation elements to maintain tissue integrity. A smaller volume exposed to injury can be more readily repaired because of diminished distances necessary for the migration of repopulating cells. Arygris and Devik[2,11] have shown that the margins of irradiated skin contain epithelial cells in accelerated kinetic states that migrate into the irradiated zone. If then, the process of injury is protracted, two factors may aid repair: less abrupt breakdown of tissue integrity, and continuous repopulation (al-

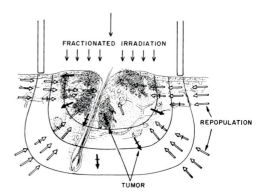

FIG. 3-23. Schematic portrayal of the kinetics of tissue restitution in a cross section of a basal cell carcinoma by means of repopulation from peripheral (unirradiated) tissue. Each arrow signifies an arbitrary time unit of radiation or repopulation. Each crossed arrow indicates a time unit of repopulation inhibited by a corresponding time unit of irradiation. Tumor cells are located entirely within the radiation zone and, therefore, are selectively destroyed by protraction of irradiation.

perimental laboratory data have explained only a relative small part of this complex problem which involves at least two dynamic cell systems (host and neoplasm) as well as the variables of irradiation dose-rate and area or volume.

To date it has not been possible to explain on the basis of *in vitro* experiments the differential slope of normal and neoplastic cell response to protracted radiation. An explanation can be sought in the actual though inhibited by the injury process) during the time of exposure to injury. Thus, larger volumes of injury may be repaired if the injury process is protracted.

These factors benefit host repair. Tumor tissue repair by repopulation is not possible if all of the tumor is within the volume of irradiation. Figure 3-23 depicts the kinetics of these processes. Thus it is not necessary to postulate differences either in radiosensitivity or in repair rates between tumor and normal cells, and, in fact, very little evidence has yet been shown to suggest that these differences exist or are significant.

Such a model can serve to explain both the advantages and limitations of radiation sterilization of tumors in man. Even with long time periods of radiation, the ability to sterilize very large tumor volumes and yet permit host repair is severely curtailed.

Practical Applications of the Dose-Time-Area Model

The three-dimensional model (Fig. 3-21), although useful for teaching purposes to give a visual appreciation of the relationships of dose, time and tissue area, is impractical for purposes of readily available computation of dosage under clinical conditions. For these purposes the nomogram has been reduced to an equation that can be readily calculated on a slide-rule.[38] This equation relates skin tolerance to the curative dose as a function of radiation depth dose (assuming single field treatment), mean diameter of the radiated field, and overall time in days, counting the first treatment as one day. The fractionation is five or six daily treatments per week. The introduction of fractionation other than daily necessitates modification of the equation using Ellis's method.[14]

The equation is employed in the following way: the radiation therapist selects the diameter and depth of the radiation field in order to adequately surround the tumor dimensions. The radiation physical factors are then selected in order to give an acceptable depth

dose fraction, f, following which the minimum overall time, T, is solved by the following:

$$T = \left(\frac{k_2}{k_1} \cdot \frac{\sqrt{L}}{f} \right)^6$$

The single dose equivalents for 1 cm diameter fields are represented by k_1 (for skin tolerance) and k_2 (for tumor cure). From previous data[34] the value for a probability of less than 3 per cent late severe skin damage is 3,100 rads (k_1) and for more than 99 per cent probability of cure is 2,150 rads (k_2). The mean diameter, L, and the depth dose fraction, f, complete the equation. Following the solution of T to the next largest whole number the tumor curative dose D_c, is solved:

$$D_c = 2150 \sqrt{TL}$$

and the skin tolerance dose:

$$D_t = f\, 3{,}100 \sqrt[3]{\frac{T}{L}}$$

may be checked to confirm that the given dose does not exceed that amount.

Figure 3-24 shows the values for T as related to field diameter and the depth dose fraction, f, following the values $k_2 = 2{,}150$ rads and $k_1 = 3{,}100$ rads. It is seen that as the field size increases the value of T rapidly exceeds the limits of clinical experience (about 6 weeks) and indicates that modifications of k_1 and k_2 to less stringent therapeutic ratios must be made in the case of larger tumors (and skin areas). This also points out the limitation of curing very large tumors with radiation therapy alone and still preserving normal tissue integrity.

Physical Considerations

EXTERNAL X-RADIATION

Cutaneous cancer grows on the body surface and only rarely is it accessible from an opposing surface (such as earlobe). The majority of techniques, therefore, depend upon a single incident beam of radiation. Massive

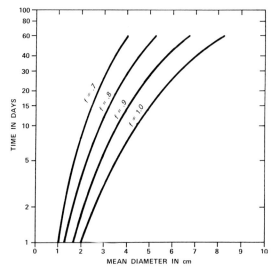

FIG. 3-24. Curves relating minimum overall time of radiation therapy in days, *T,* to field diameter, *L,* for various depth dose fractions, *f.* *T* rapidly increases with *L* and exceeds the limits of clinical experience unless a reduced therapeutic ratio is accepted. Reducing the number of fractions in a given overall time will also lead to reduction of the therapeutic ratio.

involvement may justify angled beams with wedges. The ideal goal is to limit the radiation entirely to the tumor bearing area; a practical compromise is to select those physical factors, including radiation quality, source-tumor distance, and radiation area which will encompass the lateral limits of the tumor with its estimated microscopic extension and limit transmitted radiation to underlying structures to a minimum. To accomplish this aim requires an accurate assessment of gross tumor extent by means of measurement with ruler or caliper, estimation of microscopic invasion and depth by examination of an adequate biopsy of margins, and other clinical aids such as roentgenograms. Electron beams have the practical possibility of achieving this aim with greatest success when lesions are limited to within a few centimeters of the surface. At the present, however, only x-ray and gamma

beams of selected energy and focal distance are available in the majority of radiotherapy departments.

Beginning with the energy range of about 30 Kv a fairly continuous spectrum of x-ray beams of energy ranging up to the megavoltage region should provide an adequate armamentarium for all possible situations. Lesions ranging in depth from a few millimeters to several centimeters could thus be effectively radiated with fair homogeneity of dose within tumor and with reasonable limitation of transmitted dose. These modalities are shown in Table 3-19 and Figure 3-25.

The ideal conditions of limiting the radiation to the tumor volume alone cannot be achieved by external x-irradiation. The judicious selection of treatment factors will minimize transmitted irradiation. However, the eye, middle ear, and brain must be considered special problems and elaborate measures should be undertaken to reduce the dose to the absolute minimum in these sites. The generally accepted maximally tolerated dose to the lens is 200 rads, to the middle ear is 1,000 rads, and to the brain is 5,000 rads over a protracted course of treatment up to 5 or 6 weeks. If adequate protection to these or other vital structures is not possible

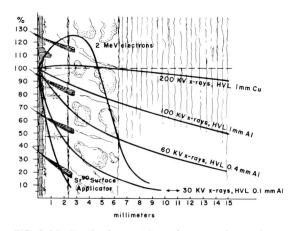

FIG. 3-25. Depth dose curves of commonly used forms of irradiation superimposed upon a section of skin drawn to the same scale.

Table 3-19. *Optimum Factors for Radiation Therapy of Superficial Cutaneous Tumors**

Tumor Depth (mm)	Field Area (cm²)	Kv	F.S.D. (cm)	HVL mm Al	% D.D.
2	5	43	15	0.40	75
4	5	50	15	0.75	71
6	5	80	15	1.00	75
8	5	100	15	3.00	75
10	5	125	15	8.00	77
2	5–15	43	15	0.40	76
4	5–15	50	15	0.75	80
6	5–15	80	15	1.00	76
8	5–15	80–100	15	2.00	73
10	5–15	80–100	30	2.00	75
12	5–15	100	30	3.00	75
16	5–15	125	30	4.00	76
20	5–15	200	50	0.5 mm Cu	78
2	15–50	29	30	0.15	71
4	15–50	50	30	0.75	80
6	15–50	50	30	0.75	74
8	15–50	80	30	1.00	75
10	15–50	100	30	2.00	79
12	15–50	100	30	2.00	74
16	15–50	125	30	3.00	71
20	15–50	125	30	3.00	71
24	15–50	125	30	8.00	73
28	15–50	200	50	0.5 mm Cu.	75

*Data obtained from numerous sources and given in approximate values.

then a relative contraindication to radiation therapy exists.

Other irradiation modalities include interstitial gamma irradiation, external short distance gamma radiation, and electron beam irradiation. Only the last agent is likely to demonstrate physical advantages over external x-irradiation of a suitable combination of factors.

Electron Beams

Up to the present, the main applications sought for superficially penetrating electron beams have been in the treatment of widespread cutaneous diseases such as mycosis fungoides, cutaneous lymphomas, exfoliative dermatitis, and psoriasis.[3,31,33]

The M.I.T. technique is by means of a 2 Mev Van de Graaff generator with a narrow slit beam of electrons delivered during the linear transit of the entire patient's body surface in both anterior and posterior aspects. The Cambridge method exposes the entire body surface to electrons emitted from a large ⁹⁰Sr source.[19] Recent refinements have been achieved by means of scattered beams of electrons which are suitably attenuated for the desired depth dose generated by megavoltage linear accelerators.[3,29] Figure 3-26 shows such depth dose curves which consequently can be tailored to the clinical findings.

The obvious advantage of these whole body surface beams is the lack of significant internal irradiation which could lead, in the

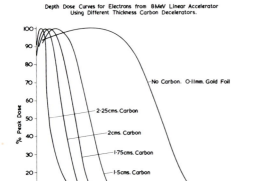

FIG. **3-26**. The relative depth dose curves of electrons of varying energy. (Courtesy: Szur, *Lancet,* 1, 1373, 1962.)

range of doses used, to bone marrow and gastrointestinal cellular depletion and death. The majority of patients, in fact, demonstrate no peripheral leukocyte or platelet depressions, even following doses of over 1,000 rads. It has also been shown that retreatment is feasible but, in general, the fatal outcome of the disease has limited the possibility to know the limits of normal tissue tolerance to this selective form of irradiation.

The consensus appears to be that a therapeutic course of irradiation for mycosis fungoides or cutaneous lymphomatosis is approximately 1,000 rads in 2 to 3 weeks with fractionation of twice or three times weekly. Repeated courses at monthly or longer intervals have been performed when indicated.

The Stanford group has gradually increased the dosage to 3,000 rads in 40 days using 2.5 Mev electrons in a 6 field distribution over nearly the entire integument.[17]

The palliative benefits to the disseminated eczematoid pruritic form of mycosis fungoides can be dramatic. The application of this form of irradiation to more localized problems such as chest wall metastases, carcinoma *en cuirasse*, and even single carcinomas may well be feasible.

COLLIMATION OF EXTERNAL BEAMS

The irradiation margins should be determined by clinical judgment. A fixed margin around visible or palpable tumors such as 0.5 or 1 cm may needlessly irradiate normal tissue in some instances of small and non-infiltrating tumors while undertreating others that may be large and widely infiltrating as determined by clinical and histological examination.

It makes good sense, radiobiologically to deliver two-thirds to three-fourths of the dosage to the tumor and its margin, then to reduce the treatment area to circumscribe only the clinical tumor for the full dosage. This is based upon the anticipated higher sensitivity of microscopic nests of tumor cells because of lower cell number and better oxygenation. This "controlled penumbra" form of treatment reduces the normal tissue dosage and, therefore, should give improved cosmetic results.

It is of vital importance to shield underlying structures whenever possible as shown in Figure 3-27. This should be done even

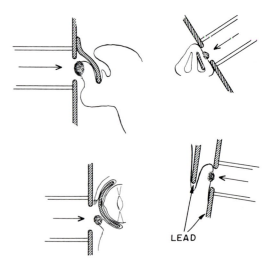

FIG. **3-27**. Diagrams showing the possibilities of underlying as well as peripheral protection in radiation therapy of tumors of the eyelid, lip, nose and ear. The lead shielding should be coated with paraffin or plastic. Lead rubber is also useful.

when optimum depth dose distribution can be obtained because any transmitted irradiation is unnecessary radiation. In sites where underlying structures cannot be shielded special precautions should be made to select the best possible quality of irradiation which will minimize the transmitted dose. Late brain damage has been reported by Pendergrass[26] following irradiation of skin tumors overlying the cranial vault.

The treatment volume should be shaped to the tumor and its margin. This is most easily accomplished by tracing the field on transparent film or cellophane and transferring the pattern to a lead shield of a thickness not transmitting more than 5 per cent irradiation.

A treatment cone alone should not be used because patient movement may result in geometric miss. It is far better to construct a special shield, or a lead face mask which is fixed to the patient, and to treat through the resulting aperture with a generously wide beam.

INTERSTITIAL METHODS

The insertion of temporary or permanent radiation sources into skin cancer, particularly epithelial tumors, has been occasionally advocated. The advantages lie in the ability to deliver a very high but localized dose when needed, such as in cases of recurrent and unresectable neoplasm. This can be accomplished, in the case of temporary (removable) implants with radium or ^{60}Co needles, ^{90}Ta wire, or ^{192}Ir ribbons and with permanent implants with ^{198}Au or radon seeds. The implants are carried out according to the volume and shape of the neoplasm. Dosage will depend somewhat on previous treatment and on the sensitivity of surrounding structures. The optimum dose-time relationships are not fully known for interstitial methods of continuous irradiation but usually dosage ranges from 5,000 rads in 3 days to about 7,000 rads in 7 days. Volume is important both with respect to tolerance and curability: larger volume implants should be given higher cumulative doses over longer time periods than small volume implants.

The disadvantages of interstitial methods are the hazards of exposure to medical personnel, the operative trauma and expense to the patient, and the uncertainty of geometric uniformity of dosage.

These considerations apply also to mold techniques with short-distance gamma ray emitting sources. These methods have some importance in the "sandwich mold" treatment of bulky lesions of the lip or of the ear, but generally a satisfactory substitute can be appropriate external irradiation with shielding of underlying structures.

Carcinoma of the Lip

Epidermoid carcinoma arising on the exposed mucosa of the lip (vermillion) can be considered for practical purposes similar in behavior and therapeutic principles to skin cancer. The management of lymphatic submental metastases (which are relatively rare) remains a surgical problem divorced from consideration of the treatment of the primary lesion. Where the lip exhibits severe actinic keratotic changes adjacent to carcinoma it is advisable to perform surgical extirpation along with vermillionectomy for cancer prophylaxis.[5] Radiation is of unique advantage in those lesions exhibiting bulky extension through much of the length and thickness of the lip without extensive ulcerative destruction. These lesions may regress leaving a surprisingly intact lip.[36] Because of the local anatomical situation many techniques have been advocated. The most common is by external radiation with adequate underlying protection. However, the "sandwich" method of local gamma irradiation may be advantageous in cases where extensive infiltration has occurred (see section on Special Gamma-ray Techniques Chapter 1).

Results of Treatment

ACUTE REACTIONS

The epithelial reactions can be classified into four groups: first degree or erythema, second degree or dry desquamative epidermitis, third degree or moist desquamative epidermitis, and fourth degree or necrosis. Necrosis naturally is to be entirely avoided. These acute reactions should be treated on the basis of general dermatological principles. When the epithelium remains intact the surface should be kept dry; greasy ointments will produce maceration of the superficial cell layers. Dryness can be achieved by application of corn starch (never talcum which may contain heavy metal compounds). However, if a third degree reaction develops the surface should be treated by saline wet soaks to remove crusts and debris and followed by plain Vaseline or antibiotic ointment if a tumor ulcer is present. Any ulcerated tumor should be carefully and gently debrided mechanically and with hydrogen peroxide and all crusts repeatedly removed. Infection very likely interferes with therapeutic results by inhibiting host repair.

LATE REACTIONS

Necrosis may occur after trauma or thermal extremes some 2 to 4 years after treatment.[32] This is an untoward reaction which should be avoided by correct treatment factors and good judgment in the selection of original treatment and modality. These reactions are self-limited and generally heal with conservative measures.

TUMOR CURABILITY

Mortality statistics have little significance in evaluating the results of skin carcinoma. The important criteria are freedom from recurrence and cosmetic appearance. The latter is hard to evaluate in a quantitative sense. Comparative data from the results of various treatment modalities show little difference when curability is evaluated.[16]

Long term control of radiation therapy in general exceeds 90 per cent[1,12,23,24,25,29,34] and those tumors that are not controlled by irradiation are generally large, invasive cancers or tumors having received previously unsuccessful treatment.

The treatment which will yield the most favorable results will be that based upon good clinical judgment and the judicious selection of optimum treatment factors.

BIBLIOGRAPHY

1. Allen, K. D. A., and Freed, J. H.: Skin cancer: Correlation of field size and cancerocidal dose in roentgen treatment, *Amer. J. Roentgen.,* 75, 581, 1956.
2. Argyris, T. S.: *Advances in Biology of Skin,* Vol. 5, W. Montagna and R. E. Billingham, Eds., Oxford, England, Pergamon Press, Inc., p. 231, 1965.
3. Bagshaw, M. A., Schneidman, H. M., Farber, E. M., and Kaplan, H. S.: Electron beam therapy of mycosis fungoides, *Calif. Med.,* 95, 292, 1961.
4. Battle, R. J. V., and Patterson, T. J. S.: The surgical treatment of basal-celled carcinoma, *Brit. J. Plast. Surg.,* 13, 118, 1960.
5. Bennett, J. E., Lynch, J. B., Lewis, S. R., and Blocker, T. G., Jr.: The operative treatment of cancer of the lip, *Amer. Surg.,* 28, 537, 1962.
6. Block, J. B., Edgcomb, J., Eisen, A., Van Scott, E. J.: Mycosis fungoides: Natural history and aspects of its relationship to other malignant lymphomas, *Amer. J. Med.,* 34, 228, 1963.
7. Bowers, R. E., Graham, E. A., Tomlinson, K. M.: The natural history of the strawberry nevus, *Arch. Derm.* (Chicago), 82, 667, 1960.
8. Cohen, L.: Clinical radiation dosage. II. Interrelation of time, area and therapeutic ratio, *Brit. J. Radiol.,* 22, 706, 1949.
9. Cohen, L.: The statistical prognosis in radiation therapy. A study of optimal dosage in relation to physical and biologic parameters for epidermoid cancer, *Amer. J. Roentgen.,* 84, 741, 1960.
10. Cohen, L.: Dose, time and volume parameters in irradiation therapy of Kaposi's sarcoma, *Brit. J. Radiol.,* 35, 485, 1962.

11. Devik, F.: Studies on cell population kinetics of x-irradiated and shielded mouse epidermis by autoradiography after administration of tritiated thymidine, *Acta. Path. Microbiol. Scand.*, 148, 35, Supp., 1961.

12. Dick, D. A. L.: Clinical and cosmetic results in squamous cancer of the lip treated by 140 Kv radiation therapy, *Clin. Radiol.*, 13, 304, 1962.

13. deNouy, P. L.: Cicatrization of wounds. III. Relation between age of the patient, the area of the wound and the index of cicatrization, *J. Exp. Med.*, 24, 461, 1916.

14. Ellis, F.: Fractionation in Radiotherapy. In: *Modern Trends in Radiotherapy*, London, Butterworths, p. 34. 1967.

15. Evans, W. G., and Mabbs, D. V.: Treatment of superficial benign lesions with x-rays, *Brit. J. Radiol.*, 35, 866, 1962.

16. Freeman, R. G., Knox, J. M., and Heaton, C. L.: The treatment of skin cancer. A statistical study of 1,341 skin tumors comparing results obtained with irradiation, surgery, and curettage followed by electrodesiccation, *Cancer*, 17, 535, 1964.

17. Fuks, Z., and Bagshaw, M. A.: Total skin electron treatment of mycosis fungoides, *Radiology*, 100, 145, 1971.

18. Graham, P. G., and McGavran, M. H.: Basal cell carcinomas and sebaceous glands, *Cancer*, 17, 803, 1964.

19. Haybittle, J. L.: A 10 curie strontium betaray therapy unit, *Brit. J. Radiol.*, 33, 52, 1960.

20. Hellriegel, W.: Radiation therapy of primary and metastatic melanoma, *Ann. N. Y. Acad. Sci.*, 100, 131, 1963.

21. Jolles, B., and Mitchell, R. G.: Optimal skin tolerance dose levels, *Brit. J. Radiol.*, 20, 405, 1947.

22. Joyet, G., and Hohl, K.: Die biologische hautreaktion in der tiefentherapie als funktion der feldgrobe; ein gesetz der strahlentherapie, *Fortschr. Rontgenpr., Rontgenpr.*, 82, 387, 1955.

23. Lederman, M.: *Ocular and Adnexal Tumors*, St. Louis, C. V. Mosby Company, p. 104, 1964.

24. MacKay, E. N., and Sellers, A. H.: A statistical review of carcinoma of the lip, *Canad. Med. Ass. J.*, 90, 670, 1964.

25. Miescher, G.: Neuere erfahrungen auf dem gebiet der strahlentherapie der hautcarcinoma, *Radiol. Clin.* (Basel), 16, 343, 1947.

26. Pendergrass, E. P., Hodes, P. J., and Groff, R. A.: Intracranial complications following irradiation for carcinoma of the scalp, *Amer. J. Roentgen.*, 43, 214, 1940.

27. Peterkin, G. A. G., MacMillan, M. B., and Maclean, A.: Pseudocarcinoma of the skin, a follow-up of cases of kerato-acanthoma seen in the 10 years 1951–60, *Scot. Med. J.*, 7, 27, 1962.

28. Reitman, P. H.: Radiation therapy of malignant melanoma, *Amer. J. Roentgen.*, 67, 286, 1952.

29. Strandqvist, M.: Studien uber die kumulative wirkung der rontgenstrahlen bei fraktionierung; erfahrungen aus dem radiumhemmet an 280 haut- und lippenkarzinomen, *Acta Radiol.* (Ther.) (Stockholm), Supp. 55, 1944.

30. Sulzberger, M. B., Baer, R. L., and Borota, A.: Do roentgenray treatment as given by skin specialists produce cancers or other sequelae? *Arch. Derm. Syph.*, (Chicago), 65, 639, 1952.

31. Szur, L., Silvester, J. A., and Bewley, D. K.: Treatment of the whole body surface with electrons, *Lancet*, 1, 1373, 1962.

32. Traenkle, H. L., and Mulay, D.: Further observations on late radiation necrosis following therapy of skin cancer, *Arch. Derm.* (Chicago), 81, 908, 1960.

33. Trump, J. G., Wright, K. A., Evans, W. W., and Anson, J. H.: High energy electrons for the treatment of extensive superficial malignant lesions, *Amer. J. Roentgen.*, 69, 623, 1953.

34. von Essen, C. F.: Roentgen therapy of skin and lip carcinoma: Factors influencing success and failure, *Amer. J. Roentgen.*, 83, 556, 1960.

35. von Essen, C. F.: A spatial model of time-dose-area relationships in radiation therapy, *Radiology*, 81, 881, 1963.

36. von Essen, C. F.: *Tumors of the Skin*, Chicago, Year Book Medical Publishers, Inc., p. 285, 1964.

37. von Essen, C. F.: Radiation tolerance of the skin, *Acta Radiol.* (Ther.) 8, 311, 1969.

38. von Essen, C. F.: A practical time-dose formula for x-ray therapy of skin cancer, *Brit. J. Radiol.*, 42, 474, 1969.

Oral Cavity and Oropharynx

General Introduction

Anatomical Site of Origin

The careful assignment of a site of origin, despite some degree of arbitrariness at times, is more than an academic exercise because it has therapeutic consequences. The assignment of a site of origin for advanced lesions of the oral cavity and oropharynx, when several contiguous structures are involved, is based on the criteria which represent the biologic characteristics of the tumors of a site. These criteria include: 1) the structure most involved and the routes of contiguous spread, 2) the histology of the lesion, *i.e.,* a lymphoepithelioma of the tonsillar region is more likely to have its origin in the tonsillar fossa than on the anterior faucial pillar where the tumors usually are keratinizing squamous cell carcinomas, and 3) the incidence, location, and bilateralism of nodes follow patterns which are specific to the anatomical sites.

Histology

With rare exceptions, the malignant tumors encountered in the oral cavity and oropharynx are: 1) squamous cell carcinomas, 2) lymphosarcomas, usually of the reticulum cell variety, found on the base of the tongue and the tonsillar bed, and 3) glandular carcinomas. Glandular carcinomas of minor salivary gland origin are most often located on the hard palate and buccal mucosa.

Grading of the squamous cell carcinomas is meaningful, although not the main determinant in the choice of therapy. The so-called verrucous keratinizing Grade I squamous cell carcinoma merits special consideration.[1] Surgical resection may be preferable as they tend to recur after irradiation.

There is some correlation between the histological differentiation and the incidence of metastases; bilateral neck nodes are twice as common with Grade III as with Grade I tumors.[8] Lymphoepithelioma metastasizes more often and has a great tendency to metastasize to remote organs.[8]

The fast clinical disappearance of the histologically undifferentiated tumors, for instance those of the tonsillar fossa, has led to the belief that they require a lower dose than the more differentiated tumors. In an experiment on regression rate in an animal tumor system, it was shown that differentiation has little bearing on control of disease.[17]

Histologic grading and the site of origin are significant in considering the advisability of comprehensive irradiation of the primary lesion and neck nodes. The response to radiation of metastatic nodes varies with the site of origin of the primary lesion. For example, metastatic nodes from tumors of the tonsillar fossa respond better than those of the base of the tongue.

Clinical Variety of the Tumor

The clinical variety of the tumor is an important factor regarding response to radiation. The best response to radiation is obtained in the well-vascularized exophytic tumors in which the cells are adequately oxygenated. Ulcerative lesions, often infected, have less radioresponse; the infiltrative nodular lesions are the least responsive.

The infiltrating lesions are often much larger than is apparent at first. Planning of treatment must be preceded by careful assessment of the actual extent of the growth, which is often only fully appreciated when the patient is under general anesthesia.

STAGING

A "T, N, M" staging system is useful for analysis of results and determining causes of failure. The staging of the primary lesion used since July 1965 is as follows:

T_1: Tumors less than 2 cm* in diameter.

T_2: Tumors 2 to 4 cm* in diameter, no invasion of surrounding tissue.

T_3: Tumors more than 4 cm* in diameter, and/or invasion of surrounding structures.

T_4: Massive tumor or bone involvement.

Multiple Primary Tumors and Recurrences

Patients who have had one squamous cell carcinoma of the upper respiratory and digestive tract are likely to develop subsequent primary lesions. Leukoplakia represents a general dysplasia of the mucous membranes producing multiple foci of *in situ* and invasive carcinomas. The buccal mucosa, gums, faucial pillars and soft palate are most often the sites of multiple primaries, concomitant or sequential. Multiple primaries cause special problems of definitive therapy. The treatment of choice for a single lesion is different than that for multiple concomitant or sequential lesions.

As a general rule, a new lesion peripheral to one previously treated by irradiation, irrespective of whether it is a new primary or a marginal recurrence, is best managed by surgical excision. Overlap of the two irradiated areas entails serious risk of necrosis.

General Condition of the Patient

Squamous cell carcinoma of the mouth and oropharynx develops in the later decades of life; the average age of occurrence is 65 with one third of patients above 70.

With modern medical care including high protein feeding, if necessary by tube, blood transfusions and antibiotics, high-dose therapy is well tolerated in patients close to 80 years of age. At or above that age, extra radical treatments are seldom worthwhile. At times surgical excision is preferred because

*Prior to July 1965, 3 and 5 cm were used instead of 2 and 4 cm. The lesions have been restaged accordingly.

it is less taxing. In younger patients, greater risks are justified in attempting to save a life.

Tuberculosis, if the sputum is positive, necessitates modifications of treatment for protection of personnel.

Chronic alcoholism, common in patients with lesions of the floor of the mouth and oropharynx, is a real problem. The reaction to alcohol withdrawal during a radium implant must be managed. Postirradiation care in chronic alcoholics is often unsatisfactory because they do not follow instructions. Nutritional deficiencies may be conducive to frequent breakdown of the mucous membrane. Unquestionably, there is a higher incidence of necrosis among chronic alcoholics, and spontaneous healing with conservative care is not as common as in nonalcoholic patients. A primary surgical procedure may be preferred for the patient who is an alcoholic.

Radiation Reactions

A fibrinous exudate is produced by the dead cells of either the epithelium or the tumor. The fibrinous exudate that covers an exophytic (Fig. 3-28) or ulcerative tumor appears sooner than mucositis (as early as 4 or 5 days after the beginning of treatment) because tumor cells disintegrate faster than normal epithelium cells; epithelitis appears 12 to 17 days after the beginning of treatment. The exudate affords a clearcut check of treatment coverage. Production of fibrinous exudate of the mucous membranes can be avoided by using a low weekly rate (850 rads) or by temporarily stopping the treatment in order to let a studded mucositis start regressing. A 5 to 10 per cent change in dosage estimation produces clinically detectable differences in reactions.[9]

As healing progresses, the thick, slightly yellowish fibrinous exudate is replaced by a thin white film on a pinkish base. The surrounding mucous membrane has a pale appearance instead of the angry red that characterizes increasing reactions.

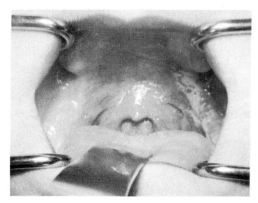

FIG. 3-28. Female, age 50, seen in February 1964 with a superficial squamous cell carinoma of the foot of the left anterior faucial pillar. Histology: squamous cell carcinoma, Grade II. No nodes. After 1,000 rads tumor dose given in a week, a fibrinous exudate covered somewhat more of the anterior faucial pillar toward the soft palate than did the visible tumor. Such tumoritis at the end of the first week of treatment is helpful in delineating the early superficial mucosal spread. The patient was NED 3-30-72.

The mucositis produced by 6 to 7 days interstitial radium implants begins when the needles are removed, and is maximal 14 to 17 days after the date of implantation. The healing time averages 6 or 8 weeks.

Patient Care

Patients must be told that there will be painful reactions. They will then be able to accept them as an unavoidable discomfort accompanying the disappearance of the tumor.

Prevention of infection and good nutritional status are essential during irradiation and afterward to allow recovery. Later breakdown of the mucous membranes and necroses can be minimized by proper care. Antibiotics should not be used routinely but reserved for infected lesions.

The hemoglobin and red cell count must be watched carefully. If the hemoglobin drops below 11 grams, blood transfusions must be given.

Smoking must be stopped. After each meal, the mouth should be irrigated. Mouthwashing and gargling with local anesthetics must be prescribed cautiously only in cases of extreme swallowing difficulties and only prior to meals, not as a routine pain relief because of danger of addiction. Cleansing with a spray kit or even power spray is a necessity in all patients with lesions of the floor of the mouth and lower gums.

A good nutritional status is not easy to maintain. Patients with larger lesions of the oral cavity necessitating irradiation of a great part of the mouth, or with lesions of the palatine arch and oropharynx, have great difficulty in swallowing from the second week on. Very old people, patients in poor general condition, and chronic alcoholics who already have an inadequate diet, require intensive care as in-patients.

Skin care, with megavoltage radiation, is seldom required. If the lower neck is irradiated, a soft cloth should be used around the neck to avoid friction. Lanolin, Borofax, or similar compounds are used in the rare instances of moist desquamation. Male patients must be advised not to shave within the irradiated areas. The beard outside of the irradiated area is best cut with clippers.

Postirradiation Care

The care associated with treatment must be continued until acute reactions have subsided. When patients are discharged, they, as well as the family, are carefully instructed in the irrigating procedure, cleaning of teeth, diet, and medications. Frequent salt and soda irrigations, cleansing of unepithelized areas by power spray, or zinc peroxide packing is beneficial in delayed healing resulting either from large denuded areas in extensive lesions or from overdose. If local anesthetics must be used for pain, care should be taken not to produce additional delay or even prevention of healing by excessive use of the anesthetics.

The progressive diminution of symptoms must be explained to the patient and family, as well as late symptoms such as some degree of tenderness, alteration of the sense of taste, and dryness of the mouth. Food acquires a salty and unpleasant taste, which may necessitate dietary advice. It is essential that patients understand that these symptoms cannot be altered by a particular mean, but will decrease with time. Tenderness of the tongue may take months to disappear. Dryness of the mouth is sometimes a severe complication. It is most common in patients whose lesions were treated by parallel opposing portals including large areas of the mucous membrane and the parotids. Whenever applicable, preference must be given to some combination of a local form of therapy (intraoral cone or interstitial gamma-ray therapy) with external irradiation, or wedge, or use of half photons and half electrons.

Minor irritations must be avoided in order not to initiate a mucous membrane breakdown. Irrigation after meals may prevent stagnation of food and infection.

If large areas of the neck have been treated, a certain amount of edema of the neck will become visible in the submental region, forming a "dewlap." This is of no significance, causes no discomfort, but should be explained to the patient to allay fright.

Complications

Bone exposure occurs in the patients in whom the radiation therapy necessarily included bone and the mucous membrane covering it. Trauma from illfitting dentures, alcohol, tobacco, heat, cold, and condiments may cause this fragile mucous membrane to erode, exposing the bone. If the erosion is small, it will usually heal. If, however, the bone is exposed for any length of time, it may become infected, and, because of the reduced blood supply, an uncontrollable osteitis sets in. Pain is always present, with varying degrees of severity.

Necrosis of soft tissues, characterized by a yellowish ulcer and induration, is usually seen in the tongue.

Necrosis of either soft tissue or bone has not been associated with active disease[7] contradicting the concept of supralethal dose.

The risk of transverse myelitis is present when long areas of spinal cords are given doses of 5,000 rads or more in 5 to 6 weeks. The spinal cord should be removed from the treatment fields at 4,500 rads.

Severe muscular or subcutaneous fibrosis can occur when doses higher than 7,000 rads in 7 weeks have been given.

Treatment for Recurrences

Recurrences may follow a surgical excision, a well-planned full course of radiation therapy, or inadequate irradiation. The recurrence may be located within the irradiated area or at the edge of the treatment zone. In the latter instance, the growth may be a new primary, or be the result of a technical error, or misjudgment of the extent of the tumor.

Recurrences following radical irradiation should be excised, if possible, otherwise, no further treatment is to be given. In our experience, radiation therapy for postradiation recurrences following a full dosage is contraindicated since it will almost invariably cause necrosis and failure to control the disease. In the oropharynx, necrosis following a retreatment is more painful than growing cancer, and causes death because of intractable pain and malnutrition.

When the original radiation treatment has been obviously inadequate, a surgical excision is preferable. Irradiation with a full dosage is employed only if surgical removal is not feasible, but a satisfactory result is rarely achieved. The same policy of surgical excision applies to either a recurrence or a new primary close to a previously irradiated zone.

Palliation for Incurable Advanced Lesions

The concept of palliation has to be clearly defined for the head and neck area. The purpose of palliative therapy is to provide the patient with a comfortable life for a period of time long enough to warrant the unavoidable acute discomfort of a semiradical treatment. Ideally, palliative treatment should result in sufficient regression of the disease at the primary site and in the neck until the patient dies from distant metastases or intercurrent disease. Death from liver or even lung metastases is less distressing.

Each surgeon or therapist has his own ideas about the boundaries between cure and palliation. Early or moderately advanced lesions, both at the primary site and in the neck, are treated for cure. Formidable lesions at the primary site and/or the neck are usually not altered by any treatment and therefore are best left alone. For instance, even if there is temporary growth restraint of massive infiltrative and ulcerative tumors on the posterior wall of the pharynx, the persistent ulceration is associated with excruciating pain. Pain is rarely relieved by irradiation.

The problem of deciding between palliative and definitive therapy is present in two groups of lesions: 1) those extensive tumors still localized both at the primary site and in the neck for which only a small hope of permanent control can be entertained, and 2) locally curable lesions with distant metastases as yet producing no clinical symptoms. The management of such lesions is determined on grounds of medical merit, on the philosophy of radicalism, and on the means available. Generally, in this country, definitive therapy for cure is chosen, although the yield of cure is low.

Age is an important factor in palliation. For patients approaching or past 80, less radical treatments are in order as irradiation may initiate a fast downhill course.

Lasting control of disease above the clavicle is only achieved with doses employed in the most radical therapy. The tumor doses and techniques are the same as those for curative therapy. Additional treatments through narrow portals or interstitial gamma-ray therapy increase the risk of complications and are not justified in palliative cases.

With megavoltage, 850 rads per week are well tolerated even by elderly people.

Intraoral Therapy

Intraoral therapy has its place when generous coverage of the lesion can be achieved with a cone and there is no risk of motion out of the aperture. Best managed by intraoral therapy are: 1) superficial lesions on the floor of the mouth close to the gum in edentulous patients (the floor of the mouth is flat), 2) some lesions on the gums the lower gingivobuccal sulcus, and 3) small lesions of the soft palate or on the ascending ramus of the mandible. Silk sutures around the lesion are often useful for guidance in positioning the cone because early lesions regress rapidly.

Six Mev electron beam is optimal for superficial lesions which are no more than 3 or 4 mm deep. The usual dose is 5,500 to 6,000 rads at the aperture of the cone given in about 3 to 4 weeks. Late mucous membrane changes are minor because underlying tissues have minimal damage.

For more infiltrative lesions, a 150 Kv beam is best using 1.5 mm Cu HVL, 40 cm FSD, and beveled cones 3 to 5 cm in diameter. Chair, patient, and cone form a rigid unit instead of relying solely on a periscopic attachment to verify coverage of the lesion (Fig. 3-29). An effective dose range is 5,000 to 5,500 rads given dose in 3 to 4 weeks at mid-distance of the bevel.

For lesions which are marginally encompassed by a cone, one may choose to give with intraoral cone therapy 1,000 to 1,500 rads to minimize the dose to be given later through the external beam; this reduces the volume of tissues brought up to a high level of radiation. The rationale is that the main bulk of the lesion is more radioresistant and should not be given less than 6,000 or 6,500 rads in 5 to 5½ weeks; the microscopic peripheral extensions will be controlled with 5,000 rads in 4 to 5 weeks.

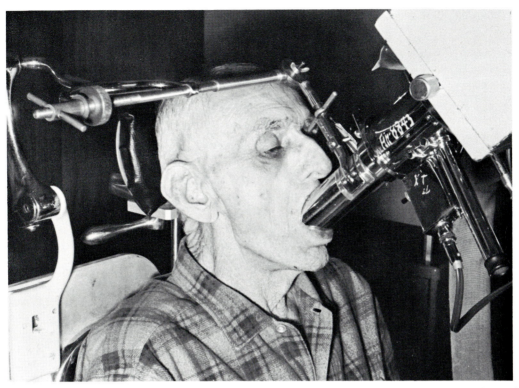

FIG. 3-29. A method of assuring coverage and lack of motion in intraoral therapy. After local anesthesia, if necessary, the cone is inserted using a flashlight for checking the coverage of the lesion. The various joints are locked and then patient, cone, cone attachment, and chair form a rigid unit. The tube housing and the cone are then brought together.

Surface Molds

The use of surface molds requires experience which can be gained only from abundant clinical material. A specialized mold room with trained personnel must be available. Lacking these aids, failures are almost inevitable. When proper facilities are available, superficial lesions of the floor of the mouth, gums, or hard palate can be suitable for surface mold therapy.

Intersitital Gamma-Ray Therapy

Interstitial gamma-ray therapy necessitates a diversified stock of radium needles (Table 3-20), experience, and some surgical skill.[4] [192]Ir should also be available (Table 3-21).

The mucous membrane should be dried by premedication with scopolamine. With exceptions, implants should be done under endotracheal anesthesia. Not only should the patient be under deep anesthesia, but a muscle relaxant should be used to enable the mouth to remain wide open without strain. Mouth openers do not fit if the teeth are absent. Tracheostomy should be done for large implants or even single plane implants if posterior, because of edema of the tongue.

A feeding tube should be inserted, before the implant. The patient must be kept comfortable by sufficient sedation. In the alcoholic patient, it is sometimes advisable to give intravenous alcohol or, if they can swallow, wine or whiskey.

Table 3-20. *Oral Cavity and Oropharynx. Radium Needle Stock*

Linear Activity (mg/cm)	Active Length (cm)	Number Needed	Total Length (cm)	Filtra- tion (mm Pt)	Milli- grams	Milligrams (Corrected to 0.5 mm Pt Filter)
0.66	4.5	10	5.8	0.65	3.00	2.91
0.66	3.5	10	4.5	0.60	2.33	2.28
0.66	3.0	10	4.2	0.60	2.00	1.96
0.66	2.0	5	3.2	0.50	1.33	1.33
0.33	4.5	15	5.8	0.65	1.50	1.45
0.33	4.0	10	5.0	0.65	1.33	1.29
0.33	3.5	10	4.5	0.60	1.16	1.14
0.33	3.0	10	4.2	0.60	1.00	0.98
Indian Club	4.5	12	5.8	0.65	1.75	1.70
Indian Club	4.0	8	5.0	0.65	1.66	1.61
Indian Club	3.5	8	4.5	0.60	1.50	1.47
Indian Club	3.0	8	4.2	0.60	1.25	1.22
0.50	4.5	12	5.8	0.65	2.25	2.18
0.50	4.0	12	5.0	0.65	2.00	1.94
0.50	3.5	12	4.5	0.60	1.75	1.71
0.25	4.5	12	5.8	0.65	1.125	1.09
0.25	4.0	12	5.0	0.65	1.000	0.97
0.25	3.5	12	4.5	0.60	0.875	0.86
0.165	4.5	12	5.9	0.50	0.75	0.75
0.165	3.5	12	4.8	0.50	0.58	0.58

For optimal adaptation to each case one should have, for oral cavity implants, active length needles of 2, 3, 3.5, and 4.5 cm; Indian club needles from 3 to 4.5 cm active length, and some 3.5 and 4.5 cm needles of quite low intensity such as 0.165 mg/cm. Dumbbell needles are not necessary.

The minimum number of needles necessary for a variety of implants is shown.

Table 3-21. ^{192}*Ir Wire Stock*

		Length	Amount on Hand	Activity	Diameter
Iridium Wire (continuous)		14 cm	140 cm	1.0–1.5 mc/cm	0.3 mm
		14 cm	140 cm	~3.0 mc/cm	0.3 mm
Iridium Pins (Epingles)	Single	5.0 cm	4	1.0–1.5 mc/cm	0.5 mm
		(may be cut to any length)	2	3.0 mc/cm	0.5 mm
	Double	5.0 cm	5	1.0–1.5 mc/cm	0.5 mm
		(may be cut to any length)	2	3.0 mc/cm	0.5 mm

Supplies are ordered sufficiently often to make available the above amounts in the usable intensity range of 1.0–1.5 mc/cm. Purchased from: Commissariat al'Energie Atomique B.P. N⁰2, 91, Gif-sur-Yvette, France

Linear Intensity of the Needles

Classically, the full intensity needles have been 0.66 mg/cm and half intensity, 0.33 mg/cm but 0.5 mg/cm and 0.25 mg/cm needles give a more satisfactory dose rate.

Dumbbell needles are constructed with 0.33 mg/cm source in the center and 0.66 mg/cm at both ends. Indian club needles are constructed with 1 mg/cm concentrated in a very short distance at one end with the remaining linear intensity 0.33 mg/cm (Fig. 3-30).

For multiplanar and volume implants, 0.33 or 0.25 mg/cm will give a dosage rate close to 1,000 rads per day.

Needles with 0.165 mg/cm are also useful in combination with 0.33 mg/cm or 0.25 mg/cm for large volume implants.

Method of Calculation

For single plane implant, using the same intensity needles throughout, or using Indian club with crossing at one end, the stated dose from Paterson and Parker tables and graphs is, for clinical purposes, close enough to the actual dose. The Paterson and Parker tables can also be used for volume implants.

For double plane implants it is often preferable to calculate the dose at every 0.5 cm of distance for each plane and then add the contribution from both planes. These calculations have the advantage of showing the variation in doses between the planes and also the dose lateral to each plane—which may be important.

In many situations, primarily when the lesion is on the anterior floor of the mouth or undersurface of the tongue, the curvature of the plane is too great for use of Paterson and Parker tables. If a back row of needles is utilized the only way to obtain the dose is by point calculation. One chooses several points representative of the distribution of the tumor in and outside the curvature and calculates the contribution of each needle to each of these points.

Cross sections of the implant are obtained

RADIUM NEEDLES

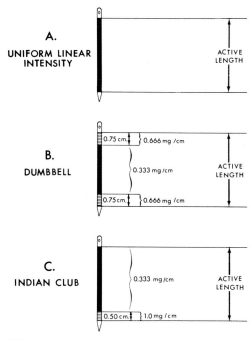

FIG. 3-30. Linear intensity of radium needles.

best with transverse tomograms. If a transverse tomograph is not available, the perpendicular section technique can be used in simple planar implants. A three-dimensional reconstruction technique must be used to obtain cross sections in the desired planes in volume or in complex implants.

Explicit calculations with the computer are done after the coordinates of the cross section of the implant in the planes of interest have been determined.[5,10,16]

Since 1961 at the University of Texas M. D. Anderson Hospital the minimal tumor dose in rads (90 rads = 100 roentgens) has been determined from computed isodose curves.

The following parameters are of importance:

1) In planar implants, a more uniform dose is achieved when all the needles are of the same intensity, and a better dose distribution is obtained when double plane implants have a separation of 1.5 cm.

2) The complication rate decreased with low dose rate implants (less than 40 rads per hour) which are easier to accomplish using low intensity (0.25 or 0.33 mg per cm) needles throughout the implant.[10]

3) The amount of external preneedling irradiation is increased in larger tumors with corresponding adjustment in the time-dose relationships for the radium implant.

4) Less generous selection of minimum tumor dose from computer isodoses. A selection of an isodose curve encompassing all the needles, although a natural first choice, usually leads to overdosage. This is particularly important in implants of the floor of the mouth where the necrosis rate is higher.

5) Attention must be directed to the clinical type of lesion. In infiltrative lesions it may be necessary to risk a necrosis in order to have an acceptable control rate[5].

Single Plane Implants

(Figs. 3-31 and 3-32)

With Paterson and Parker rules of distribution, full intensity of peripheral needles and half intensity of center needles, there is a lower dose at the center of the implant than at the periphery and the actual dose is lower than the dose calculated from the Paterson and Parker tables. Furthermore, the isodose curves are cigar-shaped which clinically fits the fact that tumors are thickest at their center.

For large single plane implants, 0.66 mg/cm may give too high a dosage rate; if so, then it may be preferable to use 0.5 mg/cm.

EFFECT OF CROSSING

With crossing needles, the isodose curves are cigar-shaped. Crossing at the active ends produces a flatness of the isodose curves. However, the inactive ends of the needles may be in the tumor as in squamous cell carcinomas of the lateral border of the tongue reaching the dorsum of the tongue.

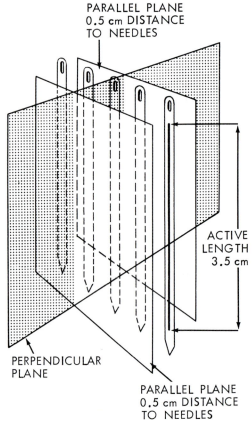

FIG. 3-31. Perspective of a planar implant with needles 3.5 cm active length. The planes of calculation of the Paterson and Parker system are parallel to the needles at 0.5 cm distance.
Isodose curves in the plane perpendicular to the implant are useful to demonstrate characteristics of the implants.

It is preferable to cross at the physical end of the needles to encompass the disease better. One crossing needle elongates the area of high dose irradiation, but on a narrower width (Fig. 3-33). It may be preferable to use one half intensity needle on each side of the dead end of the plane needles.

Implants with dumbbell needles are not equivalent to crossing. Implants with Indian club needles have a better dose distribution on the Indian club end than do dumbbells. However, with both Indian club and dumbbell needles, one must be careful that disease is not in the vicinity of or, even worse,

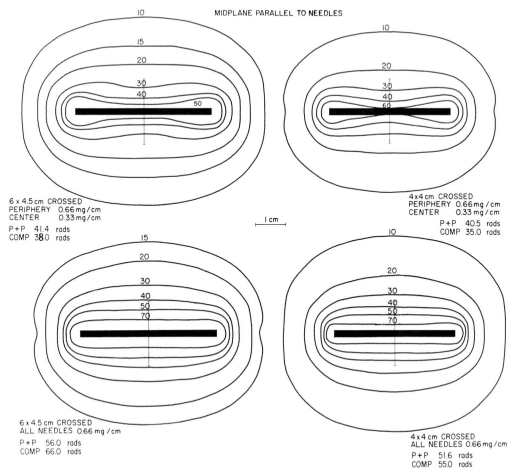

FIG. 3-32. The dose delivered actually (calculated by computer) may be lower than the Paterson and Parker dose by 15 per cent for a 4 × 4 cm implant and by 20 per cent for a 6 × 4.5 cm implant. This difference between the calculated dose and the actual dose applied to crossed implants and dumbbell implants. Using the same intensity needles for an implant 4 × 4 cm the actual dose is only 5 per cent more than the calculated dose and in a 6 × 4.5 cm implant 15 per cent more.

around the inactive ends. Only actual crossing can avoid an area of underdosage.

For lesions of the lateral border of the tongue, Indian club needles are preferable. As a rule, with proper length needles, the lower aspect of the lesion is well within the implant; then the upper aspect of the implant is crossed accordingly at the inactive ends with one or even two needles.

For tumors of the anterior undersurface of the tongue or tumors of the floor of the mouth with implants through the dorsum of the tongue, one may use half intensity need-

les if the lesion is small and well within the implanted area. If there is infiltration into the submental space, Indian club needles are preferable.

Curved Planar Implants
(Fig. 3-34)

The volume distribution is better for the curved planar implants using the same intensity needles. Otherwise, there is not sufficient width of adequate dosage.

There is great curvature of implant for

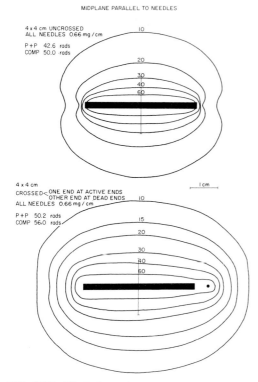

MIDPLANE PARALLEL TO NEEDLES

4 x 4 cm UNCROSSED
ALL NEEDLES 0.66 mg/cm

P+P 42.6 rads
COMP 50.0 rads

4 x 4 cm
CROSSED < ONE END AT ACTIVE ENDS
          OTHER END AT DEAD ENDS
ALL NEEDLES 0.66 mg/cm

P+P 50.2 rads
COMP 56.0 rads

FIG. 3-33. Effect of crossing.

lesions of the anterior floor of the mouth. Further, the slant of the jaw is conducive to irregular geometry. Gaps occur if needles are placed 1 cm apart. It is preferable to place needles 0.5 cm to 0.75 cm apart, using 0.25 mg/cm needles, because 0.33 mg/cm may give too high a dosage rate.

With implants which have marked curvature, if disease goes into the root of the tongue, three or four needles are implanted back within the implant's curvature.

Double Plane Implants

(Fig. 3-35)

With a 1 cm separation, the dose between the planes is greater than the dose 0.5 cm lateral to each plane; if there is disease laterally, this is conducive to underdosage.

With a 1.5 cm separation, the dose 0.5 cm lateral to the planes is closest to the dose between the planes. Actually, 1.5 cm separation is good separation for double plane implants.

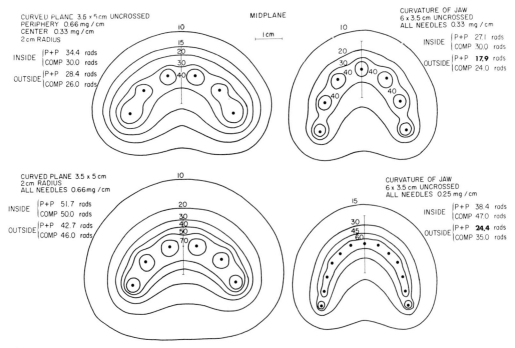

CURVED PLANE 3.5 x 5 cm UNCROSSED
PERIPHERY 0.66 mg/cm
CENTER 0.33 mg/cm
2 cm RADIUS

INSIDE { P+P 34.4 rads
        { COMP 30.0 rads

OUTSIDE { P+P 28.4 rads
         { COMP 26.0 rads

MIDPLANE

CURVATURE OF JAW
6 x 3.5 cm UNCROSSED
ALL NEEDLES 0.33 mg/cm

INSIDE { P+P 27.1 rads
        { COMP 30.0 rads

OUTSIDE { P+P 17.9 rads
         { COMP 24.0 rads

CURVED PLANE 3.5 x 5 cm
2 cm RADIUS
ALL NEEDLES 0.66 mg/cm

INSIDE { P+P 51.7 rads
        { COMP 50.0 rads

OUTSIDE { P+P 42.7 rads
         { COMP 46.0 rads

CURVATURE OF JAW
6 x 3.5 cm UNCROSSED
ALL NEEDLES 0.25 mg/cm

INSIDE { P+P 38.4 rads
        { COMP 47.0 rads

OUTSIDE { P+P 24.4 rads
         { COMP 35.0 rads

FIG. 3-34. Curved implants.

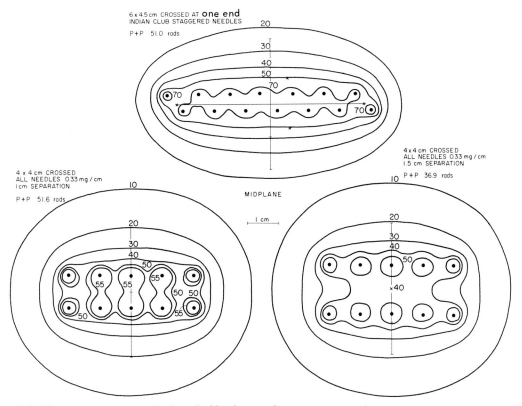

FIG. 3-35. Dosage rates are too high in double plane implants using 0.66 mg/cm.

It is advisable to use all 0.33 mg/cm for a separation of 1.5 cm and 0.25 mg/cm for a separation of 1 cm.

Assuming, for calculation, that all the needles of a staggered implant are in one plane between the two planes, the dose over a thickness of 1 cm is 40 per cent more than the calculated dose.

Staggered Implants

(Fig. 3-35)

When a lesion is too thick for a planar implant but not thick enough for a double plane implant, occasionally staggered needles with 0.5 cm between the two planes may be used.

If the lesion is too thick for one single plane implant, it is preferable to use at least 1 cm separation although it may not seem necessary.

Volume Implants

(Fig. 3-36)

For small volume implants, there is considerable ripple of the dose at the physical shell. This ripple is not great for the larger implants.

Such ripples must be kept in mind if there is disease at the physical shell. In clinical situations encountered in tumors of the tongue (and those of the female urethra) where the tumor is eccentric to the implant, one must reinforce the implant where the disease is.

In the tongue lesions, needles must also be implanted medially to palpable infiltration. Because of the fall-off dose on and beyond the shell, great care must be exercised in using a volume implant if needles cannot be inserted outside the tumor. The same considerations apply to double plane or multiple plane implants. The distance to the most lateral aspect of the tumor must be

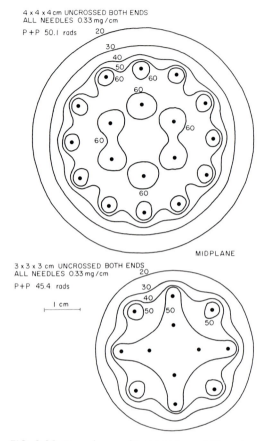

4 x 4 x 4 cm UNCROSSED BOTH ENDS
ALL NEEDLES 0.33 mg/cm

P + P 50.1 rads

3 x 3 x 3 cm UNCROSSED BOTH ENDS
ALL NEEDLES 0.33 mg/cm

P + P 45.4 rads

FIG. 3-36. For volumes of 3 × 3 × 3 cm, 0.33 mg/cm will give a dosage rate of 45 rads per hour. For a volume 4 × 4 × 4 cm, 0.33 mg/cm will give a dosage rate of 50 to 60 rads per hour. Therefore, 0.25 mg/cm is preferable; this gives a dose rate of 40 to 50 rads per hour.

carefully evaluated and the dose calculated at that point.

Combination of External Beams and Interstitial Gamma-Ray Implants

For larger lesions, volume implants or multiplanar implants are necessary. Uneven distribution of the needles is the rule even in the most skillful hands; a half and half technique of external irradiation and interstitial radium implant buffers the swings of dose within the implant.[9] One may often

resort to such a combination (Table 3-22) in lesions which are not well located for assured implant coverage, for instance those lesions of the posterolateral border of the tongue.

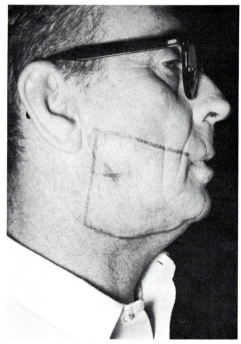

FIG. 3-37. Patient seen on 7-7-70 for a lesion measuring about 2.5 cm in diameter on the right anterior undersurface of the tongue. No palpable nodes. Biopsy: Squamous cell carcinoma.

The patient received a tumor dose of 2,000 rads in 5 consecutive treatments with the 22 Mev betatron. The subdigastric area was well covered. In actual treatment position, the patient has a cork in the mouth to depress the tongue and avoid irradiating the palate. This was followed with an interstitial radium implant which delivered 5,100 rads in 133 hours. The dose to the subdigastric area of the neck was 1,800 rads on the ipsilateral side and 1,700 rads on the opposite side. On 2-23-71 a node was palpated close to the margin of the external beam portal. A radical neck dissection was performed and squamous cell carcinoma was found in connective tissue. With 9 Mev electron beam 5,000 rads were given from 3-26-71 to 4-26-71.

The patient was doing well in February 1972.

Table 3-22. *Combinations of External Irradiation with Interstitial Gamma-Ray Therapy*

I. 2,000 rads *TD*, preneedling dose, to be given in 5-6 treatments (single field if *TD* is not less than 80% of *GD*; daily *GD* 400 rads)

Lesion selection: Lesion that may be encompassed by a small size implant and no clinically positive nodes.

Radium dosage: Use dose-time relationship of Table 3-23.

II. 3,000–5,000 rads, preneedling dose, to be given at a *TD* rate of 1,000 rads/week (parallel opposing fields, 2:1 loading or homolateral with $\geq$ 20 Mev if available.

Lesion selection: Moderate to large sized lesions, or small lesions or location which may produce a poor geometrical implant and/or desirability to give 5,000 rads to first level lymphatics.

External Beam	Radium dosage
4,000 rads	4,000 rads/5 days
5,000 rads	3,000 rads/4 days
	20–25 rads/hr. with low intensity
	(0.33, 0.25 or even 0.165 mg/cm)

In a previous publication[9] interstitial radium implant first was advocated but presently external irradiation is used first because of the risk of spreading tumor cells with the needles as they are driven through disease.[6] Unless the lesion is very small, 2,000 rads tumor dose in 5 treatments are given prior to needling (Fig. 3-37). The first relay of regional lymphatics, i.e., the subdigastric nodes, must be generously covered in the portal or portals with 1:1 loading if 3 to 6 Mev beam is used; if 20 to 25 Mev beam is available, one single homolateral portal can be used.

The adjusted dosages from the interstitial implant are shown in Table 3-23.

With increasing size of the tumor more of the treatment is given with external beam

Table 3-23. *Dose-Time Relationships for Radium Needlings (Minimum Tumor Dose Obtained from Computed Isodose Curves)*

Hours of Implant	No External Beam				2,000 rads *TD* External Beam in Five Treatments			
	Tongue		Floor of Mouth		Tongue		Floor of Mouth	
	rads/hr.	rads	rads/hr.	rads	rads/hr.	rads	rads/hr.	rads
40	107.5	4,300	100.0	4,000	86.2	3,450	80.0	3,200
50	94.0	4,700	87.0	4,350	75.0	3,250	70.0	3,500
60	83.75	5,025	77.5	4,650	66.7	4,000	63.8	3,825
70	76.1	5,325	70.4	4,925	60.7	4,250	56.4	3,950
80	70.25	5,625	65.0	5,200	56.3	4,500	52.5	4,200
90	65.1	5,860	60.3	5,425	52.2	4,700	48.6	4,375
100	60.5	6,050	56.5	5,650	48.8	4,880	45.5	4,550
110	57.5	6,225	53.2	5,850	45.9	5,050	42.7	4,700
120	54.1	6,500	50.0	6,000	43.3	5,200	40.4	4,850
130	51.9	6,750	48.1	6,250	41.5	5,400	38.5	5,000
140	49.6	6,950	45.7	6,400	39.6	5,550	36.8	5,150
150	47.3	7,100	44.0	6,600	38.0	5,700	35.3	5,300
160	45.6	7,300	42.3	6,775	36.4	5,825	33.8	5,450
170	43.8	7,450	40.9	6,950	35.1	5,975	32.6	5,550

with diminished dosage with interstitial, using low dosage rate (20 to 25 rads per hour) obtained with low linear intensity, 0.25 or even 0.165 mg/cm.

External Beam

There are two basic principles involved in radiation of cancers of the oral cavity and oropharynx.

1) Limitation of volume without risking a geographical miss. This applies to any form of radiation therapy—intraoral cone, surface mold, interstitial gamma-ray therapy or external beam therapy. In the latter, for instance, the incidence of bone exposures and necroses is function of the length of jaw irradiated.[13]

2) Easily duplicable treatment setups. Preference is to be given to anatomically simple planning over perhaps ideal volume distribution on the planning sheet. One cannot rely only on surface anatomy. Verification films taken on the machine or with a simulator must be used to make sure of coverage.

Preferably, portals should be either straight lateral or straight anterior with the exception of the wedge filter technique which requires oblique portals. Some therapists prefer to have the patient lying on the back or side, others prefer to have him sitting on a chair. For lateral portals, we believe that, using an adjustable head rest, the head extends better with the patient on the side than when in the supine position. Verification films are easily taken with the head rest which includes a slot in which to place the films (Fig. 3-38). Dead seeds or silver clips are inserted at the periphery, at least anteriorly, of the lesion to determine proper coverage (Fig. 3-39).

The therapist should familiarize himself with one method and with the means of checking the daily duplication of treatment and the accuracy of anatomical coverage by verification films.

Megavoltage External Beam Therapy

There are two commercial types of energy levels available for megavoltage therapy. One level is 2 to 6 Mev, which includes the ^{60}Co units, and the other level is 20 to 30 Mev. There are also units which can be used for electron beam therapy with levels from 6 Mev to 35 Mev.

There are physical characteristics of the 2 to 6 Mev level versus the 20 to 25 Mev level which are clinically important. The first characteristic is that the depth of maximum build-up for the 2 to 4 Mev level, is at 3 to 4 mm, whereas it is at 2.5 to 3 cm at the 20 to 30 Mev level. When nodes are immediately under the skin, wax must be used for build-up with the higher energy levels. This nullifies the skin-sparing effect and is a great disadvantage. Therefore, in practice, the 2 to 4 Mev level is preferable for most lesions of the oropharynx when extensive treatment of the neck is carried out.

The use of glancing fields partially nullifies the skin-sparing because it brings the maximum dose close to the surface. In using glancing fields, moist desquamation may be produced. If a neck dissection is contemplated and high doses are to be given, the use of glancing fields must be carefully avoided.

Dosage Rate with the Parallel Opposing Technique

If the surface coverage is not more than 50 sq cm, 6,000 rads can be given in 5 weeks. With a surface coverage from 50 to 100 sq cm, 6,000 rads are given in 5 to 6 weeks preferably in 6 weeks when it approaches 100 sq cm; for large areas or for old or debilitated or severely alcoholic patients, 850 rads per week is better tolerated; then the total dose is increased by 10 per cent giving the last 1,000 to 2,000 rads at 1,000 rads through reduced fields.

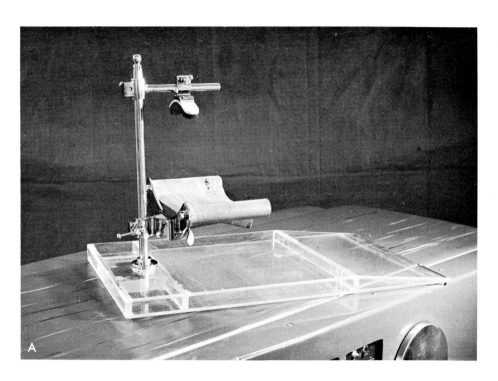

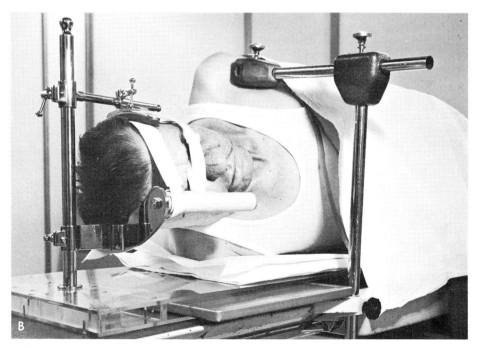

FIG. 3-38. Head rest with accessories to help secure immobility. There is a slot to take verification films. (Courtesy: Luis Delclos, M.D., Head, Department of Radiotherapy, Hospital General De Asturias Oviedo, Spain.)

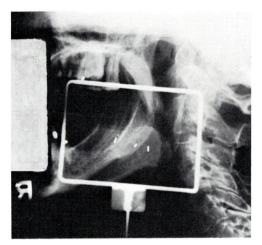

FIG. 3-39. Female, age 74, seen in 1964 with a squamous cell carcinoma of the posterolateral border of the tongue. (Dead seeds indicate area of tumor.) Because of the inadvisability of general anesthesia, the management was entirely by external beam therapy. A tumor dose of 7,000 rads was given in 5 weeks by a combination of lateral portal with the 22 Mev x-ray beam and a submental portal with the 18 Mev electron beam.

The patient did not come for followup. She died in September 1969 of what was called carcinomatosis of the lung.

Wedge Filter Techniques

(Fig. 3-40)

Using lead wedge filters, one can skew the isodose curves and use oblique portals with homogeneous distribution.

With wedge filters, 6,000 rads can be delivered with ease in 5 weeks. The sharpness of the fibrinous mucositis is striking, giving assurance of the exact areas covered by the beam. The use of wedge pair for anterior faucial pillar-retromolar trigone resulted in a significant incidence of bone necrosis.[13] With 60-degree wedge, 15 to 20 per cent more is given to bone, with 45-degree wedge and wide separation, there is a homogeneous dose but a much longer length of jaw is irradiated; both situations result in more complications. A wedge pair arrangement is useful for lesions located anteriorly (Fig. 3-41).

Oral Cavity

The anatomical sites of the oral cavity are: 1) The anterior two thirds of the tongue, which is the portion anterior to the circum-

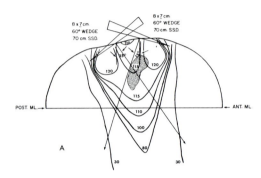

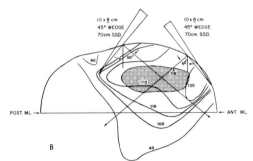

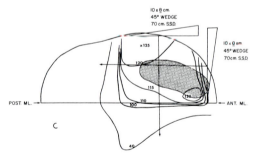

FIG. 3-40. Wedge-pair filter patterns. The patterns from top to bottom are for: **A.** a tumor of the faucial pillar where narrow portals are used with a 60-degree wedge. Small volume but 15 to 20 per cent more dose to bone; **B.** a tumor of the faucial pillar involving the buccal mucosa, gum, floor of mouth, and posterolateral border of the tongue; **C.** an extensive tumor of the floor of the mouth and tongue close to the midline anteriorly and reaching far back.

By varying the angles, the width of the portals, and the wedge thickness, one can adapt to any individual situation.

teriorly. The calculated dose in taking an average of the lengths of the needles is sufficiently accurate.

In tumors of the posterolateral border, the posterior needles must be placed in the base of the tongue. If there is the slightest suspicion of extension in the direction of the sulcus, a needle is placed under the mucous membrane of the sulcus (Fig. 3-42) or a small plane is implanted through the floor of mouth and anterior faucial pillar. There will be a small zone of high dosage between the two planes, but, being small, it is well tolerated.

Lesions of the undersurface of the tongue require adaptation if the location is anterior. Implants similar to those for the floor of the mouth (Fig. 3-43) are used.

For lesions invading more than half of the tongue or massively involving the floor of the mouth, external irradiation is the main component of the treatment with a tumor dose of 6,000 to 7,000 rads delivered with 850 rads per week. Following this, various types of treatment are used depending upon the status of the lesion.

If a radical neck dissection is to be performed 6 to 8 weeks following treatment and a residual area of induration is present at the primary site, a composite operation may be

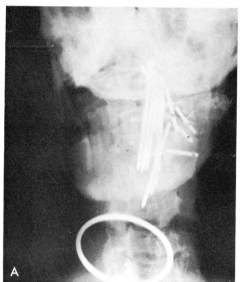

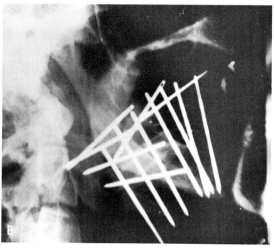

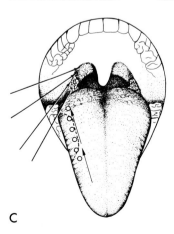

FIG. 3-42. Male, age 58, seen in December 1966 with a T_2N_0 squamous cell carcinoma of the medial and posterior lateral border of the tongue with slight impingement upon the anterior faucial pillar.

The first 4,000 rads in 4 weeks were given with external beam, homolateral portal with 22 Mev. The subdigastric area is well covered. A plastic stent depressing the tongue was used to save the hard palate; barium coating outlines dorsum of tongue. Then, an implant with one plane in the tongue (vertical plane) and another plane in the floor of the mouth and the tonsillar area (horizontal plane) giving, halfway between the horizontal and vertical planes, a dose of 3,150 rads with a dose rate of 35 rads per hour, calculated from the computer calculated curves. The horizontal plane was removed at 90 hours and the vertical plane left in place for 122 hours.

The patient was *NED* on 4-9-72.

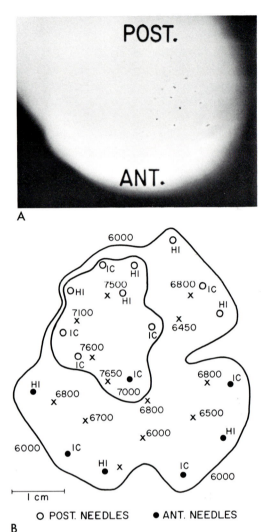

POST.

ANT.

A

6000

O HI

O IC   O HI

7500

O HI   6800 O IC

x O HI   x

HI

7100   O

x   IC

O IC   x 6450

7600

O x

IC

7650 ● IC   6800   IC

x   x   ●

HI   7000

●   6800   x

6800   x   x 6500

x   6800

x 6700

x 6000   HI

O

6000   IC   ●

●

HI   x   IC   6000

●   ●

|—————|
I cm

O POST. NEEDLES   ● ANT. NEEDLES

B

FIG. 3-43. Patient with a T_3 squamous cell carcinoma
of the undersurface of the tongue involving
the root of the tongue and the floor of the
mouth.

The implant was performed with 17
needles, 4.5 cm active length, alternating
Indian club (*IC*) and half intensity (*HI*). **A.**
Tomogram of the implant. **B.** The posterior
needles (white circles) were removed at 85
hours and anterior needles (black circles)
were left for a total of 170 hours in order
to produce the volume distribution seen.

contemplated instead of additional local irradiation (2,000 to 3,000 rads with interstitial
implants). In all cases in which the floor of
the mouth and the mandible are involved,
a composite operation is preferable.

ANALYSIS OF FAILURES

Table 3-24 shows the percentage by *T*
stages of excised or irradiated lesions, the
failure rates of irradiation by *T* staging, the
number of failures salvaged by a surgical
procedure and the ultimate failure rates.
There is a rapid increase in the incidence of
failures from T_1 to T_3 lesions.

The analysis of failures by modality of
irradiation showed that external irradiation
alone is not an effective method of treatment
for lesions of the oral tongue.[6] Because of the
tumor bed, interstitial therapy is an essential
part of the treatment of the squamous cell
carcinoma of the mobile tongue. Patients
with T_4 lesions have a high incidence of
failures irrespective of the technique used.

Floor of Mouth

The floor of the mouth is a U-shaped area
between the lower gum and the tongue. The
anatomical structures which direct the extension of cancer are the loose submucosal tissues of the submental and submandibular
spaces, the periosteum of the mandible, and
the muscles of the tongue. Cancers of the
floor of the mouth may grow centrifugally
to reach the gum, tongue, and genioglossus
muscles. Once the gum has been reached, the
disease tends to spread along the periosteum
of the mandible. Invasion of the root of the
tongue darkens the prognosis considerably.

The infiltrative lesion may be deceptive,
often presenting only a small surface ulceration. Only bimanual palpation under general
anesthesia can disclose the true extent of
infiltration into the submental space or the
root of the tongue.

The reasons for the choice of treatment of
the primary lesion for the floor of the mouth
are subtle. By and large, irradiation is preferred as floor of the mouth lesions are very
readily controlled by irradiation. Very small
lesions are simply excised. For a variety of
anatomical reasons (a very narrow arch, a
forward slant of the arch or tori precluding
a good radium implant) and in the alcoholic

Table 3-24. *Anterior Two Thirds of Tongue—Failure to Control the Primary Lesion in Patients Treated by Definitive Irradiation (Unlimited Follow-up*) January 1948–December 1968, (Analysis April 1971)*

	Percentage of Pts by Stages and Modality of Treatment		Local Results in Patients Treated with Irradiation			
	Surgical Excision	Irrad.	% of Failures Following Irradiation		Pts. Salvaged by Surgical Excision**	% of Ultimate Local Failures
T_1	53%	21%	5.7%	(3/52)	1/3	5.5%
T_2	24%	40%	17%	(17/100)	5/17	12%
T_3	19%	27%	41%	(27/66)	6/27	32%
T_4	4%	12%	67%	(20/30)	2/20	60%
Total No. of Pts.	64†	248††	27%	(67/248)		21.5% (53/248)

*Squamous cell carcinoma developing at any time in the follow-up in the vicinity of the initial lesion is counted as recurrence.
** NED at 2 years after treatment of failure.

		Surgery†	Irrad.††
5-year survival:	Absolute	60%	45%
	Determinate	72%	52%

(Adapted from: Chu and Fletcher, *Amer. J. Roentgen.*, 117, 502, 1973.)

(a high percentage of patients with floor of the mouth lesions are inveterate alcoholics) a surgical procedure may be preferred.

In extensive lesions involving bone, radiation is usually a preoperative measure. A surgical procedure is often necessary to remove either residuum of cancer or necrosis.

TECHNIQUES

Superficial lesions contiguous to the alveolus in edentulous patients, in whom the floor of the mouth is flat, are treated efficiently with intraoral therapy. Either with 6 to 9 Mev electron beam or 150 Kv, depending upon tumor thickness, 5,500 to 6,000 rads are given in 4 to 5 weeks.

The lesions close to the undersurface of the tongue are not suitable for intraoral therapy because of the motion of the tongue.

A radium implant through the dorsum of the tongue is the safest way to cover clinically demonstrable disease and the possible extensions along the periosteum, submucosal areolar tissue, and root of the tongue.

In order to keep the needles in place and in particular to maintain the lower ends of the needles deep in the submental region, the tongue must be immobilized. The tongue is sutured to the mucosa of the anterior bucco-gingival sulcus (Fig. 3-44).

Lesions of the lateral aspect of the floor of the mouth are treated with a single plane implant. The needles are threaded submucosally through the lateral aspect of the tongue, emerge into the floor of the mouth and then are directed along the inner aspect of the gum. A template may be used (Fig. 3-45).

Needles tend to be separated by the tongue's swelling. Therefore curved palisade implants with half intensity needles placed 0.5 to 0.75 cm apart to avoid gaps may be used; one row is against the arch of the mandible and a second, less extensive row, covers the lesion posteriorly (Fig. 3-46 and 3-47).

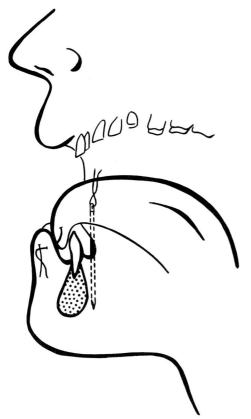

FIG. 3-44. To treat tumors of the floor of the mouth, the needles are inserted through the dorsum of the tongue, emerge on the undersurface, and are reinserted at the junction of the floor of the mouth with the gum, keeping the tip of the needle in contact with the mandible. The needles are pushed deep into the tongue so that there is only mechanical trauma to the mucosa of the dorsum of the tongue.

When more than one row of needles is used, the posterior row is implanted first since the lesion cannot be seen after the needles have been implanted against the arch of the mandible.

Implants deviate considerably from geometrical patterns for which tables have been made. Calculations of the contribution of each needle are made for selected points. Using a calculated dose of 7,000 rads, the control rate has been high, but the incidence of necrosis has also been quite significant. In using this type of palisade implant, the dose given should be 5,500 to 6,000 rads. Transverse tomograms are useful for determining the exact location of the needles and for calculations. Explicit calculation with computer is best.

When the disease extends onto the gum, intraoral therapy may be used as a supplement (Fig. 3-48). When the lateral border of the tongue is involved, crossing needles are used on the dorsum of the tongue.

In the more advanced lesion in which the root of the tongue and the periosteum is involved, a combination of external radiation and interstitial radium therapy has been used. The implant is at times weighted by the addition of quarter intensity needles in the part of the shell where the disease is present. The complication rate is high.

In the very advanced lesion with extension to the bone and root to tongue, external radiation is the primary treatment with additional local therapy as circumstances indicate.

Electron beam therapy through a submental portal has proven effective in delivering part of the radiation dose treatment, combined with parallel opposing photon beam or interstitial gamma ray therapy depending upon the size of the lesion.

COMBINATION WITH SURGERY

In the advanced cases, a sequential use of radiation and surgery is planned because an unhealed ulcer often remains even if the tumor is eradicated. The main purpose of the radiation is sterilization of the tumor within the tongue where surgical clearance is difficult to obtain. The surgical procedure varies, depending upon the evolution of the lesion, and may be performed 6 to 8 weeks after the irradiation. If there is unexpectedly good regression and apparent healing, surgical treatment is withheld until a recurrence or late necrosis necessitates intervention.

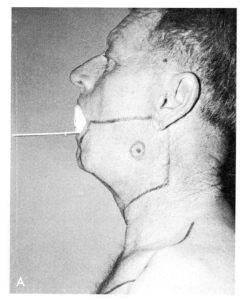

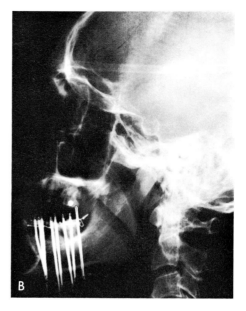

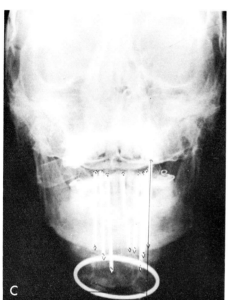

COMPUTER ISODOSE DISTRIBUTION — MIDPLANE CUT
RA Needling

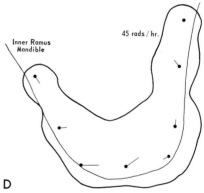

45 rads / hr.

Inner Ramus
Mandible

D

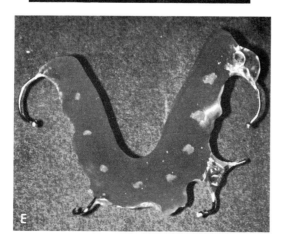

FIG. 3-45. Male, age 47, seen in March 1970 with a squamous cell carcinoma (Grade II) of the floor of mouth fixed to the periosteum. There was a 4 cm bilobe mass in the left submaxillary area. With ^{60}Co, irradiation was started on 3-24-70 delivering 5,000 rads tumor dose in 5 weeks to the floor of the mouth and upper neck through parallel opposed portals. The lower neck received 5,000 rads given dose in 5 weeks through anterior split ^{60}Co portals.

On 5-20-70, a radium needle implant was done which delivered 3,500 rads in 77.7 hours.

A left radical neck dissection was done on 7-3-70. There were no positive nodes in the surgical specimen.

On 2-10-71 the patient was NED with a small necrosis over the sublingual area.

On 9-27-71 a complete odontectomy, alveoloplasty and saucerization of lingual plate of the left mandible was performed with a forehead pedicle flap inserted in the floor of the mouth.

The patient is well on 12-10-71.

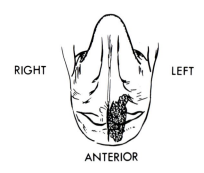

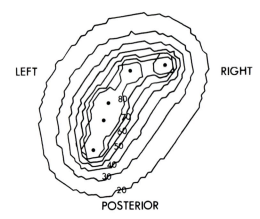

RIGHT   LEFT

ANTERIOR

LEFT   RIGHT

POSTERIOR

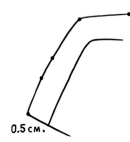

0.5 CM.

FIG. 3-46. Male, age 79, seen in October 1961 with a squamous cell carcinoma at the junction of the floor of the mouth and the undersurface of the tongue, approximately 2.5 cm in length and 1.5 cm wide.

A curved implant was performed through the dorsum of the tongue with 5 needles (4 cm active length, 0.66 mg/cm). Using the Paterson and Parker table for curved implants, dosage rate was calculated to be 56 rads per hour at 0.5 cm within the implant. This agreed with the computer data. Seven thousand rads were given in 125 hours.

The patient expired in December 1961 following a paralytic stroke.

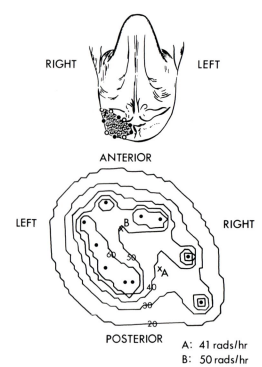

RIGHT   LEFT

ANTERIOR

LEFT   RIGHT

POSTERIOR   A: 41 rads/hr
                   B: 50 rads/hr

FIG. 3-47. Patient with a squamous cell carcinoma of the floor of the mouth with some invasion of the root of the tongue and attachment to the gingiva.

A radium implant was done with 4.5 cm active length needles going through the dorsum of the tongue. Top: cross section of the implant at the level of the floor of the mouth with alternating Indian club (*IC*) needles (white circles) and 1.33 cm (*HI*) needles (black circles). Bottom: isodose curves from computer calculation.

The implant was left for 170 hours, giving approximately 6,000 rads.

Calculations at points A and B were made from the individual contributions of the needles.

Needles		A		B	
		Dist.	r/hr.	Dist.	r/hr.
IC	1	1.35	4.27	3.0	1.36
HI	2	0.7	9.6	2.1	2.1
IC	3	1.2	4.85	1.2	4.85
HI	4	1.5	3.5	0.7	9.6
IC	5	2.25	2.04	0.7	9.9
HI	6	2.4	1.7	0.9	7.2
HI	7	1.8	2.6	0.8	8.2
IC	8	1.5	3.78	1.2	4.85
HI	9	1.1	5.6	1.4	3.9
IC	10	0.9	7.4	1.6	3.4
r/hr. Total			45.34		55.36
rads/hr. × 0.90			40.8		49.82

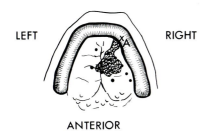

ANTERIOR

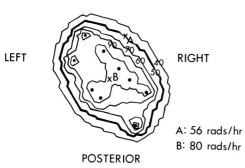

A: 56 rads/hr
B: 80 rads/hr

POSTERIOR

FIG. 3-48. Male, age 75, seen in August 1962, with a squamous cell carcinoma of the inner surface of the tongue close to the midline, extending into the floor of the mouth and to within 3 mm of the gum.

An implant through the dorsum of the tongue was done using an anterior row of 4.5 cm active length needles with 3 back Indian club needles 4.5 cm active length, half intensity (0.33 mg/cm). Manual calculation showed 80 rads per hour at point B and 56 rads per hour at point A on the gum.

From the computer data, the dose at point A was 59 rads per hour and at point B, 88 rads per hour, which closely matches the manual calculation of 56 and 80 rads per hour.

The implant was left for 90 hours. The dose between the rows was 5,600 rads with only about 4,500 rads at point A on the gum.

To make up for the difference, 2 × 500 rads were given on the gum in 2 consecutive days with a 2 cm intraoral cone using 250 Kv, 0.5 Cu plus 1 Al, 40 FSD.

The implant was performed on September 11, 1962. A necrosis developed in 1963.

The patient expired on 8-26-64 from intercurrent disease with no evidence of cancer at death.

NECROSIS

Because the mucous membrane is stretched thinly over bone, there is a significant incidence of breakdown of the mucous membrane. When a radium implant alone has been used, healing will usually occur after local sequestration. If the bone has been extensively irradiated by external irradiation, defense mechanisms are poor, and a segment of the mandible ultimately will have to be resected. Unhealed necrosis with progressive osteitis has been common when 3,000 to 4,000 rads have been given with external irradiation, even with megavoltage.

RESULTS

Table 3-25 shows the percentage by T stages of excised or irradiated lesions, the failure rates of irradiation by T staging, the number of failures salvaged by a surgical procedure, and the ultimate failure rates. The increase in the incidence of failures is not as steep from the T_1 to T_3 lesions as for those of the oral tongue. There is a high salvage rate by surgery and the ultimate failure rates are very low, even in the T_3 lesions.

Buccal Mucosa

The tumors originating on or involving the upper or lower gingivobuccal sulcus are assigned to either the buccal mucosa or the gums depending upon which structure is most involved. Lesions of the buccal mucosa are often associated with leukoplakia and there is a tendency to multiple primaries.

Small, superficial lesions are best excised. The middle-sized lesions of the buccal mucosa are often irradiated because of the extensiveness of the surgical procedure. Extension to the upper or lower sulcus, with or without invasion of bone, brings specific problems. Careful planning of surgical excision or radiation alone or both combined has to be made for each case. The unresectable infiltrative lesions are treated by radiotherapy, usually for palliation.

Table 3-25. *Floor of Mouth—Failure to Control the Primary Lesion in Patients Treated by Definitive Irradiation (Unlimited Follow-up*) January 1948–December 1968, (Analysis April 1971)*

	Percentage of Pts by Stages and Modality of Treatment		Local Results in Patients Treated with Irradiation			
	Surgical Excision	Irrad.	% of Failures Following Irradiation		Pts. Salvaged by Surgical Excision**	% of Ultimate Local Failures
T_1	35%	23%	2%	(1/49)	1/1	0%
T_2	24%	36%	11.5%	(9/77)	4/9	6.5%
T_3	28%	30%	23%	(14/60)	11/14	5%
T_4	13%	11%	79%	(19/24)	0/19	79%
Total No. of Pts.	68†	210††	20.5%	(43/210)		13% (27/210)

*Squamous cell carcinoma developing at any time in the follow-up in the vicinity of the initial lesion is counted as recurrence.
**NED at 2 years after treatment of failure.

		Surgery †	Irrad. ††
5-year survival:	Absolute	48.5%	56%
	Determinate	62%	67.5%

(Adapted from: Chu and Fletcher, *Amer. J. Roentgen.*, 117, 502, 1973.)

TECHNIQUES

Interstitial radium implants are an efficient method of management of the infiltrating lesions which have not invaded the gums, the pterygoid fossa, or the antrum.

The needles are inserted from the outside of the cheek with a guiding finger in the mouth (Fig. 3-49). If the implant is made from within the open mouth, the needles are often crowded when the mouth is closed. It is often necessary to place needles above or below the lower sulcus in order to cover lesions which involve the sulci. Usually the needles are horizontal, and the implant crossed at both ends. When two planes are used, the outer plane is larger, inserted from outside and the smaller plane is inserted from the inside.

Wedge filter technique produces a good volume distribution and should be used if a radium implant cannot encompass the lesion. Electron beam therapy is a useful

modality of treatment. With both modalities, unless the lesion is too extensive, after 5,000 or 6,000 rads, a supplement is given with an implant; ^{192}Ir being a flexible source in nylon threads.

When a lesion involves the sulcus and also extends to the alveolar ridge, the innermost extension may be far from the plane of needles. This necessitates treatment adjustment either by inserting extra needles or giving supplementary irradiation through a cone. When the commissure is involved, a curved implant is made after suturing the lips together. Lesions invading the posterior sulcus, retromolar trigone, or the mucous membrane of the ascending ramus require a plane through the tonsillar fossa. Wedge filter technique is easier and safer.

The tolerance of the buccal mucosa to irradiation is excellent, allowing radical therapy for very advanced cases. Large implants can be performed, sometimes successfully. Combining implants and external radiation

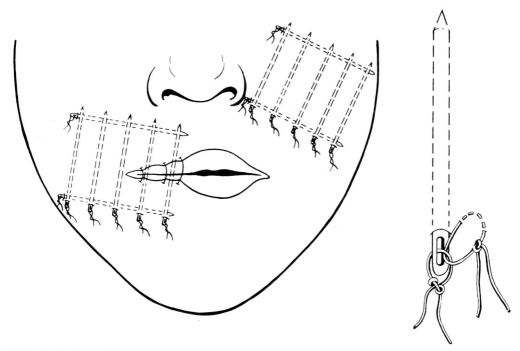

FIG. 3-49. Implants of the buccal mucosa. For a lesion in the center of the buccal mucosa, the needles are inserted from outside, with a guiding hand in the mouth; in that way there is no collapse of the needles and better geometry is obtained.

For a lesion of the commissure, the lips are sutured and an implant with crossing is performed. A method of suturing the needles so that they do not pull out is illustrated.

can be a solution for complex cases where surrounding structures are involved.

Teeth should be removed prior to the irradiation of lesions involving the sulci, but at times the lesion is so extensive that the teeth cannot be removed without cutting through disease. Treatment, however, has to be carried out and complications can be expected.

RESULTS

Table 3-26 shows the percentage by *T* stages of excised or irradiated lesions, the failure rates of irradiation by *T* staging, the number of failures salvaged by a surgical procedure, and the ultimate failure rates. New primary lesions, often at the margin of a treated area, are frequent.

Complications are uncommon with the use of radium implants. Mucous membrane breakdown appears when the commissure has been involved, but usually heals with simple conservative measures. In the more advanced cases, severe complications occur and bone resection may have to be done.

Lower Gum

The most common site of origin is in the region of the molar teeth. Leukoplakia is often present and the lesions appear usually as the verrucous type. There is a tendency toward multiple sites of origin.

Even when good healing follows radiation, dentures can cause breakdown of the mucous membrane and, despite good fit, cannot be worn. Simple excision, or marginal resection with a skin graft, is the treatment of choice for superficial lesions.

Table 3-26. *Buccal Mucosa—Failure to Control the Primary Lesion in Patients Treated by Definitive Irradiation (Unlimited Follow-up*) January 1948–December 1968, (Analysis June 1972)*

	Percentage of Pts by Stages and Modality of Treatment		Local Results in Patients Treated with Irradiation			
	Surgical Excision	Irrad.	% of Failures Following Irradiation		Pts. Salvaged by Surgical Excision**	% of Ultimate Local Failures
T_1	23%	7%	14%	(1/7)	1/1	0%
T_2	45%	34%	22%	(7/32)	2/7	16%
T_3	16%	29%	18.5%	(5/27)	2/5	11%
T_4	16%	30%	48%	(14/29)	5/14	31%
Total No. of Pts.	62†	97††	28%	(27/97)		17.5% (17/97)

*Squamous cell carcinoma developing at any time in the follow-up in the vicinity of the initial lesion is counted as recurrence.
**NED at 2 years after treatment of failure.

		Surgery †	Irrad. ††
5-year survival:	Absolute	53%	53%
	Determinate	66%	65%

The saucer type of bone involvement, caused by expanding tumor, must be differentiated from the moth-eaten type, which is caused by diffuse and far-reaching invasion. Good response to irradiation can be expected with the saucer type. When bone is truly invaded, radiation may be used as a preoperative measure to diminish the incidence of local recurrence. In those lesions with bone involvement, the combination of radiation and surgical resection may diminish the incidence of local failures, which are common when only one discipline is used alone.

TECHNIQUES

Superficial lesions can be managed by intraoral cone therapy. Tumor doses of 5,500 to 6,000 rads in 3 to 4 weeks are usually effective.

A wedge pair arrangement produces anatomically suitable volume distributions for lesions located anteriorly. The tumor doses are usually 5,500 to 6,000 rads in 3 to 4 weeks.

With electron beam, adequate doses can be delivered through a single homolateral portal without excessive dose to the rest of the oral cavity.

For preoperative irradiation, the tumor dose is 5,000 rads delivered in 4 to 5 weeks, followed by the composite operation 6 to 8 weeks later.

RESULTS

Table 3-27 shows the percentage of T stages of excised or irradiated lesions of the lower gum, the failure rates of irradiation by T staging, the number of failures salvaged by a surgical procedure, and the ultimate failure rates.

Lesions without bone involvement yield good results to radiation therapy. Because of the shift to advanced stages, there is a rather high recurrence rate. In those with bone involvement, the combination of radiation and surgical resection may diminish the incidence of local failures, which are common when only one discipline is used alone.

Table 3-27. *Lower Gum—Failure to Control the Primary Lesion in Patients Treated by Definitive Irradiation (Unlimited Follow-up*) January 1948–December 1968, (Analysis June 1972)*

Percentages of Pts by Stages and Modality of Treatment		Local Results in Patients Treated with Irradiation			
Surgical Excision	Irrad.	% of Failures Following Irradiation		Pts. Salvaged by Surgical Excision**	% of Ultimate Local Failures
T_1	13%	15%	28.5%	(2/7)	0/2	28.5%
T_2	30%	21%	30%	(3/10)	1/3	20%
T_3	31%	34%	41%	(7/17)	3/7	23.5%
T_4	26%	30%	71%	(10/14)	0/10	71%
Total No. of Pts.	105†	48††	46%	(22/48)		37.5% (18/48)

*Squamous cell carcinoma developing at any time in the follow-up in the vicinity of the initial lesion is counted as recurrence.
**NED at 2 years after treatment of failure.

		Surgery †	Irrad. ††
5-year survival:	Absolute	46%	45%
	Determinate	54.5%	53%

Tumors of the Upper Gum and Hard Palate

Tumors of the upper gums are rare. Early involvement of the maxillary antrum is common; it is difficult to estimate the degree of extension, and it is often impossible to determine whether the tumor originated in the infrastructure of the maxillary antrum or the gum. Therefore, squamous cell carcinomas of the upper gum are often included with those of the maxillary antrum under the heading of cancers of the upper jaw.

Surgical resection is the treatment of choice for patients with tumors of the upper gum. If very early, a limited resection of the bone is adequate and, if more advanced, the surgical procedure is the only way to determine the extension of the disease. The same reasoning is applied to the rare squamous cell carcinoma of the hard palate. When the lesion is extensive and involves the soft palate, irradiation may be preferred in order to include parapharyngeal lymphatics in the treatment field (Fig. 3-50). The tumors most commonly found on the hard palate are glandular tumors, which are themselves uncommon.

In the occasional tumor of the upper gum which is to be treated by irradiation, administration of irradiation by intraoral cone alone is satisfactory for early lesions, and for more advanced lesions, a combination with external irradiation is used.

If a surgical excision cannot be performed, the very extensive tumors are managed like tumors of the maxillary antrum with external irradiation, using a wedge filter arrangement.

Surface molds can be used for superficial lesions of the hard palate. For more extensive lesions, a multiple field arrangement must be designed with ^{60}Co to cover lesions of varying size and location with 18 to 22 Mev beam parallel opposing portals (Fig. 3-50).

RESULTS

The number of patients is too small for meaningful analysis.

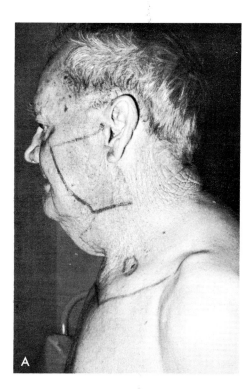

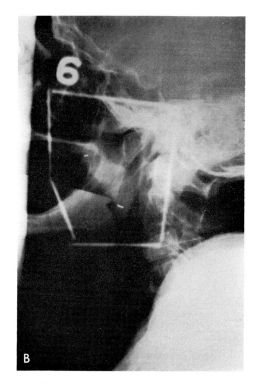

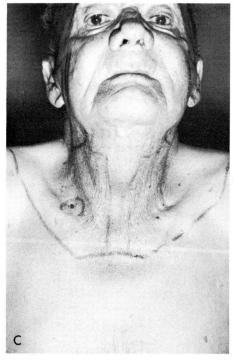

FIG. 3-50. Male, age 77, with a squamous cell carcinoma, Grade II, of the hard palate approximately 4.5 cm in diameter extending posteriorly on the soft palate. The anterior and posterior aspects of the lesion were identified with dead seeds and the treatment carried out with 18 Mev photon beam from 3-30-70 to 5-15-70. After 5,000 rads, the fields were slightly reduced to carry the final tumor dose to 7,000 rads in 7 weeks. Although there were no palpable nodes, the subdigastric area was carefully covered and the lower neck treated with one anterior portal to a given dose of 5,000 rads in 5 weeks with ^{60}Co.

It is to be noted that the parapharyngeal lymphatics area is well covered as lesions at that site do metastasize to that chain of nodes.

The patient tolerated the treatment quite well having lost no weight.

The patient was *NED* in March 1971 but died in April 1971 probably from a stroke.

Oropharynx

The tonsillar fossa, the posterior faucial pillars (including the posterior pillar component of the soft palate), and the base of the tongue are embryologically derived from the oropharyngeal segment. The anterior faucial pillar and the retromolar trigone are embryologically connected with the oral cavity.

The biological behavior of the tumors originating on the palatine arch shares some of the characteristics of tumors of the oral cavity and of some tumors of the oropharynx. For instance, the soft palate, which is made up of the anterior and posterior faucial pillars has a high incidence of nodal metastases. It is preferable, although somewhat arbitrary from the standpoint of either surgical or radiotherapeutic management, to include the tumors of soft palate, the anterior faucial pillar, and the retromolar trigone in with the oropharyngeal cancers.

There is, as a rule, in the literature, no distinction between the tumors originating on the anterior faucial pillar, the retromolar trigone, the tonsillar fossa and the glossopalatine sulcus which are referred to as the tonsillar region. Although these various anatomical sites are very close, only in early lesions is just one structure involved. It is important to assign as site of origin an individual anatomic structure because the spread patterns and the natural history of the disease vary.

By taking into consideration the lines of spread, relative degrees of extension, the histology of the tumor, the incidence and distribution of neck node metastases, a site of origin can almost always be assigned. But there are some peculiarities of cancers of this anatomical region, *i.e.*, the high incidence of the lesions in alcoholics and the fact that women have a better prognosis than men.

On the palatine arch, in addition to the three main clinical varieties of exophytic, ulcerative, or infiltrative tumors and their combinations, there is a reddish, velvety type of *in situ* carcinoma.[15] This diffuse spread

may cause a new disease. The fibrinous exudate covering the tumor delineates it at the end of the first week of irradiation.

There is a tendency to multiple primary tumors. It is a common occurrence that at least two positive biopsies may be taken from areas which are grossly not part of the same tumor. Subsequent primary tumors in the pharynx and larynx are common. Follow-up examinations must include careful examination of the entire upper respiratory tract.

Tumors of the palatine arch interfere with the buccopharyngeal sphincter; the palatine arch contains a larger number of pain fibers, and lesions in this location exhibit symptoms while still small; in addition they are easily visible to the patient. Tumors of the palatine arch do not metastasize as early as tonsillar bed or base of tongue tumors in which palpable neck nodes often are the first sign. When searching for an occult primary tumor in a patient with palpable neck nodes, if the nasopharynx has been eliminated as tumor site, a careful investigation of the base of the tongue, glossopalatine sulcus, and tonsillar bed may reveal a small primary tumor.

Since the advent of megavoltage therapy and the closer integration of radiation and surgical modalities, very definite policies of management have emerged, both for the primary lesions and diseased neck nodes varying with the anatomical site where the primary lesion occurs.

The following anatomical sites will be considered (Fig. 3-51):

1) Anterior faucial pillar-retromolar trigone.

2) Soft palate including the uvula.

3) Tonsillar fossa.

4) Posterior faucial pillar.

5) Base of the tongue (that portion of the tongue behind the circumvallate papillae).

6) Valleculae.

7) Lateral and posterior pharyngeal walls from the level of the soft palate to the hyoid.

Tumors of the glossopalatine sulci between the base of the tongue and the tonsillar area

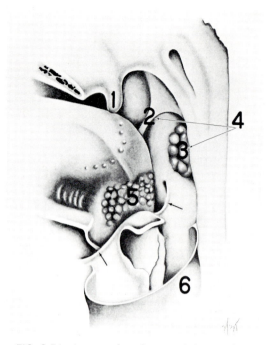

FIG. 3-51. A posterolateral view of the oropharynx showing subsites: 1) uvula, 2) anterior faucial pillar, 3) tonsillar fossa, 4) tonsillar region (2 and 3) and posterior faucial pillar (not shown), 5) base of tongue, 6) posterior pharyngeal wall. The pharyngo-epiglottic folds are clearly seen (arrows). (Modified from: Ackerman, L. V. and del Regato, J. A., *Cancer: Diagnosis, Treatment, and Prognosis,* 3 Ed. C. V. Mosby, 1962.)

are assigned to the group of tonsillar area or base of tongue tumors depending upon involvement.

TREATMENT PLANNING FOR THE PRIMARY LESION

T_1 and T_2 exophytic lesions yield a sterilization rate of 80 to 90 per cent to definite tumor dose-time formulae with specific geometric arrangements. For instance, provided the surface coverage is no more than 50 sq. cm, 6,000 rads in 5 weeks can be given. Careful localization is essential.

When the lesions are extensive (T_3 and T_4) with components in bones or muscles, and/

or there are multiple neck nodes necessitating the irradiation of large volumes, 850 rads per week is often preferred with re-evaluation at 5,500 rads to rearrange the geometry or stop treatment to carry out a surgical resection. If the lesions are to be managed by radiation only, the total dose is not less than 7,000 rads in 7 weeks for T_3 lesions and 7,500 rads in $7\frac{1}{2}$ weeks for T_4 lesions if 1,000 rads are given per week; the dose is 7,500 rads to 8,000 rads if 850 rads are given per week. The longer treatment time technique is better tolerated when a large volume is irradiated.

Soft Palate

The soft palate begins at the junction of the anterior and posterior faucial pillars, both of which contribute to the central structure, the uvula. Queyrat's erythroplasia is a common finding. Nodal metastases can be bilateral because of a rich lymphatic network.

Early lesions, which can be encompassed by an intraoral cone, are treated entirely with that modality, delivering 5,500 to 6,000 rads in 4 weeks.

The 22 Mev betatron beam is preferable for the two parallel opposing portals technique (Fig. 3-52). For lesions limited to the palate, the portals are 7 × 5 cm or 6 × 5 cm and 6,000 rads are given in 5 weeks. If a ^{60}Co unit is available, it would be preferable whenever feasible to give only 5,000 rads by the parallel opposing portals and 1,000 rads with an intraoral cone.

Lesions of the uvula often extend along the posterior faucial pillars down into the posterior aspect of the tonsillar fossa and the glossopalatine sulci. In that instance, the portals must be longer to adequately cover these downward extensions. These advanced lesions will respond satisfactorily to radiation therapy as they do not have, as a rule, infiltrative components.

If nodes are palpable, the entire neck is irradiated with the same pattern as the one

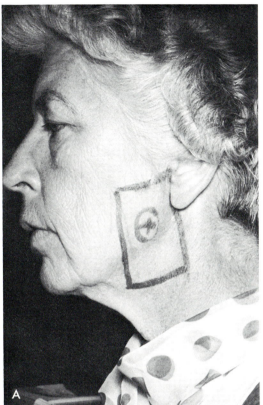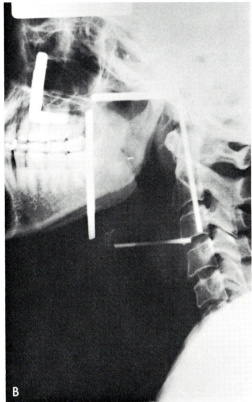

FIG. 3-52. Female, age 55, seen in October 1969 with squamous cell carcinoma of the right soft palate and uvula, T_2N_0. The patient received through intraoral cone at 6 Mev, 1,500 rads initially, and then with parallel opposing portals, 7 × 5 cm, 5,000 rads in 4 weeks with 22 Mev. Total treatment time to the primary was 5 weeks with a total tumor dose of 6,500 rads. The lower neck received 5,000 rads by ^{60}Co unit through an anterior split portal. **A.** Lateral portals. The subdigastric areas were well covered. The lower neck received 5,000 rads given dose in 5 weeks. **B.** Verification film. A dead seed has been inserted into the anterior aspect of the lesion.
    The patient is *NED* 3-23-72.

described for the tonsillar fossa and the base of the tongue.

Tonsillar Region

The tonsillar region consists of the tonsillar fossa and the anterior and posterior faucial pillars. Except for early lesions, more than one structure are involved. However in most cases, the site of origin can be ascribed to the anterior faucial pillar or the tonsillar fossa.[11] It is a rare occasion in which the posterior faucial pillar can be designated as the site of origin.

ANTERIOR FAUCIAL PILLAR
RETROMOLAR TRIGONE

The tumors originating on the anterior tonsillar pillar are better differentiated than those originating in the tonsillar fossa and exhibit less tendency toward widespread nodal metastases. The mucosa in this area blends with part of the retromolar trigone, gum, the tongue, and the palate. Therefore, the tumors originating in the anterior tonsillar pillar usually extend into the soft palate and the tongue. When very extensive, they invade the tonsillar fossa, the retromolar trigone, and the upper and lower gums.

The retromolar trigone is a roughly triangular space, posterior to the last lower molar tooth, with the base in the lower gum and the apex behind the maxillary tuberosity. The mucosa blends laterally with the buccal mucosa and medially with the anterior tonsillar pillar.

Early lesions located high on the faucial pillar or easily exposed on the retromolar trigone can be treated entirely by intraoral cone therapy.

The early lesions of the faucial arch are often reddish, velvety with ill-defined lines and at times can spread quite a distance. Often the best way to determine the extent of the lesion is to observe the tumor's fibrinous exudate, (superficial tumor cells are dead with a tumor dose of 1,000 rads; the caking produces that false membrane) at the end of the first week of treatment. On several occasions the entire palatine arch has been irradiated because of the tissues' redness which is suggestive of multiple lesions.

Most of the T_1 and T_2 lesions are presently treated with 18 to 22 Mev photon; if N_0, one-half of the treatment is by 18 Mev electron and the other half of treatment 18 or 22 Mev photon to avoid overirradiation of the opposite side of the pharynx and opposite parotid. The upper digastric and jugular region is included in the treatment field to deliver up to 5,000 rads (Figs. 3-53, 3-54). If a node is palpable at the angle of the jaw, it will be in the reduced field treating the primary. When the tongue or palate are involved to the midline, parallel opposing portals, usually with 2:1 loading favoring the diseased side, are used. If radical irradiation is given, the portals are reduced at 5,000 rads (or 5,500 rads); an extra 2,000 to 2,500 rads are given at the depth of the center of the primary lesion.

Lesions invading bone are treated with a combined surgical resection and neck dissection carried out 6 to 8 weeks later after the delivery of 5,000 rads in 5 weeks (5,500 rads if 850 rads per week). If extensive disease has not markedly regressed by the end of the 5th

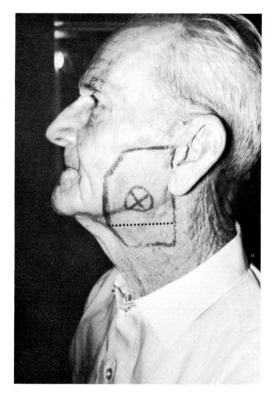

FIG. 3-53. Male, age 69, was seen on 1-2-70 with squamous cell carcinoma, Grade I, of the retromolar trigone, T_2N_0. There was an ulcerative lesion in the left retromolar trigone area extending into the soft palate and back onto the anterior faucial pillar. It extended anteriorly into the gingiva and the glossogingival sulcus, but not to the floor of the mouth. Because of the amount of ulceration and the low grade, only the primary lesion was treated to include generously the subdigastric area.

The patient was treated using half electron and half photon units, both 18 Mev, to a total dose of 6,500 rads in 44 days at 5 cm depth and 7,100 rads at 2 cm depth which was actually the depth of the ulceration on the retromolar trigone. There was marked mucositis on the side involved and barely discernible reddening of the mucous membrane on the opposite side of the mouth. This is because of the electron beam component. From 5,500 rads, the original field had been shrunk, particularly moving up the lower margin as by then the subdigastric area had received 5,500 rads which is adequate for subclinical disease.

The patient is *NED* 3-1-72.

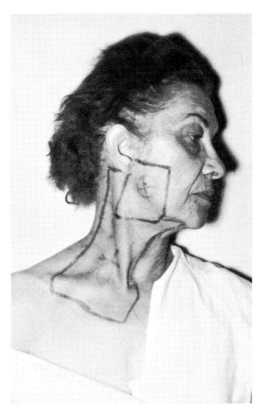

FIG. 3-54. This female, age 61, was seen with a retromolar trigone-anterior faucial pillar squamous cell carcinoma, Grade III. There were no nodes. From 11-2-69 to 12-19-69, 6,400 rads tumor dose were given at 5 cm; 7,400 rads tumor dose at 3 cm was given in $4\frac{1}{2}$ weeks with 1:1 loading 18 Mev x-rays and electron beam. There was a portal reduction at 6,000 rads at 3 cm depth. The entire right neck received 5,500 rads *BED* in $4\frac{1}{2}$ weeks with 9 Mev electron beam.

At completion of treatment there was confluent exudate over the retromolar trigone on the right side with no reaction to the opposite side of the pharynx. Because it was an N_0 lesion, essentially of the retromolar trigone, there was no need to irradiate the opposite subdigastric area.

The patient had no evidence of disease in February 1972.

week, the treatment may be stopped, at 5,000 rads (5,500 rads if 850 rads per week) and a combined operation is performed 6 to 8 weeks later.

The combination of a modified tongue-pterygoid implant[8] with external irradiation is at times an effective method for managing moderately extensive lesions, primarily those with a significant component in the tongue. Five thousand rads are given in 5 weeks at a depth of 3.5 cm to 4.5 cm with external beam followed by 2,500 to 3,000 rads with the implant.

When there are large unilateral nodes extending posteriorly, the 2 parallel opposing portals are not the same size. The portal on the diseased side covers the spinal cord, but the one from the opposite side is aimed to cover only the primary lesion and the jugular digastric area. Even if 6,000 rads are given to the homolateral portal, the spinal cord will not receive an excessive dose.

Extensive lesions which have broken through the superior constrictor muscle and invaded the pterygomandibular space are rarely controlled by radiation therapy. The surgical procedure should be carried out as primary treatment because even if preoperative radiation is given the surgical procedure is one of great radicalism. Better healing will be obtained if radiation therapy has not been given. Postoperative irradiation may be given including both necks and parapharyngeal nodes.

Tonsillar Fossa

The tonsillar bed or fossa is made of the palatine tonsil, a lymphoid organ lying between the two tonsillar pillars. Laterally, the tonsil lies on the superior constrictor muscle of the pharynx which separates it from the internal pterygoid muscle. The relationships of mucosa and musculature explain the commonly observed tendency of tonsillar tumors to extend laterally into the tonsillar pillars and thence towards the soft palate, medially into musculature of the base of the tongue and laterally into the pharyngeal constrictors and internal pterygoid muscles. The extension into the base of the tongue and the lateral pharyngeal wall carries a bad prognosis. Lymphoepithelioma and lymphosarcoma are seen with little break of the mucous membrane.

There are two basic therapy plans for the carcinomas of the tonsillar fossa:

1) Two to one loading: This is the most commonly used arrangement. If 6,000 rads tumor dose is delivered to the primary, the homolateral nodes will receive approxi-

mately 6,500 rads and the contralateral sub-digastric area about 5,000 rads. The hetero-lateral portal may be smaller if there are no large nodes on that side (Fig. 3-55).

2) One to one loading: This is used when there is extensive invasion of the tongue and/or bilateral upper neck nodes.

After 5,000 rads (5,500 rads), fields may

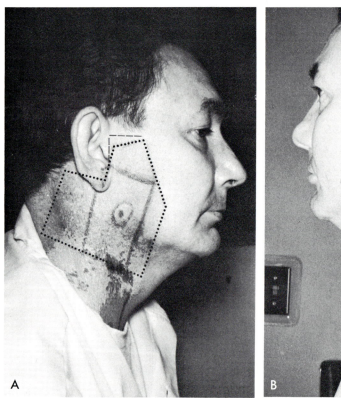
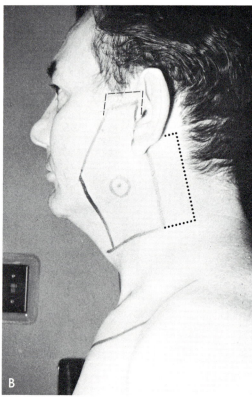

FIG. 3-55. Male, age 36, seen on 8-22-69 with a T_3N_1 lesion of the right tonsillar fossa, squamous cell carcinoma, Grade III. The node was at the angle of the jaw measuring 3×3 cm in diameter.

The basic plan was to give 5,000 rads tumor dose in 5 weeks with 2:1 loading in favor of the right side with ^{60}Co. On the right side, the field extended to include the spinal accessory chain (Fig. A, dotted lines) on the left the posterior margin avoids the spinal cord (Fig. B) and a small strip where the spinal accessory chain was treated with 9 Mev electron beam giving 2,250 rads.

In 5 weeks, 5,000 rads were given to the primary with a given dose of 4,900 rads on the right side and 2,325 rads on the left. Through an anterior split field, a 5,000 rads given dose was delivered in 5 weeks to the lower neck. Then using photon beam, 18 Mev, and electron beam, 18 Mev, 1,000 rads were given by each unit to the primary through a reduced portal to cover only the tonsillar fossa. The node at the angle of the jaw was included in the field. At the completion of treatment there was complete disappearance of the primary and the neck node. The patient has not had any neck dissection because of the high dose given to the node.

In January 1972 the patient had destruction of the base of the skull, *NED* at the primary site and in the neck. Retrospectively the coverage at the base of the skull was not adequate and should have been as indicated by the interrupted lines.

be reduced; 2,000 to 2,500 rads are added at the depth of the center of the primary lesion.

Base of Tongue

The base of the tongue can be defined as that portion of the tongue which is behind the circumvallate papillae; the mucous membrane has lymphoid tissue embedded in it. The base of the tongue is contiguous posteriorly with the valleculae; laterally, the mucosa blends with the pharyngeal walls and curves up to the tonsillar area through the glosso-palatine sulcus.

The lesions of the base of the tongue can clinically be silent until very extensive. The first sign may be nodes in the neck. Occasionally a tumor on the base of the tongue can be so small that it is undetected or at times discovered by biopsy taken almost blindly from an area which appears clinically suspicious. Lateral soft tissue films are essential for the recognition of deep ulcerations which may not be detected by mirror examination (Fig. 3-56). The infiltration of the tumors is usually more diffuse and disseminated than is evidenced by inspection and palpation.

Base of tongue tumors extend into the valleculae or the pharyngoepiglottic fold through the glossopalatine sulcus to the tonsillar area and the lateral pharyngeal wall.

The tumors are usually anaplastic squamous cell carcinomas and occasionally lymphoepitheliomas.

The valleculae are the loose connective tissue area which attaches the lingual epiglottis to the base of the tongue. Tumors can originate in that area. Although their clinical behavior may be slightly different from those of the base of the tongue, they share a great many characteristics. These tumors are best grouped with the tumors of the base of the tongue.

The base of the tongue and nodes on both sides of the upper neck are encompassed by parallel opposing portals with equal loading (Fig. 3-57). Both sides of the neck must be

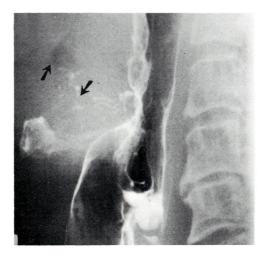

FIG. 3-56. Male, age 61, with a massive tumor of the base of the tongue and bilateral neck nodes. Coating the oral cavity and oropharynx with contrast media shows the dye deep in the base of the tongue and air trapped in a cavity.

irradiated in view of the high incidence of bilateral nodes, except for early keratinizing lesions. Then, the primary site and the sub-digastric areas only are irradiated.

With moderate size fields, a dose of 1,000 rads per week is given and at 5,000 rads reassessment is made to determine if the treatment is to be carried on to 6,000 rads with the same fields. Additional dosage is given through reduced portals for a final tumor dose of 7,000 rads. With large fields for an extensive primary lesion and/or neck disease (or in debilitated or alcoholic patients) 850 rads per week is used. The total dose is then 7,500 to 8,000 rads with reduction of field size at appropriate time.

Pharyngeal Walls

The tumors originating on the pharyngeal walls from the level of the soft palate to the level of the hyoid bone form a clinical group separate from those of the nasopharynx and the hypopharynx. For instance, their metastatic aggressiveness is somewhat less.

Often the tumors of the pharyngeal walls

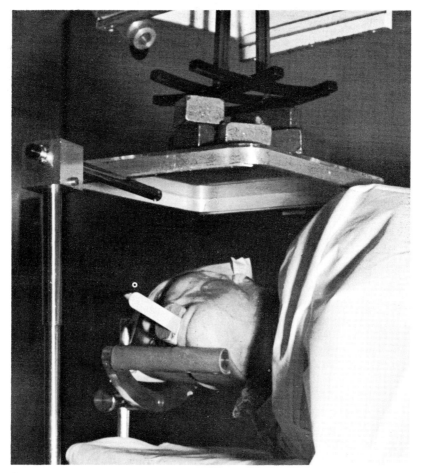

A

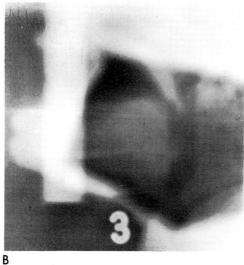

B

FIG. 3-57. A—Female, age 66, with an extensive tumor of the base of the tongue, invading the root and the oral portion of the tongue. Because of the massive disease, treatment was carried out in conjunction with intraarterial injection of 5-Fluorouracil. The portals had to be extended anteriorly. In order to spare as much of the palate as possible, a cork taped to a tongue depressor was used to hold the tongue down.

The verification films are taken by placing the film in the slot which is under the head rest.

B—Verification film.

are ulcerative and the exact extensions of the tumor upward (Fig. 3-58) or downward (Fig. 3-59) are difficult to determine because palpation of only part of the tumor is possible. Microscopic disease can extend a great distance beyond clinically demonstrable tumor. Lateral soft tissue radiographs are essential to determine the extent of the lesion on the posterior pharyngeal wall. Laryngograms can show irregularity of the mucous membrane or lack of motility and can add to the information needed to determine proper therapy. Portals, giving up to 5,500 to 6,000 rads, are usually from the base of the skull (para-pharyngeal lymphatics must be covered) to the mouth of the esophagus.

Never less than 7,000 rads are given in 7 weeks or 7,500 to 8,000 rads if 850 rads per week. The last 1,500 or 2,500 rads are given through reduced portals.

In the pharyngeal lesions, no attempt is made to cover the neck as systematically as is done when the primary lesion is in the tonsillar fossa or the base of the tongue. Nodes located along the jugular chain are included in the portals.

The lesions on the lateral pharyngeal walls are also treated by two parallel opposing

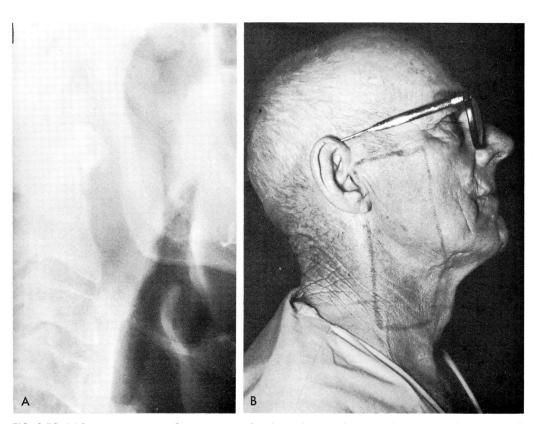

A   B

FIG. 3-58. Male, age 66, seen April 1970, presented with an ulcerative lesion on the posterior pharyngeal wall. Soft tissue of the oropharynx showed extension upward to the base of the skull and downward to the level of the hyoid bone.

From 4-22-70 to 6-9-70, a tumor dose of 7,000 rads was delivered in 7 weeks with 22 Mev beam through parallel opposed fields. The fields were reduced at 5,000 rads and again reduced at 6,000 rads.

On 9-17-70, an ulcer was seen high on the posterior pharyngeal wall. A biopsy from the superior aspect of the ulcer was positive for cancer.

The patient died on 11-24-70.

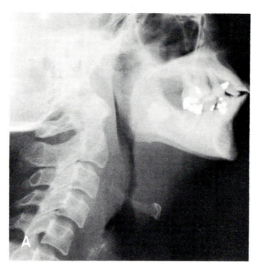
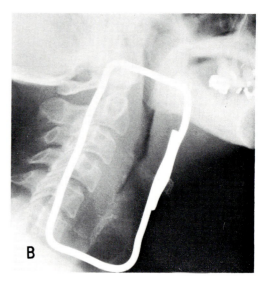

FIG. 3-59. Female, age 53, with a squamous cell carcinoma of the posterior pharyngeal wall, almost impossible to examine with a mirror. The palpating finger felt only the upper aspect of the tumor (Fig. A). In addition, the patient had a node on the left side behind the sternocleidomastoid muscle.

The patient was treated on the 22 Mev betatron with a 10 × 6 cm field, with 1,000 rads per week. In order to include the node, the spinal cord was in the beam.

At the fifth week of treatment a lateral soft tissue film was taken with a metal frame (Fig. B). Marked shrinkage was demonstrated. In order not to exceed 5,000 rads to the spinal cord, the node was no longer completely included in the reduced field which was 8 cm long and 4 cm wide. The upper aspect of the cervical esophagus was still included.

The total dose on the 22 Mev betatron was 7,000 rads in 44 days. The node received an additional 2,700 rads with a 12 Mev electron beam. The patient expired from uncontrolled disease on 8-22-64.

portals as a rule, but with a 2:1 loading favoring the diseased side if ^{60}Co is used.

Results in Faucial Arch and Oropharynx Lesions

Because of age and a high incidence of second primaries in the hypopharynx, lung and esophagus patients will die from other causes despite freedom from disease above the clavicle.[14] Absolute 5-year survival rates are, therefore, no reflections of the results achieved; determinate survival rates are a better gauge of the effectiveness of treatment (Table 3-28).

Table 3-29 shows the incidence of failures following irradiation with the surgical capability for salvage.[12] The differences in results by T staging between the various anatomical sites are probably due to differences in tumor bed and tumor cells composition. The best surgical salvage is accomplished for the retromolar trigone-anterior faucial pillar lesions (the majority of recurrences are on the buccal mucosa or gum) and the least for the pharyngeal wall lesions.[3]

Practically all the patients who developed

Table 3-28. *Squamous Cell Carcinoma of the Faucial Arch and Oropharynx Treated by Primary Irradiation January 1954–December 1965, Determinate 5-Year Survival Rates*

Retromolar Trigone-Anterior Faucial Pillar	61.0%
Soft Palate	67.0%
Tonsillar Fossa	47.5%
Base of Tongue	37.0%
Oropharyngeal Walls	26.5%

Table 3-29. Incidence of Failures at the Primary Site Following Irradiation by Stages and Anatomical Sites of the Oropharynx (Unlimited Follow-up) January 1954–December 1967, (Analysis November 1971)

Stage	Anterior Faucial Pillar Retromolar Trigone			Soft Palate			Tonsillar Fossa			Base of Tongue		
	Failure of XRT	Salvage by Surgery	Ultimate Failure	Failure of XRT	Salvage by Surgery	Ultimate Failure	Failure of XRT	Salvage by Surgery	Ultimate Failure	Failure of XRT	Salvage by Surgery	Ultimate Failure
T_1	15.0% (4/27)	3/4	4.0% (1/27)	0.0% (0/18)	0/0	0.0% (0/18)	0.0% (0/15)	0/0	0.0% (0/15)	7.0% (2/28)	2/2	0.0% (0/28)
T_2	18.5% (16/87)	6/16	11.5% (10/87)	0.0% (0/30)	0/0	0.0% (0/30)	3.0% (1/32)	0/1	3.0% (1/32)	25.0% (9/36)	2/9	19.5% (7/36)
T_3	19.5% (13/67)	9/13	6.0% (4/67)	18.0% (4/22)	0/4	18.0% (4/22)	24.0% (14/58)	6/14	14.0% (8/58)	22.5% (13/58)	1/13	20.5% (12/58)
T_4	26.0% (5/19)	1/5	21.0% (4/19)	50.0% (2/4)	1/2	25.0% (1/4)	40.0% (8/20)	1/8	35.0% (7/20)	45.5% (15/33)	2/15	39.5% (13/33)
Total	19.0% (38/200)	19/38	9.5% (19/200)	8.0% (6/74)	1/6	7.0% (5/74)	18.5% (23/125)	7/23	13.0% (16/125)	25.0% (39/155)	7/39	20.5% (32/155)
Incompletely Treated*	3			2			4			10		

*Excluded from series. (Courtesy: Gelinas and Fletcher: Radiology, publication pending.)

a necrosis were free from disease above the clavicles.[7] This is in conflict with the concept of the supralethal dose.

Malignant Tumors other than Squamous Cell Carcinoma

Lymphomas, usually reticulum cell sarcoma, are seen in the tonsillar fossa and base of tongue. The tumor dose is never less than 5,000 rads in 5 weeks (or 5,500 rads if 850 rads are given per week). Both sides of the neck are treated to 4,000 rads in 4 weeks with a boost dose to initially clinically positive nodes.

Tumors of salivary gland origin are usually mucoepidermoid, presenting often as a well-encapsulated tumor. If the tumor is low grade with a clear margin, postoperative irradiation is not indicated. If there is no clear margin or the tumor is high grade, postoperative irradiation is indicated. The technique varies with the anatomical sites. For the high grade tumor the neck should be treated electively.

The nonresected lesions are treated like squamous cell carcinomas of similar size and location. Actually there seems to be no difference in radiosensitivity.

BIBLIOGRAPHY

1. Ackerman, L. V.: Verrucous carcinoma of the oral cavity, Surgery, 23, 670, 1948.
2. Ackerman, L. V., and del Regato, J. A.: Cancer: Diagnosis, Treatment and Prognosis, 3rd Edition, St. Louis, C. V. Mosby Company, 1962.
3. Ballantyne, A. J., and Fletcher, G. H.: Management of residual or recurrent carcinoma of the oropharynx, Amer. J. Roentgen., 93, 29, 1965.
4. Cade, S.: Malignant Disease and its Treatment by Radium, II, 2nd Edition, Bristol J. Wright & Sons, Ltd., 1949.
5. Castro, J. R., Lindberg, R. D., and Fletcher, G. H.: Clinical application of computer dosimetry in interstitial radium therapy, Amer. J. Roentgen., 105, 165, 1969.
6. Chu, A. M., and Fletcher, G. H.: Incidence and causes of failure to control by irradiation the primary lesions in squamous cell carcinomas of the anterior two thirds of the tongue and floor of mouth, Amer. J. Roentgen., 117, 502, 1973.
7. Crews, Q. E., and Fletcher, G. H.: Comparative evaluation of the sequential use of radiation and surgery in primary tumors of the oral cavity, oropharynx, larynx, and hypopharynx, Amer. J. Roentgen., 111, 73, 1971.
8. Ennuyer, A. and Bataini, J.: Les Tumeurs de l'Amygdale et de la Region Velopalatine, Paris, Masson et Cie., 1956.
9. Fletcher, G. H., MacComb, W. H., and Shalek, R. J.: Radiation Therapy of the Oral Cavity and Oropharynx, Springfield, Charles C Thomas, 1962.
10. Fletcher, G. H., and Stovall, M.: A study of the explicit distribution of radiation in interstitial implantations. I. Correlation with clinical results in squamous cell carcinomas of the anterior two-thirds of the tongue and floor of mouth, Radiology, 78, 766, 1962.
11. Fletcher, G. H., and Lindberg, R. D.: Squamous cell carcinomas of the tonsillar area and palatine arch, Amer. J. Roentgen., 96, 574, 1966.
12. Gelinas, M., and Fletcher, G. H.: Incidence and causes of local failures after irradiation in squamous cell carcinomas of the faucial arch, tonsillar fossa, and base of tongue, Radiology, publication pending.
13. Grant, B. P. and Fletcher, G. H.: Analysis of complications following megavoltage therapy for squamous cell carcinomas of the tonsillar area, Amer. J. Roentgen., 96, 28, 1966.
14. MacComb, W. S., and Fletcher, G. H.: Cancer of the Head and Neck, Baltimore Maryland, Williams and Wilkins Co, 1967.
15. Shedd, D. P., Hukill, P. B., Kligerman, M. M., and Gowen, G. F.: A clincopathologic study of oral carcinoma in situ, Amer. J. Surg., 106, 791, 1963.
16. Stovall, M., and Shalek, R. J.: A study of the explicit distribution of radiation in interstitial implantations, I. A method of calculation with an automatic digital computer, Radiology, 78, 951, 1962.
17. Suit, H. D., Lindberg, R. D., and Fletcher, G. H.: Prognostic significance of tumor regression at completion of radiation therapy, Radiology, 84, 100, 1965.

Larynx and Pyriform Sinus

Introduction

Prior to making a decision on definitive therapy for patients with cancer of the larynx, one must use all possible means to determine the site of origin, the extensions of the disease and the clinical variety of the tumor.

The anatomic structures of the larynx, with the current nomenclature, are shown in Figure 3-60A. In Figure 3-60B, the laryngeal and surrounding structures are shown on the lateral soft tissue film. Although the pyriform sinus is a part of the hypopharynx, it is included in this section because tumors originating at this site present problems of management similar to those originating on the margin of the vestibulum. With the exception of an occasional sarcoma, all laryngeal tumors are squamous cell carcinomas.

The choice of therapy may be surgical resection, radiation therapy, or the sequential use of both methods, depending upon the clinical situation. To decide if radiation therapy is preferable to surgical resection, the radiation therapy must be able to eradicate the disease in a high percentage of the patients and preserve a good voice. A recurrence following radiation therapy is best managed by surgical resection. A recurrence after a surgical resection usually is not amenable to further surgical resection.

Exophytic tumors, even bulky ones, on the vocal cords, on the supraglottic structures, and high on the walls of the pyriform sinus can be controlled with a high frequency of success by radiation therapy. At the third or fourth week of treatment, all visible tumor usually has disappeared. The laryngeal structures return to normal appearance at the end of the radiation therapy. Follow-up examinations can detect early reactivation of the disease, provided no complicating edema has developed.

When there is deeply infiltrating tumor in the subglottic area, cartilage, the pre-epiglottic fossa, or into the thickness of the laryngopharyngeal walls tumor cells are in poorly vascularized myxomatous connective tissue and are, therefore, in a state of almost complete anoxia. The cells' radioresistance is considerable. Furthermore, at the end of radiation therapy, laryngeal structures and motility never return to normal; hence the follow-up examination is difficult since one cannot tell if one is dealing with residual distortion or with active disease.

X-Ray Diagnosis

Palpation of the neck and/or direct and indirect laryngoscopy cannot supply the necessary information on many of the extensions and clinical varieties of the disease. Since 1922, the lateral soft tissue film of the neck[6] and since the 1930's, frontal tomograms of the larynx[17] have been an integral part of a complete laryngeal examination to determine the site of origin and extensions of the tumor. Infiltration of the pre-epiglottic space or cartilage destruction are essentially roentgenographic findings. Infiltrating subglottic extension may be overlooked on direct and indirect laryngoscopy, but is well visualized on the x-ray film.[16] The extent of subglottic extension along the trachea can also be determined by x-ray films.

More recently, the laryngogram,[8,19,20,23] a film showing a coating of the laryngeal structures by radiopaque media, has added a dynamic element to the examination. One can observe during fluoroscopy and record on spot films taken during various maneuvers (Valsalva, modified Valsalva, phonation, inspiration, reverse phonation) changes in position of the laryngeal structures and so determine normalcy or fixation by disease.

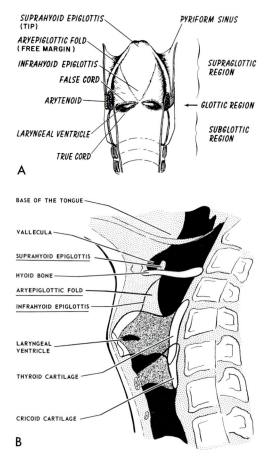

SUPRAHYOID EPIGLOTTIS (TIP)
ARYEPIGLOTTIC FOLD (FREE MARGIN)
INFRAHYOID EPIGLOTTIS
FALSE CORD
ARYTENOID
LARYNGEAL VENTRICLE
TRUE CORD
PYRIFORM SINUS
SUPRAGLOTTIC REGION
GLOTTIC REGION
SUBGLOTTIC REGION

A

BASE OF THE TONGUE
VALLECULA
SUPRAHYOID EPIGLOTTIS
HYOID BONE
ARYEPIGLOTTIC FOLD
INFRAHYOID EPIGLOTTIS
LARYNGEAL VENTRICLE
THYROID CARTILAGE
CRICOID CARTILAGE

B

FIG. 3-60. **A.** Drawing of the larynx, opened posteriorly. The nomenclature now commonly employed is as follows: glottic region (vocal cords), subglottic region (undersurface of the cord and the angle with the trachea), and supraglottic region (vestibulum).

The supraglottic region is composed essentially of the false cords, epiglottis, and the aryepiglottic folds. The ventricle is not a true structure; it is a cavity which opens only when pressure is expanding it. The roof is the false cord; the floor is the true cord. The lateral wall of the ventricle, the false cord, and the aryepiglottic fold comprise the laryngopharyngeal wall, which divides the vestibulum from the hypopharynx and the pyriform sinus. **B.** Line drawing of the lateral soft tissue film of the neck. The hyoid bone projects at the level of the valleculae, which separate the lingual epiglottis (suprahyoid epiglottis) from the laryngeal epiglottis (infrahyoid epiglottis).

Impaired motility of the laryngeal structures in bulky noninfiltrative tumors is at times erroneously observed by laryngoscopy. In such cases, motility is shown on the spot films taken during phonation and inspiration.

With very extensive tumors, a differential diagnosis between a site of origin on the vocal cords, the supraglottic region, or in the pyriform sinus cannot be made by clinical examination. The lateral soft tissue film, tomograms, and laryngogram usually help determine the site of origin. Extensive vocal cord tumors rarely spread superiorly into the laryngopharyngeal wall without there being associated subglottic disease. By contrast, extensive tumors of the supraglottic region rarely extend to the vocal cords and even less often spread to the subglottic area. This criterion, well established by Baclesse,[1,2] is reliable in most cases. The exception occurs with the rare tumor of the foot of the epiglottis which may involve the subglottic space at the anterior commissure.

The importance of diagnosing subglottic disease before definitive treatment cannot be overemphasized. If a laryngectomy is necessary, the surgeon is considerably aided by preoperative demonstration of the extent of the disease so that he may include in the resection the necessary number of tracheal rings. If there is a medical contraindication to laryngectomy, the radiotherapist must adjust the lower margin of the treatment fields to include an adequate length of trachea. Pretreatment diagnosis will also alert the pathologist to study carefully the lower aspect of the surgical specimen to determine if there is an adequate margin between the lesion and the plane of resection.

A lack of symmetry of the subglottic angle on the tomograms does not necessarily imply subglottic disease. A slight rotation of the

The pre-epiglottic space consists of a fat pad, connective tissue, and the upper loop of the "figure 8" portion of the thyroid cartilage. (Courtesy: Klein and Fletcher, *Amer. J. Roentgen.*, 92, 43, 1964.)

patient while making the tomograms, angulation of the beam, or small anatomic variations may be responsible for the lack of symmetry. If there is complete or partial preservation of cord motility, significant subglottic disease is not apt to be present. Extensive subglottic disease is almost invariably associated with upward spread into the laryngopharyngeal wall.

Asymmetry of subglottic angles, caused by minimal subglottic invasion, may be indistinguishable from distortion produced by a bulky tumor limited to the cord. The laryngogram, which allows evaluation of cord motility on inspiration and phonation views and of cord pliability on reverse phonation view,[19] demonstrates unequivocally the presence or absence of significant infiltrating subglottic disease.

Vocal Cord Tumors

Delineation of Extensions

The sparse lymphatic supply is limited to the anterior commissure and the vocal processes. Furthermore, tumors are, with exception, well differentiated. These two facts explain the low incidence of metastatic nodes even in advanced tumors.

Squamous cell carcinoma arises most often on the membranous portion, less often at the anterior commissure, and rarely on the cartilagenous portion of the cord. The tumor may arise on the upper surface, the free margin, or the undersurface (Fig. 3-61). Bulky exophytic tumors limit cord motility by their size; they may fill the laryngeal ventricle, or project into the subglottic space. The more invasive tumors cause cord fixation by extension into the adjacent structures (Fig. 3-61). They may extend laterally into the attachment of the cord, distally into the subglottic region, and superiorly into the false cords. The tumor may spread from the anterior commissure to the opposite cord, to the thyroid cartilage, or to the anterior subglottic space.

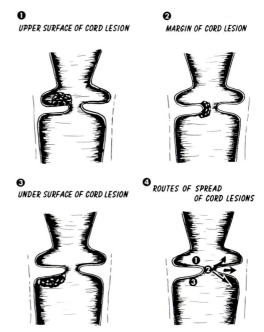

FIG. 3-61. Selective location of growth of early vocal cord tumors in drawings 1, 2, and 3. The arrows in drawing 4 indicate the lines of infiltration of vocal cord lesions. (Courtesy: Klein and Fletcher, *Amer. J. Roentgen.*, 92, 43, 1964.)

Delineation of tumors of the vocal cords requires evaluation of all adjacent structures. Superior extension into the false cord can be excluded when the ventricle is outlined by contrast material on the laryngogram (Fig. 3-62). Anterior commissure extension is well determined on the laryngograms by the irregularity of the mucosal surface and an increased distance between the anterior opaque outline and the thyroid cartilage on the lateral inspiration laryngogram (Fig. 3-63). Positive diagnosis of involvement should be made only on the inspiration view, since during the other maneuvers the commissure may bulge because of cord tension.

The squamous cell carcinomas, as well as the lesions with borderline histology, are most often lesions of the anterior third or middle third of the cords (Fig. 3-64). Rarely are they on the posterior third reaching the vocal process at the interarytenoid region

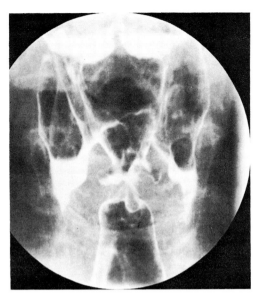

FIG. 3-62. Mirror examination and direct laryngoscopy showed a tumor occupying the entire
left cord and ventricle with limitation of
motility.
Laryngogram shows a bulky tumor of
the left cord with outlining of the ventricle
by dionysil.
Histology: Squamous cell carcinoma.
In 42 days, 6,500 rads were given; the
last 1,000 rads through a reduced portal in
July 1962. The patient had no evidence of
disease in July 1971 and had a good voice.

(Fig. 3-65). They may develop on the free
margin upper surface or the under surface
of the cord.

The laryngogram has shown that our classical concept of subglottic disease has to be
revised. There are tumors which arise in the
subglottic space and which essentially are
tracheal tumors. However, there also are
tumors which arise on the undersurface of
the cord which must be differentiated from
the deep infiltrative extensions into the subglottic structures. The laryngogram has
shown that exophytic disease will grow more
often on the undersurface at the immediate
subglottic space than on the upper surface.
These lesions are lesions with disease outside
of the cord without the serious prognosis of
infiltrative subglottic extension. In 400 vocal

cord lesions, there was no instance of exophytic anterior commissure disease growing
on the foot of the epiglottis.

STAGING

A useful staging of vocal cord cancer is as
follows:

T_1: Superficial lesions involving one or
both cords with normal motility.

T_2: Bulky lesion extending outside the
cord or cords with partial motility.

T_3: Extension to subglottic and/or supraglottic levels with complete fixation of
cord or cords.

T_4: Invasion of cartilage and/or massive
subglottic extension.

TREATMENT FOR T_1 AND T_2 LESIONS

When on the laryngogram an exophytic
subglottic lesion is seen close to the lower
aspect of the thyroid cartilage (Fig. 3-66), the

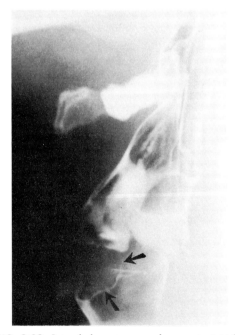

FIG. 3-63. Lateral laryngogram shows an anterior
subglottic mass. Its lower part reaches the
level of the thyrocricoid groove.

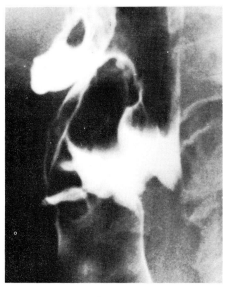
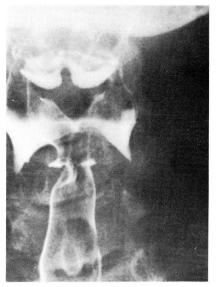

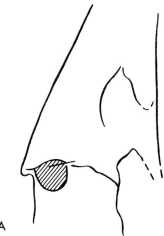
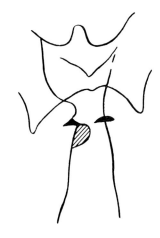

A

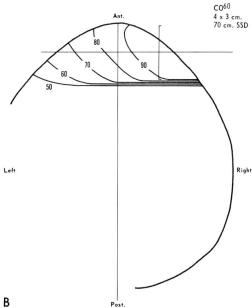

CO⁶⁰
4 x 3 cm.
70 cm. SSD

B

FIG. 3-64. **A.** The sagittal laryngograms shows a small polypoid lesion on the anterior third of the cord. On the frontal laryngogram, the lesion reaches close to the lower border of the thyroid cartilage. In 37 days, 6,000 rads were given through one homolateral field. The patient is *NED* with perfect voice in July 1971. **B.** Volume distribution; 85 per cent of the given dose was chosen for tumor dose calculation.

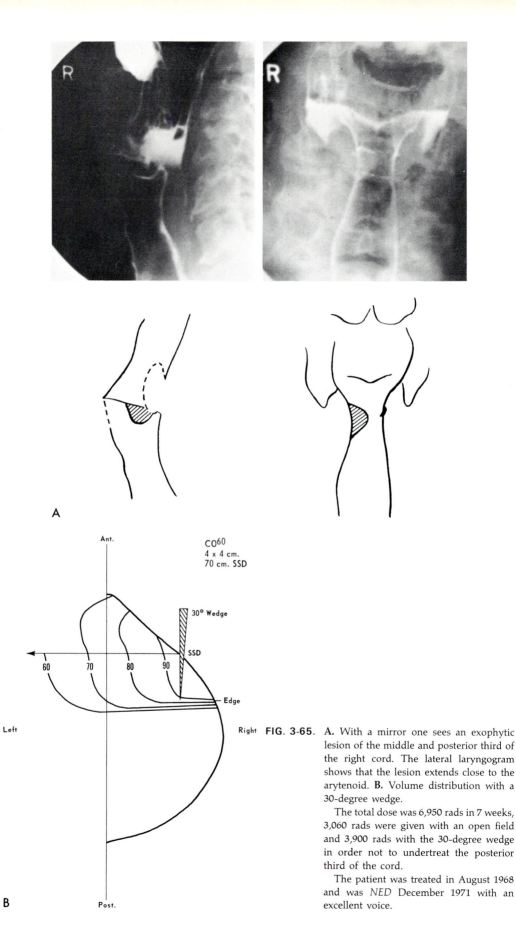

A

B

Ant.

Co^{60}
4 x 4 cm.
70 cm. SSD

30° Wedge

SSD

60   70   80   90

Edge

Left   Right

Post.

FIG. 3-65. A. With a mirror one sees an exophytic lesion of the middle and posterior third of the right cord. The lateral laryngogram shows that the lesion extends close to the arytenoid. **B.** Volume distribution with a 30-degree wedge.

The total dose was 6,950 rads in 7 weeks, 3,060 rads were given with an open field and 3,900 rads with the 30-degree wedge in order not to undertreat the posterior third of the cord.

The patient was treated in August 1968 and was *NED* December 1971 with an excellent voice.

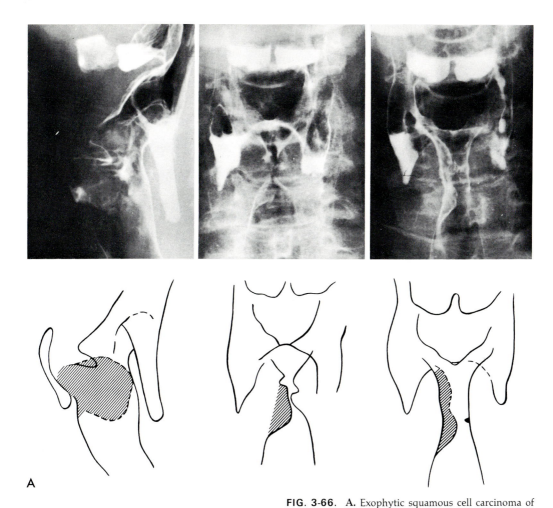

A

FIG. 3-66. **A.** Exophytic squamous cell carcinoma of the right vocal cord extending the entire length. **B.** Volume distribution with parallel opposing portals. Wedges are not used because subglottic disease is more extensive anteriorly so that the 5 to 10 per cent higher dose anteriorly is desirable.

Because of a protrusion of the tumor into the glottic space, in spite of preserved motility, the subglottic space could not be seen. The lateral laryngogram as well as the frontal one shows that the lesion has an important subglottic extension demonstrating the importance of laryngograms to demonstrate exophytic subglottic disease. The lesion extends below the level of the lower aspect of the thyroid cartilage. Motility is preserved.

The patient was treated by 2 parallel opposing portals because of the anterior subglottic disease. No wedge was used to give a higher dose anteriorly where there is more disease.

The TD at midcord was 6,700 rads in 49 days.

The patient was treated in July 1968, and was *NED* in October 1971.

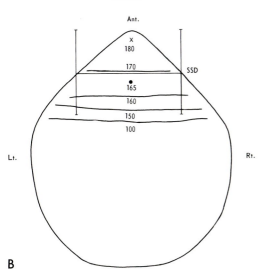

CO-60 5 x 4.5 cm
70 cm SSD

Ant.

x
180
170   SSD
165
160
150
100

Lt.   Rt.

B

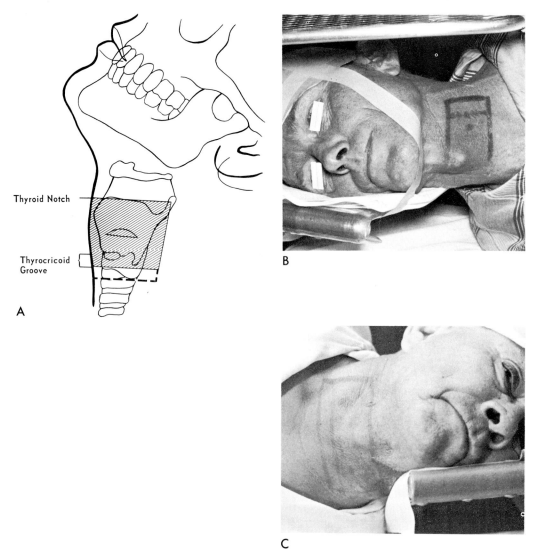

Thyroid Notch

Thyrocricoid
Groove

A

B

C

FIG. 3-67. **A.** The upper margin of the portal is at the thyroid notch. The lower margin includes only the thyrocricoid groove if there is no evidence of anterior commissure involvement and no evidence of exophytic subglottic disease. If there is radiographic or clinical evidence of anterior commissure involvement of subglottic disease, the cricoid at least is included and, at times a length of trachea. The posterior margin is marked by palpating the horn of the thyroid cartilage. The arytenoids are partially behind but need not be in full beam unless there is interarytenoid disease. Anteriorly, there is fall-off on the skin. The SSD is taken at mid-distance between the posterior and the anterior aspect of the portal. **B.** Patient is in treatment position for vocal cord cancer. A head holder is used to maintain the head and neck in a horizontal position. Masking tape is used to ensure immobilization.

The length of the portal is measured from the upper to the lower margin and the width on the projection onto the horizontal plane. The average portal size is 20 to 25 sq cm.

If the lesion does not involve the posterior third of the cord, the posterior margin is moved 1 to 1.5 cm forward to minimize irradiation of the arytenoids after a tumor dose of 5,000 rads has been given.

C. Parallel opposing portals are used for anterior commissure involvement. The lower margin includes the cricoid. The other line with arrow shows the lower margin going through the cricoid if there is no subglottic disease. (Courtesy: Fletcher and Klein: *Radiology, 82*, 1032, 1964.)

entire cricoid is included in the treatment field (Fig. 3-67). This lower coverage does not include vital structures such as the arytenoids and does not seem to be fraught with complications.

The head and neck are fixed on the head rest in the lateral position. Portals are determined superiorly by the thyroid notch, posteriorly by the horn of the thyroid cartilage, inferiorly by the cricoid, and anteriorly by "fall-off" on the skin. In lesions involving the anterior commissure or for exophytic subglottic disease, the cricoid is generously included in the beam (Fig. 3-67).

The geometry with a ^{60}Cobalt unit consists of one single homolateral portal for lesions involving one cord (Fig. 3-64), or perhaps reaching, but not grossly involving, the anterior commissure. For lesions involving both cords, or the anterior commissure (Fig. 3-66), parallel opposing portals are used; if there is disease on the posterior third of the cord(s) (Fig. 3-65) the first half of treatment may be given with open fields and the second half with wedge filter. For the rare tumors of the posterior third of the cord, a single homolateral field with a wedge filter is used for part or for the whole treatment in order to increase the dose posteriorly. Figure 3-68 shows various volume distributions. If a node is present, a larger field is used on that side with 2:1 loading (Fig. 3-69). When the node has received 5,000 rads, if a radical neck dissection is planned, the portals are adjusted to cover the lesion on the cord(s) to the desired dose.

The tumor dose increases with the volume of the tumor (Clinical Parameters, Ch. 2):

6,000 rads for the superficial lesions
6,500 rads for the small exophytic lesions
7,000 rads for the bulky lesions

If the lesion is unilateral, the tumor dose is delivered through a homolateral portal. The treatment time is $5\frac{1}{2}$ weeks for 6,000 rads; 6 weeks for 6,500 rads; and $6\frac{1}{2}$ weeks for 7,000 rads.

If the lesion reaches the other side of the anterior commissure, if there is anterior sub-

glottic disease or bilateral disease two parallel opposing portals are used. The treatment time is slightly longer because the volume brought to maximum dose is larger, 6 weeks for 6,000 rads; $6\frac{1}{2}$ weeks for 6,500 rads; and 7 weeks for 7,000 rads.

At 5,000 or 5,500 rads tumor dose the posterior margin is moved forward, unless posterior disease is present and from 6,000 rads to 6,500 rads or to 7,000 rads, fields are further reduced on the anterior larynx.

Usually by the third or fourth week all disease has disappeared, even in the bulky lesions, because exophytic tumors regress rapidly. A laryngectomy is considered if there is poor regression because it signifies deeply infiltrating disease in the laryngopharyngeal wall.

Fibrinous epithelitis is seen during treatment in only a small percentage of cases, and usually only when the portal size is 35 sq cm or more. When fibrinous epithelitis appears, it usually is on the mucosa of the pyriform sinuses, the false cords, and the interarytenoid region. A fibrinous exudate on the vocal cords has been seen in the occasional patient. Edema of the arytenoids during treatment has been almost unknown.

RESULTS

With some variation between centers, the local recurrence rate for T_1 or T_2 vocal cord tumors is 10 to 15 per cent when the tumor dose is around 6,000 roentgens given in about six weeks.[5,7,18,21,22]

In Table 3-30 is tabulated the incidence of recurrences by stages. In contradistinction to the squamous cell carcinomas of the other sites of the upper respiratory and digestive tract, only 68.5 per cent of the recurrences appear within two years. Because of the dysplasia of the epithelium, some of the lesions are new cancers. A dose-response curve has not been elicited.[15]

Clinical factors which might be common denominations in recurrences have not been elicited from our material. Although com-

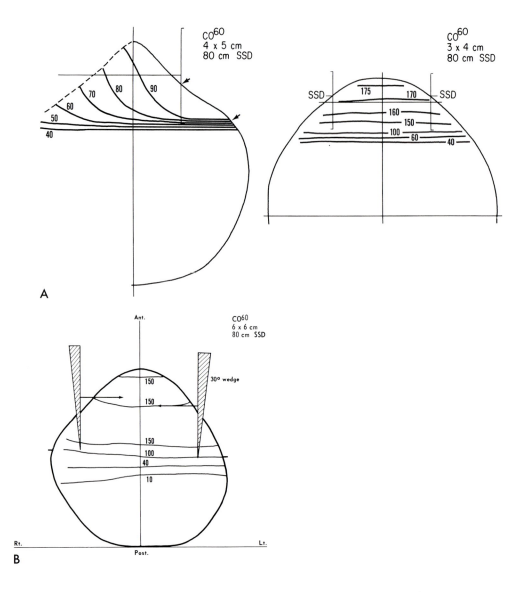

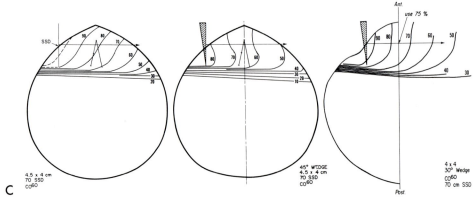

mon, leukoplakic changes in addition to invasive squamous carcinoma have not been a universal factor. In some patients, disease recurred subglottically or on the opposite cord suggesting the possibility that new disease had developed in the tracheal mucosa below the treatment field. The involvement of the anterior commissure does not affect control rate.

The ultimate failure rate is almost zero for T_1 lesions and still low for T_2 lesions. Approximately 16 per cent of the recurrences were salvaged by cordectomy or partial laryngectomy.[3]

Complications are sensitive to small variations in dosage.[15] Most laryngeal edemas and necroses appeared within a year; half of them within 6 months, usually in patients whose treatment utilized large portals. More than half of the cases of laryngeal edemas stabilized after antibiotics and voice rest, but the voice never returned to a satisfactory level. In about one-third of the patients, either permanent tracheostomy or laryngectomy had to be performed.

Treatment of T_3 and T_4 Carcinomas

When there are contraindications to laryngectomy, usually medical, radiation therapy is used. Portals are determined by the extensions of the tumor upward and subglottically.

The tumor dose is 1,000 rads per week. After the delivery of 6,000 rads in 6 weeks, 1,000 or even 1,500 rads are given in 1 week to 10 days through reduced portals. Because no operative procedure can be contemplated, the therapist will accept a higher risk of complications in order to achieve control.

The laryngeal structures rarely return to normal, making evaluation of control difficult at follow-up examinations.

BORDERLINE HISTOLOGY LESIONS

As the epithelium of the vocal cord is a stratified squamous epithelium, the carcinomas are well differentiated with all the phases from leukoplakia, atypical hyperplasia, *in situ* carcinoma.[9,23] In the verrucal cancers, it is difficult to obtain a biopsy spec-

---

FIG. 3-68. Volume distributions for vocal cord cancers. **A.** Single homolateral portal. On the left, volume distribution in a patient with a thin neck and on the right a rounded neck. The 85 or 90 per cent curve is chosen depending upon the location of the tumor on the cord. **B.** Parallel opposing portals are used when the anterior commissure or both cords are involved. In the particular cases shown, there is little difference in dose from the anterior commissure to the posterior aspect of the cord. Wedge filters are never used with parallel opposing portals because as a rule there is more anterior disease which is best treated with a higher dose. When wedge filters are used, the first part of the treatment is given with open portals and the second part with wedge filters; if wedge filters were used for the entire treatment, there would be an underdose anteriorly. **C.** Comparison of open 45-degree and 30-degree wedge volume distribution. A 45-degree wedge produces an unnecessarily high dose to the arytenoids. A 30-degree wedge is usually used for half the treatments.

Example of Calculations:

Aim 6,500 rads in 6 weeks
No Wedge—4,350 rads GD
With Wedge—4,350 rads GD

	Open	Wedge	Total
Anterior Commissure	88%—3820	61%—2650	6470
Mid-cord	85%—3690	64%—2780	6470
Posterior cord	82%—3560	67%—2910	6470

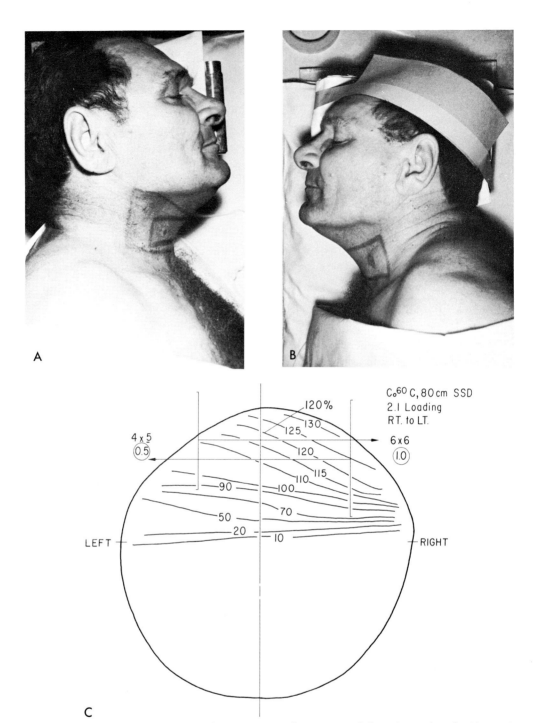

A

B

C₀⁶⁰ C, 80 cm SSD
2.1 Loading
RT. to LT.

4 x 5
(0.5)

6 x 6
(1.0)

120%
130
125
120
115
110
100
90
70
50
20
10

LEFT

RIGHT

C

FIG. 3-69. The patient was seen 2-3-70 with a squamous cell carcinoma of the right vocal cord with anterior commissure involvement. There was a palpable node in the right subdigastric area. The plan was to treat with parallel opposing portals, the right field to include node **(A)** and then a 2:1 loading in favor of the right side; when the treatment had reached 5,000 rads given dose to the right subdigastric area this was considered sufficient as a growth restraint dose to the node. At the same time, the tumor dose to the cord was 6,000 rads. From there on the field used on the right side was as on the left **(B).** Final dose to the primary tumor on the cord was 7,000 rads in 7 weeks. At completion of therapy, the tumor had disappeared at the primary site and the node on the right neck was no longer palpable. The volume distribution over the primary is shown in **(C)**; 120 per cent was taken as the tumor dose. The subdigastric node was no longer palpable on 7-10-70. The initially planned radical neck dissection was not carried out. The patient 9 months later developed recurrences in the larynx, trachea, and in the suprasternal area.

Table 3-30. *Vocal Cord—Failures by Stage and Extensions—Borderline Histology and Invasive Squamous Cell Carcinoma (415 Patients) 1948–1967, (Analysis June 1971)*

Staging	Histology	No. Pts.	Failures	Control of Failures by Surgery	Percentage Ultimate Failures
T_1					
	Borderline Histology	42	4 (9.5%)	4 (100%)	0%
No visible lesion	Invasive S.C.C.	27	3 (11.0%)	3 (100%)	0%
Post cord stripping	Invasive S.C.C.	7	1	0	
Visible—one cord	Invasive S.C.C.	148	20 (13.5%)	17/19* (89.5%)	2%
Bulky lesion	Invasive S.C.C.	21	2 (9.5%)	2 (100%)	0%
Anterior commissure involved	Invasive S.C.C.	36	3 (8.5%)	3 (100%)	0%
T_2					
Partial mobility, extension beyond cord(s) or anterior	Borderline Histology	4	1	1	0%
commissure involvement outside cord(s)	Invasive S.C.C.	109	22 (20.0%)	14/19† (73.5%)	7.5%
Combination of above features	Borderline Histology	3	0	—	0%
	Invasive S.C.C.	18	11 (61.0%)	7/10§ (70.0%)	22%

*One patient refused treatment
†Three patients refused treatment
§One patient refused treatment; one patient died postradical neck dissection (15 months after laryngectomy)—NED at autopsy.
Cumulative recurrence rate: 68.5% at 2 years; 85% at 3 yrs.
(Courtesy: Horiot, Fletcher, Ballantyne, and Lindberg; *Radiology,* 103, 663, 1972.)

imen showing frank invasion. Some lesions are bulky, extending outside the cord(s).

The diagnosis of these borderline histologies vary if several biopsies are taken or with the interpretations of several pathologists (Table 3-31). In some lesions initially diagnosed *in situ* or leukoplakia, further biopsies show invasive squamous carcinoma as demonstrated in the case of Fig. 3-70.

Stripping of the cords can at times secure material for a definitive diagnosis, often at the expense of a good voice because too much of the cord(s) has been removed by the procedure. In instances where bulky lesions are in the anterior subglottic space or laterally subglottic only a borderline diagnosis can be made despite repeated biopsies (Fig. 3-71). A practical course of action must be taken. Repeated biopsies through the years are psychologically and physically traumatic to the patient.

The lesions with a borderline diagnosis are treated, like the invasive carcinomas, according to their volume with the same treatment schedule as described under squamous cell carcinomas.

As shown in Table 3-30 the percentage of malignant recurrences is the same (10 per cent) as in the T_1 invasive squamous cell carcinomas. Of 42 patients, there are only 2 who had a recurrence of the leukoplakia; in the other patients the vocal cords are smooth and glossy (F + D). The first patient so treated is now 19 years posttreatment and has absolutely smooth cords.

Postoperative Radiation Therapy

In extensive vocal cord tumors, there are two areas where surgical clearance may be inadequate: 1) the anterior aspect of the neck when there is cartilage invasion, and 2) the

Table 3-31. *"Borderline Histology" Lesions of the Vocal Cords—Forty-Seven Biopsies (42 patients)*

Leukoplakia	1
Carcinoma *in situ*	12
Carcinoma *in situ* with foci of superficial invasion	5
Marked atypism but not definitely squamous cell carcinoma	3
Difference in successive biopsies (*in situ* ↔ atypical hyperplasia ↔ squamous cell carcinoma)	8
Different interpretations between pathologists (*in situ* ↔ leukoplakia ↔ squamous cell carcinoma)	18

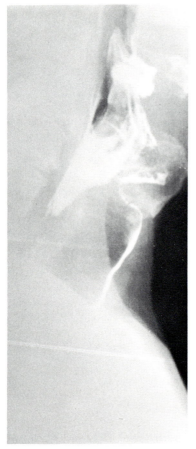

FIG. 3-70. Prior to coming to M. D. Anderson Hospital the patient had had repeated biopsies including stripping of the left cord. The slides the patient brought with him were reviewed

tracheal stoma when there is subglottic extension. Of 54 patients with confirmed tomographic evidence of subglottic disease prior to operation and not having had postoperative irradiation, 13 (24 per cent) have had a stomal recurrence after laryngectomy.[16] All died from uncontrolled disease within a year of the operation.

In these two situations, elective postoperative radiation is indicated. The technique is similar to the one used in the postoperative radiation of supraglottic tumors except that the stoma is not shielded to prevent recurrence at this site.

In the instance of massive disease with perforation through the thyroid cartilage, the dose anteriorly may be up to 7,000 rads in 7 weeks.

Radiation Therapy for Recurrences after Laryngectomy

The most common site of recurrence is around the stoma. This area of recurrent

as squamous cell carcinoma, superficial, Grade II, the tumor being predominately carcinoma *in situ*. Small foci were interpreted as presence of superficial invasion. The left cord on 11-28-67 was edematous. Laryngogram showed very marked enlargement subglottically. The patient was told that there was no rush and that after the edema had subsided the irradiation results would be functionally better. A direct laryngoscopy and, if necessary, a diagnostic laryngofissure would be performed to establish an unequivocal diagnosis.

On direct laryngoscopy, the anterior third of the left cord was enlarged but without ulceration. Both cords were normally mobile. With questionable involvement of the anterior commissure, a biopsy was taken from the main mass on the left cord proximal to the anterior commissure. This was read at frozen section as showing invasive carcinoma and was confirmed on the permanent section. There also were both superficial and invasive carcinoma.

The patient received 7,000 rads in 7 weeks through a homolateral portal including the cricoid. The patient is *NED* with a good voice in November of 1971.

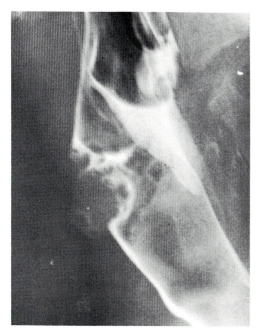

FIG. 3-71. Patient seen in July, 1968 with granular lesions on both cords. The laryngogram shows a bulky, exophytic subglottic mass below the anterior commissure extending to the inferior border of the thyroid cartilage. Biopsies taken from 3 areas at the level of the anterior commissure and the right and the left cord show *in situ* carcinoma with leukoplakia on the right cord.

The treatment consisted of 7,000 rads in 7 weeks through 2 parallel opposing portals including the cricoid and the first tracheal ring to cover adequately the inferior extent of the visible tumor on the laryngogram.

The patient is *NED* in January 1972.

disease is best irradiated with a single appositional portal which includes the lower neck, the stomas, and the upper mediastinum. A plastic tracheostomy tube is inserted during the treatment as build-up material since the disease is often superficial in the upper part of the trachea.

Supraglottic Region

Tumors of the supraglottic region (the epiglottis, false cords, and aryepiglottic folds) have specific patterns of spread which re-

quire adaptation of both surgical and radiotherapeutic management.

Delineation of Extensions

The visibility of the larynx may be impaired by the exophytic component of the tumor or by distortion of laryngeal structures because of infiltration and the frequently associated edema. Hence, extension of disease to the surrounding structures often is not detectable on direct and indirect laryngoscopy.

The epiglottis is a single continuous structure. However, the tumors originating on the free margin above the level of the hyoid, and the epiglottis below the hyoid have different patterns of spread and response to treatment.

Early tumors of the suprahyoid epiglottis can either be exophytic or invade the underlying cartilage. The erosion often seems serrated, as if cut with pinking scissors. More advanced tumors invade the pharyngoepiglottic folds, the pharyngeal walls (Fig. 3-72), the valleculae and the base of the tongue anteriorly, or may extend lower into the upper aspect of the pre-epiglottic fossa (Fig. 3-73).

Since a bulky tumor may preclude direct laryngoscopy, the lateral soft tissue film is invaluable for determining involvement of the infrahyoid epiglottis. Extension into the base of the tongue can, at times, be seen as a deep ulceration; extension into the pre-epiglottic fossa may be seen as an ulceration or a thickening of that part. The laryngogram may provide the most accurate information about the integrity of the lower mucosal surface.

Exophytic tumors of the infrahyoid epiglottis can spread superficially on the false cords and aryepiglottic folds. The exophytic type of lesion is identified on the lateral soft tissue film as a protruding tumor; on the laryngogram, there is normal motility of the epiglottis and adjacent structures of the vestibulum. Occasionally, during phonation, the normal prominence of the lower epiglottis

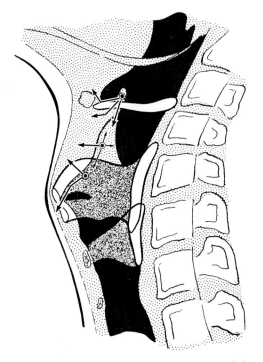

FIG. 3-72. Routes of tumor spread of lesions of the epiglottis. The upper group of arrows shows extensions of the tumors of the suprahyoid epiglottis into the base of the tongue, the upper aspect of the pre-epiglottic fossa, and along the infrahyoid epiglottis. They extend laterally to the pharyngoepiglottic folds and pharyngeal walls. The lower group of arrows on the infrahyoid epiglottis indicates invasion of the pre-epiglottic fossa, and, if low, destruction of the cartilage anteriorly, frequently resulting in a separation of the "figure 8." (Courtesy: Klein and Fletcher, *Amer. J. Roentgen.*, 92, 43, 1964.)

may be mistaken for an exophytic tumor. If fairly extensive, invasion of the pre-epiglottic space can be recognized on the lateral film. Presence of motility of the epiglottis and hyoid bone, shown on the laryngogram, helps to rule out this anterior invasion.

More extensive, primarily ulcerative tumors invade the epiglottic cartilage or its membranous attachment, then penetrate the fat pad and loose connective tissue between the epiglottis and the strap muscles (Fig. 3-72). From there, they may extend to the

anterior aspect of the thyroid cartilage. Depending upon the level of the invasion (Fig. 3-72), widening of the pre-epiglottic tissue may be seen at the level of the fat pad or closer to the "8-shaped" calcification of the thyroid cartilage.

Tumors which invade primarily downward may involve the thyroid cartilage. This can be demonstrated by disappearance of the upper half of the "figure 8" or, as is often seen, the two loops of the "figure 8" separate, the upper half being displaced upward. The tumors generally do not extend below the laryngeal ventricles. Occasionally a tumor, particularly one at the foot of the epiglottis may extend through the anterior commissure into the subglottic region. Radiological diagnosis of pre-epiglottic fossa invasion has a high correlation with the operative findings.[16]

The false cords form the roof of the ventricles, blending anteriorly with the laryngeal surface of the epiglottis and superiorly with the aryepiglottic folds. The pattern of spread is to the aryepiglottic fold and the lateral wall of the ventricle forming the laryngopharyngeal wall between the vestibulum of the larynx and the pyriform sinus (Fig. 3-73).

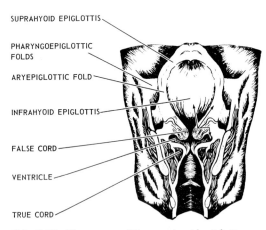

SUPRAHYOID EPIGLOTTIS

PHARYNGOEPIGLOTTIC FOLDS

ARYEPIGLOTTIC FOLD

INFRAHYOID EPIGLOTTIS

FALSE CORD

VENTRICLE

TRUE CORD

FIG. 3-73. The tumors of the suprahyoid epiglottis can early invade laterally the pharyngoepiglottic folds. Those of the false cords can extend medially and anteriorly to the epiglottis, upward into the aryepiglottic folds, or downward through the wall of the ventricle to the true cords, or into the pyriform sinus.

Tomograms demonstrate the thickened false cord and enlargement of the adjacent structures when they are invaded by tumor or are edematous. Unless the tumor is extensive or associated with ulceration, spread to the epiglottis is not evident on the lateral film. Since the laryngogram allows differentiation of the tumor from edema, an accurate estimate of the extent of tumor is possible. If there is extension into the aryepiglottic fold it appears distorted and thickened.

Tumors can arise on the free margin of the aryepiglottic folds or at the junction of the aryepiglottic folds, epiglottis, and pharyngoepiglottic folds. These tumors form a transition between those arising from the vestibulum and those arising from the pyriform sinus or other hypopharyngeal sites. Determining the site of origin of extensive lesions in this area may be difficult.

Exophytic growths arising on the free margin may project into either the vestibulum or pyriform sinus. Radiographic studies are necessary to evaluate the status of surrounding structures.

Invasive growths are usually extensive before clinically detected. They involve the laryngeal surface of the epiglottis and the upper pyriform sinus by anterior spread and large areas of the lower pyriform sinus and external arytenoid surface of the larynx by posterior spread.

An exophytic tumor may be recognized on the tomograms and lateral soft tissue films. The laryngogram, demonstrating motility of the tumor and intact adjacent structures, confirms these findings. An air-filled pyriform sinus on the tomogram helps identify the aryepiglottic fold origin of the tumor.[8]

Tumors originating on the arytenoids are rare; of 287 supraglottic tumors reviewed, only 4 were found. Little is known of their manner of spread.

Staging of Supraglottic Tumors

A useful staging of supraglottic and laryngopharyngeal tumors is as follows:

T_1: Exophytic lesion limited to the anatomical site of origin without invasion of underlying structures or loss of motility.

T_2: Exophytic lesion extending slightly to surrounding anatomical sites with questionable invasion of underlying structures and/or slight impairment of motility.

T_3: Lesions with invasion of underlying structures (cartilage, pre-epiglottic fossa, depth of laryngopharyngeal walls) with considerable loss of motility or complete fixation.

T_4: Massive disease.

The staging of neck nodes is the same as for other sites in the head and neck.

Policy of Treatment

Radiation therapy has been employed in patients with:

1. Small lesions with no palpable nodes in the neck.

2. It is the treatment of choice for advanced cancers originating on the suprahyoid epiglottis.

3. It is used for moderate-sized lesions, if the mobility of the larynx is normal, whereas a surgical procedure is used if the tumor is infiltrative and the larynx is fixed.

In some T_2 lesions where there is question of deep invasion, one can start with radiation therapy and by the fourth week of treatment be reasonably assured of the exophytic nature of the disease because in this instance all tumor should have disappeared and normal motility returned. If at 4 weeks there is evidence of deeper infiltration or persistent partial impairment of motility, it is often preferable to consider this treatment as preoperative and carry on with a laryngectomy.

In those patients with a small primary cancer with nodal metastases, permanent control of the primary cancer is sought by radiation therapy while neck disease is managed by a moderate dose of irradiation followed by radical neck dissection (Fig. 3-74). Patients with large cancers or with extensive metastasis to the nodes in the neck are treated surgically or by both surgical procedures and postoperative irradiation. A few patients with massive disease were treated palliatively by radiation therapy.

Postoperative irradiation therapy has been used for a variety of clinical situations: 1) a massive primary cancer and/or extensive nodal metastasis, 2) an incomplete surgical excision indicated by pathological study of the resected specimen, 3) proved cancer cells close to the margin of surgical resection, 4) cancer cells in connective tissue adjacent to positive lymph nodes, and 5) carcinoma *in situ* in the pharyngeal mucosa adjacent to the original cancer.

The surgical procedure employed for the primary cancer is total laryngectomy. A wide-field procedure removing the adjacent jugular lymph nodes has been performed in the last 6 years of the study. Radical neck dissection, unilateral or bilateral as indicated, is performed on the patients with clinically positive lymph nodes. A modified neck dissection is done occasionally on the least involved side if both sides of the neck are dissected.

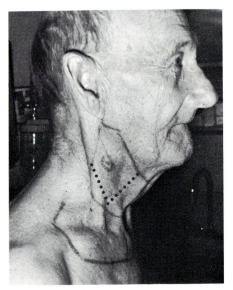

FIG. 3-74. This 75-year-old patient was seen in February 1970 with a T_2 lesion of the suprahyoid epiglottis with a 3 cm node in the upper midjugular area of the right neck.

A tumor dose of 7,000 rads through parallel opposed ^{60}Co fields to the epiglottis was delivered in 7 weeks and 5,000 rads given dose to the lower neck in 5 weeks with an anterior split Cobalt field. At 5,000 rads, the fields were reduced to cover only the suprahyoid epiglottis (dotted lines). Six weeks later a right radical neck dissection was done. Examination of the tissue removed showed squamous cell carcinoma and foreign body reaction in the connective tissue of the subdigastric area. His postoperative course was completely uneventful and on the sixth postoperative day he was discharged from the hospital to have his sutures removed at home.

The patient is *NED* in April 1971.

Treatment Technique

The portal size necessary to cover these lesions varies with the anatomical site of origin. The size is always larger than those covering vocal cord lesions. Surface landmarks cannot, as a rule, be as sharply defined as for vocal cords, so that immediate surrounding structures must be included to avoid a geographical miss. Two parallel opposing portals are usually used for satisfactory distribution (Fig. 3-75) sometimes with 2:1 loading for asymmetrical tumor.

Even early exophytic supraglottic tumors have a tendency to metastasize. In some patients, nodes are palpable and must be included in the treatment field, at least to restrain growth, until a radical neck dissection can be performed 5 to 6 weeks after the completion of treatment. The portal is larger on the node side with 2:1 loading. When the node has received 5,000 rads, the portals are trimmed to cover the primary to achieve a tumor dose of 7,000 rads in 7 weeks.

For the N_0 patients, the subdigastric and midjugular nodes are irradiated to 5,000 rads because of the probability of infestation of the lymph nodes in that area (Fig. 3-76). After 5,000 rads, the treatment fields cover

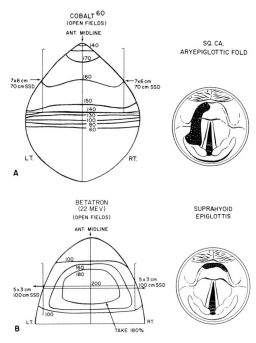

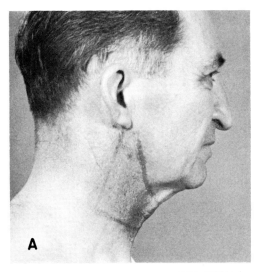

FIG. 3-75. Volume distributions for supraglottic lesions. **A.** For tumors of the infrahyoid epiglottis, the false cords, or aryepiglottic folds, the portals are larger than for vocal cord tumors. As a rule, 2 parallel opposing portals are used unless the lesion is strictly unilateral. The difference between the maximum (anterior) and minimum (posterior) tumor dose is somewhat more than for the vocal cords. However, wedge filters are not usually used. When a minimum tumor dose of 5,000 rads has been given, the fields are drastically reduced over the site of origin. **B.** For tumors of the suprahyoid epiglottis, the 22 Mev beam may be used if there are no palpable nodes. (Courtesy: Fletcher and Klein: *Radiology*, 82, 1032, 1964.)

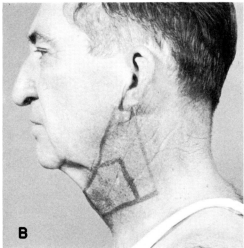

FIG. 3-76. **A.** Right lateral portal in patient with a left aryepiglottic fold tumor. Although no nodes were palpable both subdigastric areas were included. **B.** Left lateral portal. The last 1,500 rads of a total dose of 6,500 rads in 6 weeks to the primary were given through a reduced portal.

The patient died in 1972 from another primary cancer, *NED* from the larynx cancer. (Courtesy: Fletcher and Klein, *Radiology, 82,* 1032, 1964.)

only the involved anatomic structures as economically as possible because of the risk of severe laryngeal edema resulting from large volume irradiated to high doses. Risk of a geographical miss is avoided by weekly verification films (Fig. 3-77 and 3-78). For very small tumors, one may choose to use minimum coverage fields from the beginning.

An analysis of the correlation of tumor dose versus controls and complications showed that there is a dose response curve for T_2 and T_3 lesions,[21] with an optimal tumor dose of 7,000 rads in 7 weeks. After

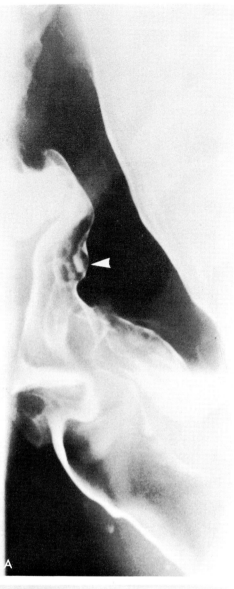

FIG. 3-77. **A.** The laryngogram shows an exophytic tumor on the free margin of the aryepiglottic fold (arrow). **B.** A portal film shows coverage limited to the structure involved. **C.** A *TD* of 6,500 rads was given in 6½ weeks through one single left lateral portal. Minimal edema of the left arytenoid developed during treatment. The patient was treated in June 1965 and is *NED* with a good voice in 1971.

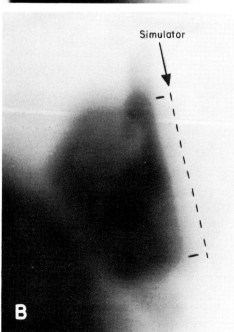

Simulator

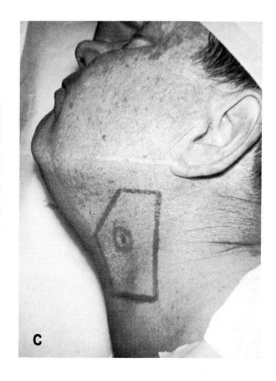

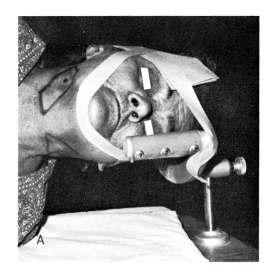

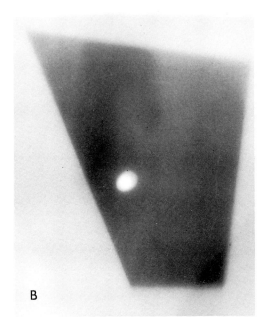

FIG. 3-78. **A.** Patient in treatment position for a tiny tumor located on the free margin of the epiglottis. The epiglottis is covered by a narrow portal, sparing the arytenoids. Six thousand five hundred rads were given in 42 days with the 22 Mev photon beam in 1962. Patient was *NED* in 1970, aged 75 and in poor medical condition. **B.** The verification film shows the top of the epiglottis and the laryngeal epiglottis well within the field. A verification film was taken weekly. (Courtesy: Fletcher and Klein, *Radiology, 82,* 1032, 1964.)

5,000 rads given in 5 weeks, the field sizes may be reduced and further reduced after 6,000 rads. The volume receiving the maximum dose is less in the 7 weeks treatment, diminishing the likelihood of complications.

In all cases, a fibrinous exudate develops in the treated area, and the weekly dose rate may be slowed because of excessive discomfort or edema of the arytenoids. Then, either the daily dose is reduced or, occasionally, the treatment stopped for a few days. When large fields are used, 850 rads per week is advisable. The total dose is then 7,500 to 8,000 rads with gradual field shrinking, if feasible, when 5,500 rads have been given.

If nodes are palpable and the treatment of the primary lesion is by irradiation, the nodes are irradiated to 5,000 or 5,500 rads, then the fields are reduced to cover only the primary. A neck dissection is performed 6 to 8 weeks after. The extent of neck irradiated varies with the initial degree of neck disease and site of origin, e.g. with a false cord and only one subdigastric node only the subdigastric areas are irradiated; with a primary on the suprahyoid epiglottis or aryepiglottic fold, the whole neck is irradiated because of the likelihood of diffuse bilateral spread.

Bilaterally opposing shaped fields are used, for the primary in the larynx and the upper neck. Unequal loading (3:2, 2:1) may be used. The lower neck is treated with a given dose of 5,000 rads in 5 weeks through a single anterior field with a narrow midline shield over the trachea.

Postoperative Irradiation

For postoperative irradiation a midline dose of 6,000 rads is given to the upper neck through 2 parallel opposing portals (the amount of disease left behind beyond the margins of resection being uncertain), and 5,000 rads given dose are delivered to the lower neck with shielding of the stoma. The stoma can be shielded because, in tumors of the supraglottic structures disease extends below the vocal cords only rarely. The para-pharyngeal lymphatics are not included in the field. In recent years there is a tendency not to perform bilateral neck dissection (Fig. 3-79) but modified dissections (Fig. 3-80). The squelae and discomfort are less for the patient. The irradiation technique is much facilitated.

RADIATION TREATMENT FOR T_3 AND T_4 TUMORS OF THE SUPRAGLOTTIC AREA WITH NECK DISEASE

These patients with such tumors usually are unsuitable for surgical excision because of extent of primary and/or neck disease, a few because of refusal of laryngectomy, or associated medical conditions. As a rule, clinically positive nodes are present and the fields have to be large, often including the entire neck bilaterally. High doses must be given to large volumes of tissue with a resulting risk of massive edemas and necroses.

The tumors of the suprahyoid epiglottis are an exception because tumors at that site, even when cartilage is destroyed, respond well to radiation, provided the base of the tongue or the pre-epiglottic fossa are not too deeply invaded. After successful irradiation,

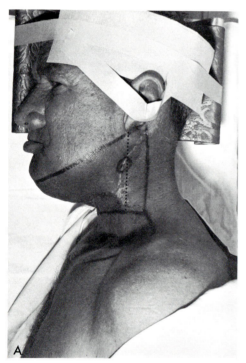
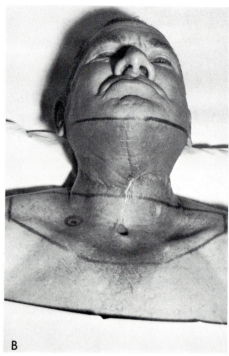

FIG. 3-79. Patient seen on 5-1-68 with a marble-size mass in the left submaxillary region. On the laryngeal surface of the epiglottis a raised ulcerated lesion was seen extending to the left false and true cords. In the right midjugular chain, there was a node 3 cm in diameter and in the left one a 4 to 5 cm node. Biopsy: Grade IV squamous cell carcinoma.

On 5-7-68 a laryngectomy and a bilateral neck dissection was done. There were positive nodes in both sides of the neck. Irradiation was delayed for 2 months because of slow wound healing. A midline dose of 6,000 rads was given to the upper neck; after 4,500 rads, the posterior margin of the parallel opposing portals was moved forward to exclude the spinal cord **(A)**. Additional therapy with the 9 Mev electron beam was used to supplement the dose to 6,000 rads. The lower neck received 5,000 rads given dose in 5 weeks with an anterior portal, the stoma being shielded **(B)**.

Without the availability of an electron beam, adequate irradiation of the surgical area, which extended to the mastoid, would not have been possible. (Courtesy: Fletcher, Lindberg and Jesse, In *Surgical Oncology*, Hans Huber Publishers, Bern, Switzerland, p. 347, 1970.)

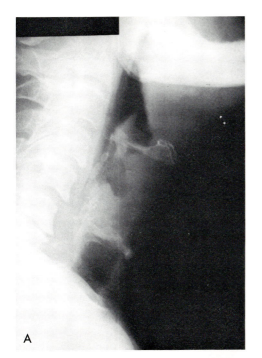

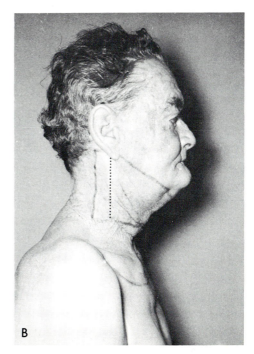

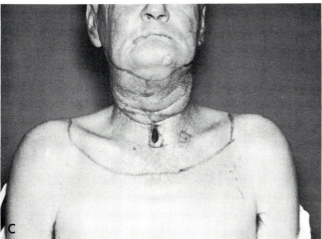

FIG. 3-80. Patient seen in June 1970 with an ulcerated lesion of the infrahyoid epiglottis. Clinical examination and lateral soft tissue film showed involvement of the pre-epiglottic space and of the valleculum. A 1.3 cm node was palpable in the left subdigastric area and two 3.0 cm subdigastric nodes were present in the right subdigastric area. Biopsy: Squamous cell carcinoma.

The plan of treatment was total wide-field laryngectomy with bilateral modified radical neck dissection and postoperative irradiation therapy.

A wide-field laryngectomy (including larynx, strap muscles, and a generous portion of the base of the tongue) was done 11-12-70. The sternocleidomastoid muscle was not removed on either side. Of 13 nodes recovered from the right modified neck dissection, 3 were positive by microscopic examination. On the left side, one node was attached to the jugular vein which was resected. Of 17 nodes removed, 2 were positive. Pathological diagnosis was squamous carcinoma, Grade II, involving the epiglottis with perforation of the epiglottic cartilage to the pre-epiglottic space, with extension to the right and left aryepiglottic folds, right and left false cords, and right and left arytenoid regions (margins of surgical excision free of tumor). The wound was closed primarily and the patient was ready for postoperative irradiation 12 days after the surgical procedure.

A. Lateral soft tissue film showing an extensive tumor of the infrahyoid epiglottis. **B.** Lateral portal covering upper neck. A midline dose of 6,000 rads was given in 6 weeks to the upper neck. The posterior margins of the parallel opposing portals were moved forward at 4,500 rads without need of a supplement because the scar was limited. **C.** Anterior portal over lower neck. A given dose of 5,000 rads in 5 weeks were delivered to the lower neck with an anterior portal, shielding the stoma of the tracheostomy. The patient died in September 1971 from distant metastases. *NED* in the neck.

the epiglottis is partially or completely self-amputated, allowing good visibility at follow-up examinations.

A basic tumor dose of 5,000 rads is attempted in 5 to 5½ weeks but, if reactions are severe, it may take 6 weeks to deliver 5,000 rads. The lower neck is irradiated with an anterior split field giving at least 5,000 rads. Through reduced portals, 2,000 rads are added in 2 weeks covering the primary site and palpable nodes. When there is invasion of the pre-epiglottic fossa, no less than 7,500 to 8,000 rads must be given in 7 to 7½ weeks.

Palliative Radiation Therapy of Advanced Tumors of the Supraglottic Area

When extensive local disease or extensive bilateral disease precludes any surgical procedure, the whole neck including the larynx and pharynx is treated. Palliation is not achieved by small doses and the treatment is radical; 6,000 rads are given, 850 rads per week. Depending upon the status of the primary disease and neck disease, additional treatment may be given through reduced portals to the primary and neck nodes. If distant metastases are present, at least 6,000 rads still must be given. Sometimes additional doses are needed to restrain growth.

Occasionally, palliative irradiation given for inoperable disease may produce permanent control. This is another reason to use radical treatment in such patients.

Results

More than 90 per cent of recurrences at the primary site are seen within 24 months of treatment (whether surgical or irradiation). Therefore, two-year *NED* rates are reliable for the purpose of comparing the various modalities. Table 3-32 tabulates *NED* rates at 2 years for *T* staging and modalities of treatment.

The treatment of choice, either surgical excision, irradiation, or a combination of both, is not the same for the various anatomical sites; therefore, there is no general statement to be made concerning the supraglottic region, except that exophytic lesions anywhere on those structures respond well to radiation therapy.

The combined treatment, which in our experience has primarily involved postoperative irradiation, is most useful for those lesions originating in sites in which it is difficult to secure a surgical margin, *i.e.*, primarily the suprahyoid epiglottic and the aryepiglottic areas, *i.e.*, the structures forming the margin of the vestibulum directly attached to the pharynx making uncertain a surgical margin in addition to more neck disease. There seems to be a notable superiority of the combined treatment for the T_3 and T_4 lesions of these two structures (Table 3-33).

Of the 115 patients treated with radiation alone, there were 37 (25 per cent) in whom permanent control of the primary lesion was not achieved. Twenty-three failures were noted in 84 patients with T_1 through T_3 lesions. Seventeen of the 23 patients later had a surgical resection which was successful in 14 instances. This emphasizes the basic principle that irradiation can be attempted if the lesion is not extensive and is on a site that can be examined readily. By this policy, maximum preservation of laryngeal function is achieved.

Fourteen per cent of the patients treated by planned combined radiation and surgical therapy had recurrence of their cancer along the pharyngeal walls. Since the patients selected for this type of treatment often had advanced disease, this percentage of recurrent disease is low. Of the patients who had a recurrence, only one was salvaged by a subsequent surgical procedure.

The fact that patients with surgical recurrences along the pharyngeal walls often are not salvaged by any form of treatment is another reason to use routinely postoperative

Table 3-32. *Supraglottic Larynx (1948–1965) NED* at Two Years*

Suprahyoid Epiglottis

Stage	Surgical Excision	Radiation	Combination Surgical Excision and Radiation
T_1	—	5/5	—
T_2	1/1	5/8	—
T_3	1/3	3/7	2/3
T_4	0/3	9/14	3/3

Infrahyoid Epiglottis

T_1	—	3/6	2/2
T_2	8/11	4/8	3/4
T_3	9/16	2/6	2/4
T_4	8/17	2/9†	8/10

Aryepiglottic Folds

T_1§	—	4/7	—
T_2	4/4	11/14	—
T_3	0/8	4/6	3/6
T_4	2/6	3/6	2/2

False Cords

T_1	—	1/1	—
T_2	5/9	8/10	5/5
T_3	15/18	1/1	1/6
T_4	1/5	1/2	1/1

Arytenoids

T_1	1/1	2/2	—
T_2	—	2/2	0/1
T_3	1/1	0/1	2/2
T_4	—	—	—

*NED at the follow-up examination immediately after the cut-off time. For instance, a patient with disease at 18 months treated, NED at 24 months, and disease again at 30 months is scored as NED at two years.

† Six N_3

§Includes the two *in situ* lesions.

(Courtesy: Fletcher, Jesse, Lindberg and Koons, *Amer. J. Roentgen.*, 108, 19, 1970.)

radiation for those lesions with indefinite surgical margin.[8]

The more diffuse and multiple the initial neck disease, the more likely there is to be recurrent disease in the radically dissected neck. When only a unilateral radical neck dissection is performed for extensive neck metastasis, disease is likely to appear in the other neck, mostly in the lesions of the suprahyoid epiglottis and the aryepiglottic folds.

The advantages of postoperative radio-therapy are seen clearly in the patients with N_2 and N_3 metastases (Table 3-33). Post-operative radiotherapy prevents appearance of recurrences in the radically dissected neck and appearance of new disease in the opposite neck.

Distant Metastases

Distant metastases were the cause of death in 20 per cent of the patients, most of whom were in the T_3 and T_4 groups. Four-fifths of

Table 3-33. *Patients with Advanced Tumors of the Epiglottis and Aryepiglottic Folds or N_2–N_3 Neck Disease—February 1948– December 1965, NED at 2 Years*

	Surgery Alone	Surgery + Postop. Irrad.
T_3-T_4 Suprahyoid Epiglottis and Aryepiglottic folds	3/20 (15.0%)	10/14 (71.5%)
T_4 Infrahyoid Epiglottis	8/17 (47.0%)	8/10 (80.0%)
N_2-N_3	13/34 (38.0%)	15/21 (71.0%)

Courtesy: Fletcher and Jesse: *Current Problems in Radiology,* Chicago, Year Book Medical Publishers, 1, 4, 1971.

the distant metastases appeared before the end of the second year. There were, however, instances in which they did not appear until after the fifth year. The lung was the most common site of metastases, followed by bone, gastrointestinal tract, and central nervous system, respectively.

Complications of Irradiation

Complications of irradiation increase with the increased size of the primary tumor.[23] The treatment portals always include the arytenoids; thus, moderate transient edema during or after radiation is common. There is a correlation between complications and dose-time and volume (Clinical Parameters, Chapter 2).[23] Severe edema or necrosis which caused seriously impaired function occurred in 12 of 115 irradiated patients. One total laryngectomy and one permanent tracheostomy were required in these patients. Several factors seem to be related to the severe edema. Patients in whom persistent edema developed almost always continued smoking cigarettes.

Voice rest and antibiotics may subdue the infection, edema may recede, and the laryngeal structures return to a semi-normal condition. A permanent tracheostomy may be needed if the edema produces an inadequate airway. If ulceration persists, a laryngectomy may be required for relief of pain.

Preservation of Laryngeal Function

Of the group of 70 patients alive and free of disease at 2 years, 50 have normal voices. Of the remaining 20 patients, 15 had a total laryngectomy because of recurrent cancer, one had a laryngectomy because of necrosis; in one patient a tracheostomy was performed because of inadequate airway caused by edema; in three others, the voice was impaired by severe laryngeal edema.

Radiation Therapy for Postsurgical Recurrences

Recurrences can appear anywhere. Treatment should include the whole neck. If the recurrence is in the middle of the neck, the entire neck is irradiated as in the postoperative radiation treatment. After 6,000 rads have been given, an additional 1,000 or 1,500 rads may be given through small portals covering the area of gross recurrence.

Follow-up after Radiation Therapy

Early recognition of reactivation of the disease is possible only if the laryngeal structures return to normal after radiation therapy. If there is residual fixation or considerable distortion of the laryngeal structures, follow-up is very difficult. The most difficult follow-up is for tumors of the laryngeal surface of the epiglottis.

The laryngogram which demonstrates irregularity of the mucous membrane helps differentiate between edema and recurrence. Usually motility is not impaired if there is edema. Fixation of the laryngeal structures during the various maneuvers indicates active disease.

When massive edema occurs after radiation therapy, follow-up is difficult. Ulcerations caused by necrosis should be biopsied; a report of inflammatory tissue may be misleading since there may be active disease underneath. A laryngectomy should be performed instead of watching the patient for too long.

PYRIFORM SINUS AND HYPOPHARYNX

Tumors arising in the pyriform sinus often defy identification by ordinary clinical means. Indeed, nothing may be seen but a swollen, bluish arytenoid. In such instances, tomograms and laryngograms may prove invaluable. Lesions of the pyriform sinus may arise (Fig. 3-81).

I. At the bottom of the pyriform sinus
  1 and may extend to:
  A. The false cord and aryepiglottic fold and the arytenoid.
  B. Posterior aspect of the ventricle at the attachment of the true cord.
  C. The subglottic area.
II. In the lateral wall of the pyriform sinus
  2 , which is the lateral wall of the pharynx.
III. On the medial wall of the pyriform sinus 3 , which is the lateral aspect of the aryepiglottic fold.

Exophytic tumors originating high on the walls of the pyriform sinus may be classified for curative radiotherapy. Similarly tumors of the posterior wall of the hypopharynx and retrocricoid tumor can be localized and be exophytic. However, the lower aspect of the lesions is never ascertained with certainty.

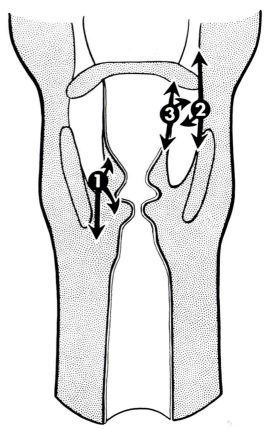

FIG. 3-81. Exophytic tumors originating high on the walls of the pyriform sinus may be selected for curative radiotherapy. Most tumors originate low in the pyriform sinus, invade medially the laryngopharyngeal wall, extend anterolaterally through the thyroid cartilage or thyrohyoid membrane into the neck and laterally fix the lateral pharyngeal wall.

An early tumor without palpable nodes is treated locally because, if large fields were used to include the node areas, arytenoid edema would be more common. In some lateral tumors, provided the neck is thin, electron beam therapy with 15 Mev alone or in combination with 60 Cobalt is the treatment of choice. The tumor dose is 6,500 rads in 6½ weeks or 7,000 rads in 7 weeks with reduction of the field size after 5,500 rads.

Early lesions are often associated with nodes. In that situation, as demonstrated in

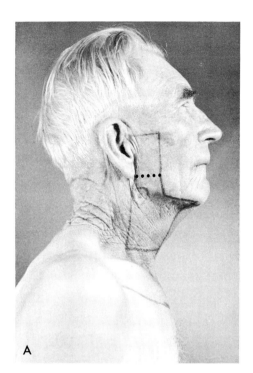

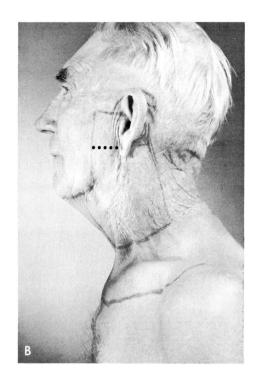

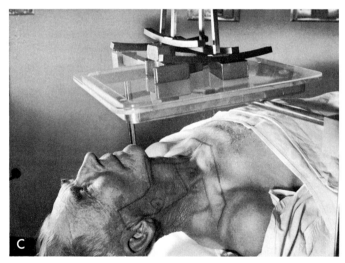

FIG. 3-82. Male, age 67, seen in October 1967 with a squamous cell carcinoma of the left pyriform sinus with a large left node. The lesion was relatively small on the medial wall. The plan was to treat the primary lesion by irradiation and the neck by radical neck dissection with 5,000 rads to the whole neck from both sides.

The first 5,000 rads in 5 weeks were given to the upper neck including the parapharyngeal lymphatics. The lower neck was given 5,000 rads given dose. Then using electron beam, 12 Mev, 1,500 rads were given through a reduced field to cover only the primary; 6,500 rads were given in 6½ weeks. Four weeks later a left radical neck dissection was done with foci of identifiable residual degenerating squamous carcinoma cells.

The patient was *NED* in January 1972.

Figure 3-82, the side of the neck with a large node is treated to include the posterior aspect of the neck whereas the other side the portal excludes the spinal cord. The parapharyngeal lymphatics are irradiated with parallel opposing portals and the lower neck with a straight anterior portal to 5,000 rads given dose. When a minimal tumor dose of 5,000 rads has been given to that comprehensive area, the fields are reduced over the primary lesion to deliver a tumor dose of 6,500 rads in 6½ weeks or 7,000 rads in 7 weeks depending upon the size of the primary lesion. A radical neck dissection is performed 6 to 8 weeks later. More advanced primary lesions with aggressive neck disease are treated with irradiation (Fig. 3-83).

The lesions of the posterior wall of the hypopharynx are treated in a similar way to include a generous portion of the cervical esophagus (Fig. 3-84), as the extent in the direction of esophagus cannot be determined with accuracy. After 5,000 rads, 2,000 rads are given through stepwise reduced fields over the area of gross disease with generous margins as tumors of the pharyngeal walls extend at great distance from palpable or visible disease.

POSTOPERATIVE IRRADIATION

In distinction to the supraglottic laryngeal structures, the parapharyngeal lymphatics (Fig. 3-85) are included in postoperative radiotherapy to a dose of 5,000 rads, the upper neck is treated (the amount of disease left behind beyond the margin of resection being uncertain) with parallel opposing por-

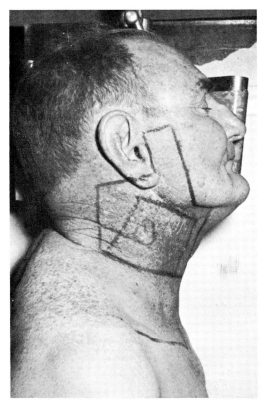

FIG. 3-83. This 68 year old patient seen with a squamous cell carcinoma of the right pyriform sinus and a large right subdigastric area. During work-up preliminary to surgical resection, the node enlarged becoming al-

most fixed. A small node appeared on the left side.

When radiation therapy was started on 5-25-70, it was a Stage T_3N_3B. The patient received an estimated 7,510 rads tumor dose in 6½ weeks to primary when calculated to a depth of 3 cm and 6,950 rads tumor dose in 6½ weeks to right subdigastric node when calculated at a depth of 1 cm. The delivery rate to the primary and upper neck was 850 rads per week. Because of the fast growth of the node, 1,500 rads BED were given twice a week during the first 3 weeks to the right node with the 12 Mev using a field-in-a-field plan. 5,000 rads given dose were delivered in 5 weeks to both lower necks. An additional 1,000 rads given dose boost was given to the left midjugular node in 4 treatments through a single left anterior field.

At the completion of treatment there was total regression of primary pyriform sinus lesion. The right subdigastric node was still palpable and measured approximately 2 × 2 cm and was mobile. The left midjugular node could no longer be palpated towards completion of therapy. The patient is without evidence of disease above the clavicles in October 1971, with possible metastasis to the left hip.

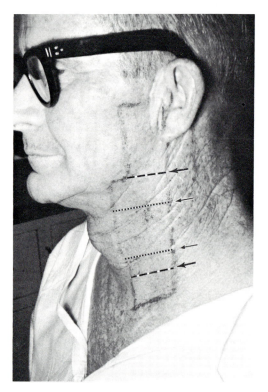

FIG. 3-84. Patient, age 54, with an exophytic tumor arising on the posterior hypopharyngeal wall extending to the left pyriform sinus. Biopsy showed squamous cell carcinoma; the biopsy from the anterior aspect of the left pyriform sinus showed *in situ* carcinoma.

From 8-22-69 to 10-13-69 using an 18 Mev photon beam, 5,000 rads were administered in 5 weeks, 5 days a week through parallel opposed portals from the base of the skull to close to the sternum. The extension to the base of the skull was to treat the parapharyngeal lymphatics and the lower extension was generous not to miss nondetectable extension into the cervical esophagus. At 5,000 rads, portals were diminished (outside dotted lines) to include segment of the pharynx and esophagus above and below the initially observed lesion; from 6,000 to 7,000 rads the portals were further reduced (inside dotted lines).

During treatment, moderate edema of the arytenoid developed. Only a patchy mucositis was seen at the level of the hypopharynx; the patient did not lose any weight.

Gross tumor had disappeared at 4,000 rads. The patient is *NED* in September, 1971.

tals to 6,000 rads given dose shielding the stoma. A given dose of 5,500 rads may be given on the side of a radical neck dissection.

Results

Because of the small number of patients with early disease treated by irradiation, statistics are meaningless. One can only say that approximately three fourths of these early lesions are permanently controlled. The evaluation of postoperative irradiation in the over-all survival rates is difficult to assess because of a marked tendency to develop distant metastases and intercurrent disease. The value of postoperative irradiation is better assessed by the freedom of disease above the clavicle.

Until 1960, most patients with lesions of the pyriform sinus were treated by laryngectomy and partial pharyngectomy with unilateral or bilateral neck dissection, the pharynx being closed primarily. Of 56 patients so treated from 1954 through 1961, 21 had postoperative irradiation (Table 3-34). The incidence of pharyngeal recurrence, in the radically dissected neck, or new disease in the opposite neck was 57 per cent in the 35 patients who had no postoperative irradiation, while the rate was 28.5 per cent in those having postoperative irradiation. The 5-year survival rates were 23 and 24 per cent for surgery alone and surgery plus irradiation respectively.[3]

From 1960 on, extended surgical procedures were done, including circumferential pharyngectomy, ipsilateral radical neck dissection and parapharyngeal lymphatic dissection. From 1962 to 1965, 57 patients were treated by surgery alone and 9 patients had surgery and postoperative irradiation. The incidence of recurrences or new disease above the clavicles was 49 per cent in the 57 patients having surgery only; none of the 9 patients having postoperative irradiation had recurrent disease above the clavicle.[4] The 5-year survival rate of the patients having had the extended radical surgical

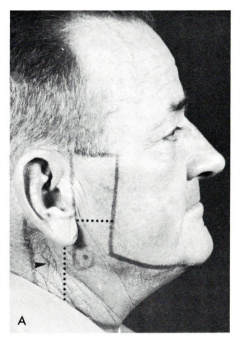 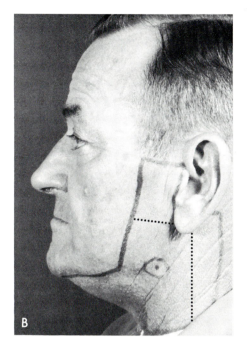

FIG. 3-85. Male, age 52, seen on 7-18-66 with a lesion of the posterior pharyngeal wall extending from the level of the posterior tonsillar pillar to below the arytenoid. There is a 4 cm node freely moveable at the low midjugular position on the right. It was staged T_3N_2 pharyngeal wall lesion.

On 7-20-66 a pharyngectomy and right radical neck dissection were done. There was squamous cell carcinoma in the excised tissue from bifurcation of right carotid artery and fibrous connective tissue adjacent to nerve.

From 9-29-66 to 11-9-66, 6,000 rads midline were given in 6 weeks to the upper neck with 5,000 rads to the lower neck with shielding of the stoma. At 4,500 rads, the posterior margin of the upper neck fields were moved forward to exclude the spinal cord. With 6 Mev electron beam, 1,000 rads were given in one week to the right posterior strip (arrow). At 5,000 rads tumor dose, the extension to irradiate the parapharyngeal lymphatics was excluded.

The patient died of distant metastases free from disease above the clavicles.

procedures was 25 per cent, no better than the survival rates for the more conservative procedures.

The diffuseness of the disease is such that resection of more of the pharynx and dissection of the parapharyngeal lymphatics does not appreciably change either the local or regional recurrence rates or the survival. The addition of postoperative irradiation clearly diminishes the incidence of surgical failures above the clavicle, but patients continue to die because of distant metastases, second primaries, and intercurrent disease. The importance of control of cancer above the clavicle is to keep patients free of the

pain, odor, and loss of function, which result from the cancer. A preferable way to die, if it is inevitable, is by distant metastases.

TREATMENT OF RECURRENCES

Recurrences may be identified as masses along the pharyngeal wall or in the radically dissected neck or it may be new disease appearing on the opposite side. In all instances, one will treat the whole neck to a tumor dose of 5,000 rads and then give an extra 2,000 rads with various modalities to the area of recurrent disease.

A common site of recurrence following

Table 3-34. *Pyriform Sinus—Analysis December 1969—January 1954–December 1961* [*]

January 1954–December 1961

	Recurrence Above Clavicle	5-Yr. Absolute Survival Rate	Compli-cation	DM	ID + SP	Unkwn
Surgery Alone 35						
	57%	23%	11.5%	17%	28.5%	
	(20)	(8)	(4)	(6)	(10)	
Surgery + Megavoltage Irradiation 21						
	28.5%	24%	5%	33%	9.5%	9.5%
	(6)	(5)	(1)	(7)	(2)	(2)

January 1962–December 1965 [*]

	Recurrence Above Clavicle	5-Yr. Absolute Survival Rate	Compli-cation	DM	ID + SP	Unkwn
Surgery Alone 57						
	49%	25%	9%	21%	17.5%	5%
	(28)	(11/44)†	(5)	(12)	(10)	(3)
Surgery + Megavoltage Irradiation 9						
	(0)	(0/5)†	(1)	(2)	(1)	(2)

[*] The distribution by T and N is the same in the four groups.
† Number of patients with 5-year follow-up.
DM—Distant Metastases
SP—Second Primary
ID—Intercurrent Disease
(Courtesy: Fletcher and Jesse, *Current Problems in Radiology*, Chicago, Year Book Medical Publishers, 1, 4, 1971.)

surgery without postoperative irradiation is a parapharyngeal node at the level or somewhat above the tonsillar fossa; the node can easily be palpated. Pain in the temporofrontal area is typical of these nodes; ear pain is also common.[20] The treatment consists of irradiating the whole neck with 5,000 rads with a dose to the node of 7,000 rads. When a parapharyngeal node appears after 2 years of the initial treatment, one may be satisfied to treat it including only a generous portion of the base of the skull to make sure that one can trace disease along the lymphatics of the vessel; there are a few patients who have been cured by this limited field irradiation.

BIBLIOGRAPHY

1. Baclesse, F.: Carcinoma of the larynx, *Brit. J. Radiol.*, Suppl. 3, 1949.
2. Baclesse, F.: Roentgentherapy in carcinoma of the larynx, *J. Fac. Radiol.*, 3, 3, 1951.
3. Ballantyne, A. J., Fletcher, G. H., Horiot, J-C, and Lindberg, R. D.: Surgical salvage of irradiation failures in squamous cell carcinoma of the vocal cords, In preparation.
4. Caderao, J. B., Fletcher, G. H., Jesse, R. H., and Lindberg, R. D.: Squamous cell carcinoma of the pyriform sinus, In preparation.
5. Cantril, S. T.: Radiation therapy in cancer of the larynx, *Amer. J. Roentgen.*, 81, 456, 1959.
6. Coutard, H.: Note preliminaire sur la radiographie du larynx normal et du larynx cancereux, *J. belge de radiol.*, 13, 287, 1922.
7. Fletcher, G. H., and Klein, R.: Dose-time-volume relationship in squamous cell carcinomas of the larynx, *Radiology*, 82, 1032, 1964.
8. Fletcher, G. H., and Jing, B. S.: In *The Head and Neck, An Atlas of Tumor Radiology*, P. Hodes, Editor, Chicago, Year Book Medical Publishers, 1968.
9. Fletcher, G. H., and Dana, M.: La Radiothèrapie des Èpitheliomas *In Situ* Lèsions, Limite, des Cordes Vocales. *Journal de Radiologie et d'Electrologie*, 51, 241, 1970.
10. Fletcher, G. H., Jesse, R. H., Lindberg, R. D., and Koons, C. R.: The place of radiotherapy in the management of the squamous cell carcinoma of the supraglottic larynx, *Amer. J. Roentgen.*, 108, 19, 1970.
11. Fletcher, G. H., Lindberg, R. D., and Jesse, R. H.: The combination of radiation and surgery in oropharynx and laryngopharynx squamous cell carcinomas, In *Surgical Oncology*, Frederic Saegesser and Jacques Pettavel, Editors, Hans Huber Publishers, Bern, Switzerland, p. 347, 1970.
12. Fletcher, G. H., and Jesse, R. H.: Interaction of surgery and irradiation in head and neck cancers, In *Current Problems in Radiology*, Robert D. Moseley, Editor, Year Book Medical Publishers, Inc., Chicago, Illinois, 1, 3, 1971.
13. Horiot, J-C, Fletcher, G. H., Ballantyne, A. J., and Lindberg, R. D.: Analysis of failures of vocal cord cancers, *Radiology*, 103, 663, 1972.
14. Klein, R., and Fletcher, G. H.: Evaluation of clinical usefulness of radiological findings in squamous cell carcinomas of the larynx, *Amer. J. Roentgen.*, 92, 43, 1964.
15. Leborgne, F.: Tomographic study of cancer of larynx, *Amer. J. Roentgen.*, 43, 493, 1940.
16. Lederman, M.: Place de la radiotherapie dans le traitement du cancer du larynx, *Ann. Radiol.*, 4, 433, 1951.
17. Lehman, Q. H.: Reverse phonation—a new maneuver for examining the larynx, *Radiology*, 84, 215, 1965.
18. Lehman, Q. H., and Fletcher, G. H.: Contribution of the laryngogram to the management of malignant laryngeal tumors, *Radiology*, 83, 486, 1964.
19. MacComb, W. S., and Fletcher, G. H.: *Cancer of the Head and Neck*, Williams and Wilkins Co., Baltimore, Maryland, 1967.
20. Nielsen, J.: Functional results and permanence of cure following roentgentherapy in intralaryngeal carcinomas, *J. Fac. Radiol.*, 3, 145, 1962.
21. Powers, W. E., McGee, H. H., and Seaman, W. B.: Contrast examination of the larynx and pharynx, *Radiology*, 68, 169, 1957.
22. Shukovsky, L. J.: Dose, time, volume relationships in squamous cell carcinoma of the supraglottic larynx, *Amer. J. Roentgen.*, 108, 27, 1970.
23. Stout, A. P.: Intramucosal epithelioma of the larynx, *Amer. J. Roentgen.*, 69, 1, 1953.

Nasopharynx

In Collaboration with
RODNEY R. MILLION

Anatomy

Nasopharynx

The nasopharynx roughly is cuboidal in shape. It is in direct continuity frontally with the nose, inferiorly with the oropharynx, and laterally with the middle ears via the eustachian tubes.

The mucosa of the roof and posterior wall is often irregular due to the pharyngeal bursa, pharyngeal tonsil (adenoids), and the pharyngeal hypophysis (Figs. 3-86 and 3-87). The mucosa tends to become smooth with age, but many folds may remain in the later years of life to add to the examiner's confusion as to whether tumor is present. Adenoids may persist well past puberty and may even be present in elderly people. Following successful irradiation these irregularities usually give way to a smooth appearance.

The lateral walls include the eustachian openings with the fossa of Rosenmuller (pharyngeal recess) located behind the torus tubarius. The superior lateral muscular wall of the nasopharynx is incomplete and provides a meager barrier to tumor spread. Once tumor has penetrated the lateral wall, it enters the lateral pharyngeal space and its contents. The floor of the nasopharynx consists of the upper surface of the soft palate, which is rarely the origin of nasopharyngeal tumors and uncommonly is invaded, even with extensive local disease.

Lymphatic Drainage

The lymphoid aggregates in the pharyngeal tonsil and the tubal tonsil are responsible for extensive submucosal lymphatic capillary plexus, attested to by the high inci-

dence of neck metastases. Tumor cells commonly spread to three different lymph node collecting stations: 1) lateral retropharyngeal node of Rouviere, 2) the jugular chain (selectively, the upper lateral jugular), and 3) spinal accessory.[10]

The lateral retropharyngeal nodes lie in the lateral pharyngeal space near the lateral border of the posterior pharyngeal wall and medial to the carotid artery (Fig. 3-88). Directly behind the nodes are the lateral masses of the atlas. According to Rouviere, there is usually one node on each side, but occasionally two and rarely three nodes are

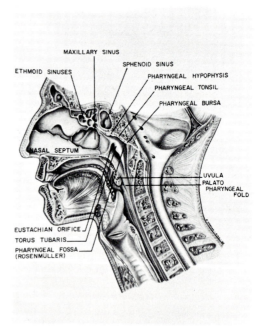

FIG. 3-86. Midsagittal section of the head showing the nasopharynx and related structures. (Courtesy: MacComb and Fletcher, *Cancer of the Head and Neck,* The Williams & Wilkins Company, Baltimore, Maryland, 1967.)

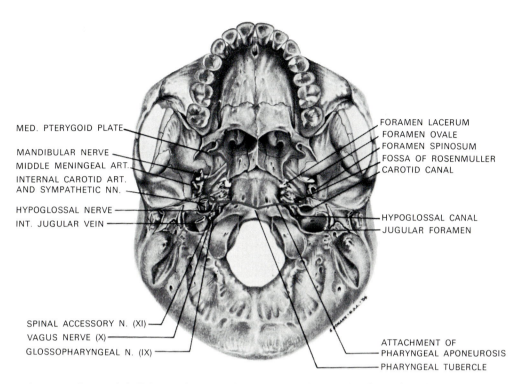

MED. PTERYGOID PLATE

MANDIBULAR NERVE
MIDDLE MENINGEAL ART.
INTERNAL CAROTID ART.
AND SYMPATHETIC NN.

HYPOGLOSSAL NERVE
INT. JUGULAR VEIN

FORAMEN LACERUM
FORAMEN OVALE
FORAMEN SPINOSUM
FOSSA OF ROSENMULLER
CAROTID CANAL

HYPOGLOSSAL CANAL
JUGULAR FORAMEN

SPINAL ACCESSORY N. (XI)
VAGUS NERVE (X)
GLOSSOPHARYNGEAL N. (IX)

ATTACHMENT OF
PHARYNGEAL APONEUROSIS
PHARYNGEAL TUBERCLE

FIG. 3-87. Basal view of skull showing bony attachments of nasopharyngeal wall. The bony foramina of the base of the skull are shown on the right and structures occupying these foramina, on the left. (Courtesy: MacComb and Fletcher, *Cancer of the Head and Neck,* The Williams & Wilkins Company, Baltimore, Maryland, 1967.)

found. These nodes atrophy with age and may be absent on one side, but rarely entirely are absent. The clinical appreciation of enlarged retropharyngeal nodes usually requires peroral palpation of the high posterolateral pharyngeal wall. Marked nodal enlargement, such as that which occurs in lymphoma, may distort the posterior tonsillar pillar, shifting it medially and anteriorly. The actual incidence of spread to these nodes is unknown, but the nodes are always included in the irradiated volume covering the primary lesion.

Lymphatic channels may bypass the retropharyngeal lymph nodes and empty directly into either the jugulodigastric or the upper lateral jugular node. Inconstant lymphatic vessels are described as draining directly to the nodes below the bifurcation of the ca-

rotid (midjugular nodes) and to the spinal accessory nodes.[10]

The so-called classic nasopharyngeal nodes refers to 3 or 4, high lateral internal jugular nodes which lie deep to the sternocleidomastoid at its insertion into the tip of the mastoid and lateral to the internal jugular vein at its exit from the jugular foramen. Carcinomas involving the soft palate and the posterior tonsillar pillar may also spread to this particular group of nodes. The high lateral jugular nodes may be a technical problem to the surgeon because they lie in juxtaposition to the base of the skull and the internal jugular vein as it exits from the jugular foramen; these nodes are not always removed in the "standard" radical neck dissection as shown by postradical neck cervical lymphangiograms.[5]

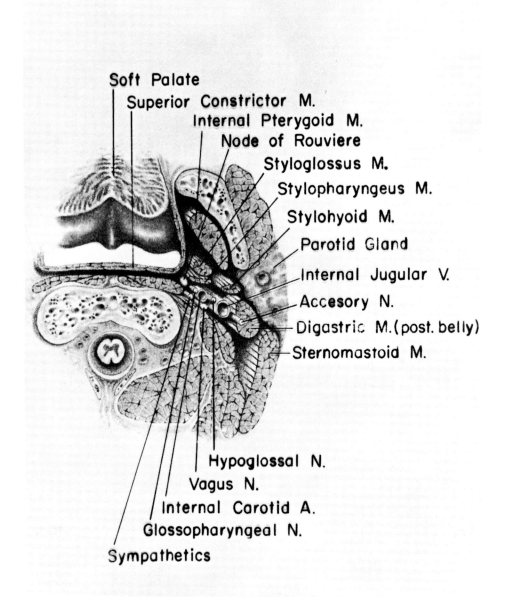

FIG. 3-88. The poststyloid portion of the lateral pharyngeal space and its contents. (Courtesy: MacComb and Fletcher, *Cancer of the Head and Neck*, The Williams & Wilkins Company, Baltimore, Maryland, 1967.)

The superior node(s) of the spinal accessory chain and the superior node(s) of the lateral internal jugular chain actually blend together, but the mid and low spinal accessory node chain then diverges inferiorly and posteriorly along the course of the spinal accessory nerve.

In the upper and mid neck the jugular vein nodes lie either lateral or anterior to the vein, but in the low neck they gradually assume a more medial position in relation to the jugular vein. In the low neck, the jugular vein and sternocleidomastoid muscle converge toward the midline so that the jugular nodes lie quite close to the lateral border of the trachea. This relationship is important in the midline blocking of the lower neck fields, as described under treatment planning.

An occasional patient may present with a clinically involved preauricular node. This route of spread is via lymphatics of the eustachian tube, some of which drain directly to the preauricular nodes.

Pathology

Most histological varieties of malignant tumors have been reported as arising from the nasopharynx and its immediate supporting structures. Tumors arising from surface epithelium comprise about 85 per cent and lymphomas about 10 per cent of the total number of malignant lesions. The remaining 5 per cent include melanoma, plasmacytoma, adenocarcinoma, carcinosarcoma, all connective tissue sarcomas, nonchromaffin paraganglionic tumors, and a few malignancies which simply defy classification.

Clinical Picture

The symptoms and signs are important to the therapist in outlining potential areas of involvement which may influence the design of his treatment.

Sore throat occurred in about 15 per cent of patients and is nearly always related to spread into the oropharyngeal wall or tonsillar bed.[6] Facial pain may be referred from any of the 3 divisions of the trigeminal nerve, usually the mandibular division. Occipital or temporal headache is frequently seen with malignant disease of the nasopharynx, but no specific pattern of spread has been uncovered to relate to the location of the headache. Pain in the scalp over the left mastoid area may be related to invasion of the high lateral internal jugular node.

Pain created by lifting the head and extending the neck is related to posterior infiltration of the prevertebral muscles and possibly the basiocciput and atlas.

Nasal obstruction requires the determination of the degree of anterior spread into the nasal cavity. Proptosis is due to posterior orbital invasion and usually displaces the eyeball straight forward, according to Ho.[11] Trismus is usually related to invasion of the pterygoid musculature and should direct adequate therapeutic coverage to this area. Obstructive ear symptoms are related to obstruction at the eustachian opening, as tumor rarely spreads very far along the eustachian tube.

Neurological symptoms and signs indicate precise areas of involvement. Involvement of cranial nerves II through VI indicates intracranial extension into the cavernous sinus and pituitary region. Cranial nerves IX through XII and the sympathetic chain usually are involved in the lateral pharyngeal space by direct invasion.

The diagnostic x-ray work-up should consist of routine skull series including a submental view, a lateral soft tissue film, and sagittal and frontal tomograms. The reader is referred to Fletcher and Jing, *The Head and Neck,* for a comprehensive review of the x-ray findings in patients with nasopharyngeal cancer.[7]

Spread Patterns

Spread to Contiguous Structures

The location of the primary lesion and types of contiguous extensions influence the arrangement and weighting of the fields used to treat the primary lesion.

Table 3-35 shows the recognized spread to contiguous structures on admission prior to treatment in 99 patients with epithelial lesions.[6]

INFERIOR EXTENSION

Inferior extension along the pharyngeal walls and tonsils was recognized in almost a third of these patients. When submucosal infiltration is felt at the junction of the posterior and lateral pharyngeal walls, it is a moot question whether one is dealing with an extension of the primary lesion or an enlarged retropharyngeal node. Infiltration down the posterior pharyngeal wall may result in invasion of the prevertebral muscles in the retropharyngeal space, in which case extension of the cervical spine is restricted and painful.

ANTERIOR EXTENSION

Extension into the posterior nasal cavity is difficult to determine by indirect mirror examination since the nasopharyngeal mass frequently occludes the view. Similarly, it is

Table 3-35. *Malignant Tumors of the Nasopharynx—Incidence of Spread to Contiguous Structures on Admission—August 1948–December 1960*

Oropharyngeal wall	29
Base of skull (sphenoid sinus—11)	25
Tonsillar bed	15
Cranial nerves	12
Pterygoid fossa	9
Nasal cavity	5
Maxillary antrum	4
Orbit	3
Soft palate	3
Hard palate	2
Ethmoids	2
Hypopharynx	1

In several cases more than one structure was involved. (Courtesy: Fletcher and Million, *Amer. J. Roentgen.*, 93, 44, 1965.)

difficult to examine the posterior nares by direct examination through the anterior nares, though shrinking of the nasal mucosa may improve visualization. Lateral soft tissue films and coronal tomograms are most useful to determine soft tissue extension into the posterior nose.

Invasion of the posterior ethmoids, the posterior maxillary antrum, and the anterior cranial fossa is recognized infrequently. However, anterior extension is important to suspect or demonstrate, since it dictates a modification of the treatment technique. The 4-field technique described in the neck section effectively treats only about 2 cm anterior to the posterior border of the nasal septum, and extension anterior to this level must be covered by adjustment of the paired anterior facial fields or by substituting a single anterior field.

SUPERIOR EXTENSION

Invasion into or through the base of the skull was recognized radiographically or clinically in at least 25 per cent of patients prior to treatment.[3,6] Early, unrecognized invasion presumably occurs in a far greater number of patients. The base of the skull, brain, and cranial nerves were the second most frequent sites of local recurrence. The reader may refer to MacComb and Fletcher[9] and to Lederman[8] for their descriptions of potential routes of spread from the nasopharynx to the intracranial cavity.

Spread to Lymphatics of the Neck

The high frequency of metastatic neck disease is one of the characteristics of nasopharyngeal malignancy. Figure 3-11 shows the incidence and distribution of metastases to the various node areas in the epithelial tumors of the nasopharynx.[1] Bilateral neck metastases occur in about half of the cases. Although the lymphatics usually drain to the nodes on the same side as the lesion, there are abundant anastomoses crossing the midline; even small, well-lateralized lesions may present with contralateral metastases.

Low-grade squamous lesions produce slightly fewer metastases (73 per cent) as opposed to more anaplastic lesions (Grade III and IV squamous and lymphoepitheliomas) which show an incidence of 92 per cent. The occasional low-grade lesions are more likely to produce unilateral and fewer neck nodes than the more anaplastic lesions.[6]

Metastases to submental and occipital nodes may appear when there is blockage of the common lymphatic pathways either by massive neck disease or by an untimely neck dissection.

Lymphomas of the nasopharynx show similar neck node patterns of spread; however, their patterns of distant spread beyond the neck differ from the carcinomas.

Staging

The staging of the primary tumor used at M. D. Anderson Hospital is as follows:

T_1: Primary tumor invisible, but biopsy positive, or tumor less than 1 cm in greatest diameter.

T_2: Tumor larger than 1 cm in diameter, but confined to the nasopharynx.

T_3: Tumor extends beyond nasopharynx, but no evidence of invasion of base of skull or cranial nerves.

T_4: Tumor involving the base of the skull and/or cranial nerves, regardless of the size of the tumor.

Analysis of Results

Table 3-36 compares some of the clinical characteristics and results of treatment for the three common histologies.

Recent re-examination of our data now shows that there is a difference in the dose required for local and regional control of the lymphoepithelioma as compared to squamous carcinoma.[3] Figure 3-89 shows the observed local recurrence rate of the primary lesion by T stage of squamous and lymphoepithelioma carcinomas. The local failure rate in the squamous group is almost 3 times higher than for lymphoepithelioma, although the distribution by T stage is approximately the same. Only a single local failure was observed above 1,750 rets[4] (5,950 rads/30 fractions/40 days) in the lymphoepithelioma group.

However, a high failure rate develops with doses less than 5,500 rads (Fig. 3-89). No

Table 3-36. *Clinical Parameters of the Three Most Common Malignant Histological Types—M. D. Anderson Hospital 1948–1965*

	Squamous	Lymphoepithelioma	Primary Lymphoma
Average Age	54	42	50
Base of skull and/or cranial nerve (T_4)	26%	27%	0–9%
Incidence of local failure	31%	12%	9%
Time of local recurrence	93% at 2 years	80% at 4 years	Insufficient data
Dose for local control	Minimum dose not established	5,950 rads 30 fractions–40 days	4,000–5,000 *R* in 4–5 weeks
No palpable nodes	16%	8%	45%
Bilateral nodes	42%	55%	27%
Incidence of neck failure	23%	12%	9%
Incidence of distant metastases	23%	35%	45%
5-year survival (*NED*-absolute) (MDAH)	27.5% (23/83)	45% (27/60)	54.5% (6/11)

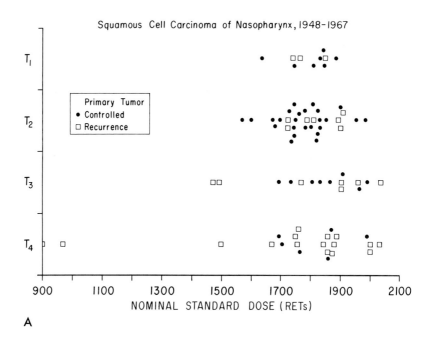

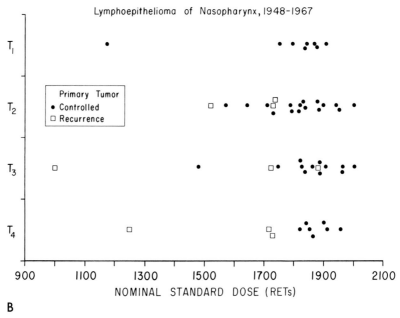

FIG. 3-89. 1,687 rets = 5,600 rads — 28 fractions in 37 days 1,750 rets = 5,950 rads — 30 fractions in 40 days 1,800 rets = 6,250 rads — 32 fractions in 43 days 1,900 rets = 7,000 rads — 35 fractions in 49 days (Courtesy: Chen and Fletcher, Malignant tumors of the nasopharynx, *Radiology,* 99, 165, 1971.)

minimal dose was elicited for the squamous cell carcinoma.

In the analysis of our data in 1965, there was only one patient with local control of disease out of 25 patients with base of skull involvement.[6] The treatment technique was adjusted in 1961 to supplement the dose to the base of skull and brain in patients with T_4 lesions. As a result, 5 patients who had unequivocal destruction of the base of the skull are alive 5 to 9 years. A sixth patient had a sixth nerve paralysis, but no observed

bony changes; he is also free of disease at 7 years. Five additional survivors had T_4 lesions but the changes on the skull films are minimal.

Analysis of neck failures shows a 23 per cent over-all neck failure for squamous cell carcinoma versus 12 per cent for lymphoepithelioma in spite of the fact that lymphoepithelioma had somewhat more advanced neck disease (Table 3-37). Failure to control neck disease as the only cause of failure is rare. When the primary lesion was controlled, neck failure occurred in only 2 of 107 patients with squamous cell carcinoma and in none of 74 patients with lymphoepithelioma (minimum 3-year follow-up).[3] Usually when there is a neck failure the primary lesion had recurred or distant metastases had appeared simultaneously.

Table 3-37. *Carcinoma of Nasopharynx-Neck Disease Uncontrolled—1948–1967*

Stage	Squamous Carcinoma		Lympho-epithelioma	
	Number	% Failure	Number	% Failure
N_0	0/18*	0	0/6*	0
N_1	2/12	16.5	0/5	0
N_2A	0/11	0	1/9	11
N_2B	5/15	33.5	1/11	9
N_3A	1/6	16.5	0/2	0
N_3B	17/45	40	7/41	17
Total	25/107†	23.5	9/74	12

*Nine patients had no treatment to the neck.
†Five patients had surgical treatment before radiotherapy, a radical neck dissection being performed before the primary lesion was found; one patient developed a recurrence in the submandibular area after radiotherapy but remained *NED* at 21 months after surgical excision of the recurrent node. (Courtesy: Chen and Fletcher, *Radiology, 99*, 165, 1971.)

Treatment Planning

Primary Lesion

The anatomical planning is the same for the various grades of squamous cell carcinoma, the transitional cell carcinomas, and the lymphoepitheliomas. Table 3-38 summarizes recommended doses by T stage and histology.

For the occasional connective tissue sarcoma, adenocarcinoma, plasmacytoma, and nonchromaffin paraganglioma, treatment is planned on an individual basis.

Table 3-38. *Guide to Dosage for Primary**

	Squamous Cell Carcinoma	Lympho-epithelioma	Lympho-sarcoma	Reticulum Cell Sarcoma
T_1, T_2, early T_3	6,500	6,000	4,000	5,000
Late T_3, T_4	7,000	6,500	4,500	6,000

*1,000 rads/week TD. If the weekly TD is 850 rads then the total dose is increased by 10 per cent.

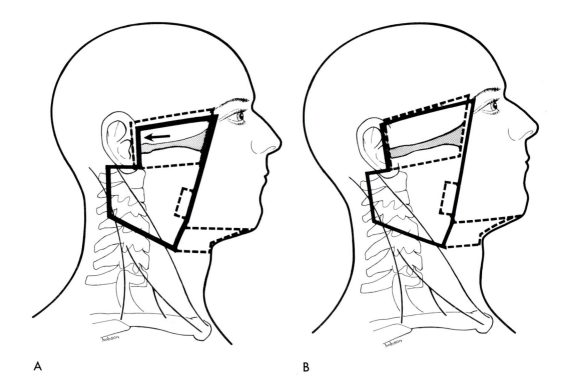

A   B

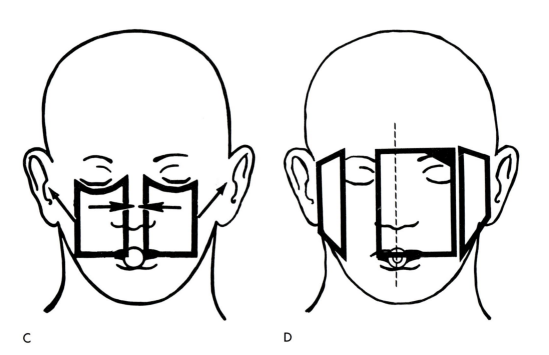

C   D

TREATMENT PLANNING FOR T_1, T_2
AND EARLY T_3

There is no place for small volume irradiation even for an early epithelial tumor of the nasopharynx. If, after complete clinical and x-ray work-up, the tumor is thought to be limited to the nasopharynx (T_1 or T_2) or has minimal soft tissue extension (early T_3), the following areas are enclosed in the treatment volume:

1) Nasopharynx proper, 2) posterior 2.0 cm of the nasal cavity, 3) posterior ethmoid sinuses, 4) entire sphenoid sinus and basiocciput, 5) cavernous sinus, 6) base of skull (7 to 8 cm width encompassing foramen ovale, carotid canal, and foramen spinosum laterally), 7) pterygoid fossae, 8) posterior one third of orbit, 9) posterior one third of maxillary sinus, 10) lateral and posterior oropharyngeal wall to level of midtonsillar fossa, and 11) retropharyngeal nodes.

The high-dose volume, roughly cuboidal in shape, is about 230 cc (5.5 cm AP, 7.0 cm wide, 6.0 cm superior-inferior).

We advocate the use of a 4-field arrangement (Fig. 3-90) with ^{60}Co or 3 to 6 Mev to cover this central volume. This technique prevents overdosage which would be approximately 5 to 10 per cent higher than the tumor dose to the temporomandibular joints, middle and external ears, and subcutaneous tissues which results from opposed lateral fields, unless a high energy beam is available ($\geq$ 20 Mev). The lateral fields deliver about two thirds and the anterior fields about one third of the tumor dose.

The lateral fields are angled 5 to 10 degrees posteriorly to ensure adequate posterior margins while avoiding direct ipsilateral irradiation of the external and middle ear. The posterior tilt also reduces irradiation to the contralateral eye. A 5-degree posterior tilt only shifts the field edge 0.5 cm backward at the midline and a 10-degree tilt moves it 1.2 cm at the midline (Fig. 3-91).

FIG. 3-90. Portals for irradiation of the primary tumor. **A.** Lateral portal for T_1, T_2, and early T_3. The upper margin of the portal is drawn from the outer canthus to the upper margin of the tragus, usually 1 to 2 cm above the zygomatic arch. The port film will show half of the pituitary fossa included in the treatment field. The posterior margin is immediately adjacent to the anterior aspect of the external auditory canal. The posterior margin is drawn posteriorly through the inferior ear lobe to about a centimeter back of the tip of the mastoid. The posterior margin is then drawn just behind the sternocleidomastoid muscle unless enlarged nodes are located further posteriorly. The inferior margin of the portal is at the level of the thyroid notch. The anterior margin slopes from the external canthus inferiorly until it reaches the neck posterior to the submaxillary gland. A small mandible block may be introduced to protect the cheek. The submandibular and submental areas are included (dashed lines) when they contain clinically positive nodes or there is massive upper neck disease.

The beam is angled 5 degrees to 10 degrees posteriorly, as determined by verification films. The reduced portal for the boost to the base of skull is indicated by dashed lines and is *not* angled posteriorly. The posterior and superior borders may be outside the original margins to ensure adequate compensation for the low dosage.

B. Lateral portal used for late T_3 and T_4. The upper margin of the lateral portal is 1 to 2 cm higher than in A and on the verification film usually extends a centimeter above the pituitary fossa. The posterior margin of the portal is either the same as in A with tilt or may be located just behind the external auditory canal, in which case no tilt of the beam is necessary. The base of skull compensating portal is located according to individual requirements.

C. Anterior portals. A cork and tongue blade are placed in the mouth to depress the tongue as far as possible out of the treatment fields. The beam is tilted medially an average of 20 to 30 degrees. The beam axis is aimed superiorly with the aid of the collimator light as seen in Figure 3-92. The superior margins glance the eyeballs. The medial margins are usually 1 cm from the midline. The inferior borders are normally at the commissure of the lip, and the fields are usually about 6 cm wide.

D. Example of a 3-field arrangement for lateralized anterior spread into the left orbit, ethmoid sinus, and posterior nose. The anterior field projects 2 cm across the midline and thus spares one eye. A lacrimal gland shield is used when possible. Wedges are used as necessary to produce the required volume distribution.

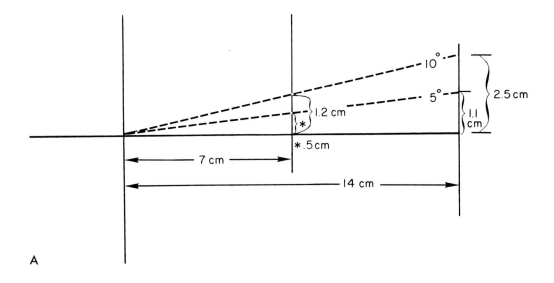

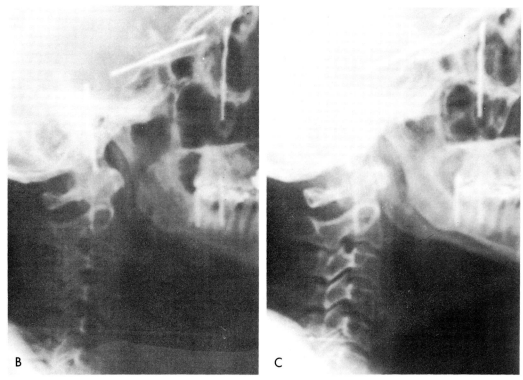

FIG. 3-91. A. Shows schematically the change in the beam edge at a depth of 7 cm (corresponding to the midline skull) resulting from both 5-degree and 10-degree posterior tilt. The 5-degree tilt results in only ½ cm displacement, and the 10-degree tilt, a 1.2 cm displacement at the midline. Note the relatively greater displacement of the exit beam at 14 cm. **B.** A simulator film using lateral portals as described without tilt, shows marginal coverage of the posterior wall of the nasopharynx. **C.** A 5-degree tilt increases posterior coverage with the entire basiocciput enclosed in the field. Note the protection of the third molar area when the small mandible block is used with the lateral portals.

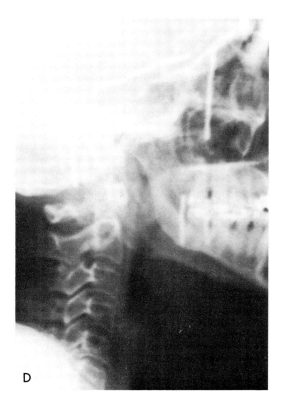

D

FIG. 3-91. **D.** A 10-degree posterior tilt produces less coverage in the posterior nares, posterior ethmoid sinuses, and orbit with slight additional posterior coverage to about 1 cm behind the basiocciput. **E.** Verification film of the small portal used to compensate for underdosage. The roof of the nasopharynx is in the center of the portal. Five hundred to 1,000 rads midline dose is added.

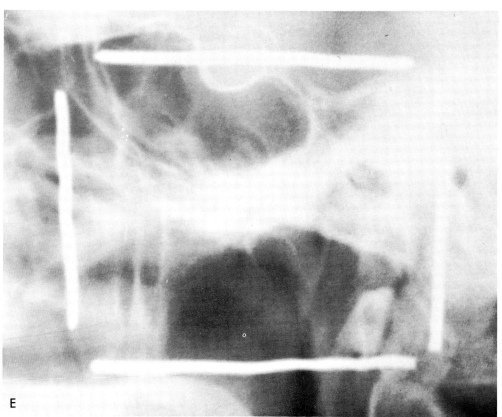

E

The anterior facial fields are angled 20 to 30 degrees. Some radiotherapists object to the anterior angled fields as being difficult to set up and reproduce. However, by opening the collimator light as shown in Figure 3-92, one can visualize the direction of the beam to determine the superior tilt and accurately reproduce this set-up each day. The anterior facial fields with their inferior border at the level of the anterior commissure of the lip provide adequate inferior coverage to about the level of the midtonsillar fossa (angle of mandible). When this technique becomes inadequate to cover low oropharyngeal extensions, by necessity one treats entirely with lateral fields. If a 20 Mev beam is available, its distribution for opposing fields (Fig. 3-93) is ideal and may be used for all or part of the treatment course.

Figure 3-93 shows six examples of volume distributions. A minimum dosage of 6,500 rads is delivered for the squamous cell carcinomas and 6,000 rads for the lymphoepitheliomas.

Examination of the local control data for the squamous carcinomas shows 10 local failures in patients with T_1 and T_2 lesions at levels of 6,500 to 7,000 rads. Failures might be related to underdosage in the posterior and superior aspect of the nasopharynx and base of skull.

1) The posterior and superior aspect of the nasopharynx, base of skull, and cavernous sinuses are on the edge or corner of the fields and thus the dose is approximately 10 per cent less than the dose at the central axis (Fig. 3-94).

2) Bone: There is an almost continuous slab of dense bone at the level of the base of the skull, and even with high energies there is differential absorption (^{60}Co—3.5 per cent/cm bone).

3) Dosimetric errors: The contour is taken at a level through the upper lip and the external auditory meatus. However, most patients are about a centimeter thicker at the level of the zygomatic arch, which causes an

underdosage of about 5 per cent from the lateral fields.

4) The anterior fields are angled superiorly, which is not allowed for in the contour. This adds about another 1 cm which is not taken into consideration in the volume distribution of the anterior fields.

The "true tumor dose," is still adequate for lymphoepitheliomas; but for squamous cell carcinoma, a compensating midline supplement of 500 to 1,000 rads is now given to the base of skull and nasopharynx through 5×4 cm opposed lateral fields (Fig. 3-94B).

TREATMENT PLANNING FOR LATE T_3 OR T_4

Base of Skull and/or Intracranial Nerve Involvement. Extension to the base of skull and/or cranial nerve involvement II-VI, requires that the superior border be raised to include all the pituitary, base of the brain in the suprasellar area, the adjacent middle cranial fossa, and the posterior portion of the anterior cranial fossa. At the completion of the basic treatment with the 4 fields, one again supplements the nasopharynx and base of skull/brain with a reduced field to compensate for undertreatment as outlined in the last section. If a 22 Mev beam is available, it is preferred for the whole treatment.

A minimum dosage of 7,000 rads is planned in late T_3 and T_4 squamous and 6,500 rads minimum in lymphoepithelioma (Table 3-38).

Split-course technique (3,000 rads/3 weeks—2 weeks rest—4,000 rads/4 weeks) or reduced weekly dose rate (850 rads per week; total dose 7,000 rads) is useful when high dose-large volume irradiation is planned in the advanced lesions.

Anterior Extension. In patients with anterior invasion to the orbit, ethmoids, or maxillary sinus, the paired anterior fields may be discarded in favor of a single straight-on anterior field. A 3-field arrangement which re-

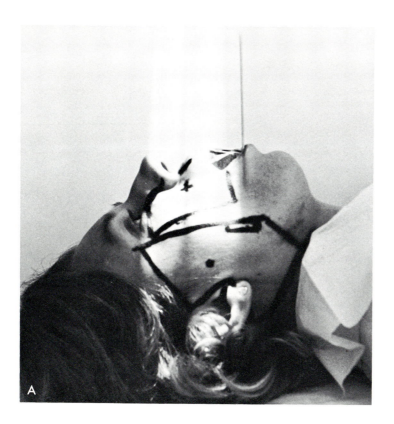

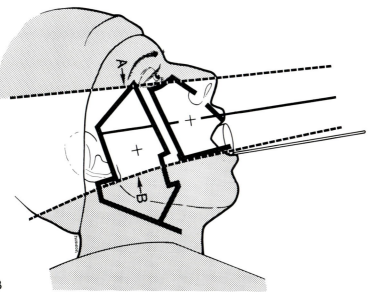

FIG. 3-92. A. Shows the use of the collimator light to adjust the superior tilt of the facial fields. The collimator light is adjusted to the superior and inferior margin of the fields and then the collimator is opened laterally to allow the light beam to glance along the lateral aspect of the face. The head position is then adjusted so that the superior margin encloses all of the superior margin of the lateral portal. The head is then fixed in position. This technique is simple and quick. The inferior margin usually projects across the angle of the mandible, indicating coverage to about the midtonsillar fossa. B. Schematic drawing of A. The facial fields are more efficient than the calculations indicate because the nostrils and maxillary antra are air filled cavities.

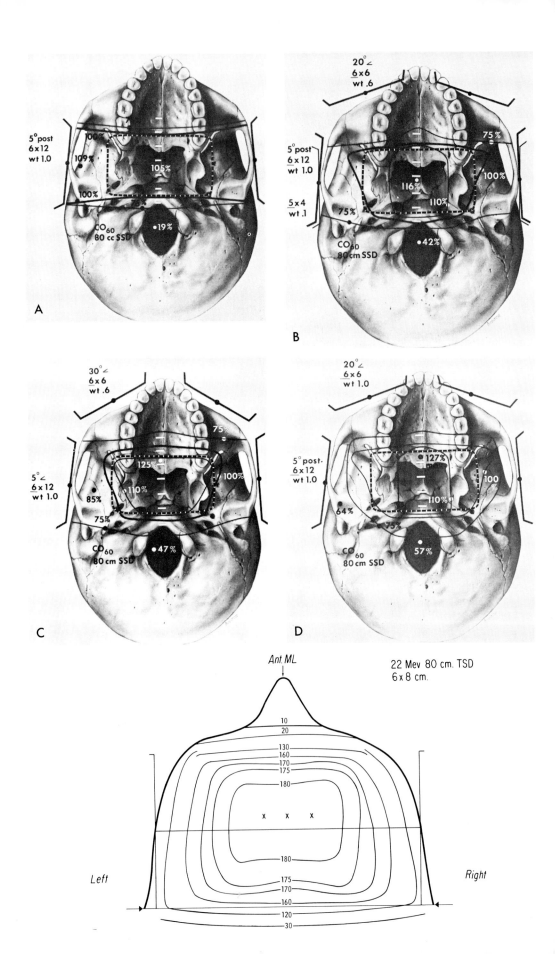

quires the combination of wedges on the lateral fields and partial use of wedge on the anterior field will produce a satisfactory volume distribution (Fig. 3-95). The lacrimal gland should be shielded if possible to retain tears and help prevent development of a painful eye. When wedge fields are used on the lateral portals, it is not feasible to include the upper neck in the primary fields; the neck is then irradiated through separate portals. One such patient with an extensive destructive lesion of the base of the skull and unilateral orbital involvement is living $7\frac{1}{2}$ years following treatment, free of disease and with good vision.

Neck Nodes

A comprehensive *en bloc* plan must be developed to irradiate the neck to the level of the clavicles for both the epithelial lesions and the lymphomas. Even patients with no palpable disease in the neck should have full neck irradiation.[1]

UPPER NECK

The retropharyngeal nodes are included in the treatment of the local lesion. The upper neck nodes are included in the lateral primary fields to the level of the thyroid notch.

FIG. 3-93. ^{60}Co isodose distributions related to base of skull anatomy. The dashed line encompasses the usual treatment volume. All isodose distributions are normalized so that the 100 per cent isodose encloses the dashed line. Weights (*wt*) refer to the relative given dose to each field.

A. Opposed lateral portals result in 5 to 9 per cent greater dose to the subcutaneous tissues, parotid, and temporomandibular joints. Posterior and anterior coverage is marginal. **B, C,** and **D.** The volume distribution from 4 fields produces a maximum dose in the anterior midline of the nasopharynx. For the T_1, T_2, and early T_3 the point of dose specification is the volume which roughly encompasses the nasopharynx and would correspond to the 110 per cent normalized isodose on the illustrations; thus, the maximum dose to a very small volume would be from 5 to 10 per cent more and the dose to the volume enclosed by the dashed line would be about 10 per cent less than the specified dose.

This differential is acceptable, since minimal spread outside the nasopharynx requires less dose than the bulky disease within the nasopharynx and its immediate vicinity.

For late T_3 and T_4 lesions the point of dose specification encompasses the larger volume outlined by the dashed line. This area usually measures about 7 to 8 cm wide and 4 to 5 cm anteroposterior. The 100 per cent normalized isodose encloses this volume. In this case, the nasopharynx proper would receive doses 10 per cent higher than the specified dose and the maximum dose to a very small volume in the middle of the nasopharynx would be 15 to 25 per cent more than the specified dose, depending upon which distribution was used.

The difference in distribution between 20-degree and 30-degree angle of facial fields is minimal (Figs. 3-91B and 91C). **D.** Equal weighting of lateral and anterior portals produces about the same distribution in the central area compared to Figures B and C. However, the dose to the brain stem and CNS is greater while the lateral subcutaneous dose is less.

Calculations for **B.** The 110 per cent normalized isodose is equivalent to 190 per cent actual depth dose, ^{60}Co, 80 SSD, including the contribution from a small portal covering only the base of the skull.

Aim: 6,500 rads minimum TD

Lateral portals   Wt. 1.0 $= \dfrac{6{,}500}{1.90} = 3{,}425$ GD (each field wt. 1.0)

Anterior portals   Wt. 0.6 $= \dfrac{6{,}500}{1.90} \times 0.6 = 2{,}050$ GD (each field wt. 0.6)

Small portals   Wt. 0.1 $= \dfrac{6{,}500}{1.90} \times 0.1 = 342$ GD (each field wt. 0.1)

E. Parallel opposed portals with a 22 Mev photon beam produces maximum irradiation to the central volume with reduced dosage to the peripheral structures.

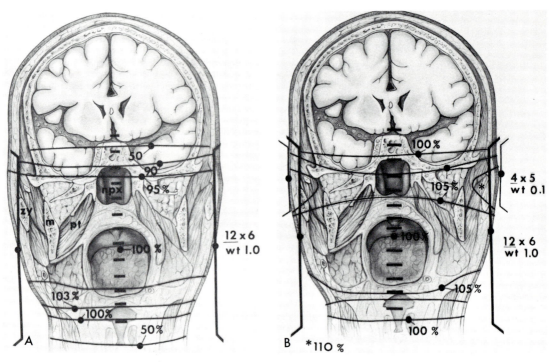

FIG. 3-94. Coronal section at the level of the mid nasopharynx with superimposed volume distribution.
A. This is a 2 cm wide area at the base of the skull which receives less dose from the opposed lateral fields due to field edge effect plus slightly increased thickness of the head at this level, not counting bone absorption. The superior margin of the lateral fields must be high enough; to compensate for this low dose, a supplement is added at the end of treatment to the base of the skull **B.** *Npx*—nasopharynx; *Zy*—Zygomatic arch; *m* = mandible, *pt* = pterygoid muscle and lateral pterygoid plate.

With no palpable nodes, the posterior margin needs to be about one centimeter behind the posterior border of the sternocleidomastoid in order to encompass the high spinal accessory nodes and upper lateral internal jugular nodes. The portals are extended anteriorly into the submental area only if there is disease in the submaxillary triangle or if the patient had an untimely neck dissection prior to irradiation.

When the treatment to the primary is shifted to the anterior facial fields, the lower neck fields are raised to encompass all the neck nodes (Fig. 3-96). Completion of upper neck irradiation usually follows two geometrical plans. The most common situation occurs after the upper neck nodes have received 4,500 rads from the lateral portals plus 500 to 1,000 rads given dose from the raised anterior portal. The final dosage to nodes is then obtained by balancing the given doses as shown in Figure 3-97A to achieve the desired dose distribution. The second situation occurs when the primary is treated with the 22 Mev beam through parallel opposed portals. Figure 3-97B shows samples of volume distribution.

LOWER NECK

The lower neck is treated through an anterior partly split field which allows protection of the larynx, part of the cervical spinal cord, part of the trachea, and the upper cervical esophagus. The lower border of the midline tapered split is drawn 1 to 2 cm below the

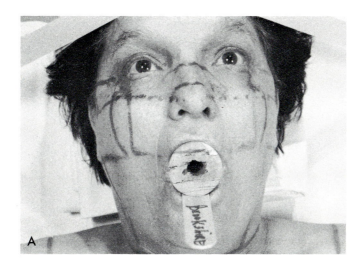

A

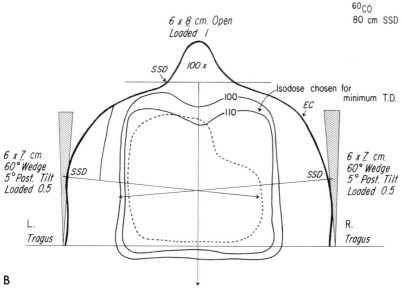

B

FIG. 3-95. Female, age 53, seen in March 1971 had poorly differentiated squamous carcinoma of nasopharynx invading left naris. There was a right upper lesion neck node, 2 cm in diameter.

Stage: T_3N_1

Treatment Plan: Nasopharynx: 3-field arrangement—6,500 rads calculated at 110 per cent isodose of **B.** One-thousand rads TD added to base of skull and nasopharynx with opposing 22 Mev lateral portals.

Neck: Upper neck, bilaterally   5,500 rads TD
        Lower neck, bilaterally   5,000 rads GD

Right upper neck node boost with anterior glancing ^{60}Co beam 1,500 rads GD

A. Photograph of patient in treatment position for anterior portal. **B.** Volume distribution.

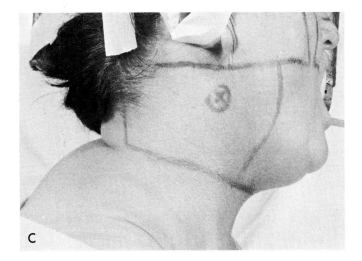

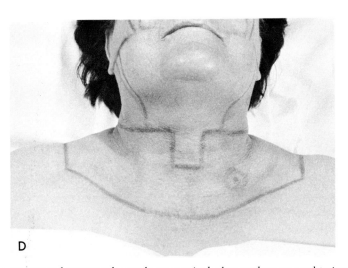

FIG. 3-95. C. Separate opposed upper neck portals are required when wedges are used to irradiate the primary. D. Lower neck field.

inferior border of the cricoid cartilage. The inferior jugular nodes move to a medial position in relation to the jugular vein in the low neck, and since the vein also assumes a paratracheal position in the lower neck, it is not usually advisable to block the midline more than 2 cm below the cricoid cartilage (Fig. 3-96A).

The junction of the upper and lower neck fields is a single line. By convention, the line is included when the upper portals are irradiated and blocked out when the lower portals are treated. Occasionally one sees a small strip of moist desquamation at this junction. The junction may occasionally divide a large node, but this is not serious since there is a slight overdose at the junction site. Occasionally one will feel a small strip of induration in the neck during follow-up at the junction areas, but this has not created a symptomatic problem. Overdosage is more acceptable than attempting to calculate the field separation and risking underdosage.

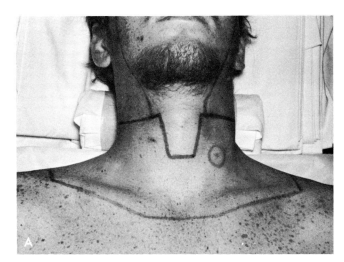

FIG. 3-96. Portals for irradiation of the neck. **A.** *En face* field used to irradiate lower neck in conjunction with the lateral nasopharynx fields. The larynx, cricoid, and 2 cm of trachea are blocked. **B.** The upper border of the lower neck field is raised to include the upper jugular and subdigastric areas when one switches from the lateral portals to the anterior fields. The superior margin usually includes 1 to 2 cm of the angle of the mandible and then continues through the ear lobe and ends 1 cm above the mastoid tip.

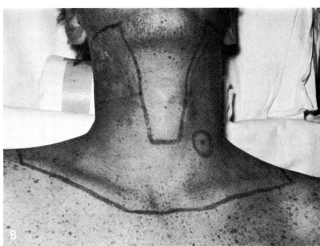

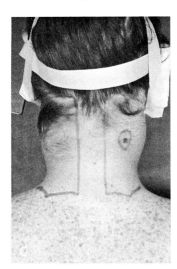

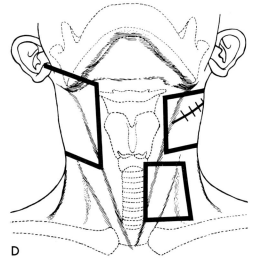

D

FIG. 3-96. **C.** Posterior split field used to supplement treatment to upper neck nodes. The lower margin is at the level of the trapezius, as the supraclavicular, posterior cervical triangle and mid- and low jugular nodes are under the skin and therefore best entirely irradiated through the anterior lower field. **D.** Examples of reduced fields for boosting residual disease are shown. If there has been biopsy of a node, the scar is a potential site of recurrence and should receive additional irradiation.

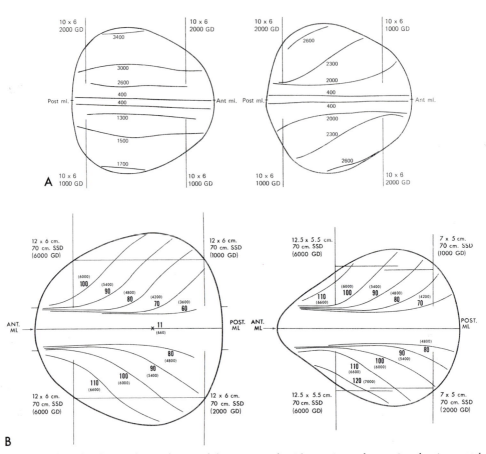

FIG. 3-97. Isodose distribution for irradiation of the upper neck with anterior and posterior glancing portals.
The upper jugular and upper posterior cervical nodes cannot be irradiated adequately through an anterior portal only.

After 4,500 to 5,000 rads to the upper neck either by lateral portals or only an anterior portal (in some selected situations, like treatment of the primary through paralled opposed portals with 22 Mev), a posterior split portal is added. Depending upon the clinical situation, the respective loading of the anterior and posterior portals varies, taking into consideration the original size and location of palpable nodes. **A.** Examples of dose distributions in a thick area on thin patients resulting from opposing anterior and posterior split portals to the upper neck, after 4,000 to 4,500 rads TD through parallel opposed portals. **B.** Volume distribution in a thick and a thin patient when 6,000 rads given dose has been delivered through anterior portal. By adding 2,000 rads given dose to the posterior portal, one raises the dose to the high jugular and spinal accessory chain nodes.

DOSAGE TO NODES

Table 3-39 gives guidelines for selecting dosage depending on the histology and size of nodes. Large neck nodes from a lympho-epithelioma frequently are just barely palpable on a Monday after 400 to 500 rads given the week before; conversely, they may still on occasion be palpable after 5,000 rads in 5 weeks. Squamous cell carcinoma nodes have a slower, more predictable regression rate. The skin over small nodes should be tattooed before they disappear to allow accurate "boost" therapy.

RADICAL NECK DISSECTION

Radical neck dissection has little place in the management of neck disease in naso- pharyngeal cancer. The classical radical neck dissection does not remove the retropharyn- geal nodes. The superior spinal accessory chain of nodes and the high deep lateral internal jugular node(s) lie in juxtaposition to the internal jugular vein as it emerges from the jugular foramen and are difficult to completely excise.[5]

Six patients had a radical neck dissection 2 months after irradiation for "incomplete resolution" of palpable node(s). No viable tumor cells were found in the specimens. Neck dissection should be reserved for re- currence or persistence after irradiation. Neck dissection for recurrent neck disease was successful in 2 of 6 patients.

Lymphomas

The local spread of the lymphomas of the nasopharynx differs from the carcinomas in that bone and cavernous sinus invasion and cranial nerve palsy are far less common. The entirety of Waldeyer's ring should be in- cluded in the lymphoma treatment volume since the disease may involve multiple areas.[12] Therefore opposed lateral fields are used.

The dose to the primary lesion has been 4,000 rads for the lymphosarcomas and 5,000 rads to occasionally 6,000 rads for the reticu- lum cell sarcomas. The pathologist often has difficulty discerning between reticulum cell sarcoma and a poorly differentiated carci- noma; a minimum dose of 6,500 rads is rec- ommended for these cases. Of 16 cases, there has been only one failure (local and regional) in a lymphosarcoma patient who received 4,000 rads in $3\frac{1}{2}$ weeks to the primary and 4,500 rads in $4\frac{1}{2}$ weeks to the neck.

The entire neck is irradiated even if there are no palpable nodes.[12] The basic dose to the nodes has been on the average 4,000 rads for the lymphosarcomas and for the reticu- lum cell sarcomas; large or residual nodes are boosted as indicated in Table 3-39.

Retreatment of Local Recurrences

Retreatment for recurrence may be re- warding, particularly in the lymphoepithelio- mas. Patients have been kept locally free of disease for various lengths of time with 4,000 rads in 4 weeks, at times 5,000 rads in 5 weeks, usually given with a 22 Mev beam.[3]

Complications of Treatment

Because of the large volume irradiated, patients experience a variety of problems

Table 3-39. *Guide to Dose for Neck Nodes*

	Squamous Cell Carcinoma		Lymphoepithelioma		Lymphosarcoma, Reticulum Sarcoma	
	Minimum TD	*Boost to Residual	Minimum TD	*Boost to Residual	Minimum TD	*Boost to Residual
No palpable nodes	4,500†	—	4,500	—	4,000	—
Small nodes, 1–2 cm	6,000	500–1,000	6,000	500–1,000	4,000	—
Nodes 3–5 cm	6,000	1,500–2,000	6,000	1,000–1,500	4,000	500
Massive fixed nodes	6,000	2,000–3,000	6,000	1,500–2,000	4,000	1,000–1,500

* Boost to residual: Boost dose added through portal just covering palpable residual disease. Neck dissection may be substituted for boost in selected cases (e.g., Grade II squamous, solitary 5 cm subdigastric node).
† Doses in rads, usually 850–1,000 rads/week.

connected with mucous membrane, muscle, bone, central nervous system, and subcutaneous tissues. Mucosal dryness of varying severity is always present. Dental problems are frequent but reduced by special care.

The auditory tube is in the high-dose area and obstruction may occur with secondary otitis media and hearing loss. This condition can be corrected by polyethylene tubes inserted through the ear drums to drain the middle ears. The obstruction often improves or clears completely following mucosal healing of the nasopharynx. Politzerization of the eustachian tubes may remove adhesions and reopen the canal.

Trismus occurs to varying degrees in about 10 per cent of the patients. This is usually due to fibrosis and contracture of the pterygoid muscles rather than temporomandibular joint fibrosis. Mandible exercises may help prevent progression of the trismus. Severe trismus may require surgical correction by detaching the pterygoid muscles from the mandible.

The unavoidable irradiation of part of the brain including the hypothalamus, temporal lobes, and pituitary to doses between 6,000 and 7,000 rads has not produced a single example of brain necrosis or hypopituitarism. Some patients show a transitory central nervous system syndrome about 2 to 3 months after irradiation.[2] The greater the volume of the central nervous system irradiated, the longer it takes the patient to recover his sense of well-being; some patients require 6 months to a year to regain their general strength. Radiation myelitis of the cervical cord or brain stem is the most severe CNS complication, 3 out of 4 patients who experienced it having died from it.

BIBLIOGRAPHY

1. Berger, D. S., Fletcher, G. H., Lindberg, R. D., and Jesse, R. H.: Elective irradiation of the neck lymphatics for squamous cell carcinomas of the nasopharynx and oropharynx, *Amer. J. Roentgen.*, 111, 66, 1971.
2. Boldrey, E., and Sheline, G.: Delayed transitory clinical manifestations after radiation treatment of intracranial tumors, *Acta Radiol.*, (Ther.) (Stockholm), 5, 5, 1966.
3. Chen, K. Y., and Fletcher, G. H.: Malignant tumors of the nasopharynx, *Radiology*, 99, 165, 1971.
4. Ellis, F.: Relationship of biologic effect to dose-time-fractionation factors in radiotherapy, In *Current Topics in Radiation Research*, M. Ebert and A. Howard, Editors, North Holland Publishing Co., Amsterdam, p. 382, 1968.
5. Fisch, U.: *Lymphography of the cervical lymphatic system*, W. B. Saunders, Co., Philadelphia, Pennsylvania, 1968.
6. Fletcher, G. H., and Million, R. R.: Malignant tumors of the nasopharynx, *Amer. J. Roentgen.*, 93, 44, 1965.
7. Fletcher, G. H., and Jing, B.: *The Head and Neck*, Year Book Medical Publishers, Inc., Chicago, Illinois, 1968.
8. Lederman, M.: *Cancer of the nasopharynx, its natural history and treatment*, Charles C Thomas, Publisher, Springfield, Illinois, 1961.
9. MacComb, W. S., and Fletcher, G. H.: *Cancer of the Head and Neck*, The Williams & Wilkins Company, Baltimore, Maryland, 1967.
10. Rouviere, H.: *Anatomy of the human lymphatic system*, translated by M. J. Tobias, J. W. Edwards, Publisher, Inc., Ann Arbor, Michigan, 1938.
11. *UICC Monograph Series, Vol. 1: Cancer of the nasopharynx*, edited by C. S. Muir and K. Shanmugaratnam, Medical Examination Publishing Company, Inc., Flushing, New York, 1967.
12. Wang, C. C.: Malignant lymphoma of Waldeyer's ring, *Radiology*, 92, 1335, 1969.

The Role and Techniques of External Irradiation Therapy in the Treatment of Carcinoma of the Thyroid

LILLIAN M. FULLER

Papillary and Follicular Carcinomas

With the exception of the rare anaplastic carcinomas and sarcomas, malignant neoplasms of the thyroid gland are usually papillary or follicular carcinomas. Papillary and follicular carcinomas are well-differentiated, relatively slow growing neoplasms, which are generally amenable to radical resection combined with unilateral or bilateral radical neck dissection for cervical metastases. Because these carcinomas are radioresistant, tumor doses in the order of 6,000 rads administered in a short period of time (4 to 5 weeks) are required to eradicate even small foci of disease. Request for radiotherapy for papillary and follicular carcinomas is usually because lesions have recurred in the operative site, and are not amenable to total surgical excision, due to dense fixation to the trachea, uncontrolled disease in the neck, etc. Because of the volume of tissue involved, these lesions are not immediately suited to an attempt at eradication by radiotherapy. It is the opinion of several authors[1,2,3] experienced in the over-all management of thyroid carcinomas that external beam therapy is most effective if it is preceded by meticulous surgical removal of all possible tumor, the rationale being to reduce the amount of tumor to be irradiated to the smallest possible volume. Care should be taken during dissection not to enter the trachea or the esophagus, to preserve the integrity of the recurrent laryngeal nerves, and to obtain primary closure of the skin flaps. Our own material indicates that when radical radiation therapy is given for a relatively small area of persistent disease after radical resection, the possibility of local control is good. Of 9 patients treated for localized, well-differentiated residual carcinoma, 8 have been followed for more than 5 years without evidence of local recurrence or distant metastases. One patient died at 2 years of other causes.

Anaplastic Carcinomas

Radiation therapy is the most effective method for the palliation of tracheal compression caused by massive anaplastic carcinomas originating from the thyroid gland. Although the immediate response may be striking, radical doses are usually required when the clinical situation warrants an attempt at complete eradication of local disease. In Smedal's report[4] of 44 cases of anaplastic carcinomas of the thyroid, a tumor dose of 4,800 r to the neck and to the mediastinum was attempted with rotational treatment using two million volts. This dose was not achieved in a large number of cases because of the development of distant metastases. Local recurrences occurred in 6 patients, all of whom received tumor doses of 4,800 r or more. However, 10 patients survived 5 years or better without evidence of local recurrence or distant metastases following radical radiation therapy to the neck and the mediastinum. Megavoltage has permitted treatment for very diffuse anaplastic carcinomas, not previously treatable by kilovoltage. Regardless of the over-all survival, the possibility of preventing death from local disease justifies radical treatment for diffuse anaplastic carcinomata.

Technique

For papillary and follicular carcinomas and other well-differentiated carcinomas, in the most favorable situations, that is, when the major portion of the carcinoma has been resected and the residual tumor is limited to a small area, the volume of tissue irradiated should be very circumspect. Tumor doses of 6,000 rads in 4 to 5 weeks are frequently required to eradicate residual disease. For residual disease situated laterally in the thyro-cricoid region, a single lateral megavoltage field is indicated (Fig. 3-98). An electron beam with voltage adjustment for the desired

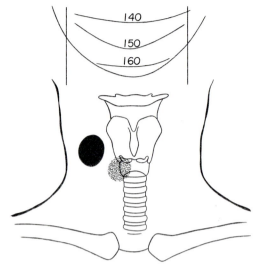

FIG. 3-99. Isodose distribution for parallel opposing ^{60}Co 7 × 4 cm lateral fields (*FSD* 50 cm) covering residual disease (shown in solid black) with associated induration (stipple) in the thyrocridoid area following a total thyroidectomy for a papillary follicular carcinoma.

A maximum tumor dose of 6,300 rads (minimum 5,600 rads) was delivered in 4½ weeks.

The patient has been followed for 8 years without evidence of local recurrence or distant metastases.

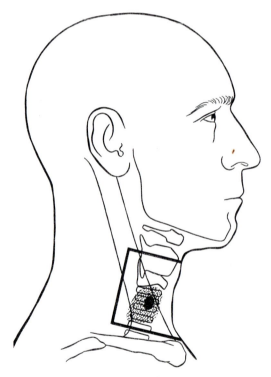

FIG. 3-98. Lateral 8 × 8 cm ^{60}Co field (*SSD* 70 cm) covering residual disease (shown in solid black) in the second tracheal ring and the surrounding induration (stipple) following a subtotal thyroidectomy for a papillary follicular carcinoma.

A given dose of 5,750 rads was delivered in 3½ weeks.

The patient has been under observation for 7 years without evidence of local recurrence or distant metastases.

depth dose is ideal. For midline involvement extending bilaterally, parallel opposing fields are required (Fig. 3-99). More diffuse but unilateral recurrences may be treated with a single large field (Fig. 3-100).

Anaplastic inoperable carcinomas of the thyroid require large volume irradiation to cover not only the obvious disease but also the potential areas of spread. Treatment is usually directed to both necks, the upper mediastinum (or the entire mediastinum) in continuity. In planning the treatment to the neck consideration should be given to the fact that anaplastic carcinomas tend to surround the trachea and the esophagus so that these structures are frequently pushed anteriorly by the disease in the retropharyngeal and esophageal spaces. The local and general tolerance for irradiation to such a large vol-

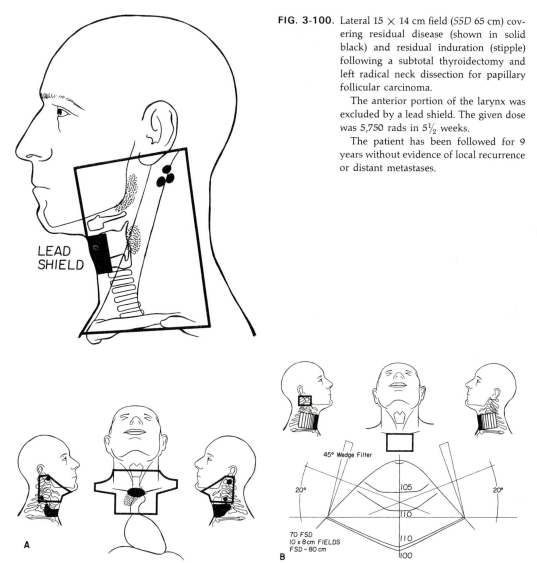

FIG. 3-100. Lateral 15 × 14 cm field (*SSD* 65 cm) covering residual disease (shown in solid black) and residual induration (stipple) following a subtotal thyroidectomy and left radical neck dissection for papillary follicular carcinoma.

The anterior portion of the larynx was excluded by a lead shield. The given dose was 5,750 rads in 5½ weeks.

The patient has been followed for 9 years without evidence of local recurrence or distant metastases.

LEAD SHIELD

45° Wedge Filter

20° 105 20°

110

70 FSD
10 x 8 cm FIELDS
FSD - 80 cm

110

100

A

B

FIG. 3-101. **A.** Schematic drawing of the basic therapy fields covering an inoperable small cell carcinoma of the thyroid (solid black and stipple). Treatment to the upper neck was delivered through lateral parallel opposing ^{60}Co (approximately 7 × 11 cm) fields (*FSD* 70 cm). A midline tumor dose of 5,000 rads was delivered in 4½ weeks. Treatment to the lower neck and the supraclavicular fossae was delivered through an anterior ^{60}Co field (80 cm *FSD*). A given dose of 4,000 rads was delivered in 3½ weeks. The minimum tumor dose calculated to the thyroid area and the upper mediastinum was 3,300 rads. **B.** Schematic drawing of the therapy fields used in administering additional treatment for residual disease. A minimum additional tumor dose of 3,000 rads, calculated on the 100 per cent isodose line, was administered to the thyroid area in 2½ weeks through anterior oblique wedge filtered fields. *The total tumor dose to the thyroid area was 6,300 rads.* An additional 1,500 rads tumor dose was administered in 3 days on the ^{137}Cs unit through a 4 × 4 cm field for residual disease in the right mastoid area. (*FSD* 22 cm). Additional treatment to the upper mediastinum was administered with the 22 Mev betatron x-ray beam (*FSD* 80 cm) through an 8 × 8 cm anterior field. The calculated additional tumor dose was 2,700 rads delivered in 2½ weeks. *The total tumor dose to the anterior superior mediastinum was 6,000 rads.* This patient has been followed for 3½ years without evidence of local recurrence or distant metastases.

ume is limited to 4,000 to 4,500 rads tumor dose delivered in a period of 4 to 5 weeks. Some anaplastic carcinomas are sufficiently radiosensitive to disappear clinically at this dosage level. Additional treatment through very sharply reduced fields may be required for residual disease in the neck. Additional treatment for residual disease in the mediastinum is a more serious problem. Because of the risk of inducing a crippling mediastinitis with doses to the entire mediastinum in excess of 4,000 to 4,500 rads, it is imperative that additional treatment be given through very restrictive fields. Additional treatment to the neck or mediastinum must be tailored to the clinical situation. An example is given in Figure 3-101A and 3-101B.

Treatment for Metastases

The pulmonary parenchyma, skeletal system, and brain are commonly sites of symptomatic metastases from carcinoma of the thyroid. External irradiation is of little or no value in treatment for pulmonary metastases. Metastases to the skeletal system tend to be voluminous. Fractures may occur in weight bearing bones. Increased intracranial pressure may be a symptom of large metastases in the skull. Metastases to the skeletal system are relatively radioresistant. Tumor doses in the order of 4,000 rads or more are required for the relief of pain or prevention of fracture. Even with such doses, massive metastatic disease in the cranial bones may be only reduced in size rather than eradicated. Curiously, with even modest reduction in size, growth restraint may persist for worthwhile periods of time.

Techniques of treatment for metastases will depend on the clinical situation. As for most metastatic lesions, the margins of the treatment fields should be as generous as possible, since new areas of metastatic disease tend to occur at the margins of previously treated areas.

BIBLIOGRAPHY

1. Carpender, J. W. J.: The place of radiation therapy and the use of isotopes in the treatment of carcinoma of the thyroid, *Proc. North Amer. Cancer Conf.*, 4, 663, 1960.
2. Dobyns, B. M.: Cancer of the thyroid: radical surgery, radiation or hormonal suppression therapy, *Surg. Clin. N. Amer.*, 42, 481, 1962.
3. Mabille, J. P.: Therapeutic results of thyroid cancers, statistics of the Fondation Curie, *Ann. Radiol.* (Paris), 4, 447, 1961.
4. Smedal, M. I., and Meisner, W. A.: The results of radiation treatment in undifferentiated carcinoma of the thyroid, *Radiology*, 76, 927, 1961.

Miscellaneous Malignant Tumors of the Head and Neck

ROBERT D. LINDBERG

This section contains a brief review of a variety of malignant tumors of the head and neck region. Some lesions are found only in this region, whereas others occur throughout the entire body. Included are: 1) esthesioneuroepithelioma, 2) Ewing's sarcoma, 3) solitary plasmacytoma of bone and soft tissue, and 4) rhabdomyosarcoma.

Individual Tumor Types

Esthesioneuroepithelioma

The pathological entity "esthesioneuroepithelioma" was first described as an olfactory nerve tumor which histologically resembled retinoblastoma.[2]

Esthesioneuroepitheliomas usually grow slowly; they invade bone locally, and finally extend into the paranasal sinuses. Although earlier authors[11] had denied metastatic spread, more recent investigators[8] confirm both lymphatic and blood-borne metastases. The usual areas of metastasis are the cervical lymph nodes and lungs.

TREATMENT

Esthesioneuroepithelioma is a moderately radioresponsive tumor, as can be predicted by its close histological resemblence to neuroblastoma and retinoblastoma.

Before a treatment plan can be established, the full anatomical extent of the disease must be appraised utilizing roentgenographic examination of the paranasal sinuses, nasopharynx, and base of skull.

The minimum treatment volume should include the entire nasal cavity, the base of the skull superiorly, the palate inferiorly, and the medial wall of the ethmoid sinus of the involved side laterally. The depth of volume includes the anterior aspect of the nasopharynx. The actual depth in centimeters can be obtained from a lateral roentgenogram of the skull. A metal ruler, notched every centimeter, is placed on the forehead and on the nose in the midline when the film is taken. The distance from the surface of the nose to any point in the nasopharynx is then measured and easily demagnified. The depth may vary from 6 to 10 cm—the average being approximately 8 cm. Six thousand rads are delivered in 6 weeks. If the orbit is invaded,

the eye must be included in the irradiated volume to insure covering adequate margins around the tumor.

Tomograms are necessary for proper treatment planning as demonstrated in Figure 3-102, which shows tumor invasion of the medial wall of the left orbit.

RESULTS

Becker and Jacox[1] report a 5-year free of disease rate of 47 per cent (8 of 17 cases). Interestingly, 7 of the 8 local recurrences were subsequently controlled by radiotherapy or extensive surgical procedures. Five patients have been irradiated at M. D. Anderson Hospital; 3 are living free of disease more than 5 years. One patient died of intercurrent disease at $4\frac{1}{2}$ years postirradiation.

Surgical resection should be reserved for radiation failures. One of our patients who had received 6,000 rads tumor dose in 6 weeks had definite regrowth of the tumor, confirmed histologically, $2\frac{1}{2}$ months following the completion of therapy. A resection of the antrum and ethmoid sinus was performed and the patient is now free of disease 6 years postoperatively.

Plasmacytoma

Extramedullary plasmacytoma should be considered a separate entity because of its behavior pattern. Ninety per cent of the solitary lesions arise in the paranasal sinuses, nasal fossa, or nasopharynx. All solitary plasmacytomas should be regarded as malignant.[3] Metastases to the regional lymph nodes occur in 20 per cent of the cases[6], whereas bone metastases occur in 29 per cent. The clinical course is of long duration, as contrasted to that of multiple myeloma.[6]

TREATMENT

Pedunculated lesions are treated by surgical excision, since the chance of recurrence

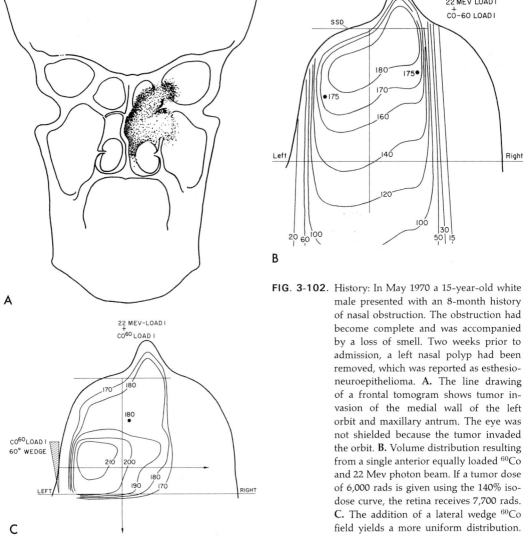

A

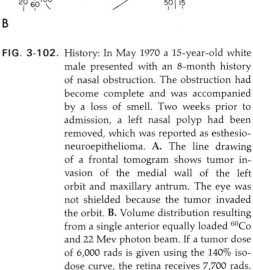

B

C

FIG. 3-102. History: In May 1970 a 15-year-old white male presented with an 8-month history of nasal obstruction. The obstruction had become complete and was accompanied by a loss of smell. Two weeks prior to admission, a left nasal polyp had been removed, which was reported as esthesioneuroepithelioma. **A.** The line drawing of a frontal tomogram shows tumor invasion of the medial wall of the left orbit and maxillary antrum. The eye was not shielded because the tumor invaded the orbit. **B.** Volume distribution resulting from a single anterior equally loaded ^{60}Co and 22 Mev photon beam. If a tumor dose of 6,000 rads is given using the 140% isodose curve, the retina receives 7,700 rads. **C.** The addition of a lateral wedge ^{60}Co field yields a more uniform distribution.

is slight.[6,7] The treatment of choice for all other lesions is radiotherapy. The aim is 5,000 rads tumor dose in 5 weeks. For extensive tumors, an additional 1,000 rads tumor dose in one week is given using reduced fields. A slow regression rate is not cause for alarm. The tumor may not disappear until 2 or 3 months after the completion of radiotherapy. In one case, a positive biopsy was obtained 2 months after completion of therapy, but no further treatment was given. The patient is now living without disease 21 years after therapy.

Lesions in the paranasal sinuses or nasal fossa are treated with the same technique as other tumors. Surgical drainage of the maxillary antrum prior to radiotherapy is not necessary.

In Waldeyer's ring, plasmacytoma has a tendency to be multiple. The best technique is parallel opposing, equally loaded fields which include all of Waldeyer's ring. The treatment aim is 5,000 rads midline tumor dose in 5 weeks. For extensive tumors, a boost is given with a lateral ^{60}Co or 22 Mev photon field.

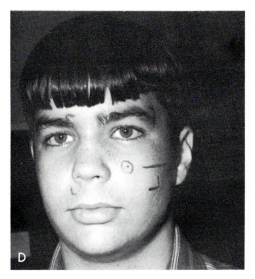

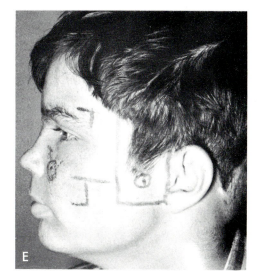

FIG. 3-102. D. Outline of anterior ⁶⁰Co and 22 Mev field. **E.** Location of the small lateral ⁶⁰Co 60° wedge field anterior to the tragus. The patient is *NED* at 20 months (January 1972).

RESULTS

Of 8 patients, 5 were treated by radiotherapy and 3 by surgery. There have been no further manifestations of disease, either local or metastatic. Four patients treated by radiotherapy are living free of disease at 3, 4, 16, and 21 years. One patient died of intercurrent disease at 11 years. Of 3 patients treated by surgery, 2 are living at 5 and 8 years, and one died of intercurrent disease at 4 months.

Ewing's Sarcoma

Ewing's sarcoma can occur in the bones of the head and neck region. Ewing's sarcoma tends to infiltrate locally and thus produces a soft tissue mass adjacent to the involved bone.

TREATMENT

Since Ewing's sarcoma usually extends well beyond the limits of the radiological defect, the entire bone and a generous margin of adjacent soft tissue should be included in the irradiated volume. A tumor dose of 5,000 rads in 5 weeks is given, plus an additional boost of 1,000 rads through reduced fields.

In order to spare the underlying brain tissues, skull lesions are best treated with an electron beam. A single appositional field using the proper energy (Mev) should include the local area of bony involvement with a generous margin. No attempt is made to treat the entire calvarium. If an electron beam is not available, widely angled wedge filters are used to minimize the volume of brain tissue irradiated.

Lesions arising in the maxilla are treated with anterior and oblique lateral fields using 60-degree wedge filters. The resulting volume distribution is homogeneous.

If a lesion presents in one side of the mandible, the entire hemimandible should be irradiated; otherwise the chance for further manifestations in the untreated portion of the bone is high. The entire mandible need not be irradiated unless the lesion involves the symphysis. Wide angle wedge fields are used to irradiate the hemimandible to 5,000 rads in 5 weeks. An appositional field is used to deliver the boost.

Lesions of the cervical spine may be treated with a wedged pair arrangement or by a single posterior field using a combination of ^{60}Co and 22 Mev photons. Such a field obviously encompasses the cervical portion of the spinal cord, but it is impossible to avoid the cord and treat the entire vertebrae irrespective of the field arrangement. The dose to the cord should not exceed 5,000 rads in 5 weeks.

RESULTS

The prognosis of patients with Ewing's sarcoma is very poor.[5,9]

Four patients with Ewing's sarcoma of bones in the head and neck area have been irradiated at M. D. Anderson Hospital. Two patients died with local recurrences. One is living free of disease at 15 years. In this patient, there was no evidence of tumor regression, therefore a surgical resection of the maxillary sinus was performed. The pathological study of the resected tissue, however, showed no evidence of tumor. The fourth patient developed an extradural metastasis at L_{4-5} 8 years posttreatment, which was confirmed histologically. This area was irradiated to 5,000 rads tumor dose. Ten years posttreatment the patient is receiving chemotherapy for bony and pulmonary metastases. There is no evidence of local recurrence in the head and neck area.

Rhabdomyosarcoma

Rhabdomyosarcomas are classified as: 1) pleomorphic, 2) alveolar, and 3) embryonal, with sarcoma botryoides as a subdivision of the third group. The pleomorphic variety usually occurs in the adult, the alveolar variety in the adolescent, and the embryonal variety in the child.

Rhabdomyosarcomas are locally invasive, extending along fascial planes for a great distance. These extensions account for the high incidence of local recurrences after surgery alone (50 to 60 per cent).[10] Metastasis occurs early in the disease, both by the bloodstream and lymphatic channels (52 per cent in our series).

CLINICAL VARIETIES

The behavior pattern of rhabdomyosarcomas of the head and neck region varies with the site of origin. The orbital primary, which is usually diagnosed early because of the symptoms, tends to remain confined to the orbit, apparently limited by the bony structures. Nerves in the orbit may be invaded, but significant extension along the nerves is unusual. Orbital lesions can be controlled by irradiation alone.

Lesions arising in the upper air passages including the nasal cavity, nasopharynx, and paranasal sinuses are usually extensive when first diagnosed. To be effective radiotherapy must be radical; therefore, one must be prepared to accept the late radiation sequelae when treating children. Chemotherapy (Actinomycin-D and Vincristine given concurrently with radiotherapy and Cytoxan after radiotherapy) is used to improve the local control rate and to prevent clinical distant metastases. Surgical resection is added when indicated, i.e., localized lesions arising in the infrastructure of the maxillary antrum.

Surgical resection as the only modality of treatment for primary lesions originating in the soft tissues is ineffective (6 of 7 patients in our series had local recurrence). The treatment is combined radiotherapy and chemotherapy with surgical resection if indicated.

TREATMENT

A tumor dose of 5,000 rads is delivered in 5 weeks plus a boost of 500 to 1,000 rads through reduced fields.

Orbital lesions are treated using anterior and lateral wedge filtered fields. The lateral field is angled posteriorly to avoid the contralateral eye and 60-degree wedges are used to compensate for this angulation. Cassidy et al have described a technique of delivering 5,000 rads tumor dose in 5 weeks using a single anterior field with 22.5 Mev x-rays.[4] Two of the 6 patients so treated have developed cataracts, but both have adequate vision in the affected eye.

The radiotherapy techniques used for lesions of the upper air passages are the same as for the other tumors of the same anatomical sites.

Rhabdomyosarcomas arising in the soft tissues, i.e., cheek or temple, are treated with an appositional electron beam field. Lesions arising in the neck are irradiated by an anterior ^{60}Co field with the head in an extended position. This field may be opposed with a posterior field to deliver a more uniform dose. Thus the cervical and supraclavicular lymph node-bearing areas can be easily covered while the larynx and spinal cord are avoided.

Because of the incidence of cervical node metastasis (35 per cent at initial examination and an additional 9 per cent during or after original treatment), the homolateral cervical nodes should be irradiated in all cases of head and neck rhabdomyosarcomas except for primaries arising in the orbit, paranasal sinuses, and nasal cavity, as the incidence of cervical node metastasis from these sites is low—7 of 32 (22 per cent). The neck receives 5,000 rads given dose in 5 weeks through a single anterior field. If clinically metastatic nodes were present initially, a radical neck dissection is done 4 to 6 weeks later.

RESULTS

From 1948 to September 1969, 40 previously untreated cases of rhabdomyosarcoma of the head and neck region were treated by radiation therapy alone or in combination with chemotherapy and/or surgery. The locations of these lesions were: orbital, 10; upper air passages, 19 (nasal cavity, 2; nasopharynx, 8; and paranasal sinuses 9); and 11 in other head and neck sites.

The prognosis is markedly influenced by the location of the primary lesion (Table 3-40). Orbital lesions have a good prognosis, lesions of the upper air passages the worst, and the remaining lesions are intermediate. Nine of the 40 patients died with distant metastasis but were free of disease above the clavicle. The control rate in the head and neck area is 65 per cent (26/40); 8 patients had uncontrolled primaries, 4 patients had uncontrolled primary and neck disease, 1 patient had uncontrolled neck disease and 1 patient died of unknown causes.

Table 3-40. *Results of Treatment—Rhabdomyosarcoma—1948 to September 1969, Unlimited Follow-up (Minimum 30 months)*

Site	Total Cases	NED	P	P + N	N	DM	Unk.	ID
Orbit	10	7	1*	1*				1
Upper Air Passages								
Nasal Cavity	2					1	1	
Nasopharynx	8	3**	4†	1*				
Paranasal Sinuses	9	1	2†		1*	5		
Other Sites	11	5	1*	2*		3		
Total	40	16	8	4	1	9	1	1

*Pt also had DM
**Patients received Actinomycin-D and Vincristine during radiotherapy and Cytoxan posttreatment
†One of the patients also had DM
NED—No evidence of disease
P—Primary uncontrolled
N—Neck uncontrolled
DM—Distant metastasis
Unk.—Dead of unknown causes
ID—Dead of intercurrent disease

The prognosis is also influenced by other factors: the presence of cervical node metastasis (only 2 of 17 patients with cervical node metastasis are living free of disease) and the histology and age of the patient (embryonal lesions in young patients have a better prognosis).

BIBLIOGRAPHY

1. Becker, M. H., and Jacox, H. W.: Olfactory esthesioneuroepithelioma, *Radiology*, 82, 77, 1964.
2. Berger, L., and Luc, Richard: L'esthesioneuroepitheliome olfactif, *Bulletin de l'association pour l'etude du cancer*, 13, 410, 1924.
3. Carson, C. P., Ackerman, L. V., and Maltby, J. D.: Plasma cell myeloma. A clinical pathological and roentgenologic review of 90 cases, *Amer. J. Clin. Path.*, 25, 849, 1955.
4. Cassidy, J. R., Sagerman, R. H., Tretter, P., and Ellsworth, R. M.: Radiation therapy for rhabdomyosarcoma, *Radiology*, 91, 116, 1968.
5. Dahlin, D. C., Coventry, M. D., and Scanlon, P. W.: Ewing's sarcoma, a critical analysis of 165 cases, *J. Bone Joint Surg.*, 43A, 185, 1961.
6. Ennuyer, A., Bataini, P., Chavanne, G., and Helary, J.: Les plasmacytomes des voies acro-digestives superieures. A propos de 248 cas dont 19 traites a la Foundation Curie, *Ann. Radiol.*, 6, 742, 1963.
7. McCall, J. W., and Bailey, C. H., Jr.: Extramedullary plasmacytoma of the upper air passages, *Ann. Otol.*, 69, 906, 1960.
8. Russell, D. S. and Rubenstein, L. J.: *Pathology of Tumors of the Nervous System*, 2 ed., Baltimore, Williams & Wilkins Company, 1963.
9. Scanlon, P. W.: Radiotherapy of Ewing's sarcoma, *Amer. J. Roentgen.*, 87, 504, 1962.
10. Stout, A. P.: Rhabdomyosarcoma of the skeletal muscles, *Ann. Surg.*, 123, 447, 1946.
11. Stout, A. P.: *Tumors of the Peripheral Nervous System*, Washington, Armed Forces Institute of Pathology, 1949.

Carotid Body and Glomus Jugulare

LOWELL S. MILLER

Carotid body and glomus jugulare tumors are histologically identical, and not infrequently occur in association with each other. Because of their highly vascular nature, profuse hemorrhage commonly complicates even biopsy. Complete surgical removal is possible but difficult for the same reason and because of their intimate respective relationships with the carotid and jugular bulbs. A high mortality rate notwithstanding, management of carotid body tumors has traditionally been surgical and has been discussed by MacComb.[3]

The minute structures from which glomus jugulare tumors arise were not named until 1941, when Guild[2] described them as located in the adventitia of the dome of the jugular bulb just below the floor of the middle ear. Such tumors are usually benign but locally invasive, and tend to have a progressive course, producing deafness, tinnitus, vertigo, bloody discharge, destruction of adjacent bone, and dysfunction of cranial nerves, especially cranial nerves number 7, 8, 9, 10, 11, and 12. Metastases to cervical lymph nodes and more distant structures are rare but have been reported. Common or external carotid arteriograms are reputedly more apt to demonstrate glomus jugulare tumors than are vertebral arteriograms, but no one of these is uniformly successful.

The first published account of an irradiated set of glomus jugulare tumors was in 1957, when I. G. Williams[4] reported a series of 12 patients treated with external irradiation. Tumor doses ranged between 4,000 and 5,000 roentgens in 28 to 40 days. There was shrinkage of tumor and at least partial relief of symptoms in all 12, but local persistence of tumor in 3. Survival rates were not stated nor were complications listed. In 1961, Bradshaw[1] reported the results of external irradiation in another series of 12 patients, only one of whom failed to benefit from treatment. Five patients were living and clinically tumor-free (2 for more than 5 years) at the time of the report. Of the remaining 7, 3 died with tumor, 2 of brain necroses, and 2 of unrelated disease. The author recommended a dose of 4,500 to 5,000 rads in 3 weeks, though noting "no definite evidence that a smaller dose is not effective".

Precise information as to medial extent of glomus jugulare tumors often is lacking, so that the minimum tumor dose usually must be carried to within approximately 2 cm of the midline of the base of the skull. This can easily be accomplished with wedge filtered fields converging in the superoinferior axis (Fig. 3-103). Fields also may be arranged in the anteroposterior axis without significant irradiation of the contralateral eye simply by employing an acute beam intersection, *i.e.,* overlapping fields, though care must be exercised to avoid unnecessarily deep projection of the high dose region. An electron beam through a single lateral field at appropriate voltage would seem a satisfactory alternative.

From 1944 through the end of 1964, a total of 14 patients with glomus jugulare tumors have been irradiated at The University of Texas M. D. Anderson Hospital and Tumor Institute. Of these, 13 are still living. In 5 cases, associated masses in the neck (3 ipsilateral, 1 contralateral, 1 bilateral) were considered probable carotid body tumors.

The usual form of treatment was telecobalt 60 irradiation through a converging pair of

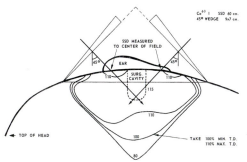

FIG. 3-103. Dose distribution obtained with superoinferior pair of converging wedge filtered ^{60}Co fields in the case of a 35-year-old woman, who 4 weeks earlier had undergone radical mastoidectomy on the right with subtotal excision of a glomus jugulare tumor. Minimum tumor dose was 5,000 rads in 35 days. There has been permanent partial epilation of the treatment fields, but at 3 years 11½ months after irradiation she leads an active life and is clinically tumor-free.

wedge filtered fields, more often along a superoinferior axis than an anteroposterior one. Minimum tumor doses have ranged from 3,450 rads in 25 days to 5,075 rads in 33 days.

All 5 of the patients who were treated 5 or more years ago received minimum tumor doses of not more than 4,500 rads in 35 days and all 5 are alive and clinically free of tumor. The one complication has been a late brain necrosis terminating fatally 38 months after delivery of a minimum dose of 4,975 rads in 38 days to an extensive tumor destroying the base of the skull and involving multiple cranial nerves. A few microscopic foci of residual tumor were found at autopsy. This is the sole known instance in our series of failure to control local tumor.

Both of the fatal brain necroses reported by Bradshaw[1] occurred at the 5,500 r level, ours at approximately the 5,000 rad level. In view of this and the clinically tumor-free long-term courses of our patients treated at the 3,450 to 4,500 rad level, the currently recommended aim is a minimum tumor dose of 4,500 rads in 5 weeks.

BIBLIOGRAPHY

1. Bradshaw, J. D.: Radiotherapy in glomus jugulare tumors. A review of cases seen at the Christie Hospital, Manchester, from 1943 to 1959, *Clin. Radiol.,* 12, 227, 1961.
2. Guild, S. R.: Hitherto unrecognized structure, the glomus jugularis in man, *Anat. Rec.* 79, Supp., 28, 1941.
3. MacComb, W. S.: The treatment of tumors of the carotid body, *Ann. Surg.,* 127, 269, 1948.
4. Williams, I. G.: Radiotherapy of tumours of glomus jugulare, *J. Fac. Radiol.,* 8, 335, 1957.

Tumors Involving the Middle Ear and Mastoid

ELEANOR D. MONTAGUE

The neoplasms involving the auditory canal are primarily squamous cell carcinomas, with basal cell carcinoma the second in frequency. Lesions of the external canal and concha can, by direct extension, reach the middle ear through a previous perforation of the tympanic membrane or by direct involvement of the membrane.[5] In addition, the middle ear may be the site of primary neoplastic disease or it may be involved by secondary extension from adjacent structures such as the petrous pyramid or the mastoid process. A primary neoplasm of the middle ear may also spread by direct extension to the mastoid process and the petrous pyramid. When extension is medial to the mastoid process, the neoplasm quickly breaks through the bone and involves the transverse process of the cervical spine and often the bodies of the first two cervical vertebra.

Whatever may be the site of the primary tumor, one is dealing with a neoplasm which has invaded the temporal bone, mastoid cells, petrous pyramid, cartilage, and a cavity, the middle ear, which is either partially or completely filled by tumor or debris. Almost certainly an element of infection is present.

The guidelines of management are the same whether the tumor originates in the middle ear or has invaded the middle ear from a primary of the external ear.

Treatment for a tumor originating in the middle ear has varied. Published data favor radical surgery alone,[4] radical irradiation alone,[1] or a combination of radical surgery followed by irradiation therapy.[3,6,7] Regardless of the type of treatment selected, the percentage of patients free of disease at 5 years is low—reported as 15 per cent of 143 patients gathered from data published by Ennuyer and Leroux-Robert,[2] and 20 per cent following radical temporal bone resection[4] reported by Lewis and Parsons.

Subtotal surgical removal of tumor (without radical temporal bone and mastoid resection) with or without postoperative irradiation leads to prolonged pain and disability. Occasionally, when irradiation has been given after extirpation, the symptoms are thought to be complications of treatment and, at death, active growing disease is found. For these reasons, surgical exploration and radical tumor extirpation are first indicated in tumors already invading contiguous bone structures: 1) surgical exploration can determine the true extent of disease; 2) radical surgery generally relieves the disabling pain, even when there is known foci of residual tumor; 3) postoperative healing is rapid; and 4) surgery provides adequate drainage of the area. Radiation therapy is better tolerated with less likelihood of symptoms resulting from infection and necrotic tumor when radiation therapy is given after the surgical cavity is covered by a skin graft and the saucerlike cavity has healed.

For lesions extending to a depth of 5 cm, irradiation is effectively accomplished by means of electron beam therapy with a single lateral field. If this modality of therapy is not available, or if the disease is at a greater than 5 cm depth, a pair of 45-degree wedge filtered portals either placed in anteroposterior or superoinferior positions have been utilized. If total treatment volumes are small, 6,000 rads tumor dose delivered to a proper depth, depending on the findings at operation, is well tolerated in 4 weeks; with larger volumes, the treatment time is extended to 5 to 6 weeks (Fig. 3-104).

Twenty-four patients were seen for definitive treatment; one had definitive surgery at an outside institution, but has been followed at M. D. Anderson Hospital. As Table 3-41 indicates, a total of 5 of 11 patients treated with radical surgery are free of disease, but 2 of the 5 were lost to follow-up at 2 years.

Three of 11 patients treated with incomplete excision and postoperative irradiation have survived 2 years without evidence of disease (one adenoacanthoma, one basal, and one squamous cell carcinoma with neck disease treated with irradiation).

Eight patients presented with recurrent disease after definitive treatment failed. Regardless of the selection of definitive treatment or, indeed, selection of treatment for recurrent disease, all 8 patients died within one year of disease of the primary neoplasm.

Even from this limited series, a few conclusions can probably be made:

1) Recurrent neoplasm after definitive treatment establishes very poor prognosis regardless of treatment. Palliative treatment, regardless of modality, is unsuccessful in symptom or pain control.

2) Surgery alone is probably the better treatment for patients with limited lesions. Our experience with irradiation alone for early tumors is too limited for conclusion. For extensive lesions, surgery is still indicated for pain relief and drainage; primary radiotherapy will lead to infection, necrosis, and continuation of pain and symptoms.

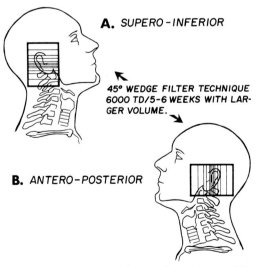

A. SUPERO-INFERIOR

45° WEDGE FILTER TECHNIQUE 6000 TD/5-6 WEEKS WITH LARGER VOLUME.

B. ANTERO-POSTERIOR

FIG. 3-104. Treatment techniques for carcinoma of the middle ear.

BIBLIOGRAPHY

1. Boland, J.: The management of carcinoma of the middle ear, *Radiology,* 80, 285, 1963.
2. Ennuyer, A., and Leroux-Robert, J.: Indications therapeutiques et resultats concernant les epitheliomas du conduit auditif externe et de 1-Oreille Moyen, *J. Radiol. Electr.,* 40, 170, 1959.
3. Frew, I., and Finney, R.: Neoplasms of the middle ear, *J. Laryng.,* 77, 415, 1963.
4. Lewis, J. S., and Parsons, H.: Surgery for advanced ear cancer, *Ann. Otol.,* 67, 364, 1958.
5. Schall, L. A.: In *Diseases of the Nose, Throat, and Ear,* 2nd ed., C. Jackson and C. L. Jackson, Eds., Philadelphia, W. B. Saunders Company, p. 457, 1959.
6. Sorensen, H.: Cancer of the middle ear and mastoid, *Acta Radiol.,* 54, 460, 1960.
7. Tucker, W. N.: Cancer of the middle ear, *Cancer,* 18, 642, 1965.

Table 3-41. Results of Definitive Treatment Attempts for Middle Ear Neoplasms—1944–August, 1969

Primary Treatment	No. of Patients	Dead of Disease or Complications P	N	Dead Other Cancer	Lost to F-U 1 Year	Lost to F-U NED 2+ Years	NED
Radical Surgery: Mastoidectomy Temporal Bone Resection ± Parotidectomy	11	3	1	1*	1	2	1* + 2**
Complete Excision + Postop XRT	1	1-brain necrosis					
Incomplete Excision + Postop XRT	11	8				1*EB 1 adeno-acanthoma ⁶⁰Co wedges	1→N→ XRT→NED
XRT Alone	2	(1***)					1 (probably no bone destruction?)
TOTAL	25	14		1	1	4	5

*Basal carcinoma
**One patient-temporal resection outside institution followed at MDAH
***Residual disease after full-course→S→postop infarct.
All others—squamous cell
P: Primary uncontrolled
N: Neck disease
XRT: Irradiation
EB: Electron beam

Cervical Lymph Node Metastasis: Unknown Primary Cancer

In Collaboration with

RICHARD H. JESSE, JR., and CARLOS A. PEREZ

Introduction

Guidelines for the optimal management of patients with cervical lymph node cancer associated with an unknown primary lesion were outlined in 1966.[1] Radical treatment was advocated employing either a surgical procedure, or radiation therapy, or a combination of the two in relation to the position, size, multiplicity, and histologic features of the nodes in the neck. Since that report, more patients have become available for study, the follow-up period is longer, and a more careful search for potential sites of primary disease has been employed.

The present policies of treatment are based on the results obtained in 210 patients who received definitive treatment for cancer in the neck for which no primary lesion could be determined at the time of the initial treatment. All patients have been followed a minimum of 3 years, almost 90 per cent of them having 5 years or more follow-up.

DIAGNOSTIC WORKUP

The diagnosis of cancer in the cervical nodes was made by surgical biopsy or excision before admission to our institution in 114 (52 per cent) of the patients. If the initial examination at M. D. Anderson Hospital failed to determine the primary site, almost all patients had, under general anesthesia, direct examination and palpation of the mucosal surfaces of the upper respiratory and alimentary tract. Biopsies were performed on any mucosal areas which were slightly abnormal. Random biopsy samples of apparently normal mucosa were usually

taken from the nasopharynx and less often from the base of tongue, tonsillar area, and pyriform sinus. If the primary cancer was found before definitive treatment for the cervical mass was started, the patient was excluded from this study.

The topographical distribution of the nodes according to whether single or multiple, unilateral or bilateral, is shown in Figure 3-105. Twenty-six of 210 patients who had cancer in their supraclavicular nodes are analyzed separately. Disease in the necks of the remaining 184 patients was staged retrospectively according to the following classification.

N_x: Previously excised node, no gross residual cancer.

N_1: Single, mobile, clinically positive node less than 3 cm in diameter.

N_2: Single, mobile, clinically positive node greater than 3 cm in diameter or multiple, mobile, clinically positive, ipsilateral nodes.

N_3: Unilateral, fixed node(s), or bilateral nodes fixed or nonfixed.

TREATMENT

Surgical Operation. One hundred four patients underwent a surgical procedure as initial treatment at the M. D. Anderson Hospital (Table 3-42). Radical neck dissection was most often used with the addition of parotidectomy, or mandibular resection, or subtotal thyroidectomy as indicated. Bilateral radical neck dissection was performed in some patients with bilateral nodal metastases. The majority of the bilateral neck dissections were staged rather than simulta-

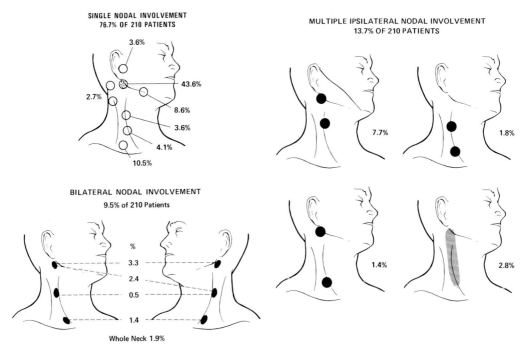

FIG. 3-105. Topographical distribution of nodes on admission. Courtesy: Jesse, Perez, and Fletcher, *Cancer,* 31, 854, 1973.

neously performed, and the jugular vein was preserved on one side, if possible.

Of the 104 patients, 29 had secondary treatment later for disease appearing at the primary site, recurrence in the treated side of the neck, or new disease in the untreated contralateral side of the neck. Of these 29 patients, radiation therapy was given as

Table 3-42. *Type of Surgical Operation in 104 Patients—January 1948–June 1968, (Analysis August 1971)*

Radical neck dissection (RND)	
Unilateral	51
Bilateral	9*
RND with parotidectomy	28
RND with thyroidectomy	4
Wide local excision	5
Partial neck dissection	4
Partial neck dissection	
with parotidectomy	3

*Of the 9, one underwent thyroidectomy and 5 underwent resection of the mandible.

additional treatment to 22, 9 of whom had no evidence of disease (*NED*) 3 years or more after the second treatment. A surgical procedure was chosen as the secondary treatment in 7 of the 29 patients, with 6 having no further cancer for an additional 3 years or more.

Radiation Therapy. Radiation therapy was the initial treatment in 52 patients, 45 of whom had portals covering the nasopharynx, tonsil, base of tongue, and the entire neck. Megavoltage irradiation has been used since 1954. Radiation therapy of the upper portion of the neck and the nasopharynx was given through parallel opposing lateral portals delivering a minimum midline dose of 5,000 rads. If the clinically positive lymph nodes were in the posterior cervical chain, a high probability of a nasopharyngeal primary site existed, and 6,000 rads were given to the nasopharynx. The posterior margin of the portals were moved forward after 4,500 rads were delivered in order to exclude the spinal cord from the field of the beam. Patients with large posterior cervical nodes received a supplemental dose of irradiation employing a posterior split field, the dose then being calculated in the sagittal midplane. Patients with palpable nodes after this dosage received an additional 1,000 to 2,000 rads through small portals covering the residual mass(es) with ^{60}Co glancing fields or appositional portals with 9 to 15 Mev electron beam (Fig. 3-106). If the patient had no node(s) anterior to the subdigastric area, the submaxillary glands were excluded to avoid excessive dryness of the mouth. The lower portion of the neck was irradiated through an anterior field with a midline block to protect the larynx. If no palpable nodes were present, only 5,000 rads given dose was delivered.

Nine of the 52 irradiated patients were treated with techniques less comprehensive than the irradiation outlined above.

Four of the 52 patients had secondary treatment for recurrent disease in the neck (Fig. 3-107) or appearance of cancer at the primary site. One patient treated surgically was free of cancer 3 years following the surgical treatment.

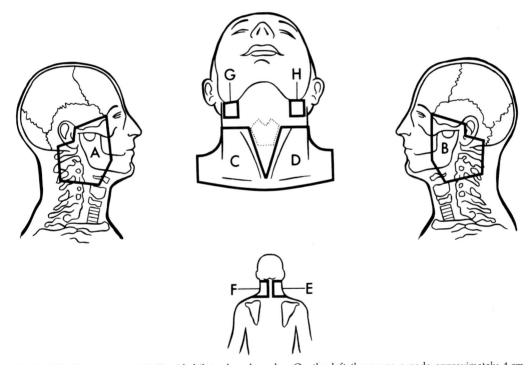

FIG. 3-106. Patient seen 1-19-62 with bilateral neck nodes. On the left there was a node approximately 4 cm in its longest diameter partially underlying the upper end of the sternocleidomastoid muscle. There was an incision over this mass.

On the right there were 3 nodes in the subdigastric and midjugular areas.

The diagnosis was anaplastic squamous cell carcinoma.

Because the right subdigastric node was high and somewhat posterior, the nasopharynx was included and a dose of 5,000 rads in 5 weeks was first given to the nasopharynx and the whole neck.

Further additional therapy was given to the nodes by the use of posterior split field and glancing fields on the ^{60}Co unit. The total dose was 7,000 rads in 7 weeks on the left. On the right the dose was 8,500 rads in 8½ weeks because a node was still palpable at the 7,000 rad dose level.

Six weeks later induration was still felt on the right which took almost 6 months to disappear. The patient was alive and well in January 1971.

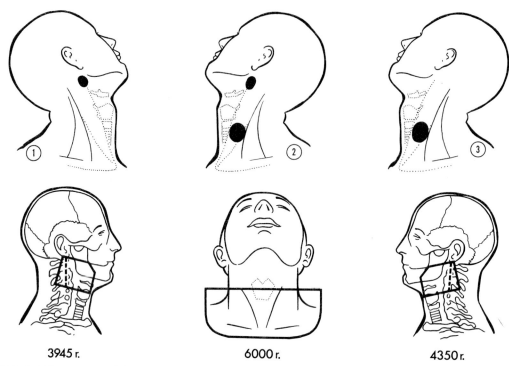

3945 r. 6000 r. 4350 r.

FIG. 3-107. A 70-year-old white male admitted to M. D. Anderson Hospital 7-16-58. He had had a mass overlying the angle of the right mandible for 1 month (1). This had recently been excised at a different institution and reported as undifferentiated squamous carcinoma. No other disease was palpable in the neck and no primary lesion was found on thorough examination. There was one suspicious area in the right valleculum which was biopsied and reported as negative for cancer. On 8-5-58 a right radical neck dissection was performed. The pathology report showed no residual cancer in the specimen. The patient was well for 1 year when he returned with 2 nodes in the opposite side of the neck (2), one subdigastric and the other low jugular in position. Examination at this time revealed the same suspicious area in the right valleculum, and a biopsy taken at this time was positive. The patient was given radiation to the whole neck and to the primary region (lower drawings). ^{60}Co was the unit used and 6,000 rads were given in 35 days. The patient remained well for one more year (until July 1960), at which time he returned with a mass in the low left jugular region (3). This was interpreted to be the same lymph node which had been present at the time of radiation therapy. On 8-5-60 a left radical neck dissection was done. There were two midjugular nodes positive for squamous carcinoma. The patient died July 1970 from a cancer of the sigmoid colon without evidence of disease from his initial tumor.

Treatment for patient with bilateral neck nodes

Field Position	Size	Given Dose	Modality
A—Right lateral	15 × 10 cm	3,900 *r*	
B—Left lateral	15 × 10 cm	4,350 *r*	
C—Right supraclavicular	6 × 16 cm	6,200 *r*	^{60}Co
D—Left supraclavicular		6,200 *r*	
E—Right posterior neck	9 × 9 cm	625 *r*	
F—Left posterior neck		625 *r*	
G—Right glancing on node	6 × 3.5 cm	2,000 *r*	^{137}Cs
H—Left glancing on node	5.5 × 5.5 cm	1,000 *r*	

Planned Combined Therapy. Preoperative irradiation of 2,000 rads in 5 fractions to the involved portion of the neck was employed in 6 patients. Eleven patients received a minimum of 5,000 rads in 5 weeks prior to radical neck dissection. Postoperative irradiation delivering a minimum of 5,000 rads to the entire neck was employed in 11 patients.

Secondary treatment was administered to 5 patients who had recurrence in the treated neck or appearance of cancer at the primary site and was successful in producing an additional 3-year arrest in one surgically treated patient.

RESULTS

The composition of each of the treatment groups according to the staging of the cervical lymph nodes is shown in Figure 3-108. The group treated surgically has a greater proportion of patients with more favorable nodal staging, whereas a greater proportion of less favorably staged patients were in the 2 groups in which radiation therapy was all or part of the treatment. Histologic diagnosis of the nodes was squamous carcinoma in 62 per cent, undifferentiated carcinoma in 28 per cent, and glandular carcinoma of salivary origin in 10 per cent of the patients. Each initial treatment category contained the same proportion of the 3 histologic types.

The incidence of failures of the initial treatment in the treated neck(s) in the 184 patients is tabulated in Table 3-43 according to whether neck disease was early or advanced. In all stages, the combination of radiation therapy and surgical operation was superior to either modality alone. Surgical

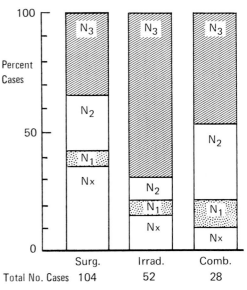

DISTRIBUTION BY CLINICAL STAGE IN 184 PATIENTS TREATED FOR CURE
(Excluding Supraclavicular)

FIG. 3-108. Distribution by clinical stage in 184 patients treated for cure (excluding supraclavicular). January 1948 through June 1968. Analysis August 1971. Unlimited follow-up. (Courtesy: Jesse, Perez, and Fletcher, *Cancer,* 31, 854, 1973.

therapy or radiation therapy were equally effective in controlling early cervical disease. Some superiority of radiotherapy over the surgical procedure was demonstrated in those patients with nodal disease in the advanced stages. If initial treatment to the neck failed, additional therapy was not effective (with one exception) in producing a further disease-free interval.

Only patients having had a unilateral neck

Table 3-43. *Failure of Initial Treatment in the Treated Side of the Neck—184 Patients (3-Years to Unlimited Follow-up) January 1948– June 1968, (Analysis August 1971)*

Stage	Surgery		Radiation Therapy		Combination	
N_x–N_1	13.0%	(6/45)	17.0%	(2/12)	0.0%	(0/6)
N_2–N_3	32.0%	(19/59)	22.0%	(9/40)	18.0%	(4/22)

Table 3-44. *Appearance of Nodes in the Contralateral Side of Neck—164* Patients (3-Years to Unlimited Follow-up)*

	Radiation	
Surgery	Therapy	Combination
16.0% (16/97)	0.0% (0/39)	0.0% (0/28)

*20 patients had initial bilateral neck disease.

dissection as their initial therapy developed nodes in the contralateral side of the neck (Table 3-44). In contrast, no patient having radiation alone or as a portion of treatment developed contralateral metastasis, because the entire neck was included in the initial radiation portals.

Thirty-seven patients developed a primary lesion at some time after the initial treatment to the neck (Table 3-45). The hypopharynx and oropharynx were the most common sites. The majority of the patients who developed primary cancers in the head and neck sites were in the surgically treated groups. The primary cancer in 14 of the 21 patients originally treated surgically was subsequently controlled—in 8 patients by radiotherapy and in 6 patients by surgical methods. The primary cancer in 2 of 7 patients (3 originally treated by radiotherapy and 4 originally treated by combined

methods) was controlled by subsequent surgical excision.

Patients who developed a primary lesion above the clavicle had only a 31 per cent chance of living 3 years, as opposed to 58 per cent for those who never developed a primary lesion in the head and neck area. For the 184 patients, the 3-year absolute cure rate was 53 per cent, tabulated by stage and by initial treatment category in Table 3-46. Also shown are the number of patients who required subsequent treatment to effect this cure. The absolute cure rate in the 151 patients eligible for 5-year follow-up indicates a cure rate of approximately 43 per cent for each treatment category.

SUPRACLAVICULAR NODES

Few of the 26 patients with disease in the supraclavicular nodes survived regardless of the treatment. Two of the 3 surviving patients had a single involved node, whereas only one having multiple, diseased nodes survived. The incidence of later appearance of a primary lesion is higher in this group of patients than in the groups in which the nodes are in the upper portion of the neck. Palliative irradiation only is usually indicated (Chapter 14, Palliation).

Table 3-45. *Location of Primary Lesions Appearing Posttreatment— 37 Patients (3-Years to Unlimited Follow-up)*

	Surg.	Irradiation	Combination Rx.
Nasopharynx	2	—	—
Maxillary antrum	—	—	1
Tonsil or faucial arch	4	—	1
Base of tongue, valleculum	4	—	—
Oral cavity, salivary glands	2	2	—
A-R fold, epiglottis	1	—	1
Hypopharynx	6	1	1
Cervical esophagus	1	—	—
Thyroid	1	—	—
Total Head and Neck	21/104	3/52	4/28
New Primaries	(20%)	(6%)	(14%)
Primaries Below Clavicle	5	3	1

Table 3-46. *Three-Year Absolute Survival: Free of Cancer—184 Patients*

	Surgery		Radiation Therapy		Combination	
N_x	79.0%	(31/39)	89.0%	(8/9)	—	(3/3)
N_1	67.0%	(4/6)	—	(1/3)	—	(1/3)
N_2	45.0%	(10/22)	75.0%	(3/4)	55.0%	(5/9)
N_3	38.0%	(14/37)	36.0%	(13/36)	31.0%	(4/13)
Total	57.0%	(59/104)*	48.0%	(25/52)**	47.0%	(13/28)***

*Includes 8 patients salvaged by XRT and 6 patients salvaged by surgery
**Includes 1 patient salvaged by surgery
***Includes 1 patient salvaged by surgery

PRESENT POLICIES

Radiation therapy and surgical operation are not competing modalities in the treatment of the patients with cervical node(s) associated with an unknown primary cancer. Based on the clinical presentation of the node(s), the treatment team must select the therapy which will give the highest control while providing the patient with an optimal quality of life. Partial or radical neck dissection appears to be an adequate treatment for the single node in the submaxillary triangle and the low subdigastric node(s). The data show that radiation therapy will produce an equal result. Which is chosen for a patient is a matter of philosophy. We would prefer not to maximalize radiation therapy treatment to produce just a few more patients free of cancer, if the alternative is to make all treated patients uncomfortable because of severe dryness. In the patient with a single node in the submaxillary triangle, a great deal of the mucosa of the oral cavity and upper pharynx would be included in the irradiation portals. The dose necessary to successfully prevent the appearance of a primary and contralateral metastases produces a dryness which may not be worthwhile to this patient since a surgical procedure can easily manage an oral cavity primary and also salvage contralateral metastases.

A surgical procedure is also preferred for a single moveable node in the low subdigastric or midjugular region, since the radiation fields must cover also the larynx and hypopharynx. Even though these sites are likely to harbor a primary lesion, we would prefer not to treat them electively with irradiation when the node is single.

Radiation therapy covering the nasopharynx, tonsillar fossa, base of tongue, and the entire lymph node-bearing area of the neck through fields which spare the larynx and hypopharynx is preferred as the only treatment for patients with small high jugular nodes, and those who have posterior cervical nodes. Patients with mobile, multiple level, ipsilateral nodes, bilateral nodes, or fixed nodes receive a high dose (5,000 rads) of irradiation to the pharynx, larynx, and the whole neck. A radical or partial neck dissection is indicated 3 to 6 weeks later.

Postoperative radiotherapy is usually reserved for those patients originally selected for surgery, but in whom the specimen shows more cancer in the neck than was appreciated on the clinical examination.

The number of patients in the surgically treated group whose primary lesion subsequently is found to be in the oropharynx or hypopharynx is disturbing and indicates that random biopsies of these areas should be routinely performed. Our reluctance to include the larynx in the radiation fields also accounts for some of the hypopharyngeal primaries manifested later. The risk, while not great, of having the primary appear later in the patient who does not receive high dose irradiation to the larynx has to be balanced against the possible undesirable complications of such treatment. The practices of routine blind biopsies of the nasopharynx plus irradiation of the nasopharynx when nodes are typically located in the high posterior triangle have almost eliminated the nasopharynx as being a site of subsequently appearing primary lesions.

BIBLIOGRAPHY

1. Jesse, R. H., Neff, L. E.: Metastatic carcinoma in cervical nodes with an unknown primary lesion, *Amer. J. Surg.,* 112, 547, 1966.
2. Jesse, R. H., Perez, C. A., and Fletcher, G. H.: Cervical lymph node metastasis: Unknown primary cancer, *Cancer,* 31, 854, 1973.

Nasal and Paranasal Sinus Carcinoma

In Collaboration with

HELMUTH GOEPFERT, and RICHARD H. JESSE, JR.

The symptoms of early nasal and paranasal sinus carcinoma are unspecific and mimic inflammatory disease. Often patients have a long history of sinus trouble and it is the sudden dramatic change in their symptomatology which brings them to seek medical attention with more or less advanced lesions.[6,8,10]

The great majority of malignant tumors are squamous cell carcinomas and their varieties including lymphoepithelioma, transitional cell carcinoma and the spindle cell carcinoma variant. Next in frequency are different types of minor salivary gland carcinomas and the adenocarcinomas, primary mucosal malignant melanomas, nonclassified or undifferentiated carcinomas and metastatic carcinomas. The nonepithelial malignant neoplasms include rhabdomyosarcomas of embryonal and alveolar variety, hemangiosarcoma, osteogenic sarcomas, chondrosarcomas, Ewing's sarcomas, the varieties of malignant lymphomas, plasmacytomas and esthesioneuroblastomas.[2,11,13]

Accurate histological diagnosis is important to decide on the proper modality of treatment for tumors with different biological behavior. The exact site of origin and extension of the disease have to be determined with accuracy based on clinical examination and the radiographic studies.

After the completion of treatment, patients need to be followed for an extended time as some tumors, notoriously the adenocarcinomas and the salivary gland carcinomas, can recur after prolonged periods of apparent control of the disease process.

Paranasal Sinuses

The site of origin can be within the ethmoid cell complex, within the maxillary antrum, in the frontal and the sphenoid sinuses. The pattern of local extension is different for each of these locations. Different methods of staging of the disease are available. Baclesse, Öhngren, Sisson, and Lederman have presented modes of classifications by anatomical site of origin and extension.[1,11,12,16] In very extensive lesions, the primary site of origin is difficult to determine.

The radiologic examination is indispensable to establish the site of origin and routes of spread of the primary tumor. Radiographs in Caldwell Waters, lateral submentovertical projections and frontal tomograms are routine. Lateral and oblique tomograms are used in certain circumstances.[3,4,8]

In selected cases, contrast studies of the sinuses and nasopharynx are helpful. Angiography is reserved for those cases in which intracranial extension is suspected.

Maxillary Antrum

Within the maxillary antrum (Fig. 3-109), there are two main sites of origin.

1) Lesions originating in the suprastructure: these can extend into nasal cavity, ethmoid cells, orbit, the pterygopalatine fossa, and the base of the skull, the zygoma, and infratemporal fossa, the inferior orbital rim, and the soft tissues of the cheek. The infraorbital nerve is of special importance as a route of spread in this location.

2) Lesions originating in the infrastructure: these can be confused with those originating in the upper gum. The routes of local extension include the alveolar process and gingivobuccal sulcus, the soft tissues of the cheek and masseter muscle, the palate and nose, the pterygoid fossa, and the pterygopalatine space.

Frontal and Sphenoid Sinuses

Primary carcinoma of the frontal and sphenoid sinuses (Fig. 3-109) is extremely rare. Sphenoid sinus carcinomas may present as intracranial tumors or as nasopharyngeal carcinoma by virtue of the pattern of local spread.

Ethmoid Cells

Tumors of the ethmoid cells (Fig. 3-110) are predominantly undifferentiated squamous cell carcinomas. The spread is into the contralateral ethmoid complex, through the ethmoidomaxillary plate into the antrum, through the lamina papyracea into the orbit and into the nasal cavity invading septum and turbinates. Posteriorly they may penetrate into the sphenoid sinus and nasopharynx, superiorly into the anterior cranial fossa and frontal sinus, and anteriorly into the frontonasal angle.

Nasal Carcinoma

The nasal cavity (Fig. 3-110) can be divided into three regions:

1) The vestibule is the portion in front of the limen nasi limited by the alae, the corresponding portion of the membraneous septum, the caudal end of the cartilaginous septum, columnella and adjacent floor of the nasal cavity. Tumors in this area are essentially skin cancers and although very often localized and amenable to simple therapy, they can present difficult problems when infiltrating into the floor of the nose and the upper lip.

2) The olfactory region is at the apex of the nasal cavity and extends as a narrow strip along the roof and lamina cribosa plus adjoining septum and lateral walls. This is the site of origin of the esthesioneuroblastoma and some adenocarcinomas.

3) In the respiratory portion of the nasal cavity behind the limen nasi, two sites of tumor origin can be established. The superior group lies above the horizontal plane at the level of insertion of the middle turbinate. The local extension in this area can occur into the opposite nasal cavity, into the ethmoid cell complex and the orbit, into the superior-medial part of the antrum, and into the anterior cranial fossa. The inferior group can spread into the opposite side, into the antrum, into the nasopharynx through the posterior choana, into the vestibule and into the hard palate.

Treatment Planning

The few patients with very small lesions, without bone destruction may require treatment with only one modality of treatment, either surgery, or radiation therapy. For most of the patients, close team work between the

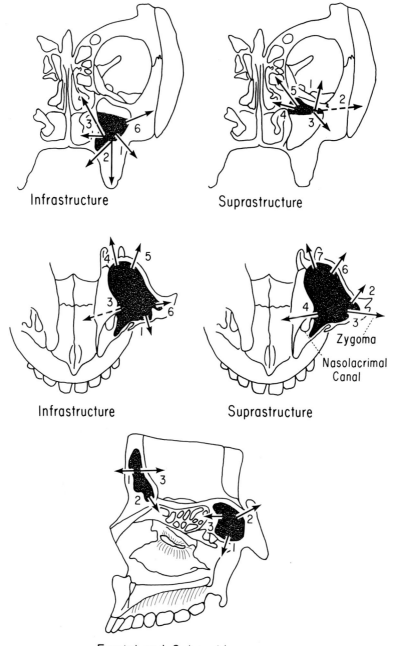

Infrastructure **Suprastructure**

Infrastructure **Suprastructure**

Zygoma

Nasolacrimal Canal

Frontal and Sphenoid

FIG. 3-109. Routes of spread, paranasal sinus carcinomas.

Antral Infrastructure Origin: 1. Into the alveolar process, gingivobuccal sulcus and soft tissues of the cheek below the zygoma. 2. Into the nasal cavity and hard palate. 3. Into the pterygoid plates and pterygopalatine space.

Antral Suprastructure Origin: 1. Into the zygoma, posterolaterally into the infratemporal fossa, and into the orbit. 2. Into the nasal cavity, ethmoid sinuses and orbit. 3. Into the pterygopalatine space and base of skull. This occurs more commonly than it does in infrastructure lesions.

Frontal Sinus Origin: 1. Anteriorly producing mass in the region of the bregna and nasion, often with secondary infection. 2. Into the ethmoid sinuses and through the superior medial wall of the orbit. 3. Into the dura and frontal lobes.

Sphenoid Sinus Origin: 1. Into the nasopharynx. 2. Through the floor of the middle cranial fossa and sella turcica. 3. Into the posterior ethmoid cells and nasal cavity. (Adapted from: Boone, Harle, and Higholt, In *Head and Neck, An Atlas of Tumor Radiology,* Vol. I, Fletcher and Jing, Chicago, Year Book Medical Publishers, Inc., p. 239, 1968.)

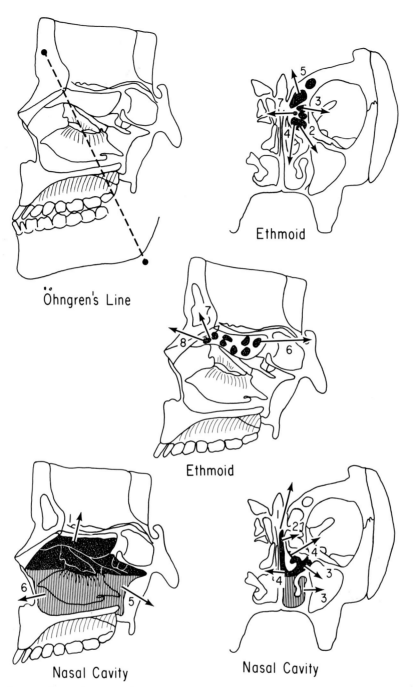

FIG. 3-110. Routes of spread, paranasal sinus carcinomas.

Öhngren's line separates the favorable lesions of the infrastructure from the less curable ones of the suprastructure, ethmoids and posterior nasal cavity.

Ethmoid Sinus Origin: 1. Into contralateral ethmoid sinuses. 2. Into the antrum with erosion of the ethmoidomaxillary plate. 3. Into the orbit. 4. Into the nasal cavity with invasion of the septum and turbinates. 5. Into the sphenoid sinus, nasopharynx and base of the skull. 6. Into the frontal sinus, cribriform plate and anterior cranial fossa. 7. Forward into the frontonasal angle (excluding vestibule).

Nasal Cavity Origin: 1. Into the anterior cranial fossa, ethmoid cells, orbit, antrum and commonly posteriorly into the sphenoid sinus and along the base of the skull and roof of the nasopharynx. 2. Posteriorly to protrude through the posterior choana, superiorly into the upper nasal cavity and occasionally to the other side of the nose. (Adapted from: Boone, Harle, and Higholt, In *Head and Neck, An Atlas of Tumor Radiology,* Vol. I, Fletcher and Jing, Chicago, Year Book Medical Publishers, p. 239, 1968.)

surgeon and the radiotherapist is of paramount importance in order to achieve the best results with a combined therapeutic approach.

Lymphomas, rhabdomyosarcomas, Ewing's sarcomas, malignant midline reticulosis, and esthesioneuroblastomas are managed essentially by radiation therapy alone. Systemic chemotherapy is used as an adjuvant for rhabdomyosarcomas and Ewing's sarcomas and occasionally it is used in lymphomas.

Radiation therapy for squamous cell carcinoma can be used preoperatively or postoperatively. Theoretically, preoperative radiotherapy is superior to postoperative, because it decreases the number of cancer cells in the field. If the preoperative dose is high, however, an increased morbidity and mortality rate can be expected, which will negate the beneficial effects of preoperative therapy. We therefore use the preoperative approach in the younger age group and in patients with a balanced metabolic status and in good general health. Patients over the age of 70 and those with a negative nutritional balance and a history of recent weight loss are best treated with surgical resection and postoperative radiotherapy because of impaired healing. Experience has shown that survival is equal for both combinations of treatment when the patients are selected for therapy this way.[7] For most patients we presently prefer surgical operation followed by radiation therapy.

Radiation Therapy Techniques

A variety of geometrical patterns according to anatomical sites and extensions are shown in Figure 3-111.

The paranasal sinuses and nasal cavity are an anatomic area where sophisticated wedge filter techniques are especially useful. Because of the rounded contour of the face, a right angle pair of wedge filtered portals may seem to be optimal but this is rarely, if ever, used because the opposite eye is in the treatment field. Furthermore, in practice, overlap-

ping or missing is not easy to avoid at the junction of portals at right angle. A dose distribution which is superior to right angle wedges in several respects may be achieved by posterior angulation of the lateral field. Care must be taken to be sure that the lateral angulated field extends posteriorly far enough to encompass lateral disease. This reduces the dose to the contralateral eye and also raises the dose posteromedially in the region of the pterygopalatine space.

For tumors originating and extending largely in the midline (ethmoid, frontal, sphenoid, nasal), an appropriately shaped anterior open field is used (Fig. 3-112). Figure 3-113 shows the portal film in a patient with a squamous cell carcinoma of the ethmoids. The anterior field may be L-shaped if disease has extended into a maxillary sinus (Fig. 3-114). Addition of a pair of lateral wedge filtered portals yields a homogeneous dose pattern extending posteriorly as far as required. If disease extends far anteriorly, 6,000 rads are given through an anterior portal with dose build-up posteriorly with wedged lateral portals. Often the anterior field can be reduced near the conclusion of treatment and the additional radiation given as a "boost." High energy electrons, because of their limited depth of penetration, may be used to an advantage for a portion of the anterior radiation and may be tailored to spare the underlying frontal lobes and brain stem. A combination of 22 Mev and ^{60}Co irradiation to an anterior field gives a satisfactory dose distribution.

Tumor doses are in the range of 5,000 rads in 5 weeks preoperatively; 5,000 rads in 5 weeks to 6,000 rads in 6 weeks are given postoperatively. When irradiation alone is used, 6,000 rads are given in 6 weeks with the treatment plans described above and an additional 500 to 1,000 rads may be given through reduced fields to areas of probable extension of the disease, such as the pterygoid space, zygomatic-temporal area, etc.

When orbital involvement has not been demonstrated, it is tempting to avoid irradia-

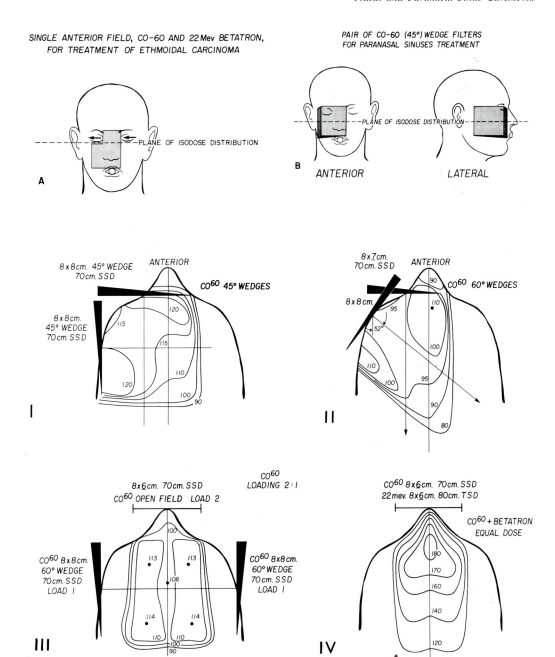

FIG. 3-111. **A.** Portal for a tumor of the ethmoid cells extending to the homolateral nasal cavity and antrum. The eyes are turned to the side involved. The homolateral margin transects the homolateral eyeball, avoiding the cornea. On the uninvolved side the margin is at the inner canthus. **B.** Wedge filter portals at 90-degrees for tumor of the maxillary antrum. The eyes may or may not be shielded depending upon invasion of the orbit. **C.** Volume distributions. I, 45-degree wedge filtered portals at right angle; II, 60-degree wedge filtered portals sparing completely the opposite eye; III, three fields, one anterior open field and two parallel opposing portals with wedge filters for a tumor involving ethmoids, antra, sphenoid sinus, and nasal cavity. A tilt of 5 to 10 degrees posteriorly of the lateral portals avoids irradiating the eyes; IV, half of the treatment with ^{60}Co and 22 Mev.

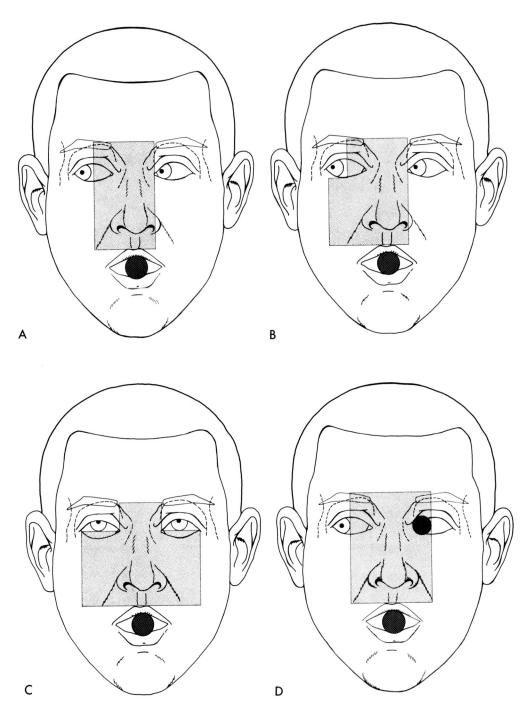

FIG. 3-112. Portals employed in the irradiation of tumors of the ethmoids and nasal cavity.
A. Coverage for unilateral ethmoid/nasal cavity involvement. **B.** Field for ethmoid/nasal cavity tumor with spread to the ipsilateral maxillary antrum. **C.** Portal for ethmoid/nasal cavity tumor with invasion of the maxillary antra bilaterally. **D.** Portal for bilateral ethmoid/nasal cavity tumor or with involvement of the sphenoid sinus. (Note left corneal eye block). (Courtesy: Shukovsky and Fletcher, *Radiology,* 104, 629, 1972.)

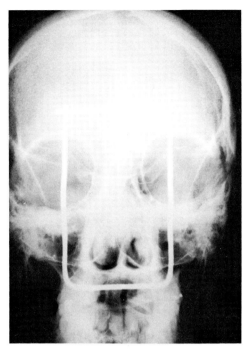

FIG. 3-113. Simulated portal film of a 54-year-old man who was first seen in February 1962, with a squamous cell carcinoma of the right ethmoid involving the nasal cavity and sphenoid sinus. The patient was treated with an anterior I-shaped field while gazing to the right. In addition, a tungsten corneal block was used over the left cornea. The optic foramen (and, therefore, part of the optic nerve) was not shielded by this block. The minimum tumor dose was 6,025 rads in 34 days, taken at 8 cm depth to cover the sphenoid sinus. The estimated dose to the right retina was 7,450 rads in 34 days. The left retina was outside the treatment field, but the left optic nerve received 7,330 rads in 34 days.

The patient had diminishing vision in the right eye progressing from March 1963 to right unilateral blindness in June 1965. Ophthalmologists reported multiple retinal hemorrhages and atrophy in the right eye. The left eye was normal to visual field and acuity testing and funduscopic examination. The right eye was enucleated in December 1965 for intractable pain.

In September 1966, the patient noted decreasing visual acuity in the left eye. This progressed to total blindness within one month. The ophthalmologist reported a normal funduscopic examination with

tion of the ipsilateral eye, but this may lead to inadequate irradiation of disease.[3,15] The roof of the antrum rises posteromedially and the use of an eye shield may produce an unwitting reduction in dose to disease in this region since the antral roof often rises to the level of the cornea (Fig. 3-115). There is marked anatomic variation in this respect, however, and evaluation of the individual case is required. Shielding of the eye may also result in decreased dose to the floor of the middle cranial fossa and foramen rotundum. When the eye is shielded, the floor of the anterior cranial fossa and ethmoidal regions may receive insufficient irradiation if these areas receive no dose contribution from lateral fields and an inadequate dose from a narrow upward prolongation of the anterior field.

Shielding of the homolateral eye from irradiation should be done only with great care to ensure adequate dosage to all known or probable disease extension adjacent to the orbit.[15] With shielding, a 5-degree upward tilt should be used.

Regional Infusion Chemotherapy and External Irradiation

The association of intra-arterial infusion and external irradiation is used for the treatment of advanced local disease. Unilateral or bilateral external carotid artery cannulation is done through the superficial temporal route. In the majority of cases, we use 5-fluorouracil, 4 to 6 mg/kg per day in a continuous infusion over 2 weeks. If methotrexate is to be used, 50 mg per day with the concomitant use of systemic citrovorium fac-

the exception of a slightly pale disc. However, six months later the same physician noted "the classical white disc of optic atrophy."

This patient also had sensory loss of the olfactory nerves. He is without evidence of disease 8 years after treatment. (Courtesy: Shukovsky and Fletcher, *Radiology* 104, 629, 1972.)

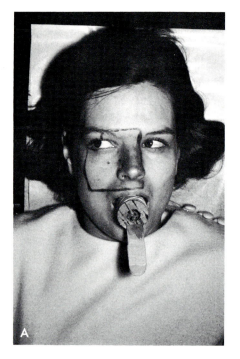

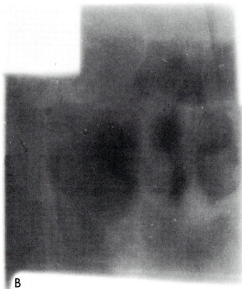

tor (Leucovorin) 6 mg IM q 6 hours. Radio-therapy is started on the second day of infusion at a rate of 1,000 rads per week. After completion of the infusion the radiation therapy is continued to a total dose of 5,000 to 6,000 rads.[9]

The combined treatment brings about an intense local reaction, sometimes severe and disabling. On the skin, dry and often moist desquamating dermatitis is seen during the second week of treatment. Fibrinous mucositis with shallow ulceration is always seen on the palate and sometimes extends to the nonirradiated portion of the oral cavity, mucosa, and to part of the pharynx. The eye in the treatment field can present conjunctivitis and variable degrees of keratitis, which may progress to a corneal ulceration and require proper ophthalmologic care.

The late complications of this combined treatment include soft part ulceration and osteoradionecrosis, which has been an important side effect in 2 of 20 patients but has required a major surgical procedure in only one patient. Four patients out of 20 became blind in the treated eye between 7 and 13 months following treatment; 2 of these, who had a unilateral infusion, developed optic neuritis on the opposite eye and subsequent total blindness at 11 and 18 months following treatment, respectively.

Surgical Treatment

A variety of surgical procedures are available to eradicate the tumor.[8] Fundamentally,

FIG. 3-114. Twenty-eight-year-old woman seen in January 1970, with a history of nasal bleeding. A sinus tumor survey demonstrated partial absence of the middle turbinate on the right and partial absence of the lower turbinate on the right. There were changes in the right maxillary and right ethmoid sinuses due to obstructive phenomena. Biopsy from the right nostril showed poorly differentiated malignant neoplasm.

Using ^{60}Co for half of the treatment and the 22 Mev beam for the other half, 6,000 rads were delivered in 40 days at a depth of 7 cm.

The patient is *NED* in August 1972.

A. Patient in treatment position with lateral eye gaze. **B.** Portal film of **A** taken with 22 Mev x-rays. The orbit is vertically bisected. (Courtesy: Shukovsky and Fletcher, *Radiology,* 104, 629, 1972.)

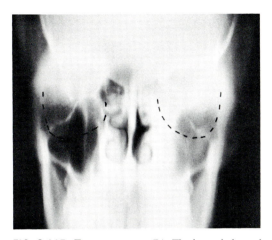

FIG. 3-115. Tomogram: 5 cm PA: The lower halves of the bony orbits have been outlined by use of the 3 cm PA tomogram. Note that approximately one third of the right maxillary antrum projects above the inferior orbital rim. Shielding the right eye in such a case could result in inadequate irradiation of tumor if it occupied the region of the antral roof, especially medially. There is considerable variability in the degree of upward slope of the posterior antral roof, even from one side to the other in the same individual as shown in this case. (Courtesy: Boone, Harle, Higholt, and Fletcher, *Amer. J. Roentgen.,* 102, 627, 1968.)

the procedures are tailored to the extent of the disease. In the majority of cases, the minimal procedure is a radical maxillectomy through a Weber-Ferguson incision and the entire antrum is removed without entering the cavity. If the cancer has spread beyond the antrum, the procedure has to be extended accordingly.

If cancer has broken through the orbital wall, it is advisable to remove the eye. The removal of the orbital floor without removing the orbital contents is very often associated with uncompensated diplopia in spite of reconstructive or prosthetic attempts to keep both eyes level. The ethmoid cells and the anterior wall of the sphenoid sinus are usually exposed and curetted if not partially removed in the extended resections.

The head and neck surgeon and the neurosurgeon must combine talents if the lesion dictates the necessity of removing part of the floor of the anterior fossa, the cribiform plate, or tumor growth along the maxillary nerve and the gasserian ganglion.[10]

The nasal septum and the nasal bones are included in the resection whenever there is extension into the nasal cavity.

When there is invasion of the pterygoid fossa, the ascending ramus of the mandible is included in the dissection to get adequate exposure to this area.[5] The pterygoid muscles are resected in their entirety along with the whole pterygoid process which is taken off at its base at the level of the pterygoid canal.

Resection of the ethmoid sinuses and the walls of the upper part of the nasal cavity, without removal of the whole maxillary antrum is occasionally done for disease exclusively confined to these areas.[14] The infraorbital nerve is resected in the foramen rotundum at the level of the dural envelope. If the nerve is involved at this point, the neurosurgeon will resect the gasserian ganglion through a temporal fossa approach after an interval of 7 to 14 days.

A split-thickness skin graft is used to cover all surfaces. When part of the palate is removed, an immediate prothesis or temporary obturator is inserted.[8] If large areas of skin of the cheek and buccal wall have to be removed, soft tissue reconstruction is done in subsequent operative sessions.

NASAL VESTIBULE

Squamous cell carcinoma of the nasal vestibule and of the anteroinferior part of the nasal septum can be equally well eradicated by external radiotherapy in the form of electron beam, ^{60}Co, by radium needle implant (Fig. 3-116), or by radium molds (Fig. 1-30).

The surgical excision and immediate repair is used only for limited lesions which can be repaired by split-thickness skin or small pedicle grafts. More extensive lesions growing into the floor of the nose and into the upper lip require a large removal of tissue

1.0 mg. x 3 = 3.0 mg.
2.0 mg. x 2 = 4.0 mg.
1.33 mg. x 2 = 2.66 mg.

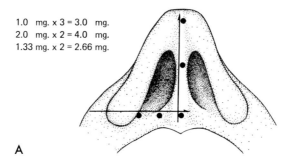

A

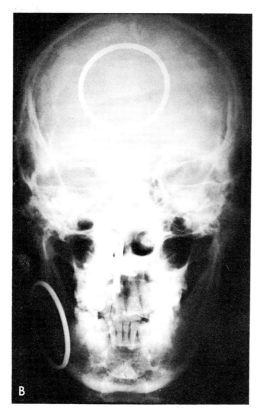

B

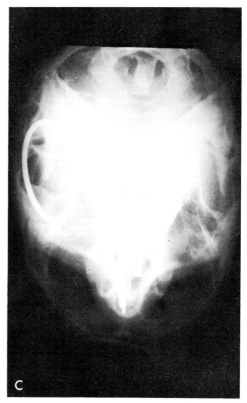

C

FIG. 3-116. Thirty-seven-year-old male seen in October 1956 with a history of having had a lesion removed from the right nasal cavity some 20 months previously which was reported malignant but no further therapy given. He began having bloody discharge from the nose and on admission to M. D. Anderson Hospital, biopsy of the right columella showed mixed squamous and basal cell carcinoma.

The patient had a single L-shape plane radium implant which covered the septum and the floor of the right nostril for the 1 × 1.5 cm lesion. The implant delivered, at 4 and 5 cm on the inside of the curvature, a dose of 6,200 rads in 5 days.

The patient was *NED* in September 1971.

and often necessitate complicated surgical repairs. These large lesions are treated by radiotherapy, since the results are excellent and the cosmetic results outweigh the minor complaint of dryness of the mucous membranes.

If surgical resection of an extensive primary lesion or the rarely recurrent lesion after radiotherapy is necessary, a temporary prosthesis of soft acrylic is used and the eventual repair of the defect is deferred.

When the disease extends into the upper lip, the incidence of ipsilateral and also contralateral cervical lymph node metastases is high. If nodes are present, a radical neck dissection is done and the lymphatics of the face and the cheek are included in the treatment field of postoperative radiotherapy.

Results of Treatment

Between January 1954 and December 1968, a total of 226 patients with a variety of tumors of the paranasal sinus, 31 patients with tumors of the nasal cavity proper and 20 patients with squamous cell carcinoma of the nasal vestibule were observed at MDAH (Table 3-47).

One hundred forty-nine patients with squamous cell carcinoma of the paranasal

Table 3-47. *Histology—January 1954– December 1968*

Histology	No. of Patients	
	Paranasal Sinus	Nasal Cavity
Squamous cell carcinoma	149	15
Adenocarcinoma	12	5
Salivary gland	12	3
Malignant melanoma	1	5
Unclassified + miscella.	52	3
Total	226	31

Table 3-48. *Paranasal Sinus—Cumulative Recurrence Rate—Squamous Cell Carcinoma*

<6 months	<1 year	<2 years	<5 years
66%	76%	95%	100%

sinuses were seen. Of this group, 124 patients completed definitive therapy. Eight of the remaining 25 patients refused therapy, 8 did not complete therapy, 7 had disease too advanced for treatment and 2 had only systemic chemotherapy because of their advanced disease. None of these 25 survived over 1 year.

A cumulative recurrence rate of the treated patients is seen in Table 3-48. Of the recurrences from squamous cell carcinoma, 66 per cent present within the first year and only 5 per cent occur later then the second year after definitive treatment.

Of the treated group, 95 patients with squamous cell carcinoma of the paranasal sinuses were eligible for a 5-year follow-up. These were staged according to the method outlined by Sisson et al.[15] T_1 and T_2 type tumors have a considerably better 5-year absolute survival rate than the more advanced T_3 and T_4 lesions (Table 3-49). For 95 patients treated for cure, the absolute 5-year survival was 37 per cent and the determinate survival was 42 per cent.

Cause of failure are slightly different depending on the primary site of involvement (Fig. 3-117). Squamous cell carcinomas of ethmoid sinus origin show a higher propensity to present distant metastases, when compared to this lesion originating within the maxillary antrum (Table 3-50). Death caused from ethmoid carcinoma can occur later than 2 years after treatment and very often a combination of local recurrence, regional lymph node and distant metastases is the cause of treatment failure. If a maxillary antrum carcinoma fails to respond to treatment, it will more often be because of local recurrence or persistence of disease at the site of the primary.

Table 3-49. *Paranasal Sinus—Squamous Cell Carcinoma—Survival According to T Staging of 95 Patients—Eligible for 5-Year Follow-up*

	Absolute Survival—5-Year		
	T_1 & T_2	T_3 & T_4	Total
Radiation	0/3	1/13	
Radiation + Infusion	—	3/9	
Surgery	7/11	6/19	
Radiation + Surgery	8/11	10/29	
Total Absolute	60%	28%	37%
Total Determinate	68%	33%	42%

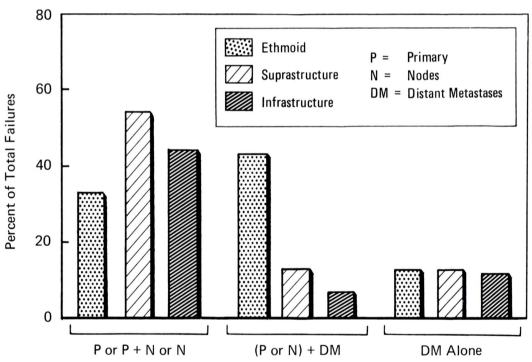

CAUSES OF FAILURE
Squamous Cell Carcinoma of Paranasal Sinuses

FIG. 3-117. Recurrent or persistent disease at the site of primary tumor is the principal reason for failure in the treatment of paranasal squamous cell carcinoma.

Primary tumors of the ethmoid sinuses have a higher incidence of clinically apparent distant metastases.

Table 3-50. *Ethmoid Sinuses—Squamous Cell Carcinoma*

	Primary Site Failure	Absolute Survival	
		2-Year	5-Year
Radiation	4	4/7	1/5
Radiation + Infusion	1	0/1	0/1
Surgery	0	1/1	0/0
Surgery + Radiation	1	4/6	2/5
Total Absolute		60%	27%
Total Determinate		69%	37%

Frontal and Sphenoidal Sinuses

All of these patients were treated by radiotherapy. Two patients were treated for squamous carcinoma of the frontal sinus; neither survived 2 years. Two patients were treated for squamous carcinoma of the sphenoid sinus; although one survived 2 years, neither survived 5 years.

Ethmoid Cells (Table 3-50)

Sixty per cent of patients with primary tumors within the ethmoid sinuses are alive at 2 years.

Patient survival decreases to 27 per cent by 5-year periods due, in part, to recurrences of the primary site but to a greater extent to the development of distant metastases. The combination of radiation and surgery offers a better control of the disease at the primary site.

Maxillary Antrum (Tables 3-51 and 3-52)

Early lesions can be handled properly by surgical therapy alone in both locations, the suprastructure and the infrastructure. This is reflected in the tables and in the very satisfactory survival by this modality of treatment. Combined treatment, either by irradiation and surgery or irradiation and infusion, is reserved for the more advanced-type lesions. For the suprastructure lesions, the absolute 2-year survival of 53 per cent and a 5-year survival of 37 per cent have been achieved, respectively. Satisfactory results are obtained by combining radiation therapy

Table 3-51. *Suprastructure—Squamous Cell Carcinoma*

	Primary Site Failure	Absolute Survival	
		2-Year	5-Year
Radiation	4	1/7	0/4
Radiation + Infusion	4	5/10	1/6
Surgery*	11	13/25	7/14
Surgery + Radiation	6	16/24	9/22
Total Absolute		53%	37%
Total Determinate		55%	42%

*Surgery alone is reserved for the more localized or earlier lesions thus giving adequate control of the disease process.

Table 3-52. *Infrastructure—Squamous Cell Carcinoma*

	Primary Site Failure	Absolute Survival	
		2-Year	5-Year
Radiation	2	1/5	0/3
Radiation + Infusion	0	2/2	2/2
Surgery*	5	9/18	6/16
Surgery + Radiation	4	9/14	7/13
Total Absolute		54%	44%
Total Determinate		60%	48%

*Surgery alone is reserved for the more localized or earlier lesions thus giving adequate control of the disease process.

with infusion, provided the disease does not extend too far into the area supplied by the internal carotid artery (ethmoid cells, olfactory area, and orbit).

Within the infrastructure a 2-year survival of 54 per cent and a 5-year survival of 44 per cent is observed. Here again, surgery is reserved for the more limited lesions and the combination of radiation and surgery or radiation and infusion is used for the more advanced lesions.

Neck Nodes

Neck node metastases were present upon admission in 10 patients and developed at a later date during the follow-up in another 18 patients. Twenty-one patients were treated; 4 with radiation therapy and 17 with surgery alone or a combination of surgery and postoperative radiotherapy. Eight of the 21 treated patients survived 2 years (38 per cent); only one patient survived 5 years.

Nasal Cavity Proper

Squamous cell carcinoma of the nasal cavity proper was treated in 15 patients. The survival rate is 90 per cent at 5 years (Table 3-53). This good survival reflects in part the fact that lesions in this area become symptomatic at an earlier stage and therefore the patient seeks medical attention early.

Table 3-53. *Nasal Cavity Proper—Squamous Cell Carcinoma*

	Absolute Survival	
	2-Year	5-Year
Radiation	6/6	4/5
Radiation + Infusion	1/1	0/0
Surgery	5/6	5/5
Surgery + Radiation	1/2	1/1
Total Absolute and Determinate	87%	91%

Nasal Vestibule

Squamous cell carcinoma of the nasal vestibule has a 2-year survival of 95 per cent and a 5-year survival of 76 per cent (Table 3-54). Failures are due predominantly to large primary or recurrent lesions invading the upper lip with subsequent lymph node metastases.

Table 3-54. *Nasal Vestibule—Squamous Cell Carcinoma*

	Absolute Survival	
	2-Year	5-Year
Radiation	9/10	8/10
Surgery	10/10	5/7
Absolute Survival	95%	76%
Determinate Survival	95%	87%

Malignant Melanoma

Only 1 of 5 patients survived 5 years. This patient had a primary lesion of the nasal cavity treated by radiation therapy alone. The other 4 patients died of local recurrent disease plus a combination of lymph node metastases and distant metastases.

Adenocarcinomas and Malignant Salivary Gland Tumors (Table 3-55)

Good control has been obtained with both groups of tumors if the lesion is in the nasal cavity. This is probably due to the early diagnosis of tumors in this location. Control of these lesions is less satisfactory if the primary is in the paranasal sinuses since the tumor is more advanced before it becomes symptomatic. Prolonged follow-up is important in patients with these tumors since local recurrences occur after several years of apparent cure.

Treatment of Recurrences

For recurrent lesions, very often no treatment is offered or the patient refuses any further therapy. Depending upon the circumstances, we have used surgical procedures, x-ray treatment, and chemotherapy alone or in combination.

The salvage rate for those patients treated for the recurrence of squamous cell carcinoma is 23 per cent at 2 years (8/35) and 10 per cent at 5 years (3/29) after the treatment of the recurrent disease.

BIBLIOGRAPHY

1. Baclesse, F.: Les cancers du sinuses maxillaire, de l'ethmoid et des fosse nasales, *Ann. Otolaryngol.,* (Paris), 69, 464, 1952.
2. Batsakis, J. G., Holtz, F., Sueper, R. H.: Adenocarcinoma of nasal and paranasal cavities, *Arch. Otol.,* 77, 71, 1963.
3. Boone, M. L. M., Harle, T. S., Higholt, H. W., Fletcher, G. H.: Malignant disease of paranasal sinuses and nasal cavity, *Amer. J. Roentgen.,* 102, 627, 1968.
4. Boone, M. L. M., Harle, T. S., and Higholt, H. W.: In *Head and Neck, An Atlas of Tumor Radiology,* Vol. I, G. H. Fletcher and B. Jing, Year Book Medical Publishers, Inc., Chicago, p. 239, 1968.
5. Fairbanks-Barbosa, J.: Surgery of extensive cancer of paranasal sinuses, *Arch. Otol.,* (Chicago), 73, 129, 1961.
6. Frazell, E. L., and Lewis, J. S.: Cancer of the nasal cavity and accessory sinuses, *Cancer,* 16, 1293, 1963.
7. Jesse, R. H.: Preoperative versus postoperative radiation in the treatment of squamous carcinoma of the paranasal sinuses, *Amer. J. Surg.,* 110, 552, 1965.
8. Jesse, R. H., Butler, J. J., Healey, J. E., Fletcher, G. H., and Chau, P. M.: In *Cancer of the Head and Neck,* Williams and Wilkins Co., Baltimore, p. 329, 1967.

Table 3-55. *Adenocarcinomas and Malignant Salivary Gland Tumors* *

Site	Absolute Survival			
	2-Years		5-Years	
	Adeno-carcinoma	Salivary Gland	Adeno-carcinoma	Salivary Gland
Nasal Cavity	3/4	3/3	2/3	1/1
Paranasal Sinus	3/9	7/12	2/7	4/9

* Adenoidcystic carcinoma—8
Mucoepidermoid carcinoma—4
Malignant mixed—3

9. Jesse, R. H., Goepfert, H., Lindberg, R. D., and Johnson, R. H.: Combined intra-arterial infusion and radiotherapy for the treatment of advanced cancer of the head and neck, *Amer. J. Roentgen.*, 105, 20, 1969.

10. Ketcham, A. S., Wilkins, R. H., Van Buren, J. M., and Smith, R. R.: A combined intra-cranial facial approach to the paranasal sinuses, *Amer. J. Surg.*, 106, 698, 1963.

11. Lederman, M.: Tumours of the upper jaw, *J. Laryng.*, 84, 369, 1970.

12. Öhngren, L. G.: Malignant tumors of the maxillo-ethmoidal region, *Acta Otolaryng.*, (Stockholm) Suppl. 19, 1, 1933.

13. Ringertz, N.: Pathology of malignant tumors arising in the nasal and paranasal cavities and maxilla, *Arch. Otolaryng.*, Suppl. 27, 1, 1938.

14. Ross, R. E.: Radical en bloc ethmoidectomy for cancer, *Surg. Gynec. & Obstec.*, 108, 109, 1959.

15. Shukovsky, L. J., and Fletcher, G. H.: Retinal and optic nerve complications in a high dose irradiation technique of ethmoid sinus and nasal cavity, *Radiology*, 104, 629, 1972.

16. Sisson, G. A., Johnson, N. E., Amiri, C. S.: Cancer of the maxillary sinus: Clinical classification and management, *Ann. Otol.*, 72, 1050, 1963.

Malignant Tumors of Salivary Glands

OSCAR GUILLAMONDEGUI, ROBERT M. BYERS, and NORAH duV. TAPLEY

Introduction

Malignant tumors arise in both the major and minor salivary glands. While 70 to 80 per cent of all salivary gland tumors occur in the parotid salivary gland, most parotid tumors are benign.[3,4] A tumor arising in the submaxillary gland or minor salivary glands is more likely to be malignant than is a parotid tumor. The minor salivary glands are scattered within the mucosal lining of the oral cavity, oropharynx, hypopharynx, larynx and paranasal sinuses. Malignant tumors of minor salivary gland origin may occur in any of these sites, but are more common in the mucous membrane of the oral cavity.

The traditional treatment of malignant salivary gland lesions has been surgical, based on the supposition that they are not responsive to radiation therapy. Data showing that adjunctive radiation therapy has a place in the treatment of salivary gland cancer is beginning to emerge.

Classification

Malignant salivary gland tumors are derived from the cell types comprising the glandular structures. The currently widely accepted classification for salivary gland tumors is that of Foote and Frazell.[7] This classification divides the malignant salivary gland tumors into malignant mixed tumors, mucoepidermoid tumors (low and high grade), squamous carcinoma, unclassified malignant tumors, and the adenocarcinoma group which includes adenoidcystic carcinoma, acinic cell carcinoma, and a miscellaneous adenocarcinoma group. The classification used at MDAH differs only in separating the acinic cell and adenoidcystic carcinomas from the remaining adenocarcinomas. Additionally, malignant lymphomas and sarcomas may arise in the salivary gland but clear histological evidence of transition from salivary gland to mesenchymal tumors of these types is rare in the experience of most pathologists. Squamous cell carcinoma without mucin production must be differentiated if possible from metastatic squamous carcinoma of skin origin. This is particularly important in geographical areas where a high incidence of squamous cell cancer of the skin exists.

The relative frequency of the malignant salivary gland tumors depends on the site in question. Beahrs,[4] in reporting 162 patients with malignant parotid tumors, indicated that mucoepidermoid carcinomas comprised approximately 25 per cent of his series whereas adenoidcystic carcinoma, acinic cell carcinoma, malignant mixed tumors, and adenocarcinomas otherwise unclassified comprised 16, 15, 11, and 8 per cent of the group respectively. Adenoidcystic adenocarcinoma is the most common malignant tumor in the submaxillary gland and the minor salivary gland sites, comprising 60 per cent of the M. D. Anderson Hospital series (Byers, R. M., Personal communication) and 38 per cent of other series.[5] Mucoepidermoid carcinoma, malignant mixed tumor, and adenocarcinoma occur in the minor salivary gland sites, each comprising approximately 20 per cent of most series. Acinic cell carcinoma and squamous carcinoma rarely are seen outside of the parotid gland.

Growth Characteristics

Review articles concerned with the surgical treatment of salivary gland tumors delineate two groups of histological lesions based on the favorability of prognosis in the patient. The group usually listed as low to moderate grade of malignancy includes the mucoepidermoid carcinomas (low grade), the acinic cell carcinomas, and the adenoidcystic carcinomas. The group in the highly malignant category is comprised of the high grade mucoepidermoid carcinomas, the malignant mixed tumors, the squamous cell carcinomas, the adenocarcinomas otherwise unclassified, and the undifferentiated carcinomas. These categories are based on the survival statistics

in patients at 5 years and do not necessarily reflect a disease-free interval. Approximately 25 per cent of patients with a diagnosis of adenoidcystic carcinoma and approximately 15 per cent of those with high grade mucoepidermoid tumors will pass their 5-year anniversary with demonstrable recurrent tumor. Adenoidcystic carcinoma properly belongs in the highly malignant group because of the high rate of local recurrences after surgical resection even though it may be delayed for many years.

Salivary Gland Tumors of Low to Moderate Malignancy

MUCOEPIDERMOID CARCINOMA (LOW GRADE)

Low grade mucoepidermoid tumors develop slowly. Often there is a long period of observation between the time the patient first notices the tumor and the time he seeks treatment. The growth is usually very gradual, often with periods of minimal to no growth. A painless mass is the presenting sign and 7th nerve involvement does not occur. The lesion is more common in females.

ACINIC CELL CARCINOMA

Two thirds of the patients are female. This tumor is almost entirely limited to the parotid gland. Tumor growth is slow and there is usually a long history. Facial nerve involvement does not occur. These tumors very rarely metastasize to cervical nodes and spread is usually to contiguous structures.

ADENOIDCYSTIC CARCINOMA

This tumor occurs equally in males and females. It is the most common malignant lesion in the submaxillary and minor salivary gland sites. Approximately half of the patients have symptoms of a slowly growing mass. These tumors are submucosal in the minor salivary gland sites and ulceration does not occur until the lesion attains great size or a biopsy has been performed.

In approximately half of the patients symptoms of pain are a prominent feature. This cancer has a high propensity for invasion of nerves and perineural spaces. Cervical lymph node metastasis occurs in 30 to 40 per cent of the patients during the course of the disease, and distant metastasis is common with or without local recurrence. A number of patients with demonstrable local, regional, or distant disease are living relatively symptom free 10 to 20 years after the original treatment.

Malignant Salivary Gland Tumors of High Grade Malignancy

MUCOEPIDERMOID CARCINOMA (HIGH GRADE)

Mucoepidermoid tumors of high grade malignancy usually present as rapidly growing masses which often cause pain early in the disease. Local invasion, cervical lymph node metastasis, and distant metastasis occur regularly.

MALIGNANT MIXED TUMORS

Malignant mixed tumors may be present for many years, existing as a small, painless lesion which changes into a rapidly growing cancer. Some tumors exhibit a steady slow growth, eventually attaining large size. Pain and interference with facial nerve function occur in approximately one half of the patients. Local recurrence predominates, but metastasis to cervical lymph nodes occurs in about one third of the patients with parotid primaries and about one half of the patients with submaxillary primaries. Distant metastasis is common. Malignant mixed tumors, as contrasted to adenoidcystic carcinoma, infrequently have a prolonged course and the fate of the patient is usually decided prior to the fifth year.

ADENOCARCINOMA (OTHERWISE UNCLASSIFIED)

With few exceptions the adenocarcinomas not otherwise classified are highly malignant tumors. These rapidly developing tumors are associated with cervical lymph node metastasis in one half of the patients. Characteristically the course of the disease is rapid with nerve paralysis and distant metastasis within 3 years of initial treatment.

SQUAMOUS CARCINOMA

These tumors are rapidly growing, hard, and cause pain and nerve palsy early in the course of the disease. Extensive cervical node metastasis is a prominent feature. The patients often succumb to local and regional disease before distant metastasis can occur.

Anatomy

PAROTID GLAND

The parotid, largest of the salivary glands, is surrounded by a layer of fibroconnective tissue which is an extension of the cervical fascia. The gland occupies an irregular space behind the ascending ramus of the mandible near the external auditory canal, known as the parotid compartment or cell (Fig. 3-118). The lateral aspect of the parotid gland where the capsule is thick and well-defined, is covered by skin and subcutaneous tissue. Posteroinferiorly the gland extends to the mastoid process and is covered by the tendonous insertion of the sternocleidomastoid muscle, often becoming adherent to the upper anterior border of the muscle.

Posteromedially it is in contact with the cartilaginous and osseous portion of the external auditory canal. Posterosuperiorly it extends over the temporomandibular joint and covers the lower portion of the zygoma. Anteriorly the deep portion of the gland conforms to the shape of the posterior border of the ascending ramus of the mandible and

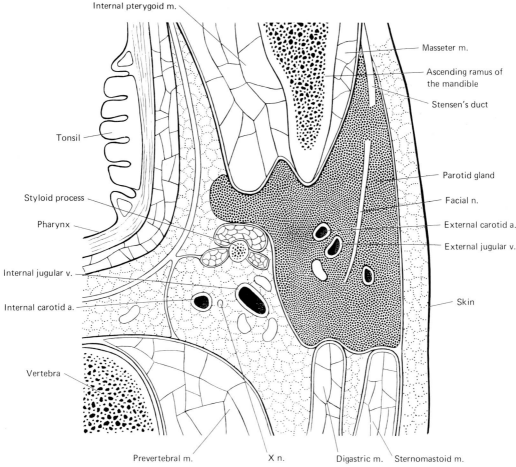

FIG. 3-118. View of horizontal cut through level of tonsillar fossa.

Internal pterygoid m.

Masseter m.

Ascending ramus of the mandible

Stensen's duct

Tonsil

Parotid gland

Facial n.

Styloid process

External carotid a.

Pharynx

External jugular v.

Internal jugular v.

Internal carotid a.

Skin

Vertebra

Prevertebral m.   X n.   Digastric m.   Sternomastoid m.

is loosely adherent to it. The superficial part of the gland extends over the masseter muscle to its anterior border where it is in relationship to Stenson's duct. Anteroinferiorly the parotid covers a portion of the subdigastric area where it is separated from the submaxillary gland by the stylomandibular ligament or intraglandular septum, a usually well-defined fascial structure. The inferior-posterior aspect of the gland comes in contact with the posterior belly of the digastric muscle, the styloid process, the styloglossus and stylopharyngeus muscle and the stylomandibular and stylohyoid ligaments. Medially, there are usually 2 extensions of the gland; one between the internal pterygoid muscle and the ascending ramus of the mandible while the majority of the gland extends into the lateral pharyngeal space in front of the styloid process and sometimes reaches the superior constricter muscle of the pharynx. In the depths of the lateral pharyngeal region the parotid is close to the internal carotid artery, the internal jugular vein, the glossopharyngeal, vagus, spinal accessory, and hypoglossal nerves and the cervical sympathetic chain.

The parotid compartment is entered by several important vascular and neural structures that become incorporated into the glandular tissue. Unquestionably the most significant anatomical element in this area is the facial nerve which supplies motor fibers to all the facial muscles. The facial nerve leaves the temporal bone through the stylo-mastoid foramen and proceeds obliquely forward and laterally penetrating the parotid gland. Within the gland, the facial nerve bifurcates into 2 terminal divisions, the tem-poral-facial and cervical-facial. These 2 major divisions subdivide into many branches which are variable, inconsistent, and have numerous anastomoses with each other. The 7th nerve divides the gland into very arbi-trary and indistinct divisions or lobes, the larger superficial lobe and the smaller deep lobe. The auriculo-temporal nerve, a branch of the mandibular division of the 5th nerve, arises in the pterygo-maxillary fossa at the level of the foramen ovale and enters the parotid compartment after circling behind the condylar process of the mandible. This nerve divides into several branches, the upper ones following the superficial temporal artery and other smaller branches perforating the gland and extending to the skin of the ear, the temporomandibular joint, and in the parotid substance itself where some cross-over to 7th nerve branches occurs.

Most neoplasms, benign or malignant, occur in the more superficial portion of the parotid gland, although anterior deep lobe tumors do occur. Malignant tumors are, therefore, anatomically close to the facial and auriculo-temporal nerves early in their de-velopment. Extension into these nerves or perineural spaces can carry the disease into the peripheral branches of the nerves and back through the facial nerve canal into the mastoid bone.

When the 7th nerve is involved in the canal, tumor pressure usually causes paraly-sis of the entire face, whereas if the nerve is involved peripherally the muscles ener-vated by only one division or branch may be paralyzed.

Invasion of the auriculo-temporal nerve peripherally causes pain referred to the ear, ear canal, or superficial temporal region. If it is involved proximally, extension through

the foramen ovale can invade the gasserian ganglion and thereby all branches of the 5th nerve.

Numerous lymphatic vessels drain into the parotid lymph nodes. The lymph nodes within the parotid gland are usually multiple and small. The superficial parotid lymph nodes are located in the lateral aspect of the gland and receive the afferent vessels from the skin and subcutaneous tissue of the tem-poral area, eyebrows, eyelids, part of the cheek, auricle, external auditory canal, and middle ear. The deep parotid lymph nodes course along the external carotid artery and drain portions of the external auditory canal, eustachian tube, and the gland itself. The afferent vessels from the parotid lymph nodes drain into nodes at the angle of the mandible, the upper posterior cervical area, or the subdigastric (jugulo-digastric) group of nodes.

SUBMAXILLARY GLAND

The submaxillary gland is an irregular structure 4 to 5 cm in greatest diameter situ-ated in the submaxillary triangle of the neck (Fig. 3-119 and 3-120). The upper portion of the lateral surface of the gland lies against the inner surface of the mandible and the insertion of the internal pterygoid muscle. The lower portion of the lateral surface is covered by skin, superficial fascia, the facial vein, the marginal branch of the 7th nerve, and lymph nodes. Anteriorly, the gland overlies the mylohyoid muscle and usually touches the anterior belly of the digastric muscle. Posteriorly, the gland is in direct contact with the stylomandibular ligament and the tractus angularis. Inferiorly, the gland overlies the tendon of the digastric and stylohyoid muscles thereby being in close approximation to the hyoid bone. The deep surface of the gland is in close contact with the mylohyoid, hyoglossus, styloglossus, and stylohyoid muscles and also the posterior belly of the digastric muscle. An uncinate process extends between the mylohyoid and

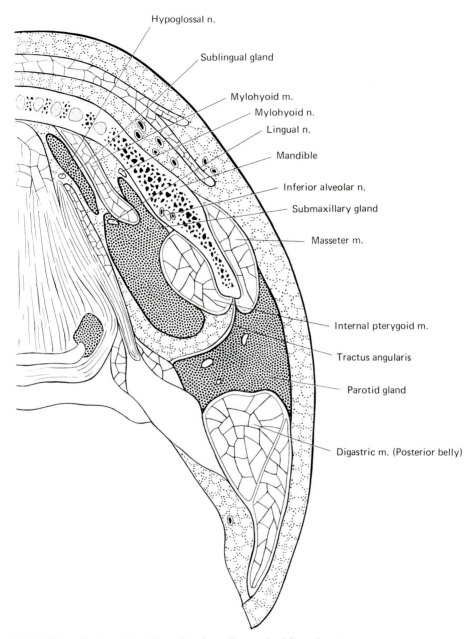

FIG. 3-119. View of horizontal cut through submaxillary and sublingual region.

Labels (top to bottom, left to right):
- Hypoglossal n.
- Sublingual gland
- Mylohyoid m.
- Mylohyoid n.
- Lingual n.
- Mandible
- Inferior alveolar n.
- Submaxillary gland
- Masseter m.
- Internal pterygoid m.
- Tractus angularis
- Parotid gland
- Digastric m. (Posterior belly)

hyoglossus muscles along the submaxillary duct. The lingual nerve passes between the hyoglossus muscle and the deep portion of the submaxillary gland and is lateral and superior to the submaxillary duct. The submaxillary ganglion coming off the lingual nerve is in close communication with the gland. The mylohyoid nerve, a branch of the inferior alveolar nerve, lies in contact with the gland on its way to innervate the mylohyoid muscle and the anterior belly of the digastric. This nerve joins the inferior alveo-

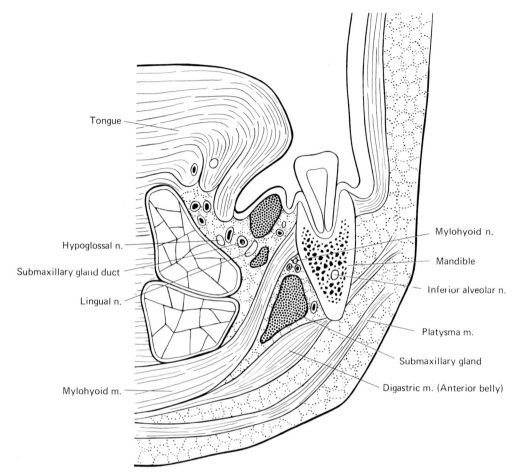

Tongue

Hypoglossal n.

Submaxillary gland duct

Lingual n.

Mylohyoid m.

Mylohyoid n.

Mandible

Inferior alveolar n.

Platysma m.

Submaxillary gland

Digastric m. (Anterior belly)

FIG. 3-120. View of frontal section through tongue, sublingual and submaxillary region.

lar nerve just prior to the entrance of the latter into the inferior alveolar canal of the mandible. The hypoglossal nerve courses along the deep surface of the gland.

Most malignant tumors of the submaxillary gland invade the thin fascial covering and involve local structures by direct extension. The mylohyoid and digastric muscles, the periosteum of the mandible and the subcutaneous tissue overlying the gland are the most common sites for direct extension. Some malignant tumors, particularly the adenoidcystic carcinomas, may remain within the capsule of the submaxillary gland, but extensively invade the perineural lymphatics of the mylohyoid, lingual, and hypo-

glossal nerves. Extension can occur via the perineural invasion of the mylohyoid nerve to the inferior alveolar nerve and thus to the mandible or through the other 2 nerves to the base of the skull.

Lymphatic channels are also frequently invaded, particularly by the high grade mucoepidermoid tumors, the malignant mixed tumors, and the undifferentiated lesions. The first level of nodal metastasis is usually to the nodes overlying the submaxillary gland and thus to the subdigastric and high midjugular lymph nodes. Nerve invasion was proven in 50 per cent of the previously untreated series of submaxillary gland malignant tumors in the MDAH series, while the incidence of nodal metastasis in the same group was 44 per cent.

Control by Irradiation

The role of irradiation in the management of malignant tumors of the salivary glands has been considered negligible because of the misconception that these tumors are uniquely radioresistant. The treatment of choice primarily has been surgical removal with radicalism of the surgery being dictated by the local extent of the tumor. Sacrifice of the facial nerve for tumors in the parotid gland, removal of the lingual and hypoglossal nerve and the mandible for tumors in the submaxillary gland, and functional defects in the palate or other areas for minor salivary gland tumors are often necessary aftermaths of radical surgical procedures.

Review of our material[2,8] and reports in the literature[9,11] have shown that irradiation is effective in some clinical situations for local control when used alone or as adjuvant treatment to surgical excision. Two clinical situations are encountered which dictate consideration of radiation therapy in patients with malignant salivary gland tumors.

1) *Patients with gross tumor*

a) The patient is inoperable because of the extent of the primary cancer, the patient refuses surgical treatment, or the patient has a medical contraindication to surgical treatment.

b) Recurrent disease after primary surgical therapy is inoperable.

2) *Probable subclinical disease*

a) cancer is demonstrated histologically at the surgical resection margin; the majority of the lesion has been removed.

b) microscopic cancer is assumed to be at or close to the surgical margin or in nerve sheaths after all gross tumor has been removed.

The efficacy of postoperative irradiation is indicated by the very low rate of recurrence in those patients receiving radiation therapy for definite or probable subclinical disease (Table 3-56). Only 6.5 per cent of the patients living 3 years or more developed local recur-

Table 3-56. *Carcinoma in Salivary Glands—Local Failures by Histology in Patients Irradiated after Surgical Excision for Definite* or Probable Subclinical Disease—January 1948–December 1968, (Analysis March 1970)*

(Patients who died from intercurrent disease or distant metastases in less than 3 years NED locally are excluded)

Histology	Number of Patients	Number of Recurrences
Malignant mixed tumor	3	1**
Mucoepidermoid carcinoma (high grade)	4	0
Adenoidcystic carcinoma	9	1**
Adenocarcinoma	4	0
Squamous cell carcinoma	7	0
Undifferentiated carcinoma	1	0
Unclassified neoplasm	2	0
Total	30†	2 (6.5%)††

* Approximately half of the patients had definite residual disease left after surgical excision.
** At 7 and 31 months
† 2 submaxillary glands
†† Beahrs (4)   Moderately malignant tumors of the parotid gland 37.5%
    Recurrences <3 years   Highly malignant tumors of the parotid gland 72.5%

rence. The various histologic types of tumor seem to be controlled equally well by irradiation. Radiation therapy is also helpful in the control of neck metastases. Only 2 of 48 patients receiving irradiation to the neck developed recurrence in the irradiated field.[8] New disease did develop in the neck outside the irradiated field in 6 patients not receiving irradiation to the entire ipsilateral neck.

Irradiation treatment to the major salivary glands is given principally with the external beam. [60]Co wedge pairs or combined electron and photon beams are used to deliver 5,000 rads in 5 weeks to 6,000 rads in 6 weeks. If treatment is being given to a primary inoperable lesion or recurrent tumor, the total tumor dose reaches 7,000 or 7,500 rads through a reduced portal. With positive cervical nodes or when there is a high statistical risk of infested nodes, ^{60}Co or the electron beam is used to irradiate the ipsilateral neck.

Treatment Policies

PAROTID GLAND

A high local recurrence rate after surgical procedures performed for malignant parotid gland tumors is recognized in the literature.[1,3,4,6,10] Most authors described the highest rates of recurrence in patients with adenocarcinoma, high grade mucoepidermoid carcinoma, adenoidcystic carcinoma, and squamous carcinoma. Some of the series quoted include patients who have already had a definitive procedure and have had at least one recurrence prior to their inclusion in the data.[4,6]

None of these series includes previously untreated patients only who were treated by modern surgical techniques as dictated by the histology and extent of the lesion. Most tumors of low grade malignant potential can be successfully removed surgically with minimal deformity of the parotid area and rarely require total resection of all branches of the 7th nerve. Postoperative radiation therapy is infrequently required for these patients.

A surgical resection is adequate for selected, previously untreated, lesions of the high grade mucoepidermoid, adenoidcystic, and malignant mixed varieties if it completely encompasses the lesion with a wide margin. Radiation therapy in these cases is unnecessary. Moderate sized previously untreated lesions of the high grade malignant mucoepidermoid, adenoidcystic, or malignant mixed varieties in which the surgeon has difficulty obtaining wide surgical margins should be irradiated postoperatively. Previously untreated lesions classified as squamous or undifferentiated carcinomas often recur after secondary surgical procedures and all should receive postoperative radiation therapy. Radiation therapy is given in patients who have had a recent definitive surgical procedure elsewhere, with all gross disease removed, but the surgeon doubtful that all microscopic cancer has been eradicated.

A surgical procedure for recurrent lesions of the highly malignant types tend to be less successful than the same procedure for an untouched lesion. In most instances, radiation therapy should be considered after these secondary operations.

Regardless of cell type or whether previously treated, all patients whose removed specimen shows disease beyond the confines of the parotid gland, nerve or perineural invasion, invasion into muscles, bone or cartilage, or who have extensive cervical node metastasis, should receive immediate postoperative irradiation.

There is some evidence that an alternative plan of management which preserves nerve function and offers an equal chance of local control, should be considered. With this procedure, all macroscopic tumor is removed along with those branches of the facial nerve which are grossly invaded by tumor. The surgeon may stop at this point without trying to remove a wide margin of supposedly normal tissue, preferring to treat the patient with immediate postoperative irradiation.

Patients with gross recurrent tumor occurring sometime after the original surgical procedure should have an additional surgical procedure to remove all gross tumor, if possible. This should be followed by radiation therapy.

Metastatic Squamous Cell Carcinoma

Squamous cell cancers of the skin of the face, in particular the temple and ear, and of the upper neck, may metastasize to the parotid lymph nodes or to the parotid gland. The exact skin lesion of origin may not be easily determined if many areas of the skin have been previously treated, particularly if the specimen was not subjected to histological examination.

Metastatic carcinoma to the salivary gland must be suspected in any patient with a history of skin cancer in the head and neck area. Unless the metastatic lesion is limited to an easily removable parotid node, the treatment should be essentially as for a primary salivary gland tumor. After biopsy or excision of the tumor, the parotid area is irradiated and the entire ipsilateral neck because of the high probability of cervical node metastases.

Techniques of Treatment

PAROTID TUMOR

The area to be irradiated includes the entire parotid bed and the full extent of the surgical scar (Fig. 3-121). The fields extend from the ridge of the zygoma superiorly down to below the angle and horizontal ramus of the mandible. The height of the field will vary from 8 to 10 cm. The anterior margin of the field is at least to the anterior border of the masseter or approximately 6 cm anterior to the external auditory meatus. The posterior margin is placed sufficiently behind the auricle to provide complete coverage of the posterior edge of the parotid and the surgical scar with an adequate margin. The mastoid should always be covered in patients with perineural invasion or a high grade malignant tumor.

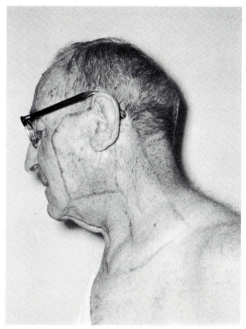

FIG. 3-121. This 75-year-old male was admitted in June 1971 with a long history of multiple skin lesions of the face treated by fulguration and surgery. Two months prior to admission he noticed a lump in the left cheek in front of the ear which gradually increased in size. The superficial lobe of the parotid was resected and the histological report was poorly differentiated carcinoma. It was considered that the patient had metastatic carcinoma to the parotid gland with a high probability of spread to the cervical lymph nodes.

The entire parotid area was treated through a single lateral portal with 18 Mev photon and electron beams to a tumor dose of 6,000 rads at a depth of 5 cm in 6 weeks. The entire ipsilateral neck received 5,500 rads given dose in 4½ weeks with 9 Mev electrons. A brisk skin erythema developed with dry desquamation and rapid healing.

On 7-28-72 there is no evidence of disease in the parotid area but the patient has a metastasis to the right femur.

When there is known residual disease demonstrated in the ear canal, temporal bone, or base of skull, or there is potential extension into the middle cranial fossa, the best treatment technique is provided by ^{60}Co 45- to 65-degree wedge pairs. This technique provides a satisfactory and relatively homogeneous dose distribution to a large volume and a depth approaching the midline (Fig. 3-122). The entire auricle and scalp in the lateral occipital area and most of the ipsilateral mandible will be included in the high-dose zone. This large volume is treated to a depth of 5 to 6 cm and to a dose of 6,000 rads in 6 weeks or 6,500 rads in 6½ weeks.

In treating inoperable or recurrent bulky tumors, an additional 1,000 to 1,500 rads in 5 to 7 treatments is given through a reduced field. Individualization of treatment is necessary in many patients because of the extensions of the primary inoperable tumor, or the location of the recurrent disease.

Irradiation of the tumor bed after removal of a lesion of limited extent without facial nerve involvement, requires treatment to a smaller volume. A good treatment technique, if available, is a combination of high energy

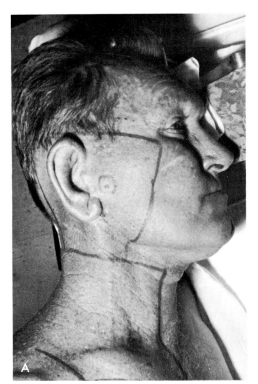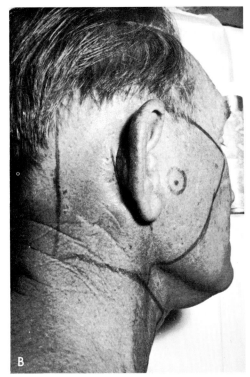

FIG. 3-122. This 52-year-old male was admitted to MDAH June 1970 with a 3-year history of pain in the right mastoid area. Some months before admission he noticed a swelling behind the ear which increased in size. Just prior to admission the postauricular mass was removed. The pathology report was adenoidcystic carcinoma with perineural invasion. On admission here the patient was noted to have slight 7th nerve weakness and x-ray examination of the mastoid showed bone destruction. The parotid area was treated with ^{60}Co 45-degree wedge fields and received 6,000 rads tumor dose at 6 cm depth in 6 weeks. The ipsilateral neck received 5,000 rads given dose in 5 weeks with an anterior ^{60}Co field. The patient showed no evidence of disease in August 1972.

    A & B. Patient in position for treatment of parotid area. The ^{60}Co wedges include the preauricular area, the entire ear, and the mastoid and postauricular tissues with a wide margin.

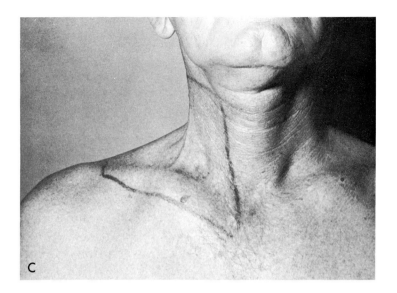

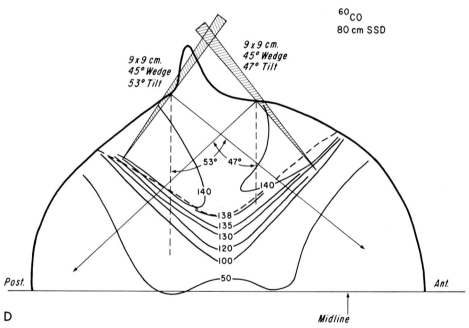

FIG. 3-122. C. Treatment for the ipsilateral neck. The anterior ^{60}Co field extends from the lower border of the parotid field.

D. Isodose distribution of ^{60}Co wedges. The tumor dose is taken at the 138 per cent curve. The tissue volume included in the high dose range is not excessive.

electron and photon beams, both in the range of 18 to 22 Mev. The total irradiated volume is reduced while providing excellent coverage of the parotid bed area (Fig. 3-123). With equal given doses, homogeneous dose distribution is achieved from the surface to a 5 cm depth. The superior and inferior margins are essentially as described for the ^{60}Co fields but the anterior and posterior margins are less widely separated and a more economical

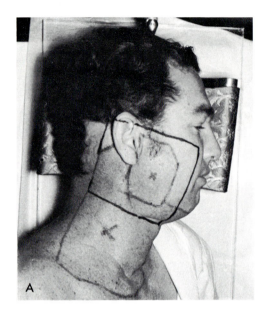

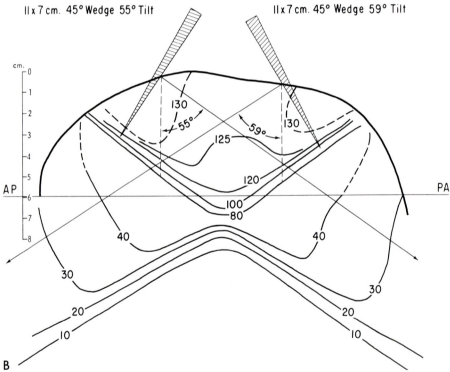

FIG. 3-123. This 35-year-old male was admitted January 1970 with a history of a mass presenting below the right ear 10 months previously. Approximately 3 months before admission the right parotid gland began to swell and a mass the size of a golf ball was present just prior to surgery. The superficial lobe of the parotid gland was resected and a radical neck dissection was done. The histologic report was high grade mucoepidermoid carcinoma with metastasis to one subdigastric lymph node. Radiation therapy was started 6 weeks after surgery. The patient showed no evidence of disease in August 1972.

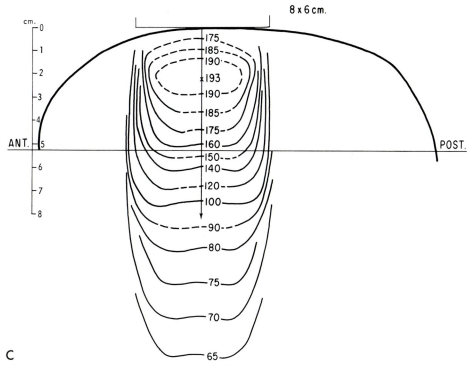

The original treatment plan included ^{60}Co wedges for the parotid area and an anterior ^{60}Co field for the lower ipsilateral neck. After the fields were drawn and the isodose distribution was obtained, it was decided to treat the parotid area with combined 18 Mev photon and electron beams. Since the gross tumor apparently was confined to the superficial lobe, it was not considered necessary to treat the large volume of tissue which would be encompassed by the wedge pair fields in order to obtain the desired depth dose.

A. Patient with fields drawn both for ^{60}Co and for the photon and electron beams. The heavy dark lines delineate the area included by the ^{60}Co wedges. The lighter lines drawn within the heavy lines delineate the field covered by the electron and photon beam field which extends to the angle of the mandible and to the vertebral bodies posteriorly. The entire neck, including the submental tissues and the posterior cervical lymph node chain, is covered by the 9 Mev electron beam field. **B.** Isodose distribution for ^{60}Co wedge fields. The 120 per cent curve would have to be used to provide a satisfactory depth dose. A large volume of tissue is included in the high dose range. **C.** Isodose distribution of combined photon and electron beams. The high dose area is much more economical than with ^{60}Co wedges. The tumor dose is taken at the 5 cm depth and the field receives equal given doses from the 18 Mev photon and electron beams.

treatment volume results. Since the field usually extends posteriorly over the spinal cord, the field is moved off the cord, at 4,500 rads. The 9 Mev electron beam is then used to give 1,000 to 1,500 rads to the posterior portion of the field, particularly to include the surgical scar which extends behind the ear.

The entire ipsilateral neck is treated with an anterior ^{60}Co field (Figure 3-122C) which is aligned with the inferior margin of the ^{60}Co wedge fields. The given dose is 5,000 rads in 5 weeks after radical neck dissection or 6,000 rads in 6 weeks in the unoperated neck. The electron beam may be used to treat the entire neck including the posterior cervical chain, the field being defined by a lead cut-out (Fig. 3-123A). Nine Mev is used for the unoperated neck with a given dose of 5,000 rads in 4 weeks or 6,000 rads in 5 weeks. Six Mev must be used after radical neck dissection because of the thinness of the tissues overlying the hypopharynx and larynx and the cervical cord. The given dose is 5,000 rads in 4 weeks.

Treatment Policies

SUBMAXILLARY GLAND

Malignant tumors of the submaxillary gland occur in a higher ratio of malignant to benign than in tumors of the parotid gland. In addition malignant tumors of the submaxillary gland appear to behave in a more aggressive manner than those of a similar cell type in the parotid. The most logical explanation for this fact is the usually inadequate surgical treatment performed for submaxillary gland tumors. Ideally the surgeon should approach any submaxillary mass as a possible malignant tumor and do a submaxillary gland resection as a biopsy. If, on frozen section, the mass is malignant, the minimal surgical procedure necessary to remove the most likely sites of spread should include removal of the surrounding muscles, nerves, periosteum, occasionally the mandible itself and completion of the radical neck dissection.

All patients with high grade malignant tumors, those with nerve or perineural invasion, or nodal metastases, or in whom the disease is demonstrated outside the capsule of the submaxillary gland should receive postoperative irradiation. This includes coverage of the neck, the mandible, and the nerve pathways to the base of the skull.

TECHNIQUES OF IRRADIATION

Radiation therapy should be administered as soon as healing is complete after the surgical procedure. When there is no gross residual tumor and no perineural invasion, an appositional 18 Mev electron beam portal can be used to provide 5,000 rads tumor dose in 5 weeks at the 80 per cent depth (4.7 cm).

Treatment is given with ^{60}Co wedge pairs when disease is extensive and particularly if there is perineural invasion (Fig. 3-124). The tumor dose is 5,000 rads in 5 weeks for elective treatment and 6,000 to 6,500 rads in 6 weeks for known residual disease.

If a neck dissection has not been done, treatment to the ipsilateral side of the neck should always be given unless the lesion was a well-encapsulated, low-grade tumor. The ipsilateral neck should be treated after radical neck dissection if tumor is present in connective tissue or if many nodes contain tumor deposits. The low neck may be treated with an anterior ^{60}Co portal. If an electron beam is available, an appositional field contiguous to the primary treatment field can be used with 6 Mev after surgery and 9 Mev when a radical neck dissection has not been done. The given dose is 5,000 rads in 5 weeks with ^{60}Co.

Treatment Policies

MINOR SALIVARY GLANDS

The treatment policy relative to malignant minor salivary gland tumors varies greatly depending upon the histopathology and the anatomical site of the lesion. Tumors in some sites such as the nasopharynx and to a lesser extent the base of tongue, are unresectable and require radiation therapy as the only modality of treatment. For those sites in which surgical resection is possible, macroscopic tumor should be removed. Rarely, however, can the surgeon be confident that microscopic disease has been completely eradicated from muscle sheaths and perineural spaces. Postoperative irradiation should be given after the surgical procedure in all patients with a high grade malignant neoplasm. Radiation therapy should be used after surgery if tumor is close to the line resection when there is known residual disease or if the specimen shows perineural invasion. The radiation technique is selected for the area to be treated (Fig. 3-125). The

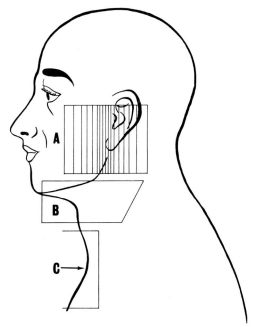

POST-OP IRRADIATION FOR
MUCOEPIDERMOID CA. INFILTRATING
SHEATH OF MANDIBULAR NERVE
(A) 45° Co⁶⁰ A-P WEDGES 6000 RADS
(B) Cs¹³⁷ 7500 RADS G.D.
(C) Cs¹³⁷ 5100 RADS G.D.

FIG. 3-124. This 54-year-old male was seen in February 1963 after excision of the left submaxillary gland and contents of the submaxillary triangle. The histological diagnosis was high grade mucoepidermoid carcinoma of the submaxillary gland. No tumor was palpable on admission, but the surgical report stated that residual tumor was left in the pterygoid region. The pathologist reported many areas showing infiltrative sheets of poorly differentiated mucoepidermoid carcinoma, some in nerve sheaths.

From 2-12-63 to 3-18-63, treatment was given to include the submaxillary triangle (7,500 rads given dose in 5 weeks) and the pterygoid fossa, to trace the nerve to the base of the skull (6,000 rads tumor dose in 5 weeks). The ipsilateral neck received 5,100 rads given dose in 4 weeks.

The patient was without evidence of disease in October 1970. No radiation complications had occurred. He was killed in a traffic accident in 1971. (Courtesy: Alaniz and Fletcher, *Radiology,* 84, 412, 1965.)

ipsilateral neck may require treatment as well as the primary site when nodal metastases are present or suspected. If the specimen shows a well-differentiated tumor, as in low-grade mucoepidermoid carcinoma, a limited field may be irradiated after surgery and an intraoral cone may provide a satisfactory technique (Fig. 3-126).

Complications

Irradiation of the parotid area and surrounding structures produces specific complications. Radiation sequelae of sufficient degree to affect the normal tissue functions are uncommon. A dry mouth is usually minimal to moderate. The degree of fibrosis which may occur is partially dependent on the extent of the cancer which controls the extent of the surgical procedure and the size of the radiation field. Trismus may develop because of radiation-induced fibrosis in muscles or the temporo-mandibular joint. This usually is seen with extensive tumor infiltrating the masseter muscle.

The ear may present quite severe problems. There is usually dryness and scaling of the epithelium lining of the external auditory canal. Chrondritis is uncommon but a tender painful ear can occur. This is not seen when treatment is given with combined electron and photon beams since the entire auricle is not irradiated. The ear drum may thicken and hearing may be affected. The most disturbing complication is a serous otitis externa or media with pain and partial deafness. Occasionally surgical drainage through the tympanic membrane is necessary.

Facial nerve palsies associated with parotid tumor may slowly improve after irradiation if the reason for the defect was partial compression by the tumor mass. If nerve invasion has occurred irradiation will not improve the paralysis. If nerve resection and grafting are done, irradiation usually does not interfere with the full extent of recovery that could be expected.

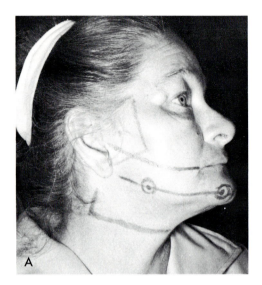

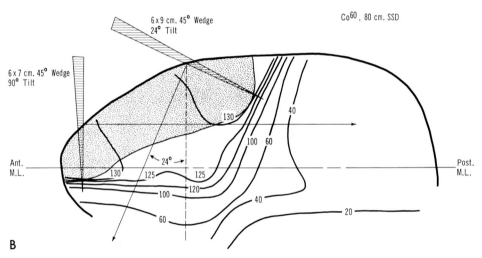

FIG. 3-125. This 48-year-old female had noticed discomfort with her lower dentures for about one year before admission to MDAH in April 1970. Three weeks before admission a lesion was removed from the right lower gum in the right cuspid area. On examination no abnormalities of the mucous membrane were observed and there was no mass on palpation. X-ray examination of the mandible showed an area of destruction with a smooth margin in the body of the right mandible. The histological diagnosis was mucoepidermoid carcinoma with invasion of nerves.

Treatment was radiation therapy to the entire right mandible from the midline of the chin to behind the angle of the mandible. The ascending ramus of the mandible and the pterygoid fossa were included in the treatment field to irradiate the mandibular branch of the facial nerve to the base of the skull. The tumor dose to the mandible was 6,500 rads in 6½ weeks and 6,000 rads to the ascending ramus.

The patient showed no evidence of disease in August 1972.

A. Treatment fields—^{60}Co wedges to mandible. Combined 18 Mev photon and electron beams to a 5 × 4 cm field over ascending ramus of mandible. **B.** Isodose distribution of ^{60}Co wedges showing a homogeneous high dose throughout the right mandible.

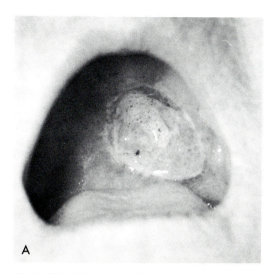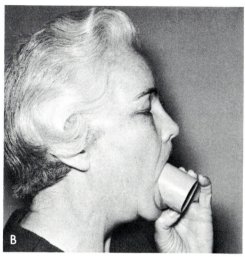

FIG. 3-126. This 57-year-old female was first seen at MDAH in September 1970 after excision and cautery of a 1 cm lesion at the junction of the hard and soft palate. The histological diagnosis was low grade mucoepidermoid carcinoma originating in minor salivary glands. Radiation therapy was recommended because the tumor was close to the surgical margins. The area of the surgical defect was well encompassed by a 4 cm intraoral cone. The patient received a given dose of 5,500 rads in 4½ weeks using 6 and 9 Mev electrons. The patient showed no evidence of disease in August 1972. **A.** Area of lesion in palate. **B.** Intraoral stent to aid in positioning intraoral cone.

BIBLIOGRAPHY

1. Abrams, A. M., Cornyn, J., Scofield, H. H., and Hansen, L. S.: Acinic cell adenocarcinoma of the major salivary glands, *Cancer*, 18 1145, 1965.
2. Alaniz, F., and Fletcher, G. H.: Place and technics of radiation therapy in the management of malignant tumors of the major salivary glands, *Radiology*, 84, 412, 1965.
3. Bardwil, J. M., Luna, M. A., and Healey, J. E., Jr.: Salivary Glands, In *Cancer of the Head and Neck*, Maccomb, W. S., and Fletcher, G. H., editors, The Williams & Wilkins Co., Baltimore, Maryland, 1967.
4. Beahrs, O. H., Woolner, L. B., Carveth, S. W., and Devine, K. D.: Surgical management of parotid lesions. *Arch. Surg.*, 80, 890, 1960.
5. Conley, John: In *Concepts in Head and Neck Surgery*, Grune and Stratton, New York, New York, 1970.
6. Dockerty, M. B., and Mayo, C. W.: Primary tumors of the submaxillary gland with special reference to mixed tumors, *Surg., Gynec., Obstet.*, 74, 1033, 1942.
7. Foote, F. W. Jr., and Frazell, E. L.: *Tumors of the Major Salivary Glands*, Armed Forces Institute of Pathology, Washington, D. C., 1954.
8. King, J. J., and Fletcher, G. H.: Malignant tumors of the major salivary glands, *Radiology*, 100, 381, 1971.
9. Lott, J. S.: Clinical experience with radiation therapy in the management of parotid tumors, *J. Canad. Assoc. Radiol.*, 14, 70, 1963.
10. Robinson, D. W. and Masters, F. W.: Tumors of the parotid gland, In *Reconstructive Plastic Surgery*, Converse, F. M., editor, W. B. Saunders Company, Philadelphia, Pennsylvania, 1964.
11. Stewart, J. G., Jackson, A. W., and Chew, M. K., Role of radiotherapy in the management of malignant tumors of the salivary glands, *Amer. J. Roentgen.*, 102, 100, 1968.

4. Central Nervous System

JEAN BOUCHARD

Introduction

The use of ionizing radiation and high energy ionizing particles is a valid method of treatment in the management of tumors of the central nervous system either primary or metastatic. Radiation therapy may be efficaicious also in a few selected lesions affecting the peripheral nervous system.

It should be stated from the onset of this chapter that adequate irradiation of tumors involving the brain or other intracranial structures, the pons, and the spinal cord can be accomplished with minimal risks of damage to the adjacent tissues and intervening normal anatomical structures. The beneficial effects of radiation therapy in the management of lesions of the central and peripheral nervous system have been considerably greater, in our experience, than the rare actual or potential adverse effects. Such observation is also relevant to the use of radiation therapy in pituitary tumors. It is valid not only for adults but for infants and children as well.

Analysis of our long-term results has demonstrated that the length and quality of survival of patients irradiated in the treatment of most types of primary intracranial neoplasms are generally better than expected. It has also proved that children affected with malignant brain tumors can be exposed to intensive irradiation without significant risk of undue physical or mental sequelae. Radiation therapy can be and often is of considerable value as a palliative measure against cerebral metastases.

In pituitary tumors, irradiation alone has arrested tumor growth over long periods of time.

Irradiation of primary tumors of the spinal cord appears to be of definite value although it is sometimes difficult to assess. It is a very effective therapeutic measure in the treatment of most of the extradural tumors pressing on the cord. The controversial usefulness of radiation in the treatment of non-neoplastic conditions such as syringomyelia and arachnoiditis will be discussed.

A brief reference will be made at the end of this chapter regarding the role of radiation therapy in the management of neoplastic and non-neoplastic diseases affecting the peripheral nervous system including the cranial nerves. Consideration will be given to the value of radiation therapy for the relief of pain in neuritis and neuralgia, or pain and pruritus when associated with scars and keloids. The analgesic effect of irradiation is of paramount importance in the control of pain related to primary or metastatic neoplastic manifestations involving nerve roots, trunks or endings, or else affecting visceral and skeletal structures.

The role of radiation therapy in the management of lesions involving the nervous system will be discussed under the following headings: 1) Primary intracranial neoplasms, 2) Metastatic intracranial tumors, 3) Tumors involving the hypophysis, 4) Spinal cord tumors and other lesions, and 5) Lesions of the peripheral nervous system.

Primary Intracranial Neoplasms

Natural History and Special Characteristics

The growth and extension of the majority of primary intracranial tumors is essentially a localized and regional neoplastic process from beginning to end. As the tumor grows intracranially it also exerts direct local and regional pressure on the adjacent normal nervous tissue, disturbing its normal functions and causing various neurological signs. Disturbances in the blood circulation occur at least at the site of the tumor and localized edema is often observed at the same time at its periphery. Occasionally secondary cystic gliosis and sometimes necrosis may be observed. The tumor by its growth may also cause pressure upon cranial nerves which may become atrophied. The existence of such tissue reactions and complications, primarily caused by the tumor growth, must be recognized when present. Too often such reactions are ignored as initial manifestations of intracranial tumors and are subsequently attributed to the surgical or radiotherapeutic treatment employed to control the intracranial neoplasm itself.

A very significant anatomical factor in keeping most of the primary intracranial tumors within the cranial cavity is the absence of lymphatic channels in the central nervous system. The possibility of dissemination of tumor cells by lymphatics to other parts of the body does not exist in brain tumors. This is a rare and highly favorable feature in the treatment of neoplastic conditions. Spontaneous dissemination of primary brain tumors through the blood stream appears to be extremely uncommon.

The only natural anatomical avenue of dissemination for tumor cells detached from primary intracranial neoplasms is along the subarachnoid spaces where cerebrospinal fluid is circulating. This mode of spread seems to occur spontaneously mostly in medulloblastomas, and occasionally in the less common ependymoblastomas and sarcomas of the brain. The tumor implants, which may result from such shedding of cells by the primary tumor, are usually found first distally to the tumor itself in the direction of the cerebrospinal fluid flow along the spinal axis. However, once the cerebrospinal flow is blocked by the tumor it may reverse its direction so that circulating tumor cells can ascend into the ventricles and the subarachnoid spaces around the cerebral hemispheres. This is an adverse factor which must be taken into serious account in the management and treatment of tumors in which it occurs.

Tumor implants in operative wounds or scars are extremely rare following removal of even the most malignant intracranial neoplasms. We have yet to observe a single direct surgical transplantation of human glioma arising from an operative scar.

The intracranial behavior of the primary brain tumors must be clearly known and understood. The gliomas, which represent approximately 50 per cent of all primary intracranial tumors, usually grow as a single tumor mass but may be multicentric and form more than one tumor when they originate simultaneously either in one or in both cerebral hemispheres, or in some other anatomic part of the central nervous tissue. Infiltrating types of gliomatous tumors may extend to the opposite side of the brain under the falx cerebri through the corpus callosum, a finding which is not too unusual when one is aware of this and seeks for it. Infiltrating gliomas may also extend down into the brain-stem or the basal ganglia, or else they may originate in the brain-stem and extend upwards into the midbrain and beyond, in either way always by direct neoplastic invasion of the adjacent central nervous structures.

Meningeal tumors may occasionally extend directly through the dura and calvarium under the scalp or through the base of the skull into adjacent cavities. Chordomas and craniopharyngiomas also extend at times directly outside of the cranial cavity proper into the sphenoid sinuses and the nasopharynx.

Diagnosis and Localization

The therapeutic radiologist cannot judiciously use ionizing radiation in the treatment of primary intracranial neoplasms unless he has full knowledge of the localization and extent of the tumor to be irradiated in each individual case.

The advances made in neurologic diagnostic procedures in the last 20 years have been so considerable that the diagnosis of intracranial neoplasms can be made with increasing precision. Radiotherapists must be conversant with the degree of valid information which may be derived from each procedure and used for guidance in the planning of individual treatment. Special radiologic x-ray examinations with contrast media provide radiation therapists with more adequate practical information than any other group of diagnostic procedures for the planning of treatment with ionizing radiation.

Brain tumors can be accurately diagnosed and localized by pneumograms in more than 90 per cent of the cases. Cerebral angiography has become an extremely useful method of radiological examination capable of establishing the presence of an intracranial tumor and its exact location by the extent and character of the modifications of the normal vascular pattern. Gamma encephalography, the localization of intracranial neoplasms with radioactive isotopes, is another radiologic method with an accuracy which appears to be reliable as yet in not more than 50 per cent of the cases. The best results have been reported in meningiomas and also in glioblastomas, that is, in tumors with increased vascularization.

Considering that the majority of primary intracranial tumors are irradiated postoperatively, the surgeons' observations recorded in the operative report should provide most valuable information concerning the identi-

fication, location and extent of the tumor. Initial surgical management also has the advantage of making tissue available for histopathological studies permitting the identification of the type of tumor and its classification. In many cases in which craniotomy and surgical removal is not advisable, biopsy material adequate for pathologic studies and classification is obtained by needle biopsy taken through twist drill holes made in the calvarium.

Classification and Pathology of Intracranial Neoplasms

The histopathological classification followed in our institution has been largely the one proposed by Baley and Cushing.[2] The terminology used by pathologists in the classification of gliomas can be and often is very confusing.

Intracranial gliomas are primary brain tumors arising from the glial cells of which three different types are generally recognized: the astrocytes, the oligodendrocytes and the ependymal cells. Gliomas arising from the astrocytic group of cells represent approximately three-quarters of all primary intracranial gliomatous tumors. Tumors originating from the oligodendroglial cells appear to be identified easily. Gliomas derived from the ependymal cells are relatively uncommon just like the oligodendrogliomas.

Medulloblastomas are still classified with the gliomas by the majority of neuropathologists.

Irradiation of Primary Intracranial Neoplasms

Unquestionable clinical and histologic evidence has demonstrated that the majority of primary intracranial tumors are radiosensitive to some degree. Medulloblastomas are the most sensitive to radiation in contrast with glioblastomas whose radiosensitivity is minimal and radiocurability very low.

When radiation therapy is used for primary intracranial neoplasms, it is mostly in combination with surgical treatment as a postoperative procedure. Surgical methods are and continue to be the most important in the management of those tumors. Various surgical techniques are used to obtain tissue for histopathologic studies to arrive at a firm diagnosis. The relief of increased intracranial pressure by shunt or other surgical decompression means is imperative in many cases, especially prior to initiation of radiation therapy and particularly when it is intended to use irradiation alone for treatment. Certain types of tumors like meningiomas, cerebellar astrocytomas, hemangioblastomas and others occasionally can be removed surgically in toto and the rate of recurrence is low. In the majority of the gliomas compressing adjacent structures, craniotomy and partial removal of neoplastic tissue by suction or electrocoagulation are indicated primarily. However, surgical removal no longer needs to be radical, since neurosurgeons know that they can preserve or restore function by partial removal only and may depend upon postoperative radiation therapy to complete treatment.

As yet, surgery and radiation, used alone or jointly are the only methods of treatment which have accomplished lasting results or apparent cures in the control of intracranial neoplasms.

INDICATIONS FOR RADIATION THERAPY

The indications for radiation therapy in the management of primary intracranial tumors must be clearly enunciated. All cases of primary intracranial neoplasm are not requiring radiation therapy. Irradiation should be considered when a case presents certain requirements. In our opinion, the indications for irradiation bring the patients into 5 categories:

1) Patients whose tumor has been treated surgically but could not be extirpated completely should receive adequate postoperative irradiation. Although certain tumors may be removed satisfactorily, time and ex-

perience have shown that in most of the gliomata actual removal in toto is rarely possible so that additional treatment with irradiation is required following operation in the majority of gliomas.

2) Patients whose brain tumor was not removed at the time of craniotomy and surgical exploration must be treated by irradiation alone. In this second category of patients, a biopsy is obtained in some so that a definite histologic diagnosis might be established, although this is not always the case. This occurs when a tumor is located in a highly critical area like the midbrain, the pons, the motor area of the cerebral cortex, because its surgical extirpation is then considered too hazardous for the patient's like or for a useful recovery.

3) Patients with a proven diagnosis of brain tumor obtained by needle biopsy who are not considered suitable cases for craniotomy and surgical removal should be treated with radiation only. Cases in that category may be medulloblastomas, cerebellar sarcomas, pinealomas or other midbrain tumors, and occasionally gliomas involving the cerebral motor area.

4) Those presenting with definite clinical evidence but without histologic proof of a tumor growing in the pons or brain-stem should be treated with radiation only. Too many patients are denied treatment. No attempt at surgical removal is made because of the high operative mortality rate, and irradiation is excluded because histological proof is lacking, and yet the diagnosis is established on otherwise sound evidence.

5) Those whose tumor has recurred after a surgical removal, considered complete at the time of operation, should have external radiation therapy, unless another operation is considered more advisable. Irradiation may be preferable in recurrent brain tumors. Further surgery is rather indicated for cystic tumors and some meningiomas.

Indications 2, 3, and 4 for treatment by irradiation alone are applicable to a minority of patients with primary intracranial tumors.

Actually there are only 16.8 per cent of our patients for whom radiation therapy only was indicated and utilized.

CONTRAINDICATIONS TO RADIATION THERAPY

Contraindications to the treatment of intracranial tumors by irradiation may be absolute and decisive when they preclude the use of radiation therapy in a majority of cases. They may be relative and transitory when they merely prevent initiation of irradiation until certain prohibitive conditions have been corrected satisfactorily or removed completely.

The following should be considered absolute contraindications:

1) The inadequate diagnosis or localization of a primary intracranial tumor.

2) The identification of a diffuse degenerative encephalitis such as reported in toxic conditions like uremia or severe anorexia, or observed occasionally in lymphosarcoma.

Diffuse gliosis involving one or two cerebral hemispheres may at times simulate an astrocytoma and it should not be treated with radiation therapy. Cerebral atrophy either unilateral or bilateral may contraindicate the use of radiation therapy or at least should caution against the administration of dosage which may exceed the minimum level of brain tolerance.

3) The presumptive recurrence of a brain tumor without adequate proof of neoplastic reactivation, irrelevant of the treatment procedures previously used.

4) The previous intensive irradiation of an intracranial tumor should preclude the use of further irradiation in the event of neoplastic reactivation because of the considerable risk of postradiation damage and brain necrosis when a second course is administered.

Exceptionally, we have reirradiated a brain tumor, providing that satisfactory evidence of tumor reactivation was available, that the patient has made a good recovery and that the period of remission from initial irradiation to the time of recurrence was not less than 6 months and preferably longer. It must be emphasized that recurrence of a brain tumor may easily be simulated by distension of residual cystic areas or a hemorrhage within the previously treated region.

Adequate reirradiation of an intracranial neoplasm is always hazardous in regard to postradiation injury, a risk which must be clearly understood and accepted by all concerned. Some patients have tolerated a second tumor dose as large as the initial one without subsequent complication but this is unpredictable. Nevertheless, our only case of postradiation brain necrosis has developed 3 years after reirradiation of a sarcoma which has recurred nearly 3 years after initial treatment. When a second course of radiation therapy is administered adequate protraction of dose is imperative.

5) Routine or prophylactic postoperative radiation therapy is not advocated for tumors which ordinarily can be eradicated completely by surgery, when the neurosurgeon feels certain that he has extirpated the neoplasm in toto.

This contraindication must be determined for each individual patient. It mostly applies to the "benign" types qualified by Horrax as favorable tumors which consist of the majority of meningeal tumors in adults, and of the cerebellar cystic astrocytomas and the few hemangiomatous cysts in children.

We consider the following conditions as relative contraindications:

1) Uncontrolled severe intracranial pressure with probable cerebral edema, until the increased pressure is under control through adequate and persistent decompressive measures including, if necessary, suitable medication such as diuretics and steroids.

Patients should not be denied radiation therapy if their condition appears critical providing that their intracranial pressure can be controlled. In many instances patients who were accepted for treatment despite their critical condition eventually recovered and enjoyed long useful survival.

2) The lack of histopathologic diagnosis to indicate the exact type of an intracranial tumor, when this can be determined without undue risk for the patient's life, should be considered as a relative contraindication.

Treatment Planning

Our experience has demonstrated conclusively that primary intracranial neoplasms can be treated adequately and safely with ionizing radiation generated at energy level of 200 to 250 Kv.

Megavoltage offers certain technical, biological, and clinical advantages even though the survival and recovery rates may not necessarily be superior to those attained with kilovoltage.

In the treatment of intracranial neoplasms, the main technical advantage of radiation in the megavoltage range consists of a greater penetrating power such that better depth dose distribution can be obtained, particularly when cross-firing in the anteroposterior direction through deep intracranial neoplasms or when tumors of small volume are irradiated. The increased depth dose is accompanied by lesser absorption by bone so that the use of high energy radiation should minimize the potential danger of postradiation aseptic bone necrosis in the calvarium or in the base of the skull. The radiobiological effects on the other intervening cephalic structures should be attenuated with high energy radiation. Scalp reactions should barely exceed the degree of mild erythema so that late changes consisting of telangiectasis and atrophy are rarely observed. The incidence of permanent epilation has diminished markedly, an advantage which is not negligible but is of no major importance.

Because of the multiple advantages just mentioned above, megavoltage radiation should be used in the treatment of intracranial tumors in preference to kilovoltage radiation. Since 1955, we have increasingly utilized the high energy radiation of ^{60}Co teletherapy sources to the extent that we are now using it exclusively. This must be clearly understood and applies to the treatment planning and the tumor doses recommended hereafter in the treatment of different types of intracranial tumors. The tumor doses recommended are expressed in rads and represent the minimal dose of radiation energy absorbed in the tumor itself from ^{60}Co radiation beams.

The natural tendency of certain cerebral gliomata to spread by direct invasion along known anatomic paths and even to cross midline at times has already been mentioned because this must be taken into consideration in the planning of treatment by irradiation. It has been demonstrated by Concannon *et al.*[9] that brain tumors are almost invariably larger and more extensive than suspected by clinical and roentgenologic examinations. Concannon *et al.* have concluded that there is no place for small or medium volume radiation therapy in the more malignant gliomata. It means that localized irradiation can be effective only insofar as the radiotherapist in planning treatment is reasonably certain that the fields will be large enough to include all of the intracranial neoplasm in each individual case.

For accurate localization and demarcation of the tumor-bearing area it is essential to make a topographic reconstitution of each tumor. To accomplish this most important part of treatment planning one must use fully all the information available from the clinical picture, the neuroradiologic and many other special investigative examinations which may be indicated, together with the operative findings of the neurosurgeon. If pin-point localization of primary brain tumors should be avoided because of the risk of not irradiating part of the tumor and jeopardizing a patient's chances for a cure, I believe that intensive irradiation of the entire intracranial content without specific reasons is an extreme solution to the problem of accurate localization and beam direction.

Once we are satisfied that the localization and extent of a brain tumor is confined to part of one cerebral hemisphere, a suitable technical plan of irradiation is devised for each patient individually. It is essential to circumscribe the tumor from every direction. This can be accomplished most efficiently by an arrangement of fields such that growth may be controlled primarily in both antero-posterior and vertical directions: opposing beams of ^{60}Co radiation are directed from the front and from the back of the calvarium through the affected hemisphere only. Tumor extension in the transverse direction towards and possibly beyond midline is the rationale for opposing lateral fields being placed not only on the homolateral side of the tumor-bearing area, but also on the contralateral side (Figs. 4-1A and 4-1B). Field size varies from 6 × 8 cm to 6 × 10 cm in the antero-posterior direction, and 8 × 8 cm to 10 × 10 cm laterally.

When there is evidence that a hemispheral glioma actually extends beyond midline or there is a suspicion that the tumor might cross over, the field size and arrangement in the anteroposterior direction must be such that the beam of ^{60}Co radiation will include part or all of the opposite hemisphere (Figs. 4-2A and 4-2B), including the third ventricle. In some cases, the tumor may be so extensive that the entire cranial content must be irradiated homogeneously.

In medulloblastomas the entire intracranial content must be irradiated because of their natural tendency to spread to the ventricles and all the subarachnoid spaces within the skull and the spinal canal. This illustrates the importance of knowing the histopathology of a tumor for adequate planning of its treatment with ionizing radiation. The treatment technique in medulloblastomas will be discussed and illustrated further in this chapter in the section devoted to the medulloblastomas.

Treatment planning of tumors growing in the midbrain and pontine regions usually depends more upon the critical anatomic

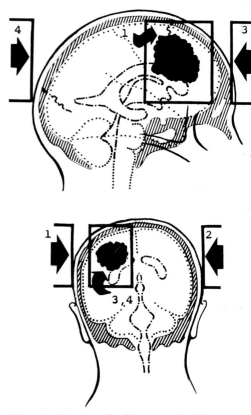

FIG. 4-1. Glioma confined to one cerebral hemisphere.

location of the primary tumor than its exact pathology, because these are not commonly accessible for biopsy or surgical extirpation. The technique of irradiation will be presented in the section on results of treatment of gliomatous tumors.

CLINICAL CONSIDERATIONS IN THE TREATMENT OF PATIENTS WITH IONIZING RADIATION

Whether the patient will be irradiated postoperatively or will be treated with radiation alone for a primary intracranial tumor, irradiation must not be initiated unless increased intracranial pressure is under control. The fear that cerebral edema might develop and become so severe as to cause death must not be so great that a patient will be deprived from adequate radiation therapy

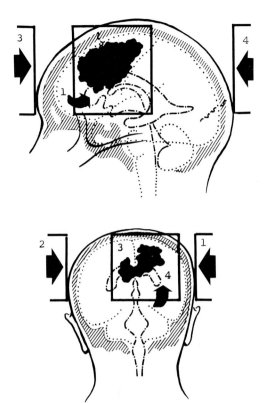

FIG. 4-2. Glioma of left frontal lobe crossing midline to right hemisphere.

when indicated in the management of a primary intracranial tumor. It must be realized that some degree of cerebral edema may be present before treatment is initiated, either because of increased intracranial pressure or due to the size of the tumor itself. Cerebral edema can be aggravated by excessive initial doses of radiation, unless it is relieved first by decompressive surgical procedures or by adequate medication. The risk of lethal cerebral edema is greater for patients who will be treated with radiation alone, without decompression, than for those exposed to postoperative irradiation after a craniotomy has been performed and the bulk of the tumor removed. Edema may occasionally develop during the initial part of the course of radiation therapy, even after decompression has been accomplished with shunts or other procedures. Cerebral edema can be identified by

aggravation of the neurologic symptoms and signs, particularly by headache of increasing severity. When severe edema develops after completion of treatment, a rare occurrence in our experience, it may simulate reactivation of the tumor growth. From a practical standpoint, in order to obviate any complication from existing or potential cerebral edema, regardless of whether or not the patient has had a decompression prior to treatment, it is my practice to administer only 50 to 100 rads tumor dose through but one port for the first 3 or 4 treatments at the onset of a course of radiation therapy. By protracting total tumor doses of 5,000 to 6,000 rads or more over a period of 50 to 60 days, cerebral edema has been avoided in nearly all cases.

In postoperative irradiation, treatment is usually initiated approximately 2 weeks after operation when the incision of the scalp is well healed and local subcutaneous fluid collection or edema have regressed.

Radiation sickness is uncommon in the treatment of intracranial neoplasms when protracted fractionated doses adding up to not more than 800 to 900 rads tumor dose per week are administered. So much so that if a patient vomits under such treatment, it is more often related to developing increased intracranial pressure or to some complication other than radiation sickness.

It is essential that both the neurosurgeon and the radiation therapist observe the patient closely during the first few days of treatment and, if indicated, they reassess the case and modify the plan of treatment. The necessity for periodic decompression has become negligible in recent years, probably because of careful planning and cautious administration of radiation therapy.

POSTRADIATION EFFECTS ON NORMAL BRAIN TISSUE AND OTHER INTRACRANIAL STRUCTURES IN HUMANS

The true effects of ionizing radiation on the normal human brain and the rest of the intracranial content cannot be determined accurately by studying the tissue reactions which may be observed in patients irradiated for primary intracranial neoplasms. The main reason is that, when a patient is subjected to radiation therapy for an intracranial neoplasm, the brain and adjacent tissues are no longer in their normal state but are diseased in some degree.

In humans, the radiation tolerance of the normal brain and other intracranial structures can be studied with strict scientific objectivity only from patients whose intracranial content presumably was normal at the time that a zone of their brain happened to be irradiated because it was located directly beneath an extracranial lesion treated with ionizing radiation. Lampe[19] has noted that, with few exceptions, the non-nervous tissue lesions treated, "when parts of the central nervous system have been included in the irradiated zone, have been neoplastic lesions requiring the therapeutic administration of relatively large radiation doses." Several authors have reported damage to the brain and other intracranial structures following irradiation of malignant tumors of the scalp.

Sizable single doses of ionizing radiation have been administered in the treatment of extracranial lesions. The radiation tolerance of the underlying normal human brain tissue should be commensurate with that of the normal animal brain tissue investigated under similar conditions of exposure to radiation. Observations[22,26] suggest that single tissue doses in the range of 2,400 to 3,000 r or more exceed the radiation tolerance of the normal brain in man. In animal experiments, single doses of comparable magnitude (2,400 r) have been reported to exceed the radiation tolerance of normal brain and single tissue doses of 3,000 r have invariably induced brain necrosis.

Several reports[11,22] have illustrated the danger of irradiating normal human brain with total doses which are relatively large when administered over a short period of time even in divided and multiple exposures, especially when a fair volume of tissue is irradiated so that the amount of radiation absorbed is high. A second course of irradiation may be a decisive factor in producing brain necrosis particularly when the initial course had been administered intensively. The length of the latent periods before brain necrosis may manifest itself can vary considerably. The initial acute reactions, which may occur after massive single doses or following intensive irradiation in divided doses, apparently caused no detectable symptoms and clinically passed unnoticed in the latter cases of late necrosis of the normal brain.

POSTRADIATION EFFECTS ON CEREBRAL AND OTHER INTRACRANIAL TISSUES INVOLVED IN THE TREATMENT OF MALIGNANT INTRACRANIAL NEOPLASMS

It is difficult to evaluate postradiation changes in the human brain following the treatment of intracranial tumors with large doses of ionizing radiation. One has to try to differentiate between morphologic changes which are practically identical, whether they have been induced by generalized increased intracranial pressure or by the local tumor growth or possibly by radiation. The fact that the brain adjacent to a tumor is already diseased to some degree, in part or in toto, at the onset of irradiation must render the brain tissue more vulnerable to large doses of radiation than if it were normal to begin with. In other words, in the presence of a primary intracranial neoplasm the radiation tolerance of the surrounding central nervous tissue must be less than that of the normal human brain.

Wachowski and Cheneault[31] published their experience in 6 cases of brain tumor which showed postradiation degenerative effects following radiation therapy with tumor doses of 6,100 to 8,800 r in 85 to 100 days. The tissue changes described were affecting all the cellular elements.

Arnold *et al.*[1] have reported delayed necrosis of the brain-stem and hypothalamus in 2 patients 1 year or more following the treatment of brain-stem gliomas, having used tumor doses of 4,500 *r* of 400 Kv x-rays in 30 days.

Lampe[19] has reported his experience in relation to late radiation damage of the brain in cases of medulloblastoma of the cerebellum. Of 26 patients, 7 survived beyond 5 years. Brain damage has occurred in 4 of the 7 survivors. Two were perfectly normal approximately 12 and 13 years after irradiation. The 7th patient presented questionable signs of radiation damage 15 years after irradiation. In 1950, Lampe[19] altered his method of irradiation to a fractional technique protracted over 55 to 65 days using an estimated dose of 5,000 to 6,000 *r*. At the time of his report (1957) he had treated 7 patients who could be observed for 3 years or longer. Four of the 7 had already survived from 3 to 6 years and all 4 were in good health.

The only identified case of postradiation brain necrosis in our own series showed extensive bilateral necrosis of the occipital lobes, with evidence of residual or recurrent tumor at the site of the primary lesion in the right cerebellum. This resulted from two intensive courses of roentgen therapy administered for a perithelial sarcoma located in the right cerebellar lobe. In the first course of irradiation, the patient received postoperatively a tumor dose of 6,500 *r* in 38 days to the entire intracranial content, and 2,000 *r* in 18 days to the spinal axis as the diagnosis of medulloblastoma was considered just as probable as that of sarcoma. She then presented nearly 3 years later with signs of recurrence, and the tumor-bearing area received a further dose of 5,300 rads over a period of 60 days.

A clinical pattern appears to be more or less identical and constant in all patients who have developed postradiation brain necrosis. Following treatment, a period of improvement and even total recovery usually happens and this condition may persist for 1 to 5 years or longer. Sudden or gradual deterioration of the patient's clinical condition will develop without signs of increased intracranial pressure, *i.e.*, without papilledema or increased tension at level of the osteoplastic flap, or even with depression at level of the operative wound. Neurologic signs are also present, but obviously they vary in relation to the cerebral territory directly damaged by radiation. Such clinical pattern has been considered by most observers as evidence of postradiation damage of the central nervous tissue. The overall picture must be differentiated from deterioration of clinical condition associated with evidence of tumor reactivation or progression, thrombosis, or hemorrhage, abscess or other inflammatory process.

The majority of immediate complications or late sequelae are attributable to the tumor itself rather than to the use of radiation alone or in combination with surgery in the course of treatment. Too often, residual clinical manifestations which have not regressed following treatment are also considered as sequelae of the treatment applied, especially when radiation has been used. Reactivation of tumor and concomitant deterioration of a patient's condition is often attributed unduly to postradiation damage.

In reviewing reports of the proven cases of postradiation necrosis observed at various sites of the central nervous system in humans, one is impressed with the fact that such complications appear to have developed mostly under two sets of circumstances, either of which may have been sufficient to play a paramount role in inducing such complication. The first hazard seems to be the administration of large tumor doses, which may be excessive when delivered over a relatively short period of time (3,000 to 5,000 rads in 2 to 3 weeks) or even when protracted over longer periods of time if the doses are very high. The second hazard, and often the most common, appears to be the repetition of series of treatment over a period of 1 year or even much longer, in which moderate to large doses of ionizing radiation are directed to the same regions of the central nervous system during each course of treatment with radiation.

We have accumulated considerable evidence that postradiation injury of the brain can be avoided by fractionation and protraction of radiation doses in a continuous series. Aside from the technical and physical factors of irradiation, adequate control of increased intracranial pressure is probably the most important safety factor, since this may allow brain tissue damaged under pressure effects to recover before or soon after initiating irradiation of an intracranial neoplasm.

The importance of protraction and fractionation of the dose in the treatment of intracranial neoplasms by irradiation has been demonstrated by the absence of immediate histopathologic changes in the peritumoral neurones, glial cells, blood vessels and meninges. In the cases in which the dose has been fractionated within the range of accepted tissue doses (approximately 5,000 rads over periods varying from 30 to 50 days), there were no appreciable postradiation tissue changes observed beyond the tumor-bearing area, either immediately or even months to years later.

Several workers have attempted to determine dose levels which might be used safely in the treatment of primary intracranial neoplasms. Most of the radiation tolerance doses suggested have been expressed in terms of definite time periods for the administration of radiation therapy, since it is recognized that dose and time are the basic factors combining to determine the true magnitude of irradiation intensity and of all radiobiologic effects. Boden[4] has emphasized the importance of a third major factor in relation to the radiation tolerance of the central nervous tissue. This factor is the magnitude of the volume of tissue exposed to radiation. He has demonstrated that the dose tolerance of brain tissue is inversely proportional with the volume of tissue subjected to irradiation: the smaller the volume the greater the tolerance

to radiation, and the larger the volume the lesser the tolerance.

The limits of radiation tolerance of brain tissue have been studied by several investigators who have suggested levels of irradiation intensity that could be considered safe. Boden gave an upper limit of 3,500 r depth dose in 17 days when large field techniques were used and 4,500 r in 17 days with small field techniques. Effectively, Boden[5] was first to publish radiation tolerance curves applicable to the brain-stem and the rest of the human brain. From Boden's tolerance curves, dosage biologically equivalent can be obtained readily in relation to the highest dose that the brain-stem and the rest of the brain may tolerate over certain periods of time and in consideration also of the volume of brain tissue exposed to radiation. Boden used Strandqvist's curves for skin necrosis and, on the basis of the depth doses that the brain and cord could tolerate in 17 days (3,500 to 4,500 r), he arrived at the following biological equivalents for the central nervous tissue: 3,650 to 4,700 r in 21 days, 3,900 to 5,000 r in 28 days, 4,100 to 5,300 r in 35 days, 4,300 to 5,500 r in 42 days, 4,500 to 5,800 r in 49 days, and 4,700 to 6,100 r in 56 days. McWhirter and Dott[23] have stated that 5,500 r tumor dose in 4 weeks is at the upper limit of brain tolerance, but they also indicated that it is desirable not to exceed 5,000 r over the same period of time.

Lindgren[21] published time-dose relationship curves in respect to the incidence of radionecrosis in the human brain. Using all the data available, Lindgren drew up a modified Strandqvist's diagram showing two logarithmic curves: 1) the upper line corresponds to the maximum dosage level above which the risk of cerebral necrosis is considerable; 2) the lower line shows the lowest level of dosage at which brain necrosis has been induced. The dose given is that received in the center of the irradiated region. Of the 17 cases used by Lindgren in the making of his diagram of brain tolerance to irradiation, 10 lie above the line of maximum tolerance and 7 lie between the lines of maximum and minimum tolerance.

Lindgren has compared his dose level curves with the ones published by Boden and by Zeman and he has observed that the limits of brain tolerance to radiation that each of them has shown individually lie below the upper limits obtained in his investigation, and therefore lie within the dosage range where the risk of necrosis is less pronounced. Furthermore, Lindgren has plotted the focal doses received by 5 of his patients still living in comfort 4 to 10 years after irradiation of brain tumors, and in 4 of the 5 the dose levels were lying on or below the lowest level producing necrosis, whereas the dose in the remaining cases was between the lines of minimum and maximum tolerance.

The time-dose relationship curves (Fig. 4-3) for radionecrosis in human brains that Lindgren has calculated from collective precise data are the result of a considerable endeavor to assess the radiosensitivity of human brain tissue. These curves could serve as a safety guide in the management of any patient whose brain will be irradiated for an intracranial neoplasm or perhaps for some extracranial lesion. The use of Lindgren's curves might prevent one from exceeding the safe limits of exposure to ionizing radiation at both the high and low levels of brain tolerance. In Lindgren's opinion, of the two curves of his modified Strandqvist's diagram the lower is the more important because it indicates the lowest dosage level capable of producing cerebral necrosis in patients.

The dose-time range that we have considered and are still considering within the limits of brain tolerance in the irradiation of primary intracranial tumors consists of 5,000 to 6,000 rads tumor dose, administered over a period of approximately 50 days with a quality of radiation corresponding to that produced by kilovoltage x-ray apparatus.

It is generally agreed that the relative biological effects of high energy radiation are less intense than those of the lower energy level corresponding to kilovoltage. This

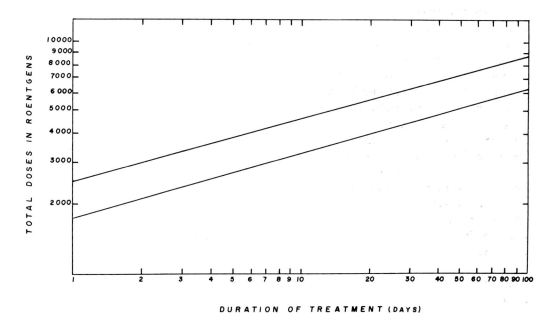

DURATION OF TREATMENT (DAYS)

FIG. 4-3. Time dose curves made by Lindgren in relation to radionecrosis in human brains. The upper line corresponds to the maximum dosage level above which the risk of cerebral necrosis is considerable. The lower line shows the lowest level of dosage at which brain necrosis may occur. The dose given is that received in the center of the irradiated region.

difference in tissue reaction should be compensated by increasing tumor doses by 20 per cent when using ^{60}Co gamma radiation or 4 Mev x-radiation. However, we never exceed total tumor doses of 6,500 rads over 50 days.

The tumor doses just mentioned are in agreement with Boden's upper limits of brain tolerance to radiation and fall below the upper and lower limits in Lindgren's curves. In view of our long-standing experience with irradiation of the brain surrounding primary cerebral gliomas and with exposure at the same time of the other intracranial structures, our long-term results strongly suggest that the time-dose relation used in the treatment of our patients probably represents an optimum range of tissue tolerance for the brain and the entire intracranial content.

The possibility of postradiation damage to the pituitary in the treatment of intracranial neoplasms not arising from the gland itself must be considered. The hypothysis and its stalk are often damaged indirectly by an intracranial neoplasm causing erosion and enlargement of the sella turcica together with compression of the gland within the sella. In such cases the pituitary gland is no longer normal and may be more vulnerable to irradiation when it happens to lie in the path of one or more beams of ionizing radiation directed primarily to a malignant intracranial tumor. Under the circumstances radiation injury may occur, but it must be rare within the range of tumor doses to which the pituitary may be exposed when the irradiated tumors are located in proximity to the sella turcica. To damage the normal pituitary as result of irradiation of an intracranial neoplasm, brain tolerance doses would have to be exceeded considerably. It has been suggested that doses as high as 25,000 to 30,000 rads may be required to destroy the normal pituitary gland, as desired in the management of advanced carcinoma.

The potential consequences that, in the treatment of intracranial neoplasms, the incidental but inherent irradiation of the normal pituitary gland might have on the mental and physiologic development of children so exposed are a legitimate concern. Any fear in that respect might be dissipated by considering the long-term results that will be presented for 119 children whose pituitary glands inevitably were irradiated 5 to 25 years ago in the treatment of primary brain tumors.

POSTRADIATION EFFECTS ON MALIGNANT INTRACRANIAL NEOPLASMS

It is our opinion that adequate radiation therapy may be effective in all types of glioma, but not to the same degree in all. There is universal agreement that medulloblastomas are the most radiosensitive of all primary intracranial tumors, although they may be curable only in a proportion which varies from 1 to 2 out of 5. Malignant ependymomas or ependyblastomas are also very radiosensitive and usually exhibit a higher degree of radiocurability than medulloblastomas, since at least 1 of 2 patients with ependymal cell tumors may be expected to survive 5 years or longer.

Gliomas originating from the astrocytes represent by far the majority of the gliomatous tumors. Considerable differences of opinion are prevailing in respect to the relative degrees of radiosensitivity within the broad group of malignant gliomas generally regarded as being of astrocytic origin. Glioblastoma multiforme is the most malignant of all intracranial neoplasms and it is considered as radioresistant by most people. Although it is recognized that its radiosensitivity is low, in our experience, glioblastomas seem to respond to radiation therapy in the majority of cases even though its growth restraint is usually of short duration. Consequently radiocurability of glioblastomas is poor, but there is always the odd case which will respond better than anticipated, if adequately irradiated, so that patients may survive for 5 years or longer in the proportion of 1 out of 15.[7]

In the intermediate type of astrocytoma, which appears in our own material as unclassified glioma, tumors usually show a moderate degree of radiosensitivity. Results indicate that we may anticipate that approximately 1 of 3 malignant gliomas classified in this group will remain under control for 5 years or longer.[6]

The low grade and well-differentiated astrocytomas are generally considered as tumors of low radiosensitivity. Our opinion differs appreciably. In contrasting survival rates between a first group of patients who were believed not to require irradiation following surgical removal and a second group of patients irradiated postoperatively because of evidence of residual tumor, it appears clearly that our results at 5 years and 10 years after treatment have been superior in the group of irradiated patients.[6]

The usually slowly growing oligodendroglioma and the low malignancy oligodendroglioblastoma are also tumors of limited radiosensitivity. When irradiated, the oligodendroglial tumors require doses which approach or sometimes exceed the dose tolerance of the normal brain tissue. Adequate protracted irradiation seems to be helpful in controlling tumors of this histologic type when removed incompletely or showing malignant characters. Our postoperative results in the oligodendroglioma group have shown that in 1 of 2 patients the condition has remained under control for 5 years or longer.

Outside of the glioma group, practically all other histologic types of intracranial tumors are capable of responding in some degree to radiation therapy. However, the degree of radiosensitivity is variable and it must be determined for each individual group of tumors. Only in a limited way should the selection of cases suitable for irradiation be made purely on the basis of known radiosensitivity. Such selection should be made primarily on the basis of other factors that we have discussed above in the section on indications and contraindications for radiation therapy.

The histologic assessment of the degree of tumor damage as a direct radiobiologic effect on gliomas is difficult. When gliomas which have been treated by irradiation are examined histologically, the amount of tissue changes which may be attributed to radiation therapy alone can hardly be differentiated from variable degrees of necrosis, hemorrhage and vascular changes which often occur spontaneously in the nonirradiated tumors, particularly in the most malignant.

Nearly all the histopathologic studies on the effects of radiation therapy on primary brain tumors reveal consistently the finding of microscopic evidence of residual tumor cells at the site of the primary neoplastic lesion. Whether these cells may be viable or not is a biological character which cannot be determined with any degree of certainty from their morphology. Our experience coincides with that of the majority of observers.[25] From a series of 130 patients with glioblastomas, irradiated with tumor doses averaging 6,500 r up to 7,500 r in approximately 6 to 8 weeks, tumor cells were found at the site of the primary neoplasm in all cases reoperated upon (24 cases) or autopsied (30 cases). Very recently, I have reviewed the autopsy findings in 63 of 564 patients who were exposed to intensive irradiation for all types of primary intracranial neoplasms, and there is not a single case in which complete disappearance of all tumor cells has been observed.

In an outstanding study on the tolerance of brain tissue and the sensitivity of brain tumors to irradiation, Lindgren[21] has reported 10 cases in which no residual tumor cells could be found at autopsy. His study is based upon 71 cases of intracranial gliomas treated with radiation which were carefully studied postmortem and of which 18 proved to be highly informative.

The radiobiologic effects on primary intracranial gliomata and other neoplasms, following radiation of adequate intensity can be best appraised on the basis of the immediate clinical results observed during the course of treatment and subsequent months, and far more from the long-term results estimated by the survival and recovery rates.

Results of Treatment

In discussing the role of radiation therapy in the management of primary intracranial neoplasms, it is my intention to use our own results to a large extent.

Over a period of 25 years, from 1939 to 1963 inclusive, we have treated with external irradiation 788 patients with primary intracranial tumors, of which 668 were classified with the gliomata and 120 or 15.2 per cent with the nongliomatous tumors (Table 4-1).

From 1939 to 1958, a period of 20 years, 564 primary brain tumors have been irradiated in our department under constant conditions with radiation in the kilovoltage range, except for 17 cases exposed to the higher energy of ^{60}Co. These 564 cases are available for full assessment 5 to 25 years following irradiation.

In our series of 494 irradiated gliomata, histological confirmation is available in 449 cases, nearly 91 per cent.

The program of radiation therapy applied to the management of the 564 primary intracranial neoplasms under review has consisted of a single protracted series of exposures with 220 to 250 Kv or kilovoltage radiation. In general, tumor doses in the range of 5,000 to 6,000 r have been delivered over a period of approximately 50 days. During the initial years of our program, various dose levels have been tried. However, it can be stated that the dosage intensity has been fairly consistent through the years, since it has not varied much from an average of 800 to 1,000 r per week (tumor dose) over a period of 6 to 8 consecutive weeks. At the onset of treatment, small daily tumor doses of 50 to 100 rads are used over 4 or 5 days.

Table 4-1. *Primary Intracranial Neoplasms (Adequately Irradiated)*
Author's Experience Over 25 Years, 1939–1963

Type or Location	Number of Cases		
	1939–58	1959–63	Total
Gliomata:			
Glioblastoma	176	49	225
Glioma—unclassified	40	42	82
Astrocytoma	123	54	177
Oligodendroglioblastoma	14	3	17
Ependymoblastoma	20	3	23
Medulloblastoma	50	13	63
Midbrain tumors	37	4	41
Brain-stem or pontine tumors	34	6	40
	494	174	668
Nongliomatous Tumors:			
Sarcomas	16	4	20
Meningeal tumors	25	13	38
Vascular tumors	15	7	22
Congenital tumors	8	7	15
Miscellaneous	6	19	25
	70	50	120
Total	564	224	788

Subsequently, tumor doses are gradually increased to 150 to 200 rads per sitting, on a basis of 5 treatment visits per week.

Once irradiation is initiated, it is important to persist and persevere until treatment has been completed. Occasionally a course of treatment may have to be slowed down and perhaps interrupted for a few days but, inasmuch as radiation effect is cumulative, irradiation should be resumed soon and continued as a single course. In many instances patients have been accepted for irradiation despite their critical condition, and yet many of them have recovered eventually and survived for a long time. Close collaboration between the neurosurgeon and the therapeutic radiologist is essential during all phases of treatment. Decompressive procedures must be established and maintained with effectiveness in all cases in which there is marked increase in intracranial pressure at the onset of treatment. Symptomatic treatment must be used as required.

Patients who were not adequately irradiated have been omitted from this series of primary intracranial neoplasms. These were patients who, for some reason or another, had received less than 50 per cent of the average tumor dose usually administered in this series. Accordingly, a total of 45 patients, 19 of whom were more or less terminal with glioblastoma, have been classified as inadequately irradiated on the basis that radiation had little or no opportunity to influence the course of their disease. For all practical purposes, irrespective of the outcome of their illness, such patients had to be regarded as untreated with radiation.

The majority of our patients (83.2 per cent) were irradiated postoperatively, because of tumors which admittedly had not been removed completely. Exceptionally, postoperative irradiation was administered despite the presumably complete extirpation of a glioma, because the relatives were insisting for radiation therapy. This was probably the proper thing to do when considering that so many neurosurgeons have expressed the opinion that it is almost impossible to remove gliomatous tumors completely. Some patients were not irradiated early after a surgical removal which was believed to be complete, but had radiation therapy later when they showed unquestionable evidence of tumor recurrence. There are 29 patients, or 5.1 per cent of our 564 cases, who were subjected to postoperative irradiation only at the time of recurrence (21 gliomas and 8 malignant meningeal tumors). It must be noted that in these cases the period of survival has been calculated from the onset of irradiation and not from the time of previous surgical management.

Results of treatment of intracranial neoplasms must be assessed under two essential aspects: 1) the length of survival and 2) the quality of survival expressed by recovery rates. In evaluating the methods of treatment of intracranial tumors, high survival rates are meaningful inasmuch as the majority of survivors are capable of resuming an active useful life or at least of caring for themselves, whereas only a low minority are remaining totally disabled, mentally or physically, or both.

The length of survival has been calculated in all our cases from the first day of treatment with radiation. No allowance has been made for correction on account of death resulting from unrelated diseases or accidents. Not a single case had to be recorded as deceased during the first 5 years following treatment because of lack of follow-up information.

In evaluating the quality of survival, the degree of clinical recovery is estimated and recorded as good, fair or poor corresponding to a grading in categories I, II or III as shown in Table 4-2. The quality of survival is good when the patient has returned to an active useful life; it is fair, if some degree of partial disability has persisted more than 3 to 6 months after completion of treatment; it is poor, when total disability has developed and the patient has remained completely incapable physically or mentally or both. A valid

Table 4-2. *Primary Intracranial Neoplasms—Long Term Survival and Recovery Rates* Subsequent to Adequate Irradiation Used Postoperatively or Alone*

Survival Over	Length of Survival			Quality of Survival		
	Total Possible	No. of Survivors	Per Cent of Survivals	Percentile Recovery Grade†		
				I	II	III
5 Years	564	196	35	80	15	5
10 Years	412	106	26	82	16	2
15 Years	258	51	20	84	14	2
20 Years	111	21	19	90	10	—

*From patients adequately irradiated, 83.2 per cent postoperatively, 1939–1958.—Follow-up complete to 1964.
† Grading of Recovery: Grade I—Good—Active useful life
                     Grade II—Fair—Partial disability
                     Grade III—Poor—Total disability: physical and/or mental.

and objective assessment of the degree of recovery has been relatively facile in the present series because of the accumulated clinical follow-up information which could lend itself to very little subjective interpretation.

It is important to know the degree of recovery obtained during the major part of the survival of the 368 patients who have lived less than 5 years following irradiation, considering that 65 per cent of the 564 patients that we have irradiated for primary intracranial neoplasms have not survived 5 years following treatment. Regardless of the length of survival of the individual patient, whether it was just a few months or a few years, it is estimated that only 9 per cent of the patients who have survived less than 5 years after irradiation have shown no improvement whatsoever; 19 per cent have remained with some degree of partial disability, whereas 72 per cent were well for the major part of their survival. This overall assessment of the quality of survival among those who have survived less than 5 years has applied to all age groups of patients, both adults and children. Such results are gratifying enough to encourage and stimulate anyone to continue to use radiation therapy when indicated in the management of primary intracranial neoplasms.

Many are skeptical regarding the quality of survival of patients who have been irradiated for primary brain tumors and have survived over long periods of time. In order to arrive at true recovery rates, expressed by the percentage of those whose recovery grading was good, fair or poor more than 5, 10, 15, or 20 years after irradiation of their brain and intracranial content, we have recently reviewed and reassessed the degree of recovery in the case of each patient who has survived more than 5 years.

Long-term survival and recovery rates, based upon 564 primary intracranial neoplasms of all types, have been tabulated and presented side-by-side in Tables 4-2 and 4-3. All cases have been observed clinically and followed up for not less than 5 years subsequent to adequate irradiation, administered postoperatively or alone. Table 4-2 clearly reveals that the proportion of long-term survivals and good recoveries is higher than most people would dare to predict among patients whose brain and other intracranial tissues were exposed to intensive irradiation more than 10, 15 or 20 years ago. The longer the survival, the higher the proportion of good recovery among the survivors. It is significant that only 11 or 5.5 per cent of the 196 patients who have survived over 5 years were totally disabled 5 years after irradiation. The rate of total disability is only 2 per cent among the 10- and 15-year survivors, whereas it is nil in the group of 21 who have survived more than 20 years following radiation therapy of adequate intensity.

In the course of management of patients with intracranial neoplasms, the referring specialist, the family physician, the relatives and others often inquire as to what might be the life expectancy of a patient who is irradiated for a certain type of brain tumor. For that purpose the primary intracranial gliomata have been separated from the nongliomatous intracranial tumors and assembled by histological groups.

The nongliomatous primary intracranial neoplasms are a very mixed group in which the role of radiation therapy may vary considerably. Intracranial sarcomas represent a rather heterogeneous histologic group of tumors which often respond to radiation therapy better than most would presume. The majority of meningeal tumors can be extirpated completely by surgical removal, so that the number of cases for which radiation therapy is indicated may be relatively small. Many of the blood vessel tumors consist of relatively benign hemangiomas which, whether treated or not, are compatible with a good life expectancy. The majority of

hemangioblastomas, particularly those arising from the cerebellum, may be controlled fully by surgical removal so that postoperative irradiation is required only in the few tumors which have not been extirpated completely. Congenital tumors other than those of vascular origin are not numerous and consist mostly of craniopharyngiomas and chordomas. Several tumors in our series were diagnosed pinealomas on a clinical basis but in final analysis there is not a single pinealoma proven by histology among the miscellaneous nongliomatous tumors which have been irradiated.

In the present series of 70 nongliomatous intracranial tumors, the life expectancy of patients who have been exposed to irradiation, alone or postoperatively, has been tabulated. Of the 70 patients irradiated more than 5 years ago and followed up completely to 1964 (Table 4-4), 45 were treated over 10 years ago; 29 over 15 years ago; and 17 over 20 years ago. In 55 or 79 per cent of the 70 cases, irradiation was used postoperatively either because of incomplete surgical removal or else postoperative recurrence (8 meningeal tumors). Irradiation was used alone in the treatment of 15 patients or 21

Table 4-3. *Primary Intracranial Gliomata—Life Expectancy of Patients Treated with Surgery and Irradiation or Irradiation Alone*

Type or Location of Glioma	Percentile Life Expectancy Greater Than					
	1 Year	3 Years	5 Years	10 Years	15 Years	20 Years
Glioblastoma	44	13	7	4	2	0
Glioma—unclassified	71	48	30	20	13	13
Astrocytoma	86	65	52	31	24	21
Oligodendroglioblastoma	100	79	50	33	18	15
Ependymoblastoma	90	75	70	56	52	43
Medulloblastoma	74	36	26	17	9	8
Midbrain tumors	70	54	46	39	30	20
Brain-stem tumors	56	29	29	24	23	20
Average Rates	66	40	30	20	15	15

Table drawn up from actual survival rates of 494 patients irradiated adequately, 1939–1958 inclusive.
Clinical follow-up complete to 1964, ranging from a minimum of 5 years up to 25 years.
Of the 494 patients, 367 were treated over 10 years ago; 229, over 15 years; and 94, over 20 years.
Surgical removal plus postoperative irradiation: 414 gliomata or 83.8 per cent.—Irradiation alone: 80 or 16.2 per cent.

Table 4-4. *Primary Intracranial Neoplasms—Nongliomatous—Life Expectancy of Patients Treated with Surgery Plus Irradiation or Irradiation Alone*

Types of Tumor	Proportion of Survivals Over					
	1 Year	3 Years	5 Years	10 Years	15 Years	20 Years
Sarcomas	11/16	9/16	7/16	4/14	2/5	0/2
Meningeal	24/25	18/25	17/25	11/17	6/10	2/5
Vascular	15/15	15/15	13/15	12/14	8/10	4/7
Congenital	6/8	6/8	5/8	1/4	0/2	0/1
Miscellaneous	5/6	4/6	4/6	4/6	1/2	1/2
All Types	61/70	52/70	46/70	32/45	17/29	7/17

Table drawn up from actual survivors among 70 patients irradiated adequately, 1939 to 1958 inclusive.
Clinical follow-up complete to 1964, ranging from a minimum of 5 years up to 25 years.
Of the 70 patients, 45 were treated over 10 years ago; 29, over 15 years; and 17, over 20 years.
Surgical removal (incomplete) plus postoperative irradiation: 55 patients or 79 per cent.—Irradiation alone: 15 or 21 per cent.

per cent of the nongliomatous intracranial neoplasms irradiated more than 5 years ago. In preparing Table 4-4 we have merely attempted to obtain some idea as to what the life expectancy might be in each category of nongliomatous intracranial neoplasms by considering the proportion of those who have survived over 1, 3, 5, 10, 15, and 20 years in relation to the total number of patients irradiated. Because of the predominance in our series of meningeal and vascular tumors, which usually carry a good prognosis, the proportion of long-term survivals over 5, 10, 15, and 20 years following irradiation is relatively high, and this could be anticipated.

The results of adequate treatment with irradiation alone in the management of primary intracranial neoplasms deserve to be reviewed with particular attention, since there is very scanty information in that respect in the current medical literature. Of the 564 primary intracranial neoplasms that we have irradiated more than 5 years ago, a total of 95 patients (80 with gliomata and 15 with nongliomatous tumors) had no surgical removal of their tumor and were treated only with radiation. In regard to the life expect-

Table 4-5. *Primary Intracranial Neoplasms—Long Term Survival and Recovery Rates* Subsequent to Treatment with Adequate Irradiation Alone*

Survival Over	Length of Survival			Quality of Survival		
	Total Possible	No. of Survivors	Per Cent of Survivals	Percentile Recovery Grade†		
				I	II	III
5 Years	95	34	36	85	6	9
10 Years	59	22	37	95	—	5
15 Years	30	11	37	100	—	—
20 Years	13	3	23	100	—	—

* From 80 gliomata and 15 nongliomatous tumors treated without surgical removal, a total of 95 or 16.8 per cent of all primary intracranial tumors adequately irradiated, 1939–1958. Follow-up complete to 1964.
† Grading of Recovery: Grade I—Good—Active useful life
  Grade II—Fair—Partial disability
  Grade III—Poor—Total disability: physical and/or mental.

ancy of patients so treated, the long-term survival and recovery rates subsequent to the treatment with irradiation alone of 95 primary intracranial neoplasms of different types have been tabulated side-by-side (Table 4-5). The actual degree of recovery at 5 and 10 years has been quite good when considering that only 3 of the 34 survivors or 9 per cent of the patients treated with irradiation alone were totally disabled at 5 years, and only 1 or 5 per cent of the 22 survivors at 10 years was totally incapacitated. The 11 patients who survived over 15 years, and among them the 3 who were alive over 20 years after irradiation were all in perfect condition.

Because of the relatively small number of patients so treated, the life expectancy of patients treated with irradiation alone for a variety of intracranial gliomata, grouped by histologic types or according to their particular location, is not presented on a percentile basis in Table 4-6.

Among the patients treated with irradiation alone in the management of medulloblastomas, midbrain and brain-stem tumors (Table 4-6), the relatively high proportion of long-term survivals may be somewhat surprising. Considering that some type of surgi-

cal decompression was effected in 24 of the 80 cases classified as gliomata and treated with irradiation alone, one wonders to what extent the decompressive procedures might be responsible for better results. Although there was no surgical removal of tumor in any of those cases, the surgical exploration performed in 3 cases, the establishment of shunts alone in 15 cases, or the combination of surgical exploration and insertion of shunts in 6 others are all surgical procedures which must have influenced the course of the disease considerably. In the immediate management of patients treated for inoperable intracranial tumors, decompressive measures, in our opinion, have been most useful during and after their course of irradiation. In several cases dramatic improvement of patient's condition has been observed before irradiation was even initiated. Shunts have the advantage of being relatively simple procedures and seem to be particularly indicated in the management of tumors located in a region from which they can rarely be extirpated like in the midbrain area and to a lesser extent in the brain-stem. Shunts are often useful in the management of medulloblastomas located in the posterior fossa. The various surgical procedures used for reliev-

Table 4-6. *Life Expectancy of Patients Treated with Irradiation Alone in Primary Intracranial Neoplasms*

Gliomata (80 cases)	Proportion of Survivals Over*					
	1 Year	3 Years	5 Years	10 Years	15 Years	20 Years
Glioblastoma	2/5	1/5	0/5	—	—	—
Glioma-unclassified	2/3	1/3	0/3	0/1	0/1	0/1
Astrocytoma	2/3	0/3	0/3	0/1	—	—
Medulloblastoma	8/10	4/10	4/10	2/7	1/4	0/1
Midbrain	20/29	15/29	12/29	7/17	1/5	0/2
Brain-stem	15/30	8/30	8/30	5/20	4/12	1/5
All Types	49/80	29/80	24/80	14/46	6/22	1/9
Average Rates	61%	36%	30%	30%	27%	11%
Nongliomatous Tumors (15 cases)	14/15	13/15	10/15	8/13	5/8	2/4

*Table drawn up by showing the actual proportion of survivors over the total number of patients who, by the end of each period of time indicated above, had been treated only with radiation—a total of 95 patients from 1939 to 1958 inclusive. Clinical follow-up complete to 1964, ranging from a minimum of 5 years up to 25.

ing increased intracranial pressure must have influenced the length of survival in some cases just as much as the radiation therapy administered. Of the group of 24 patients who had some type of surgical decompression without surgical extirpation of tumor prior to irradiation, 11 are among those who have survived 5 years or longer from the 80 patients whose gliomas were directly treated only with radiation. Various types of shunts were used in 9 of the 11 survivors who were decompressed intracranially and went on to survive 5 years or longer after irradiation. No decompression had been required in 13 of the 24 5-year survivors who were treated by irradiation alone. In the nongliomatous tumors, decompression was needed prior to irradiation in 7 of 15 cases, but it was not in the remaining 8 patients who had presented no significant evidence of increased intracranial pressure before they were irradiated for cerebral vascular tumors.

Results by Histologic Group or Location

RADIATION THERAPY OF GLIOMATOUS TUMORS

Glioblastoma Multiforme. Irrespective of its location in the central nervous system, glioblastoma multiforme is universally recognized as the most malignant type of glioma. Its incidence is the highest of all malignant gliomata in nearly every large series of cases. Judging from the duration of symptoms prior to diagnosis it is usually a type of fast growing tumor.

Of the 176 patients that we irradiated with kilovoltage x-radiation in the management of their glioblastoma multiforme, 171 were irradiated postoperatively and 5 were treated only with radiation. Both the short- and long-term results have demonstrated a low life expectancy in glioblastomas. Results indicate (Table 4-3) that 44 per cent of our 176 patients have survived over 1 year as compared with 13 per cent of the 183 patients

of Fraenkel and German treated only surgically.[13] Their longest survival was 48 months, whereas 7 per cent or 13 of our patients who had intensive postoperative irradiation have survived over 5 years. The quality of recovery was graded as good, with return to normal life for most of the duration of their survival in 75 per cent of the patients who survived less than 5 years. In the 13 patients who survived over 5 years, the degree of recovery was such that 10 were in excellent condition, 3 had partial disability, and not a single patient was totally disabled.

Only 5 patients, when the diagnosis had been established by needle biopsy, were treated by irradiation alone; 2 have survived over 1 year and only 1 of these over 3 years.

After reviewing and comparing the results of treatment by various methods, we are convinced that the treatment of choice of glioblastoma multiforme should consist primarily of surgical decompression and removal followed with intensive irradiation. The extent of surgical extirpation should be such as to provide a good decompression by removing the bulk of the tumor and thus reduce the volume of tissue whose neoplastic activity may be controlled by irradiation. Such surgical removal is justifiable inasmuch as it can be performed with a minimum risk that the patient may remain with a serious deficit of the normal functions, particularly when the tumor is located in the motor area of the dominant hemisphere. Protraction is most important. In the irradiation of glioblastoma multiforme the optimum time-dose relationship would seem to be of the order of 6,500 rads tumor dose, over a period of approximately 50 to 60 days, and using ^{60}Co radiation.

Unclassified Gliomata. They are mixed gliomas which histologically show a mixture of a variety of glial cells so dispersed within the tumor that no predominant pattern is distinguishable.

Of the 40 patients with unclassified gliomas in our series, 37 have been treated with craniotomy, decompression and surgical removal followed by irradiation, whereas 3 have been treated with irradiation alone.

The results of treatment are presented in Table 4-3 and also in Table 4-6. Comparison of results reveals that both the short- and long-term survivals are decidedly better in unclassified gliomata than in glioblastomas, but they are not as good as in the astrocytoma group. It is difficult to compare the results of treatment of unclassified gliomas in relation with the method of treatment, whether this was by surgical removal alone or surgery and postoperative irradiation. Long-term recovery rates have been remarkably good, as only 1 of 12 patients has survived with partial disability at 5 years, and not one with total disability among those who have survived over 5, 10, 15, or 20 years after treatment.

Because of the moderately malignant character of most unclassified gliomata and their natural tendency to be infiltrating in type, our aim is to irradiate postoperatively up to an average tumor dose of 6,000 rads over a period of 50 to 60 days.

Astrocytoma. This category of gliomas is grouping tumors which are relatively well differentiated histologically and can be readily identified as being of astrocytic origin.

Intracranial astrocytomas involve the cerebral hemispheres in about 65 or 75 per cent of the cases and the cerebellum in 20 to 25 per cent. They may be found in the midbrain, brain-stem or pons, and occasionally in the optic chiasm and nerves. The prognosis varies markedly with the anatomic location, whether it is supratentorial in the cerebrum or infratentorial in the cerebellum. Astrocytomas involving the midbrain or the pons should be considered separately from the majority of intracranial gliomata of astrocytic origin; they should be grouped with other tumors located in the same critical areas, where the hazard to the patient's life is related probably more to the location of the new growth than to its histopathology.

Astrocytomas arising from the optic chiasm and nerves are few and should be discussed at the same time as other histologic varieties of tumors developing from the same anatomic structures.

Supratentorial astrocytomas represent the largest group of cerebral gliomata after glioblastomas multiforme. The majority of astrocytomas involve the frontal lobes, and many in that region have been seen to have crossed the midline to the other side. The diffuse type is observed predominantly in the temporal region. Most of the cerebral astrocytomas are slowly growing. The average duration prior to diagnosis and treatment seems to vary from 2 to 4 years and even longer, with the result that tumors in that category are often sizable.

In cerebral astrocytomas, surgical treatment consisting of craniotomy is indicated primarily to accomplish decompression and obtain tissue for histologic diagnosis, and then to remove the bulk of the tumor if not all of it. However, it seems that surgical extirpation in toto may be feasible in approximately one-third of the cases only. According to Levy and Elvidge,[20] the fact that the removal of an astrocytoma is known to be incomplete does not necessarily indicate a poor prognosis, but merely that it was difficult for the surgeon to determine the limits of the tumor at the time of operation.

Of the 105 patients (Table 4-7) whom we have irradiated more than 5 years ago, following surgical removal of astrocytomas located in the cerebral hemispheres exclusively, 51 or 49 per cent have survived over 5 years. Considering all that evidence, it appears that from the standpoint of longevity, patients who were irradiated postoperatively have done increasingly better than those treated by surgical removal only.

Clinically, subjective and objective improvement has been observed in the majority of patients who survived operation following surgical decompression and tumor extirpation, including partial lobectomy of frontal, temporal or even occipital lobes. Several pa-

Table 4-7. *Cerebral Astrocytomas—Comparison of Survival Rates in Relation to Treatment‡*

Survival Over	Surgery Only (42 cases)*		Surgery and Irradiation (45 cases)*		Surgery and Irradiation (105 cases)†	
	No. of Survivors	Per Cent	No. of Survivors	Per Cent	No. of Survivors	Per Cent
1 Year	34	81	37	82	90	86
3 Years	22	52	28	62	67	64
5 Years	11	26	16	36	51	49

* Table prepared from analysis of data presented by Levy and Elvidge (1956) in study of 87 patients followed up after surgical treatment—42 of these had surgery only—and 45 had postoperative irradiation.
† Author's series, comprising 105 patients irradiated postoperatively from 1939–1958. Follow-up complete to 1964.
‡ All three series above include astrocytomas (Grade I and II) involving cerebral hemispheres only.—Midbrain and pontine astrocytomas have been excluded.

tients have made a slow immediate recovery and were not in very good condition when postoperative irradiation was initiated within a couple of weeks after operation. By the time that adequate irradiation has been completed most patients usually have made a satisfactory recovery. The maximum degree of recovery may not be fully appreciable for 3 to 6 and possibly up to 12 months after completion of treatment.

Of all the patients that we have irradiated and followed up for various types of primary intracranial gliomata, those treated for cerebral astrocytomas have shown the lowest rate of complete recovery. Actually 60 to 65 per cent of the patients among our 5-, 10-, 15-, and 20-year survivors have made a Grade I recovery and remained perfectly well following surgical removal and irradiation of their hemispheral astrocytomas. The corollary is that the proportion of 5- and 10-year survivors with disability, partial in 23 per cent and total in 12 per cent, is higher than in any other group of patients that we have treated for intracranial tumors and reviewed for evaluation of the quality of survival.

Radiation therapy may be used advantageously in the management of patients with recurrences of cerebral astrocytomas. Our series of 105 cases of hemispheral cerebral astrocytomas comprises 12 patients who were irradiated for tumor recurrences. Initially 9 of these 12 patients had been treated by surgery alone and had radiation therapy only later after their tumor had recurred. Clinical improvement occurs during and after treatment.

When cerebral astrocytomas have recurred subsequent to previous combined treatment with surgical extirpation and intensive postoperative irradiation, further remission of symptoms and perhaps prolongation of life might be accomplished. When a second course of intensive radiation therapy is administered, there is a potential risk of postradiation necrosis, should the patient survive long enough.

Technically, in our series, cerebral astrocytomas have been irradiated with kilovoltage, at tumor doses ordinarily averaging 5,000 rads in 45 to 50 days, and perhaps slightly higher doses in recurrences. We are now treating cerebral astrocytomas with ^{60}Co high energy radiation delivering tumor doses of 5,500 to 6,000 rads over a period of 45 to 50 days. In 11 patients who were autopsied, residual tumor cells could be identified in all cases.

Infratentorial astrocytomas are gliomata which consist almost exclusively of cerebellar tumors found in children, adolescents, and few young adults.

Astrocytomas arising from the cerebellum usually carry a better prognosis than those arising from the cerebrum. This is probably due to the fact that cerebellar astrocytomas give rise to symptoms earlier. Furthermore these are predominantly of the piloid variety in which approximately 75 per cent tend to be cystic tumors relatively not invasive. In view of such characteristics, cerebellar astrocytomas often lend themselves to complete surgical eradication. The operative mortality is low, often nil. Recurrences are relatively infrequent. Following surgical removal alone, long-term survivals of 5 years or longer may be expected in approximately 75 to 80 per cent of the patients.

Postoperative irradiation of cerebellar astrocytomas might be indicated in 15 to 20 per cent of all cases, particularly in the cases of solid tumors which may not be completely eradicated surgically. Considering the localized nature, the small volume, and low depth of cerebral astrocytomas, small fields 5×5 to 6×8 cm in size are usually adequate. The portal arrangement consists of two lateral and one posterior occipital fields. Cross firing with ^{60}Co radiation beams, tumor doses of 4,500 to 5,000 rads are administered over periods of 40 to 45 days.

Cystic tumors in which the astrocytic neoplasm is usually attached to the wall of the cyst can be controlled by surgery alone.

It is difficult to elicit the value of postoperative irradiation in the treatment of cerebellar astrocytomas in consideration of the high rate of long survivals (76 per cent of 29 patients) and satisfactory recoveries following surgical removal alone.

Expanding lesions in the posterior fossa should not be irradiated unless a histological diagnosis is available prior to irradiation. This is particularly important because tumors in that location are largely found in the young under 15 years of age, their nature is variable and the therapeutic management differs with the type of tumor. Once a diagnosis of cerebellar astrocytoma is made or suspected, surgical management is indicated primarily.

Oligodendrogliomas. Tumors arising from the oligodendrogliocytes are far from common. These tumors are found mostly in the cerebellar hemispheres of young adults, occasionally in middle-aged people, rarely in children. Oligodendrogliomas have the lowest incidence of all primary intracranial gliomata. These tumors are known to be usually slow growing, well circumscribed and relatively benign. Oligodendrogliomas often contain numerous deposits of calcium which can be identified frequently on plain x-ray films of the skull. Some of these tumors are classified as oligodendroglioblastomas because of their more malignant appearance since they grow faster and histologically exhibit larger round cells with occasional mitoses.

Our series of cases irradiated postoperatively comprises only 14 patients. These received roentgen therapy following surgical removal either because of the more malignant histological appearance than usual or in view of surgical extirpation definitely incomplete. Actual survivals show that one-half of the patients (7 patients) irradiated, all postoperatively, have survived over 5 years. From these, 3 of 9 patients irradiated over 10 years ago are still living and 1 of them treated more than 20 years ago is alive and well. All patients surviving over 5 years have made a good recovery and remained well from the time of irradiation.

Considering that oligodendrogliocytic tumors usually are well differentiated and are probably not overly radiosensitive, they should be treated with megavoltage radiation and tumor doses of approximately 6,500 rads in 50 to 60 days.

From our limited experience in dealing with oligodendrogliomas and oligodendroglioblastomas I find it difficult to determine to what extent postoperative irradiation may contribute to longer and better survivals in comparison with surgical removal alone. The number of cases is too small (only 9 patients irradiated more than 10 years ago) to allow for any comparison which might be truly significant and reveal more than a trend.

Ependymomas and Ependymoblastomas. These tumors represent a group of neoplasms arising from the ependymal lining of the ventricular system. Tumors developing from ependymal cells and tissue may be found anywhere along the ventricular system. The majority of them are histologically benign. The minority, approximately 15 to 20 per cent, are classed as ependymoblastomas when histologically they show tumor cells of embryonal type with increased mitotic activity, and biologically they appear to grow faster than usual. Zimmerman *et al.*[33] consider that ependymal cell tumors are usually not completely removable and that recurrence is frequent even after surgical removal is considered complete. French[14] is of the opinion that all ependymomas, except the papillomas, are fundamentally malignant because of their invasive tendencies. The incidence of intracranial ependymal tumors is low.

Ependymomas are seen mostly in children and young adults, and also in the fifth decade of life. The duration of symptoms prior to diagnosis and treatment varies with their location, since these tumors grow slowly and predominantly within the ventricular cavities that the tumor may fill.

The exact diagnosis of ependymal tumors cannot be made ordinarily without surgical exploration. At the same time, extirpation of as much tumor as feasible should constitute the initial treatment in all cases. There seems to be general agreement among neurosurgeons to the effect that in the majority of cases complete surgical removal of ependymomas and ependymoblastomas, whether supratentorial or infratentorial, cannot be accomplished safely because of their anatomical location and invasive tendency.

Ependymal cell tumors are reported to spread along the cerebrospinal spaces just like medulloblastomas do. On that basis, Dyke and Davidoff[12] have advocated prophylactic doses of radiation to the entire spinal axis in the treatment of histologically verified ependymomas, either of the cerebrum or the cerebellum. In previous articles[6,7] we have stated that in the management of ependymomas our practice has been not to irradiate routinely the spinal axis. Postoperative irradiation was concentrated at the site of the primary tumor. At present our series comprises 20 patients and in 2 cases only the spinal axis was irradiated prophylactically in the manner suggested by Dyke and Davidoff.[12] Clinical evidence of such potential neoplastic dissemination and implant along the spinal subarachnoid spaces has not been observed as yet in any of the 20 patients that we have irradiated postoperatively for histologically proven intracranial ependymomas and ependymoblastomas. All our patients have been followed longer than 5 years from the onset of radiation therapy. The primary location was supratentorial in 17 and infratentorial in the remaining 3 cases.

Our own series comprises 20 patients who were also treated with surgery and adequate irradiation for intracranial ependymomas and ependymoblastomas. All were followed for at least 5 years from the onset of postoperative irradiation. From 17 patients treated for supratentorial tumors, 11 or 65 per cent have survived over 5 years (Table 4-8). The 3 patients treated for infratentorial tumors are still living, 18, 19, and 22 years respectively. The overall 5-year survival rate is 70 per cent, since 14 of 20 patients have survived over 5 years from the onset of postoperative irradiation (Table 4-3). It should be added that 10 of 18 have survived over 10 years, 7 of 12 have exceeded 15 years of survival, and 3 of 7 are living over 20 years. Of the patients now deceased, 2 did not improve following treatment and 6 died from local recurrences. The quality of survival was good (Grade I) 5 years or longer in 11 of 14 survivors and remained such for those among the 11 who have survived over 10, 15, or 20 years. The remaining 3 patients were partially disabled from the time they were irradiated, 2 over 15 years and the other over 20 years. One of these 3 patients has

Table 4-8. *Intracranial Ependymomas—Comparison of 5-Year Survival Rates in Relation to Location of Tumor and Method of Treatment*

Method of Treatment	Supratentorial			Infratentorial			Total		
3 series of cases	No. of Patients	5-Year Survivors	Per Cent	No. of Patients	5-Year Survivors	Per Cent	No. of Patients	5-Year Survivors	Per Cent
Surgical removal alone									
Ringertz and Reymond	13	2	15	15	5	35	28	7	25
Surgical removal and adequate irradiation									
(*a*) Kricheff, Becker, Schneck and Taveras	9	2	22	33	15	45	42	17	41
(*b*) Bouchard and associates	17	11	65	3	3	100	20	14	70

recently become totally disabled from local recurrence.

Ependymomas and ependymoblastomas have been treated in our series with kilovoltage x-radiation. We have been using a cross firing arrangement consisting of anterior and lateral pairs of opposing fields. In a single course of daily treatments, 5 days a week, tumor doses of 5,000 rads delivered over 45 to 50 days have been administered. The younger children have received tumor doses of 4,500 to 5,000 rads and the older were given depth doses equal to those administered to adults over the same average period of time. With megavoltage, total tumor doses should be increased by 500 to 1,000 rads over the same period of time for treatment.

Medulloblastoma. Of all primary intracranial tumors, medulloblastomas are recognized as the most common type in children and also the most sensitive to ionizing radiation. Microscopically, medulloblastomas often are difficult to differentiate from cerebellar sarcomas and at times from ependymoblastomas. Medulloblastomas are known to have a natural tendency to spread within the subarachnoid and ventricular spaces.

Irradiation should not be administered upon a presumptive diagnosis of medulloblastoma. Histopathologic proof is essential to guide the surgeon in determining the procedure to follow and the radiotherapist in selecting the appropriate method of irradiation. It is generally considered that radiation therapy should follow an operation at which histological verification is obtained and decompression accomplished by removal of tumor tissue to a degree which may vary with the extent of the tumor and the wisdom of the neurosurgeon. Other surgical procedures are being used for obtaining histological diagnosis and decompression without craniotomy prior to irradiation.

Our series of cerebellar medulloblastomas comprises a total of 50 patients, all irradiated more than 5 years ago; 37 children aged 15 or less, and 13 patients over 15 years of age.

In our series of 37 children with histologically proven cerebellar medulloblastoma, treatment in 27 cases has consisted of surgical removal, more or less radical, followed by irradiation of the entire cerebrospinal axis. Irradiation alone was used in 10 children who, prior to initiation of radiation therapy, had an aspiration biopsy and histological verification of their tumor. The 13 patients classed in the adult group were all treated by surgery plus postoperative irradiation.

Results in children are shown (Table 4-9) by the proportion of survivors after 1, 3, 5, 10, 15, and 20 years in relation to the method of treatment, either by surgery plus irradiation or by irradiation alone following aspiration biopsy. It is true that the number of

Table 4-9. *Cerebellar Medulloblastomas in Children*—Results of Treatment by Surgery and Irradiation or Irradiation Alone—Results by Method of Treatment and Survival*

	Proportion of Survivors Over					
	1 Year	3 Years	5 Years	10 Years	15 Years	20 Years
Surgical Removal and Irradiation	17/27	9/27	6/27	3/23	1/17	0/5
Needle Biopsy and Irradiation Only	8/10	4/10	4/10	2/7	1/4	0/1
Overall Survivals	25/37	13/37	10/37	5/30	2/21	0/6
Average Rates	70%	35%	27%	17%	10%	0%

* All patients of 15 years of age or under—every case verified histologically.
At the end of each 5-year period, Grade I recovery in all survivors except for one partially disabled at 5 years.

children treated by irradiation alone for cerebellar medulloblastomas is relatively small (10 patients) but the proportion of long-term survivors among these is twice as high as it is among children treated by irradiation postoperatively. As yet, not 1 of the 10 children who had radiation therapy alone has developed clinical evidence of seeding and implant of tumor cells along the subarachnoid cerebrospinal spaces. Among the 27 children irradiated postoperatively, 5 had to be treated because of tumor dissemination along the spinal cord. Our overall survival rates are 27 per cent at 5 years, 17 per cent at 10 years, and 10 per cent at 15 years. Of 6 potential 20-year survivors none have survived that long. The degree of clinical recovery is such that 9 out of the 10 children followed more than 5 years from the onset of irradiation have grown and were living normally at the 5-year period of follow-up. One was partially disabled and died from cardiac disease without evidence of recurrence of her medulloblastoma. The quality of survival of those living at 10 and 15 years after treatment has remained excellent all along, without recurrence.

In the group of 13 patients who were exceeding 15 years of age when treated for proven medulloblastoma, the results of treatment estimated by survival rates are practically identical to those obtained in children. Every patient in this adult group was irradiated postoperatively and followed for at least 5 years from the onset of radiation therapy. Three of the 13 patients have survived over 5 years, 2 having died 7 and 10 years respectively after treatment, whereas the other is still living and working 22 years following postoperative irradiation. The 2 who died had made a good recovery and remained well for the major part of their survival.

If we share the view that cerebellar sarcomas belong to the same histological class of tumors as medulloblastomas and accordingly group them all together (Table 4-10), the survival rates from our 12 cerebellar sarcomas (5 in children and 7 in adults) are definitely higher than those from medulloblastomas although the number of sarcomas is relatively small. Obviously the effect of merging all cerebellar sarcomas with medulloblastomas would seem to result into better survival rates.

If it should be agreed that cerebellar sarcomas may not be different from medulloblastomas in children and they might all be classed in the same histopathologic group, this means that logically the entire cerebrospinal axis should be irradiated by those who may continue to consider and classify cerebellar sarcomas independently from medulloblastomas. The natural tendency for cerebellar sarcomas to metastasize along the cerebrospinal fluid pathway has been observed by many and considered as a characteristic that these tumors have in common

Table 4-10. *Cerebellar Medulloblastomas and Sarcomas*—Comparison of Combined Survival Rates in Children and Adults*

	No. of Cases	Survival Rates Over					
		1 Year	3 Years	5 Years	10 Years	15 Years	20 Years
Medulloblastomas	50	74	36	26	17	9	8
Cerebellar Sarcomas	12	83	75	58	30	66	0
Medullos and Sarcomas Combined	62	76	44	32	20	14	7
(*a*) in Children Only	42	70	40	30	18	14	0
(*b*) in Adults Only	20	90	50	40	24	15	15

*All verified histologically—Surgical removal plus Irradiation in 40 medulloblastomas and 10 sarcomas. Irradiation alone in 10 medulloblastomas and 2 sarcomas.

with medulloblastomas. The cerebrospinal axis was irradiated in 3 of our 5 patients now classed in the cerebellar sarcoma group. Irradiation of the spinal axis happened by chance and not by design, since these children were originally diagnosed as medulloblastomas and treated as such before revision of diagnosis.

Treatment should be delivered in a single course of protracted doses over a total period of 45 to 50 days. During that period of time tumor doses of 5,000 rads through the entire intracranial content and 2,000 rads over the entire spinal canal are administered with ^{60}Co teletherapy units.

A modification of the technique used by Paterson and Farr[24] has been devised in which the entire cerebrospinal axis is irradiated at once, in one stretch, through a single and properly shaped field. The patient is lying in the prone position below a shielded screen resting on top of the treatment table. In that screen a window has been cut which measures 9×9 cm over the posterior part of the head and narrows to a width of 4 cm below the occiput in order to expose the spinal cord and subarachnoid spaces down to the level of the first sacral segment. Lead bricks are used to maintain the exposed field to the desired width. A multicurie ^{60}Co source exposes the entire cerebrospinal axis at a focus skin distance of 125 cm (Fig. 4-4A).

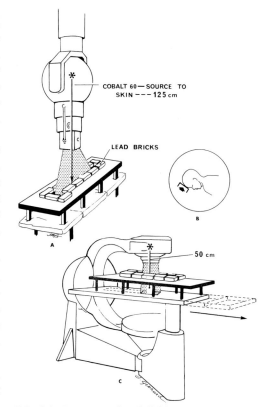

FIG. 4-4. Treatment of medulloblastoma by irradiation of the entire cerebrospinal axis.

A. Fixed field technique exposing the entire area in one stretch. **B.** Anterior cranial field to complete adequate irradiation of cranial content. **C.** Moving field technique with the table and the patient being displaced along its longitudinal axis in a stationary field.

The exposure of the intracranial content to the desired tumor dose level is completed by adding an anterior field as shown in Figure 4-4B. This is introduced as a separate field starting from the time that the spinal axis has received the full tumor dose contemplated at that level.

We also use at times a moving field technique (Fig. 4-4C) in which both the table and the patient move longitudinally in relation to a perpendicular ^{60}Co radiation beam which is stationary at a 50 cm focal skin distance. While the other technical factors are identical to those described with the previous technique, the content of the skull and entire spinal canal is exposed to radiation.

Midbrain and Brain-Stem Tumors. When intracranial tumors develop in the midbrain or in the brain-stem regions, the prognosis is considered unfavorable because of their anatomic location. Midbrain tumors consist of neoplastic lesions arising in the anatomic region extending from the posterior portion of the third ventricle down to the pontine protuberance. The midbrain is the cross-road of nearly every important motor and sensory nerve fibers where they converge on their way through the pons to the medulla. It also contains the aqueduct of Sylvius which controls the circulation of the cerebrospinal fluid within the brain itself. Nerve pathways emerge from the midbrain into the brain-stem or pons through which they establish a close anatomic liaison between the cerebrum, cerebellum, and upper part of the medulla. There is not true anatomic division between the midbrain and the pons, or between the pons and the upper part of the medulla.

Tumors growing in the midbrain and pontine regions represent 14 per cent of all primary intracranial gliomata in our series of 494 primary intracranial gliomas. These tumors are infrequently accessible for biopsy and ordinarily they cannot be extirpated surgically when explored, except at the cost of a high operative mortality. Unless the tumor

should happen to be a glioblastoma multiforme, the important prognostic element is more the anatomic location of tumor growth than its histopathologic type. Untreated midbrain and pontine tumors are invariably fatal, although in a few patients with midbrain tumors life may be prolonged merely as a result of decompression through shunts.

If the decision is made to treat, this may be accomplished by surgical exploration to try and obtain a biopsy and possibly risk surgical removal or else treatment might consist of irradiation alone without the benefit of histologic confirmation and tumor classification. Occasionally an aspiration biopsy may provide tissue diagnosis, otherwise histologic verification might become available only later should there be a postmortem examination. There is considerable surgical and necropsic evidence that tumors growing in midbrain and pons are nearly always gliomata. Gradually, through the years, a policy of compromise was adopted. I accept patients with midbrain tumors for treatment by irradiation alone when a firm clinical diagnosis and a definite localization of the lesion are available, rather than risking a fatality. The use of shunts to restore intraventricular circulation of cerebrospinal fluid and thus relieve increased intracranial pressure has contributed to reduce the incidence of complications. This is applicable particularly in the management of midbrain tumors, perhaps not so much in pontine tumors. Our results suggest that adequate radiation therapy alone is capable of improving markedly the prognosis of midbrain and pontine tumors.

Our series comprises 37 midbrain and 34 brain-stem or pontine tumors treated largely by irradiation alone. Surgery plus irradiation was used in 12 cases altogether. All patients could be followed for 5 years at least, and up to 20 years or longer for some (Table 4-11).

In our group of 37 patients with midbrain tumors, 29 were treated by irradiation alone and 8 by irradiation postoperatively. All veri-

Table 4-11. *Midbrain and Brain-stem Tumors—Life Expectancy of Patients Treated with Irradiation Alone or Surgery Plus Irradiation**

Location of Tumors	Proportion of Survivals Over					
	1 Year	3 Years	5 Years	10 Years	15 Years	20 Years
Midbrain	26/37	20/37	17/37	9/23	3/10	2/6
Brain-stem	19/34	10/34	10/34	5/21	4/13	1/5
Overall survivals	45/71	30/71	27/71	14/44	7/23	3/11
Average Rates	63%	42%	38%	32%	30%	27%

* Irradiation alone in 59 patients with midbrain and 30 with brain-stem tumors.

fied tumors were gliomata. Five of the 8 patients irradiated postoperatively survived over 5 years and 2 of these have exceeded 20 years of useful survival without recurrence.

Decompression procedures were accomplished in 18 of the 29 midbrain tumors treated by irradiation alone, and this consisted of shunts only in 11 patients, surgical exploration with shunts in 5, and in 2, surgical exploration alone. No decompression procedure was used in 11 patients. Of the 12 patients who have survived over 5 years following treatment by irradiation, without surgical removal, 7 had decompression all by shunts except for 1.

The life expectancy of patients with midbrain tumors treated by adequate irradiation, used alone or postoperatively, is presented in Table 4-3 on a percentile basis derived from the actual survival rates of the patients whom we have treated. It must be emphasized that the length of survival among the 29 patients treated by irradiation alone (Table 4-6) over 5 years ago is such that 12 or 41 per cent have survived longer than 5 years, 7 of 17 patients treated over 10 years ago (41 per cent) have exceeded 19 years, whereas 1 out of 5 potential survivors has lived over 15 years.

The majority of patients irradiated for midbrain tumors have shown clinical improvement at least temporarily. The long-term quality of survival, expressed by the degree of clinical recovery has shown that of

the 17 5-year survivors 13 had returned to active useful life, whereas the degree of recovery was fair in 2 and poor in the other 2. The quality of survival has remained good in the 9 patients who survived over 10 years, and among these in the 2 who have survived over 20 years.

Pontine tumors consist largely of infiltrative gliomas. In our series there are 34 cases of brain-stem tumors in which intensive irradiation, considered adequate, has been used. Twenty were children from 3 to 15 years of age. In the period under review a radical change has occurred at the Montreal Neurological Institute in the management of patients with brain-stem tumors. From 1939 to 1947, only 5 patients were treated with radiation, but 2 of these responded to irradiation alone beyond expectation. In 1947 we began to accept the responsibility of treating by irradiation alone patients with a firm diagnosis of brain-stem tumor, without demanding a pathological diagnosis. From 1947 to 1958, 29 patients with pontine tumors have been treated with intensive radiation therapy.

All patients improved clinically for at least 6 to 12 months, and 19 survived 1 year in good condition most of the time. It is very gratifying to report that 10 of 34 have survived over 5 years, 5 of 21 over 10 years, 4 of 13 over 15 years, and 1 over 20 years after treatment (Table 4-11). The degree of clinical recovery and the quality of survival, both under and over 5 years, have been most satisfactory for the major part of life duration following treatment.

Treatment planning must be individualized to some degree, particularly in relation to the direction of radiation beams and size of fields. In view of the factors mentioned in previous paragraphs, we must be fully aware that tumors arising in the midbrain may infiltrate not only into the direction of its vertical axis but also in forward and lateral directions. Necropsy material has shown this in a few cases in which we failed to restrain and control tumor growth by irradiation because such factors were ignored in the planning of treatment. Fields must therefore be long enough in the vertical axis of the midbrain and pons to exceed by an adequate margin any probable extension above and below the apparent level of neoplastic infiltration. One posterior and two lateral fields should be used in all cases (Figs. 4-5A and 4-5B). These fields may be narrow (approximately 6 cm in width) below the level of the foramen magnum, but above this level they must be wide enough to include the posterior part of the third ventricle and the hypothalamic region, together with the supratentorial and infratentorial parts of the posterior cranial content, because of possible infiltration via the cerebral and cerebellar peduncles. When the anterior limit of gliomatous infiltration may be quite indefinite, like in midbrain tumors involving the posterior thalamic and hypothalamic regions, it is wise to cross-fire the tumor-bearing region with an anterior field in addition to the other fields just indicated (Figs. 4-6A and 4-6B). Midbrain and brain-stem tumors are not to be pin-pointed with sharply demarcated fields of invariable size or tailored to cover just the apparent area of tumefaction. Gliomata involving those midline structures of the central nervous system are nearly always more extensive than they seem to be.

Exceptionally, patients will develop in the posterior and superior region of the third ventricle small tumors which appear to be well circumscribed. These usually consist of

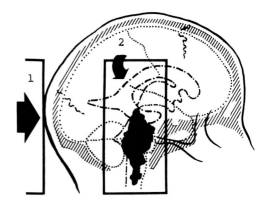

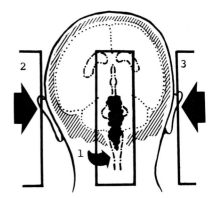

FIG. 4-5. Pontine or brain stem tumor extending upward and downward.

tumors arising from the choroid plexus (cyst or ependymoma) or may represent a pinealoma. Tumors in that anatomic location are generally considered inaccessible for surgical extirpation. We treat such tumors using a small field technique, and megavoltage (^{60}Co), with tumor doses of 5,000 rads in 40 to 45 days (Figs. 4-7A and 4-7B).

The midbrain and pons may have been damaged by the tumor itself and are most vulnerable to irradiation under such conditions. Edema is ordinarily present to some degree and this must not be increased by irradiation. Against edema corticosteroids may be effective adjuvants, associated with

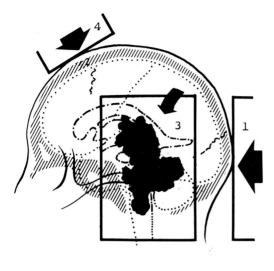

practice on smaller doses over shorter periods of time in the treatment of midbrain and brain-stem tumors because the surrounding brain tissue is usually compressed and infiltrated by the growing glioma and probably more vulnerable to radiation than can be estimated.

NONGLIOMATOUS TUMORS

Intracranial Sarcomas. Malignant tumors may arise intracranially from various tissues of mesenchymal origin and make up the heterogeneous group of sarcomas of the brain. These intracranial sarcomas are not common and comprise tumors of different histopathologic types: fibrosarcomas, reticulum cell sarcomas, perithelial sarcomas, and cerebellar or alveolar sarcomas.

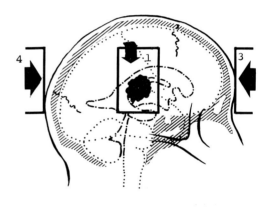

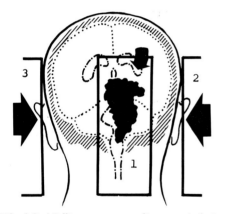

FIG. 4-6. Midline tumor extending superiorly into the third ventricle, laterally into the left cerebral hemisphere, and inferiorly into the pons and upper medulla.

small initial doses of radiation. By and large irradiation is the only therapeutic agent capable of restraining and controlling tumor growth, and it must be administered without exceeding radiation tolerance of the adjacent brain tissue. Using ^{60}Co radiation beams, we aim to deliver tumor doses of not less than 5,000 rads to the pons and upper medulla and 6,000 rads to the midbrain region always in a single course, on a long protracted basis of 50 to 60 days. Even though radiobiologic effects on normal brain tissue might be equivalent in principle, I would not rely in

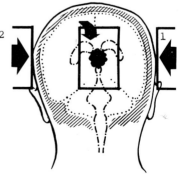

FIG. 4-7. Small glioma in upper posterior part of third ventricle.

The prognosis of patients with intracranial sarcomas is less severe than with sarcomatous growths arising in other parts of the body, unless they are diffuse and then invade or replace the brain tissue. Certain intracranial sarcomas originate from the leptomeninges in the posterior cranial fossa and morphologically are practically undistinguishable from medulloblastomas.

Our total series of intracranial sarcomas comprises 16 cases: 7 children and 9 adults. In 4 cases the sarcomatous lesions arose from the cerebral hemispheres, whereas in 12 these appeared to originate from the cerebellum or the cerebellopontine angle. The diagnosis of intracranial sarcoma was made at operation at the same time as surgical removal and this was followed by intensive postoperative irradiation in 14 patients. In the 2 remaining cases a tissue diagnosis was obtained by needle biopsy and treatment consisted of irradiation only. Localized irradiation was administered in all sarcomas which were considered circumscribed lesions, using tumor doses equivalent to 6,000 rads in 50 to 60 days.

The overall survivals in that broad variety of intracranial sarcomas are presented in Table 4-4. It should be noted that there were only 2 patients treated more than 20 years ago, but none have lived that long in our group. The 2 patients treated by irradiation only improved dramatically following treatment, but their tumors recurred and they survived 18 and 52 months respectively from the onset of treatment. Recovery rates of patients who have survived 5, 10, and 15 years after treatment have been satisfactory.

A brief mention should be made of the fact that metastases to the brain from systemic Hodgkin's sarcoma and lymphosarcoma of the small or lymphocytic cell type have not been observed by Kernohan and Uihlein.[16] This confirms our personal experience in the management of a substantial number of patients with such lymphomatous sarcomas.

Meningeal Tumors. Intracranial tumors arising from the meninges consist in general of slow growing, sharply circumscribed benign neoplasms. Meningiomas comprise about 15 per cent of all primary intracranial tumors. They occur mostly in middle-aged adults, rarely in children. The prognosis depends more upon the location of meningeal tumors than the histologic appearance. The natural history of meningeal tumors is favorable because their growth is usually long and slowly progressive.

The majority of meningeal tumors may be treated successfully by surgical extirpation alone. Surgical results are usually good. Long survivals without recurrences have been reported by many neurosurgeons.

Radiation therapy is not indicated following surgical removal of meningiomas, unless the neurosurgeon's observations at operation and the histopathologic evidence are such that certain tumors are properly identified as malignant meningiomas or meningeal sarcomas. If in that respect a case is considered borderline we usually abstain and withhold the use of radiation for later should it ever be needed, and it seems that many never do. The degree of radiosensitivity of malignant meningiomas is variable. This could be predicted merely from the tremendous histological differences in the types of meningeal tumors. Malignant fibroblastomas have shown a degree of radiosensitivity which is variable, from moderate to low. Doses approaching the normal brain tolerance must be administered. When malignant meningiomas are irradiated, tumor doses equivalent to 6,000 to 6,500 rads in 50 to 60 days are usually administered with ^{60}Co, using cross-firing technique with four fields. Wedge field technique may be suitable in properly selected cases.

Our experience is based upon a group of 25 patients treated postoperatively for malignant meningeal tumors. Of these 25 patients, 17 were irradiated 10 to 15 days following a first operation. The remaining 8 patients were irradiated for postoperative recurrences, 3 without another operation and the others after a second or even a third surgical removal. We have irradiated 2 benign meningiomas on account of partial removal only.

It is not easy to make a valid objective appraisal of the effects of radiation therapy on meningeal tumors showing malignant characters microscopically or clinically by their invasive behavior. Survival rates are not necessarily a true yardstick, because of the natural tendency of meningeal tumors to grow slowly and recur, when they do, many years after surgical extirpation. The ability of patients to recover from the neurologic signs caused by meningiomas should be almost entirely due to the surgical removal. The duration of recovery may be related to a more complete tumor eradication than estimated or else it might be due to the control of actual residual tumor by irradiation resulting in prevention of tumor recurrence.

It seems reasonable to consider that the low recurrence rate (11 per cent) in our small series represents objective evidence that radiation therapy plays a useful role in the combined treatment of malignant meningeal tumors by surgery and irradiation. Further evidence may be derived from the clinical improvement and long survivals, without additional recurrence, that we have observed in several patients irradiated for postoperative recurrence.

Vascular Tumors. Intracranial expanding lesions of vascular origin consist essentially of two separate pathologic entities: 1) angiomas which represent congenital malformations and 2) hemangioblastomas which are true neoplastic lesions.

Cerebral angiomas are classified with tumors merely because they are space-occupying lesions. These are not new growths in the true sense of the word. They are vascular anomalies representing congenital malformations which involve arteries and veins. Intracranial angiomas are supratentorial lesions, being located almost exclusively in cerebral hemispheres, rarely in the cerebellum. Such lesions may be present for years without clinical manifestations of their existence. When cerebral angiomas ever cause trouble,

this occurs in the third or fourth decades of life and even later. Cerebral angiomas rarely manifest themselves during infancy and childhood. Our youngest patient was 17 years of age. Cerebral angiomas cause clinical manifestations when they affect the adjacent cerebral tissue or else they hemorrhage. These lesions seldom endanger a patient's life so that survival rates are not an indication of the value of the method of treatment employed.

With the increasing use of cerebral angiography, the discovery of angiomatous anomalies may be fortuitous. Treatment should be considered only when such vascular lesions are causing symptoms. The treatment of intracranial angiomas may consist of surgical excision of the lesion when it is located near the surface of a cerebral hemisphere. In deeper locations it may be feasible to ligate the major feeding vessel of a cerebral angioma.

The majority of deeply seated cerebral angiomas should be managed conservatively, and radiation therapy is indicated in them. The objective is to induce with radiation a reaction of endarteritis obliterans in the smaller blood vessels and capillaries, which may eventually occlude sufficiently to relieve the patient's symptoms and prevent repeated episodes of bleeding or even massive hemorrhage. Radiation therapy may not bring correction of the neurologic deficit present at the onset of treatment and caused by the vascular lesion. We have previously[7] suggested that a tumor dose of 3,500 rads over a period of 30 to 35 days should be adequate to induce the desired radiobiological effect. With ^{60}Co high energy radiation, tumor doses of 4,000 to 4,500 rads over the same period of time are recommended.

Hemangioblastomas represent true neoplastic lesions arising almost exclusively from the cerebellar hemispheres. These are tumors of low grade malignancy growing slowly in the infratentorial region. Hemangioblastomas are usually well-demarcated neoplasms growing with a cyst in which they form a solid nodule attached to some part of the wall of the cyst. Histologically these tumors are formed of abundant capillaries and more or less cystic vascular spaces containing blood with strands of endothelial cells lying between them. Hemangioendotheliomas are a histologic variant in which the basic cell is also endothelial in origin with proliferation of capillaries of a more or less invasive character, often showing nodular tumor masses in the periphery of the cysts. The diagnosis of hemangioblastomas is usually made at operation once the cyst is opened and the blood supply to the neoplasm is interrupted. The diagnosis is confirmed by microscopic examination.

Complete surgical removal can be accomplished successfully in a high proportion of the cases. Irradiation is indicated postoperatively in these tumors when they cannot be removed completely.

Because of the potential malignant character of hemangioblastomas, tumor doses varying between 3,000 and 5,000 rads in 35 to 50 days have been administered. Since hemangioendotheliomas are considered more malignant in character, tumor doses equivalent to 5,000 to 6,000 rads have been given over a period of 45 to 50 days. Now that ^{60}Co high energy radiation is readily available, it should be used in the treatment of these tumors, aiming at the maximal tumor doses just mentioned.

Congenital Tumors

There are several expanding lesions occurring intracranially which are considered primary neoplasms of congenital origin. Those of vascular origin, like angiomas, have already been discussed. The most common is probably the group of craniopharyngiomas. Chordomas are less common.

CRANIOPHARYNGIOMAS

Craniopharyngiomas are histologically benign intracranial tumors, considered malignant on account of their location and their natural behavior inducing severe disturbances often difficult to control. The term craniopharyngioma designates all intracranial growths that arise in the hypophyseal region and are composed of cystic formation whose cavities are lined with squamous epithelium and filled with pale yellow oily fluid containing cellular debris including cholesterol crystals. These tumors may be solid and consist of squamous epithelium. The term craniopharyngioma was coined by Cushing. The majority of these tumors are found above the sella turcica but others may arise within the sella itself.

The incidence of craniopharyngiomas in large series of intracranial tumors varies between 2 and 4 per cent. These tumors occur most frequently in children and young adolescents who present with the adiposogenitalis or Fröhlich's syndrome. Craniopharyngiomas may also be found in adults in whom they often simulate chromophobe adenomas or suprasellar meningiomas. Symptoms are those of pituitary suppression and compression of adjacent structures, in particular the optic chiasm and the floor of the third ventricle.

In view of the cystic component present in the majority of craniopharyngiomas, the ideal treatment would consist of craniotomy, emptying of the cystic cavity and surgical extirpation of the wall of the cyst. This is a hazardous procedure to perform in that anatomic location because of the vicinity of highly vulnerable structures. Solid tumors in principle could be extirpated, but this is difficult to accomplish successfully in practice without serious complications.

In recent years, Kramer *et al.*[17] have recommended that patients with craniopharyngiomas be subjected to combined surgery and radiation therapy. Their experience seemed to indicate that such combined treatment is likely to produce the best results. Of 10 patients treated in that fashion, 9 were alive and well for over 6 years after treatment and none of them were showing any evidence of damage of the brain as a result of irradiation.

Kramer *et al.* have suggested that surgery be limited to the minimum necessary to prove the diagnosis and evacuate the cyst. The rest of the treatment should consist of high energy radiation (2 Mev, *HVL* 11 mm Pb) delivered by external beams, carefully directed to the tumor, aiming to deliver doses varying in children from 5,000 rads in 37 days to 6,500 rads in 57 days, and in adults from 5,580 rads in 39 days to 6,950 rads in 51 days.

CHORDOMAS

Chordomas are congenital tumors originating from embryonic rests of the notochord. These neoplasms may be found anywhere along the vertebral column, but they occur predominantly at the base of the skull and in the sacrococcygeal region.

Intracranial chordomas are rare. Such tumors arise ordinarily from the posterior region of the basisphenoid, below the dorsum sellae, at level of the clivus. Chordomas may bulge posteriorly within the base of the cranial cavity where they stretch the basilar artery and press upon the pons. These tumors may also extend upward through the sella turcica, compressing the pituitary gland before emerging above the sella where they expand in the hypothalamic region more or less in a spherical fashion and induce pressure symptoms by involvement of the adjacent structures. At times, chordomas developing from the basisphenoid erode the base of the skull, invade the sphenoidal sinuses and finally break into the nasopharynx.

Histologically, chordomas can be identified readily. Microscopically, they resemble tissue of the embryonic notochord. These neoplasms are considered malignant not because of their histologic appearance but on account of their tendency to invade and destroy bone, soft tissue, and brain. For these reasons chordomas are virtually impossible to eradicate and tend to regrow rapidly after surgical removal with or without postoperative irradiation. Intracranial chordomas do not tend to metastasize.

Intracranial chordomas clinically behave like highly malignant tumors from the time they are discovered and the diagnosis is firmly established. Neurosurgeons and therapeutic radiologists agree that the majority of these tumors carry a bad prognosis. The role of surgical procedures is largely to assist in making a diagnosis rather than contribute to the treatment of chordomas. The evidence presented above indicates that even with high doses of radiation, chordomas are rather radioresistant. Irradiation, however, is capable of inducing some degree of growth restraint and palliation of symptoms. If radiation therapy may be considered responsible for prolongation of life in the few patients who have long survivals, it might be used in all cases of intracranial chordomas for whatever beneficial effects it might achieve.

Miscellaneous Tumors

Under this heading it is intended to discuss briefly a few uncommon intracranial tumors.

PINEALOMAS

Pinealomas are tumors originating from the parenchyma of the pineal gland. Because of the high operative mortality associated with attempt at surgical removal, microscopic verification is not obtained very often. Other tumors in the same location may resemble and mimic pinealomas. In general, surgical removal of pinealomas is not done and the treatment consists of shunts plus external radiation therapy. Pinealomas are said to be radiosensitive and capable of giving a good percentage of long survivals. Personally, I am unable to assess the value of radiation in the treatment of pinealomas for lack of accurate data both from my own clinical material or from the current literature. Brain tumors, which are presumed to be pinealomas, have been treated empirically by cross-firing the tumor with small beams of ^{60}Co radiation, aiming at a tumor dose of 5,000 rads over 40 to 45 days (Figs. 4-7A and 4-7B).

GLIOMAS OF THE OPTIC CHIASM AND NERVES

These are tumors, which are rather uncommon, are considered congenital in nature. Tumors involving the optic chiasm and nerves are found mostly in children, but may appear in adults. These tumors that are usually growing slowly may become very large and fill the third ventricle. Histologically, chiasmatic tumors belong to the astrocytoma group and ordinarily are well differentiated. Because of their anatomic location, gliomas of the optic chiasm and nerves are not easily accessible for surgery.

Our own experience with gliomas arising from the optic chiasm and nerves is limited to 3 patients treated more than 5 years ago, 2 children and 1 adult. One of the children is alive and well 10 years following combined treatment by surgical removal and postoperative intensive irradiation. The other child was found to have a very large tumor at the base of the brain, obstructing the aqueduct. At operation, biopsy only could be taken and this revealed an astrocytoma. A shunt was established and a tumor dose of nearly 5,000 rads was administered in 45 days. The child survived 27 months but was almost completely blind. At autopsy, an astrocytoma of the optic chiasm and nerves was found. The adult patient survived only 10 months after treatment. Not included in our present series is the recent case of a large chiasmatic glioma in a child who survived only 2 years after removal and irradiation.

Treatment planning must vary according to the size of the lesion, insofar as the position and size of the fields are concerned, but we rely largely on opposing lateral fields. Tumor doses must be adequate but well protracted because of the vulnerability of adjacent hypothalamic and thalamic structures. High energy radiation should be used and tumor doses of not less than 6,000 rads over 50 to 60 days should be administered.

Radiation Therapy of Brain Tumors in Children

In view of the potential late repercussions which might occur and effect the mental development and somatic growth of children irradiated for brain tumors, it is imperative that every aspect of this problem be thoroughly scrutinized. Considerable apprehension exists concerning the exposure to ionizing radiation of the brain and skull of children. This is because their central nervous system is being irradiated during the latter period of its anatomic and physiologic development. The central nervous system is believed not to reach its complete development before the age of 15. There is a strong and persistent belief that the pituitary gland may be affected adversely by direct or indirect exposure to radiation during treatment of brain tumors in children, and that serious interference might result in somatic growth.

Radiation therapy of brain tumors in children is considered hazardous by many. It is particularly so in consideration of the tumor doses that are required in our opinion for treatment to be considered adequate and were actually the doses used in the infants and children whom we have irradiated for brain tumors over the last 25 years.

Over the years, the continued observation of our cases, through periodic follow-up examinations, has allowed us to make some evaluation of the effects of irradiation of the central nervous system in the young. The usefulness and relative safety of intensive ionizing radiation therapy in the management of intracranial neoplasms in children can be evaluated best not only by analysis of the results observed during the first few months or even years after treatment, but better still by long-term recovery and survival rates.

INCIDENCE OF PRIMARY BRAIN TUMORS IN CHILDREN

Our total experience is based upon 119 children of ages ranging from a few months to 15 years at the time of irradiation of their skull and intracranial content in the management of their tumors. Brain tumors are rare in the first year of life, gradually increase in frequency to reach their peak incidence between the ages of 6 and 10 and then decrease to the incidence level attained at 5 years. The classification of our material has been made according either to the histologic type of primary neoplasms or to their location in the midbrain and brainstem (Table 4-12).

All children with the diagnosis of primary intracranial tumor were not subjected to radiation therapy. Indications and contraindications for irradiation have been determined upon the basis outlined above in this chapter. These are the same for children as for adults. In many instances, children were accepted for treatment despite their critical condition, and yet several eventually recovered. Some of our long-term survivals belong to this group of cases.

The majority (65 per cent) of children have been treated by surgery followed with intensive irradiation, usually initiated 2 to 3 weeks after operation. Actually, 78 of the 119 children were treated by surgical removal followed by intensive irradiation. Irradiation was the sole therapeutic agent applied directly for the control of tumor growth in 41 (35 per cent) of the 119 patients. Nearly all children in this series were treated with conventional or kilovoltage irradiation. The high energy radiation from ^{60}Co beam therapy units was used in just a few selected cases that were treated between 1955 and 1958.

Our program of radiation therapy in children is almost the same as in adults except that tumor doses administered in children are usually lower by a factor of approximately 20 per cent. Accordingly, average tumor doses of 4,500 to 5,000 rads in 45 to 50 days have been rarely exceeded in this age group. High energy radiation or megavoltage should be used. In children treated by irradiation only, treatment is ordinarily initiated as soon as the diagnosis has been established. When a child is first subjected to craniotomy and surgical removal of his tumor, irradiation is commenced approximately 2 weeks later.

Table 4-12. *Primary Brain Tumors Irradiated in Children**

	Children in Series		5-Year Survivors	
	No.	Per Cent	No.	Per Cent
Gliomata				
Glioblastoma	3	2	3	—
Glioma, unclassified	11	9	4	36
Astrocytoma	16	14	12	75
Ependymoma	7	6	5	71
Medulloblastoma	37	31	10	27
Midbrain	14	12	8	57
Brain-stem	20	17	5	25
Non-gliomatous tumors				
Sarcoma	7	6	2	28
Craniopharyngioma	3	2	3	100
Meningeal fibroblastoma	1	1	1	100
	119	100.0	50	42

* All children were treated under 15 years of age, 78 postoperatively and 41 with irradiation alone 1939-1958.
Clinical follow-up complete to 1964.

RESULTS FOLLOWING IRRADIATION
OF BRAIN TUMORS IN CHILDREN

Primary brain tumors initially are all radiosensitive, more or less like most primary malignancies are in children. The younger they are, the more radiosensitive. However, it must be noted that radiosensitivity is not synonymous of radiocurability. Immediate clinical improvement is usually observed early after the onset of treatment, an amelioration often dramatic. When a child's condition is critical because of increased intracranial pressure, decompression is urgent. Radiation therapy should be initiated immediately after decompression and must be considered an emergency procedure in some cases. Most children respond quickly and improve to such degree that by the time radiation therapy is completed, a full clinical recovery ordinarily can be observed.

The length and the quality of survivals are presented side-by-side (Table 4-13). The rates are shown on a quinquennial basis at the end of 5, 10, 15, and 20 years after treatment. This is a global assessment for all types of primary brain tumors treated by adequate irradiation, either after surgery or alone, in children 15 years of age or under from the time of their treatment.

In children, irradiation was administered postoperatively in 65 per cent of all cases.

Brain tumors irradiated postoperatively consisted of all glioblastomas, unclassified gliomas, astrocytomas, ependymomas, the majority of medulloblastomas, and the minority of midbrain and brain-stem tumors. Most of the few nongliomatous tumors were treated by combined surgical removal and postoperative irradiation.

Radiation alone was used to treat 41 or 35 per cent of our 119 children. Primary brain tumors treated by irradiation alone consisted of the majority of brain-stem and midbrain tumors, plus 10 medulloblastomas and 2 cerebellar sarcomas. Comparison of survival rates was made between the children treated by irradiation alone and those treated for gliomas of the same categories with surgery followed by irradiation. The two groups were comparable in size, 37 and 34 children, and composed of the same types of tumors. The results of this comparison clearly reveal that survival rates between the two groups are identical at 5 years, but are appreciably higher at 10, 15, and 20 years among those who were treated solely by irradiation more than 10, 15, and 20 years ago. Therefore, our experience indicates that children who have been treated for medulloblastomas, midbrain, and brain-stem tumors have survived longer and have attained long survivals in a higher proportion when actively treated solely by adequate irradiation.

Table 4-13. *Primary Intracranial Neoplasms in Children—Long Term Survival and Recovery Rates* Subsequent to Adequate Irradiation Used Postoperatively or Alone*

Survival Over	Length of Survival			Quality of Survival		
	Total Possible	No. of Survivors	Per Cent of Survivals	Recovery Grade by Ratio†		
				I	II	III
5 Years	119	50	42	39/50	8/50	3/50
10 Years	86	31	36	25/31	5/31	1/31
15 Years	45	14	31	10/14	3/14	1/14
20 Years	14	6	43	5/6	1/6	—

*From Children adequately irradiated under 15 years of age, 66 per cent postoperatively, 1939–1958.—Follow-up complete to 1964.
† Grading of Recovery: Grade I—Good—Active useful life
                       Grade II—Fair—Partial disability
                       Grade III—Poor—Total disability: physical and/or mental.

Of the 37 children treated by irradiation alone 12 or 33 per cent have survived over 5 years. All of these 12 children who have survived over 5 years up to 23 are still living: 6 between 5 and 10 years, 3 between 10 and 15 years, 2 between 15 and 20 years, and 1 over 20 years. None have developed tumor recurrence as yet. All have grown normally from the somatic standpoint. Not one is mentally disabled or insane. Only 2 have not recovered fully from the symptoms and neurologic deficit that they presented prior to irradiation, even though they have shown some improvement. Both have to move around in a wheelchair in which one is taken to school. They were treated 6 and 7 years ago by irradiation alone for midbrain tumors, at the ages of 2 and 5 respectively.

The 5-year survival rates are shown for all children by histologic type and anatomic location (Table 4-12). It is obvious that the highest 5-year survival rate, 75 per cent, occurred in the astrocytoma group of primary intracranial tumors.

In the treatment of midbrain tumors in children we are depending, in our center, more and more upon the effects of adequate irradiation.

We were curious to try and find out whether there might be any difference in 5-year survival rates in relation to the age of infants and children when they were irradiated for their brain tumors. This analysis suggests that the older a child is at the time of diagnosis and treatment of an intracranial glioma, the better the prognosis as determined by the higher survival rates, regardless of the treatment used in our series (Table 4-14). The favorable difference in 5-year survival rates appears to be particularly significant in the group of children who were treated between the ages of 11 to 15.

In general, children can be expected to do as well and probably better than adults in terms of longevity and useful survivals. We believe that the number of cases studied in Table 4-15 is large enough to be statistically significant. From a close scrutiny of this difference it appears that different factors may be accounting for it. One of these factors is the difference in incidence of glioblastomas which is low in children and high in adults, so that the latter group has sustained

Table 4-14. *Primary Intracranial Tumors Irradiated in Children Under 15 Years of Age Age Distribution and Survival Rates*

Age Group	No. of Children	5-Year Survivals	
		No.	Per Cent
6 months—5 years	35	12	34
6 years—10 years	53	20	39
11 years—15 years	31	18	58
	119	50	42

Table 4-15. *Irradiation of Primary Intracranial Neoplasms—Comparison of Postradiation Survival Rates in Adults and Children*

Survival Over	Adults			Children		
	Total Possible	No. of Survivors	Per Cent	Total Possible	No. of Survivors	Per Cent
5 Years	445	146	32	119	50	42
10 Years	326	75	23	86	31	36
15 Years	213	37	17	45	14	31
20 Years	97	15	16	14	6	43

From a total of 564 patients adequately irradiated in the treatment of their intracranial neoplasms, 1939–1958.
Among these, 119 or 21.1 per cent were children under 15 years of age at the onset of irradiation.
Clinical follow-up complete to 1964, ranging from a minimum of 5 up to 25 years.

heavy losses from these highly malignant tumors. Another factor which has contributed to a higher salvage rate in the group of children in our series seems to be directly related to the increasingly better results that were achieved in the management of medulloblastomas as well as midbrain and pontine tumors, in which losses of life can be so heavy in children. There can be no doubt in our minds that such reversal in the prognosis of children affected with brain tumors, still considered hopeless by many, is mainly attributable to adequate irradiation in the management of their tumors.

Metastatic Intracranial Tumors

The incidence of brain metastases is increasing steadily. The site of primary malignant neoplasms which metastasize to the brain most frequently is changing from time to time, and perhaps from one part of the world to another. In countries where bronchogenic carcinoma is detected with an increasing frequency, metastases to the brain may be identified more often than ever before. The problem of clinical management of cerebral metastases must be considered. Relief or improvement of the mental and physical condition of patients affected with brain metastases may be achieved by radiation therapy, often most dramatically. In some cases craniotomy and surgical extirpation might be considered. Chemotherapeutic agents may be employed with efficacy in a small proportion of the cases, particularly in the fast growing anaplastic malignant lesions.

Brain metastases are multiple in the majority of cases, approximately 80 per cent. A single metastatic nodule may be the only manifestation of cerebral metastasis in other cases. Evidence of an expanding intracranial lesion not uncommonly may be the first and sole manifestation of a distant primary malignant lesion which has not manifested itself as yet at the primary site. In such cases the metastatic lesion may be undistinguishable

by its symptoms and signs from any other intracranial tumor. Some metastatic brain tumors have infiltrated the brain and other intracranial structures in a way such as to simulate a primary brain tumor, not only grossly but microscopically as well. We have reported[7] such incidence in 10 cases of metastases which simulated primary intracranial tumors so completely that these were diagnosed and treated as primary tumors of various histological types.

The diagnosis of brain metastasis can be made on a clinical basis only. It may also result from histologic verification when a biopsy has been obtained at craniotomy or by needle aspiration. The selection of the method of treatment must be judicious. If the lesion is singular and the patient is apparently free of other distant metastases, craniotomy and attempt at extirpation should be preferred to other methods of treatment. This approach is particularly indicated should the metastasis originate from a primary malignancy which is well differentiated and presumably radioresistant.

Radiation therapy alone is indicated in preference to surgery in brain metastases under the following circumstances: 1) when the primary tumor is not under control and the presence of metastases can be demonstrated in other parts of the body particularly in vital organs; 2) when clinical investigation shows objective evidence of multiple cerebral metastases; and 3) when the brain metastases are deemed radiosensitive.

Combined radiation therapy and chemotherapeutic agents may be more effective in certain cases particularly when metastases are multiple not only in the brain but elsewhere in the body.

Chao *et al.*[8] reported observations on 38 patients treated for palliative purposes with x-radiation. They listed the common sources of brain metastases as being: 1) carcinoma of the lung; 2) cancer of the breast; 3) cancer of the gastrointestinal tract; and 4) renal tumors. Because of the prevalent incidence of multiple metastatic lesions, they have used opposing lateral fields encompassing the entire area. In order to avoid excessive intracranial pressure, small initial daily doses have been used. In their experience clinical improvement became manifest after approximately 1,000 rads in the first week or 10 days. When palliation only was desired, tumor doses of approximately 2,000 *r* were delivered, but ordinarily the total dose was carried up to 3,000 *r* in the hope of preventing recurrence of neurological signs. Good palliative results were obtained in 63 per cent of the 38 patients treated.

This may be the place to recall that cerebral metastases are extremely rare in patients affected with malignant lymphomas, particularly with Hodgkin's and lymphocytic sarcomas. Reticulum cell sarcomas, however, send metastases to the brain occasionally.

Tumors Involving the Hypophysis

Radiation therapy, used alone or in combination with surgery, holds a paramount place in the control of tumors of the hypophysis. Once the tumor growth appears to be restrained, hormonal management prevails. The proper management of tumors of the pituitary gland depends largely upon the knowledge and experience of each consultant in a team of specialists which should group endocrinologists, neurologists, neurosurgeons, and radiologists.

In the treatment of patients affected with pituitary tumors, the prime objective is the suppression of adverse pressure effects on the surrounding glandular components within the hypophysis itself, and on adjacent extrasellar structures such as the optic chiasm and the hypothalamus. This must be accomplished with the minimum hazard to the patient's life and the maximum probability of correcting, in full or in part, the physiopathological disturbances created by a given type of pituitary tumor.

My experience in the use of ionizing radiation for the treatment of primary pituitary tumors consists of 151 cases. Of those, 111 were treated more than 5 years ago and followed for periods varying from 5 to over 20 years. These 111 cases comprise 59 chromophobe adenomas, 36 eosinophilic, 9 basophilic, and 7 miscellaneous tumors. There is only one primary malignant tumor in the present material. A few metastatic tumors involving the pituitary gland were treated palliatively by irradiation but these were not included in the present figures. The incidence of primary pituitary tumors represents approximately 8 per cent of all intracranial tumors. Pituitary tumors are uncommon in children and adolescents, as they usually manifest themselves between 30 and 45 years of age.

Chromophobe Adenomas

Chromophobe adenomas form the largest group of pituitary tumors under scrutiny. The onset of chromophobe adenomas is insidious. Ordinarily, diagnosis is not made until a chromophobe tumor has reached a size sufficient to cause pressure on the normal acidophil and basophil cells and induce physiopathologic disturbances resulting in hypopituitarism. Chromophobe cells produce no endocrine secretion that is known as yet. When the tumor extends outside the sella, it may press upon the optic chiasm with secondary hemianopsia demonstrable by both clinical examination and visual fields. Visual complaints are the presenting symptoms in 60 to 65 per cent of the cases and headache in approximately 40 to 50 per cent.

Hypopituitarism is more commonly associated with a chromophobe adenoma of the pituitary gland than with any other intracranial lesion. It must be emphasized, however, that the same clinical syndromes may be induced by several types of intracranial lesions which may directly or indirectly cause pressure on the pituitary gland and depress its functions.

The treatment of chromophobe adenomas may consist primarily of either surgical removal only or irradiation alone, or else a combination of both methods in which irradiation is commonly used postoperatively. Treatment of chromophobe adenomas by surgery only is capable of controlling some chromophobe adenomas. Irradiation alone has been used in the management of tumors diagnosed as chromophobe adenomas. There are several reports in the literature showing that chromophobe adenomas treated by irradiation alone may respond favorably and remain under control for long periods of time.

We have treated by irradiation alone 28 chromophobe adenomas available for review 5 years or longer after treatment. The most significant finding in our analysis is that 20 of the 28 patients initially treated by irradiation alone have never required any further treatment as they remained recurrence-free for 5 years or longer, a rate of 71 per cent. Of these 20 patients, 10 have been irradiated between 5 and 10 years ago, 8 between 10 and 15 years and 2 between 15 and 20 years (Table 4-16). In our series of pituitary tumors treated more than 5 years ago, 28 patients were treated first by surgery combined with postoperative irradiation for chromophobe

adenomas. Twenty-four have made a good recovery and have remained free of recurrence (Table 4-16).

Recurrence-free rates are valid measures in the evaluation of methods of treatment. In the treatment of chromophobe adenomas, most series found in the literature have shown that, following surgery alone, rates of recurrence have not been too high as they rarely exceed 50 to 60 per cent. The incidence of recurrences and the speed with which they develop have been reduced considerably by combining irradiation with surgery postoperatively. This has been clearly demonstrated from the reports mentioned above. Irradiation alone is of definite value since it can yield good results and allow a reasonably high number of patients to be recurrence-free for 5, 10, 15 years or longer after treatment. Correa and Lampe[10] are of the opinion that no significant difference exists in the results obtained by surgery plus irradiation and by radiotherapy alone. Our own series suggest that perhaps there is a slightly higher proportion of patients who have improved and remained recurrence-free among those treated by combined surgery and postoperative irradiation and followed

Table 4-16. *Pituitary Tumors—Patients Improved and Recurrence-free*

Follow-up Over	Chromophobe (56 cases)*		Eosinophilic (32 cases)†
	Irradiation Alone (28 Patients)	Surgery and Irradiation (28 Patients)	Irradiation Alone (32 Patients)
Over 5 Years	10	5	8
Over 10 Years	8	10	6
Over 15 Years	2	7	5
Over 20 Years	0	1	7
Total Improved and recurrence-free	20	23	26
Rate	71%	82%	81%

*Not included are 3 patients irradiated for treatment of tumor recurrence, several years after surgery only.
†Not included in this total are 4 patients treated by surgery plus irradiation, which controlled 3 of the 4.

for a long time. Richmond[27] believes that surgery followed by adequate irradiation is the method of choice and that all chromophobe adenomas should be treated in that manner and his opinion is based on 220 cases of pituitary tumors, a large proportion of which consisted of chromophobe adenomas.

Assessment of treatment results on the basis of survival rates is not considered a valid yardstick by many in the management of pituitary tumors. We have tabulated our long-term survival rates side-by-side for chromophobe and eosinophilic adenomas and the rates shown at 5, 10, 15, and 20 years following treatment revealed no great difference between the two (Table 4-17).

There appear to be substantial variations in the rates of improvement of visual field defects. Richmond has reported some form of visual improvement in 87 per cent of chromophobe adenomas following combined surgery and postoperative irradiation. The rates of nonimprovement of visual fields are relatively consistent. Correa and Lampe[10] report a 40 per cent rate of nonimprovement following irradiation alone. Sheline *et al.*[29] have reported no improvement of visual fields following operation alone in 32 per cent of the cases and 46 per cent following operation and irradiation.

The determination of endocrine improvement by hormone tests or assays continues to present some difficulties for many practical reasons. One of these reasons is the need for the administration of supplementary hormone to correct the effects of hypopituitarism in most patients.

Restoration of the sella turcica must not be expected to be an index of the efficacy of treatment of pituitary adenomas.

There are a number of reports clearly stating that there is a direct relation between the results obtained and the doses of radiation delivered to the pituitary. Doses varying between 4,500 and 5,000 rads over a period of 40 to 45 days are used presently. All patients are treated with ^{60}Co radiation beams at 50 or 80 cm focus skin distance.

Regarding the technique of irradiation, the size and number of fields directing radiation beams to pituitary adenomas preferably should be determined for each patient. This can be decided from the estimated size of the tumor, as judged from the degree of enlargement of the sella turcica and of tumor extension above it. The majority of chromophobe adenomas are well encapsulated and measure approximately 2 or 3 cm in diameter. Fields averaging 4 × 4 cm should be adequate to irradiate such volume of tissue. When appreciable suprasellar extension is clearly demonstrated by pneumoencephalography, fields 5 × 5 cm in size rarely need to be exceeded. With fixed fields the entire course of treatment may be administered by two lateral opposing fields. Positioning films are very useful to control beam direction through the tumor-bearing area. It is difficult to conceive why so many are using lateral fields measuring 6 × 8 cm covering areas of 48 sq cm to aim at tumors averaging 3 cm in diameter. In cases with suprasellar extension additional anterior and posterior fields are often used to cross-fire the pituitary

Table 4-17. *Radiation Therapy in Pituitary Adenomas—Long Term Survivals*

Survival Over	Chromophobe			Eosinophilic		
	No. of Patients	No. of Survivors	Per Cent	No. of Patients	No. of Survivors	Per Cent
5 Years	59	53	90	36	32	89
10 Years	41	32	80	28	20	71
15 Years	19	15	79	20	13	65
20 Years	11	4	36	9	4	44

tumor, in order to avoid missing possible extension in the anteroposterior direction. Many are using beam direction devices which are more or less involved.

Rotational techniques are employed by several. Personally I use these rarely for the irradiation of pituitary tumors. This is because a substantial volume of normal brain tissue is exposed unnecessarily to doses of radiation which are still relatively high, even though decreasing, at the periphery of the rotational field in relation to the central dose delivered. This may be visualized by superimposition of the isodose curves obtained when direct lateral opposing small fields are used by comparison with concentric isodose curves resulting from rotation of the radiation beam (Fig. 4-8).

The morbidity associated with treatment must be considered before making a treatment decision. The treatment of chromophobe adenomas by irradiation alone can be achieved properly with virtually and practically no complications. Even though the operative mortality has reduced considerably in most centers, it is still in the vicinity of 3 to 5 per cent. If irradiation alone is selected, it is important to repeat visual field examina-

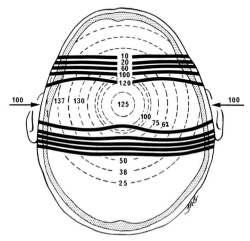

FIG. 4-8. Irradiation of pituitary tumor—superimposed isodose curves in direct lateral opposing fields, compared with concentric curves in rotational technique.

tions to determine if there is any progression or regression in the visual field defect. The results of treatment have been said to be less favorable in chromophobe adenomas. This seems to have changed considerably in the last 15 years with the use of higher doses estimated at level of the tumor. The advent of high energy radiation appears to have given more confidence to many in regard to the therapeutic potential of irradiation.

The selection as to which method of treatment should be used first, whether surgery or irradiation, should be made in each case largely on the basis of the size of the tumor and the degree of pressure that it may exert on the extrasellar structures particularly the optic chiasm. If the suprasellar components suggest the possibility of a cystic lesion or if the diagnosis of chromophobe adenoma remains doubtful, despite suitable investigation, surgical exploration and management should be considered first. This will have the advantage of verifying the diagnosis and cause decompression at the same time. It is our opinion and that of many others that cystic lesions are ordinarily not controlled as well and for so long with radiation therapy as they can be by surgical removal. When a patient is rapidly becoming blind, one should not risk that this may continue to complete and permanent atrophy of the optic nerves and chiasm. Surgery should then be used first to relieve the pressure and give the nerve tissue a chance to restore.

When the probability of a lesion other than a chromophobe adenoma is minimal and there is no significant extrasellar extension, radiation therapy should be used first. Surgery should then be withheld for future use in the event that radiation therapy alone should prove incapable of controlling permanently the pituitary adenoma. Pressure on the optic chiasm by minimal or moderate suprasellar extension may be relieved with considerable efficacy with radiation therapy alone in the majority of the cases. If the tumor appears to extend into the floor of the third ventricle or temporal lobes, surgical treatment should be preferred and used first. In our experience, surgical treatment seems to be superior to irradiation in the treatment of recurrence when adequate irradiation has been used before, either alone or postoperatively.

Eosinophilic Adenomas

Eosinophil or acidophil adenomas are small benign tumors developing in the anterior lobe of the pituitary gland. These adenomas are composed of proliferating eosinophil cells which are secreting growth hormone actively. Excessive secretion of growth hormone causes acromegaly, a syndrome of eosinophilic hyperpituitarism. This abnormal production of growth hormone does not merely affect facial bones and extremities but viscera as well.

Enlargement of the sella turcica is present in the majority of cases but may be absent in approximately 20 per cent. Visual field changes are not constant. Acidophil adenomas extend outside the sella and press upon the optic chiasm and nerves in less than one-half of the patients. As the tumor increases in size, signs of hypopituitarism begin to manifest themselves because the tumor is depressing the other pituitary functions in relation to the target glands: thyroid, gonads, adrenals.

The treatment of eosinophilic adenomas may vary according to the degree of activity of the tumor. The main objective is to control the excess of secretion of growth hormone by the adenoma. The second purpose is to control undue pressure when this exists in the acromegalic patient. Some believe that conservative treatment and symptomatic management may be sufficient as long as the tumor does not seem to be overactive and there is no pressure symptoms demanding decompression. It is not always easy to determine to what extent the adenoma is active and secreting growth hormone in excess. So far these hormonal assays have not been readily available and yet they would be most desirable. Direct treatment of the eosinophilic adenomas when indicated consists of irradiation alone or surgery plus irradiation. It seems that in most treatment centers surgery alone is no longer considered adequate.

Results of treatment in eosinophilic adenomas cannot be assessed by the length of survival of patients in view of the fact that long survivals are not uncommon among patients with this type of tumor (Table 4-17). The main criterion is the evidence of arrest of tumor growth. Secretion in excess of growth hormone may then cease and return to normal. Active signs of acromegaly should then stop progressing without, however, regressing, because these signs are considered irreversible. Relief of headache may be expected in at least 80 per cent of the patients. Swelling of the soft tissues in the face and hands may subside. Visual fields when affected may improve partially or even in toto. These are the clinical signs of tumor arrest but the salient external features of acromegaly persist.

Following irradiation, the apparent arrest of tumor growth is not an infallible criterion of efficacy of treatment. Periods of remission may occur spontaneously and periods of discrete reactivation may intervene. These might be detectable by growth hormone assays and increase in serum phosphorus. The incidence of diabetes is high in patients with acromegaly and remissions after treatment may be an indirect indication that an eosinophilic adenoma is probably in a state of remission.

Results of treatment by irradiation were reported by Correa and Lampe[10] who have shown that these were good in 63.3 per cent of 31 patients with eosinophilic adenomas. Eleven were counted as poor. Seven survived over 10 to 15 years. In their opinion, no statistically significant difference could be demonstrated between the results in the chromophobe and the eosinophilic patients. The good results following radiation therapy have increased significantly with higher doses ranging from 2,000 to 2,500 up to 4,000 rads. When delivering large doses, 4,000 rads in 28 to 32 days, they like to use the high energy radiation of ^{137}Cs or ^{60}Co.

In our experience with the treatment of eosinophilic adenomas by irradiation alone 32 patients have been treated more than 5 years ago and followed completely. Our long-term survival rates (Table 4-17) are amazingly high. Analysis of results shows that tumor growth has been apparently arrested in 26 of the 32 patients. The rate of patients who have improved and remained recurrence-free indefinitely over 5 years after treatment up to over 20 years is 81 per cent in our series (Table 4-16).

Presently we treat acromegalic patients with ^{60}Co radiation and tumor doses of 4,500 to 5,000 rads over 40 to 50 days.

Basophilic Adenomas

Adenomas consisting of basophil cells are not common. Because of their relatively small size they may be present without causing appreciable enlargement of the sella turcica, but this occurs in only a small proportion of the cases. Judging from our small series, enlargement of the sella might occur in 40 to 50 per cent of the cases.

Sosman[30] presented a classical article on Cushing's disease and pituitary basophilism. He then discussed the role of radiation therapy and its beneficial effects in 4 of 6 cases. He clearly demonstrated that this syndrome may be reversible and can be controlled completely by external irradiation of the pituitary gland, but this does not occur in all cases.

We have, in our series, 9 cases treated with external radiation therapy and followed for 5 years or longer. Clinical remission has been observed in 5 of them, whereas the 4 remaining patients did not improve and died from complications associated with their syndrome.

We give now a single course with ^{60}Co

radiation and tumor doses averaging 4,000 to 4,500 rads in 40 to 45 days.

Miscellaneous Pituitary Tumors Mixed and Others

Mixed tumors are pituitary adenomas which histologically are composed of both active elements of eosinophilic and chromophobe cells. These patients usually have a mild degree of acromegalic features with a predominant clinical picture of hypopituitarism. The exact diagnosis of mixed tumor is usually made at operation. The diagnosis was made at operation in 6 of the 7 cases comprised in our series and at autopsy in the other case. They were all treated postoperatively by external radiation and have enjoyed long and good survivals varying from 7 to 15 years except for 2 patients.

Malignant primary tumors of the pituitary gland are rare. There is one proven case of adenocarcinoma in our series. Diagnosis was made at operation. Following partial removal a tumor dose of 6,500 rads was given over a period of 68 days. We are somewhat surprised that he is alive and well 8 years after treatment. Richmond[27] has reported 7 carcinomas of a total of 220 patients who have received postoperative radiotherapy, but it appears that 4 are in the group of the malignant chromophobes. In the management of tumors of the pituitary gland he favors surgical removal followed by radiation therapy. He indicates a figure of 57 per cent 5-year survivals in carcinoma.

Metastatic tumors occasionally involve the hypophysis or develop in the sellar region. These may be suspected clinically, but they are more often found at autopsy. We have seen a few cases mostly in metastases from carcinoma of the breast involving the base of the skull and cranial nerves particularly the sixth nerve. Good palliative effect was achieved with radiation exposure of the corresponding area using lateral opposing fields and depth doses averaging 2,500 rads in approximately 4 weeks.

Spinal Cord Tumors and Other Lesions

The value of radiation therapy in the management of tumors and other lesions involving the spinal cord is difficult to assess. There must be very few observers who have irradiated and followed more than 50 cases of primary intramedullary gliomata. Extramedullary intradural tumors are far more common but these are surgical problems exclusively. Intramedullary metastases from distant malignant tumors are rare for some unknown reason. In the management of neoplastic diseases, extradural metastases are not uncommon. Through the intervertebral foramina, these invade and infiltrate the spaces between the dura mater and the rigid vertebral canal, affecting the cord indirectly by mechanical pressure. A brief mention will be made of the role of radiation therapy in the treatment of syringomyelia and arachnoiditis.

Primary Intramedullary Neoplasms

Our experience is based upon a series of 30 patients treated by irradiation postoperatively more than 5 years ago and followed completely up to 1964. In our series of primary tumors of the spinal cord, all cases were verified by surgical exploration and partial removal or biopsy. Histological diagnosis revealed the following types of tumors: 9 ependymomas, 6 astrocytomas, 8 unclassified gliomas, 1 glioblastoma, 3 meningeal tumors, and 3 miscellaneous neoplasms (recurrent glioma of the filum terminale, fibrolipoma, and teratoma). Tumor distribution showed involvement of the cervical cord in 8 patients, thoracic in 16, and lumbar including filum terminale in the 6 remaining cases. More than one segments of the cord were involved at once in 2 patients. Not included is a recent case in which an intramedullary ependymoma was found that extended the length of the entire cord. This is suggesting a multicentric origin of the neoplastic process

which developed simultaneously at every level of the cord.

Treatment of primary intramedullary tumors has consisted of surgical procedures initially. Laminectomy was performed to provide adequate decompression and exposure of the cord in every case. Some degree of surgical removal was achieved in 18 patients, whereas in the remaining 12 cases biopsy or cyst aspiration only were considered advisable.

Postoperative radiation therapy was administered in every case. The 5 initial patients in this series had short repeated courses of irradiation in the same fashion as that described by Wood[32] and his associates. At present treatment by irradiation is administered consistently in a single course with ^{60}Co and tumor doses equivalent to 4,500 to 5,000 rads over periods of 40 to 45 days. Such doses are well within the safe limits of radiation tolerance of central nervous tissue given in Boden's curves. In view of the width of the spinal canal, which seldom exceeds 3 cm, long narrow fields measuring 3 or 4 cm in width were considered suitable. Provision was made to include a good safety margin above and below the apparent extent of the intramedullary neoplasms to be exposed to radiation.

Results of treatment have revealed complete clinical improvement during the first year in 73 per cent of our patients, no improvement in 20 per cent, and partial improvement in the others. Of our 30 patients, 18 or 60 per cent have survived over 5 years and it happens that each of the survivors has actually been followed for more than 8 years. Not one of the survivors has lived less than 8 years from the onset of treatment.

The survival and recovery rates are presented side-by-side in Table 4-18. There seems to be a fairly constant pattern that we have observed. Long-term clinical improvement has been more or less a matter of all or nothing, either with complete lasting recovery or else complete paraplegia at once. An intermediate group improved at first and

Table 4-18. *Intramedullary Spinal Cord Tumors—Long Term Survival and Recovery Rates**

Survival Over	Length of Survival			Quality of Survival		
	Total Possible	No. of Survivors	Per Cent of Survivals	Proportion of Recovery Grades†		
				I	II	III
5 Years	30	18	60	11/18	2/18	5/18
10 Years	21	11	52	7/11	—	4/11
15 Years	13	7	54	4/7	—	3/7
20 Years	7	3	43	2/3	—	1/3

*From 30 patients, verified surgically and histologically—all followed over 6 years.
†Grading of Recovery: Grade I—Good—Active useful life
Grade II—Fair—Partial disability
Grade III—Poor—Paraplegia

later developed some paraplegia, between 3 to 7 years after operation and radiation therapy. Ten years after treatment, the degree of recovery has become definitive for better more often than for worse as shown in Table 4-18. Beyond 10 years following treatment very few died from reactivation of their spinal cord tumor.

Metastatic Intramedullary Tumors

These are rare findings and the diagnosis can be made only by surgical exploration and biopsy. We have seen only 2 cases, one with metastases from cancer of the breast and the other with lymphosarcoma. The treatment should consist of radiation therapy directed to the spinal cord in the same way as in the case of primary cord tumor.

Extradural Tumors

Metastases from various types of primary malignancy occur fairly frequently and are by far the most common malignant lesions affecting the spinal cord. These occur by involvement of the paravertebral soft tissues with invasion through the intervertebral foramina and infiltration between the dura itself and the vertebral canal. Once the metastatic process is within the vertebral canal it may extend in every direction including a circular fashion around the cord.

Such metastatic lesions are seen most frequently in cancer of the breast, bronchogenic carcinoma, hypernephroma, and particularly in the lymphoma group in Hodgkin's sarcoma and lymphosarcoma. This also occurs with testicular tumors and carcinoma of the prostate.

The treatment of such metastatic lesions can also occur when metastases involve the bone of vertebrae and break through the osseous barrier to extend into the vertebral canal. From the treatment standpoint, it is essential and most important that these lesions be suspected and identified early so that adequate treatment can be established before permanent damage be inflicted on the cord, with resulting paraplegia. No matter how radiosensitive the tumor may be, it is imperative to perform a surgical decompression of the cord in all cases with paraplegic symptoms of 24-hour duration. Otherwise permanent paraplegia will result. Immediate surgical decompression is imperative when extradural pressure on the cord results from the collapse of a metastatic vertebra. These lesions are usually infiltrating and can rarely be removed completely by surgical procedure at the time of decompression.

Palliative irradiation is indicated following decompression. The plan of treatment will depend on the nature and character of the metastatic process. Extradural metastatic lesions often are from types of carcinoma or sarcoma which may be radioresistant. The prognosis, the plan of treatment and radiation doses will be influenced by those factors. Hodgkin's sarcoma or small cell lymphosarcoma infiltration can be expected to respond quickly with moderate doses of radiation therapy alone. Enhancing effects may be obtained when radiation is associated with radiomimetic chemotherapeutic agents. Complete clinical evaluation of each case individually should be the most important and perhaps the only guide as to the plan of treatment either with radiation therapy alone or combined with palliative surgical procedures or chemotherapy.

Sacrococcygeal Chordoma

The diagnosis of a chordoma in that location is not common. We have seen only 4 cases in our series of tumors. Recently Kamerin et al.[15] presented 30 cases of chordomas of which 5 involved the sacrococcygeal area, and 9 were found at other levels of the spinal column. Tumors in any of these locations invade the vertebral canal and press on the cord extradurally. The diagnosis is made at operation and subtotal removal is indicated first. Tumor doses must be high and should rarely be less than 5,000 to 6,000 rads over a period of approximately 50 days using ^{60}Co. The prognosis is not good although we have seen good palliative response in some of our cases. Kamerin and associates indicate that survival from time of therapy has been 3 years' average.

Miscellaneous Benign Lesions

Syringomyelia

This is a benign condition involving the upper segment of the spinal cord. The ependymal canal is dilated and usually filled with small cystic cavities. This process tends to expand into other portions of the spinal cord. It is considered by many as a lesion of embryonal development. Dyke and Davidoff[12] have made an extensive review of the literature on this subject. They express the opinion that syringomyelia is a disease in which some cases appear to respond favorably to roentgen therapy. However, they have agreed that cures of the disease did not occur. My own experience is limited to approximately 6 cases in which improvement of symptoms, particularly of pain, was evidenced following a short course of treatment with relatively small doses totalling in depth 1,000 to 1,200 *r* over a period of 10 to 15 days. Our follow-up is practically nonexistent in this group of cases. Therefore I feel unable to offer any guidance in relation of the results of treatment of syringomyelia by irradiation.

Arachnoiditis

We have attempted to treat adhesive arachnoiditis with radiation in 4 cases. Total doses averaging 1,500 to 1,800 *r* depth dose should be administered at a slow rate over periods of 30 to 35 days. Our objective was to reduce the fibrotic adhesions existing between the surfaces of the arachnoid membrane. No definite evidence of improvement has been observed in the few cases that were treated.

Lesions of Peripheral Nervous System

Peripheral nerves are recognized as structures which normally are rather radioresistant. This does not mean that nerve fibers are immune to radiation. When nerves are injured by irradiation, this seems to be by a process of demyelinization. Primary neoplasms arising from the peripheral nerves are not common. These tumors consist almost exclusively of slowly growing benign lesions diagnosed histologically as neuromas, neurinomas, and neurofibromata. Peripheral nerve tumors are usually single and localized lesions. If they should be multiple, they nearly always are manifestations of generalized neurofibromatosis or von Recklinghausen's disease.

The management of these tumors, wherever they may be, is primarily a surgical problem. Radiation therapy should not be expected to induce regression of neuromas. At the most there might be palliation of pain of variable duration. This has been the experience of many observers through the years. Our last attempt at irradiation of a neuroma was entirely futile. A tumor dose of 6,500 rads was delivered in 50 days to a large neuroma measuring approximately 12 cm in diameter. This was a manifestation of generalized neurofibromatosis. The tumor was located in the posterior part of the pelvic cavity so it was readily accessible for clinical observation. There was no appreciable effect on the tumor at any time during or after treatment.

Occasionally small tumors involving a peripheral nerve may show partial regression under irradiation and this is accompanied with relief of pain. Such radiation effects have been observed in 2 of our patients with recurrent neuromas in which a predominance of fibrous connective tissue reaction was reported by the pathologist. These lesions were treated with tissue doses of 1,000 to 1,200 rads in small divided doses over a total period of 4 to 6 weeks. It is important to treat over a long protracted basis since our aim is to induce antifibrotic effect and not to cause more fibrosis. Total improvement may be appreciable 3 to 6 months only following completion of treatment.

Palliative irradiation still has a place in the treatment of neuritis and severe neuralgia when this cannot be relieved satisfactorily by any other method. Patients should be so treated providing only that such treatment may not prevent or unduly delay investigation which might disclose some serious cause of pain which should be treated primarily and quite differently.

Postherpetic neuralgia is the most common neuritic condition that we are still treating nowadays with a reasonable amount of success. Severe neuralgia occurs in a minority of patients afflicted with herpes zoster. It is preferable to treat such neuralgia towards the end of an acute phase of herpes zoster than once it has become chronic and may persist indefinitely without improvement. Radiation therapy directed over the corresponding nerve roots will often induce some degree of analgesic effect and at times relieve pain completely and permanently. It is wise to irradiate one or two nerve root levels above and below those apparently involved. Relief of pain may be observed towards the end of a course of treatment but improvement is slow, and complete results of treatment may not be fully appreciable until 2 to 3 months have elapsed from onset of treatment. Total relief of pain in postherpetic neuralgia may be anticipated in the majority of the acute cases and in a proportion of 40 to 50 per cent of the patients in the chronic cases. Our plan of treatment usually consists of a total incident dose of 1,500 to 1,800 r at 200 Kv in divided doses of 150 r 3 times a week over a period of approximately 4 weeks. The tissue dose at level of the nerve roots varies between 1,000 to 1,200 rads. In a few cases the amount of peripheral scarring in the skin appears to be involving the nerve endings to such an extent that these have to be treated as well as the nerve roots. This is then treated on the same basis as that used for the treatment of keloids.

Trigeminal neuralgia has been treated in the same fashion on several occasions and with highly satisfactory results. The external radiation beam is then aimed to the gasserian ganglion and the emerging nerve roots.

Painful scars, associated or not with itchiness, may be quite distressing in some patients and these symptoms may be relieved completely by localized external irradiation. Such symptoms may manifest themselves with or without keloid formation. The radiobiologic objective is then to induce an anti-fibrotic reaction which will result in analgesia by freeing nerve endings and terminal nerve branches from constriction by scar tissue. This can only be accomplished properly if treatment is administered slowly and with doses which will not increase the existing fibrosis, but bring its regression. Fibrosis is a reversible reaction which may be either induced or reduced by ionizing radiation. Since tissue inflammation is a predominant factor in causing radiation fibrosis, it is important that any plan of treatment be such as to avoid causing inflammation in the treatment of painful scars. Single skin doses of 300 r at a time are administered every 2 or 3 weeks for a total of 4 or 5 treatments. Improvement usually begins to be appreciable, and sometimes relief of pain and itchiness is complete about the time the patient returns for the third treatment.

The analgesic effect of ionizing radiation on primary or secondary malignant tumors is often dramatic. Pain relief in patients with bone metastases or metastases infiltrating soft tissues unquestionably represents one of the most useful and beneficial utilization of radiation.

Acknowledgement

I wish to express my deep appreciation to all the staff of the Montreal Neurological Institute who through the years have contributed in so many ways to the results presented here. It is through their valuable scientific assistance and support that we were able together to pursue this clinical work. I must pay tribute in particular to my outstanding colleagues Drs. W. Penfield, A. Elvidge, T. Rasmussen and the late William Cone, and also to my fellow radiologists Drs. C. B. Peirce and D. L. McRae.

My sincere gratitude to my devoted secretary, Mrs. Agnes Boudreau. It is largely due to her dedication for the last 12 years that our follow-up is complete. Clinical reports and autopsy findings have been collected all over Canada and abroad to be suitably analyzed and recorded. Her assistance in the final editing of this chapter has been splendid.

BIBLIOGRAPHY

1. Arnold, A., Bailey, P., and Harvey, R. A.: Intolerance of primate brain stem and hypothalamus to conventional and high energy radiations, *Neurology,* 4, 575, 1954.
2. Bailey, P. and Cushing, H.: *A Classification of the Tumors of the Glioma Group on a Histogenetic Basis with a Correlated Study of Prognosis,* Philadelphia, J. B. Lippincott Company, 1926.
3. Bailey, P. and Cushing, H.: Medulloblastoma cerebelli: A common type of midcerebellar glioma of childhood, *Arch. Neurol. Psychiat.,* 14, 192, 1925.
4. Boden, G.: Radiation myelitis of the brain stem, *J. Fac. Radiol.,* 2, 79, 1950.
5. Boden, G.: Radiation myelitis of the cervical spinal cord, *Brit. J. Radiol.,* 21, 464, 1948.
6. Bouchard, J.: In *The Biology and Treatment of Intracranial Tumors,* Fields, W. S. and Sharkey, P. C., eds., Springfield, Charles C Thomas, p. 371, 1962.
7. Bouchard, J. and Peirce, C. B.: Radiation therapy in the management of neoplasms of the central nervous system, with a special note in regard to children: Twenty years' experience, 1939–1958, *Amer. J. Roentgen.,* 84, 610, 1960.
8. Chao, J. H., Phillips, R., and Nickson, J. J.: Roentgen-ray therapy of cerebral metastases, *Cancer,* 7, 682, 1954.
9. Concannon, J. P., Kramer, S., and Berry, R.: The extent of intracranial gliomata at autopsy and its relationship to techniques used in radiation therapy of brain tumors, *Amer. J. Roentgen.,* 84, 99, 1960.
10. Correa, J. N. and Lampe, I.: The radiation treatment of pituitary adenomas, *J. Neurosurg.,* 19, 626, 1962.
11. Dugger, G. S., Stratford, J. G., and Bouchard, J.: Necrosis of brain following roentgen irradiation, *Amer. J. Roentgen.,* 72, 953, 1954.
12. Dyke, C. G. and Davidoff, L. M.: *Roentgen Treatment of Diseases of the Nervous System,* Philadelphia, Lea & Febiger, 1942.

13. Fraenkel, S. and German, W. J.: Glioblastoma multiforme-Review of 219 cases with regard to natural history, pathology, diagnostic methods, and treatment, *J. Neurosurg.*, 15, 489, 1958.

14. French, L. A.: In *The Biology and Treatment of Intracranial Tumors*, Fields, W. S. and Sharkey, P. C., eds., Springfield, Charles C Thomas, p. 412, 1962.

15. Kamerin, R. P., Potanos, J. N., and Pool, J. L.: An evaluation of the diagnosis and treatment of chordoma, *J. Neurol., Neurosurg., Psychiat.*, 27, 157, 1964.

16. Kernohan, J. W. and Uihlein, A.: *Sarcomas of the Brain*, Springfield, Charles C Thomas, pp. 25, 120, 154, 1962.

17. Kramer, S., McKissock, W., and Concannon, J. P.: Craniopharyngiomas. Treatment by combined surgery and radiation therapy, *J. Neurosurg.*, 18, 217, 1960.

18. Kricheff, I. I., Becker, M., Schneck, S. A., and Taveras, J. M.: Intracranial ependymomas: A study of survival in 65 cases treated by surgery and irradiation, *Amer. J. Roentgen.*, 91, 167, 1964.

19. Lampe, I.: In *Progress in Radiation Therapy*, New York, Grune & Stratton, p. 224, 1958.

20. Levy, L. F. and Elvidge, A. R.: Astrocytomas of the brain and spinal cord. A review of 176 cases, 1940–1949, *J. Neurosurg.*, 13, 413, 1956.

21. Lindgren, M.: On tolerance of brain tissue and sensitivity of brain tumors to irradiation, *Acta Radiol.*, supp. 170, 1958.

22. Lowenberg-Scharenberg, K. and Basset, R. C.: Amyloid degeneration of human brain following x-ray therapy, *J. Neuropath. Exp. Neurol.*, 9, 93, 1950.

23. McWhirter, R. and Dott, N. M.: *Practice in Radiotherapy*, St. Louis, C. V. Mosby Company, p. 330, 1955.

24. Paterson, E. and Farr, R. F.: Cerebellar medulloblastoma: Treatment by irradiation of whole central nervous system, *Acta Radiol.*, 39, 323, 1953.

25. Peirce, C. B. and Bouchard, J.: Role of radiation therapy in the control of malignant neoplasms of the brain and brain stem, *Radiology*, 55, 337, 1950.

26. Pennybacker, J. and Russell, D.: Necrosis of the brain due to radiation therapy. Clinical and pathological observations, *J. Neurol. and Psychiat.*, 11, 183, 1948.

27. Richmond, J. J.: Section of Radiology; Discussion on pituitary tumors, *Proc. Roy. Soc. Med.*, 51, 911, 1958.

28. Ringertz, N. and Reymond, A.: Ependymomas and choroid plexus papillomas, *J. Neuropath. Exp. Neurol.*, 8, 355, 1949.

29. Sheline, G. E., Boldrey, E. B., and Phillips, T. L.: Chromophobe adenomas of the pituitary gland, *Amer. J. Roentgen.*, 92, 160, 1964.

30. Sosman, M. C.: Roentgen therapy of pituitary adenomas, *J.A.M.A.*, 113, 1282, 1939.

31. Wachowski, T. J. and Cheneault, H.: Degenerative effects of large doses of roentgen rays on the human brain, *Radiology*, 45, 227, 1945.

32. Wood, E. H., Berne, A. S., and Taveras, J. M.: The value of radiation therapy in the management of intrinsic tumors of the spinal cord, *Radiology*, 63, 11, 1954.

33. Zimmerman, H. M., Netsky, M. G., and Davidoff, L. M.: *Atlas of Tumors of the Nervous System*, Philadelphia, Lea & Febiger, 1956.

5. Eye and Orbit

Treatment of Retinoblastoma with Radioactive Applicators

H. B. STALLARD

The tragedy of retinoblastoma is that this highly malignant neoplasm commonly affects both eyes of infants, and if unchecked will rapidly destroy sight and endanger life. It is also tragic that the failure of doctors and nurses in infant welfare clinics to realize the significance of a mother's observation "his (or her) eye is like a cat's eye when light enters it" may so delay appropriate treatment that there remains no hope of saving the less affected eye.

Until 1929 (and regrettably in some countries today) both eyes were excised, however slightly the second eye was affected by retinoblastoma. Until 1929 attempts to destroy retinoblastoma by the crude apparatus then used for irradiation so damaged the whole eye that excision became inevitable. In 1929 Foster Moore,[2] with whom I was privileged to work as Chief Assistant, was the first to achieve success in destroying retinoblastoma by radon seeds. The first patient, a boy, thus treated lived to 32 years of age and died of bladder carcinoma.

Clinical Features

Fortunately retinoblastoma is rare. Weller[11] states that it occurs once in 34,000 live births. It is probably bilateral in about 40 per cent when the disease arises sporadically; it may occur in 100 per cent of the affected progeny of stock so tainted. Retino-blastoma is sometimes present at birth, the neoplasm completely filling one eye and affecting part of the retina in the other. In most cases, the neoplasm is evident during the first year of life, very rarely does it appear between 11 and 13 years of age.

Retinoblastoma follows a dominant hereditary character, for it is common for 100 per cent of the families of one parent tainted by this disease to be so affected; it is known to be transmitted through three generations. When it occurs sporadically, the parents being unaffected, the risk of a second child becoming a victim to this neoplasm is less than 4 per cent.

Generally, when the "cat's eye reflex" is noted, more than half the retina is affected by the neoplasm and some or all of the remainder is detached.

If the other eye is affected, the neoplasm is generally less extensive. Retinoblastoma is commonly hemispherical, white, flocculent, and resembles cream cheese in appearance and consistence (Fig. 5-1). Loops of thin-walled blood vessels are evident. Sometimes up to six islands of retinoblastoma may be present. The neoplasm grows rapidly.

Pathology

Retinoblastoma arises from "rests" of primitive retinal epithelium; its cells resemble those of the embryonic nuclear layers of

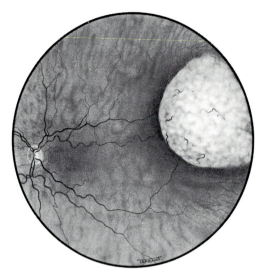

Fig. 5-1. Retinoblastoma.

the retina and are generally disposed in islands each around a central thin-walled blood vessel, and those at the periphery of each island undergo degeneration as they become remote from their blood supply (Fig. 5-2). Epithelial rosettes signify a partial differentiation and a slower rate of growth of the neoplastic cells. Flecks may break off from the neoplasm, being carried by the intraocular fluids and lodging between the ciliary processes and in the anterior crypts of the iris, filling partly the anterior chamber resemble a hypopyon. Complicated cataract

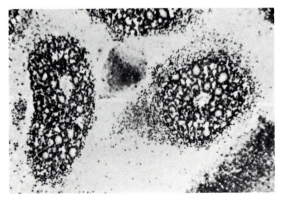

Fig. 5-2. Section through island of retinoblastoma. Central blood vessel zone of active tumor cells, peripheral degenerate cells and debris.

may occur. Calcification occurs in degenerate areas. The neoplasm infiltrates the optic disc and the optic nerve may be involved in a curious manner, islands of growth being separated by apparently healthy nerve in the earlier stages. Once retinoblastoma has reached the subarachnoid space the cells may be carried rapidly to the chiasma and floor of the skull. Retinoblastoma may penetrate the optic nerve sheaths without invading the optic nerve. Toxin from large masses of degenerate neoplastic cells may excite an iridocyclitis. The increased intraocular volume caused by the growth induces hydrophthalmia (infantile glaucoma), the eyeball enlarges and the sclera thins. Eventually the neoplasm bursts through the corneoscleral junction and rapidly forms a large fungating mass which spreads over the face.

Metastases are uncommon, but they occur in the skull, long bones, and spinal cord and also appear in the liver and regional lymph nodes. Death occurs from intracranial extension.

Very rarely spontaneous regression occurs. Such regression has coincided with a severe attack of scarlet fever.

Treatment

If the neoplasm has destroyed over half of the retina in one eye and the other eye is unaffected, excision with the full orbital length of the optic nerve is generally indicated. The optic nerve is divided at its entrance into the optic foramen. Serial sections of the nerve are cut and, if it has become infiltrated by the neoplasm, the orbit is irradiated by ^{60}Co beam, and chemotherapy with cyclophosphamide is given. When 12 mm or less of the retina is affected by retinoblastoma the prospect of destroying the neoplasm by irradiation, using ^{60}Co applicators, and conserving some useful vision is good, just over 96 per cent of the treatments are successful. The method of irradiation which seems to produce the best results to date is suturing a radioactive applicator to the sclera precisely over the base of the neoplasm. In the design of these applicators, much help was originally given by G. S. Stewart and later by Mr. G. Innes, physicists to the Radiotherapy Department of Saint Bartholomew's hospital. These applicators have been used since 1948, before which radon seeds were sutured to the sclera over the site of the neoplasm.

Radioactive ^{60}Co Applicators

The applicators are: 1) discs of 5, 7.5, 10, and 15 mm active diameter; 2) crescents of 13 × 6.5 mm, 13 × 9 mm, and 19 × 9.5 mm; 3) demidisks of 5 × 2.5 mm, 7.5 × 3.75 mm, and 15 × 10 mm. These conform with the average radius of curvature (11 mm) of an infant's sclera, have a platinum casing 0.5 mm thick and a central well 0.3 mm deep into which is placed ring-formed radioactive ^{60}Co for the small applicators and disk and rings in the larger. These arrangements of the ^{60}Co produce even isodose curves through what is commonly a hemispherical tumor arising from a concave surface (Fig. 5-3).

The loading of each applicator is such that a dose of 4,000 *r* is delivered to the summit

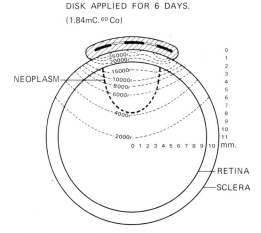

ISODOSE FOR 10mm. DIAMETER
DISK APPLIED FOR 6 DAYS.
(1.84mC. ^{60}Co)

Fig. 5-3. Diagram of a 10 mm active diameter 1.84 mc ^{60}Co disk to the sclera to show isodose curves.

of the neoplasm in 6 days. On an average, the height of the neoplasm was two-thirds the diameter of its base. It was histologically evident on cutting serial sections of irradiated eyes containing retinoblastoma that a dose of 3,500 *r* was lethal to the tumor cells.

Retinoblastoma is placed fourth in the order of tumor radiosensitivity. Moreover it is the only exception of Ellinger's law which states that the radiosensitivity of a neoplasm is relative to the radiosensitivity of the tissue from which it arises. The retina like the brain, from which it is an outgrowth, is radioinsensitive.

TECHNIQUE OF APPLICATION

The sclera over the site of the neoplasm is exposed by reflecting a flap of conjunctiva and Tenon's capsule, and if necessary, an extraocular muscle between mattress sutures is divided. The periphery of the neoplasm is marked by three of four katholysis punctures through the sclera, the string of hydrogen bubbles being seen by the ophthalmoscope. The diameter of the tumor base is measured by calipers. An applicator is chosen in which the radioactive element will overlap the periphery of the neoplasm by at least 1 mm.

The applicator is then placed in position, and through the hole in each lug the sclera is tattooed with a mapping pen dipped in gentian violet. At these two marked sites, sutures are first passed through the superficial layers of the sclera and then through the holes in the lugs and tied (Fig. 5-4). The transparent media of the eye allow a perfect ophthalmoscopic view of the regression of the neoplasm to a flat pigment-stippled scar when the neoplasm is 5 mm or less in diameter; when it is 6 to 12 mm in diameter there remains some inert dense white debris with sharp discrete edges (Fig. 5-5).

RESULTS

Statistics are mainly of value when a trend is shown. Success in saving the eye which

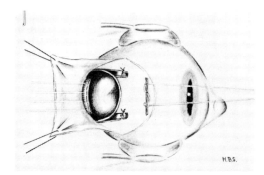

Fig. 5-4. [60]Co applicator sutured to the sclera over the marked site of retinoblastoma. (Stallard, courtesy of *Trans. Ophthal Soc. U. K.*)

has some useful vision in a little more than 96 per cent when one or two islands of retinoblastoma 12 mm or less in diameter is affected. Figure 5-6 shows the results of 162 patients (169 eyes) arranged in five groups according to Reese's classification of size, site, and number of islands of retinoblastoma, used at the 20th International Congress of Ophthalmology (Munich 1966).

Group I—An island or islands of retinoblastoma 6 mm in diameter or less.

Group II—Single or multiple islands, 6 to 15 mm in diameter.

Group III—Single tumor, 15 mm in diameter, most of it anterior to the equator.

Group IV—Multiple retinoblastoma islands. The sum total of affected retina well over 15 mm in diameter.

Group V—More than half the retina destroyed by retinoblastoma. Vitreous seedings.

In Group I the success rate was high, 100 per cent for ^{60}Co applicators. Three had previously failed with deep x-ray therapy and 8 with light coagulation. One in this group and 8 in Group II had a successfully irradiated remaining eye but died of recurrence from the orbit of the excised eye in which it seemed likely that the surgeon had not removed the full orbital length of the optic nerve. In Group II for a neoplastic mass or masses amounting to 15 mm in diameter it would seem preferable to treat by ^{60}Co beam and if there is any residue of doubtful activity to use a ^{60}Co applicator sutured to the sclera over the site of the neoplasm. It is probable that 10 of the failures in this group might have been prevented by using this technique instead of the reverse order (^{60}Co applicator first and ^{60}Co beam later). It is evident that the results of radiotherapy are

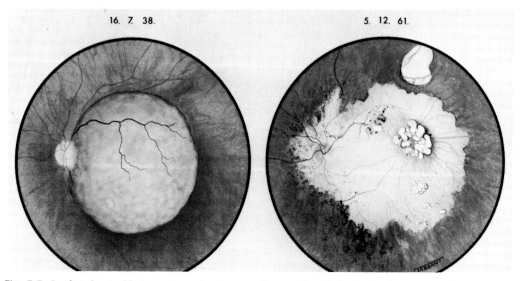

Fig. 5-5. Irradiated retinoblastoma, 8 mm in diameter, dense white debris. (Stallard, courtesy of *Trans. Ophthal Soc. U. K.*)

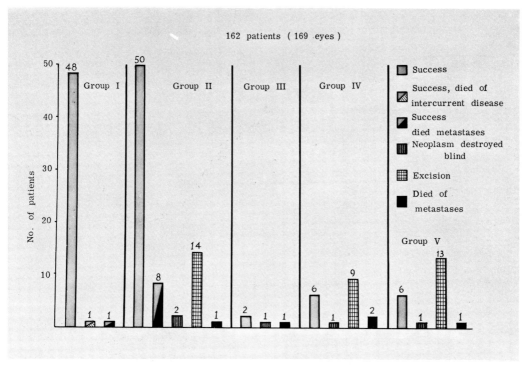

Fig. 5-6. Comparison of results of treatment of 162 children (169 eyes) in 5 groups.

poor in Groups III, IV and V. In 22 of these such serious complications as late vitreous hemorrhage, glaucoma and retinal detachment destroyed any remaining vision and necessitated excision of the eye. Serial sections through some of these showed no evidence of active retinoblastoma cells 5 years after treatment.

Table 5-1 shows the visual results of 110

Table 5-1

Vision	Groups				
	I	II	III	IV	V
6/6	29	14			
6/9	13	6	1		
6/12	1	2	1	2	
6/18	2	3			1
6/24	1	3			
6/36				2	3
6/60		7			
4/60-2/60	3	13		1	2

children classified in Reese's Groups I–V. Those with with vision 4/60–2/60 had neoplastic involvement of the macula in 13 and irradiation cataract, which ultimately required surgery, in 6 children. It is remarkable that a one-eyed child with the macula destroyed (Fig. 5-5) was able to train the nasal part of his retina to read J.4. without optical aid, to write well, and to draw accurately, to attend an ordinary school and eventually to become a secretary.

^{60}Co Beam Therapy and Chemotherapy

When a little less or more than a half of the retina is involved in the neoplasm and when there are more than three to six islands of the retinoblastoma and seedings are present in the vitreous ^{60}Co beam therapy is given with chemotherapy. Synergic therapy—chemotherapy and irradiation—is still in the experimental stages and at present the choice of any of the several agents under trial rests on somewhat uncertain evidence of their relative values.

In this series, 32 children have received cyclophosphamide; the majority received it orally, and a few by perfusion of the internal carotid artery. The eye is at a disadvantage in that perfusion of the ophthalmic artery to the exclusion of the internal carotid and its important collateral vessels is surgically impracticable.

To date, the less intense but more sustained effect of oral administration has been preferred. Probably in the future cyclophosphamide will be replaced by tritiated synkavit which increases the effective dose of irradiation by 40 to 60 per cent, or by some better and even less toxic alkylating agent.

Light Coagulation—Cryotherapy

For a small area, about 3 mm in diameter, of retinoblastoma behind the equator, light coagulation effectively destroys the neoplasm without serious intraocular damage if it is between the larger branches of the retinal vessels and not adjacent to either the macula or optic nerve.

Cryotherapy is effective for a neoplasm of like size between the equator and the ora serrata. For larger neoplasms, these forms of destruction by intense light and cold are often ineffective, may accelerate growth, induce endophthalmitis from the rapid breakdown of tumor cells and cause severe intraocular hemorrhage.

Prevention

Sterilization, abhorred by some religions and not publicly approved by most democratic politicians, is of course the only means at present of stopping the perpetuation of this binocular tragedy. It sometimes affects 100 per cent of the progeny of tainted stock into the third and probably more generations.

The Future

The future of radiotherapy depends on a better understanding of the interaction of ionizing irradiation with living matter, on new methods of selective irradiation of tumor cells, and on the discovery of means of increasing the radiosensitivity of these.

It is probable that the use of synergic therapeutic agents which either accelerate mitosis or render the dividing cell more vulnerable to irradiation and chemotherapy may improve considerably the results.

Ultimately, the biochemists may wrest from nature facts about organochemical and biophysical changes which effect a spontaneous cure, or it may be possible to induce specific cellular immunity to malignant cells.

To sum up—at present it seems that by use of ^{60}Co applicators there is a good chance of destroying a retinoblastoma which is 12 mm or less in diameter.[3-10] Cryotherapy applied to the surface of the sclera may be effective for a neoplasm 3 mm or less in diameter, situated at or anterior to the equator, and light coagulation is effective for those of like size in the posterior part of the eye and between the larger retinal vessels.[1] For the multiple islands of retinoblastoma scattered over the fundus, for masses larger than 12 mm in diameter and when seeding into the vitreous has occurred, ^{60}Co beam irradiation, in some cases with chemotherapy, is indicated.[10]

BIBLIOGRAPHY

1. Meyer-Schwickerath, G.: The preservation of vision by treatment of the intraocular tumors with light coagulation, *Arch. Ophthal.*, 66, 458, 1961.
2. Moore, R. F.: Glioma retinae, *Proc. Roy. Soc. Med.*, 26, 1036, 1933.
3. Stallard, H. B.: Radiotherapy of malignant intraocular neoplasms, *Brit. J. Ophthal.*, 32, 618, 1948.
4. Stallard, H. B.: The pathological study of retinoblastoma treated by radon seeds and

radium disks. The comparative value of radium and deep x-rays in the treatment of retinoblastoma, *Brit. J. Ophthal.*, 36, 245, and 3, 13, 1952.

5. Stallard, H. B.: Retinoblastoma treated by radon seeds and radioactive disks, *Ann. Roy. Coll. Surg.*, 16, 349, 1955.

6. Stallard, H. B.: *Eye Surgery*, 3rd ed. Wright & Sons, Ltd., Bristol, 1958.

7. Stallard, H. B.: Radio-active isotopes, *Acta XVIII Concil Ophthal.*, 2, 518, 1958.

8. Stallard, H. B.: Retinoblastoma treated by radioactive applicators, *Acta XVIII Concil Ophthal.*, 2, 1360, 1958.

9. Stallard, H. B.: The irradiation of retinoblastoma, *Trans. Ophthal. Soc., U.K.*, 80, 589, 1960.

10. Stallard, H. B.: The conservative treatment of retinoblastoma, *Trans. Ophthal. Soc., U.K.*, 82, 473, 1962.

11. Weller, C. V.: Inheritance of retinoblastoma and its relationship to practical eugenics, *Cancer Res.*, 1, 517, 1941.

Malignant Melanoma of the Choroid Treated by Radioactive Applicators

H. B. STALLARD

One of the saddest and grimmest decisions we have to make concerns the treatment of a malignant melanoma of the choroid in an only eye, or when the other eye is too diseased and disordered to be of any visual use. Does excision of an eye containing a malignant melanoma save life or prolong it?

Westerveld-Brandon and Zeeman,[4] believing that excision of the eye in a patient over 60 years of age does not affect the ultimate prognosis either in saving life or prolonging it, delay this radical surgery until either useful vision is lost or the pain of complicated glaucoma occurs.

As an alternative to the tragedy of radical surgery or the expectancy of inevitable defeat by taking no action, it seems justifiable to attempt conservation of the eye by radiotherapy.

It is unfortunate that some authorities have stated that malignant melanomata are radioresistant and that this comparative term should have acquired a meaning synonymous with that of unsuitability for irradiation. This attitude seems to be so widely spread that it is appropriate to present evidence that some malignant melanomata of the choroid are radiosensitive.

It is, I think, desirable to bring the source of irradiation as close as possible to the neoplasm and this is done by applicators which conform to the scleral curvature; these and the surgical technique of their fixation to the sclera over the base of the malignant melanoma are the same as used in the treatment for retinoblastoma. The diameter of the base of the neoplasm may be measured with fair accuracy by an ophthalmoscopic graticule. The height of the lenticular-shaped neoplasms before bursting through Bruch's membrane seems to average one third to one half of the diameter of the base.

The r dose is still empirical and under trial. It is at present impossible to assess precisely the r dose received throughout an intraocular neoplasm for, by no means are all these symmetrical in shape. Calculations from isodose curves suggest that, in the majority of the 107 patients in this series, the summit of the neoplasm probably received about

7,000 to 14,000 *r* and the base about 18,000 to 36,000 *r* in 10 to 14 days respectively (Table 5-2). In Table 5-2, the patient who received 108,000 *r* at the base and 42,000 *r* at the summit had three radioactive applications. The greater number of successes occurred in those who received 18,000 to 36,000 *r* at the base and 7,000 to 14,000 *r* at the summit. Success followed a single application to 66 patients and a second application to 17.

Clinical Facts

In this series of 107 patients, 22 had their only eye affected by a malignant melanoma; in 34 the other eye was almost blind, either from some gross pathological disturbance or amblyopia; 17 patients declined excision; and in the remainder it was considered justifiable to try irradiation because vision was still good, the neoplasm had not burst through Bruch's membrane and was between 4 to 9 mm in diameter. It is remarkable that among these 107 patients there was one with bilateral symmetrical malignant melanoma of the choroid at the age of 36; and two others had malignant melanoma of the iris and ciliary body in one eye and malignant melanoma of the choroid in the other.

Sex

The sex incidence in this series is 53 males, 54 females. Among the 83 patients in whom irradiation has been apparently successful to date, 45 are women and 38 men. Of the failures requiring excision of the eye, 11 were men and 7 women; of the 10 patients who died of malignant melanoma metastases 6 were men and 4 women.

MacRae[2] has stated that females tend to develop malignant melanoma earlier in life than males, but the death rate from metastases is only 31.4 per cent in females as compared with 57.6 per cent in males. Does some endocrine factor in the female check or delay the appearance of metastases, and does such a factor affect the radiosensitivity of the malignant melanoma cells?

Age

The age of onset is seldom determined with accuracy. Some relatively slow growing neoplasms may have been present and un-

Table 5-2

No. of Applications	r dose		Successes Group				Failures Group			
	Base	Summit	1	2	3	4	1	2	3	4
	18,000	7,000		6	1					
1	27,000	10,000		16	4	1			1	3
	36,000	14,000	1	8	18	11		2	4	3
	45,000	17,000		1						
2	54,000	20,000			4					
	63,000	24,000						1	3	2
	72,000	28,000			6	5			1	1
3	108,000	42,000						1		1
Total				82				23		

Approximate *r* dose

heeded by the patient a year or more before advice is sought. The age pattern in this series follows that of any large series of patients suffering from malignant melanoma, the larger number of patients are in the fifth and sixth decades of life, the youngest was 13 and the oldest 84. Does age have any effect on response to irradiation? In this series the neoplasm, 10 × 10 mm in a boy of 13 and 8 × 8 mm in a girl of 14, was more rapidly reduced to a flat plaque by irradiation than was the case in patients in the fifth and sixth decades of life. Also it seemed that irradiation was rapidly effective in 6 patients, 4 of whom are women between 32 and 41 years of age.

Site and Size of the Neoplasm

The larger diameter of the neoplasm, measured with an ophthalmoscope graticule before operation and checked by katholysis markings at operation, varied between 3 and 18 mm. In the 69 patients in whom irradiation has seemed successful to date, the diameter of the neoplasm in the majority was 7 to 8 mm. It is remarkable that successful destruction of the neoplasm was effected when the malignant melanoma was 18 mm in diameter in one patient, 16 mm in two, 14 mm in four, and 13.5 in one. The neoplasm in the 14 patients who failed to respond to irradiation measured between 4.5 and 14 mm in diameter.

The site of the neoplasm seemed to be of little consequence in achieving either success or failure by irradiation.

Results

Successes

Figure 5-7 shows the results of 107 patients arranged in four groups according to

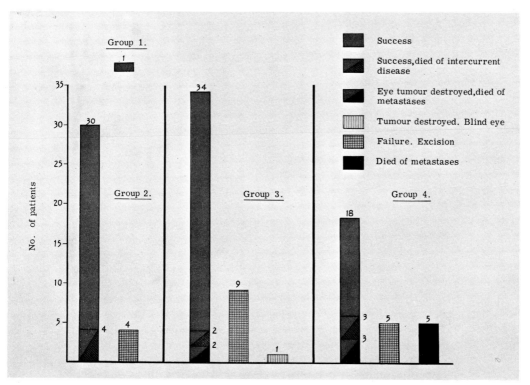

FIG. 5-7. Malignant melanoma of choroid in 107 patients treated by ^{60}Co applicators.

Reese's classification of size and site of a malignant melanoma of the choroid, used at the 20th Congress of Ophthalmology (Munich) 1966.

I—Malignant melanoma up to 3 mm in diameter.
II—Malignant melanoma between 3–7.5 mm in diameter.
III—Malignant melanoma over 7.5 mm, periphery visible.
IV—Malignant melanoma over 7.5 mm, periphery not visible.

To date 107 patients have been treated by the technique described above. Sixty-nine of these have been successful to date (Fig. 5-7) for at the site of the irradiated neoplasm there is a flat scar with pigment debris (Fig. 5-8, A and B), the adjacent fundus is stippled with white and brown dots, and the retinal vessels in the vicinity are attenuated. In 2 patients with large neoplasms, the one 13.5 mm and the other 14 mm in diameter, a cyst containing debris and much smaller than the size of the neoplasm remained at the site of irradiation, and in one of these the cyst collapsed. Nine patients with a successfully irradiated malignant melanoma of the choroid have died of causes other than malignant melanoma metastases; 3 of these died of carcinoma and 1 died in an air crash (Fig. 5-7).

One patient with a successfully irradiated malignant melanoma adjacent to the optic disc became blind from central retinal vein thrombosis, but was alive and without either recurrence or metastases 26 years after irradiation. Five patients whose choroidal malignant melanoma was destroyed by irradiation died from metastases 5 or more years after treatment. Histological examination of their irradiated eyes showed no evidence of neoplastic cells.

Failures

Among the failures the irradiated eye has been excised in 18 patients, 11 men and 7 women all of whom have survived to date, some as long as 13 years. Excision was done because it was doubtful whether the neoplasm was destroyed, the vision had become less than 6/60 and the retina detached in 5. In 3 of the patients a wait of 2 months after irradiation was probably inadequate in which to judge of effective recession of the neo-

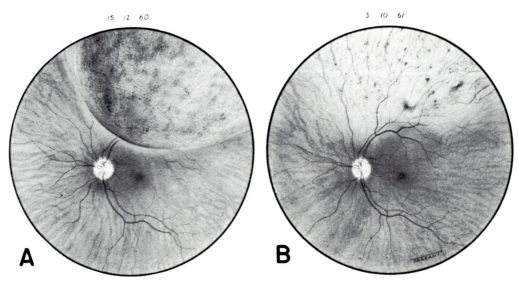

FIG. 5-8. A. Malignant melanoma of choroid upper temporal quadrant before irradiation of December 15, 1960. B. 10 months after irradiation, October 3, 1961. This appearance is the same in March, 1970.

plasm, and in the light of later experience it would seem proper to wait 4 to 6 months, provided, of course, that the neoplasm was not growing during this period of postirradiation observation.

Ten patients have died of metastases. In 2 it was evident that this was likely, for surgical exposure of the sclera over the base of the neoplasm showed that it had already extended through the sclera. One of these patients had vascular hypertension and had already suffered cerebral vascular episodes. She lived with useful vision despite occlusion of nasal retinal arteries for 2 years after irradiation. Another patient had a large neoplasm which occupied most of the lower half of the choroid. He lived 2 years after irradiation and had 6/36 vision. In a fourth the neoplasm was on the nasal side and measured 14 mm in diameter. After irradiation it

shrank to a flat scarred area with cystic debris and seemed to be destroyed. He had 6/18 vision until his death 1½ years after irradiation. A fifth patient had 6/6 vision until her end, and in a sixth the successfully irradiated neoplasm was at the macula.

Survival to Date

The only patient in Group I is alive and well 20 years after irradiation. Figures 5-9, 5-10, and 5-11 show the fates of those in Groups II, III, and IV up to 1965. It is, of course, obvious that insufficient time has elapsed to present a true picture of the results of irradiation of malignant melanomata. During a span of 20 to 25 years it is likely that some of those presented as successful results to date will have failed either through local recurrences or metastases. It is hoped

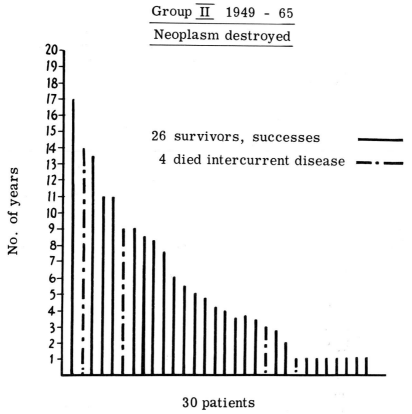

Group II 1949 - 65

Neoplasm destroyed

26 survivors, successes ⎯⎯⎯

4 died intercurrent disease ⎯•⎯

No. of years

30 patients

FIG. 5-9. Fate of 30 patients in Group II, 1949 to 1965.

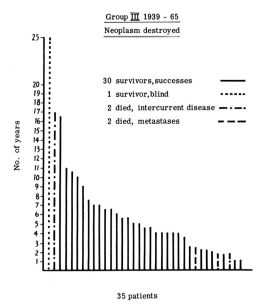

FIG. 5-10. Fate of 35 patients in Group III, 1939 to 1965.

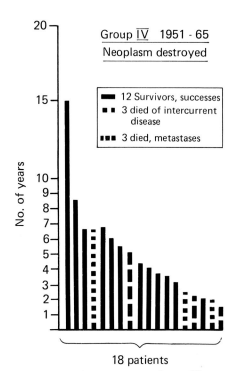

FIG. 5-11. Fate of 18 patients in Group IV, 1951 to 1965.

that by detecting melanogen precursors in 24-hour specimens of urine that in the future it will be possible to assess whether the metastases originated before treatment and lay dormant or occurred after it. Chisholm[1] has reported a patient who had metastases 36 years after excision of an eye for malignant melanoma.

Pathology

From examination of serial sections of the malignant melanomata which failed to respond to irradiation I had hoped to learn something about a pattern of histological facts common to all. It might be expected that the more malignant epitheloid and mixed-cell types would be more radiosensitive than the spindle-cell and fascicular varieties of malignant melanoma, but this has not been the case in this small series.[3]

The reticulin content, generally a good prognostic sign, was heavy in six and light in two. This heavy reticulin content in 40 per cent of these specimens may be significant or mere coincidence in this small series. Does reticulin in some way protect the cells of the neoplasm from irradiation?[3]

Complications

Perimacular exudates have appeared in 11 patients, in all of whom the irradiated growth has been successfully destroyed and is flat. The exudates appeared 5 months after irradiation in 1 case and cleared in 3 months, and in the other 10 were evident from 1 year and 7 months to 7½ years after treatment. In 6 female patients the exudates resembled circinate retinopathy. Minute petechial retinal hemorrhages were present in most of these cases. A few punctate retinal hemorrhages were evident in 4 patients, 1 occurred at 1 year and 10 months, 2 at 2 years and 9 months, and the fourth 3 years after irradiation.

Vitreous hemorrhages occurred in 2 patients. Table 5-3 shows the main clinical details about posterior cortical irradiation

Table 5-3. *Irradiation Cataract*

Patient	Age	Sex	Site of Opacity	Onset in Years	r dose Base	r dose Summit	Course
M.B.	36	♀	⊙	$7^9/_{12}$	27,000	10,000	Static
K.C.	52	♀	⊙	$7^9/_{12}$	27,000	10,000	Static
P.L.	33	♀	⊙	$2^6/_{12}$	36,000	14,000	Static
R.H.	38	♂	⊙	$3^7/_{12}$	36,000	14,000	Static
M.P.	13	♂	◓	3	36,000	14,000	Static
G.H.	35	♂	◒	$3^8/_{12}$	72,000	28,000	Static
M.E.	67	♀	◓	$3^7/_{12}$	36,000	14,000	Static
L.W.	50	♀	◓	$2^8/_{12}$	27,000	10,000	Static
T.M.	51	♂	⊛	$3^3/_{12}$	72,000	28,000 ⎫	Slowly
H.P.	49	♂	⊛	$2^{10}/_{12}$	27,000	10,000 ⎭	increasing

cataract which affected 10 patients in this series of 107.

Partial scleral sloughing occurred in 3 male patients with large neoplasms which required the application of a 15 mm active diameter radioactive disc. In one of these the defect was shelving 3 × 4 mm on the surface of the sclera and less in its deepest part. Its edges were freshened with a 6 mm trephine and the defect filled with a corneal graft. In another the defect was filled by a piece of fascia lata of double thickness. Complicated glaucoma occurred in 2 patients, one following central retinal vein thrombosis. Superficial punctate keratitis followed heavy irradiation in front of the equator of the eye in two patients.

Visual Results

Table 5-4 shows the visual results in the 69 patients successfully treated in Groups I–IV.

In 4 patients the irradiated neoplasm was at the macula and in 6 others it was adjacent to it so this accounts for a reduction of vision to between 6/24 and 1/60. In 11 patients perimacular exudates and small petechial hemorrhages lowered sight between 6/18 and 6/60. In 2 patients senile cataract caused deterioration of vision from 6/6 to 6/36 in one and to less than 6/60 in the other.

Table 5-4

Vision	Groups I	II	III	IV
6/6		6	5	
6/9		3	7	
6/12		2	1	
6/18		2	5	
6/24		1	1	
6/36		5	1	
6/60	1	5	1	1
<6/60		5	10	7
Total	1	29	31	8

Vision

Partial Choroidectomy

If irradiation fails to destroy completely a malignant melanoma in an only eye it is, I think, justifiable to reflect a lamellar scleral flap over the base of the neoplasm which is circumvallated by diathermy. A scissors incision is made in the diathermized zone and the tumor is removed.

Conclusion

To sum up, it seems evident that some malignant melanomata of the choroid are destroyed by a radioactive ^{60}Co applicator sutured to the sclera precisely over the base of the neoplasm; and that better results may be expected when the neoplasm is 8 mm or less in diameter and has not burst through Bruch's membrane. However, there have been successes when the neoplasm has been 13 to 18 mm in diameter. The prognosis seems to be better in the young and in women. Most of the successes followed a single application of radioactive ^{60}Co and a dose of about 14,000 r at the summit of the growth and 40,000 r at its base.

BIBLIOGRAPHY

1. Chisholm, J. F., Jr.: A long term follow-up on malignant melanomas of the choroid based on the Terry and Johns series, *Amer. J. Ophthal.,* 36, 61, 1953.
2. MacRae, A.: *Trans. Ophthal. Soc. U.K.,* 73, 3, 1953.
3. Stallard, H. B.: Malignant melanoma of the choroid treated with radioactive applicators, *Ann. Roy. Coll. Surg., Eng.,* 29, 170, 1961.
4. Westerveld-Brandon, E. R., and Zeeman, W. P.: *Ophthalmologica, Basel,* 134, 20, 1959.

External Irradiation of Retinoblastoma

NORAH duV. TAPLEY

Introduction

In 1933, Hayes Martin and A. B. Reese instituted the method of treating bilateral retinoblastoma with prolonged, high doses of external beam irradiation to the remaining eye following enucleation of the more extensively involved eye.[7] In 1971, at Columbia-Presbyterian Medical Center, the treatment of choice remains external beam irradiation at reduced doses. Adjuvant chemotherapy and photo-coagulation are used when indicated.

External beam therapy is preferred because cases suitable for the highly specialized techniques of radioactive surface applicators are rare. Retinoblastoma is multicentric in origin. Eighty per cent of patients with retinoblastoma seen at the Eye Institute have multiple tumors.[1] Stallard, limiting his treatment field to the lesion itself, noted the appearance of multiple islands of retinoblastoma in 26 of 43 patients following their initially successful treatment with gamma ray surface applicators.[16]

Retinoblastomas originate in the external or internal nuclear layers of the retina. The choroid is invaded in about 25 per cent of the cases and its rich blood supply permits rapid and extensive growth. Optic nerve invasion may occur and, if the eye is to be enucleated, the longest possible segment of the optic nerve should be removed.[12] Tumor extension into the periglobal soft tissues occurs via the emissary veins of the sclera, leading to orbital recurrence. Growth of the tumor is more often toward the vitreous cavity with the formation of exophytic tumor masses in the vitreous. Spread along the retina to the iris, ciliary body, and posterior surface of the cornea may occur.

Radiation Complications

Although there were only five deaths due to retinoblastoma in 68 cases of bilateral disease treated from 1938 to 1952, fair to good vision was limited to 18 patients when reviewed in 1960.[17] Treatment had been enucleation of one eye followed by 250 Kv irradiation through lateral and oblique nasal portals to the remaining eye. The tumor doses were calculated to be from 6,000 to 17,000 roentgens in 8 to 18 weeks.

Based upon descriptions of the ophthalmoscopic findings and pathology after enucleation, vision failed in approximately 40 per cent of the cases because of acute radiation damage. This was evidenced by hemorrhagic retinitis, hemorrhage into the vitreous, retinal detachment, and acute glaucoma. Similar destructive changes, as well as atrophy of the retina, phthisis bulbae, and cataract formation, occurred as late as two or three years after completion of treatment. Severe late radiation effects were seen in the skin, orbital tissues, and bone included in the treatment fields. The deformities produced often required plastic surgical repair.

Secondary tumors arising in the irradiated tissues are of concern when treating young children. In a series of 397 patients with retinoblastoma, 243 eligible for five year analysis, treated at the Columbia-Presbyterian Medical Center, the incidence of radiation induced tumors or tumors occurring in the irradiated areas was 11.6 per cent.[13] Of nine osteogenic sarcomas arising in the irradiated area, none occurred with a tumor dose of less than 8,000 r. The latent period for the entire group ranged from 4 to 30 years.

The tissues involved when irradiating retinoblastoma have an extremely wide range of radiosensitivity and degree of functional impairment from radiation injury. The skin, bony orbit, and surrounding muscle and connective tissues can tolerate high radiation doses. The sclera is a very radioresistant organ, best demonstrated by its tolerance to 30,000 to 40,000 rads delivered with the small surface applicators used by Stallard and Innes.[5] The retina is derived from the neural tube and would be expected to have the same resistance to radiation as the central nervous system which can tolerate doses up to 4,500 to 5,000 rads in 5 weeks. The doses of 6,000 to 17,000 rads given to the patients treated between 1938 and 1951 can damage the most resistant structures.

In a review of 30 patients with malignancies of the ethmoid sinuses and nasal cavity treated with irradiation at the M. D. Anderson Hospital, Shukovsky[14] described a technique that delivered high radiation doses to the retina and optic nerve while sparing the sensitive cornea and lens. Nine patients lost their sight in 12 eyes as a result of irradiation injury to the eye vasculature leading to macular and retinal degeneration in seven eyes, optic nerve atrophy in three eyes, and central retinal artery thrombosis in two eyes. The author concludes that radiation doses in excess of 6,800 rads in 6 weeks (NSD = 2,000 rets) will result in loss of sight within two to five years. The doses currently used in the treatment of retinoblastoma confined to the glove have NSD's of 1490 rets or 1570 rets.

With radiation doses to the eye above 6,000 rads, the risk of damage to the retinal vessels increases with subsequent vitreous hemorrhage and hemorrhagic retinitis. Below doses of 4,500 rads in 4 weeks this risk is practically eliminated. It is not known what amount of irradiation to the ciliary body will produce obliteration of Schlemm's canal with subsequent glaucoma. Acute glaucoma has occurred in patients with extensive eyelid tumors receiving 5,000 rads in 6 weeks when the radiation field included the globe.

Threshold radiation doses below which no damage or recoverable damage will occur in the more sensitive structures of the eye are becoming established through retrospective studies of clinical material and through animal studies. Merriam and Focht,[9] accurately reconstructing the treatment geometry and obtaining ionization chamber measurements of the radiation dose potentially delivered to the lens in a large series of patients receiving irradiation for malignant disease located in the head, demonstrated that a cataract could develop following a single lens dose of 200 rads. They noted that the incidence of cataracts increased and that more of them were progressive with increasing doses of irradiation. In 26 of 38 cases of retinoblastoma treated with heavy radiation doses, the lens was calculated to have received 900 rads or more. Cataracts, 59 per cent of which were progressive, were seen in two thirds of the patients. In retinoblastoma patients treated in recent years with lower doses of irradiation (4,250 roentgens in 5 weeks), the lens dose was calculated to be 130 to 250 rads.[10] The minimum cataractogenic dose was 400 roentgens fractionated over a period of 3 weeks to 3 months. A small, stationary posterior subcapsular opacity can result.[11]

Treatment Policies

The evidence of radiation damage has led to extensive modifications in radiation dosage plus the addition of chemotherapy and photo-coagulation when indicated. Control of disease and preservation of useful vision results from the particular characteristics of retinoblastoma.

1) In bilateral cases the rate of tumor growth is unequal in both eyes permitting salvage of useful vision in the remaining eye.

2) Retinoblastoma is sensitive to ionizing radiation and can be eradicated with doses of 3,500 rads in 3 weeks.

3) Extension of tumor beyond the cut end of the optic nerve or through the sclera into the periglobal tissue is infrequent.

Because of the young age of retinoblastoma patients, the signs and symptoms initially observed are almost invariably due to extensive tumor growth in at least one eye. The fortunate circumstance of a markedly slower rate of tumor growth in one eye compared with the other permits the currently high degree of success in achieving useful vision. Enucleation of the extensively involved eye is followed by irradiation of the entire retina of the remaining eye. Intra-arterial triethylene melamine and/or light coagulation are added dependent upon the extent of disease and the response to radiation therapy.

Staging

The method of treatment selected for retinoblastoma in the remaining eye is based upon the stage of the disease and its influence upon prognosis. The size, location, and number of tumors in the eye determine the stage[3] of disease (Table 5-5). The extent of retinal involvement and the location of the tumor are of particular significance with reference to visual acuity since tumors which have destroyed large areas of the retina will produce large defects in the visual field and tumors located in the macula will destroy the area of sharpest visual acuity. Lesions anteriorly located, from the equator to the ora serrata (Fig. 5-12), provide a greater possibility of a geographical miss in the effort to avoid radiating the lens. Results of lens extraction for radiation cataracts in this young

Table 5-5. *Staging for Method of Treatment and Prognosis*

Group I.   Very Favorable
    a. Solitary tumor, less than 4 dd in size, at or behind the equator.
    b. Multiple tumors, none over 4 dd in size, all at or behind the equator.

Group II. Favorable
    a. Solitary lesion, 4–10 dd in size, at or behind the equator.
    b. Multiple tumors, 4–10 dd in size, behind the equator.

Group III. Doubtful
    a. Any lesion anterior to the equator.
    b. Solitary tumors larger than 10 dd behind the equator.

Group IV. Unfavorable
    a. Multiple tumors, some larger than 10 dd.
    b. Any lesion extending anteriorly beyond the ora serrata.

Group V.   Very Unfavorable
    a. Massive tumors involving over half the retina.
    b. Vitreous seeding.

Courtesy: Hyman, Ellsworth, and Reese, *Acta Union Internat. contra le Cancer*, 20, 407, 1964.

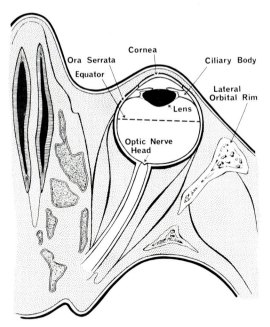

FIG. 5-12. Diagram of horizontal section through the eye and adjacent structures. The temporal portal is positioned so that the anterior margin of the radiation beam is anterior to the equator but posterior to the lens. Most of the retina will be included but the lens will be spared. It is important to remember that lesions anteriorly located, close to the ora serrata, can be incompletely irradiated in the effort to avoid the lens.

age group are far less satisfactory than for senile cataracts.

Adjuvant Treatment

CHEMOTHERAPY

With the recognition of a possible synergistic or additive effect resulting from the concomitant administration of an alkylating agent with irradiation,[6] the Retinoblastoma Study Group at Columbia-Presbyterian Medical Center in 1953 initiated the parenteral administration of triethylene melamine in all cases of bilateral retinoblastoma. A controlled study of irradiation alone randomized with irradiation plus i.m. *TEM* in favorable cases did not demonstrate that the addi-

tion of *TEM* improved the results.[17] In this favorable group, the tumor control rate was over 90 per cent.

All cases with massive and recurrent tumors received intra-arterial *TEM* (0.08 to 0.1 mgm/kg of body weight) 24 to 48 hours prior to the initiation of radiation therapy. Studies with labeled cylophosphamide have demonstrated that there is a greater concentration of the drug in the tumor when the intra-arterial rather than the intra-muscular route is used.[4] Since a controlled study has not been done, the effect of the addition of the chemical on tumor control has not been determined.

PHOTO-COAGULATION

Light coagulation permits destruction of tumor masses on the surface of the retina or obliteration of the nutrient vessels of the tumor.[2] It has been used effectively in the primary treatment of very small retinal tumors. It provides a particularly useful adjuvant treatment for those accessible retinoblastoma lesions which have responded unsatisfactorily to radiation treatment or which show signs of activity 2 to 6 months after irradiation has been completed. Since any regrowth of tumor requires retreatment of the entire retina if external beam radiation is used, the possibility of selectively treating a very limited area of the retina is highly desirable.

Technique of External Beam Irradiation

The optimal radiation technique requires accurate localization of the radiation beam to include all of the globe posterior to the lens. Doses of the order of 3,500 to 4,500 rads should be tumorocidal if retinoblastoma exhibits a radiosensitivity similar to neuroblastoma and medulloblastoma. These doses expose the vessels, lens, retina, and sclera to a negligible risk of damage. The orbital tissues, bony orbit, and radiated skin should show minimal later radiation changes.

In order to include as much of the retina as possible, the anterior margin of the beam should pass just posterior to the lens. This provides the best insurance against the appearance of second or multiple tumors following completion of therapy. Megavoltage radiation with a well-defined beam is desirable not because of the high depth dose but because of the limited side scatter and the decreased bone absorption. The late radiation sequelae with destruction of the normal orbital architecture observed in patients treated with high doses of 250 Kv radiation are not seen in patients treated with megavoltage radiation.

A single 4 × 3 cm "D" shaped temporal portal (Fig. 5-13) (the 4 cm diameter oriented in the caudad-cephalad direction), ensures that a 1.0 cm margin of irradiation surrounds the globe except anteriorly. The anterior edge of the beam is defined by a pointer and the portal is angled slightly posteriorly so that the beam will pass posterior to the lens. With every placement of the portal, the position of the cornea above the lateral orbital rim is determined (by exophthalmometry) to locate the anterior margin of the beam with reference to the posterior pole of the lens. A nasal portal (Fig. 5-14) is used only in those patients with lesions at or above the equator on the nasal aspect of the retina. It is 2.0 cm in diameter, with a rounded Lucite tip which fits snugly into the socket of the enucleated eye, and is so angled that the anterior margin of the beam does not pass through the lens.

Maintenance of optimum positioning of the eye with reference to the beam is essential if the meticulous efforts made to achieve this positioning are to be effective. Adequate

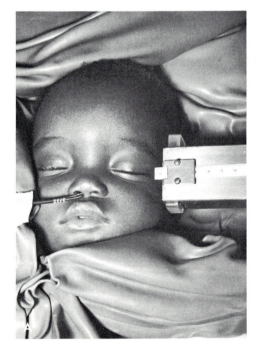
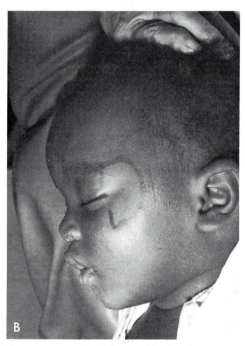

FIG. 5-13. Patient in treatment position. **A.** *Treatment Portal*. The anterior margin of the portal is placed just anterior to the lateral orbital rim. The portal is angled 3 degrees posteriorly to assist in avoiding the posterior pole of the lens. Lucite bolus 1 cm thick inserted at the end of the treatment cone places the 100 per cent dose at 2.5 cm depth. **B.** *Shape of Treatment Field*. The "D" shaped radiation beam, defined by a light beam, has been drawn on the skin. The field measures 4 × 3 cm.

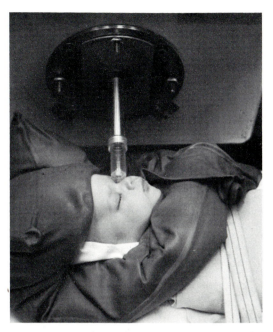

FIG. 5-14. Nasal portal in treatment position. The Lucite tip fits into the enucleated socket on the contralateral side. The angle of obliquity of the beam is selected to place the anterior margin of the beam immediately posterior to the lens. The nasal portal is used only for lesions located on the nasal aspect of the retina. Flexicast* is used around the head to maintain treatment position. *(Developed by Picker X-ray Corporation, White Plains, New York.)

immobilization can be achieved in the majority of patients. Mild sedation may be used for the particularly apprehensive patient at the onset of therapy but usually this can be discontinued. Repeated anesthesia, particularly in the child, is most undesirable and is unnecessary. It is of limited value unless the eye is sutured in position since the eye will wander in the anesthetized patient. If a child is well swaddled, providing him with a sense of security, if he is not frightened, and if there is a brightly colored moving object (such as a bird or butterfly mobile) suspended overhead for the fixation of his gaze, the treatment can be accomplished with the eye moving little, if at all.

Unilateral Disease

Approximately 70 per cent of all retinoblastoma patients have disease in one eye only, but this eye is usually extensively involved and immediate enucleation is indicated. With massive involvement of the retina, useful vision will not result even though the tumor is controlled and retinal hemorrhages and detachment are common. The eye frequently becomes painful and enucleation is necessary. The apparently uninvolved eye must be carefully examined under anesthesia and observation of this eye continued since tumor may develop in the second eye at a later date.

With enucleation an implant in the muscle funnel is cosmetically desirable but it must be remembered that this will make the early diagnosis of orbital recurrence difficult. If radiation therapy is necessary because of tumor invasion of the optic nerve or spread of tumor into the periglobal tissues, an implant of heavy metal such as gold will present a radiation dosimetry problem.

Occasionally a small tumor may be discovered when the siblings of retinoblastoma patients are routinely examined or when the tumor is located on the macula and strabismus results. Such cases may be treated by the Stallard technique of scleral ^{60}Co applicators but the incidence of new foci of tumor in the retina is as high as 60 per cent.[16] A sharply defined megavoltage beam using a single lateral field is a satisfactory way to treat these favorable cases because of limited side scatter and minimal irradiation to the lens of either eye.

Bilateral Disease

In groups I, II, and III, the dose to the retina is 3,500 rads in 3 weeks calculated at a depth 2.5 cm medial to the lateral orbit. The treatment is given in 9 fractions, 3 fractions per week, and can be equated with a tumor dose of 4,500 rads in 4 weeks or 5,000 rads in 5 weeks given in the conventional 5 times per week fractionation. These are comparable time-dose-fractionation schedules and range from an *NSD* of 1490 to 1570 rets. A nasal portal is added only if there is a nasal lesion located anteriorly in a position inaccessible to light coagulation. Group IIIa, where the lesion is anterior to the equator, will receive light coagulation at the completion of irradiation unless tumor regression is marked. When the patients of groups I, II, and III are examined under anesthesia at 4 to 6 weeks after irradiation, light coagulation will be used if tumor shrinkage and calcification are not marked. Light coagulation is repeated if the tumor still appears active or if there has been any evidence of regrowth at later examination. If regrowth of tumor occurs, a repeat course of irradiation is not worthwhile and enucleation is necessary.

In groups IV and V with large tumors extending to the ora serrata and with vitreous seeding, an anterior 4 cm portal is used to give 1,000 to 1,500 rads. With the 18-22 MeV betatron, the dose to the cornea is very low. A lateral portal is used to give the major portion of the treatment. The tumor dose to the posterior retina is 4,500 rads in 4 weeks administered in 3 fractions per week. Photocoagulation is used earlier in these groups to destroy the tumor blood supply unless there is satisfactory tumor regression at the conclusion of irradiation. Intra-arterial *TEM* is used in recurrent cases with extensive disease.

In those rare cases where the disease is limited in both eyes or where the parents refuse enucleation of one eye, treatment to both eyes is given using bilateral opposed fields. The tumor dose is 3,500 to 4,500 rads in 3 to 4 weeks calculated to the posterior retina. Slight depression of the temporal bone will be seen in later years.

Table 5-6 provides the most recently published results of treatment of bilateral retinoblastoma at the Columbia-Presbyterian Medical Center.[1] This is a review of 192 cases treated between 1960–1965 according to the policies described in the preceding pages. All patients have received radiation

Table 5-6. *Results of Treatment in Patients with Bilateral Retinoblastoma or with Orbital Disease Review of 1968*

Group	Number of Patients	Cure Rate (%)
I	20	95
II	32	87
III	24	67
IV	32	69
V	74	34
Orbital Disease	10	30

These patients were treated between 1960 and 1965, with a minimum follow-up of three years. In groups I and II the failures are frequently deaths due to distant metastases with the treated eye remaining under control and vision maintained. This series of patients was treated at Columbia-Presbyterian Medical Center in New York City.

therapy. Intra-arterial *TEM* has been administered only to patients designated unfavorable (groups IV and V) and to patients with orbital tumors. Many of these patients have been followed for more than five years and the minimum follow-up time for any patient is three years. Patients are listed as failures if dead of metastases, even though useful vision had been preserved in the remaining eye up to the time of death. Currently, irradiation without chemotherapy is used in all cases staged as groups I, II, and III. In favorable cases with single or multiple small tumors posteriorly located the tumor control rate is 85 per cent. These patients would be expected to have excellent vision. In groups III and IV, which may include very large tumors and anteriorly located tumors, the control rates are 67 and 69 per cent but visual acuity may be decreased because of the amount of retina involved by these lesions. In group V with massive tumors, tumor control is achieved in over 30 per cent of the cases.

Residual Disease

Residual disease refers to the presence of tumor cells in the cut end of the optic nerve or in the periglobal tissues. After exenteration treatment consists of intra-arterial *TEM* and irradiation of the orbit. A 3 cm anterior field and a 3 × 4 cm or 4 × 5 cm temporal field are used to deliver a tumor dose of 4,500 rads in 4 weeks to a point 2.5 cm deep to the eyelid surface and in from the lateral skin surface. Cases of orbital recurrence are treated in the same way if intracranial involvement or distant metastases are not demonstrated.

In 74 patients (Table 5-6) with residual tumor treated at Columbia-Presbyterian Medical Center prior to 1965, the salvage rate is 20 per cent.

Intracranial Disease and Distant Metastases

Retinoblastoma which has extended beyond the orbit may involve the central nervous system or the skeleton and other organs or both.[8] Radiation therapy in palliative doses is used to shrink tumor masses and to alleviate symptoms. In the treatment of distant metastases triple therapy with Actinomycin D., Chlorambucil, and Methotrexate has been tried with limited response in some patients.[15] The current regimen used at the Columbia-Presbyterian Medical Center utilizes Cytoxan 300 mgm/m^2 and Vincristine 2.0 mgm/m^2 administered intravenously once a week. One patient with a diseased bone marrow has had a normal marrow for 8 months and has developed no signs of toxicity.

If the central nervous system has been invaded, radiation therapy is administered to the base of the brain or the whole head. With tumor cells in the cerebrospinal fluid, irradiation of the spinal cord meninges can be considered. The dose will vary with the age of the patient from 3,500 rads in 4 weeks to 5,000 rads in 6 weeks. If signs and symptoms persist or recur after a course of radiation therapy, intrathecal Methotrexate is used, 0.5 mgm/kg every 2 days, until there has been a response. The intrathecal injection is repeated until there is clearing of the cells from the spinal fluid and symptoms have

improved. Up to eight or nine doses may be required.

The results of treatment of both central nervous system spread of tumor and distant metastases have been universally disappointing with no reported cures in proven disease beyond the orbit. Alleviation of symptoms and clearing of signs can be achieved for relatively short periods. With repeated courses of chemotherapy survival may be prolonged up to 18 months or 2 years.

BIBLIOGRAPHY

1. Ellsworth, R.: The practical management of retinoblastoma. *Trans. Amer. Ophthal. Soc.*, 67, 462, 1969.
2. Hopping, W., and Meyer-Schwickerath, G.: In *Ocular and Adnexal Tumors*, Boniuk, M., Ed., St. Louis, C. V. Mosby, p. 192, 1964.
3. Hyman, G. A., Ellsworth, R. M., and Reese, A. B.: The results of combination therapy of retinoblastoma. A nine year study of 250 cases. *Acta Union Inter. Contre le Cancer*, 20, 407, 1964.
4. Hyman, G. A., Feind, C. R., Spalter, H. F., and Finkel, M. P.: Chemotherapy of retinoblastoma, *Cancer*, 17, 992, 1964.
5. Innes, G. S.: In *Ocular and Adnexal Tumors*, Boniuk, M., Ed., St. Louis, C. V. Mosby, p. 142, 1964.
6. Kupfer, C.: Retinoblastoma treated with intravenous nitrogen mustard. *Amer. J. Ophthal.*, 36, 1721, 1953.
7. Martin, H. E., and Reese, A. B.: Treatment of retinal gliomas by the fractionated or divided dose principle of roentgen radiation: A preliminary report, *Arch. Ophthal.*, 16, 733, 1936.
8. Merriam, G. R., Jr.: Retinoblastoma. Analysis of seventeen autopsies, *Arch. Ophthal.*, 36, 71, 1946.
9. Merriam, G. R., Jr., and Focht, E. F.: A clinical study of radiation cataracts and the relationship to dose, *Amer. J. Roentgen.*, 77, 759, 1957.
10. Merriam, G. R., Jr., and Focht, E. F.: Radiation dose to the lens in treatment of tumors of the eye and adjacent structures, *Radiology*, 71, 357, 1958.

11. Merriam, G. R., Jr., and Focht, E. F.: A clinical and experimental study of the effect of single and divided doses of radiation on cataract production, *Trans. Amer. Ophthal. Soc.,* 60, 35, 1962.
12. Reese, A. B.: *Tumors of the Eye,* 2nd ed., New York, Hoeber Medical Division, Harper & Row, 1963.
13. Sagerman, R. H., Cassady, Jr., Tretter, P., and Ellsworth, R. M.: Radiation induced neoplasia following external beam therapy for children with retinoblastoma. *Amer. J. Roentgen.,* 105, 529, 1969.
14. Shukovsky, L. J., and Fletcher, G. H.: Retinal and optic nerve complications in a high dose technique of ethmoid sinus and nasal cavity irradiation, *Radiology,* 104, 629, 1972.
15. Sitarz, A. L., Heyn, R., Murphy, M. L., Origenes, M. L., Jr., and Severo, N.: Triple drug therapy with Actinomycin D, Chlorambucil, and Methotrexate in metastatic solid tumors in children, *Cancer Chemother.,* 45, 45, 1965.
16. Stallard, H. B.: Multiple islands of retinoblastoma, *Brit. J. Ophthal.,* 39, 241, 1955.
17. Tapley, N. duV.: In *Ocular and Adnexal Tumors,* Boniuk, M., Ed., St. Louis, C. V. Mosby, p. 158, 1964.

Radiotherapy in Eye Disease

MANUEL LEDERMAN

In Collaboration with

C. H. JONES and R. F. MOULD

Effects and Complications of Occular Irradiation

In advocating radiotherapy for the treatment of malignant tumors of the eye one must ever be conscious of the possible risks of damage to the normal as well as the pathological tissues of the eye. If the risks of radiation damage to the eye are considerable, then a case can be made out for removing the eye rather than embarking upon radiotherapy. If, however, the risks can be shown to be acceptable, then it is far better for a patient to retain a radiation damaged eye with impaired vision than suffer its removal.

The following is a summary of the clinical effects of radiation on the eye, orbit, and related structures and the postradiation complications which may ensue:

The Lids and Bulbar Conjunctivae

These react to radiation in the same way as similar tissue elsewhere, *e.g.,* the cheek.

Erythema followed by dry or moist desquamation is seen in the cutaneous aspects of the lids, while their conjunctival surface becomes red, inflamed and edematous and covered by fibrinous exudate. The following sequelae may occur:

1) Lid deformity either entropion or ectropion, associated with atrophy of the tarsal plate.

2) Epiphora following obstruction of the lacrimal punctum.

3) Epilation of the lashes.

4) Keratinization of the palpebral conjunctivae.

5) Atrophy and telangiectasis of the skin or conjunctivae.

Lid complications are seen only when the lids are directly irradiated for tumors affecting them or when radioactive sources are placed in contact with the epibulbar tissues.

The most troublesome complication is keratinization of the mucous membrane of the lid; for some obscure reason obstruction of the lacrimal papillae is rarely followed by permanent epiphora.

The use of megavoltage x-rays or an electron beam helps reduce the reactions arising in the lids and anterior ocular segment.

The Cornea

Structurally the cornea is avascular, and exposure to radiation cannot therefore produce those vascular disturbances which indicate the inflammatory changes termed "radiation reaction." However, the following corneal changes may occur after direct irradiation without special protection:

1) Pericorneal injection. The earliest sign of corneal irritation is seen at the limbus when the normally invisible pericorneal plexus of blood vessels becomes visible.

2) Corneal edema. Following pericorneal injection and congestion of the superficial conjunctival vessels, edema of the superficial layers of the cornea may occur and this is usually associated with diminution of the corneal reflex.

3) Keratitis. The edema may be followed by superficial or deep keratitis, depending on the amount of irradiation given, and corneal ulceration may ultimately ensue.

All of these complications are rare and can usually be avoided if superadded sepsis and trauma are eliminated.

Severe corneal ulceration and necrosis occur when excessive irradiation has been given, but although the normal cornea is tolerant of radiation in therapeutic doses if sepsis and trauma can be avoided, changes in the cornea are most likely to occur in the following circumstances:

1) After contact radiation of the cornea and limbus using low voltage x-rays or gamma-ray emitting isotopes.

2) As part of an exposure keratitis associated with proptosis and chemosis.

3) Secondary to lid changes in particular deformities and keratinization. The risks are greatest when these changes occur in the upper rather than the lower lid.

4) A filamentary keratitis or corneal xerosis may occur following irradiation of the lacrimal apparatus (see "Lacrimal Apparatus" below).

The Intraocular Structures

The iris and ciliary body are extremely resistant to irradiation. An iridocyclitis can be provoked by irradiation and atrophy of a segment of the iris may occur. Secondary glaucoma is exceptional after external irradiation, but may occur after contact application of radioactive materials directly to the limbus.

Of the intraocular structures, the lens is undoubtedly the most sensitive to radiation damage. In our view radiation cataract can be expected after a single dose of 600 r x-rays, or 1,500 r x- or gamma-rays fractionated over 1 month. Merriam and Focht,[5] from an analysis of 100 cases of radiation cataract, suggest that 200 r single dose; 400 r fractionated over 3 weeks or 1 month; or 550 r fractionated over 3 months can produce a cataract.

The retina is not sensitive to radiation and can tolerate large doses. Stallard records the appearance of perimacular exudates and minute petechial hemorrhages in some of his choroidal melanoma cases treated by cobalt discs.

Retinal or vitreous hemorrhage following radiotherapy should be a most exceptional complication and is nearly always due to damage to the retinal vasculature by excessive radiation. Proper control of dosage should eliminate this complication, although its spontaneous occurrence in an irradiated eye independently from causes other than radiotherapy is a rare possibility.

Lacrimal Apparatus

Irradiation of the lacrimal glands may result in an alteration both of the quantity and quality of the tears. This may result in a troublesome, dry, irritable eye, filamentary keratitis or, rarely, xerosis of xerophthalmia.

The Orbit

The normal tissues forming the orbit should not be damaged by irradiation but if already invaded by neoplasm, an osteitis with sequestration of bone may follow.

Deformities of the nasal or orbital bones and radiation-induced soft tissue sarcomata following radiation treatment of retinoblastomas have been reported by Reese.[7] These complications are entirely avoidable and are a direct consequence of the excessive dosage employed in the treatment of these children.

Socket Contraction

Atrophy of the socket is an important complication following radiation treatment and can be completely avoided by insisting on the patient wearing a glass or plastic shell from the very commencement of the treatment. These shells are tolerated very well even in the presence of a reaction and maintain the socket cavity so that a satisfactory prosthesis can be fitted later. When this precaution is neglected the socket may atrophy completely and it becomes impossible for an artificial eye to be used.

Purpose of Radiotherapy

Although it is customary to associate radiotherapy chiefly with the treatment of malignant disease, it has in practice a far wider usefulness. It can be applied in the treatment of the following:

1) Malignant tumors.
2) Benign tumors.
3) Inflammatory processes.
4) Disorders of function and miscellaneous conditions.

The purpose of radiotherapy will clearly differ from group to group.

Malignant Tumors

Radiation may be used in the treatment of malignant disease for curative purposes as an alternative to surgery; as a palliative agent; or as an ancillary agent to surgery in the form of pre- or postoperative treatment.

Benign Tumors

Benign tumors may require radiation treatment for cosmetic reasons or when the tumor is known to be predisposed to malignant change. The commonest benign tumors encountered by the radiotherapist are: angiomata, papillomata, keloids, and hyperkeratoses.

Although cure is the object, treatment must be given so as to avoid reactions and precautions taken to spare the patient cosmetically unwelcome sequelae such as cutaneous atrophy, depigmentation and telangiectasis, any of which may detract from the patient's appearance far more than the original tumor.

Inflammatory and Miscellaneous Conditions

Whereas the purpose of treating a tumor is to eradicate dangerous or unsightly tissue with which the body cannot deal, in the case of inflammatory processes or manifestations of unknown or doubtful etiology, the purpose is to assist gently a natural but ineffective process of healing and defense or to restore an organ to normal function.

Nonmalignant Diseases

The main aims of radiotherapy in the treatment of non-neoplastic diseases are:[2,4]

1) To relieve symptoms, particularly pain.
2) To promote healing by assisting: the resolution of inflammatory processes; the absorption of a hematoma or hemorrhage; the epithelization of an ulcerated surface; the organization and removal of granulation tissue.
3) To affect blood vessels: to reduce vascular engorgement and congestion accompanying inflammation; to obliterate or reduce

in size newly-formed vessels invading the cornea.

4) To reduce intraocular tension.

5) To restore function, *e.g.,* an attempt may be made to improve vision where the cornea is the seat of an opacity, dystrophy, or degenerative process.

The precise mode of action whereby radiation can favorably influence an inflammatory process is not known, but there are three possible mechanisms which may separately or together play some part in producing a favorable response:

1) A possible stimulation of antibodies.

2) An effect on the cellular elements of the exudate, particularly the leukocytes.

3) An effect upon the blood vasculature, especially the capillaries.

Indications and Selection of Cases for Radiotherapy

Radiotherapy should be considered in the following circumstances:

1) Where there is no response to recognized therapeutic methods within a reasonable time (one to two months).

2) Where no accepted method of treatment exists and there is reason to believe that radiotherapy may be of help.

3) For chronic progressive lesions accompanied by symptoms which radiotherapy may relieve without necessarily arresting the course of the disease.

4) For chronic relapsing lesions wherein periods of apparent improvement or healing are followed by repeated recurrence.

The following lesions are of the most importance and interest to the radiotherapist:

1) Mooren's ulcer.

2) Corneal vascularization.

3) Virus infections.

4) Vernal catarrh.

5) Pterygium.

In cases of Mooren's ulcer, radiotherapy is the only method of treatment known to be of value and forms the sole exception to the general rule that radiotherapy should be used only as a last resort in the treatment of non-neoplastic processes. The early use of radiotherapy in Mooren's ulceration gives the patient his only chance of cure.

The judicious use of radiation for corneal vascularization associated with keratoplasty can go far to help obtain a satisfactory functional result.

In virus infections and superficial punctate keratitis, radiotherapy is only occasionally curative but it can nevertheless effect a certain degree of symptomatic relief not to be obtained by other remedies.

A note of warning must be sounded in relation to the radiation treatment of vernal catarrh because in recent years there has been an enthusiastic revival of the beta-ray treatment of this disease, particularly in the United States. Although the sufferers are usually children and the disease is seasonal and ultimately self-limiting, high doses of beta radiation have been recommended as a method of eradicating the characteristic "cobblestone" papules that appear on the tarsal conjunctiva. To any radiotherapist conversant with the effects of beta radiation, the consequences of high doses applied to the mucosal surfaces of the lids could easily be predicted—namely, replacement fibrosis with atrophy and scarring of the palpebral conjunctival mucous membrane, so leaving the patient in a worse state than if no treatment had been given at all.

We have not practiced the beta-ray treatment of vernal catarrh using high doses; after tentative trials, when it became obvious that the papules could not be eradicated with small safe doses, beta radiation was abandoned and replaced by small doses of x-radiation. The aim of treatment has been either preventive by irradiating the eye one month before the expected onset of the seasonal attack, or to reduce the acuteness of the florid attack and so relieve symptoms until the seasonal respite occurs. Beta radiation is indicated only in the rare cases in which the bulbar conjunctiva is affected.

Most of the cases of pterygium seen by

us have been in patients coming from tropical and subtropical countries. The customary treatment is surgical removal, but the recurrence rate is by no means negligible. Radiotherapy should be reserved for the recurrent case, when excision and immediate postoperative radiation is the treatment of choice.

Factors Influencing Choice of Treatment

1) Low voltage therapy is always used for an acute or extensive lesion. The radiation is applied directly to the closed eye so that the whole of the outer eye and the eyeball are irradiated.

2) Beta radiation is reserved for chronic lesions, chiefly affecting the cornea. Beta radiation is not used in the presence of: A) Severe lid spasm, because any difficulty in inserting the beta-ray shell into the conjunctival sac may result in injury to the cornea; B) a contracted pupil, marked ciliary congestion, or other evidence of uveal irritation or inflammation, for fear of producing an exacerbation of symptoms.

3) Quite frequently x- and beta radiation may be used in combination. Thus, for an acute keratoconjunctivitis or a deep keratitis associated with an iridocyclitis, treatment can be begun with low voltage therapy and when the eye is reasonably comfortable and quiet beta rays can be applied to any persistent localized corneal lesion.

The purpose of the x-ray treatment is to assist the resolution of an acute inflammatory process affecting a part or the whole of the eye. The radiation is therefore applied in very small doses to the affected organ in its entirety on the assumption that the favorable effect of the radiation mediates through the blood supply, all of which should therefore be exposed to the radiation. In the case of beta radiation the 'anti-inflammatory effect' of radiation is not usually sought, but the purpose is to heal a corneal ulcer or obliterate unwanted blood vessels invading the cornea; to achieve this, the strictly localized

effects of high doses of beta radiation are ideal.

There are two standard techniques for treating non-neoplastic lesions of the eye:

X-Radiation: Bulbar or ''Whole Eye'' Technique (Fig. 5-15)

This is so-called because no attempt is made to protect or shield any part of the globe or lids, treatment being given through a 3 cm diameter circular field placed directly over the closed lids. Any low voltage apparatus can be used, *i.e.*, 45 Kv, 60 Kv, or 100 Kv, and the x-ray dosage employed in the treatment of an infection of the outer eye is always minimal, namely 10 *r*. It would appear that, if radiotherapy is going to help, this minute dose is perfectly adequate and there is no advantage in giving higher doses, *i.e.*, 100 *r*, as the results are the same. The smaller

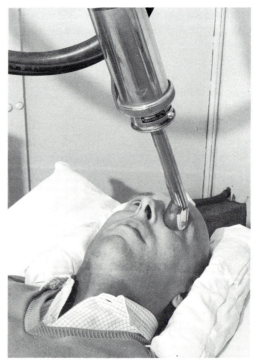

FIG. 5-15. Bulbar or whole eye technique. (Courtesy: Henry Kimpton, 1962, Duke-Elder, S., *System of Ophthalmology*, Vol. VII.)

dose is absolutely safe, does not provoke exacerbations, requires no manipulation of the lids, and can be continued for more than a month with safety. In the event of a relapse a course of low dosage treatment can be repeated two or three times a year.

X-ray treatment is given once or twice a week for 4 weeks, and the treatment can be stopped if the eye is comfortable and quiet at the end of this period. If the eye is white and corneal ulceration persists, beta radiation can be used; if no improvement is observed, radiation treatment should be abandoned completely.

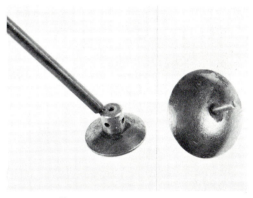

FIG. 5-17. ^{90}Sr beta-ray applicator for direct contact application to globe. (Courtesy: Henry Kimpton, 1962, Duke-Elder, S., *System of Ophthalmology*, Vol. VII.)

Beta Radiation

This forms the mainstay of the treatment of corneal lesions. Two types of apparatus are available: one in which a silver loaded radioactive strontium shell is inserted into the conjunctival sac so that the radioactive surface comes into contact with the cornea and the surface of the globe. A range of such shells is available (Fig. 5-16). The second type consists of a radioactive strontium disc with a screw cap into which a rod fits and so allows the shell to be held in place on the cornea (Fig. 5-17). The dosage required depends on the lesion being treated; for Mooren's ulcer single doses of 500 *r* to 1,000 *r* are given at weekly intervals for 4 weeks. For corneal ulceration of dendritic or rosacea origin a dose of 600 *r* is given weekly

for 4 weeks. For corneal vascularization after grafting treatment may be begun as soon after operation as possible, and 600 *r* given twice weekly for 2 weeks. The dose and the type of applicator used depend on the state of the eye when seen, and the extent, age, and depth of the vessels to be treated; the treatment is the same whether the graft be lamellar or fullthickness. For preoperative corneal irradiation, the same dosage of 600 *r* is given, and operation is advised 10 to 14 days after the last treatment. Preoperative radiation can be followed by postoperative treatment in the more heavily vascularized cases. It is advisable not to exceed 5,000 *r* beta rays from a radioactive strontium source as a cataract may occur if larger doses are given.

For vernal catarrh, the patient should ideally be treated 1 month before the expected onset of the attack. A lead shield is placed in the conjunctival sac to protect the eye and the size of field used will depend on whether one or both lids are to be treated; in each case the fornices must be irradiated and the field extended to the bony orbital margin. A dose of 100 *r* is given once weekly for 4 weeks. If the patient is seen during an attack, the same treatment should be given.

It is advisable when treating any bilateral

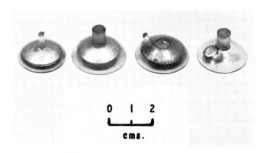

FIG. 5-16. ^{90}Sr beta-ray applicators for insertion into conjunctival sac. (Courtesy: Henry Kimpton, 1962, Duke-Elder, S., *System of Ophthalmology*, Vol. VII.)

eye condition to begin by treating the worse eye first and to treat both eyes only if no exacerbation of symptoms has occurred. For bulbar lesions, beta radiation should be used in order to avoid lens damage, a dose of 600 *r* being given once a week for 4 weeks.

Recurrent pterygium can be treated by beta radiation, a single dose of 2,400 *r* being given at or as soon after the operation as possible.

The doses used in beta-ray therapy bear little relation to the doses employed in low voltage x-ray therapy, for the following reasons:

1) The marked difference in penetration of the two types of radiation. Under the treatment conditions described, the dose of x-radiation incident on the anterior surface of the lids falls to half its intensity at a depth of 1.1 cm. In contrast, the dose of strontium beta radiation incident on the surface of the cornea falls to half its intensity at a depth of 1.3 mm.

2) The volumes of tissue irradiated by each method vary greatly. With low voltage therapy the lids and the eye itself are irradiated, whereas with beta radiation only tissues in close contact with the source are irradiated. There is an inverse relationship between the volume of tissue irradiated and the quantity of radiation given, *i.e.*, the larger the volume the smaller the dose that can be safely given.

Any attempt to imitate the high single doses used in beta-ray therapy with low voltage x-ray therapy would almost certainly be harmful to the inflamed eye. Conversely, to imitate the small doses used in x-ray therapy with a beta-ray source would be pointless and ineffective.

Benign Tumors

The nonmalignant tumors of the outer eye for which radiotherapy may be indicated are hemangiomata, papillomata, hyperkeratoses, and keloids. The need for and value of radiotherapy varies for each lesion.

Hemangiomata

While most hemangiomata occurring in infancy disappear spontaneously without treatment, there are nevertheless certain medical indications for active treatment:

1) The presence of hemorrhage or infection.

2) The situation of the hemangioma in a region exposed to irritation, *i.e.*, the scalp, lips, or the napkin area, or where its presence predisposes to infection of a neighboring organ, *e.g.*, infection may take place in the conjunctival sac where the lids are closed by an angioma.

In addition to these medical indications there is one further important indication: namely, the child has to be treated for the mother's sake. Many of the sufferers are first-born baby girls, and it is unreasonable to expect the mother to accept verbal reassurance that all will be well, particularly during the period when the angioma apparently increases in size with the growth of the infant. Radiotherapy is the treatment of choice for lid angiomata. There is no indication in these cases for excisional surgery, which can only result in unnecessary mutilation and should be avoided at all costs. Radiotherapy offers a simple and safe remedy, the judicious use of which can arrest the growth of the angioma and restore confidence and peace of mind to the parents.

It is our general policy: not to give large doses of irradiation to these tumors; to avoid radon seed or other implantation methods; to repeat treatment only once or twice with the longest possible intervals between treatments.

Gamma radiation is to be preferred but, because of the greater ease in protecting the eye, contact therapy (60 Kv) is usually employed for lid angiomata, and the child is anesthetized for the treatment in most cases. A single dose of 250 to 400 *r* is given, depending on the age of the patient and the thickness of the lesion, the lower dose never being exceeded in a newborn infant. The treatment is not repeated as long as regression continues, but if the improvement is not maintained a further treatment is given after 6 months, and very rarely a third treatment after 18 months. The child should be treated as soon after birth as possible and the parents warned that complete regression may not be obtained for from 3 to 5 years or even until adolescence is attained.

Papillomata

The treatment of choice for either the true papilloma, or the infective wart is surgical removal. Such warts may be single or multiple and may affect the lids or the conjunctiva. It is rarely possible to cause true papillomata to disappear by using small safe doses of radiation, and an adequately effective dose of radiation must inevitably be accompanied by a local tissue reaction. Such reactions occurring in regions away from the eye may be reasonably free from risk, but this is not so in the case of the eyelid or conjunctiva.

In spite of the desire to use surgery whenever possible, there are nevertheless some indications for radiotherapy in the treatment of papillomata:

1) For a solitary sessile papilloma affecting more than one third of the lid margin, when surgery would involve plastic repair of the lid.

2) Multiple papillomata of the lids and conjunctiva.

3) Repeated recurrences after surgery.

X-ray therapy is used for a solitary papilloma, a single dose of 2,000 *r* at 60 Kv being given. Infective or multiple papillomata in children are treated by x-ray therapy to the lid lesions, a single dose of 600 *r* being given, and beta-ray therapy to any bulbar conjunctival lesions, a single dose of 1,000 *r* being given. These doses can be repeated at the end of 3 months if necessary.

Keratoses

The senile type of keratosis is usually a precancerous lesion and when affecting the lid margin is best treated by radiotherapy, because a wider area of tissue can be irradiated than can be excised. The need to irradiate or excise a wide area of tissue surrounding the lesion is due to the presumed 'instability' of the tissues from which the keratosis arises. The technique is the same as for solitary papilloma.

Keloids

These may form in a scar on the lid, or may occur after injury or postoperatively. If the keloid is of the raised, red, fleshy type, radiotherapy should be undertaken but if the lesion is of the hard, white, linear variety, excision associated with pre- or postoperative irradiation is indicated. A single dose of 600 *r* x-rays at 60 Kv to 100 Kv can be given and repeated at 6-week intervals on two further occasions.

Epibulbar Tumors

The term epibulbar is used here to include the lids, conjunctival sac, limbus, and cornea. Lid tumors have been dealt with elsewhere and reference will be made here to the remaining sites.

Malignant Melanoma

We believe the epibulbar malignant melanomata are radiosensitive tumors of slow growth, their radiosensitivity depending on:

THE SITE OF THE TUMOR

There appears to be a gradient of sensitivity varying from the limbus across the fornix and lid onto the cutaneous surface of the latter. As a rule the nearer the tumor lies to the limbus the more radiosensitive it is and the better the prognosis with radiotherapy. Tumors of the cutaneous aspect of the lid are the least radiosensitive and often resemble the other skin melanomata in their response.

MACROSCOPIC APPEARANCES

As a rule the more pronounced the tumor formation the more satisfactory is the response. The degree of pigmentation is also important since a moderately pigmented patch near the limbus can be made to disappear but a densely pigmented lesion affecting the fornices and lids may show only limited change after radiotherapy, although it may persist in an apparently harmless fashion for some time. Pigment associated with tumor formation need not necessarily form an integral part of the tumor and after radiation treatment it may disappear leaving a residuum, which disappears later. The radiotherapist's aim is not to depigment the eye but to bring about the disappearance of the tumor, and persistent pigmentation if unaccompanied by tumor is not as a rule an indication for any active measures.

HISTOLOGY

The malignant melanomata encountered may fall into the following groups:

A) Malignant melanomata arising from a pre-existing mole.

B) Malignant melanomata arising spontaneously or *de novo*.

C) Cancerous or precancerous melanosis.

It is difficult to assess accurately the true radiosensitivity of malignant melanomata arising from a pre-existing mole since wide surgical excision is usually performed as a preliminary in all the lid cases, but for the limbal and conjunctival melanomata the surgery employed is often in the nature of a biopsy and any satisfactory result must be attributed mainly to the postoperative radiotherapy.

The malignant melanomata arising *de novo* without any apparent relationship to a pre-existing mole or cancerous melanosis have nearly all proved highly radiosensitive.

The view originally advanced by Reese[7] that precancerous melanosis is radiosensitive and that cancerous melanosis is radioresistant has not been supported by experience, and has in fact now been retracted by Reese.[8] Both lesions are radiosensitive, the latter more than the former as would be expected since a frankly cancerous cell is usually more radiosensitive the more it deviates in character from its precancerous or normal precursor cell.

Radiotherapy can be recommended in the following circumstances:

Where malignant change can be demonstrated histologically.

Where a lesion presents "aggressive" features clinically suggestive of malignancy, even though the biopsy is negative.

Any circumstances where sight is threatened.

Treatment Policy

When the tumor primarily affects the lid, particularly its cutaneous surface, or where the bulk of a cancerous melanosis is related to the lid, surgery is preferable.

The treatment of a small limbal melanoma must embrace the cornea and much of the bulbar conjunctiva, while for cancerous melanosis the whole conjunctival sac and both lids require attention.

Technique of Radiation Treatment

Local excision of any exuberant tumor masses is an essential preliminary to radiation treatment. By this means biopsy material is obtained and a reasonably flat surface provided for the application of radioactive materials or appliances. Where there is little elevation of the tumor a biopsy alone should be undertaken and the tumor left undisturbed.

To date three technical methods of treatment have been employed:

1) Beta radiation.
2) Gamma radiation.
3) X-radiation.

The precise method used depends on the site, extent, and nature of the tumor.

Beta radiation is used when the tumor is confined to the limbus or bulbar conjunctiva and is histologically a malignant melanoma unrelated to cancerous melanosis. Radioactive strontium is used as the source of beta radiation and standard applicators are available. For special cases applicators can be individually constructed.[9] Single doses of the order of 2,000 r to 2,500 r are given at weekly intervals for a period of 4 to 6 weeks, the total dose given varying between 9,000 r and 12,000 r. It is possible to construct these applicators so that both bulbar and palpebral conjunctivae can be simultaneously irradiated; but it is difficult to irradiate the fornices and lid margins by this method, hence its restricted use.

When the whole conjunctival sac requires irradiation as is necessary in most cases of cancerous melanosis, or when any other malignant melanotic process affects the conjunctiva of the globe, lids and particularly the fornices, some form of gamma radiation is indicated. After trying various techniques, the method at present employed is the implantation of radon seeds into the lids, which are previously sewn together and used as a holder for the seeds. Each seed has a single black thread at one end and contains 1 mc of radon. The dose given is 3,000 to 4,000 r in 3 to 4 days. In a previous radon technique the seeds were sewn directly onto the bulbar conjunctiva, but this has now been abandoned. This gamma-ray technique inevitably means that much of the eye as well as the lids, conjunctiva and cornea has to be irradiated and the resulting risks of ocular damage have to be accepted.

Low or medium voltage x-ray therapy has been used postoperatively for melanomata and for some of the localized tumors arising from the lid conjunctiva. A protective shield is inserted into the conjunctival sac and a surface dose of 5,000 to 6,000 r is given in 2 to 3 weeks.

High voltage x-ray therapy and telecurietherapy are generally reserved for the treatment of socket or orbital recurrences follow-ing surgery, or for lymph node metastases, and have therefore found little indication in this series of epibulbar tumors.

The treatment of precancerous melanosis at a stage before malignant changes can be histologically demonstrated is exceptional and presents special problems since it is difficult to justify the use of gamma-ray techniques which carry a high rate of radiation cataract for a condition which is not definitely malignant. In these circumstances beta radiation can be used for limited lesions of the limbus or the bulbar conjunctiva, but if there is very extensive pigmentation involving the lids and fornices then gamma-ray techniques have to be employed in exactly the same manner as for cancerous melanosis.

Complications

While beta radiation is almost free of serious complications and reactions are rarely severe, in the development of gamma-ray techniques unpleasant reactions and complications have been encountered and permanent ocular damage can occur. The most serious damage was found in the more resistant cases where repeated treatments or very high doses were given. If serious ocular damage is to be avoided, it is wise not to repeat radiation treatments. If the first radical attempt at radiation treatment fails, surgery is indicated since further radiation will give no renewed promise of success and defeats its main purpose, which is to save vision as well as to control the disease.

Epithelioma

Epithelioma of the limbus and bulbar conjunctiva is rare. It may occur spontaneously, or be preceded by a papilloma, or be associated with xeroderma pigmentosa. It is a radiosensitive tumor and the eye should only be sacrificed if it is blind. In all other cases the treatment of choice is local excision and radiotherapy, and when beta radiation is employed the chance of retaining good vision is excellent. Using a radioactive strontium source, 8,000 *to* 10,000 *r* beta radiation is given, 2,000 *r* weekly for 4 to 6 weeks. In an elderly patient who already has a lens opacity low voltage x-radiation, 45 to 60 Kv, can be employed, the dosage being 5,000 *r* in 21 days.

Regional lymph node metastases are most unusual and these areas require no special treatment in the absence of frank deposits, for which block dissection should be performed.

Bowen's Disease

This condition, also known as intraepithelial or *in situ* carcinoma, is rare and differs from an epithelioma in being noninvasive for a long time and often multifocal in origin. It is generally a disease of elderly men and occurs at the limbus and may involve the cornea and adjacent bulbar conjunctiva. The lesion is slow growing and may ultimately take on invasive characters and when this happens lymph node metastases may exceptionally occur.

The treatment of choice if the eye has useful vision is local excision of the tumor and beta radiation. Unlike the epithelioma, where the irradiation can be limited to the obviously diseased area, in the case of Bowen's disease the whole of the cornea and bulbar conjunctiva should be treated irrespective of the precise site and extent of the lesion.

This disease with its curious multicentricity is the epithelial counterpart of cancerous melanosis, behaving locally in a similar fashion but not possessing its metastatic tendencies.

The dosage employed should be as for epithelioma; in the event of recurrence or in the presence of an extensive lesion a gamma-ray technique (see cancerous melanosis) is justified since it is better for the patient to accept the risk of a cataract rather than forfeit a useful eye.

Orbital Tumors

Primary malignant tumors of the orbit are rare, the tumors being seen by the radiotherapist tending to be those regarded by the surgeon as unsuitable for operation.

The commonest tumors seen are the sarcomas of lymphoid tissue, the lacrimal gland tumors that cannot be totally removed, and finally the group of rare, rapidly growing sarcomata affecting children and young adults.

Sarcomas of Lymphoid Tissue

These are the commonest primary orbital tumors; they are generally radiosensitive and radiotherapy is the treatment of choice.

The sarcomas affecting the orbit and head and neck region can be divided into two main groups:

1) Those tumors which are truly of extranodal origin.

2) Those tumors that start primarily as generalized lymphnodal sarcomas, but where secondary manifestations may occur in the region of the eye, orbit, or head and neck.

These secondary manifestations may so dominate the clinical picture that the patient is forced to consult the ophthalmologist or otolaryngologist. In these cases evidence of generalization may be found on careful clinical search at the time the patient is first seen, or such generalization may occur some time later, usually within a year of onset.

The true extranodal primary lesions have an excellent prognosis as far as survival is concerned. Any lymph node enlargement associated with these lesions tends to occur in the immediate lymph drainage territory, *i.e.,* the cervical lymph node region alone, and are amenable to therapy.

This type of lymphoma is not necessarily highly radiosensitive and not infrequently doses approximating those required for the eradication of squamous cancers are required. It would seem that the less dramatic the response and the higher the dose required, the less virulent is the disease and the better the prognosis.

By contrast the highly radiosensitive lymphomas are those which are primarily of lymphnodal origin and are already generalized or will generalize at an early stage.

There is one common feature of the natural history of the tumors of lymphoid tissue of the head and neck region, namely there seems to be a critical period 10 to 20 years after treatment when the disease may recur, not necessarily locally but in some other extranodal site and thereafter generalization may take place.

Although in many cases the ultimate fate of the patient may seem to depend on a capricious providence, the following clinical pictures are of prognostic importance in an adverse sense:

1) Bilateral tumors.

2) The presence of an associated enlargement of some part or all of Waldeyer's ring.

3) Lymph node involvement outside the cervical lymph node regions.

4) The presence of skin deposits or deposits in the larynx.

5) An associated blood abnormality.

Lacrimal Gland Tumors

These are rare, the commonest being the adenocarcinoma, followed by the "mixed" tumor which appears to be analogous both clinically and histologically to the mixed tumor affecting the major and minor salivary glands of the buccal cavity and pharynx. These tumors have a common epithelial origin but because of their cellular pleomorphism the histological appearances may range from the benign adenoma to the adenocarcinoma, and a tumor may sometimes be completely anaplastic. These wide variations in morphology are reflected in their clinical behavior, which may vary from apparent simplicity to high malignancy with widespread metastases.

With the so-called mixed tumors of the lacrimal gland, the tempo of recurrence and spread is usually more rapid than with the corresponding tumors of the main salivary glands and the prognosis is therefore much graver. Reese[7] attributes the high proportion of recurrences and the high mortality from lacrimal gland tumors to the difficulties of surgical approach and removal, the tendency to invasion of the capsule, and particularly the early invasion of bone.

It is a common observation that mixed salivary gland tumors are relatively radioresistent. Radiotherapy can help reduce the recurrence rate within the limitation and fallacies imposed by the 5-year period of observation, and should therefore be routinely used in association with surgery. Radiotherapy is, of course, the method of choice for the inoperable, recurrent or highly malignant tumors and the lymphosarcomata.

Malignant mesodermal tumors, connective tissue, nerve tissue or bone, are best treated surgically, but there is one rare tumor, the rhabdomyosarcoma, that should be treated by radiation. It is generally agreed that these tumors are exceedingly rare, occur in children, and are highly lethal. There is evidence to show that these tumors remain localized to the orbit and are highly radiosensitive, but unfortunately are only exceptionally radiocurable, since prompt recurrence is nearly always the rule.

The rhabdomyosarcoma or, when typical cells cannot be demonstrated, the embryonal sarcoma, should always be treated by radiotherapy in the first instance. If, as is often the case, recurrence takes place exenteration can be performed. There is no evidence to show that immediate exenteration has any advantage for cases behaving in this fashion, and as these tumors appear to remain localized, any delay in operation because of the preliminary attempt at cure by radiotherapy is not apparently associated with an increased risk of metastases.

Radiation Treatment Techniques

The technique of treating an orbital tumor depends mainly on whether the eye is present and whether the tumor is primary or secondary. If a sound eye is present, no effort should be spared in its protection, whereas if the eye has been removed, techniques can be much simplified. With a primary orbital tumor treatment can be localized to the orbit with consequent limitation in general and local reactions; whereas in secondary invasion of the orbit, particularly from the paranasal sinuses, the need to irradiate the orbit complicates to a great extent the technique of treatment of the primary site, and imposes an extra and often severe burden upon the patient.

Technique of Treating a Primary Orbital Tumor with the Sound Eye Present

The factors influencing the technique are as follows:

GENERAL FACTORS

A) The age and general condition of the patient do not matter greatly provided the patient is neither too senile nor too young and fractious to cooperate in treatment. Occasionally young children may require sedation at the beginning of treatment but as a rule they quickly learn to cooperate.

B) The state of the eye and orbit. It may be stated quite categorically that it should never be necessary to remove a sound eye prior to radiation treatment since under proper treatment conditions the risks of serious postradiation ocular damage are small.

C) The purpose of treatment. Radiation treatment is usually employed as a curative measure, but palliative treatment alone may be indicated in the following circumstances:

a) Where the local disease is very widespread and associated with active destruction of the orbital or facial bones.

b) Where there are bilateral or fixed secondary lymph node metastases.

c) Where distant metastases are present.

d) Cases recurrent after previous treatment.

The purpose of treatment in these cases is to relieve symptoms, particularly pain and proptosis, so as to enable the patient to die without having to undergo an operation on the eye or to endure the miseries of uncontrolled proptosis.

LOCAL FACTORS

Of the local factors affecting the technique, the chief ones are the nature and extent of the tumor and its situation within the orbit.

A) The histology of a tumor is of vital importance in the selection of treatment technique, since the variations in radiosensitivity which exist among normal tissues are also found among the malignant tumors to which these tissues may give rise. A biopsy is therefore an essential preliminary to radiation treatment and should be performed routinely in all cases. There are few risks associated with this procedure provided adequate treatment is instituted promptly after the diagnosis of malignancy is established.

B) The situation of the tumor within the orbit. When dealing with these tumors the technique of treatment must be such that the whole orbit is irradiated, with the following two exceptions:

a) The pre- or postoperative treatment of a lacrimal gland tumor, when treatment can be localized to the region of the lacrimal fossa, care being taken to irradiate a wide zone of the surrounding bone because of the known tendency of these tumors to produce widespread bone invasion.

b) In the treatment of glioma of the optic nerve or other rare tumors affecting the posterior part of the orbital cavity, the radiation can be largely concentrated in the retro-ocular segment of the orbit, the posterior part of the globe related to the nerve head alone being included in the field of radiation.

In all other cases where the whole orbit has to be irradiated the inclusion of the eye to a greater or lesser extent is unavoidable unless one is prepared to run the risk of leaving some part of the tumor inadequately irradiated.

External radiation is the method of choice for treating an orbital sarcoma. In all cases the attempt must always be made to protect as much of the eye as is consistent with adequate irradiation of the tumor. Two fields (anterior and lateral) are usually necessary for treating a primary orbital tumor. Occasionally a single anterior field can be employed for some of the very sensitive sarcomas of lymphoid tissue. The field sizes used are 4×4 cm minimum, the exact size depending on the extent of the tumor. The lateral field is always placed behind the lateral bony orbital margin so that the anterior edge of the beam is placed behind the plane of the lens and at the same time the irradiation of the lacrimal gland and fornix is avoided. The lateral field is of great importance since its use helps compensate the deficiencies in the radiation field within the orbit caused by the shielding of the eye against anterior direct irradiation. This field is also of great value in treating the retro-ocular segment of the orbit (which is the larger segment) without having specially to protect the eye. It is important to ensure that the lateral field is placed suitably to avoid irradiation of the contralateral eye. The dosages recommended are as follows:

1) Sarcomas of the lymphoid tissue: 3,000 to 4,000 rads in 3 to 4 weeks.

2) All other tumors, including the pre- and postoperative radiation of lacrimal gland tumors: 6,000 rads in 6 to 8 weeks.

Bilateral Orbital Tumors

The rare bilateral tumors of the orbit are usually radiosensitive sarcomas of lymphoid tissue, and the technique of treatment should be the same for both orbits. It is wise to begin treatment on the most seriously affected side and allow a few days' interval before beginning treatment to the second tumor.

Protective Devices Available

Various devices are available for protecting the eye so as to minimize the risks of radiation damage without jeopardizing the patient's chance of cure. The reduction of dose to the anterior segment of the eye can be effected by the absorption of the primary beam with specially shaped lead or tungsten inserts. There are two devices of this kind:

A) Direct protection when a lead shield is placed directly over the part of the eye to be protected.

B) Indirect protection, an absorbing material such as lead or tungsten interposed in the beam of radiation so as to absorb that part of the beam which would otherwise reach the eye.

Direct ocular protection however can only be employed for treating orbital tumors with kilovoltage x-radiation.

The indirect method consists of the insertion in the beam of radiation of an absorbing material (2 mm lead in the case of 250 Kv radiation; 7 cm lead in the case of 2 Mev and ^{60}Co radiation; 5 to 6 cm tungsten for 4 Mev radiation) so that the part of the eye to be protected is brought within the shadow produced by the interposed absorbing material.

It is of value when:

1) The eye is severely proptosed and the lids cannot be closed.

2) The eye is abnormally displaced or immobile owing to an associated ophthalmoplegia.

3) Gross chemosis and edema of the lids are present.

4) There is neoplastic invasion of the conjunctival sac.

5) When megavoltage radiation is employed.

This method can be termed the "shadow method" and can only be used with radiation fields delineated by a light beam. The region of total protection produced on the front surface of the eye in this method will depend on the geometrical size of the radiation source, the position, shape, and size of the absorbing insert, and the amount of scattered radiation reaching the shielded area from the open field. For high energy sources with small focal spots (of diameter about 0.5 cm) such as 2 Mev Van de Graaff generators and 4 to 6 Mev linear accelerators, a very sharp cut-off can be obtained and the amount of radiation reaching tissues deep to the cornea can be as little as 2 per cent of the incidence dose in the open field.

The technical details of a device providing

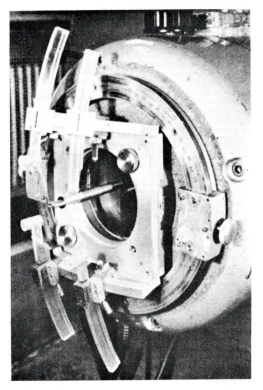

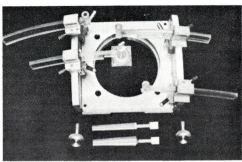

FIG. 5-18. Ocular protective devices for 2 Mev.

indirect shielding, designed and used at the Royal Marsden Hospital are described by Lederman[3] (Fig. 5-18). The inserted lead or tungsten cut-out is held in the primary beam in such a way that it always lies along some ray through the target, whatever its position in the field. For 2 Mev x-rays about 7 cm lead are necessary to reduce the primary intensity to 1 per cent. The inserts are tapered so as to make allowance for the approximate size of the focal spot.

^{60}Co gamma ray beams are less easily shaped due to the larger source diameter which casts a penumbra around the protected area. Although the magnitude of the penumbra can be reduced by placing the shield close to the patient, this distance is best kept at a minimum of 15 cm to avoid secondary electron contamination of the treatment beam.

Treatment Techniques

In practice the value of such protective measures as those described above depends upon the immobilization of the patient and the use of accurate beam direction techniques. To this end it is often advantageous to use a perspex or plaster cast of the patient as this permits accurate delineation of the treatment volume, fixation of the patient during treatment, and it can act as a reliable aid to beam direction (Fig. 5-19). Furthermore, it enables any protective devices to be applied accurately with minimal inconvenience to patient and radiotherapist.

2 MEV X-RAYS

High energy beams of x-rays produced in Van de Graaff generators have the following advantages:

1) The small focal spot (5 mm diameter) casts only a small radiation penumbra both at the edges of the treatment field and around any protective device inserted directly in the beam.

2) The amount of side scattered radiation

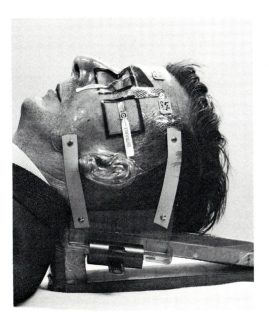

FIG. 5-19. Treatment case and head rest.

beneath the shaded area of the cornea and underlying intraocular tissues is small.

3) The maximum dose occurs at 5 mm below the skin surface, permitting higher total exposure doses to be given without severe skin reaction ensuing.

4) There is no differential absorption of the radiation by bone as compared with tissue.

In order to maintain maximum skin sparing, after treatment planning has been completed the field areas on the cast are cut out. A typical treatment plan is shown in Figure 5-20.

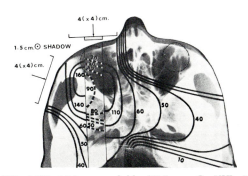

FIG. 5-20. 2 Mev open fields. (11.7 mm, Cu *HVL*, 67 cm, *FSD*).

^{60}Co GAMMA RAYS

It is usual for cobalt teletherapy units to have sources of about 1 to 2 cm diameter. The penumbra associated with such sources

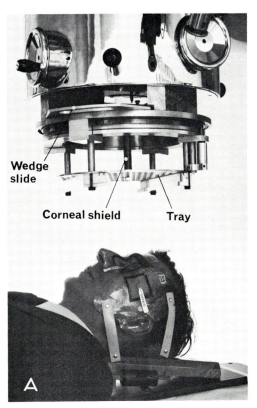

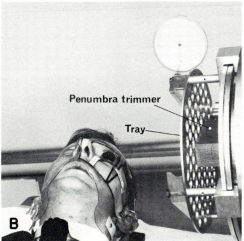

FIG. 5-21. Treatment for the orbit by ^{60}Co radiation. **A,** Direct wedge field. **B,** Lateral field.

prohibits complete protection of the cornea by lead inserts. The diffuseness of the treatment beam, however, can be conveniently trimmed with a lead block supported on a tray on the head of the unit as shown in Figure 5-21. The dural tray consists of a grid of $\frac{3}{4}$ inch holes into which various inserts can be attached. It is strong enough to support several lead cutouts and penumbra trimming blocks. Each insert is securely clamped to the tray by a brass screw passing through an anchored perspex washer. Figure 5-22 illustrates a typical treatment technique, the penumbra trimmer reducing the dose to the contralateral eye from the lateral field.

4 TO 6 MEV LINEAR ACCELERATORS

Paterson[6] has described a wedge pair treatment which is illustrated in Figure 5-23. The patient looks directly into the radiation beam through a 1.5 cm diameter cylindrical hole through the built-up wax. Although, due to the surface effect, the dose to the anterior segment of the eye is insufficient to cause an unpleasant radiation reaction, it is not claimed that cataract formation is always avoided.

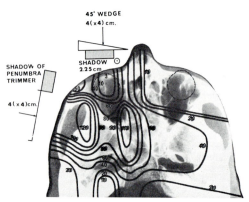

FIG. 5-22. ^{60}Co wedged and open fields (2,500 Curie 70 cm, *SSD*).

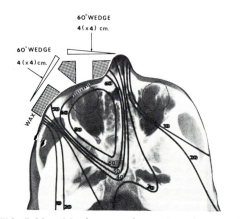

FIG. 5-23. 4 Mev linear accelerator (Manchester technique). After: Paterson, *Treatment of Malignant Disease by Radiotherapy*, Williams & Wilkins Company, 1963.

BIBLIOGRAPHY

1. Duke-Elder, S.: *System of Ophthalmology*, Vol. VII, London, Henry Kimpton, 1962.
2. Lederman, M.: Radiotherapy of non-malignant diseases of the eye, *Brit. J. Ophthal.*, 41, 1, 1957.
3. Lederman, M.: Technique of radiation treatment of orbital tumors, *Brit. J. Radiol.*, 30, 469, 1957.
4. Lederman, M.: In *Progress in Radiation Therapy*, F. Buschke, Ed., New York, Grune & Stratton, p. 256, 1958.
5. Merriam, G. R., Jr., and Focht, E. F.: A clinical study of radiation cataracts and the relationship to dose, *Amer. J. Roentgen.*, 77, 759, 1957.
6. Paterson, R.: *Treatment of Malignant Disease by Radiotherapy*, Baltimore, Williams and Wilkins Company, 1963.
7. Reese, A. B.: *Tumors of the Eye*, New York, Paul B. Hoeber Inc., 1951.
8. Reese, A. B.: In *Ocular and Adnexal Tumors*, M. Boniuk, Ed., St. Louis, C. V. Mosby Company, 1964.
9. Ridley, F.: Applicators for irradiation of conjunctival sac, *Trans. Ophthal. Soc., U. K.*, 78, 171, 1958.

6. Breast

Management of Localized Breast Cancer

In Collaboration with

NORAH duV. TAPLEY, ELEANOR D. MONTAGUE, and GEORGE R. BROWN

Characteristics of Breast Cancer

Histology

Few histological types of breast cancer have a specific natural history. Adenocarcinoma is the most common malignant lesion in the breast. Grading of adenocarcinomas is worthwhile according to some pathologists[6] and lack of differentiation is considered to connote a poorer prognosis. However, the majority of pathologists do not believe that the common variety of adenocarcinomas can be graded. As a rule, the histologic type is not considered to be a factor in management.

Routes of Spread in Breast Cancer

The spread of breast cancer through the lymphatics is paramount in determining its behavior. Figure 6-1 schematically shows the pattern of spread to the regional lymph nodes. In the breast itself, the lymphatics originate in a delicate network around the mammary lobule. The connecting lymphatics accompany the ducts and terminate in the subareolar plexus. Connecting trunks from the breast flow around the outer edge of the pectoralis major, penetrate the axillary fascia and enter the axillary lymph nodes. The axillary lymphatic routes empty into the subclavian group of nodes at the apex of the axilla, but there is also the possibility of direct flow to the supraclavicular nodes. The subclavian lymphatic trunks empty into the supraclavicular group of nodes or into the jugular-subclavian venous confluence. Accessory routes of lymphatic drainage from the breast, which result in a more direct pathway to subclavian nodes than does the axillary route, are the retropectoral collecting trunks which drain both the upper and inner portions of the breast. These trunks run between the pectoralis major and minor or beneath the minor pectoralis muscle and empty into the subclavian nodes.

Lymphatic drainage from the breast into the internal mammary nodes takes place by means of the connecting lymphatic vessels in the central and medial portions of the breast. These vessels follow the perforating vasculature through the pectoralis major muscle to empty into the internal mammary chain nodes situated in the intercostal spaces at the sternal border. The nodes, measuring 2 to 4 mm in diameter, are located in the interspace between the costal cartilages and within 3 cm of the sternal edge. The internal mammary lymphatic trunks can overflow into the thoracic duct, into the supraclavicular group, or into the great veins at the jugular-subclavian vein confluence.

In the cases studied by Abrao and DaSilva Neto,[1] 56.5 per cent of nodes were located behind the costal cartilages. Retromanubrial nodes were also described between the left and right lymphatic trunks at the level of the first interspace in 21 per cent of their subjects.

The lymphatics of the dermis of the chest wall, in the entire upper anterior and lateral quadrants, have a consistent directional lym-

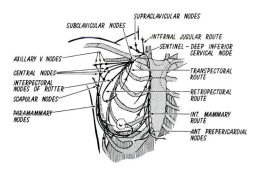

FIG. 6-1. Pattern of metastatic spread to the regional lymph nodes in carcinoma of the breast. (Courtesy: Haagensen, In *Diseases of the Breast* 2nd ed., Philadelphia, W. B. Saunders Company, 1971.)

phatic flow to the axilla; there is a dividing line at the umbilicus between the superior drainage to the axilla and the inferior drainage to the groins.

Occasionally the skin lymphatic vessels on one side of the sternum cross the midline and empty into the nodes of the opposite axilla. Another route of spread for contralateral metastases is through the deep lymphatics of the pectoral fascia beneath the opposite breast. Some studies suggest that there is a direct flow from the breast lymphatics to the intercostal lymphatics.

Primary Tumor

There is no rigid correlation between treatment and the size of the primary tumor, but accumulated data indicate that the larger the tumor size, the poorer the prognosis and the higher the incidence of local failures.[25,37]

Skin disturbance seems to carry a higher risk of chest wall recurrences. Peau d'orange, often produced by massive involvement of the dermal lymphatics, indicates a poor prognosis. Skin ulceration is not particularly significant except that it usually occurs with large tumors and therefore presents two grave signs of Haagensen.[25] The so-called inflammatory carcinoma, with skin redness, ridges, and heat, should be recognized as a clinical entity.

Location of the cancer in the axillary tail of the breast or close to the sternum or in the inframammary fold causes technical problems which influence management. It is not yet clear what the practical consequences will be of the information provided by whole organ studies[21] that a percentage of patients have multicentric tumors. However, there are indications that a secondary primary in the opposite breast is more likely in those patients with multiple foci of tumor in the first breast.

Axillary Nodes

There is a 38 per cent error, in both directions, between finding palpable nodes in the axilla and the histological findings in the surgical specimen.[10] According to Haagensen[25] axillary nodes 2.5 cm or more in diameter have a 90 per cent chance of being histologically positive. Involvement of low pectoral or midaxillary nodes does not indicate nearly as poor a prognosis as when subclavian (axillary apex) nodes are diseased.[27]

In an untreated patient, edema of the arm indicates that the disease has involved the lymphatic pathways, blocking the drainage of lymph to the axilla.[25] Patients with such symptoms have a very poor prognosis.

Supraclavicular Nodes

The incidence of occult deposits in the supraclavicular nodes is 20 to 25 per cent in patients with positive axillary nodes in the surgical specimen.[29,34] The percentage of occult deposits is very low if the axillary nodes are not involved. There have been cyclic attempts at surgical extirpation of supraclavicular nodes.[46]

Few patients with supraclavicular nodes involved with disease have been reported alive and free from disease at 5 years in any series. From 1948 through December 1967 at *MDAH*, there were 67 patients with initial supraclavicular disease treated with irradiation alone. Local control was obtained in 61

(90 per cent) of these patients. All but 6 died from disease before 5 years. Four patients died from disseminated disease at 80, 82, 89, and 90 months; 2 are alive with no evidence of disease at 73 and 80 months.

Internal Mammary Chain Nodes

It is now well established[8,11,28,42,43] that the incidence of internal mammary chain nodes is a function of the location of the tumor in the breast and of the extent of involvement of the axillary nodes.

Figure 6-2 from Handley's series shows the incidence of involvement of the internal mammary chain nodes relative to location of the tumor in the breast and the extent of involvement of the axillary nodes.[28] The frequency of involvement of the first 3 internal mammary nodes is of the order of 30 per cent in patients with lesions located in the central or inner portions of the breast or located in the outer quadrants with positive axillary nodes. The frequency of involvement is of the order of 50 per cent if the tumor is central or if the inner quadrants of the breast and the axillary nodes are positive.

According to various reported series of extended radical mastectomies, the internal mammary chain nodes when involved are, with few exceptions, minimally involved or are of small size.[8,25,27,44] Microscopic nests of cancer cells have also been described in the areolar tissues.[25,27]

There are patients with involved internal mammary chain nodes treated with extended radical mastectomy who are alive, disease free, at 10 years.[27,43,46] Sterilization of biopsy proven disease in the internal mammary chain nodes has been reported.[24] The survival rates are identical when the axillary nodes alone or the internal mammary chain nodes alone are involved.[8,46] The accumulated data seem to indicate that systematic treatment of the internal mammary chain nodes, either by extended radical mastectomy or by postoperative irradiation, can achieve actual cures.

The diagnosis of parasternal recurrence is based on the definition given by Urban of a "firm, fixed, mound-like mass arising from the depths of the intercostal space close to the sternum."[42] The incidence of parasternal nodules, although not consistent in the liter-

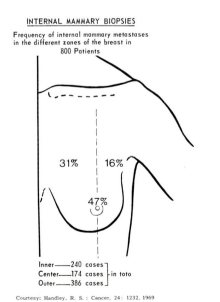

INTERNAL MAMMARY BIOPSIES

Frequency of internal mammary metastases in the different zones of the breast in 800 Patients

31%   16%

47%

Inner——240 cases
Center——174 cases } in toto
Outer——386 cases

Courtesy: Handley, R. S. : Cancer, 24 : 1232, 1969

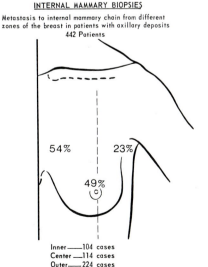

INTERNAL MAMMARY BIOPSIES

Metastasis to internal mammary chain from different zones of the breast in patients with axillary deposits 442 Patients

54%   23%

49%

Inner——104 cases
Center——114 cases
Outer——224 cases

Courtesy: Handley, R.S. : Cancer, 24 : 1232, 1969

FIG. 6-2. Incidence of internal mammary chain involvement by location of the tumor in the breast and in association with axillary deposits.

ature[34,42] can be correlated with the stage of disease.[27]

In one series[36] of 65 patients with parasternal recurrences, the majority had lesions located in the inner half of the breast; only 4 of the 65 patients had received postoperative irradiation to the internal mammary chain.

Clinical Criteria of Inoperability

If a patient has an unresectable mass in the breast, axilla, or supraclavicular area there is no choice regarding modality of treatment. When the tumor is technically resectable there are alternate methods of management. Criteria are needed to determine whether the patient is operable. If one does not use rigid criteria in the selection of patients for operation, the incidence of recurrences locally and in the regional lymph nodes is high.

In 1943, Haagensen and Stout[26] reviewed the course of 109 patients having had radical mastectomy for breast cancer. In the only 3 five-year survivors, local recurrences and distant metastases developed shortly after the five-year period. The incidence of recurrences within the operative area was 47.7 per cent. Analysis of the clinical features in this series of patients led Haagensen and Stout to define criteria of operability. These criteria are principally those shown for Category III patients.

In Spratt's series[37] of 704 patients with breast cancer treated by radical mastectomy, chest wall recurrences were seen in 40 to 45 per cent of patients with heavily infested axillary nodes. In the same series, patients with tumors larger than 8 cm had a local recurrence rate of 33 per cent.

Local and Regional Results

Categories I and II

Local results are the real index of effectiveness of treatment method and patient selection.

The clinical criteria used in the material analyzed are shown in Table 6-1.

SUPRACLAVICULAR NODES

Table 6-2 correlates the incidence of supraclavicular nodes appearing later in patients with and without postoperative irradiation when the axillary nodes were positive in the surgical specimen. Prior to ample availability of skin sparing beams (^{137}Cs and ^{60}Co), 250 Kv irradiation was used for pre- and postoperative treatment. Always using a single anterior supraclavicular portal, the skin dose was 4,000 r in 3 weeks for postoperative irradiation and 4,000 r in 4 weeks for preoperative irradiation. The highest dose to the lymph nodes was 3,500 rads in the center of the supraclavicular field, and 3,000 rads maximum under the clavicle and at the portal corners because of lack of scatter. Until 1967, 4,000 rads given dose was delivered with ^{60}Co preoperatively, the node dose being never less than 90 per cent and 100 per cent for most of the field. There are 4 supraclavicular recurrences in 121 patients so treated.

AXILLARY AND PARASTERNAL NODES

Recurrences at these 2 sites are infrequent in our material (Table 6-3). The negligible incidence of parasternal recurrences in patients with positive axillary nodes (2 of 362) is suggestive of irradiation sterilization of internal mammary chain metastases.

CHEST WALL

Chest wall recurrences have been distributed approximately evenly between single or multiple nodules close to the mastectomy scar and diffuse skin involvement.

Chest wall recurrences are more common when the axillary nodes are involved (Table 6-3), as reported many times. In patients treated at *MDAH* by radical mastectomy followed by postoperative peripheral lymphatic irradiation, the chest wall recurrence

Table 6-1. Categories* of Treatment for Localized Breast Cancer

	I	II	III	IV
	Radical Mastectomy Outer Quadrant and Axilla [-]: No Post-operative Irrad. Others: Periph. Lymph. Irradiation	Preoperative Irradiation + Radical Mastectomy†	Technically Suitable for Radical Mastectomy	Technically Unsuitable for Radical Mastectomy
Primary Size	<5 cm	>5 cm	$<$Whole Breast	Whole Breast
Skin	—	Edema or fixation over tumor only	Edema, Ulceration, / Skin fixation $<\frac{1}{2}$ breast / Satellite nodule(s) in continuity with primary	Edema / Ulceration / Skin fixation / Peripheral satellite nodule(s) / Inflammatory } $>\frac{1}{2}$ breast
Pect. Fascia + Chest Wall	—	—	Pectoral fascia fixation	Chest wall fixation
Axillary Node(s) Size	<2 cm	>2 cm	Single large node without fixation	Matted nodes,
Number	Single	or Few	or Multiple nodes	fixed or not fixed
Location	Not apical	Not apical	or Apical node(s)	
Supraclavicular Node(s)	—	—	Moveable	Fixed
Staging UICC (41)	$[T_1, T_2] \ N_0$: Stage I / $[T_1, T_2] \ N_1$: Stage II	T_2, N_1: Stage II / $T_3[N_0, N_1]$: Stage III / Or Unstaged†	$[T_3 \ [+] \ [N_0, N_1]]$ / $[T_1, T_2, T_3 \ [+]] \ N_2$ / $[T_1, T_2, T_3 \ [+]] \ N_3$ | Stage III Late	$T_3 \ [+], N_3$ / $T_4[N_0, N_1, N_2, N_3]$ | Stage III Very Late

*The worst feature places the patient in the appropriate category. Multiple features in one category do not change the category.
†Also patients with outside open biopsy and a disturbed wound.

$T_x \ [+]$: Late T_x
$T_x \ [N_y, N_z]$: $T_x N_y$ and $T_x N_z$
$[T_x T_y] \ N_z$: $T_x N_z$ and $T_y N_z$

Table 6-2. *Incidence of Disease Developing in the Supraclavicular Area After Radical Mastectomy when Axillary Nodes are Positive in the Surgical Specimen*

Christie Hospital Manchester, Eng. Memorial Center Hospital N.Y.C.*	M. D. Anderson Hospital Houston, Texas
Without Postoperative Irradiation	With Postoperative Irradiation 250 Kv $\leq$ 3,500 rads node dose/4 wks 7% (6/89) ^{137}Cs, ^{60}Co, Electron Beam 5,000–5,500 rads *GD*/ 4 wks 1.3% (4/273)
20–25%	With Preoperative Irradiation ^{60}Co 4,000 rads *GD*/4 wks. 3% (4/121)

*Jackson, *Clin. Radiol.*, 17, 107, 1966.
Robbins, et al, *Surg. Gynec. and Obstet.*, 122, 979, 1966. (Courtesy: Fletcher, *Cancer*, 29, 545, 1972.)

rates were 4.5 per cent when the axillary nodes were negative, 11 per cent with less than 50 per cent positive nodes, and 22 per cent with more than 50 per cent positive nodes. There was correlation also with the characteristics of the primary tumor, *i.e.*, the absence or presence of grave signs.

In the *MDAH* series, the lowest incidence of chest wall recurrence is in patients having had preoperative irradiation.[16,20] With this technique, the entire skin of the chest wall is irradiated in addition to the peripheral lymphatics. The data do not substantiate the conclusions of Dao and Kovaric[12] that the incidence of chest wall recurrences is greater if the chest wall skin has been irradiated.

Since 1963, the chest wall, in addition to the peripheral lymphatics, has been irradiated when a significant percentage of nodes is positive. Table 6-4 gives the status and sites of recurrence correlated with the extent of disease before radical mastectomy for 70

Table 6-3. *Recurrences in Radical Mastectomy Patients by Therapeutic Groups and Axillary Status in Surgical Specimen*
1955–Dec. 1967

	Preoperative		Postoperative		Alone	
	Positive 121	Negative 298	Positive 241	Negative 112	Positive 22	Negative 224
Chest Wall	10(8%)	9(3%)	24(10%)	5(4.5%)	2	11(5%)
Axilla	1	0	1	0	1	1
Parasternal	0	1	2	1	0	3

Courtesy: Fletcher, *Cancer*, 29, 545, 1972.

Table 6-4. *Elective Irradiation of Chest Wall—Correlation of Results of Treatment With Incidence of Involved Axillary Nodes in Operative Specimen*

May 1, 1963–December 31, 1966
Analysis of September, 1970

70 Patients*	Extent of Disease Prior to Mastectomy			Results of Treatment		
	Axillary Nodes			Chest Wall Recurrence	Disease Other Sites	Disease Other Breast
	<50% 24/70 (35%)		>50% 46/70 (65%)			
	No Grave Signs	Grave Signs				
Alive						
No Evidence of Disease (24 Patients)	3	9	12	1—in field** 1—outside field†	1§	
Alive with Disease (8 Patients)	0	3	5		8	
Dead with Disease (38 Patients) (*DID*-1)	3	6	29	5	32	4

* 44 of 70 patients developed distant metastases.
** Nodule in field at 36 months resected. *NED* at 42 months.
† Nodule outside field at 7 months treated with electron beam. *NED* at 37 months.
§ Node in opposite axilla at 36 months radical mastectomy breast negative. *NED* at 60 months. (Revised from: Tapley, and Fletcher, In *Breast Cancer, Early and Late*, Year Book Medical Publishers, Inc., Chicago, Illinois, 1970, p. 281.)

patients receiving prophylactic treatment of the chest wall followed from one and one-half to 7 years after irradiation. Seven patients developed chest wall recurrence, a recurrence rate of 10 per cent; in one patient the recurrence was outside the treatment field. Since the patients in this series either had heavily infested axillary nodes, or grave signs associated with the breast tumor, or both, a chest wall recurrence rate of 10 per cent is a significant improvement when compared with previously reported series.[25,26,37] The management of recurrences is not nearly as successful (Table 6-5), the local control rate being only 50 per cent.

SURVIVAL RATES IN RADICAL MASTECTOMY PATIENTS

Table 6-6 gives the survival rates at 10 years. The 10-year survival rate is the true index for assessing permanent success deal- ing with breast cancer patients, because at 10 years the cumulative death rate almost parallels that of patients without cancer. These survival rates compare favorably with survival rates reported for a series of patients having had extended radical mastectomy.[46] The overall survival rates were found to be as good in central or medial as in lateral lesions; this is also true on analyzing survival rates relative to negative or positive axillary nodes. These results are in definite contrast with those reported in the Memorial Hospital series[42,43] in which survival rates for outer quadrant lesions were approximately 10 per cent higher than for inner quadrant or central lesions.

The 10-year survival rate in the preoperative group (29 per cent histologically positive axillary nodes) is the same as in the radical mastectomy only group (9 per cent histologically positive axillary nodes). This suggests that irradiation of the peripheral lymphatics

Table 6-5. *Results of Treatment—Irradiation of Chest Wall Recurrences*

May 1, 1963–December 31, 1966
Analysis of September 1970

37 Patients*	Alive *NED* 5 Pts.	Alive with Disease 7 Pts.	Dead with Disease 25 Pts.
Second Chest Wall Recurrence 22/37 (59%)	1—outside field at 8 mos.†	5—in field	14—in field 2—outside field
No Recurrence Chest Wall	4	2	9
Disease Other Breast 9/37 (24%)		6—with or after recurrence 2—concomitant both breasts 1—opposite breast earlier	

*27 developed distant metastases
†Treated with electron beam, *NED* at 57 months. (Revised from: Tapley, and Fletcher, In *Breast Cancer, Early and Late,* Year Book Medical Publishers, Inc., Chicago, Illinois, 1970, pp. 281.)

cure a percentage of patients as, in all series reported, survival rates decrease with increased infestation of the axillary lymph nodes. These patients received the largest amount of irradiation when disease was still present. This contradicts the theory that irradiation diminishes the immune response, producing distant metastases, and achieving a lower survival rate than in patients who do not receive irradiation. The patients who received preoperative irradiation comprise 2 clinical groups: 1) patients referred after an incisional biopsy who presented either with apparently gross excision of the primary tumor or with extensive residual induration and various degrees of ecchymosis and infection and 2) patients who had lesions as defined in Category II with the histological

Table 6-6. *10 Year Survival Rates in Radical Mastectomy Series**

	January 1955–December 1967		
	No. Pts.	Per Cent of Ax. Nodes Histol. Pos.	Per Cent
Radical Mastectomy Only	246	9∇	+35 63† § −64
Radical Mastectomy + Postop. Irradiation	353	63∇	+40.5 50† § −68
Preop. Irradiation + Radical Mastectomy	419	29∇	+43 62† § −70

* Age adjusted survival rate—Berkson-Gage; 25% of the patients are private.
† The survival rates are the same for the patients with inner quadrants or centrally located lesions versus those with lesions in the inner quadrants.
+ Axilla histologically positive
§
− Axilla histologically negative
∇Percentage of clinically positive axillary nodes are respectively 26%, 46%, and 54%.

Table 6-7. *Results of Preoperative Irradiation in Patients with an Aspiration Biopsy*

1948–December 1967
Analysis February 1972

Size of Primary Lesion Estimated by Palpation ≥5 cm in greatest dimension	
NED ≥5 years	13 (6 ≥ 10 yrs.)
NED <5 years	2
Dead ID, no data ≤5 years	5
Dead from disease ≤5 years	26
Dead from disease >5 years	1
Total No. of Patients	47

diagnosis established by aspiration biopsy at *MDAH*. Table 6-7 shows the status of these latter patients with a minimum of 3 years follow-up. For patients with lesions 5 cm or more in greatest dimension, the *NED* rate at 5 years is slightly over 30 per cent.

Category III

Category III lesions (except with positive supraclavicular nodes) are technically suitable for radical mastectomy since the planes of dissection can encompass gross cancer, but are clinically unsuitable because of the high risk of cutting through microscopic disease with dissemination of disease in the operative area, and possible systemic dissemination.

The incidence of recurrences in the chest wall, axilla, supraclavicular area, and parasternal area are tabulated in Table 6-8. Chest wall recurrences are clearly less in those patients having had a total mastectomy than in those whose primary tumor was treated by irradiation only. Chest wall and axillary recurrences have almost been completely eliminated since 1964.[7] Only one parasternal recurrence in 467 patients with advanced disease indicates the effectiveness of irradiation in sterilizing internal mammary chain metastases.

Table 6-8 also gives 5- and 10-year survival rates with or without total mastectomy. The patients who had total mastectomy usually had lesions with a greater possibility of control. Otherwise, mastectomy would not have been feasible. The results are gratifying considering the extent of initial disease.

Table 6-8. *Local Control in Patients with Late Stage III UICC Cancer of the Breast Technically Suitable for Radical Mastectomy*

January 1955–December 1967
Analysis January 1972*

	With Simple Mastectomy		Without Simple Mastectomy 229
	1/55–12/63 103	1/64–12/67 32	1/55–12/67
Chest Wall† **	88% (91/103)	97% (31/32)	78% (179/229)
Axilla† ***	88% (91/103)	100% (32/32)	89.5% (205/229)
Supraclavicular† §	93% (96/103)	100% (32/32)	98% (224/229)
Parasternal†	99% (102/103)	100% (32/32)	—

†A patient may have a recurrence in more than one location.
* By 36 months, 90% of recurrences have developed.
** Patients treated from January 1955 through December 1963 had 4,000 to 4,500 rads to the chest wall and from 1964 on, 5,000 rads minimum.
*** Axilla: January 1955 through December 1963, 4,400 to 5,000 rads usually with no boost. Since 1964 after 5,000 rads, 1,000 to 2,000 rads boost to palpable nodes.
§ Two of the 7 supraclavicular failures were in the 4 patients with initial supraclavicular nodes.

Survival rates: (Modified life table method)	With Simple Mastectomy	5 yrs.—45.5% 10 yrs.—21.5%
	Without Simple Mastectomy (Irradiation alone)	5 yrs.—30.0% 10 yrs.—12.5%

Table 6-9. *Incidence of Disease Appearing in Clinically Negative Axillae* after 5,000 rads Tumor Dose Given in 5 weeks with* *[60]Cobalt in Patients with Late Stage III (UICC Staging) Cancer of the Breast* *January 1955–December 1967*

No Evidence of Disease on Chest Wall or Retained Breast	
Number of patients	65
Axillary failure	1

* 38 per cent expected to be positive (Courtesy: Fletcher, Cancer, 29, 545, 1972.)

Table 6-9 shows the incidence of axillary failures in the Category III patients with clinically negative axillary nodes. There is only one failure to control axillary disease in 69 patients. In all reported series of patients treated with radical mastectomy, approximately 38 per cent of the patients with clinically negative axillary nodes have histologically positive nodes in the surgical specimen.[10] One would expect to find at least that same percentage in patients with tumors which are large and/or associated with grave signs.

Table 6-10 shows the incidence of axillary failures in patients with clinically positive axillary nodes. There was 4.3 per cent failure in the axilla in the 161 patients who had no active disease in the chest wall or the retained breast. Assuming that 40 per cent of the patients with these clinically positive

Table 6-10. *Category III Patients—6,000 rads TD in 6 wks. to 7,000 rads TD in 7 wks. with* *[60]Co—Clinically Positive Axillary Nodes* *January 1955–December 1967*

	NED C.W.*	Residual or Recurrent Disease in C.W.*
Number of Patients	161**	26
Axillary Failure	7 (4.3%)	13 (50%)

* C.W. = Chest wall or retained breast
** 62 per cent expected to be histologically positive.[9] (Courtesy: Fletcher, Cancer, 29, 545, 1972.)

nodes would have histologically negative nodes, as in the reported radical mastectomy series,[10] one would expect at least 100 of the patients to have histologically positive nodes.

The radiotherapy technique in these patients included 5,000 rads to the whole axilla, and usually 1,000 rads added through a small appositional portal over the node(s) if they had disappeared at the end of 5 weeks. If the nodes were still palpable, 2,000 rads were added.

Supraclavicular disease developed in less than 3 per cent of the patients, a very low incidence considering that these patients had advanced tumors locally and/or in the axilla. In this group, the skin dose to the supraclavicular area was 5,000 rads skin dose in 12 weeks with 250 Kv or 5,000 rads given dose in 5 weeks with [60]Co.

Category IV

Patients with disease which exhibits the features of inflammatory carcinoma, *i.e.,* heat, erythema, and ridges, or with lesions that have satellite nodules peripheral to the breast mass or are fixed to the chest wall, or with fixed axillary nodes and large supraclavicular disease, are not technically suitable for radical mastectomy. Selectivity must be used for radical irradiation when the prognosis is limited. If the local disease has advanced beyond a certain point, long, protracted radical irradiation is not warranted. Conversely, one should not always treat patients with palliative doses of irradiation even if the chance of survival at 10 years is almost zero; short-range palliative irradiation must be reserved for those patients whose probable survival time is very short. Table 6-11 shows the incidence of failures and the 5- and 10-year survival rates. A 65 per cent rate of freedom from disease locally and/or regionally is quite good in these advanced lesions.

The fact that there was only one parasternal recurrence in 192 patients with far-advanced disease is indicative of the effectiveness of irradiation in sterilizing internal mammary chain metastases.

Table 6-11. *Sites of Failures in Category IV Patients**
1948–December 1964

	With Total Mastectomy 48	No Total Mastectomy 144
Chest Wall†	23.0%	30.0%
Axilla†	19.0%	14.5%
Supraclavicular†	17.0%§	5.5%
Parasternal†	0	0.7%
Percentage of Pts. without local and/or regional recurrent disease	65.0%	

*Survival Rates: (Modified life table method)	With Total Mastectomy	5 yrs.—12.5% 10 yrs.—10.0%
	Without Total Mastectomy	5 yrs.—14.0% 10 yrs.— 5.0%

† A patient may have a recurrence in more than one location.
§ 8/48, no statistical significance.

Several authors[2,13,38] have indicated that local control can be achieved in a high percentage of patients when high doses are given in a few fractions. In our series, the growth restraint with this technique has averaged less than one year for massive, noninflammatory local disease and averaged less than 6 months for inflammatory disease. The few survivors are beset with complications such as multiple rib fractures and axillary and supraclavicular fibrosis with restriction of shoulder motion. Three instances of brachial plexus damage have occurred. Rapid treatment for palliation has been abandoned. A 3-weeks course of treatment supplemented with ^{198}Au seed implants in the breast mass has been found to be effective for local control during the interval of life prior to death, as long as 16–18 months.

Concepts in Management of Breast Cancer

Radiosensitivity of Breast Cancer

From the data presented one can conclude that 3,000 to 3,500 rads delivered in 4 weeks control 60 to 70 per cent, 4,000 rads in 4 weeks control 80 to 90 per cent and 4,500 to 5,000 rads in 5 weeks control more than 90 per cent of subclinical disease in adenocarcinoma of the breast.

In elective postoperative irradiation without gross disease, a tumor dose of 4,500 rads is adequate for subclinical disease. One may give 5,000 rads in some areas with a high risk of infestation.

Ninety per cent of clinically positive supraclavicular nodes have been controlled by 6,000 to 6,500 rads in 6 weeks. There is a very low incidence of axillary failures in the Category III patients with clinically positive axillary nodes and without residual or recurrent disease on the chest wall (Table 6-10) treated with doses of 6,000 rads in 6 weeks to 7,000 rads in 7 weeks. The data indicate that breast cancer, size for size, has the same radiosensitivity as squamous cell carcinoma.

It has been stated that breast cancer in lymph nodes is more radiosensitive than the primary lesion. Since the involved nodes are usually smaller than the primary lesion, they are controlled with a lower dose of irradiation. A 3 cm node in the axilla is considered a large node. Supraclavicular nodes are usually small. In general, the farther away the nodes are from the primary lesion, the smaller they are (Fig. 6-3).

Large masses in the corpus mammae re-

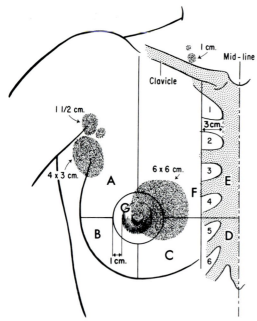

FIG. 6-3. As a rule the largest mass is the primary tumor, the next largest occurs in the axillary nodes and then in the supraclavicular nodes. The supraclavicular nodes, if palpable, are usually 1 to 2 cm in diameter.

quire 9,000 to 10,000 rads in 9 to 10 weeks for permanent control. At *MDAH,* modification of the long-protracted irradiation technique initiated by Baclesse[4,5] in the 1930's has been used. The very high doses necessary to control enormous masses in the corpus mammae can result in severe, at times excessive, fibrosis and occasional necroses.

Combination of Conservative Surgery with Irradiation

The inability of any type of superradical surgery to eradicate cancer of the breast which has advanced past a certain stage is due to the diffuse spread of disease to the lymphatics in the dermis, intercostal spaces, axilla, supraclavicular area and internal mammary chain. The additional dissection of a centimeter here or there or the thinning of the flap by one millimeter does not alter the outcome.

A conservative procedure limited to removal of the main masses without unnecessary manipulation combined with doses of the order of 5,000 rads given as soon as possible postoperatively is an effective method to deal with advanced breast disease as shown by the excellent results in freedom from disease in the chest wall, the axilla, and the supraclavicular area (Table 6-8). This experience is similar to that reported in another series.[3]

Where to Go Next?

Many series reported from the world over, including several from the United States, show that the so-called classical radical mastectomy does not improve survival rates over other varieties of mastectomy. It is discouraging that survival rates do not demonstrate the value of either surgery or irradiation in the treatment of the peripheral lymphatics. The opinion that the patient who does not have a radical mastectomy has been jeopardized in her chances to be cured is not scientifically tenable. The diagnosis of invasive adenocarcinoma in the breast should not elicit a conditioned reflex to perform a radical mastectomy.

Local treatment, whether surgical or radiotherapeutic, affects disease within the treated area and has no influence on distant metastases already present at the time of initial treatment. Survival rates can be altered only by eradicating disease which is present in the peripheral lymphatics in patients who do not as yet have distant metastases. In an individual patient, there is no way to show occult deposits in the supraclavicular area and internal mammary chain nodes or to rule out distant metastases not yet clinically detectable. Therefore, those patients who might benefit by more encompassing treatment cannot be sharply defined; they can only be loosely circumscribed by the probability of peripheral lymphatics infestation and a small risk of having distant metastases. For example, patients with a small outer quadrant tumor and histologically negative axillary nodes have a low probability of regional and distant spread whereas patients with almost all of the recovered axillary nodes histologically positive almost certainly have distant spread in addition to regional spread. Increased survival rates have been found in various groups of patients defined in between these two extremes.[9,14]

After nearly 80 years of trying, the superior treatment for carcinoma of the breast has not yet been identified. As well expressed by J. Chandler Smith,[35] the comparison of survival rates is not likely to reveal the superior treatment because survival rates do not correlate with the amount of tissue removed. There is no "superior" method of treatment for "all" patients with breast cancer but for the individual patient the superior method of treatment is the one which ablates tumor in tissues likely to be infested. This approach will secure maximum freedom from disease in the treated area.

The treatment method varies with the clinical characteristics and location of the breast tumor. Two patients, shown in Figures 6-4 and 6-5, illustrate this point. There are no rigid rules which can be used in evaluating the management of an individual patient since many parameters should be considered. The factors to be balanced are the size, characteristics, and location of the tumor in the breast and the presence or absence of clinically positive axillary nodes. There may also have been previous interference which places the management outside any predetermined pattern. Age and wishes of the patient should be considered. For a woman in her mid 40's with a lump in the outer quadrants of the breast, a wedge excision followed by irradiation preserves the breast, which has psychosexual significance. A 70-year-old patient with the same lesion would be treated best by radical mastectomy since, if the axillary nodes are negative in the surgical specimen, there is no need for postoperative irradiation. Therefore, this will be the simplest treatment.

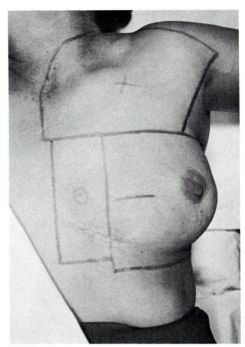

FIG. 6-4. Fifty-nine-year old patient seen on 12-17-70, with a history of an excisional biopsy on 11-23-70. By her description there was no fixation of this mass to the skin or underlying muscle and the pathology report stated that the primary lesion was 1.8 × 1.4 cm in size. At the time of her examination, she had a well-healed scar. In a patient with a tumor over the xyphoid, the risk of involvement is to the internal mammary chain which the surgical procedure does not dissect. Why dissect the axilla which is almost certainly not involved?

Patients survive with disease 5 years or more, or may evidence metastatic disease between 5 and 10 years; this emphasizes the importance of controlling local and regional lymphatic disease for long periods of time. Hormonal and chemotherapeutic management of breast cancer can control internal metastases for many months to years. Disease recurring in the local area is seldom completely eradicated by these methods; patients must live with obvious disease in the chest wall, the axilla, or the supraclavicular region. This visible disease may be the dominant event in the last period of life, and

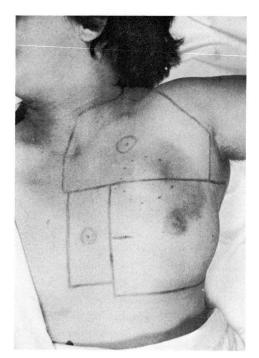

FIG. 6-5. The patient was seen with a 7 cm ill-defined mass in the upper inner quadrant of the left breast and a 2.5 cm node in the left mid-axilla. Dots have been placed around the mass. With a 7 cm tumor high on the chest wall and a 2.5 cm axillary node, in addition to the palpable disease in the corpus mammae and in the axilla, the patient had a 50 per cent chance of disease in the internal mammary chain, 25 per cent chance of having occult deposits in the supraclavicular area, and a significant risk of spread to the intercostal lymphatics. Of the 5 areas of known or probable disease, surgery removes only 2. Preoperative irradiation gives only 3,000 rads to the chest wall (which is low), whereas, after a simple mastectomy, 5,000 rads are given which is significantly more effective.

is frequently an enormously troublesome problem for the family and physician.

Wedge Excision and Irradiation Therapy

Several centers have reported on the treatment for early breast cancer by wedge excision and irradiation.[31,32,33] The survival rates at 5 and 10 years are identical with those obtained with radical mastectomy. Even if in some series there is a somewhat higher incidence of local recurrences, one must keep in mind that patients are included that have been treated since 1930 and have, therefore, received inadequate irradiation. Most recurrences were successfully excised.[33] Patients suitable for wedge excision are those with a lump in the breast without skin disturbance and a clinically negative axilla.

The records of 25 patients treated at *MDAH* with a wedge excision followed by irradiation have been reviewed. Eleven of the patients had a tumor smaller than 3 cm. The other 14 patients had large lesions excised elsewhere and presented at *MDAH* with variously sized residual induration. Fourteen patients are *NED* from 22 to 110 months. The only local recurrence was in a patient with an initial lesion apparently 6 × 7 × 8 cm in size. The 11 patients with lesions less than 3 cm received 5,000 rads in 5 weeks and are *NED*; the others received long, protracted treatment.

The fact that some breast cancers are found to be of multicentric origin on whole organ study is not a deterrent to irradiation. If 5,000 rads can eradicate subclinical disease in the axilla and supraclavicular area, there is no reason why this dose cannot do the same in the corpus mammae.

Preoperative Irradiation

A radical mastectomy can be performed 5 to 6 weeks after completion of ^{60}Co irradiation without increased difficulty for the surgeon. Surgical dissection is often aided by the interstitial edema which is present. Wound healing complications are not increased.

Preoperative irradiation with 4,000 rads in 4 weeks eradicates a high percentage of cancer cells, many of the axillary specimens being negative when the axilla was clinically positive.[22] Many breast specimens were negative after aspiration biopsies had demonstrated cancer.[22] With a decrease in the number of viable cells, the extensive surgical manipulations associated with a radical mastectomy are less likely to produce implants and distant metastases.

For locally advanced lesions, a simple mastectomy followed by irradiation seems to be a more effective method of treatment than preoperative irradiation followed by radical mastectomy (Tables 6-7 and 6-8). Because of the initial large number of cancer cells, too many viable cells remain after 4,000 rads to make the extensive manipulations of the radical mastectomy safe.

If one insists on a radical mastectomy, the use of preoperative irradiation is probably for those patients in whom the tumor size is larger than the small "lump" in the breast and less than 5 cm diameter with or without moderate clinical axillary involvement.

Simple Mastectomy Followed by Irradiation

The indication for simple mastectomy is a large mass in the breast, *e.g.,* greater than 5 cm, which can be removed without cutting through gross tumor. Clinically positive axillary nodes should be excised without performing an axillary dissection.

A simple mastectomy, not a total mastectomy (which removes all accessory mammary tissue), without thin skin flaps or dissection of axillary nodes unless easily accessible, is done with a minimum of surgical manipulation. If a radical mastectomy is done when the tumor is large or attached to the skin or if there is peau d'orange, a skin graft is necessary. Extensive surgical manipulation provides greater opportunity for local tumor implants and possibly distant metastases. After a simple mastectomy, radiotherapy can begin within 10 days to 2 weeks, whereas after radical mastectomy, radiation therapy may be delayed for 3 to 6 weeks and, with a skin graft, up to 8 weeks.

Chest wall irradiation should be reduced to 4,500 rads tumor dose in $4\frac{1}{2}$ weeks in total mastectomy patients with favorable primary tumors. Following an extensive axillary dissection, 5,000 rads given dose is delivered to the anterior supraclavicular-axillary portal, but only a given dose is delivered to the posterior axillary field that is sufficient to bring the midaxillary tumor dose to 4,000 rads.

Value of Elective Postoperative Irradiation

Even if there is no definite evidence that elective postoperative irradiation of the peripheral lymphatics or of the chest wall increases survival rates, the policy of "waiting" is not correct for patients with a significant risk of recurrence since gross disease is not as easily controlled as subclinical disease and further spread can occur during the interval of waiting. Large recurrences, particularly in the supraclavicular area, can produce severe symptoms by invasion of the brachial plexus. Once this has occurred, palliation is very difficult to obtain.

Irradiation of the peripheral lymphatics with moderate doses controls subclinical disease without producing complications or even detectable sequelae.[15,19] Therefore, it does not seem reasonable that a patient with a central lesion and positive axillary nodes who has 50 per cent chance of infestation of the internal mammary chain, and 20 to 25 per cent chance of occult deposits in the supraclavicular area (the combination of the two probably gives the patient at least a 60 per cent risk of having disease in the peripheral lymphatics) should not receive irradiation if so-called definitive surgery already has been used for the primary and axillary areas of spread.

Chest wall irradiation with the 6 Mev electron beam is free of complications and, therefore, is indicated in patients with a significant risk of chest wall recurrence.

Irradiation Following Conventional or Modified Radical Mastectomy

A modified radical mastectomy entails removal of the pectoralis minor muscle and axillary contents. The axilla is thoroughly dissected, the pectoralis fascia is removed as completely as possible but the pectoralis major muscle is left virtually intact.

Conventional and modified mastectomies entail careful axillary dissection and, if done for clinically operable axillary disease, yield similar survival and local control rates. Following either procedure, if the primary tumor is in the outer quadrants and the axillary nodes are histologically negative, the possibility of infestation of the supraclavicular and internal mammary chain nodes is low and no further treatment is indicated. If the tumor is located in the central or inner portion of the breast or if the axillary nodes are histologically positive, peripheral lymphatic irradiation should be given.

Axillary recurrences are extremely rare when the axilla has been properly dissected and if the axillary disease was not very extensive at the time of surgery. If the axilla was clinically operable and with no evidence of extranodal disease, even if many positive nodes were recovered, only the apex of the axilla requires treatment to dovetail with the surgical procedure (Line 1 of Fig. 6-6A).

After a radical or modified radical mastectomy, the whole axilla (Line 2 of Fig. 6-6A) should be treated postoperatively only if:

1) The adequacy of the axillary dissection is in question. This is decided by the number of nodes recovered as stated in the pathology report. If few nodes were recovered with some of them infested, the probability of infested nodes left behind is high.

2) The preoperative description was that of multiple large nodes (greater than 3 cm) with or without fixation.

3) Extranodal disease is identified on pathological study.

A posterior axillary portal (Fig. 6-6B) is added to bring the midline axillary tumor dose to 5,000 rads in 5 weeks.

Indications for irradiating the chest wall with the peripheral lymphatics are:

1) Twenty per cent or more positive axillary nodes recovered at surgery.

2) Primary breast tumor greater than 5 cm.

3) Fixation of tumor to pectoral fascia.

4) Skin fixation or disturbance (*i.e.,* edema or erythema).

5) Multifocal tumor in the breast.

6) Perineural or lymphatic invasion.

Not infrequently, data as to the location and characteristics of the tumor and of the clinical status of the axilla, sometimes even the pathological specimen, are not clear. One must then tend toward more extensive treatment, being guided by the thickness of the flaps, the presence or absence of the pectoral muscle, and clinical judgment of the quality of the axillary dissection.

Chest wall irradiation must not be initiated until there has been complete healing. Wound healing is not considered satisfactory if there is thick crusting along the mastectomy scar or if there is fluid collection under the chest wall flaps. If a skin graft has been used and has been slow to heal (greater than 8 weeks), chest wall irradiation carries with it considerable potential for chest wall necrosis. If irradiation is given in these circumstances, breakdown of the wound may occur during or shortly after treatment is concluded. With breakdown of the chest wall, spontaneous healing will be very slow; necrosis with persistent ulceration may develop and require surgical resection and grafting.

Irradiation Alone

Irradiation alone may be necessary for patients with contraindications to general anesthesia or who refuse surgery. The indications for irradiation alone, other than these factors, depend on the characteristics of the breast tumor. It is selected for patients who have tumors with extensive grave signs and in

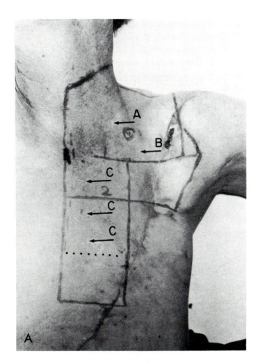

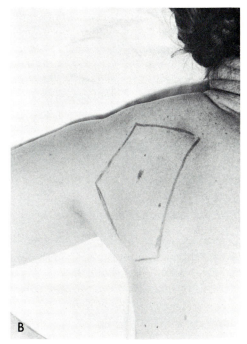

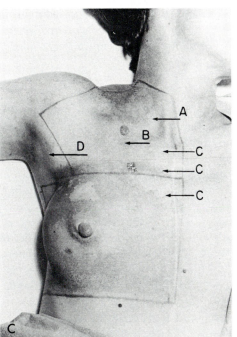

FIG. 6-6. **A.** Peripheral lymphatic technique with ^{60}Co, utilizing a single anterior L-shaped field. The interrupted line drawn within the medial border of the internal mammary portion of the field defines the midline of the sternum. The medial border of the sternal field slants upward from the midline at the xyphoid to 1 cm across the midline at the first interspace. One may irradiate only the first 3 interspaces (dotted line) as the others are rarely involved. When the axilla is not to be irradiated, the inferior border of the anterior supraclavicular portal is at the level of the medial end of the first rib (Line 1). When the entire axilla is to be irradiated, the inferior border of the anterior supraclavicular-axillary portal is at the level of the second costal cartilage (Line 2). **A.** Supraclavicular nodes—0.5 to 1 cm depth **B.** Supraclavicular apical nodes—1 cm depth **C.** Internal mammary nodes—3 cm depth.

B. Posterior axillary portal used to deliver additional irradiation to the axilla.

C. Anterior supraclavicular and axillary portal without dissection of the axilla shown to contrast the depth of the midaxillary nodes. **A.** Supraclavicular nodes—0.5 to 1 cm depth **B.** Supraclavicular apex nodes—1 cm depth **C.** Internal mammary nodes—3 cm depth **D.** Axillary nodes—average of 6–7 cm depth. (Courtesy: Montague, *Cancer, 29, 557, 1972.*)

whom a simple mastectomy cannot be done because the disease is technically unresectable, is inflammatory carcinoma, or there is extensive skin edema.

Five thousand rads given in 5 weeks does not produce a high percentage of local control,[3,23] but the protracted Baclesse technique offers excellent control of disease in the corpus mammae and in the axilla. The local control rate is less satisfactory in inflammatory carcinoma.[18]

Bilateral Breast Disease

There is an increasing awareness that breast cancer is a multifocal disease and, therefore, may affect both breasts.[45] The diagnosis of bilateral breast disease is being made with greater frequency when the initial diagnosis of one obvious breast cancer is made, or bilateral disease can become evident later after the treatment of the first breast cancer.

Bilateral breast cancer requires individualization of therapy, avoiding maximal therapy which can result in a very handicapped patient. Bilateral radical mastectomy may be truly crippling and mutilating, not only from the standpoint of appearance but because of interference with arm and shoulder function. Similarly, bilateral comprehensive and radical irradiation is too much for the patient. Therefore, one must compromise which, incidentally, will have very little effect on the over-all survival rates since the chance that distant metastases have already occurred is obviously great.

More frequent use of wedge excision or of total mastectomy with removal of all accessory breast tissues and exploration of the mid and lower axilla is in order. If there are no positive nodes in the axilla, and if the tumor is in the outer quadrant, nothing more should be done. For patients with bilateral inner quadrant tumors and demonstrated negative axillae, irradiation of both internal mammary chains only may be in order. One cannot cover all possible situations, the fore-

going being guidelines for a conservative approach to the problem.

Irradiation Techniques

There are two basic geometric patterns:
1) Postradical mastectomy peripheral lymphatics techniques (Figs. 6-6A and 6-7).
2) Irradiation of peripheral lymphatics and retained breast or chest wall (Figs. 6-8, 6-9, 6-10, 6-11).

The dose schedules and treatment fields used for the various categories of breast cancer are schematically shown in Figure 6-12.

Postradical Mastectomy Peripheral Lymphatics Techniques

^{60}CO (FIG. 6-6A)

Position of Patient. Supine, upper arm abducted 90°, the forearm supported in upright position by a vertical arm board, the head turned sharply to the contralateral side. The beam is vertical.

Field. A single "L" shaped field covers the ipsilateral internal mammary chain, supraclavicular area, and apex of the axilla. The *SSD* is taken at the subclavicular area near the sternum.

Supraclavicular area and apex of axilla: The *medial border*, drawn from the midline at the base of the xyphoid, is 1 cm on the contralateral side at the level of the sternal notch and extends superiorly to the thyrocricoid groove. The *superior border* extends laterally from the lateral border of the internal mammary field at the level of the first costal cartilage. The *lateral border* follows the curve of the shoulder, crossing the acromioclavicular joint, and meets the line of the inferior border. The apex of the axilla is included by these margins and the shoulder joint is largely excluded. The dissected axilla is not treated unless there is extranodal disease, few nodes are recovered at the time of surgery, or there is extensive infestation of axillary nodes.

Internal mammary portion: The *medial border* is drawn from the midline of the xyphoid-sternal junction at a slight angle to meet the medial border of the supraclavicular field 1 cm across the midline at the sternal notch. The *inferior border* is drawn laterally for 6 cm from the midline at the level of the xyphoid-sternal junction. The *lateral border* is drawn to intersect the inferior border of the supraclavicular portion at the level of the first costal cartilage.

Dose. Five thousand rads given dose in 4 weeks, 250 rads daily. The tumor dose in the apex of the axilla and supraclavicular area is close to 5,000 rads and is 4,500 rads at 3 cm. The first 3 interspaces are boosted to a given dose of 5,650 rads (5,000 rads tumor dose at 3 cm) in patients with a high risk of involvement (inner quadrants or central lesions with positive axillary nodes).

ELECTRON BEAM (FIG. 6-7)

Position of Patient. Supine, upper arm abducted 90°, the forearm supported in upright position by a vertical arm board, the head turned sharply to the contralateral side. The foot of the treatment table is tilted down so that the plane of the sternum is relatively parallel to the floor. (The angle of table tilt is charted for daily duplication.) The beam is vertical.

Fields. Internal mammary field: The *superior border* is placed just inferior to the sternal notch and extends laterally between the sternal end of the clavicle and first costal cartilage. The *medial border* is placed 1 cm to the contralateral side of the midline of the sternum. The *lateral border,* separated by 7 cm, parallels the medial border of the field. The *inferior border* is placed just above or at the xyphoid-sternal junction to include the first 5 internal mammary nodes. It usually measures 17 cm in length but may be 14 cm if the

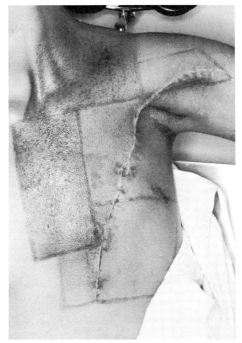

FIG. 6-7. Electron beam treatment fields after radical mastectomy. The supraclavicular field is treated with 12 Mev electrons, the internal mammary field with 15 Mev electrons and the chest wall with 6 Mev electrons.

The skin reactions are more intense in the supraclavicular and internal mammary fields because of the higher surface dose. (Courtesy: Tapley and Fletcher, *Radiologic Clinics of N. Amer.,* Vol. VII, No. 2, 301–317, 1969.)

thorax is short or 19 cm with a long thorax. If the chest wall is being treated and the mastectomy scar extends across the sternum, this portion of the scar may be included by an addition to the internal mammary field.

Supraclavicular field: The *medial border* extends upward from the upper corner of the medial border of the internal mammary field to the level of the thyrocricoid groove, parallel to the medial border of the sternal portion of the sternocleidomastoid muscle. The *superior border* extends laterally straight across the neck. The lateral border follows the curve of the shoulder and crosses the acromion process. A small portion of the shoulder joint may be included to ensure that the field extends sufficiently laterally to cover the apex of the axilla. The *inferior border* is the lateral extension of the superior border of the internal mammary field.

Separation of Fields. The fields are contiguous, with no separation. Every line is treated by at least one field but no line is treated by 2 fields.

Doses. The internal mammary field is treated with 15 Mev electrons. The given dose is 5,000 rads in 4 weeks, 250 rads daily. The tumor dose at 3 cm is 4,500 rads.

The supraclavicular field is treated with 12 Mev electrons. The given dose is 5,000 rads in 4 weeks, 250 rads daily. The tumor dose is at least 4,500 rads.

Chest Wall Irradiation after Radical Mastectomy

TANGENTIAL CHEST WALL FIELDS WITH ^{60}CO

The tangential chest wall fields include the entire mastectomy scar and operative field. Except in extremely small patients, a separate internal mammary field is used. To avoid an unirradiated wedge of skin between the internal mammary field, the medial tangential field, and the chest wall if the rib cage is unusually convex, it may be necessary to overlap the adjacent borders of the internal mammary field and the medial tangential field. The dose is 5,000 rads in 5 weeks calculated as in the treatment after total mastectomy. Bolus is used in the same fashion.

ELECTRON BEAM TECHNIQUE

A single field is used, if possible, to cover the entire chest wall scar. If the scar is not satisfactorily covered by one field, small contiguous fields are added (Fig. 6-7).

The *medial border* is provided by the lateral border of the internal mammary field. The *superior border* is provided by the inferior

border of the supraclavicular field but may extend into the axilla to cover the scar. The *inferior border* is placed at or just below the xyphoid. The *lateral border* is defined at the midaxillary line. The lateral portion of the field is treated with beam fall-off over the curve of the rib cage, resulting in a dose significantly lower than that to the chest wall close to the sternum where the *SSD* is measured.

The field is treated with 6 Mev electrons except in an occasional patient when the chest wall flaps are unusually thick and 9 Mev electrons are used. The given dose is 5,500 rads in 4 weeks, 275 rads daily.

Peripheral Lymphatics and Retained Breast or Chest Wall after Wedge Excision, Total Mastectomy or Biopsy Only

SUPRACLAVICULAR AND ANTERIOR AXILLARY FIELD (FIG. 6-8A)

Position of Patient. Supine, upper arm abducted 90°, the forearm supported in upright position by a vertical arm board. The head turned sharply to the contralateral side (no pillows are used unless convexity of upper chest is extreme).

Angle of Beam. The beam is tilted 15° laterally to avoid irradiation of part of the trachea and esophagus and still to irradiate the deep inferior cervical nodes medial to the sternocleidomastoid muscle. Additionally, the tilt usually assures that nodes close to the margin of the pectoral muscle are included without requiring fall-off of the beam which would produce a moist desquamation.

Boundaries. The field covers the entire axilla and the supraclavicular fossa, including the deep inferior cervical nodes under the medial *SCM* insertion and the lower jugular nodes. The field size averages 150 to 160 sq cm (10 × 16 cm).

The *medial border*, drawn 1 cm over the

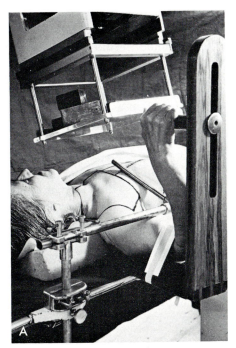
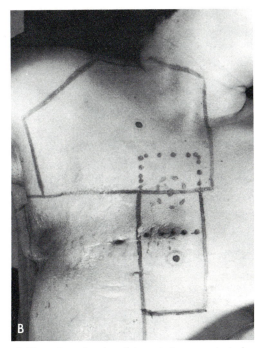

FIG. 6-8. A. Irradiation technique when the axilla is treated. The inferior border of the anterior supraclavicular-axillary portal is at the level of the second costal cartilage.

The patient is positioned with the head turned sharply to the contralateral side. The medial margin of the supraclavicular field extends 1 cm across the midline of the sternum. The lateral margin is drawn within the border of the pectoral muscle. A bar prevents the breast from flopping. The beam is tilted 15° laterally to avoid irradiation of part of the trachea and esophagus and still irradiate the deep inferior cervical nodes medial to the sternocleidomastoid muscle. Additionally, the tilt usually assures that nodes close to the margin of the pectoral muscle are included without requiring fall-off of the beam which would produce a moist desquamation.

The upper lobe of the lung, which is irradiated from the second rib upward, is not shielded. When a posterior axillary field is used, only a small strip of peripheral lung tissue is included and gross overdose is not given to the lung. Pneumonitis has been minimal and asymptomatic except for a short period of cough. Furthermore, there are possibly direct lymphatics into the intercostal spaces perforating the pectoral muscles which can be advantageously irradiated. The dose in the second interspace at 3 cm depth is increased because of the contiguity with the internal mammary chain field.

B. Supplemental field (dotted line) to first 3 interspaces. The patient had an 8 × 6.5 × 6 cm centrally located lesion with a 2 cm node in the axilla. (A—Courtesy: Delclos, Head, Department of Radiotherapy, Hospital General de Asturias, Oviedo, SPAIN.)

midline, extends superiorly to the thyrocricoid groove and inferiorly to the middle of the second costal cartilage and includes the first intercostal space. The *superior border* is drawn laterally from the medial border and extends to approximately 1–2 cm inside the margin of the pectoral muscle unless fall-off is needed. The *lateral border* is drawn across the upper arm with as much of the shoulder joint as possible being excluded. The field

margin may be sufficiently lateral to include the entire axillary contents. If the axilla is concave, the beam is kept slightly within the pectoral margin to avoid fall-off. Fall-off is needed if the axilla bulges beyond the pectoral margin (due to obesity or to enlarged nodes).

SSD. 70 cm or greater, if necessary for field size. The *SSD* point is placed near the area in the supraclavicular field where 5,000 rads *TD* is to be delivered. If the *SSD* is not at the same level as the axilla, a separate dose calculation is made for the axilla.

Dose. 5,000 rads given dose in 5 weeks, 200 rads daily.

POSTERIOR AXILLARY FIELD (FIG. 6-9)

Position of Patient. Prone, head turned to the contralateral side, without pillows, forearm rotated down, the shoulder in contact with table top, and back of hand on pelvic brim.

Beam. Vertical.

Boundaries. The *medial superior border* follows the spine of the scapula and the *lateral-superior border* bisects the humeral head. The *medial border* should include the convex lateral wall of the bony thorax and 1 to 1.5 cm of lung (as seen on verification film). The *inferior border* should, in most cases, match the lower border of the supraclavicular field anteriorly. This inferior border can be tailored to include disease in the axilla, *i.e.,* moved down to include palpable low axillary nodes. However, whether or not fall-off should occur across the latissimus dorsi depends on the location of nodes. Except where there are protruding axillary nodes, the *lower lateral border* is drawn slightly medial to the border of the latissimus dorsi.

SSD. 70 cm at the level of the apex of the axilla.

Dose. 2,500 to 3,000 rads given dose, 200 rads per treatment, usually two treatments per week, to bring the midaxilla dose to 5,000 rads.

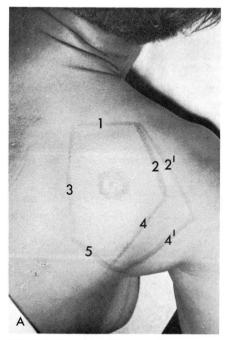
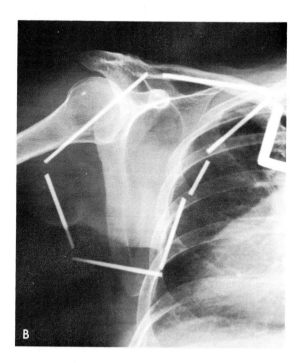

FIG. 6-9. Posterior axillary portal
    A. With protracted irradiation alone or with total mastectomy, more generous coverage of the axilla is necessary (2′ and 4′). **B.** Verification film. A thin strip of lung must be included to assure coverage of the lymphatics along the veins which skirt the chest wall.

INTERNAL MAMMARY FIELD

Boundaries. The *medial border* is drawn at the midline. The *lateral border* is drawn 6 cm from and parallel to the medial border. The *superior border* is at the level of the inferior border of the supraclavicular field. The *inferior border* crosses the base of the xyphoid.

Dose. 5,000 rads given dose in 5 weeks, 200 rads daily. In patients with high risk of infestation of the internal mammary chain nodes, the first three interspaces receive additional treatment—650 rads given dose to provide 5,000 rads tumor dose at 3 cm depth (Fig. 6-8B).

TANGENTIAL CHEST WALL FIELDS (FIG. 6-10)

Fields. The upper boundary is defined by the lower margin of the supraclavicular field which is at the level of the second costal cartilage. The medial and lateral beams are opposed. The breast bridge, with a rolling ball inclinometer, is fitted to the lateral and medial margins of the tangential fields to measure their separations and angles.

The *medial field* abuts the lateral border of the internal mammary field unless an overlap of the two fields is desired. In this case, the total dose in the area of the overlap must be taken into consideration. The *lateral field* is aligned with the midaxillary line. If the surgical scar extends beyond the midaxillary line, either the lateral field should be drawn so that there is an adequate margin beyond the scar or a ⁶⁰Co tangential field can be used to cover this part of the scar. The lower border of the supraclavicular field provides the *superior border* of the tangential fields. The *inferior border* of the tangential fields extends across the chest wall at the level of the tip of the xyphoid to include the area of the inframammary fold.

SSD. 70 cm.

Doses. The medial and lateral fields should optimally be treated every day. Using the transverse contour of the midportion of the chest wall, isodose distributions are made with bolus and without bolus (Fig. 6-11). The percentage of bolused treatment must be increased with 4 and 6 Mev linear accelerators to produce a brisk erythema with dry desquamation. The daily given dose is calculated to give 1,000 rads tumor dose per week at the following depths: a) 2–2.5 cm for postradical mastectomy chest wall irradiation, b) 3–3.5 cm for posttotal mastectomy, c) excised tumor depth for postwedge excision, and d) maximum tumor depth in irradiation alone.

IRRADIATION AFTER WEDGE EXCISION

Five thousand rads given dose are delivered in 5 weeks to the supraclavicular area and axilla, 200 rads daily. The posterior axillary portal is given sufficient dosage to provide 5,000 rads tumor dose to the midaxilla in 5 weeks. A boost through reduced fields, using the electron beam or ⁶⁰Co, is given to the axilla when axillary node(s) are palpable prior to treatment. The tumor dose is 1,000 rads in 5 treatments if the node(s) disappear during therapy, and 1,500 to 2,000 rads if the node(s) are still palpable after 5,000 rads tumor dose to the axilla.

Bolus is used for the first one or 2 weeks and alternates with treatment without bolus. A tumor dose of 5,000 rads is delivered in 5 weeks to the depth of the excised tumor. If there is known residual tumor, a boost of 1,000 rads may be given to the tumor-bearing area through a reduced field with the electron beam or ⁶⁰Co.

IRRADIATION PRIOR TO RADICAL MASTECTOMY

Coverage of the axilla (Fig. 6-9) should be kept as "economical" as possible, without compromising coverage of palpable nodes. It is advisable to avoid fall-off at the margins

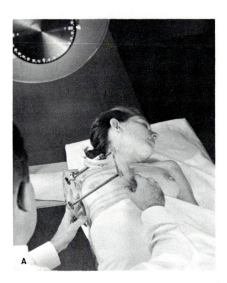

FIG. 6-10. Tangential chest wall fields. Optimally both fields should be treated every day.

The patient is supine, in the same position as that used for the anterior supraclavicular and axillary field. The medial field abuts the lateral border of the internal mammary field. The breast bridge **A** and **B,** with a rolling ball inclinometer, is fitted to the medial and lateral margins of the tangential fields to measure their separation and angles.

An applicator has been designed for the tangential portals to eliminate penumbra and divergence.

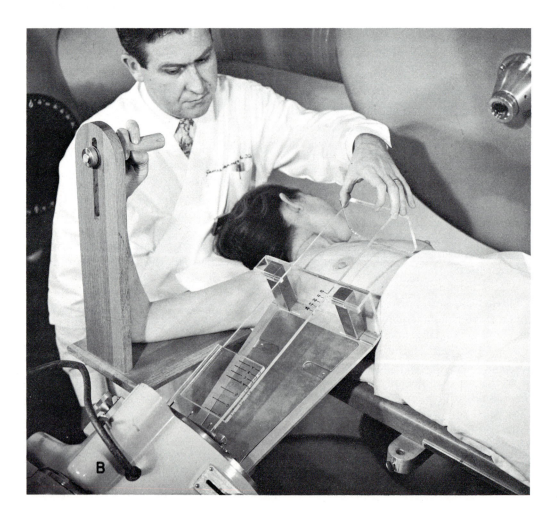

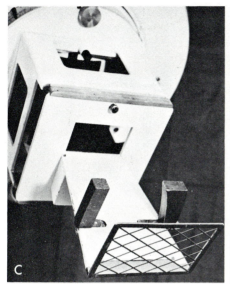

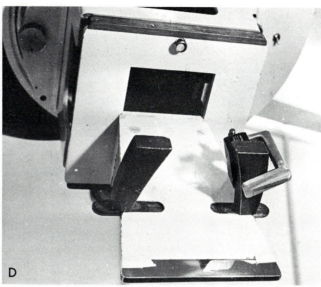

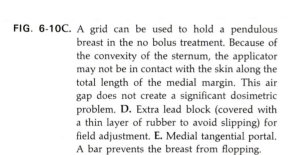

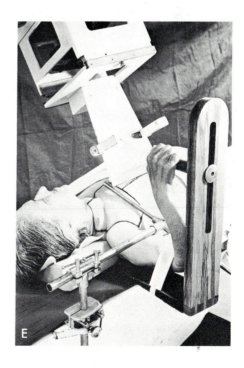

FIG. 6-10C. A grid can be used to hold a pendulous breast in the no bolus treatment. Because of the convexity of the sternum, the applicator may not be in contact with the skin along the total length of the medial margin. This air gap does not create a significant dosimetric problem. **D.** Extra lead block (covered with a thin layer of rubber to avoid slipping) for field adjustment. **E.** Medial tangential portal. A bar prevents the breast from flopping.

of the pectoral and latissimus dorsi muscles and to avoid overlap of the lateral tangential field with the posterior axillary field. The apex of the axilla, which is not treated surgically, must be well covered. The rationale for this conservatism is based on the fact that after surgery, recurrence in the axilla is not a problem.

The dose to the anterior supraclavicular-axillary field is 5,000 rads given dose in 5 weeks, 200 rads daily. Sufficient dosage is given to the posterior axillary field to give

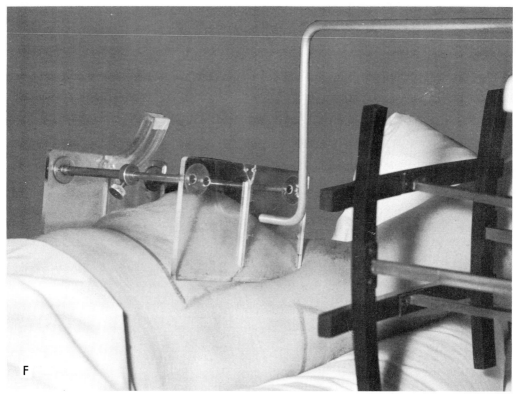

FIG. 6-10F. If the unit does not have an isocentric or rotation suspension mechanism, the patient is propped on pillows until the rolling ball inclinometer shows that the plates of the breast bridge are vertical. If the therapist does not have a breast applicator (that lack can be easily remedied and it is recommended to do so) the fields are set up with a pointer, and the trimmers are completely out. If bolus is to be used, the breast bridge is filled in with rice bags between the plates.

To avoid an unirradiated wedge of breast occurring between the internal mammary field, the medial tangential field, and the chest wall in an unusually convex rib cage and/or firm full breast, it may be necessary to overlap the adjacent borders of the internal mammary field and the medial tangential fields, in which case the total dose in the area of overlap should be taken into consideration. (Courtesy: Fletcher: *Amer. J. Roentgenol.* 84, 761, 1960. C, D and E: Courtesy: Delclos: Head, Department of Radiotherapy Hospital General de Asturias Oviedo, SPAIN.)

4,000 rads tumor dose to the midaxilla in 5 weeks. Usually 800 to 1,000 rads total given dose (200 rads per treatment) are delivered in two treatments per week.

The breast fields are treated on alternate days; 4,000 rads tumor dose in 4 weeks are given to the midbreast. To ensure maximum skin sparing, bolus is not used.

POSTTOTAL OR SIMPLE MASTECTOMY

Five thousand rads in 5 weeks are given to a depth of 2.5–3.5 cm, depending upon the extent of the disease, 200 rads daily. The number of bolus treatments for each tangential field varies from 2 to 4, depending on the depth of the isodose curve selected, the extent of initial disease, the flatness of the chest wall, and whether the scar is longitudinal or transverse.

With extensive initial disease and a high risk of chest wall recurrence, the entire mastectomy scar (Fig. 6-13) is given additional treatment with the electron beam or with tangential ^{60}Co fields. The width of the strip depends upon the initial disease. If the scar

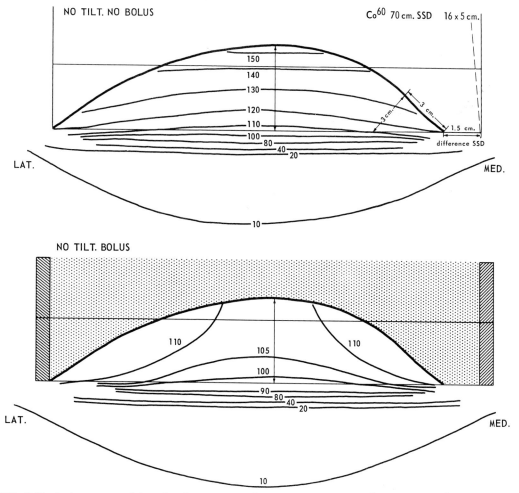

FIG. 6-11. Isodose curves of dose distribution across chest wall with tangential ^{60}Co fields.

On the medial border, although the light follows the line drawn, the applicator may not be in contact with the skin along the full length because of the convexity of the sternum. It creates a slight dosimetric variation because of *SSD* difference.

1. With the posttotal mastectomy technique, the use of alternating bolus is varied according to the depth selected for the tumor dose. It is usually excluded in the fourth and fifth weeks.

2. If the chest is very flat, little or no bolus is used because the beam is glancing with more superficial build-up.

3. The isodose selected in the no bolus volume distribution is 2–2.5 cm below the skin (130 per cent in this case). With increased disease in a thick chest wall, it may be selected at 3–3.5 cm (115 to 120 per cent in this case). In this instance, one should consider using less bolus or even no bolus because the dose to most of the skin is 10 to 20 per cent more than the selected isodose for tumor dose.

4. When there is minimal disease, the isodose at mid distance in the no bolus volume distribution (130 per cent in this case) may be chosen.

5. With the intact breast in Categories III and IV disease, one takes the isodose at the maximal depth of the tumor, never less than the midbreast.

One risks a moist desquamation because of the high skin dose if the depth dose selected results in too wide a range, *i.e.*, 150 per cent at the surface and 110 per cent at the depth.

6. When a separate internal mammary chain field is not used, the medial tangential field is tilted 10° (dotted line). The location of the internal mammary chain nodes is 3 cm from the sternal border and 3 cm deep. The same tilt and calculations are used for the treatment with bolus.

7. With 4 or 6 Mev accelerators the percentage of treatment with bolus must be increased to produce a marked erythema with dry desquamation. The radiotherapist must experiment to determine the right percentage of bolused treatment.

DOSE SCHEDULES AND TREATMENT FIELDS

FIELDS	WEDGE EXCISION Co60	POST-RADICAL MASTECTOMY — ELECTRON BEAM — PERIPHERAL LYMPHATICS	POST-RADICAL MASTECTOMY — ELECTRON BEAM — PERIPHERAL LYMPHATICS CHEST WALL	POST-RADICAL MASTECTOMY — Co60 — PERIPHERAL LYMPHATICS	POST-RADICAL MASTECTOMY — Co60 — PERIPHERAL LYMPHATICS CHEST WALL	PRE-OPERATIVE IRRADIATION Co60	PRIMARY IRRADIATION Co60 — WITH TOTAL MASTECTOMY	PRIMARY IRRADIATION Co60 — IRRADIATION ALONE
BREAST AND CHEST WALL A and B	5000 T.D./5 wks.		5500 G.D./6 Mev (275 G.D. x 20)		5000 T.D./5 wks.	4000 T.D./4 wks.	5000 T.D.	6000 T.D.
SUPRACLAVICULAR INTERNAL MAMMARY NODES** C and E	5000 G.D. (200 G.D. x 25)	5000 G.D./12 Mev (250 G.D. x 20); 5000 G.D./15 Mev (250 G.D. x 20)	5000 G.D./12 Mev (250 G.D. x 20); 5000 G.D./15 Mev (250 G.D. x 20)	5000 G.D. (250 G.D. x 20)	5000 G.D./20 Rx (250 G.D. x 20)	5000 G.D. (200 G.D. x 25)	5000 G.D. (200 G.D. x 25) See text	5000 G.D. (200 G.D. x 25) See text
POSTERIOR AXILLARY D	q.s. ad. 5000 T.D./5 wks.	—	—	—	—	q.s. ad. 4000 T.D./5 wks.	q.s. ad. 5000 T.D.	q.s. ad. 5000 T.D.
BOLUS	2 wks alternating only		Alternating depending on skin flaps			NO	Bolus - see text	Bolus - see text
TOTAL TREATMENT TIME	5 wks.	4 wks.	4 wks.	4 wks.	5 wks.-chest wall 4 wks.-peripheral lymphatics	4 wks.-Breast 5 wks.-Axilla, supraclavicular internal mammary chain	5 wks.	5 wks.-peripheral 8 wks.-breast
BOOST***	Elective Boost over primary site - 1000 T.D./5 days AXILLA--Initially clinically positive nodes 1. No longer palpable 1000 T.D. (5 x 200 T.D.) 2. Still palpable 1500-2000 T.D.						*** PRIMARY--Elective Boost to scar with ↑ risk of recurrence 1000 T.D./5 days AXILLA--As stated SUPRACLAVICULAR AREA-- Same as axilla	*** PRIMARY--Residual Disease 3000 T.D./2 weeks AXILLA AMD SUPRA CLAVICULAR AREA-- As in post total

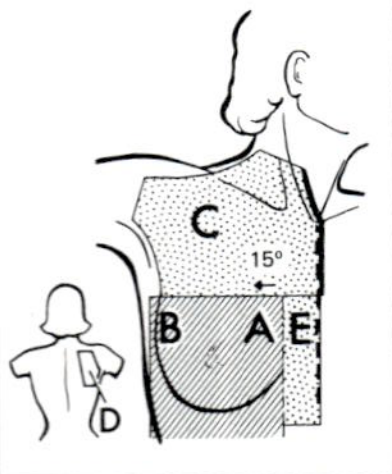

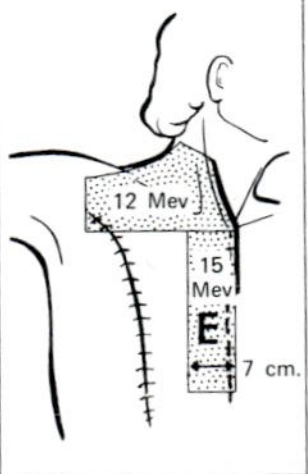

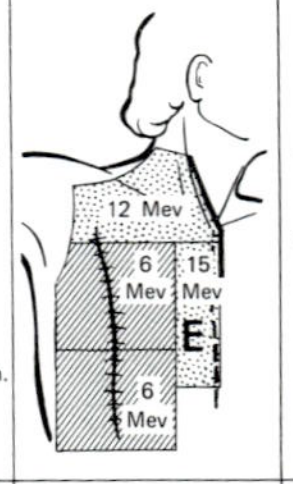

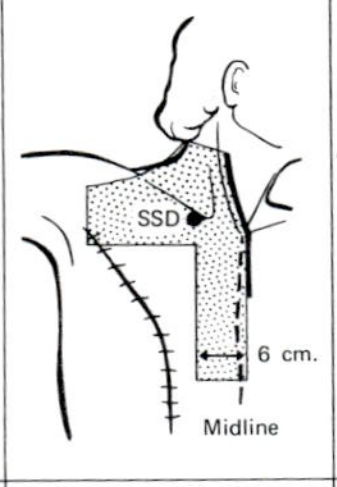

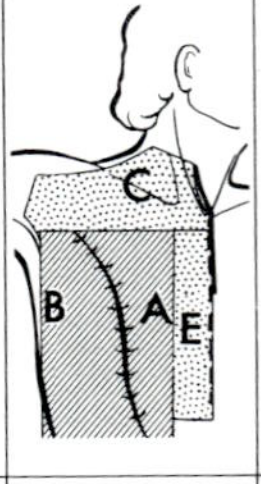

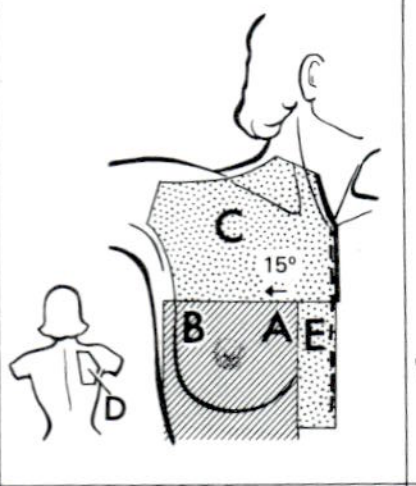

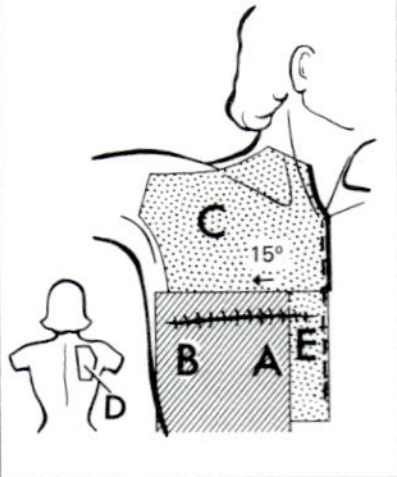

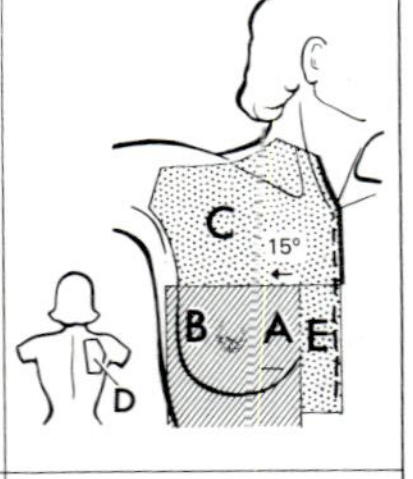

* In patients with low risk of infestation of the supraclavicular area, the given dose to the C field can be limited to 4,500 rads.

** The first three interspaces received 5,000 rads tumor dose at 3 cm. if there is a higher risk of infestation of the internal mammary chain.

*** Reduced fields.

FIG. 6-12. Schematic drawings and summary of dose schedules which do not give details of portals or dosimetry. One must refer to individual sections for details.

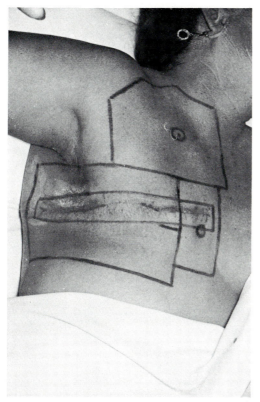

FIG. 6-13. Boost therapy may be given to a strip of the chest wall which will include the mastectomy scar. The dose, width, and length of the field varies with the initial extent of disease and the depth of the isodose curve chosen for the minimum tumor dose to the chest wall.

During ^{60}Co therapy a wet gauze strip is used every other day on the part of the scar which is in the internal mammary chain field to provide build-up depth with a direct beam.

Patients with total mastectomy for favorable primary tumors should have only 4,500 rads tumor dose to the chest wall. Those patients with extensive axillary dissection should receive 4,000 rads tumor dose to the midlevel of the axilla. The given dose to the anterior supraclavicular-axillary portal is 5,000 rads which gives 5,000 rads to the lymphatics of the supraclavicular and infraclavicular areas (apex of axilla). The given dose to the posterior portal is that which is sufficient to deliver 4,000 rads to the midaxilla.

Both tangential fields should be irradiated each treatment day to eliminate the lateral tissue effect which contributes to the development of fibrosis and rib radiation osteitis.

is vertical, only that portion which extends into the supraclavicular field requires boost treatment, as the dose to the scar given via the chest wall fields will be 10 to 20 per cent higher than the tumor dose at the selected depth. If the scar extends into the internal mammary field, a wet gauze strip is used every other day to increase the dose to the surface of the scar. If indicated, an electron beam boost is given to the entire chest wall using 6 or 9 Mev electrons. The given dose is 1,000 rads in 4 treatments to 1,500 rads in 6 treatments.

At completion of treatment, if axillary node(s) were initially palpable, additional treatment is given through a small portal, usually appositional, to cover the area of the node. Using ^{60}Co or the electron beam, 1,000 rads tumor dose is given in 5 days. The tumor dose is increased to 1,500 to 2,000 rads in 7 to 10 treatments if the node(s) are still palpable at the end of treatment.

PROTRACTED IRRADIATION ALONE (BACLESSE'S TECHNIQUE)

A tumor dose of 6,000 rads is delivered to the breast in 8 weeks (750 rads *TD* per week), selecting the isodose curve deep to the palpable mass. In order to give a satisfactory dose to the breast skin, bolus should be used alternately during the first 3 or 4 weeks and again in the seventh and eighth weeks if the skin reaction has not reached a dry desquamation.

The supraclavicular fossa receives 5,000 rads given dose in 5 weeks. Sufficient dosage is given to the posterior axillary portal to bring the midaxilla dose to 5,000 rads.

The internal mammary field receives 5,000 rads in 5 weeks, 200 rads daily. The tumor dose to the first 3 interspaces is brought up to 5,000 rads at 3 cm depth. The given dose varies according to size of the field, etc.

The additional treatment is given if indicated for residual disease in the breast, axilla, or supraclavicular fossa (Fig. 6-14). The technique used depends upon the location and

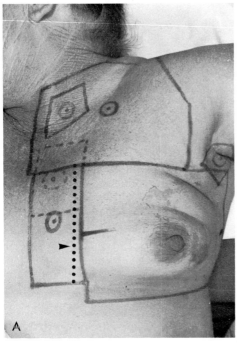
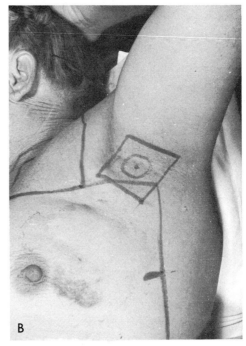

FIG. 6-14. A. Patient with a mass 6 cm in diameter, multiple axillary nodes and a hard 1 cm node in the supraclavicular area. After 5,000 rads given dose in 5 weeks to the anterior supraclavicular-axillary field, 1,800 rads were given to the posterior axillary portal for 5,000 rads tumor dose in the midaxilla. Boosts were given of 1,000 rads to the axilla through an appositional portal, 1,000 rads to the area where a supraclavicular node was palpated, and 650 rads to the first 3 interspaces to make 5,650 rads given dose to the internal mammary chain field for 5,000 rads at 3 cm depth. The corpus mammae received 6,000 rads in 8 weeks followed by 2,000 rads with a squeeze bridge.

The dotted line shown is an adjusted tangential portal border to avoid a wedge of unirradiated breast tissue if the breast is thick under the lateral border of the internal mammary chain field.

B. Appositional boost field to area of residual node in axilla.

size of the mammary lesion. The boost is given at the completion of treatment; to the supraclavicular-axillary area, after 5 weeks, and to the breast, after 8 weeks. If the skin reaction precludes immediate additional treatment, boost therapy is delayed for 3 to 4 weeks.

Additional dose to the mass in the breast can usually be given by squeeze technique with ^{60}Co. The tumor mass is compressed between the two plates of a bridge (Fig. 6-15). The dose varies from 2,000 rads *TD* in 2 weeks to 3,000 rads *TD* in 3 weeks. If an electron beam is available, it may be preferable to treat with an appositional portal. The dosage and electron energy are selected according to the size of the initial lesion and the residual disease. The dose range is 2,500 to 3,750 rads given dose; 250 or 300 rads daily, depending on the size of the field and energy used.

TECHNIQUE WITHOUT A SEPARATE INTERNAL MAMMARY CHAIN FIELD (FIG. 6-16)

Tangential chest wall fields without a separate internal mammary field are used for very small patients when the breast has not been removed and a significant portion of the corpus mammae would be included in the internal mammary chain field. One can use

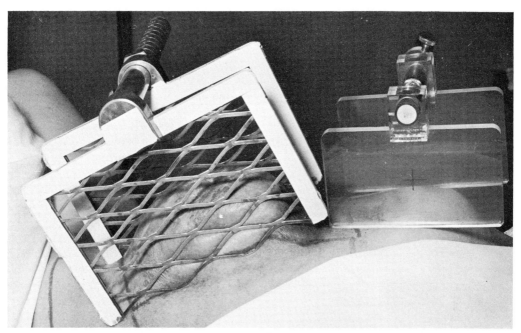

FIG. 6-15. Tangential compression bridges for delivery of additional irradiation to reduced volume. The plastic
cone is used to achieve maximum build-up if the skin is grossly involved.

    Following the basic dose of 6,000 rads to the breast through the tangential fields, residual tumor
is then given additional treatment with reduced fields eliminating as much of the uninvolved breast
as possible. The dose depends on amount of disease present, from 1,500 to 3,000 rads midline bridge
dose in 5 to 10 treatments. (Courtesy: Fletcher and Montague, *Amer. J. Roentgen.*, 93, 573, 1965.)

this technique with a bridge separation of up
to about 18–19 cm without an excessive drop
in dose to the midbreast or the midchest
wall.

    Specific changes must be made in the
placement of the tangential chest wall fields
in order to include the internal mammary
chain nodes, assumed to be located 3 cm
deep to the parasternal line and 3 cm from
the midline. In order to ensure the inclusion
of the internal mammary chain, the medial
aspect of the medial tangential portal is 1 cm
on the opposite side of the midline (Fig.
6-16A) and the medial tangential beam is
tilted 10° downward (Fig. 6-15 and 6-16B).
Thus, the tangential fields are not parallel
opposed. The lateral margin of the tangential
field is aligned with the midaxillary line.

    With a given dose of 5,000 rads to the
anterior supraclavicular-axillary portal, the
first interspace receives 4,500 rads at 3 cm.

The dose to the remaining interspaces is
approximately 110 per cent of the given dose
to the tangential fields. An appositional portal (Fig. 6-16A) to the second and third interspaces is added to bring the dose at 3 cm
depth to 4,500 rads, or up to 5,000 rads if
there is a high risk of involvement of the
internal mammary chain nodes. The latter
requires that the first interspace receive an
extra given dose to bring the tumor dose to
5,000 rads.

Palliative Irradiation for Carcinoma of Breast

    Palliative irradiation for advanced breast
cancer is given for:

    1) Growth restraint and potential growth
control with advanced local disease (Category IV) and no evidence of distant metastasis.

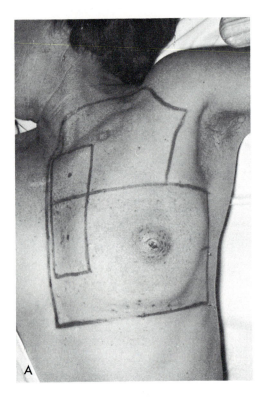

A

2) Control of pain, bleeding, or discharge in advanced local tumors in patients with distant metastases.

Four thousand rads tumor dose are delivered in 3 weeks (15 fractions) to the breast, the midaxilla, the supraclavicular, and internal mammary chain fields. Supplementary treatment, as with an [198]Au seed implant to give an additional 3,000 rads, is necessary to ensure tumor growth control. Two patients, alive at 16 months, who did not receive supplementary treatment to the primary mass have had clinical regrowth of the breast tumor.

When radiation therapy is given in conjunction with chemotherapy (usually 5-FU), the dose rate is reduced to 250 rads tumor dose per day for the first 2 weeks. If skin tolerance permits, the dose rate is increased to 275 to 300 rads tumor dose toward the last half of treatment. In these instances, 4,000 rads tumor dose may be delivered in 4 weeks instead of 3 weeks, followed by supplementary irradiation to residual tumor masses. Skin reactions have not been a problem nor has there been difficulty with the patient's tolerance to treatment.

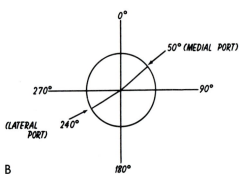

B

FIG. 6-16. Technique without a separate internal mammary chain field. **A.** The bridge separation is 18 cm and the given dose to each tangential chest wall field is 3,000 rads. To bring the dose to the second and third interspaces to 4,500 rads, the internal mammary chain field drawn within the tangential fields is given 1,350 rads. **B.** Drawing of the therapy chart record of the angles of the tangential fields. The medial tangential field is tilted 10° downward if a separate internal mammary chain field is not used. This increased tilt assures coverage of the internal mammary chain nodes.

TECHNIQUE

The same techniques are used as those described for treatment of the peripheral lymphatics and retained breast except that a separate internal mammary chain field is very rarely used. A posterior axillary field delivers additional irradiation to bring the total midaxillary doses to 4,000 rads.

BOOST

In patients who have no clinical evidence of distant metastases, supplemental treatment is given to the breast tumor and palpable nodes. There is usually a rest of one to 2 weeks after the initial treatment. If residual palpable disease is present, boosts of 1,000 to 1,500 rads are given in 3 to 5 days to reduced fields in the supraclavicular, axillary or breast areas. Frequently, the boost to the primary tumor in the breast is given by means of an ^{198}Au seed implant. This can be done on an outpatient basis under local anesthesia.

Complications

Irradiation Combined with Radical Mastectomy

With ^{137}Cs, ^{60}Co, or the electron beam, the skin reaction is usually mild; late skin changes with ^{137}Cs or ^{60}Co are almost unnoticeable, constituting only a slight difference in the texture of the skin. Electron beam therapy, with 5,000 rads given dose to the peripheral lymphatics and 5,500 rads given dose to the chest wall in 4 weeks, occasionally causes moderate telangiectasia and fibrosis but the incidence of these has decreased significantly with a 10 per cent decrease from the dose originally given.

The incidence of symptomatic radiation pneumonitis has been low, using a field 6 cm wide for the ipsilateral internal mammary chain. A streak of fibrosis in the parasternal area is seen in a small percentage of the patients.[19] Asymptomatic radiation fibrosis in the apex of the upper medial lung margin develops in almost all patients treated with either postoperative or preoperative irradiation.

Irradiation to the entire chest wall with tangential fields may result in acute and late complications. Symptomatic pneumonitis and pulmonary fibrosis are possible sequelae that can be avoided by 6 Mev electron beam fields.

Occasional arm edema is observed in radical mastectomy patients. Cardiac complications following irradiation given before or after radical mastectomy have not occurred with the techniques used.

Radical Radiation Therapy

With ^{60}Co the chest wall necrosis rate is 5 per cent. The majority of these necroses

have healed within 6 months. Long standing and troublesome necroses have been eliminated in 5 instances by simple mastectomy. The pain secondary to the necrosis is immediately alleviated with removal of the necrotic ulcer. Wound healing will be delayed after the intensive irradiation.

Approximately 10 per cent of the patients treated with total mastectomy and radical irradiation have had symptomatic pneumonitis requiring conservative treatment. The incidence is 3 per cent in protracted irradiation patients without total mastectomy. In those patients having had a total mastectomy, more lung tissue is usually included because treatment must be given to the entire length of the scar.

Arm edema is rare, having occurred in only 5 patients; in at least 2 of these there were chest wall and/or axillary recurrences of disease. Severe axillary fibrosis and chest wall fibrosis have occurred in patients treated with kilovoltage and megavoltage irradiation, but are more common with kilovoltage. With marked axillary fibrosis, limitation of motion of the involved shoulder becomes severe and can be aided only partially by physical medicine. The complication of limitation of motion has occurred less often since prophylactic physiotherapy has been started routinely at the beginning of radiation therapy.

About 5 per cent of patients treated with radical irradiation have developed rib fractures, usually in a single rib. These fractures were frequently asymptomatic or became so in several months with healing.

Symptomatic cardiac abnormalities and pericardial effusion, with 2 cases of tamponade, have been observed in 5 patients (2 with simple mastectomy) in the radical irradiation group. Following pericardiocentesis (cells positive for malignancy), additional irradiation to the mediastinum and pericardium temporarily improved the clinical status. At autopsy all 5 patients had tumor in the pericardium and myocardium.

Following total mastectomy and irradiation, 10 per cent of the patients developed rib fractures—half of them in one rib. Symptoms developed with multiple rib fractures, but were limited to 2 to 3 months in duration. Six per cent of patients had either chest wall or axillary necrosis, but 5 of these healed with conservative management in 3 to 14 months; one required surgery and grafting. Twelve per cent of patients have developed arm edema, but each patient had large either fixed or matted axillary nodes prior to surgery. The edema developed in half of the patients within 2 months of treatment. In only 2 patients was the edema severe and it was improved significantly with pneumomassage.

In an attempt to improve patient logistics by saving machine time, treatment fractionation for radical irradiation was changed from 5 days per week to 3 days per week in 1962. Doses were not altered, but the use of bolus was reduced. Immediate sequelae did not appear to increase, but with 12 to 18 months follow-up it became apparent that all complications increased in number and severity. This forced a return to 5 days per week fractionation.

Treatment for Recurrences

Chest Wall Recurrences

NO PREVIOUS IRRADIATION

A previous study[47] indicated that irradiation of the entire chest wall is the most effective treatment of chest wall recurrences, even if the initial recurrence is a single nodule. Using ^{60}Co with bolus for half of the treatment, 5,000 rads in 5 weeks are given to the chest wall. Only a brisk erythema develops. In the case of single or several small nodules recurring 5 years or more after surgery in elderly patients, it may be advisable not to use irradiation at all, treating with hormones or chemotherapy only if distant metastases eventually develop. If irradiation is used it should be limited to a small field and the peripheral lymphatics are not treated.

Surface molds carrying gamma sources are best used when the flap is thin and minimum penetration is desired (Fig. 1-32). With thicker surgical flaps, the chest wall can be treated by means of interstitial irradiation. Exposure to all personnel is minimized with afterloading techniques using ^{192}Ir wires and seeds, ^{198}Au seeds, ^{60}Co, etc. (Fig. 1-33).

If the electron beam is used for treating recurrent breast cancer in the chest wall, both the chest wall and the adjacent node-bearing areas are included if previous irradiation has not been given.[39] If the peripheral lymphatics have been irradiated, the chest wall only is treated. The given dose with the 6 or 9 Mev electron beam is 5,500 rads in 4 weeks, with an additional 1,000 to 1,500 rads through a reduced field to a residual mass. Nine Mev is used only if the soft tissues of the chest wall are thicker than 2.0 cm.

Results of treatment of 39 patients with chest wall recurrence are given in Table 6-3.[40] Five patients (13 per cent) are alive free of disease $3\frac{1}{2}$ to 7 years after treatment for recurrence. Skin nodules recurred within the irradiated field in 19 patients and outside the irradiated field in 3 patients, a local control rate in the chest wall of only 42 per cent. This is in contrast to an expected 90 per cent control rate in the chest wall after prophylactic irradiation.

PREVIOUS IRRADIATION

If the skin has received previous irradiation, further treatment will be possible for small areas only; each new group of nodules is treated as it appears. With the use of direct fields with the electron beam or with low kilovoltage and short treatment distances, doses of 3,000 to 3,500 rads in 5 days are sufficient to obtain growth restraint. If single treatments are desired, particularly in an attempt to control bleeding or odor or if disseminated disease is present, single exposures of 1,500 to 1,750 rads are used.

Peripheral Lymphatic Recurrences

In our experience, when a single peripheral lymphatic site has been treated for recurrence after mastectomy, patients surviving long enough will develop disease in the adjacent lymphatic area. In 4 parasternal recurrences with treatment only to the parasternal area, disease developed in the supraclavicular area within a period of 2 years. Conversely, 3 supraclavicular recurrences with no treatment other than to the supraclavicular area have recurred in the homolateral parasternal area. Consequently, with recurrence in one site prophylactic irradiation is delivered to the other site. The dose is 5,000 rads in 4 weeks, with an additional 1,000 to 2,000 rads (250 to 300 rads per treatment), to the initial disease area. The entire axilla may be irradiated if the axilla has not been radically dissected.

Axillary recurrences appear to be the most troublesome, mostly because they attain a large size or become painful before the patient, and frequently the doctor, are aware of them. Without previous irradiation, axillary recurrences are generally treated with 5,000 rads tumor dose through parallel opposed fields followed by an additional 1,000 to 2,000 rads tumor dose with appositional fields. There is very little that can be offered for the axillary recurrence which has received definitive radiation doses. We have found that these recurrences, in general, do not respond to chemotherapy or hormonal therapy. Occasionally patients who are incapacitated with bleeding or ulcerated masses in the axilla are best palliated with a forequarter amputation.

BIBLIOGRAPHY

1. Abrao, A., and DaSilva Neto, J. B.: Estudo anatomico de cadeia ganglionar mammana interna en 100 casos, *Rev. Paul Med.*, 45, 43, 1954.
2. Atkins, H. L.: Massive dose technique in radiation therapy of inoperable carcinoma of the breast, *Amer. J. Roentgen.*, 91, 80, 1964.
3. Atkins, H. L., and Horrigan, W. D.: Treatment of locally advanced carcinoma of the breast with roentgen therapy and simple mastectomy, *Amer. J. Roentgen.*, 85, 860, 1961.
4. Baclesse, F.: Roentgen therapy as sole method of treatment of cancer of breast, *Amer. J. Roentgen.*, 62, 311, 1949.
5. Baclesse, F.: Roentgen therapy alone in cancer in the breast, *Acta Un. Int. Cancr.*, 15, 1023, 1959.
6. Bloom, H. J. G.: III. The role of histology in the treatment of breast cancer, *Brit. J. Radiol.*, 29, 488, 1956.
7. Brown, G. R., Horiot, J-C, Fletcher, G. H., White, E. C., and Ange, D. W.: Simple mastectomy and irradiation for advanced breast cancers technically suitable for radical mastectomy, *Amer. J. Roentgen.*, publication pending.
8. Caceres, E.: An evaluation of radical mastectomy and extended radical mastectomy for cancer of the breast, *Surg. Gynec. Obstet.*, 125, 337, 1967.
9. Chu, F. C. H., Lucas, J. C., Jr., Farrow, J. H. and Nickson, J. J.: Does prophylactic radiation therapy given for cancer of the breast predispose to metastasis, *Amer. J. Roentgen.*, 99, 987, 1967.
10. Cutler, S. J. and Connelly, R. R.: Mammary cancer trends, *Cancer*, 23, 767, 1969.
11. Dahl-Iversen, E.: Recherches sur les metastases microscopiques des ganglions lymphatiques parasternaux dans le cancer due sein (recherches histologiques de 57 cas operes radicalement), *J. Internat. Chir.*, 11, 492, 1951.
12. Dao, T. L. and Kovaric, J. P.: Incidence of pulmonary and skin metastases in women with breast cancer who received postoperative irradiation, *Surgery*, 52, 203, 1962.
13. Edelman, A. H., Holtz, S. and Powers, W. E.: Rapid radiotherapy for inoperable carcinoma of breast: Benefits and complications, *Amer. J. Roentgen.*, 93, 585, 1965.
14. Edland, R. W., Maldonado, L. G., Johnson, R. O., Vermund, H.: Postoperative irradiation in breast cancer, *Radiology*, 93, 905, 1969.
15. Fletcher, G. H.: Control by irradiation of peripheral lymphatic disease in breast cancer, *Amer. J. Roentgen.*, 111, 115, 1971.
16. Fletcher, G. H.: Local results of irradiation in

the primary management of localized breast cancer, *Cancer*, 29, 545, 1972.

17. Fletcher, G. H., Braun, E. J., Moore, E. B., and Van Roosenbeek, E.: The design of a second 60Cobalt unit, based on the experience acquired with the first unit, *Amer. J. Roentgen.*, 84, 761, 1960.

18. Fletcher, G. H., and Montague, E. D.: Radical irradiation of advanced breast cancer, *Amer. J. Roentgen.*, 93, 573, 1965.

19. Fletcher, G. H., Montague, E. D., and White, E. C.: Evaluation of irradiation to the peripheral lymphatics in conjunction with radical mastectomy for breast cancer, *Cancer*, 21, 791, 1968.

20. Fletcher, G. H., Montague, E. D., and White, E. C.: Role of radiation therapy in the primary management of breast cancer. In *Progress in Clinical Cancer*, New York, Grune & Stratton, Inc., p. 242, 1970.

21. Gallager, H. S. and Martin, J. E.: The study of mammary carcinoma by mammography and whole organ sectioning, *Cancer*, 23, 855, 1969.

22. Gallager, H. S., and Hallauer, W. C.: Effects of radiation on human breast cancer (In Preparation).

23. Griscom, N. T., and Wang, C. C.: Radiation therapy of inoperable breast carcinoma, *Radiology*, 79, 18, 1962.

24. Guttman, R. J.: Effects of radiation on metastatic lymph nodes from various primary carcinomas, *Amer. J. Roentgen.*, 79, 79, 1958.

25. Haagensen, C. D.: *Disease of the Breast*, (2nd Ed.), Philadelphia, W. B. Saunders Company, 1971.

26. Haagensen, C. D. and Stout, A. P.: Carcinoma of the breast. II. Criteria of operability, *Ann. Surg.*, 118, 859, 1032, 1943.

27. Haagensen, C. D., Bhonslay, S. B., Guttman, R. J., Habif, D. V., Kister, S. J., Markowitz, A. M., Sanger, G., Tretter, P., Wiedel, P. D., and Cooley, E.: Metastasis of carcinoma of the breast to the periphery of the regional lymph node filter, *Ann. Surg.*, 169, 174, 1969.

28. Handley, R. S.: A surgeon's view of the spread of breast cancer, *Cancer*, 24, 1231, 1969.

29. Jackson, S. M.: Carcinoma of the breast—The significance of supraclavicular lymph node metastases, *Clin. Radiol.*, 17, 107, 1966.

30. Montague, E. D.: Adaptation of irradiation techniques to various types of surgical procedures for breast cancer, *Cancer*, 29, 557, 1972.

31. Peters, M. V.: Current cancer concepts— Wedge resection and irradiation, *J.A.M.A.*, 200, 134, 1967.

32. Rigby-Jones, H.: Personal Communication (1968).

33. Rissanen, P. M.: A comparison of conservative and radical surgery combined with radiotherapy in the treatment of Stage I carcinoma of the breast, *Brit. J. Radiol.*, 42, 423, 1969.

34. Robbins, G. C., Lucas, J. C., Fracchia, A. A., Farrow, J. H., and Chu, F. C. H.: An evaluation of postoperative prophylactic radiation therapy in breast cancer, *Surg. Gynec. Obstet.*, 122, 979, 1966.

35. Smith, J. C.: The superior treatment for carcinoma of the breast, *Surg. Gynec. Obstet.*, 132, 284, 1971.

36. Smithers, D. W. and Rigby-Jones, P.: Clinical evidence of parasternal lymph node involvement in neoplastic disease, *Acta Radiol.*, Suppl. 188, 235, 1959.

37. Spratt, J. S.: Locally recurrent cancer after radical mastectomy, *Cancer*, 20, 1051, 1967.

38. Stoll, B. A.: Rapid palliative irradiation of inoperable breast cancer, *Clin. Radiol.*, 15, 175, 1964.

39. Tapley, N. duV. and Fletcher, G. H.: Radiation therapy with electron beam: Current techniques, In *Radiologic Clinics of North America*, Vol. VII, Philadelphia, W. B. Saunders Company, p. 301, 1969.

40. Tapley, N. duV., and Fletcher, G. H.: Electron beam treatment of the chest wall after radical mastectomy, In *Breast Cancer—Early and Late*, Chicago, Year Book Medical Publishers, Inc., p. 281, 1970.

41. UICC (Union Internationale Contre le Cancer) TNM Classification of Malignant Tumours, Pocketbook prepared by the Committee on *TNM* Classification, Geneva, 1968, pp. 39–43. (UICC, P.O. Box 400, 1211 Geneva 2, Switzerland).

42. Urban, J. A.: Radical mastectomy in continuity with en bloc resection of internal mammary lymph node chain; new procedure for primary operable cancer of breast, *Cancer*, 5, 992, 1952.

43. Urban, J. A.: Clinical experience and results

of excision of the internal mammary lymph node chain in primary operable breast cancer, *Cancer,* 12, 14, 1959.

44. Urban, J. A.: Personal Communication, May 1967.

45. Urban, J. A.: Bilateral breast cancer, In *Breast Cancer—Early and Late,* Chicago, Year Book Medical Publishers, Inc., p. 263, 1970.

46. Veronesi, U. and Zingo, L.: Extended mastectomy for cancer of the breast, *Cancer,* 20, 677, 1967.

47. Zimmerman, K. W., Montague, E. D., and Fletcher, G. H.: Frequency, anatomical distribution and management of local recurrences after definitive therapy for breast cancer, *Cancer,* 19, 67, 1966.

Metastasis from Breast Cancer

LUIS DELCLOS, and ELEANOR D. MONTAGUE

In order to obtain satisfactory palliation in the treatment of metastatic breast cancer, it is important to differentiate between bone metastases and metastases involving soft tissues, nodes, or nerves. Bony metastases respond well to low doses of radiation, whereas, other metastases require a higher dose for significant palliation.

Bone Metastases

Up to 80 per cent of pain and disability caused by bony metastases from breast cancer responds to x-ray treatment. In many instances, treatment is followed by restoration of bone, but sometimes, although there is symptomatic relief, no changes are seen in the diagnostic x-ray films.

It may be appropriate to combine bone irradiation with other measures. For instance, in the case of fractures, one might well advocate internal fixation procedures. When there are multiple bone metastases, irradiation may be combined with exogenous or ablative hormonal therapy or, when indicated, with systemic chemotherapy. Techniques and doses for megavoltage are shown in the diagrams of Figure 6-17. Bony metastasis should be treated with large fields encompassing all

of involved bone, *e.g.,* lesions of the supra-acetabular area should be treated with hemi-pelvic fields; midthoracic vertebral disease is treated with a field encompassing all the thoracic vertebrae.

One field is used when possible. If the part to be treated is thick or in the midline, two parallel opposing fields are used. When treating the whole pelvis, one posterior square field covering the sacrum and entire pelvis is used opposed by one anterior U-field, which prevents unnecessary irradiation to the bowel. If the sacrum requires treatment because of symptomatic disease, a small block can be placed above the pubis to eliminate unnecessary irradiation to the bowel.

It is desirable to make the course of treatment short so that it does not occupy a disproportionate part of the patient's remaining life. If the patient lives a great distance from the treatment center, or if the disease is advanced and the pain is severe, a single exposure will be adequate, *i.e.,* for a painful single bony metastasis one single exposure of 1,200 rads tumor dose will be sufficient to control the pain.

Treatment to small volumes is given in one week, and to larger volumes in two weeks.

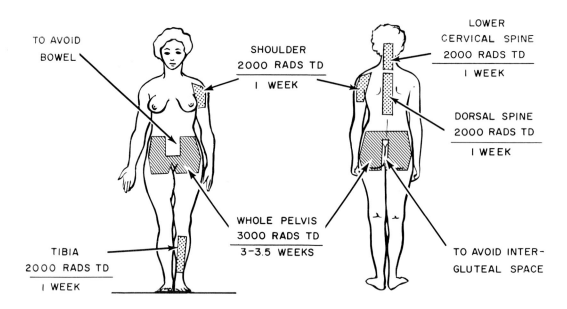

TO AVOID
BOWEL

SHOULDER
2000 RADS TD
——————
I WEEK

LOWER
CERVICAL SPINE
2000 RADS TD
——————
I WEEK

DORSAL SPINE
2000 RADS TD
——————
I WEEK

WHOLE PELVIS
3000 RADS TD
——————
3–3.5 WEEKS

TIBIA
2000 RADS TD
——————
I WEEK

TO AVOID INTER-
GLUTEAL SPACE

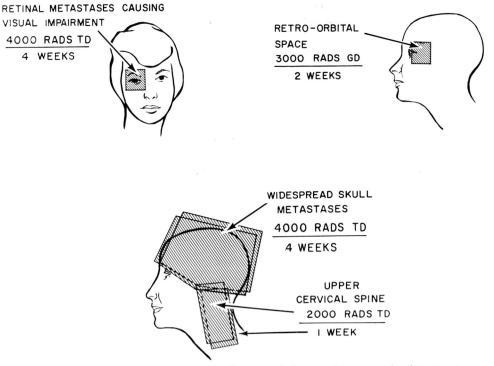

RETINAL METASTASES CAUSING
VISUAL IMPAIRMENT
4000 RADS TD
——————
4 WEEKS

RETRO-ORBITAL
SPACE
3000 RADS GD
——————
2 WEEKS

WIDESPREAD SKULL
METASTASES
4000 RADS TD
——————
4 WEEKS

UPPER
CERVICAL SPINE
2000 RADS TD
——————
I WEEK

FIG. 6-17. Selection of field arrangements, overall time, and dosages of treatment for distant metastases with megavoltage. The course of treatment is made short so that it does not occupy a disproportionate part of the patient's remaining life. It must be remembered that many patients will have to be treated several times for different metastases.

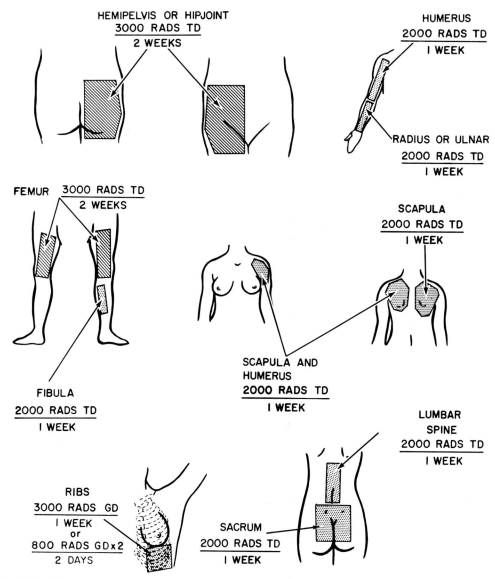

FIG. 6-17. (Cont.)

The whole pelvis is treated in three to three and one-half weeks. Megavoltage is recommended because of its skin sparing effect and the simplicity of achieving a greater depth dose.

Intrathoracic Metastases

Esophageal obstruction and/or a superior vena cava syndrome caused by mediastinal lymph node involvement may be appreciably relieved by 4,000 rads tumor dose in 4 weeks through 2 parallel opposing fields.

Orbital Metastases

A given dose of 3,000 rads in 2 weeks to a single temporal portal is, as a rule, effective for retro-orbital metastases.

Retinal or Choroid Metastases

Survival in these patients is very limited (90 per cent are dead in 2 years), but vision remains good if the metastasis is detected early. A tumor dose of 4,000 rads is delivered with an anterior field in 4 weeks; bilateral metastases are very common.

Soft Tissue Pelvic Metastases

Metastases in the "cul de sac" may call for pelvic irradiation if the cancer ulcerates through the vaginal epithelium and causes bleeding. Pain would be better managed by neurosurgical procedures than by irradiation.

Intracranial Metastases

Symptoms caused by intracranial metastases can be relieved by irradiation of the whole brain through two parallel opposing fields. A tumor dose of 3,000 rads given in two weeks is adequate if the prognosis for life is short (less than four months), but generally these patients are better treated by corticosteroids alone. If prognosis for life is greater than four months, 4,000 rads tumor dose in 4 weeks should be delivered to the whole brain. It has been the experience in some long-term survivors with metastases to the brain who presented without other vital organ metastases, such as lung or liver, that repeated courses of treatment for control of central nervous system symptoms were necessary with doses less than 4,000 rads. In these instances, it is indicated to consider 5,000 rads delivered in 5 weeks. Brain scans are helpful in determining regression of disease. High doses of corticosteroid therapy are given during the course of therapy and are gradually tapered off after completion of treatments.

Brachial Plexus Metastases

Patients who have recurrence in the supraclavicular area with brachial plexus involvement require high doses for relief of pain.

Fields include the low neck and supraclavicular area and extend medially to include the nerve roots exiting from C-5, 6, 7 and T-1 and 2. A tumor dose of 5,000 rads is delivered to the midline with parallel opposing fields followed by an additional 1,500 to 2,000 rads to residual masses through reduced fields. If skin tolerance becomes a problem, it is frequently necessary to let the patient have a rest for a week between the 5,000 rads and the boost. Even with a total dose of 6,500 to 7,000 rads, it has been our experience that only about 50 per cent of the patients experience significant pain relief.

Without involvement of brachial plexus, but with recurrent supraclavicular disease, treatment is delivered through an anterior field only and 5,000 rads given dose is delivered in 5 weeks, plus a boost of 1,500 to 2,000 rads to reduced fields.

Spinal Cord Involvement

In the event of neurological deficits related to spinal cord tumor, either by invasion or extrinsic pressure defect, doses on the order of 4,000 rads tumor dose are delivered in 4 weeks through a single posterior field.

Liver Metastases

In our experience, the patients with liver metastases are not improved measurably by x-ray therapy.

Pituitary Irradiation

With metastases to pituitary causing diabetes insipidus, irradiation has not relieved symptoms or signs.

BIBLIOGRAPHY

1. Delclos, L., and Johnson, G. C.: Palliative irradiation in breast cancer, *Radiology,* 83, 272, 1964.
2. Eckles, Nylene, and Sears, Mary: Personal communication.

Castration

LUIS DELCLOS

Irradiation of the ovaries is done to stop ovarian hormonal function. It is useful for premenopausal women and for those 1 to 2 years postmenopausal. Castration should be used preceding androgen therapy and other major ablative procedures. Irradiation is an alternate and a second choice to extirpative ovarian surgery as it is less predictable and slower to produce an effect; surgery also provides an opportunity to explore the abdomen for metastases. There occasionally has been an irradiated patient who subsequently became pregnant or who otherwise demonstrated quite overtly hormonal function; this noneffectiveness is to be attributed to either an abnormal anatomical position of the ovary, low dose, or inadequate size fields. A minimum of 1,200 rads tumor dose in 4 days or 2,200 rads tumor dose in 2 weeks are given through fields adequate to encompass the entire true pelvis with margins. Percentage wise, the over-all per cent response to castration is the same in patients castrated with irradiation as in those castrated with surgery.

7. The Lymphomatous Diseases

Introduction

RODNEY MILLION

The malignant lymphomas have recently come under considerable re-examination as to etiology, modes of spread, and new methods of treatment. In the past decade much information has been accumulated regarding Hodgkin's disease. Although there are similarities between Hodgkin's disease and the non-Hodgkin's lymphomas, one cannot extrapolate information from one group to the other. There has been an improvement in survival rates in Hodgkin's disease over the past decade,[4,5] but there is no convincing evidence that there has been any improvement for the non-Hodgkin's lymphomas.

Table 7-1 summarizes the differences in the two groups according to data gathered from the literature.

Anatomy for Treatment Planning
Head and Neck Nodes

Parapharyngeal nodes occasionally are involved in the lymphomas. These nodes lie

Table 7-1. *Comparison of Hodgkin's Disease, Lymphocytic Lymphomas, and Reticulum Cell*

	Hodgkin's Disease	Lymphocytic Lymphomas	Reticulum Cell
Age	Median 35	Median 50	Median 50
Sex	M:F = 1.7:1.0	M:F = 1.7:1.0	M:F = 1.7:1.0
Leukemic transformation	<1%	Adults 7% Children 33%	1–2%
Fever, night sweats, pruritus	39%	15%	15%
Per cent localized on admission (Stages I or II)	60%	50%	40%
Nodular pattern	50%	50%	10%
Contiguous spread on admission	80 to 90%	Unknown	Unknown
Primary nodal presentation	98%	60%	40%
Mesenteric nodes positive on admission	Rare	20–30%	Unknown
Extranodal on admission, all cases	10%	50%	70%
Primary extranodal presentation	2%	40%	60%
Waldeyer's ring	<1%	9%	12%
Gastrointestinal	<1%	12%	25%

anterior to the lateral mass of *C1* and would be on the edge of most *en face* neck treatment fields even if the submental region is not blocked; adequate treatment would depend on placement of the superior neck margin and degree of extension of the head in the treatment position, and whether the submental region or cervical cord are or are not shielded. No important nodes are left untreated by midline blocking from the thyroid notch to 1 to 2 cm below the border of the cricoid. The jugular chain lies very close to the lateral border of the thyroid cartilage and trachea, and tapered blocks are necessary to avoid low dose to this important group of nodes.

Axillary Nodes

Figure 7-1 shows two examples of axillary nodes outlined by lymphangiography. When visualized on an *AP* chest film, the low axillary nodes lie adjacent to the lateral rib cage, while the high axillary nodes are superimposed on the lateral curve of the first, second, and third ribs. The lowest axillary nodes usually will be encompassed by establishing a level even with the anterior fourth interspace. The lateral extent of the axillary nodes may be defined by the junction of the lateral margin of the pectoralis muscle with the deltoid muscle of the upper arm.

Figure 7-2 shows wire surrounding a 2.5 cm subclavicular node. The subclavicular nodes project medial to the rib cage on an *AP* simulator film, and therefore close attention must be made when drawing this portion of the line if lung blocks are traced from simulator chest x-rays. The subclavicular nodes will be encompassed if the medial axillary border of the mantle field is directed to the medial third of the clavicle.

Mediastinum

Since opposed fields are used to irradiate the mediastinum, only the lateral borders determine superior mediastinal and hilar

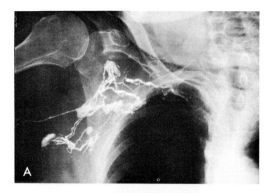

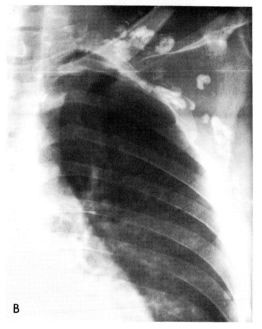

FIG. 7-1. **A.** Axillary nodes opacified by hand lymphangiogram. **B.** Axillary nodes opacified by reflux from foot lymphangiogram.

nodal inclusion. Frequent reports of marginal recurrences in the hilar and parahilar bronchopulmonary nodes dictate that these areas must be adequately treated.[7] The posterior intercostal and paraesophageal nodes in the inferior mediastinum are uncommonly involved, but nevertheless are included in the mantle for completeness.

The posterior intercostal nodes lie in a retropleural position in the crotch between the head of the ribs and the lateral border of the vertebrae. These nodes are usually

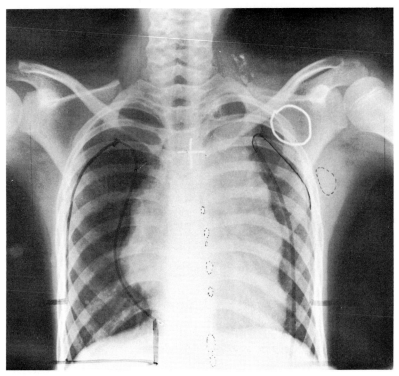

FIG. 7-2. Simulated chest x-rays on patient with bulky mediastinal nodes of Hodgkin's disease. Wire circle outlines 2.5 cm subclavicular node. Left midaxillary node circled in ink. Numerous small left paraesophageal nodes were filled on foot lymphangiogram and are outlined in ink.

small but when enlarged, they displace the pleural line laterally and can be diagnosed as a paravertebral mass on an overpenetrated film of the chest.[10] Figure 7-2 also shows left paraesophageal nodes outlined on a lymphangiogram.

The width of the lower mantle segment can usually be adjusted to about 1.5–2.0 cm lateral to the vertebral body and encompass the posterior intercostal and paraesophageal nodes. Attention to this detail is important to reduce lung and heart irradiation.

Spleen and Splenic Nodes

The spleen is situated in the left hypochondrium with its posterior superior surface against the diaphragm, which separates it from the posterior pulmonary sulcus. It is in contact with the posterior wall of the stomach, the left flexure of the colon, the left upper pole of the kidney, and generally in contact with the tail of the pancreas. In the adult, the spleen normally measures up to 16 cm in its longest axis, 7 cm in superior-inferior diameter, and about 3 to 4 cm thick. The position of the normal-sized spleen varies considerably and localization techniques such as plain film of the abdomen to show the tip of the spleen, splenic scintigram, and intravenous pyelogram are useful to avoid unnecessary irradiation of normal tissues.[6] Small nodules of splenic tissue, varying in size from that of a pea to a plum, may be found either isolated or connected to the spleen and are known as accessory spleens. They are usually found in the immediate neighborhood of the spleen, especially in the gastrosplenic ligament and greater omentum.

Several nodes lie in the hilum of the spleen

and there are usually 3 or 4 nodes scattered along the efferent lymphatic trunk which accompanies the splenic vessels along the superior margin of the pancreas to its termination in the celiac group of nodes (Fig. 7-3).[9]

The splenic vascular pedicle may retract to various positions after splenectomy, and metal clips are used to identify its position. The course of the splenic chain nodes is then an imaginary line between the pedicle and the origin of the celiac artery. The retroperitoneal position of the pedicle and splenic nodes allows treatment via a single posterior field in order to reduce irradiation of the stomach and colon.

Hepatic Nodes

The hepatic node chain includes 4 to 8 nodes located along the hepatic artery.[8] Usually there is one very large node at the origin of the hepatic artery from the celiac artery. The remainder of the hepatic nodes either accompany the horizontal part of the hepatic artery or are situated between layers of the lesser omentum in relation to the common bile duct. In the average-sized person, most of these nodes are included in 10 cm wide paraaortic node fields (Fig. 7-3).

Bone Marrow Distribution

The average estimated distribution of active red marrow for a normal 40-year-old is shown in Table 7-2.[2] Autopsy studies reveal that the marrow distribution in the femur and humerus varies considerably in adults.[3] Amos studied the pelvic marrow from both irradiated and nonirradiated areas in 8 patients with Hodgkin's disease and 4 non-Hodgkin's lymphomas from 6 to 54 months after completion of total nodal irradiation.[1] Partial recovery of the irradiated marrow occurs with a dose of 3,000 to 3,500 rads, and one patient showed recovery at 4,000 rads. Marrow from the anterior crest, outside the

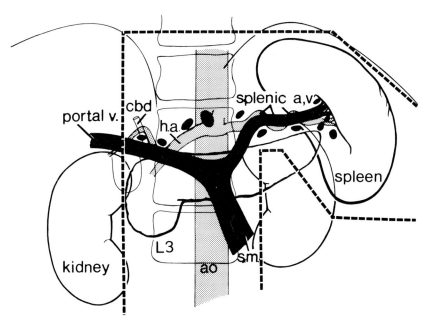

FIG. 7-3. Schematic drawing taken from a celiac angiogram showing pertinent relationships in upper abdomen. ao = aorta, cbd = common bile duct, ha = hepatic artery, sm = superior mesenteric vein.

A portal covering the spleen, celiac region and paraaortic nodes is shown with a dotted line. The paraaortic portal is 10 cm wide.

Table 7-2. *Marrow Distribution in Adults*
(40 Years Old)

Site	Per Cent
Head	13.1
Upper limb girdle (scapulae, clavicles, humeri)	8.3
Sternum	2.3
Ribs	7.9
Vertebrae	
Cervical	3.4
Thoracic	14.1
Lumbar	10.9
Sacrum	13.9
Lower girdle (pelvis, femoral head/neck)	26.1

Courtesy: Ellis, *Physics in Medicine and Biology*, 5, 255, 1961.

direct path of irradiation, appeared normal to slightly hypoplastic. Peripheral counts returned to normal in successfully treated patients.

BIBLIOGRAPHY

1. Amos, E. H., and Million, R. R.: Evaluation of the bone marrow after successful total nodal irradiation, To be published, 1972.
2. Ellis, R. E.: The distribution of active bone marrow in the adult, *Physics in Medicine and Biology*, 5, 255, 1961.
3. Hashimoto, M.: The distribution of active marrow in the bones of normal adult, *Kyushu J. Med. Sci.*, 11, 103, 1960.
4. Johnson, R. E., Thomas, L. B., Schneiderman, M., Glenn, D. W., Faw, F., and Hafermann, M. D.: Preliminary experience with total nodal irradiation in Hodgkin's disease, *Radiology*, 96, 603, 1970.
5. Kaplan, H. S.: On the natural history, treatment, and prognosis of Hodgkin's disease: *The Harvey Lectures*, Series 64, p. 215, 1968–69.
6. Kreel, L., and Mindel, S.: The radiographic position of the spleen, *Brit. J. Radiol.*, 42, 830, 1969.
7. Maruyama, Y., and Khan, F. M.: Blocking considerations in mantle therapy, *Radiology*, 101, 167, 1971.
8. Rouviere, H.: *Anatomy of the Human Lymphatic System*. Translated by M. J. Tobias, J. W. Edwards, Inc., Ann Arbor, Michigan, 1938.
9. Seydel, H. G., Bloedorn, F. G., and Wizenberg, M. J.: Results of radiotherapeutic treatment of relapsing Hodgkin's disease, *Cancer*, 23, 1033, 1969.
10. Witten, R. M., Fayos, J. V., and Lampe, I.: The dorsal paraspinal mass in Hodgkin's disease, *Amer. J. Roentgen.*, 94, 947, 1965.

Hodgkin's Disease

RODNEY R. MILLION

Pathology

At the Rye, New York, Conference on Hodgkin's Disease in 1966, a nomenclature committee proposed a workable histologic subclassification of Hodgkin's disease which has been adopted by most lymphologists.[20] Table 7-3 lists the distribution by stage of the new subclassification of Hodgkin's dis-

ease in 176 cases seen at Stanford Medical Center from 1956 to 1966.[19]

Three experienced lymphoma pathologists reviewed the 176 cases shown in Table 7-3 and all three agreed on the subtype of Hodgkin's disease in about two thirds of patients; 2 of the 3 pathologists agreed on a total of 92 per cent.[19] The attempts to evolve individualized treatment patterns based on the

Table 7-3. *Distribution of Histologic Types According to Anatomic Stage and Systemic Symptoms in 176 Previously Untreated Cases of Hodgkin's Disease*

Histology	Stage I & II		Stage III & IV		Symptoms A	B*
	No.	%	No.	%	No.	No.
Lymphocyte Predominance	8	7%	1	1%	9	0
Nodular Sclerosing	63	57%	29	45%	60	32
Mixed Cellularity	37	34%	28	43%	35	30
Lymphocyte Depletion	3	2%	7	11%	3	7
	111	100%	65	100%	107	69

*B = fever, night sweats, generalized pruritus. (Courtesy: Keller, Kaplan, Lukes, and Rappaport, *Cancer,* 22, 487, 1968.)

subtype of Hodgkin's depend on the pathologists' reliability in identifying the various patterns.

As one proceeds from lymphocyte predominance to lymphocyte depletion, fewer and fewer lymphocytes are found with, usually, a progressive increase in the number of Reed-Sternberg cells; diffuse fibrosis and reticular pattern become increasingly dominant.

Proceeding from the most favorable lymphocyte predominance group to the least favorable lymphocyte depletion group, the presenting stage becomes progressively more advanced and there is a greater likelihood of constitutional "B" symptoms, vascular invasion and extranodal involvement.

The four histologic types have different prognoses and different spread patterns, but there has been no study to date which has determined that a different radiation dosage or chemotherapeutic dosage is required for the various subhistologies.

Strum and Rappaport report 6 cases in which lymph node biopsy showed a lymph node pattern essentially preserved with only minute foci of Hodgkin's disease.[31] The difficulty in detecting minute foci reinforces the need for total nodal irradiation in the face of negative lymphangiogram and negative exploratory laparotomy.

Vascular invasion has been described in lymph node and splenic tissues by Rappaport and Strum; only veins were invaded.[24,29,32] Venous invasion occurs in about 6 per cent of Stage I and II cases and increases to 20 to 40 per cent of Stages III and IV. No vascular invasion was found in lymphocyte predominance groups, but was increasingly found in percentage as one progressed to the groups with poorer prognosis. Extranodal extension of disease after initial treatment was noted in 22 per cent of the patients with vascular invasion and in only 8 per cent of the patients without vascular invasion. Venous invasion in involved spleens was related to positive liver biopsies, suggesting a route of spread from the spleen to the liver via the portal vein.[29]

Spread Patterns

Most lymphologists accept the concept of a unifocal origin on Hodgkin's disease followed by predictable routes of spread. Spread of Hodgkin's disease follows mainly the lymphatic pathways. Evidence of vascular dissemination at the time of diagnosis is seen in about 10 per cent of cases, based on the incidence of venous invasion in nodes and of noncontiguous organ dissemination. Direct extension occurs when the tumor breaks through the nodal capsule and invades adjacent structures (*e.g.,* lung, pericardium, dura).

Lymphatic Spread Patterns

NODAL PATTERNS

Kaplan plotted the initial sites of lymphatic involvement in 340 consecutive untreated patients with Hodgkin's disease.[15] Table 7-4 outlines the distribution by site and the incidence of contiguity (the neck and paraaortic nodes are considered contiguous). In analyzing spread patterns, it is no longer tenable to think of the mediastinum as a skip area between the neck and the paraaortic nodes, since the thoracic duct usually bypasses these nodes. Excepting the right axilla, contiguous node involvement approaches 100 per cent.

Patients with bilateral neck or left neck adenopathy demonstrate a 50 per cent incidence of disease below the diaphragm, while involvement of right neck alone is associated with abdominal disease in approximately 7 per cent of cases studied.[14] These findings are consistent with the lymphatic connections between the abdomen and the neck. Johnson reports that 3 of 12 patients with

Stage I disease confined to the right neck had disease extended to the paraaortic nodes when no prophylactic irradiation was directed to the lumbar area; 3 of 8 with disease confined to the left neck later had disease extended to paraaortic nodes.[10]

Patients with Stage I disease clinically isolated to the upper neck have an exceptionally low rate of abdominal involvement.[6,23] Submental, preauricular node involvement and Waldeyer's ring involvement is slightly greater in patients with upper neck disease.

In the abdominal cavity, Hodgkin's disease selectively involves the paraaortic and splenic nodes. Inguinal and pelvic involvement is less common and usually is associated with late Stage III or Stage IV disease. Positive mesenteric nodes were documented in only 2 of 340 untreated cases of Hodgkin's disease at Stanford Medical Center.[15]

Hepatic nodes are rarely reported to be involved at exploratory laparotomy in untreated cases; fortuitously, most of the hepatic nodes are irradiated in the conventional paraaortic node fields (Fig. 7-3).

Table 7-4. *Hodgkin's Disease: Contiguity of Lymphatic Sites of Involvement in 340 Untreated Cases*

Site	Total No. instances involved	Sole site involved	Additional sites involved	Anatomic relationship to other sites		
				Non-contiguous	Contiguous	% Contiguous
1. Right axillary nodes	78	5	73	8	65	89
2. Left axillary nodes	90	3	87	3	84	97
3. Right cervical-supraclavicular nodes	199	12	187	1	186	99
4. Left cervical-supraclavicular nodes	241	23	218	6	212	97
5. Mediastinal nodes	211	5	206	1	205	99.5
6. Hilar nodes	39	0	39	0	39	100
7. Paraaortic nodes	114	1	113	1	112	99
8. Iliac, inguinal, femoral nodes	54	5	49	1	48	98
9. Spleen	44	0	44	5	39	88

(Courtesy: Kaplan, *The Harvey Lectures,* Series 64 1968, p. 215.)

NODAL SPREAD PATTERNS RELATED TO HISTOLOGY

Mediastinal involvement is characteristic of the nodular sclerosing group of Hodgkin's disease,[2] but rarely is the mediastinum the sole site of involvement (Table 7-4). Mediastinal involvement occurs over-all in 72 per cent of nodular sclerosing cases compared to 34 per cent of mixed cellularity. When preoperative assessment of the abdomen was negative or equivocal, nodular sclerosing Hodgkin's was discovered by laparotomy in only 3 of 17 cases (17 per cent) compared to about 50 per cent positive abdominal disease for mixed cellularity and lymphocyte predominance.

Lymphocyte predominance cases show a predilection for abdominal and peripheral adenopathy while rarely invading the mediastinum.

Mixed cellularity cases demonstrate a 62 per cent over-all chance of abdominal disease compared to 43 per cent of nodular sclerosing cases.[2]

SPLEEN

Based on the data gained from exploratory laparotomy in unselected cases, the clinical impression of splenomegaly does not correlate well with involvement unless the spleen is massively enlarged.[8,9] At least 15 per cent of patients with disease presenting above the diaphragm and a negative or equivocal lymphangiogram will prove to have unsuspected Hodgkin's disease in the spleen (Table 7-5). When the lymphangiogram was diagnosed as being positive, the spleen was invaded in 12 of 17 cases (70 per cent). When disease is proven in the abdomen by staging laparotomy, the spleen is positive about 90 per cent of the time.

When the spleen was positive, the splenic hilar nodes were usually found to be positive; an occasional case will have positive splenic hilar nodes with a negative spleen. Accessory spleens are occasionally involved.[2] The risk of splenic involvement correlates with the histologic type, being most frequent with mixed cellularity (62 per cent) and lymphocyte depletion (66 per cent).[2]

WALDEYER'S RING

Although Waldeyer's ring involvement is detected as a presenting site in only 1 to 2 per cent of cases, subsequent relapse in this area is seen in patients with high neck disease. Irradiation of Waldeyer's ring with Stage I upper neck disease or involvement appears justified on the basis of an estimated 5 to 10 per cent eventual relapse in that area.

Extralymphatic Spread Patterns

Primary extralymphatic Hodgkin's (*e.g.,* GI tract, lung) accounts for less than 2 per cent of all cases.

About 10 per cent of Hodgkin's cases will show secondary extranodal disease prior to treatment. Musshoff reports that one third of pretreatment extranodal extensions are con-

Table 7-5. *Relationship of Lymphangiogram Findings to Abdominal Disease at Exploratory Laparotomy in 50 Unselected Cases*

Lymphangiogram	Symptoms	Nodes +		Spleen +		Liver +	
Negative or Equivocal	A	4/19	21%	2/19	11%	0/19	> 0
	B	1/14	7%	3/14	21%	0/14	
Positive	A	7/9	78%	5/9	56%	1/9	11%
	B	8/8	100%	7/8	83%	3/8	37%

Courtesy: Glatstein, Trueblood, Enright, Rosenberg, and Kaplan, *Radiology,* 97, 425, 1970.

tiguous spread from nodal disease to an adjacent organ and the remainder are random extranodal vascular dissemination.[22]

A predictable progression of extranodal spread in some cases of Hodgkin's disease lends credence to the current treatment plans which may include not only the nodal areas, but also those contiguous extranodal areas potentially or actually involved.

LIVER

Hodgkin's involvement of the liver may be either diffuse or nodular.[7] Microscopically, the earliest site of liver involvement is within the portal triads. Jaundice accompanying Hodgkin's disease is most often related to liver involvement by Hodgkin's disease, the sequelae of liver treatment by irradiation or chemotherapy, or transfusions to an immunologically incompetent patient with resultant serum hepatitis; obstructive jaundice caused by nodes pressing on the excretory bile ducts is uncommon and is usually seen only in preterminal cases.

Liver involvement correlates best with grossly involved paraaortic nodes on lymphangiogram (Table 7-5), presence of systemic symptoms, the presence of a greatly enlarged spleen involved by Hodgkin's disease, and vascular invasion of spleen by Hodgkin's disease.[8,9,29] Liver invasion is rarely encountered without splenic involvement; when the spleen is positive, the liver is also positive in 25 per cent of the cases. Liver function studies and increased liver size are not reliable in predicting liver involvement. Liver samples are obtained at staging laparotomy by random wedge biopsies and several deep needle biopsies.

BONE MARROW

Bone marrow biopsy prior to treatment in previously untreated patients shows nearly zero incidence of marrow invasion for apparent Stages I and II and 9 per cent involvement of more advanced clinical stages. Rosen-

berg[26] reports that bone marrow invasion correlates with elevated alkaline phosphatase, older patients, "B" symptoms, and recurrent disease. The peripheral blood picture is usually normal in the untreated patient with bone marrow involvement; however, white blood cell count below 5,000, platelet count below 150,000, or hematocrit below 29 per cent were associated with either bone marrow involvement or hypersplenism. Knowledge of bone marrow involvement is important, since it dictates a change in treatment planning. A leukemic syndrome is rare in Hodgkin's disease.

BONE

Radiographically, Hodgkin's disease in bone is predominantly osteolytic. Pure osteoblastic involvement is rare and usually seen only in the vertebral bodies. The distribution of the involved bones shows the most common sites are the pelvis, especially near the sacroiliac joints, the vertebral bodies, the sternum, the medial halves of the clavicles, and the upper femurs.[5] By rough estimate, total nodal irradiation would fortuitously include most of the commonly involved bony areas.

In otherwise early stages of Hodgkin's disease, solitary bone involvement may be found adjacent to nodal involvement and under these conditions may be a favorable presentation.[22]

LUNG, PLEURA

Lung, pleural, and rib extensions occur mainly in patients who have demonstrable intrathoracic nodal disease. Patients with mediastinal adenopathy have a 10 per cent risk of lung involvement on initial evaluation; with hilar adenopathy the rate increases to 50 per cent.[15] Where the hilar lymphadenopathy is unilateral the ipsilateral lung is almost always the one involved. Direct extension to the lung or pleura (Stage IIe or IIIe) is usually suitable for irradiation and may have a favorable prognosis, especially where the histology is of the nodular sclerosing type. Some radiotherapists advocate 1,500 to 2,000 rads prophylactic irradiation to the entire ipsilateral lung where hilar disease is present, even if the lung tomograms are normal.

PERICARDIUM

The incidence of pericardial involvement is unknown. This involvement is suspected when there is involvement of the adjacent hilum and mediastinum, particularly when such involvement is bulky. Kaplan identified only 5 instances of pericardial involvement of 340 untreated, fully evaluated cases.[15]

RARE EXTRANODAL AREAS

Hodgkin's disease may spread to involve the skin, breasts, *GI* tract, and central nervous system, but these areas are so rarely involved that one cannot plan a course of radiation therapy based on this unlikely involvement.

Hodgkin's Disease in Children

The histological varieties are more often lymphocyte predominance or nodular sclerosing histology in childhood Hodgkin's disease.[32] The constitutional symptoms of pruritus are apparently less common in this age group than in adults.[33] Otherwise, there are no major differences in the disease in children and it is usually approached in a manner similar to that for adults. The concept of total nodal or mantle irradiation in very young children (under 6), of course, presents problems because of the actively growing tissues, the relatively small size of the lungs in comparison to the mediastinum, and the more medial position of the kidneys. Data on dosage in Hodgkin's disease in children are sparse, but many authors report a low recurrence rate with 3,000 rads. Splenectomy

before the age of 7 may be associated with an increased risk of serious bacterial infection, especially pneumococcal, and should not be done routinely. The consequences of splenic irradiation on the immune mechanism are unknown in the under-7 age group.

Hodgkin's in Pregnancy

Pregnancy occurring during the course of Hodgkin's disease has no direct influence on the disease, nor does the Hodgkin's disease directly influence the course of the pregnancy or the condition of the fetus. However, pregnancy indirectly influences the disease since treatment is often altered or delayed.

It may not be desirable to delay therapy to allow the fetus to reach full term. As in cancer of the cervix, these decisions become a matter of individual determination, and the patient must be appraised of the risks developing with delay of treatment. Therapeutic abortion must be considered appropriate in those patients who require irradiation. The fetal/ovarian dose from 4,000 rads mantle irradiation is estimated at 20 to 65 rads, but will depend upon the particular technique.[21]

Staging

Diagnostic Workup

A thorough workup is essential in deciding the mode of treatment (radiotherapy and/or chemotherapy) and the scope of the radiation fields.

Special attention should be directed to the following aspects of the pretreatment study.[25]

HISTORY

"B" symptoms include unexplained fever, night sweats, weight loss greater than 10 per cent. Pruritus alone no longer qualifies for "B" classification since it does not indicate a poorer prognosis.

LABORATORY

1) CBC, including platelet count, and erythrocyte sedimentation rate.

2) Serum alkaline phosphatase.

3) Evaluation of renal function.

4) Evaluation of liver function.

RADIOLOGICAL

1) Chest films, *PA* and lateral.

2) *IVP* (renal function and location of kidneys).

3) Lymphangiogram (bipedal). Note: Skeletal system can be evaluated on the lymphangiogram films.

SUPPLEMENTAL PROCEDURES WHEN ABOVE TESTS ARE EQUIVOCAL

1) Whole chest tomograms, frontal and lateral (indicated for all patients with mediastinal or hilar disease or questionable parenchymal lesion on routine chest x-ray films).

2) Inferior cavography (indirect demonstration of enlarged nodes in *L*1-2 area where the lymphangiogram visualizes few if any nodes).

3) Bone marrow biopsy guided by bone marrow scan for:

    a) unexplained anemia, leukopenia, or thrombocytopenia

    b) elevated alkaline phosphatase

    c) x-ray or scan evidence of bony disease

    d) Stage III or greater

    e) vascular invasion in biopsy specimen

4) Exploratory laparotomy. The concept of exploratory laparotomy for staging purposes was initiated at Stanford Medical Center in 1960 to more accurately define liver, spleen, and paraaortic node involvement.[8,9,14] A critical comparison of the clinical, laboratory, and lymphangiographic findings with the laparotomy findings has made us skeptical of our abilities to accurately assess the presence or absence of abdominal disease. The question remains when to use exploratory laparotomy in routine clinical settings since the procedure is occasionally accompanied by significant morbidity.

When Hodgkin's disease is clinically and radiographically confined to lymph nodes above the diaphragm, staging laparotomy rarely alters the treatment plan and is not routinely justified for the following reasons: 1) The surgical sampling of abdominal nodes when negative is unreliable and prophylactic paraaortic and pelvic node irradiation is still indicated. Only a very few nodes are usually obtained and often the specific nodes sought are not obtained for study. A false-positive error of 12 per cent and a false-negative error of 15 per cent are reported when comparing lymphangiogram diagnosis to laparotomy findings.[9] The combination of negative lymphangiogram and negative staging laparotomy will still miss 20 to 35 per cent of cases with subclinical disease in the paraaortic nodes and therefore does not significantly influence treatment decisions[15] (Table 7-6). 2) The detection or recurrence of nodal disease outside the standard paraaortic and splenic fields is rare when lymphangiogram results are normal or equivocal.[10] 3) Irradiation of a normal to slightly enlarged spleen is a safe alternative to splenectomy.[10]

Splenectomy reduces the volume of irradiation in the left upper quadrant and, of course, negates the chance of recurrence in the spleen. However, one still must irradiate the splenic chain nodes, which means the upper pole of the left kidney is incidentally irradiated. Following splenectomy, one irradiates less of the left lateral base of the lung, pericardium, and *GI* tract with the splenic pedicle field (See Johnson: Total Nodal Irradiation). The small savings in field reduction is more than offset by the over-all morbidity and cost of the laparotomy.

However, when the lymphangiogram is grossly abnormal or the spleen greatly en-

Table 7-6. *Risk of Later Spread (Extension) in the Paraaortic Nodes in Patients with Stage I and II Hodgkin's Disease Involving the Lower Cervical-Supraclavicular Lymph Nodes*

	Radiotherapeutic Fields	
	Limited Field*	Extended** "Total Lymphoid"
Number of cases at risk	80	74
Number of cases with paraaortic node extension or recurrence	29 (36%)	4 (5%)
Number of cases with extension to other sites	6 (8%)	12 (16%)
	35 (44%)	16 (21%)

*Either involved areas only or a mantle field.
**Mantle, paraaortic node, pelvic nodes, and usually the spleen. (Courtesy: Kaplan, *The Harvey Lectures*, Series 64, 1968–69, p. 215.)

larged, the risk of liver involvement (about 15 per cent) or atypical nodal spread (still uncommon) justifies laparotomy. Irradiation of a grossly enlarged spleen precludes even partial protection of the left kidney and is also justification for splenectomy. Patients with clinically isolated upper neck disease (Stage I_A) apparently have a low risk of abdominal disease; laparotomy for these patients will increase the accuracy of staging and when negative, will permit use of irradiation limited to the neck rather than total nodal irradiation as recommended for other Stage I presentations.

In institutions where the philosophy remains to treat only sites of involvement, the accuracy of staging will be improved by laparotomy done in cases of apparently early stages. Laparotomy also is indicated where a particular patient has a specific cause to avoid abdominal and/or pelvic irradiation, even though the usual plan is to treat all lymphatic regions. For instance, a negative laparotomy could help decide the necessity of pelvic irradiation in a young woman wishing to retain ovarian function. The laparotomy findings may also assist in treatment decisions of children (under 6) where it is especially desirable to reduce irradiation of actively growing structures.

Staging

The staging proposed at the Rye Conference is presently in use, but may be replaced by the Ann Arbor staging in the near future (Table 7-7).[25]

The major improvement of the Ann Arbor system is to move favorable Stage IV (Rye) cases with contiguous organ involvement into earlier stages consistent with their prognosis. The Ann Arbor classification is also easily adapted for the non-Hodgkin's lymphomas due to use of extralymphatic designations.

After extensive diagnostic evaluation of 340 consecutive untreated cases of Hodgkin's disease at Stanford Medical Center, the following distribution was found using the Ann Arbor staging system: Stage I, 16 per cent; Stage II, 44 per cent; Stage III, 26 per cent; Stage IV, 14 per cent.[15]

Guidelines for Treatment Planning

Table 7-8 outlines general guidelines for treatment planning in Hodgkin's disease (Ann Arbor staging).

Stage I: Total nodal irradiation is recommended for all sites except disease isolated

Table 7-7. *Comparison of Rye Staging and Proposed Ann Arbor Staging*

Rye Staging	Proposed Ann Arbor Staging
Stage I. Disease limited to one anatomic region or to two contiguous anatomic regions on the same side of the diaphragm.	*Stage I.* Involvement of a single lymph node region (1) or of a *single* extralymphatic organ or site (1e) excluding liver and marrow.
Stage II. Disease in more than 2 anatomic regions or in 2 noncontiguous regions on the same side of the diaphragm.	*Stage II.* Involvement of 2 or more lymph node regions on the same side of the diaphragm (II) or involvement of an extralymphatic site and of one or more lymph node regions on the same side of the diaphragm (IIe) excluding liver and bone marrow.
Stage III. Disease on both sides of the diaphragm, but not extending beyond the involvement of lymph nodes, spleen, and/or Waldeyer's ring.	*Stage III.* Involvement of lymph node regions on both sides of the diaphragm (III) which may also be accompanied by involvement of the spleen (IIIs) or by solitary involvement of an extralymphatic organ or site (IIIe) or both (IIIse).
Stage IV. Involvement of the bone marrow, lung parenchyma, pleura, liver, bone, skin, kidneys, gastrointestinal tract, or any tissue or organ in addition to lymph nodes, spleen, or Waldeyer's ring.	*Stage IV.* Multiple or disseminated foci of one or more extranodal organs or tissues with or without lymph node involvement. A *single* liver or marrow nodule.
All stages will be subclassified as "A" or "B" to indicate the absence or presence, respectively, of systemic symptoms. The following documented symptoms, otherwise unexplained are significant: (a) fever; (b) night sweats; and (c) pruritus.	"B". Night sweats, fever, weight loss greater than 10%, pruritus.

in the upper neck. The pelvis is excluded for classical supradiaphragmatic nodular sclerosing cases. When the disease is clinically limited to the upper neck (*i.e.,* above the thyroid notch), staging laparotomy and ipsilateral prescalene node biopsies will make the staging more secure. If no disease is detected by these two procedures, irradiation may be confined to the neck.

Stage II or IIe: Total nodal irradiation is recommended for all patients in this category; the pelvis is excluded for classical supradiaphragmatic nodular sclerosing cases. For the rare lymphocyte depletion case, multiple drug therapy (*MOPP*) following total nodal irradiation is to be considered.[1] If an extralymphatic site is involved, it is included in the total nodal irradiation plan on an individualized basis.

Stage III$_A$: Total nodal irradiation is recommended for Stage III$_A$ patients following staging laparotomy to rule out liver involvement and unusual nodal extensions. In the occasional lymphocyte depletion case, consideration should be given to *MOPP* following total nodal irradiation.

Stage III$_B$: Staging laparotomy is advised when possible in these patients because of high risk of liver involvement and other extensions of disease beyond the conventional irradiation fields. When the patient presents with minimal toxicity and minimal abdominal disease, total nodal irradiation seems a reasonable choice, as some of these patients appear to be curable. However, many of the patients have marked toxicity, exhibiting a rapid progression of disease; in these cases, *MOPP* is the preferable starting point.

Combinations of *TNI* and *MOPP* have been tried by various groups, and early results would suggest some improvement over the use of either modality alone. However, the combined use of *TNI* and *MOPP* is still in a trial phase and requires very careful monitoring to avoid depleting the marrow.

Stage IV: Stage IV disease resulting from positive bone marrow biopsy is treated initially with *MOPP*.

If the patient is staged IV only because of positive liver biopsies, two options are available. In a patient with minimal toxicity, minimal liver disease, and in otherwise good condition, total nodal irradiation including

irradiation of the liver should be considered. There is meager evidence that radiation will successfully eradicate minimal Hodgkin's disease in the liver. The author has selectively irradiated the entire liver to a dose of 3,000 rads in 6 to 8 weeks in combination with *TNI* in 8 patients; radiation hepatitis has not been observed. Careful attention to shielding of the kidneys is mandatory. In patients with rather advanced liver involvement, initial therapy with *MOPP* is probably more judicious.

Patients with disseminated foci are treated

Table 7-8. *Guidelines for Treatment Planning in Hodgkin's Disease*

Ann Arbor Stage	Site	Histology*	Lap.†	Management	Comment
I	Upper neck	LP NS MC	Yes	Local irradiation of entire neck	Include Waldeyer's ring and preauricular nodes
	Other	LP NS MC	No	TNI**	Exclude pelvis for nodular sclerosis
II	All sites	LP NS MC	No	TNI	Exclude pelvis for nodular sclerosis
		LD	No	TNI + MOPP	
III$_A$	All sites	LP NS MC	Yes	TNI	
		LD	Yes	TNI + MOPP	
III$_B$	All sites	LP NS MC LD	Yes	Early: TNI Advanced: MOPP	May combine TNI and MOPP
IV	Bone marrow only	All	No	MOPP	
	Liver only	All	Yes	Early: TNI + liver ± MOPP Advanced: MOPP	Liver: 3,000 R/6 wks.
	Disseminated	All	No	MOPP or palliative tx.	

*LP: lymphocyte predominance   MC: mixed cellularity
NS: nodular sclerosis   LD: lymphocyte depletion
†Lap.: staging laparotomy
**TNI: total nodal irradiation (both axillae, both necks, mediastinum, paraaortic nodes, spleen or splenic pedicle, and pelvis).

either with *MOPP* or with individualized palliative chemotherapy or radiotherapy.

Treatment for Relapsing Patients

Relapse of Hodgkin's after apparent control by radiotherapy requires careful reassessment to determine the exact extent of disease before selecting additional therapy. Local or marginal recurrence requires judicious appraisal of the original irradiation plan in order to determine the risks associated with reirradiation. It is generally inadvisable to consider curative reirradiation of the mediastinum or abdomen when the original dose was 3,000 rads or more.

If the patient has only localized extension in a previously untreated area, then irradia-

tion of the new area(s) of involvement is occasionally compatible with long survival or even cure.[28] A few patients have received total nodal irradiation when extension appeared following localized irradiation; the original area, usually the neck, is retreated when possible because of the potential for reseeding.

Patients with a picture of disseminated disease are usually approached either with chemotherapy or with a palliative treatment plan.

Dose

Figure 7-4 shows the data collected from the literature by Kaplan and arranged to show the probability of local recurrence for

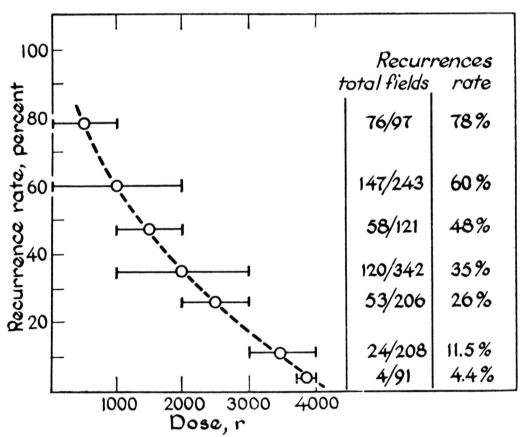

Recurrences total fields	rate
76/97	78%
147/243	60%
58/121	48%
120/342	35%
53/206	26%
24/208	11.5%
4/91	4.4%

FIG. 7-4. Correlation of percentage of local recurrences in Hodgkin's disease with doses delivered with megavoltage at 1,000 rads per week. (Courtesy: Kaplan, *Cancer Research,* 26, 1221, 1966.)

a single area when supervoltage irradiation was delivered at 1,000 rads per week.[17]

There are no data as yet to allow regulation of dose as determined by the parameters of histological subclassification or stage.

Kaplan now reports 1.4 per cent true local recurrence with doses of 4,400 rads per $4\frac{1}{2}$ weeks, 6 Mev.[18] Johnson reports only two true local recurrences in 62 patients using split dose techniques of 4,000 rads in 6 to $7\frac{1}{2}$ weeks, $^{60}Co^{11}$ (Table 7-12). The total dose seems of greater importance than over-all time. If one is to avoid serious normal tissue reactions and late complications, either split course techniques or fractionation schemes less than 1,000 rads per week (3,500 to 4,000 rads in 5 to 6 weeks) should be used. Refinement of the mantle technique to assure consistent delivery of the specified dose to all areas may allow gradual reduction of doses. The associated morbidity, especially of the lung and pericardium, with 4,000 rads in 4 weeks is high.

Controversy still exists as to whether a lesser dose is sufficient for microscopic foci in areas with no clinically detectable disease. Johnson lists only 2 recurrences in "prophylactic fields" receiving 3,000 rads[13] and Seydel reports no recurrence with doses over 2,500 rads.[29]

The mediastinum, upper abdomen, and spleen may harbor major disease that cannot be detected by very thorough workup, and therefore doses less than 4,000 rads are risky in these areas. Prudence dictates use of 4,000 rads to the neck regardless of the clinical findings. In summary, 4,000 rads is recommended as the prophylactic dose to the upper two thirds of the mediastinum, the neck, the paraaortic nodes, and the spleen, since these are areas at high risk which cannot be easily retreated (except the neck) in case of local recurrence.

However, in certain low-risk areas, 3,000 to 3,500 rads appears to be a very safe prophylactic dose; these low-risk areas include the axilla, inferior third of the mediastinum, and pelvic-inguinal nodes when adjacent areas are clinically and radiographically normal.

Table 7-9 lists the dose schemes which will produce a rate of local control approaching 100 per cent in involved areas with an acceptable risk of complications if very careful attention is paid to the details of field size, dosimetry, and fractionation. One must balance, as always, the price of serious complications and sequelae against a high local control.

Time of Recurrence or New Manifestation

Study of the relapse rate after apparent complete remission indicates that 80 to 85 per cent of relapses occur within 4 years and 90 per cent by 10 years.[4] Patients who survive 8 to 10 years following initial therapy with no evidence of relapse have about the same chance of living or dying when compared to a normal population of the same age and sex and have in excess of a 90 per cent chance of cure. A single relapse implies a drastic reduction in the expected cure rate

Table 7-9. *Hodgkin's Dosage Recommendations for Involved Areas**

	Continuous	Split
Large field—curative* (*e.g.*, mantle, Y)	4,000/5–6 weeks**	2,000/2 weeks— 2–2½ weeks' rest— 2,000/2 weeks**
Small field—palliative	3,000/2 weeks 2,300/5 days	Not applicable

* See text for recommendations for prophylactic dose.
** 5 treatments/week; an additional 500–1,000 rads may be added to large, bulky tumors.

even though a few long survivals or even cure may accrue with subsequent therapy.[4,16,28]

Extranodal relapse usually appears within the first year after treatment; patients with advanced stages tend to show recurrences sooner than those with earlier stages.[14] The extranodal relapse for "A" patients is 5 per cent, as compared to 20 per cent for the "B" patients.

Extranodal relapse occurred in 27 per cent of mixed cellularity cases (Stages I to III$_B$) and 3 of 5 with lymphocyte depletion. All other stages and histologic varieties had relatively low failure rates in extranodal areas. This information is of value if one is considering the probability of improving survival by adding chemotherapy to an irradiation scheme or deleting irradiation in favor of chemotherapy.

Prognosis

Ten-year survival rates from the orthovoltage era average about 40 per cent for localized disease (Stages I and II) and about 10 per cent for generalized disease (Stages III and IV). Predicted 6- to 8-year survivals free of relapse utilizing concepts outlined in this text approach 80 per cent for Stages I and II, 50 per cent for Stage III, and 10 per cent for Stage IV (Ann Arbor staging).

BIBLIOGRAPHY

1. DeVita, V. T., and Carbone, P. P.: Chemotherapeutic implications of staging in Hodgkin's disease, Cancer Research, 31, 1838, 1971.
2. Dorfman, R. F.: Relationship of histology to site in Hodgkin's disease, Cancer Research, 31, 1786, 1971.
3. Ellis, R. E.: The distribution of active bone marrow in the adult, Physics in Medicine and Biology, 5, 255, 1961.
4. Frei, E., and Gehan, E. A.: Definition of cure for Hodgkin's disease, Cancer Research, 31, 1828, 1971.
5. Fucilla, I. S., and Hamann, A.: Hodgkin's disease in bone, Radiology, 77, 53, 1961.

6. Fuller, L. M., Gamble, J. F., Schullenberger, C. C., Butler, J. J., and Gehan, E. A.: Prognostic factors in localized Hodgkin's disease treated with regional radiation, Radiology, 93, 641, 1971.
7. Givler, R. L., Brunk, S. F., Hass, C. A., and Gulesserian H. P.: Problems of interpretation of liver biopsy in Hodgkin's disease, Cancer, 28, 1335, 1971.
8. Glatstein, E., Guernsey, J. M., Rosenberg, S. A., and Kaplan, H. S.: The value of laparotomy and splenectomy in the staging of Hodgkin's disease, Cancer, 24, 709, 1969.
9. Glatstein, E., Trueblood, H. W., Enright, L. P., Rosenberg, S. A., and Kaplan, H. S.: Surgical staging of abdominal involvement in unselected patients with Hodgkin's disease, Radiology, 97, 425, 1970.
10. Johnson, R. E.: Is staging laparotomy routinely indicated in Hodgkin's disease? Annals of Internal Medicine, 75, 459, 1971.
11. Johnson, R. E.: To be published.
12. Johnson, R. E., Thomas, L. B., and Chretien, P.: Correlation between clinicohistologic staging and extranodal relapse in Hodgkin's disease, Cancer, 25, 1071, 1970.
13. Johnson, R. E., Thomas, L. B., Schneiderman, M., Glenn, D. W., Faw, F. and Hafermann, M. D.: Preliminary experience with total nodal irradiation in Hodgkin's disease, Radiology, 96, 603, 1970.
14. Kadin, M. E., Glatstein, E., and Dorfman, R. F.: Clinicopathologic studies of 117 untreated patients subjected to laparotomy for the staging of Hodgkin's disease, Cancer, 27, 1277, 1971.
15. Kaplan, H. S.: On the natural history, treatment, and prognosis of Hodgkin's disease, The Harvey Lectures, Series 64, p. 215, 1968–69.
16. Kaplan, H. S.: Prognostic significance of the relapse free interval after radiotherapy in Hodgkin's disease, Cancer, 22, 1131, 1968.
17. Kaplan, H. S.: Evidence for a tumoricidal dose level in the radiotherapy of Hodgkin's disease, Cancer Research, 26, (part 1), 1221, 1966.
18. Kaplan, H. S.: To be published.
19. Keller, A. R., Kaplan, H. S., Lukes, R. J., and Rappaport, H.: Correlation of histopathology with other prognostic indicators in Hodgkin's disease, Cancer, 22, 487, 1968.
20. Lukes, R. J., Chairman, Report of the nomen-

clature committee, *Cancer Research,* 26 (Part 1), 1311, 1966.

21. Meurk, M. L., Green, J. P., Nussbaum, H., and Vaeth, J. M.: Phantom dosimetry study of shaped Co-60 fields in the treatment of Hodgkin's disease, *Radiology,* 91, 554, 1968.
22. Musshoff, K., and Boutis, L.: Evaluation, principles of treatment and results of treatment in lymphogranulomatosis; in malignant lymphoma interdisciplinary discussions, German Roentgen Congress, 1968, *Stranlentherapie,* Sonderbaende, 69, 59, 1969.
23. Peters, M. V., Brown, T. C., and Rideout, D. F.: Hodgkin's disease—Prognostic influences and radiation therapy according to pattern of disease, *JAMA,* 223, 53, 1973.
24. Rappaport, H., and Strum, S. B.: Vascular invasion in Hodgkin's disease: Its incidence and relationship to the spread of the disease, *Cancer,* 25, 1304, 1970.
25. Rosenberg, Saul A. (Chairman): Report of the committee on Hodgkin's disease staging procedures, *Cancer Research,* 31, 1862, 1971.
26. Rosenberg, S. A.: Hodgkin's disease of the bone marrow, *Cancer Research,* 31, 1733, 1971.

27. Seydel, H. G., Bloedorn, F. G., and Wizenberg, M. J.: Time-dose-volume relationships in Hodgkin's disease, *Radiology,* 89, 919, 1967.
28. Seydel, H. G., Bloedorn, F. G., and Wizenberg, M. J.: Results of radiotherapeutic treatment of relapsing Hodgkin's disease, *Cancer,* 23, 1033, 1969.
29. Strum, S. B., Allen, L. W., and Rappaport, H.: Vascular invasion in Hodgkin's disease: Its relationship to involvement of the spleen and other extranodal sites, *Cancer,* 28, 1329, 1971.
30. Strum, S. B., Hutchison, G. B., Park, J. K., and Rappaport, H.: Further observations on the biologic significance of vascular invasion in Hodgkin's disease, *Cancer,* 27, 1, 1971.
31. Strum, S. B., and Rappaport, H.: Significance of focal involvement of lymph nodes for the diagnosis and staging of Hodgkin's disease, *Cancer,* 25, 1314, 1970.
32. Strum, S. B., and Rappaport, H.: Hodgkin's disease in the first decade of life, *Pediatrics,* 46, 748, 1970.
33. Teillet, F., and Schweisguth, O.: Hodgkin's disease in children, *Clinical Pediatrics,* 8, 698, 1969.

Non-Hodgkin's Lymphoma

RODNEY R. MILLION

Pathology

Most of the past American literature has utilized the terminology of reticulum cell sarcoma, lymphosarcoma, and giant follicular lymphoma, the latter sometimes included in the lymphosarcoma group. Rappaport's classification and the common synonyms are shown in Table 7-10;[19] this classification more precisely indicates the histological differences, hopefully allowing a more accurate comparison and study of the differences in the groups.

Nodular and Diffuse Forms

Rappaport's survey of 235 cases of nodular lymphoma in the files of the AFIP[19] has shown that patients with the nodular patterns have better survivals when compared with those for the diffuse forms at 5 and 10 years. Many cases with the nodular pattern, if not checked by treatment, progress to a diffuse pattern, with the original cell line either remaining the same or progressing to a less favorable prognostic group. The reverse progression from diffuse to nodular

Table 7-10. *Rappaport's Classification Matched to Common Synonyms in American Literature and Corresponding Survivals**

Synonym	Rappaport's Classification	Number of Cases	Per cent Survival 5 Years	Per cent Survival 10 Years
Giant follicular lymphoma——Lymphocytic, well differentiated . . . . nodular		18	50	—
Lymphocytic, well differentiated . . . . diffuse		118	25	2
Lymphosarcoma ——Lymphocytic, poorly differentiated . . nodular		93	54	17
Lymphocytic, poorly differentiated . . diffuse		76	3	0
Mixed cellularity . . . . nodular		46	30	—
Reticulum cell sarcoma — Mixed cellularity . . . . diffuse		No data		
Reticulum cell . . . . nodular		16	25	12%
Reticulum cell . . . . diffuse†		106	12	3%

* Table modified from Rappaport.[19]
† Combining stem cell and clasmatocytic, Gall and Mallory.[6]

does not seem to occur, although both patterns occasionally coexist. The nodular pattern is often maintained in regions of extranodal invasion.[6] Interchange between Hodgkin's and non-Hodgkin's lymphomas probably does not occur.

Leukemic Transition

The incidence of lymphosarcoma converting to chronic lymphatic leukemia is reported as 7 per cent in adult lymphosarcoma.[20] Conversion to acute lymphatic leukemia occurs in 30 per cent of childhood lymphosarcomas.[2] However, bone marrow invasion in adult lymphosarcoma on admission may, according to DeVita, run as high as 50 per cent, although only a fraction evolve to leukemia.[5] The criteria for early bone marrow involvement in the well-differentiated lymphocytic lymphomas are not difficult to define.

The pathologist cannot distinguish in a positive node between well-differentiated lymphocytic lymphoma and chronic lymphocytic leukemia; therefore, other parameters such as the peripheral smear, blood count, and bone marrow examination are necessary for differential diagnosis.

Spread Patterns

Many cases appear to be localized at onset and apparently cured by local therapy, sug-

gesting a unifocal origin. Less attention has been directed to extensive pretreatment study, and data from staging laparotomy are scanty. Spread occurs via lymphatic channels and by direct local invasion; vascular invasion has not been studied in nodal or organ specimens but patterns of dissemination suggest that it occurs frequently.

Nodal

There is diminishing likelihood of primary nodal presentation as one progresses from giant follicular to lymphosarcoma to reticulum cell sarcoma. Almost all giant follicular lymphomas, about 60 per cent of lymphosarcomas, and 40 per cent of reticulum cell sarcomas present as nodal disease. Although neck nodes are the most common nodal presenting site, the distribution of involved nodes at the time of diagnosis tends to be below the diaphragm as compared to involved nodes in Hodgkin's disease. Mediastinal nodal involvement is uncommon in early stage disease, there is a greater tendency of involvement of the more peripheral nodal chains such as preauricular, occipital, epitrochlear, and superficial inguinal nodes. Hanks[9] obtained positive mesenteric nodes in 7 of 10 patients studied by staging laparotomy; the lymphangiograms were positive in all 7 patients with positive mesenteric nodes.

Although there is considerable data to suggest that the spread patterns develop on a less predictable basis than in Hodgkin's disease, most of this data was gathered without confirmation by staging laparotomy (either before treatment or at the time of recurrence), and therefore we must await controlled studies for accurate documentation.[8, 18]

Extranodal Spread from Primary Nodal Presentation

Two types of organ extension occur: one is a direct extension from the site of nodal presentation to a neighboring organ; the second is a generalized vascular-disseminated spread. With adequate treatment, the localized organ involvement has a significantly better prognosis than the disseminated organ attack, which is virtually always fatal.

Secondary involvement of extranodal sites on admission occurs in about 20 per cent of nodal reticulum cell sarcoma and lymphosarcoma cases. For lymphosarcoma, about 25 per cent of extranodal extensions are direct continuity organ involvement and for reticulum cell sarcoma, about 10 per cent show contiguous organ involvement.

It is becoming apparent that the lymphocytic lymphomas show a predilection to involve the bone marrow, even though their spread patterns otherwise seem to follow contiguous pathways. The bone marrow involvement may be clinically dormant and be detected by random bone marrow biopsy. Amos[1] described 4 patients in whom bone marrow biopsies were obtained 11 to 54 months after total nodal irradiation when the patients were clinically in remission.

Persistent abnormalities of the peripheral count (anemia, thrombocytopenia, neutropenia, lymphocytosis) after total nodal irradiation are suggestive of lymphoma involving the bone marrow.

Primary Extranodal Presentations

Table 7-3 shows the distribution of extranodal presenting sites for lymphocytic lymphomas and reticulum cell sarcoma. About one half to two thirds of cases with primary organ involvement show a pattern of adjacent spreading either within the same system or to adjacent nodes.[16]

Waldeyer's Ring. Primary lymphoma of Waldeyer's ring accounts for about 10 per cent of nasopharynx, 5 per cent of tonsil, and 3 per cent of base of tongue malignancies.

Only 40 per cent of 74 patients with primary Waldeyer's ring, completely evaluated including lymphography, had disease apparently confined to the head and neck area. The most common site of relapse after irradiation of localized cases was to extranodal sites, especially the stomach.[3]

GI Tract. Peters reports the GI tract as the first recognized site of involvement in 12 per cent of lymphosarcoma and 25 per cent of reticulum cell sarcoma cases.[18] In adults, primary GI tract involvement occurs mainly in the stomach and small intestine, in children (16 and under), the lesions occur in the lower ileum, appendix, and ascending colon.[4, 12] Early spread occurs to contiguous mesenteric nodes. Later stages show involvement of paraaortic nodes, seeding of the mesentery and peritoneum, and direct invasion of adjacent structures.

Occult GI involvement is more frequent than realized, as evidenced by occasional unexpected disease found at staging laparotomy[10] and by routine upper GI series in Banfi's Waldeyer's ring series.[3]

Bone. Primary lymphoma originating in bone is almost always reticulum cell sarcoma. Bone presentation accounted for 7 per cent of reticulum cell sarcoma and 2 per cent of lymphosarcoma cases in Peters' analysis.[18] It presents a predominantly osteolytic picture of a tumor arising in medullary bone. It may occur in any portion of the shaft of long bones and may cross the epiphyseal line. The boundaries of the lesion are ill defined and the entire marrow cavity must be considered to be involved.

Those cases which disseminate show distant blood-borne metastases similar to other malignant bone tumor, although a few patients develop regional node involvement as the next site of involvement. Multiple bone lesions may be present when first seen, occasionally compatible with long survival.

Diagnostic Procedures

The diagnostic work-up prior to the planning of therapy is similar to that for Hodgkin's disease with the following exceptions.

1) Routine bone marrow biopsy is recommended for all lymphocytic lymphomas, regardless of the peripheral blood count or apparent early stage. Multiple marrow samples may improve the yield, according to Johnson.[13]

2) Routine *GI* radiography should be included, especially in those patients with primary Waldeyer's ring presentations and those patients with primary nodal disease in the abdomen.

3) Exploratory laparotomy has not been utilized to a great extent, so few data are available. Hass[10] reported the findings in 25 cases, Ultmann[22] in 12 cases, and Hanks[9] in 15 cases. Spleen, liver, and paraaortic node correlations parallel those for Hodgkin's disease. However, a high risk of mesenteric node involvement and an occasional unsuspected *GI* involvement are the major differences discovered to date. Staging laparotomy should include multiple sampling of mesenteric nodes and palpation of the *GI* tract.

The older age of the patients requires more restraint in selecting patients for staging laparotomy.

Staging System

The Ann Arbor staging system for Hodgkin's disease (Table 7-7) can be adapted for the non-Hodgkin's lymphomas. Staging laparotomy is recommended when possible to fully outline extent of disease; Hanks reports 6 of 15 cases and Ultmann 4 of 12 cases that had the stage advanced because of laparotomy findings while staging reduction occurred in only 2 of their combined 27 cases.[9,22]

Guidelines for Treatment Planning

Since irradiation policies are not well standardized, the minimal acceptable therapy will be described for various clinical situations; unproven extended treatment plans under trial will be mentioned. Guidelines to management are summarized in Table 7-11.

Localized Nodal (Stages I and II)

There is no statistical proof that irradiation of more than the involved areas alters the results of treatment.

Peters studied the value of prophylactic irradiation (1,200 to 2,400 rads delivered in 2 to 3 courses over a period of 4 to 5 months) in Stage I cases and could show no advantage to electively irradiating the uninvolved main lymphatic node chains compared to irradiation of the involved site only.[17] However, many therapists still prefer to electively irradiate some "uninvolved" areas, if for no other reason than to reduce the incidence of bothersome marginal and regional recurrences with little added increase in morbidity or treatment time.

Based on patterns of spread, one may predict that use of total nodal irradiation for localized nodal presentations would not significantly improve the survival rate, because of the higher risk of having positive mesenteric and peripheral nodes, *GI* involvement, and other extranodal extensions.

Studies are now underway to test the hypothesis of total lymphoid irradiation (mantle and total abdomen) with the use of higher doses in the "uninvolved" areas compared to previous studies.

Table 7-11. *Guidelines to Irradiation Planning in Non-Hodgkin's Lymphoma*

A. NODAL		
Stage/ Presenting Site	Minimum Treatment	Extended Treatment
STAGE I		
Lower neck	Both necks + mediastinum + adjacent axilla	*TLI*
Upper neck	Both necks + Waldeyer's ring	*TLI* + Waldeyer's ring
Mediastinum	Mediastinum + neck	*TLI*
Axilla	Axilla + adjacent neck	*TLI*
Paraaortic Inguinal-pelvic Mesentery	Total abdomen + inguinal	*TLI*
STAGE II Above diaphragm	Involved areas with generous margin, as above.	*TLI*
Below diaphragm	Total abdomen + inguinal	*TLI*
STAGE III WDLL, PDLL (see text)	*TBI* or Multiple drug chemotherapy	*TBI* or Multiple drug chemotherapy
Reticulum cell	*TLI* or Multiple drug chemotherapy	*TLI* and/or Multiple drug chemotherapy
STAGE IV WDLL *or* PDLL 1. Marrow	*TBI* or Multiple drug chemotherapy	*TBI* or Multiple drug chemotherapy
2. Visceral with or without positive marrow	Multiple drug chemotherapy ± local irradiation	Multiple drug chemotherapy ± local irradiation
Reticulum cell	Multiple drug chemotherapy ± local irradiation	Multiple drug chemotherapy ± local irradiation
B. WALDEYER'S RING		
STAGES I, II	Entire Waldeyer's ring + entire neck	Waldeyer's ring + *TLI*
STAGES III, IV	*See* NODAL STAGE III or IV	*See* NODAL, STAGE III or IV
C. GASTROINTESTINAL		
Stages Ie & IIe	Total abdomen	*TLI*
Stages IIIe & IV	*See* NODAL, STAGE III or IV	*See* NODAL, STAGE III or IV

TLI: Total lymphoid irradiation includes the nodes of the entire neck, both axillae, mediastinum, total abdomen, and inguinal nodes.
TBI: Total body irradiation.[11]
WDLL: Well-differentiated lymphocytic lymphoma.
PDLL: Poorly differentiated lymphocytic lymphoma.

Earlier studies combining radiation and single drug chemotherapy did not produce a measurable increase in cure rates; however, combinations of radiation and multiple drug chemotherapy appear more promising, but as yet are unproven. One must remember that the older patients will usually not tolerate extensive work-up plus comprehensive irradiation and/or multiple drug chemotherapy.

Above Diaphragm (with or without Contiguous Organ Involvement). Patients should have the area(s) of involvement treated with a generous margin. (Table 7-11, Stages I and II, Nodal.) Adjacent lymph node areas are included as outlined.

The lymphatics of the supraclavicular region and adjacent axilla are actually part of the same lymphatic chain and both areas are treated if either is involved. Both the neck and mediastinum should be treated together if either is involved since the neck-mediastinal match at a later date carries the risk of spinal cord overdose or tumor underdose.

Prophylactic irradiation of Waldeyer's ring is recommended for patients with high neck presentation, since a number of these patients will develop disease at that site if left untreated. Patients with Stage II disease will frequently require a mantle-type portal. Portal alignment should be arranged so that contiguous areas may be treated in the future without undue difficulty in matching adjacent fields. Skin tattoos are recommended for this purpose.

Trials are underway to study total lymphoid irradiation for Stages I and II disease. The high risk of mesenteric node and abdominal visceral disease lends support to this approach. Local irradiation plus multiple drug chemotherapy is also a logical plan for trial because of the early progression to extranodal sites outside total lymphoid irradiation portals (*e.g.,* bone marrow, skin, lung).

Below Diaphragm (with or without Contiguous Organ Involvement). The diagnosis is fre-

quently made at the time of exploratory laparotomy, at which time careful *GI* tract evaluation, biopsy of the liver and other nodal areas, and perhaps splenectomy, while desirable, are infrequently done. Total abdominal irradiation is recommended regardless of the extent of disease (Fig. 7-5). A dose of 3,000 rads in 6 weeks with open anterior-posterior fields to the entire peritoneal-retroperitoneal areas plus inguinal nodes is well tolerated; both portals are treated each day. An extra 500 to 1,000 rads may be added to the original areas of involvement. The dose to the kidneys should be limited to 2,300 to 2,500 rads over 6 weeks, although occasionally it may be necessary to exceed this limit to one kidney when tumor is adjacent to it. The simplest way to protect the kidneys is to shield them with 2 *HVL* of lead (2 cm lead for ^{60}Co) from posterior after 1,500 rads midline tumor dose.

The addition of mantle irradiation to total abdomen therapy (*TLI*) severely tests the bone marrow reserve, but has been successfully completed in several cases. A split course plan has been devised which allows completion of the scheme in most cases; close monitoring of the peripheral blood count, especially the platelets, is essential.

Total Lymphoid Irradiation (Split Course Scheme)

Case: 53-year-old male
    Reticulum cell, Stage II$_B$
    Epigastric mass 10 × 12 cm; 4 cm inguinal node
    Fever; 20 per cent weight loss

Total abdomen (including inguinal nodes)	1,500/3 weeks
Followed by mantle	2,000/2 weeks
6 weeks rest	
Total abdomen	1,500/3 weeks
Boost residual epigastric mass	1,000/8 days
6 weeks rest	
Mantle	2,000/2 weeks

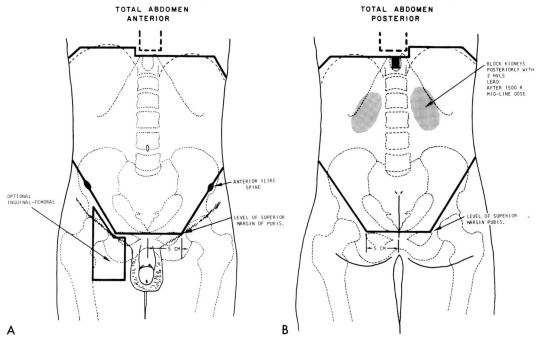

FIG. 7-5. **A.** Anterior total abdomen portal used to encompass contents of peritoneal cavity and retroperitoneal nodes. The inferior border is at the level of superior border of pubis. The superior border is irregular to conform to the outline of the diaphragm. Inguinal-femoral portals are added as indicated.

B. Posterior total abdomen portal is a mirror image. The kidneys are shielded by 2 *HVL* of lead (2 cm of lead for ^{60}Co) after 1,500 rads midline tumor dose.

Both portals are treated each day. The aim is 3,000 rads in 6 weeks, 5 treatments per week, when only the abdomen is to be treated. An additional 1,000 rads may be added to reduced area to "boost" residual disease. Inguinal-femoral nodes are treated through an anterior only; the tumor dose is usually calculated at 2 to 3 cm depth.

Peripheral count recovered by 2 months, and patient returned to full-time activity by 3 months. No evidence of disease at one year.

Disseminated Nodal Disease (Stages III and IV)

The high risk of bone marrow and visceral dissemination in Stage III lymphocytic lymphomas and of generalized dissemination in Stage III reticulum cell sarcomas does not allow for a simple irradiation policy.

Fractionated total body irradiation as outlined by Johnson[14] appears to be the most promising advance for Stages III and IV (marrow) lymphocytic lymphomas. Figure 7-6 shows current survival data following fractionated total body irradiation *(TBI).*[13]

Approximately one half the survivors remain continuously free of disease. For fractionated *TBI,* patients are treated in a sitting position to reduce field size; selective anatomical shielding is not necessary. A midrectal dose of 10 rads a day is delivered with alternate exposures from the left and right sides. Patients are treated 3 times per week to an over-all dose of about 200 rads in 7 to 11 weeks. The tumor air ratio *(TAR)* for ^{60}Co can be calculated from Figure 7-7. *In vivo* rectal dosimetry checks are recommended. Peripheral count is closely monitored and evidence of marrow depression may require a break in therapy to allow recovery. Some patients require additional localized irradiation to bulky or residual masses. Most patients may be cared for on an outpatient basis

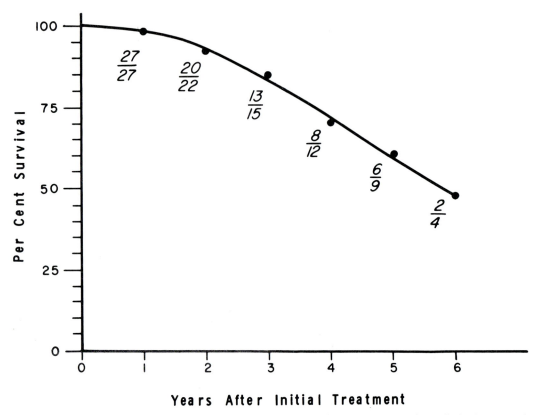

FIG. 7-6. Per cent absolute survival of Stages III and IV lymphocytic lymphoma managed initially by fractionated total body irradiation. (Courtesy: Johnson, R. E., Personal communication 1972.)

as the constitutional effects are reported to be minimal.

Split course *TLI* is recommended for favorable Stage III reticulum cell sarcoma. However, many of these patients will have a very toxic response or rapidly advancing disease. Chemotherapy is the initial treatment with irradiation added on an individualized basis.

The newer multiple drug chemotherapy protocols report complete remission in 30 to 50 per cent of reticulum cell cases, sometimes of lasting duration.[15] Gamble reports preliminary success with combination chemotherapy followed by modified total lymphoid type irradiation for localized and diffuse reticulum cell sarcoma.[7]

Fractionated total body irradiation is recommended for Stage IV lymphocytic lymphomas because of bone marrow involvement with no visceral disease.[14]

Stage IV patients with visceral involvement should be treated with multiple drug chemotherapy or selectively for palliation only.

Waldeyer's Ring

Stages I and II. Treatment for localized disease originating in Waldeyer's ring consists of irradiation of the entirety of Waldeyer's ring with inclusion of all neck nodes down to the clavicles, regardless of the absence or presence of adenopathy (Fig. 7-8). Primary

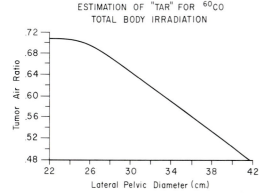

ESTIMATION OF "TAR" FOR ^{60}CO
TOTAL BODY IRRADIATION

FIG. 7-7. Estimation of tumor air ratio for ^{60}Co total body irradiation. The lateral pelvic diameter (cm) is used to compute the appropriate central axis air exposure to deliver a given tissue dose specified as the midrectal dose. Patients are treated alternately from each side.

EXAMPLE

Aim: Approximately 200 rads total body in 7 to 12 weeks; 20 to 30 rads midrectal dose per week in 2 to 3 treatments.

Calculation: Lateral pelvic diameter = 34 cm
$$TAR = 0.59$$

$$\frac{10 \text{ rads}}{0.59} = 17 \text{ rads/air to central axis.}$$

Instructions: Central axis of patient (*i.e.*, rectum) positioned at source to axis distance.

Patient placed in sitting position to reduce necessary field size.

Unit calibrated in rads/air at specified field size and source to axis distance.

Treat one side each day.

Lithium fluoride rectal *in vivo* dosimetry check.

Daily *CBC* prior to treatment; 2 to 4 week rest period for depressed blood count.

sites in oral cavity, sinuses, and orbit require individualized planning. Trials with total lymphoid irradiation or adjuvant chemotherapy may improve survival since one half of the cases originally thought to be localized eventually develop new manifestations outside the head and neck area.

Stages III and IV. If disease has already extended beyond Waldeyer's ring and the neck, then treatment planning is similar to that outlined under Stages II, III, or IV, nodal.

Gastrointestinal—Stages Ie and IIe

Surgical operations play an important part in the management of primary gastrointestinal lymphoma. Although the disease may be suspected from appropriate x-ray studies, exploratory laparotomy and biopsy are almost always necessary to make the final diagnosis and also to determine the extent of disease. The pathologist may be unable to distinguish between lymphoma and poorly differentiated carcinoma on frozen section, and the surgeon must complete his procedure knowing only that he is dealing with a malignant tumor. Local removal of limited disease and contiguous nodes is appropriate and may result in cure by itself. Heroic surgery is seldom justified, as extensive *GI* involvement can sometimes be controlled with irradiation. It is thought by most surgeons and radiotherapists that it is possible to evaluate only crudely the extent of disease in the abdomen from the surgical and pathological findings, and therefore postoperative radiation should be added regardless of the surgical findings.

Although large field irradiation of the abdomen to include the primary site and the adjacent nodal areas is often recommended according to the literature, we most often prefer total abdominal irradiation (Fig. 7-5). Frequent recurrences outside the treatment areas, multiple sites of *GI* tract involvement, mobility of the gut, inaccurate assessment of disease extent, difficulty to match portals for intraabdominal extensions, and improved success are the reasons for advocating total abdominal irradiation.[4,12]

The technique for total abdominal irradiation has been outlined. The moving strip technique is not recommended since the over-all time of dose delivery seems of rela-

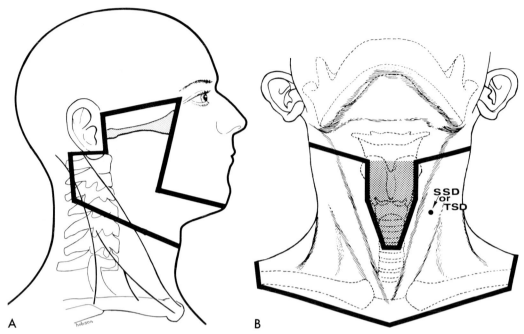

FIG. 7-8. A. Portal used to irradiate Waldeyer's ring (nasopharynx, tonsil, and base of tongue) and upper neck nodes. The lower border is located by the thyroid notch. The superior border is about 1 cm above the zygomatic arch. The posterior border coincides with the tragus and then bends posteriorly to encompass the sternocleidomastoid muscle. The anterior border extends from the orbital rim toward the second molar region; it then bends forward along the mandible so that the submental nodes are encompassed.

B. Portal used to irradiate lower neck nodes in conjunction with Waldeyer's ring—upper neck portal. The upper border coincides with the lower border of Figure A. Midline larynx shielding extends from the thyroid notch to 1 to 2 cm below the cricoid. The lateral margin is defined by the junction of the trapezius with the clavicle. The inferior extent is usually 1 to 2 cm below the clavicles.

tive unimportance for the lymphomas and the chance of bowel perforation is increased. Perforation during irradiation of *GI* lymphoma has not been observed while using the low dose of 100 rads a day at midplane.

Secondary progression of the disease to the neck and mediastinum may occur, and *TLI* should be considered.[7,18]

Bone

Localized reticulum cell sarcoma of bone is managed by irradiation of the entire involved bone. Tailored treatment portals are used in order to exclude as much soft tissue as possible. Reduction of the field to the original site of gross involvement is consid-

ered safe after 4,000 rads tumor dose; the final tumor dose is usually 5,000 rads.

Investigation of local irradiation followed by adjuvant chemotherapy is in progress, but no data are yet available.

Patients presenting with multiple bone involvement (2 or 3 lesions) should be treated aggressively, since a few of these would appear to have a good prognosis.

Dosage

Lymphocytic Lymphoma (Lymphosarcoma)

Compilation of the published dose control data for lymphocytic lymphomas (lymphosarcoma) indicates use of a dosage schedule the same as for Hodgkin's disease (Table 7-9) for 95 per cent or greater local control;[21] results with split course schemes have not been reported.

Control dose data for well-differentiated lymphocytic lymphoma (giant follicular lymphoma) are difficult to obtain because of the long natural history of the disease, the scarcity of cases, and the tendency to convert to reticulum cell sarcoma or poorly differentiated lymphocytic lymphoma. A dose of 3,000 rads in 3 weeks or its equivalent is reported by Seydel to produce a high local control rate on a short-term basis.[21]

The complete remissions and relatively long relapse-free survivals in some Stage III and Stage IV cases following 200 rads fractionated total body irradiation present a time-dose paradox since local control is almost nil with 200 rads to limited treatment fields. These data reconfirm the observation that some of the so-called Stages III and IV lymphocytic lymphomas are closer to lymphatic leukemias. (Johnson also reports similar remissions in chronic lymphocytic leukemia with 200 rads fractionated total body irradiation.)

Reticulum Cell

The data for *nodal* reticulum cell lymphoma indicate use of doses similar to those recommended for Hodgkin's disease (Table 7-9) to achieve 95 per cent greater local control. Doses of 5,000 rads are recommended for localized primary bone, the larger Waldeyer's ring lesions, and the bulky nodal presentation.

When the pathologist is undecided between reticulum cell sarcoma or undifferentiated carcinoma (*e.g.*, base of tongue), the carcinoma dose schedule must be selected.

Results of Treatment

The results of treatment for all histologies, largely from the orthovoltage era, show approximately 50 per cent 5-year and 40 per cent 10-year survival for localized pre-

sentations and approximately 10 per cent 10-year survival for generalized presentations. Separate analysis of the reticulum cell sarcomas shows a lesser survival at 5 years, but very little difference at 10 years, compared to the lymphocytic lymphomas. Nodal and extranodal presentations have similar survival rates stage for stage.[18]

Statements made relating cure to the tumor-free interval for Hodgkin's disease apply generally to non-Hodgkin's groups. There is little or no improvement in survival rates such as recently reported for Hodgkin's disease.

Lymphosarcoma in Children

The non-Hodgkin's lymphomas are relatively scarce in children and therefore scant information is available about the natural history of the various histologies. The main difference when compared to adult forms of the disease is the rather high conversion to acute leukemia, which appears in at least one third of the patients. Leukemic conversion would appear to be as common in patients presenting with localized disease as with regional involvement. Mediastinal presentations have a relatively higher risk to evolve to leukemia; Jenkins reported a 46 percent transition for mediastinal presentations compared to 4.4 per cent for *GI* tract, abdomen, or retroperitoneal presentations.[11]

Previous forms of treatment were generally unsuccessful, whether radiation and/or chemotherapy. Accumulated cases of local and regional childhood lymphosarcoma show 5-year survivals of only 9 per cent of 221 cases.[2]

However, recent improvement in prognosis has been suggested by the use of intensive multiple-drug chemotherapy similar to the schemes used for acute leukemia in childhood plus localized irradiation to clinically involved areas with modest doses. Aur reports 6 of 8 patients in complete remission from 16 to 27 months with the use of his technique.[2]

Reticulum cell sarcoma in children is generally managed in a fashion similar to that in adults.

BIBLIOGRAPHY

1. Amos, E. H., and Million, R. R.: Evaluation of the bone marrow after successful total irradiation, To be published 1972.
2. Aur, R. J. A., Hustu, H. O., Simone, J. V., Pratt, C. B., and Pinkel, D.: Therapy of localized and regional lymphosarcoma of childhood, *Cancer,* 27, 1328, 1971.
3. Banfi, A., Bonadonna, G., Carnevali, G., Milinari, R., Monfardini, S., and Salvini, E.: Lymphoreticular sarcomas with primary involvement of Waldeyer's ring; clinical evaluation of 225 cases, *Cancer,* 26, 341, 1970.
4. Bush, R. S., and Ash, C. L.: Primary lymphoma of the gastrointestinal tract, *Radiology,* 92, 1349, 1969.
5. DeVita, V. T.: Personal communication, 1971.
6. Gall, E. A., and Mallory, T. B.: Malignant lymphoma: a clinical-pathologic survey of 618 cases, *Amer. J. Path.,* 18, 381, 1942.
7. Gamble, J. F., Fuller, L. M., Butler, J. J., and Shullenberger, C. C.: Combined chemotherapy and radiotherapy for advanced Hodgkin's disease and reticulum cell sarcoma, *South. M. J.,* 64, 775, 1971.
8. Han, T., and Stutzman, L.: Mode of spread in patients with localized malignant lymphoma, *Arch. Intern. Med.,* 120, 1, 1967.
9. Hanks, G. E., Terry, L. N., Bryan, J. A., and Newsome, J. F.: Contribution of diagnostic laparotomy to staging of non-Hodgkin's lymphoma, *Cancer,* 29, 41, 1972.
10. Hass, C. A., Brunk, S. F., Gullesserian, H. P., and Givler, R. L.: The value of exploratory laparotomy in malignant lymphoma, *Radiology,* 109, 157, 1971.
11. Jenkin, R. D. T., and Sonley, M. J.: The malignant lymphoma in childhood, In *Neoplasia in Childhood,* Yearbook Medical Publishers, Inc., p. 305, 1967.
12. Jenkin, R. D. T., Sonley, M. J., Stephens, C. A., Darte, J. M. M., and Peters, M. V.: Primary gastrointestinal tract lymphoma in childhood, *Radiology,* 92, 763, 1969.
13. Johnson, R. E.: Personal communication, 1972.
14. Johnson, R. E., Foley, H. T., Swain, R. W., and O'Connor, G. T.: Treatment of lymphosarcoma with fractionated total body irradiation, *Cancer,* 20, 482, 1967.
15. Lowenbraun, J., DeVita, V. T., and Serpick, A. A.: Combination chemotherapy with nitrogen mustard, vincristine, procarbazine, and prednisone in lymphosarcoma and reticulum cell sarcoma, *Cancer,* 25, 1018, 1970.
16. Musshoff, K.: Therapy and prognosis of two different forms of organ involvement in cases of malignant lymphoma (Hodgkin's disease, reticulum cell sarcoma, lymphosarcoma) as well as a report about stage division in these diseases, *Klin. Wschr.,* 48, 673, 1970.
17. Peters, M. V.: The contribution of radiation therapy in the control of early lymphomas, *Amer. J. Roentgen.,* 90, 956, 1963.
18. Peters, M. V., Hasselback, R., and Brown, T. C.: The natural history of the lymphomas related to the clinical classification, In *Proceedings of the International Conference on Leukemia-Lymphoma,* C. J. D. Zarafonetis, editor, Lea & Febiger, Philadelphia, Pa. p. 357, 1968.
19. Rappaport, H., Winter, W. J., and Hicks, E. D.: Follicular lymphoma: a reevaluation of its position in the scheme of malignant lymphoma, based on a survey of 253 cases, *Cancer,* 9, 792, 1956.
20. Rosenberg, S. A., Diamond, H. D., and Craver, L. F.: Lymphosarcoma—survival and the effects of therapy, *Amer. J. Roentgen.,* 85, 521, 1961.
21. Seydel, H. G., Bloedorn, F. G., Wizenberg, M., and Berk, S.: Time-dose relationships in radiation therapy of lymphosarcoma and giant follicle lymphoma, *Radiology,* 98, 411, 1971.
22. Ultmann, J. E.: The management of lymphoma, *CA,* 21, 342, 1971.

Clinical and Technical Aspects of Total Nodal Irradiation for Hodgkin's Disease

RALPH E. JOHNSON

In Collaboration with

FREDERICK L. FAW, DWIGHT W. GLENN, and ROBERT W. SWAIN

Introduction

Total nodal irradiation (*TNI*) is a term coined to describe the incontinuity irradiation of all lymphatic chains which are involved by Hodgkin's disease with unexplained selectivity. The phrase, total nodal, quite obviously does not imply that all discrete lymphoid structures within the body are irradiated, a feat virtually impossible without resorting to total body irradiation. Rather, *TNI* refers to the systematic irradiation of only those major lymph nodes which are at a relatively high risk of lymphomatous involvement, whether the involvement is diagnostically evident or occult. In this sense, *TNI* is not a rigid technique. There is allowance for some degree of flexibility since not all lymph node chains in every patient require irradiation for treatment to be optimally definitive. However, the proper exploitation of this flexability demands an understanding of the biologic behavior of Hodgkin's disease, especially as it is influenced by the clinical presentation and the histopathologic subclassification.

There is a striking propensity for Hodgkin's disease to have its initial clinical manifestation in selected lymph nodes and the spleen as schematically illustrated in Figure 7-9. Collectively, these nodal sites comprise the tissue volume usually treated with *TNI*. The radiotherapy technique to be described for this purpose has evolved from the attempt to administer homogeneous tumor doses to a geometrically irregular absorber (the body) in such a manner as to minimize both acute reactions and late complications. In certain instances, optimal dose homogeneity has been compromised in order to

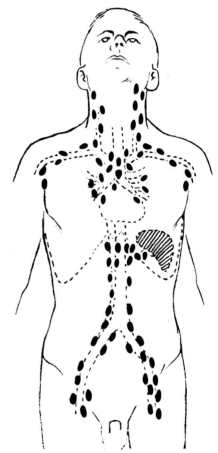

FIG. 7-9. Lymph node chains which, in addition to the spleen, are selectively involved by Hodgkin's disease at the time of initial diagnosis.

achieve increased precision in patient positioning and treatment field reproduction. While sacrifice of absolute dose homogeneity may be objectionable to "purists," experience has demonstrated that recurrence from underdosing tumor or complications resulting from overdosing normal tissues has not been a practical reality. And certain of these compromises in dosimetry have significantly reduced the frequency of error in treatment accuracy which often plagues widefield irradiation for Hodgkin's disease.

The dual rationale underlying the concept of *TNI* is to avoid the technical disadvantages inherent in "patchwork quilt" radiotherapy and to obviate the extensive dissemination of disease which may develop by the time extension to sites left untreated becomes detectable.[10] Recently, carefully controlled study[12,13] has documented the fact that radical prophylactic irradiation is mandatory for attaining optimal results, even in the earliest stages of involvement. This type of widefield radiotherapy demands meticulous treatment planning; relevant technical considerations in this regard are discussed in the following sections.

Technique

Dose Fractionation

General acceptance of an absorbed dose of 3,500 to 4,000 rads as tumoricidal for Hodgkin's disease[17] is widely associated with the misconception that such a dose must be administered within an elapsed time of 3 to 4 weeks for therapeutic effectiveness. Adoption of such fractionation ensued from the assignment of a Strandqvist-type dose-response curve[25,6] to observed clinical data. We have disparately interpreted the data reported by others as suggesting that, in fact, a tumoricidal effect is retained with more protracted irradiation, provided an adequate total dose is delivered. In general, however, protracted treatment schedules have received

scant attention for Hodgkin's disease[19] and most radiotherapists in the world persist with conventional fractionation and protraction while irradiating ever-increasing volumes of normal tissues.

Split-course and continuous schedules have been compared in our department in treatment for Hodgkin's disease. Using 200 rad fractions, tumor doses of 4,000 rads were delivered in 4 to 5 weeks and compared to 4,000 rads in 6 to $7\frac{1}{2}$ weeks for continuous and split-course irradiation respectively. There has been no indication of reduced tumoricidal effect with split-course irradiation (Table 7-12) whereas the normal tissue reactions and delayed complications have been greatly attenuated. Split-course irradiation deserves particular mention with respect to treatment to the mediastinum. Interruption of therapy after a tumor dose of 2,000 rads permits the continued regression of mediastinal lymphadenopathy during the "break" in treatment. As a result, more complete shielding of uninvolved lung and cardiac tissue during the second half of a split-course schedule will virtually eliminate radiation pericarditis and pneumonitis as being complications secondary to mediastinal irradiation. There is obvious need for others to reconsider the practice of irradiating wide fields with mean tumor doses of 4,000 rads in an elapsed time of 4 weeks, a policy which occasionally produces morbidity tolerable only to extremely stoic patients and/or their unconcerned physicians.

Table 7-12. *Therapeutic Effectiveness of Split-Course Irradiation in Hodgkin's Disease (1965–1969)*

Number of Patients Treated	=	62
Number Developing a Local Recurrence of Disease	=	2
Number of Local Recurrences per Number of Fields at Risk		
Involved Fields	=	2/168
Prophylactic Fields	=	0/317

TREATMENT OF SUPRADIAPHRAGMATIC LYMPH NODES

Perhaps the most universal theme in the radiotherapy of Hodgkin's disease has become the widely employed technique referred to as the "mantle field" for the incontinuity irradiation of lymph node chains above the diaphragm.[16,24] As depicted in Figure 7-10, the mantle field avoids the inherent disadvantages of multiple field techniques but consequently encompasses anatomic areas which are variable in terms of surface contour, thickness, and tissue density. These variables in the patient are further

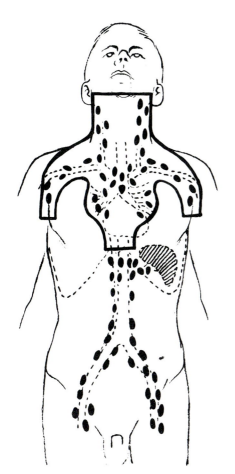

FIG. 7-10. The lymphatics encompassed by the standard "mantle field" technique are schematically shown.

compounded by factors related to the physical characteristics of the radiation beam itself, creating a compelling requirement for highly individualized treatment planning.

A major prerequisite in mantle field irradiation is an effective method for shielding the uninvolved lung and heart. An ingenious technique[27] consists of preparing styrofoam molds (Fig. 7-11) to hold lead shot or other blocking materials. The device (Fig. 7-12) employs a hot cutting wire to trace the desired block shape from a chest radiograph. This device is inexpensively constructed and permits the rapid fabrication of styrofoam molds tailored to each patient's anatomy and the presentation of his disease. The molds have beam divergent edges which reduce transmission penumbral effect which is an unavoidable defect in perpendicularly cut lung blocks. For ^{60}Co teletherapy, a 4-inch styrofoam mold filled with #7 lead shot will transmit approximately 3 per cent of the primary beam. Addition of paraffin wax to the lead shot produces a mixture which, after heating to a low temperature, can readily be poured into the styrofoam molds and subsequently can be reused with reheating. The total construction time for a set of blocks is only 3 hours, including the required cooling time (setting) of the lead-paraffin mixture. Serial retailoring of the heart-lung blocks thus is permitted for each patient as the mediastinal lymphadenopathy regresses.

A second critical necessity is the homogenization of tumor doses in various regions of the mantle field. In the absence of corrective measures, considerable inhomogeneity of absorbed dose is inevitable.[2,20] The dosimetric variation stems from three primary considerations, namely 1) intrinsic absence of beam flatness with large treatment fields, 2) surface contour irregularity which alters the source-skin distance over the treatment field, and 3) different depths of the lymph nodes in various anatomic sites. Some system for insuring uniformity of absorbed dose is thereby essential to avoid underdosage of

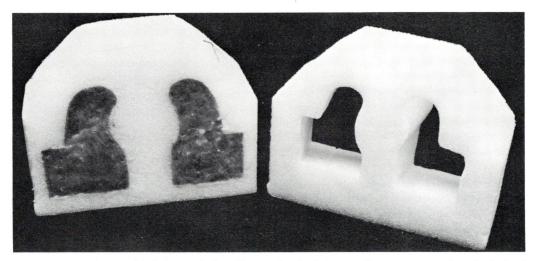

FIG. 7-11. Styrofoam molds before and after filling with a lead shot-paraffin mixture provide individualized shielding of the lungs and heart during mantle field irradiation.

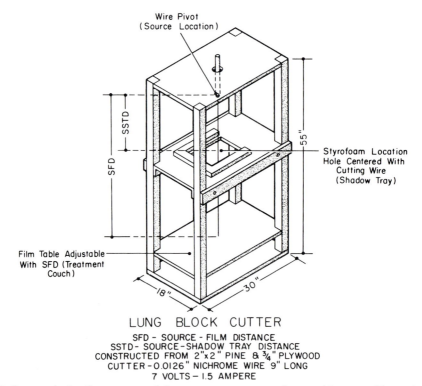

LUNG BLOCK CUTTER

SFD – SOURCE - FILM DISTANCE
SSTD – SOURCE – SHADOW TRAY DISTANCE
CONSTRUCTED FROM 2"x 2" PINE & ¾" PLYWOOD
CUTTER – 0.0126" NICHROME WIRE 9" LONG
7 VOLTS – 1.5 AMPERE

FIG. 7-12. By reproducing the geometry of the treatment setup, styrofoam molds are readily produced which customize lung-heart shielding using this device.

diseased tissue or an inadvertent overdosage of critical normal tissues.

To achieve improved dose homogeneity within the mantle field volume, we have elected to use compensating filters[5] rather than "shrinking" the field as more superficial areas are adequately (but too rapidly) dosed. These filters (Fig. 7-13) compensate for the various causes of dose inhomogeneity so that the various regions within the mantle field receive a fairly uniform (usually ±5%) daily tumor dose.

Each filter set consists of 41 brass components, 6 of which are individually selected for each patient. The filter selections are based upon a set of measurements for each patient. The patient is positioned so that the center of the field is at the sternal notch at a set distance (usually 90 cm from the source), the perpendicular distance from the source to the lower margin of the mediastinum is then measured. The anterior posterior patient thickness is also determined at the lower margin of the mediastinum, at the sternal notch, at the midaxilla, and at the upper neck (just above the thyroid cartilage). Details of this system has been described by Faw *et al*[5] and further information can be obtained from this article. A plastic plate holds filter parts which are easily assembled immediately before daily treatment. A single set of components is thus adequate for mantle field irradiation of many patients. This method of improving dose homogenization has been employed in about 150 patients over the past 5 years and the reliability of the filter design is affirmed by the results observed.

Difficulty has also been encountered with mantle field therapy in the attempt to match opposing treatment portals. Few radiotherapy units permit isocentric irradiation of such large field sizes with the patient remaining in an ideal fixed position. Many radiotherapists elect to rotate patients between prone and supine positions on alternate days; this has several disadvantages. They include shifting of internal organs[26]

and difficulty in precise duplication (within necessary millimeters rather than centimeters) of the patient's position. In addition, use of a complete posterior mantle field demands midline shielding over the cervical portion of the spinal cord. As shown in Figure 7-14, a narrow block of 1 cm in width for spinal cord shielding reduces the absorbed dose throughout the entire volume under the block, thereby underdosing lymph nodes in the anterior midcervical area. Albeit infrequently, these midline lymph nodes occasionally have been the site of disease recurrence when so shielded. Because of these factors, we have elected to maintain patients in a fixed and relatively comfortable supine position for the entire treatment with *TNI*. This offers the maximum reproducibility of both patient and treatment portal positioning which are considered to be *sine quo non* for effective mantle field irradiation.

Anterior Mantle Field. With the patient positioned (Fig. 7-15), the treatment field is centered on the suprasternal notch. The upper margin of the field passes through the chin tip and external auditory canal. Failure to routinely include the submental and uppermost cervical nodes in the irradiated volume will risk marginal recurrence and secondary reseeding of the lower neck. The cephalocaudad dimension of the field is automatically determined by the distance from the suprasternal notch to the external auditory canal. The lower margin approximates the level of the diaphragm in the average patient but this is inconsequential when the abdominal lymphatics are to be sequentially treated. With the patient in treatment position, first a chest radiograph is obtained with the film cassette located under the patient's back. This film is then centered on the suprasternal notch and a focal-skin distance identical to the treatment source-skin distance is employed. A contour for the lung blocks is then drawn free-hand on this radiograph (Fig. 7-16) for the construction of styrofoam molds as discussed above. These styro-

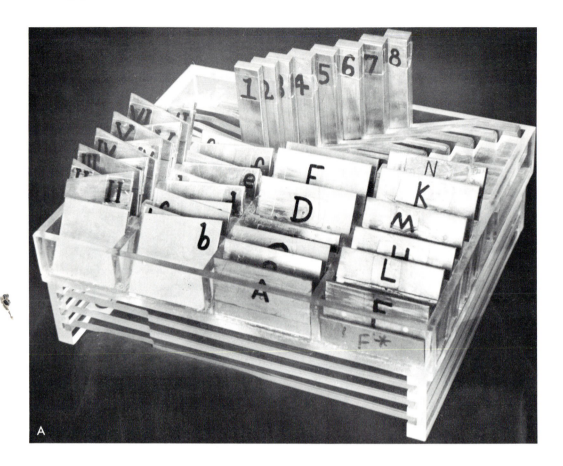

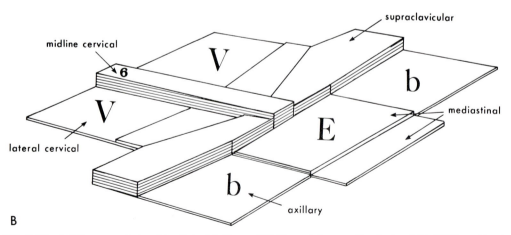

FIG. 7-13. **A.** Filters manufactured by: Poly-Fab Corp., 4230 Howard Avenue, Kensington, Md. 20795; or Atomic Development Corporation, 7 Fairchild Court, Plainview, N.Y. 11803.
   B. Compensating filter arrangement schematically represented.

ISODOSE CURVE, COBALT-60, 10 x 20 CM
AT 80 CM SSD, CORD BLOCK PROJECTS
2 CM WIDE ON SURFACE

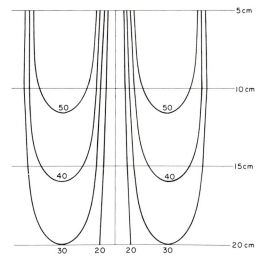

FIG. 7-14. A 1 cm wide lead block used for spinal cord shielding attenuates the absorbed dose at all depths beneath the block.

foam-lead blocks are readily fixed in the proper cephalocaudad and lateral directions on the shadow tray by cutting midline holes through the styrofoam for transmission of the light field on the central axis (suprasternal notch) and lower midmediastinum. For experienced technicians, the total setup time for an anterior mantle field averages 2 to 3 minutes, including the positioning of the compensating filters.

Posterior Mantle Field. For reasons discussed, a posterior mantle field has not been adopted. It is essential, however, to irradiate at least the mediastinal portion of the mantle field through parallel-opposed fields in order to avoid excessive exposure of the anterior cardiac structures.[15] The remainder of the mantle field volume, *i.e.* the cervical and axillary regions, is irradiated only through the anterior treatment port. This requires a modified lung block (Fig. 7-17) for alternate

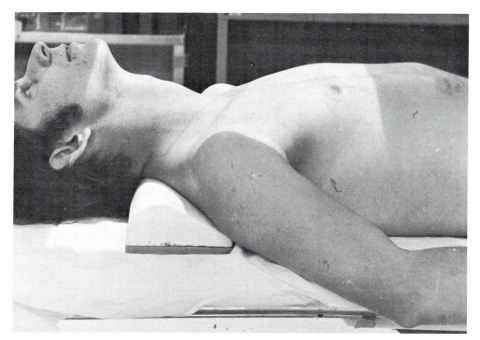

FIG. 7-15. The field for mantle field irradiation includes the submental and high cervical lymph nodes, thereby requiring moderate extension of the head.

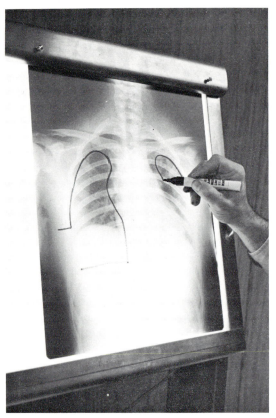

FIG. 7-16. Contours for lung-heart shielding blocks being drawn on a chest radiograph obtained when the patient is in the treatment position.

One comment is deserved regarding the hilar regions of the lung. The decreased density of overlying lung tissue increases the amount of radiation delivered to the hilar regions relative to the midmediastinum. In order to compensate for this factor, the hila are shielded during approximately one half (depending on patient thickness) of the posterior mediastinal irradiations.

TREATMENT OF INFRADIAPHRAGMATIC LYMPH NODES

In contrast to widespread adoption of some technique for mantle field irradiation, there is substantial variation in the methodology for treatment of lymph nodes below the diaphragm. For example, it has been proposed that irradiation of the entire upper abdomen to be employed[7] rather than restricting treatment to the more centrally located lymphatics and the spleen. This proposal may have merit for cases with extensive clinical involvement in the upper abdomen.[14] However, early abdominal involvement with Hodgkin's disease tends to preferentially involve the midline nodes depicted in Figure 7-9 to the relative exclusion of nodes in other sites such as the porta hepatis and mesentery. This contention is substantiated by experience[14] showing that 1) prophylactic irradiation limited to the aortic nodes and spleen prevents extension of disease to the abdomen with great consistency and 2) that with absence of prophylactic abdominal irradiation, extension of disease below the diaphragm almost invariably is limited to the midline nodes or the spleen.

There also is divergence of opinion as to the desirability of irradiating all infradiaphragmatic lymphatics in continuity with a single field (the so-called "inverted-Y" port) versus the use of individual aortic and pelvic fields. The inverted-Y type of field has been advocated in order to both expedite the completion of treatment and to avoid potential overlap or underdosage at the junction of adjoining fields, these latter considerations

days when the mediastinum is irradiated posteriorly. Whereas such treatment of the neck and axillae through an anterior field only delivers a relatively high surface dose to these areas in order to achieve an adequate depth dose, marked skin reactions and delayed fibrosis or other complications have not been observed *provided* a split-course schedule is utilized. Likewise, recurrence of disease in the posterior axilla (prescapular nodes) or in the posterior cervical region has not been observed. The major asset of maintaining patients in a fixed supine position for all treatments has been maximal reproduction of treatment geometry with the result that the incidence of local and marginal recurrence has been negligible in our experience with the mantle field technique.

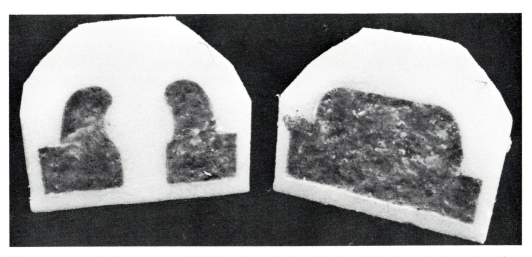

FIG. 7-17. A modified anterior mantle field lung-heart block which also shields the mediastinum is used on alternate days when the mediastinum is irradiated with a posterior treatment port.

also being applicable to the junction between the mantle field and upper abdominal treatment port. As illustrated by Figure 7-18, adjacent treatment fields may be overlapped, abutted, or separated on the surface of the body. Both overlapping and abutting fields produce "hot spots" at depth and, conversely, excessive separation of adjacent fields may result in "cold spots" within the junction volume. The correct separation for any situation (*e.g.* beam energy, source-skin distance, field sizes, tumor depth, etc.) is readily calculated from isodose curves or is measured directly with thermoluminescent or film dosimetry.[4] In this manner, tabulations can be developed (*e.g.* Table 7-13)

Table 7-13. *Separation Distance (cm) Between Fields, Theratron 80, 80 cm, SSD*

Field Lengths (cm)* \ Depth (cm)	5	6	7	8	9	10	11	12	13	14	15
10–10	.50	.50	.75	.75	1.00	1.00	1.25	1.25	1.50	1.50	1.75
10–15	.50	.75	1.00	1.00	1.25	1.25	1.50	1.75	1.75	2.00	2.00
10–20	.75	1.00	1.25	1.25	1.50	1.75	2.00	2.00	2.25	2.50	2.75
10–25	1.00	1.00	1.25	1.50	1.75	2.00	2.25	2.50	2.75	3.00	3.00
10–30	1.00	1.25	1.50	1.75	2.00	2.25	2.50	2.75	3.00	3.25	3.50
15–15	.75	.75	1.00	1.25	1.50	1.50	1.75	2.00	2.25	2.50	2.50
15–20	.75	1.00	1.25	1.50	1.75	2.00	2.25	2.50	2.75	3.00	3.00
15–25	1.00	1.25	1.50	1.75	2.00	2.25	2.50	2.75	3.00	3.25	3.50
15–30	1.00	1.25	1.75	2.00	2.25	2.50	2.75	3.00	3.25	3.50	3.75
20–20	1.00	1.25	1.50	1.75	2.00	2.25	2.50	2.75	3.00	3.25	3.50
20–25	1.25	1.50	1.75	2.00	2.25	2.50	2.75	3.25	3.50	3.75	4.00
20–30	1.25	1.50	2.00	2.25	2.50	2.75	3.00	3.50	3.75	4.00	4.25
25–25	1.25	1.50	2.00	2.25	2.50	3.00	3.25	3.50	3.75	4.25	4.50
25–30	1.50	1.75	2.00	2.50	2.75	3.25	3.50	3.75	4.00	4.50	4.75
30–30	1.50	2.00	2.25	2.50	3.00	3.50	3.50	4.00	4.25	4.75	5.00

*Lengths of fields perpendicular to their adjoining edges. A larger listing may be obtained from the senior author.

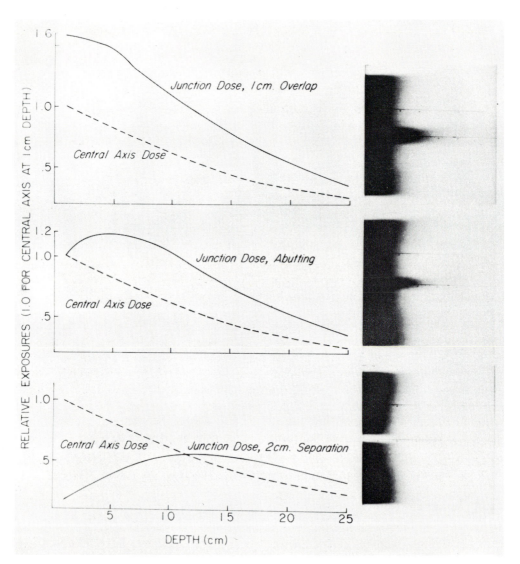

FIG. 7-18. Central axis (for each of two adjoining fields) and junction doses are shown when adjoining treatment fields overlap, abut, or are separated on the surface of the body.

which specify the appropriate surface separation for adjoining treatment fields. Appreciation that selection of the correct "gap" between adjoining ports can assure delivery of the desired dose to the junction volume allows the confident use of individual aortic and pelvic-groin fields as an alternative to the inverted-Y field.

Further, the large integral dose administered daily by an inverted-Y field is poorly tolerated by many patients. And the systemic side effects are, at times, complicated by a precipitous depression of hematologic values forcing interruption of treatment. When resumption of radiotherapy is delayed beyond several weeks, the therapeutic effectiveness of irradiation may be jeopardized. Therefore, we prefer to divide the inverted-Y field into 2 segments for most patients. When using split-course irradiation, this policy permits treatment of the upper abdomen during the "break" in mantle field irradiation (Fig. 7-19).

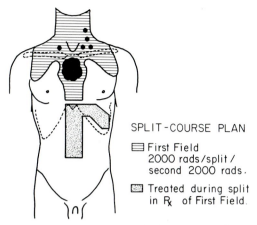

SPLIT-COURSE PLAN

▤ First Field
2000 rads/split /
second 2000 rads.

▨ Treated during split
in Rx of First Field.

FIG. 7-19. Scheme for use of split-course irradiation of the mantle field and upper abdomen.

In such a method, patients remain under continuous treatment until radiotherapy of the mantle and upper abdominal region is completed. Then after a rest interval of 4 to 8 weeks, irradiation of the pelvic and groin lymph nodes can be undertaken without hematologic complications in most cases.

IRRADIATION OF THE SPLEEN

Irradiation of a normal-sized spleen is technically feasible using a treatment port which does not excessively expose the left kidney or left lung base, contrary to the opinion of many radiotherapists. Careful field shaping and localization using intravenous pyelography (Fig. 7-20) need only be accompanied by the caution to patients that deep respiratory movements are to be avoided during treatment. Provided the spleen is not clinically enlarged, treatment is predictably effective and not a single recurrence of disease in the spleen has been clinically noted for 74 consecutive patients now observed for a median of 5 years.

In contrast, gross splenomegaly does necessitate the excessive radiation exposure of the left kidney. Splenectomy is considered indicated for these selected patients, especially since clinical splenomegaly is associated with an appreciable risk of hepatic in-

volvement by Hodgkin's disease and the latter is most reliably detected by open biopsy.[8] As previously noted,[14] occult microscopic involvement of the spleen is not similarly associated with a high incidence of liver involvement and routine staging laparotomy which detects such microscopic disease in the spleen does not justify a change in therapeutic approach. However, prophylactic irradiation of the spleen is nearly always mandatory for presentations of Hodgkin's disease above the diaphragm since at least 20 per cent of clinically normal spleens will contain occult involvement by lymphoma.

TREATMENT OF PELVIC-GROIN LYMPH NODES

The procedure illustrated in Figure 7-21 has been adopted for irradiation of the iliac

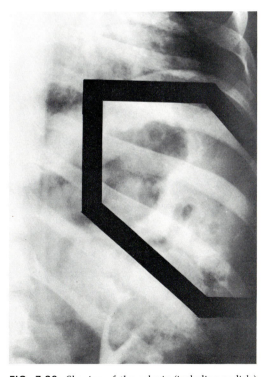

FIG. 7-20. Shaping of the splenic (including pedicle) field using pyelography avoids the complications of radiation nephritis and pneumonitis when the spleen is not grossly enlarged.

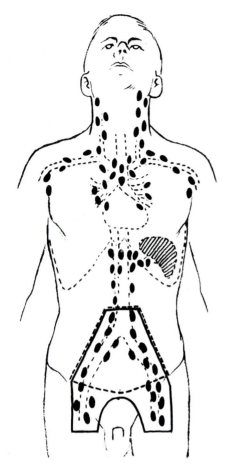

FIG. 7-21. Lymphatics in pelvis and groin are irradiated with weighted fields using 2 anterior exposures for each posterior treatment. The daily absorbed dose of 200 rads is calculated at the midpelvis avoiding the irradiation of superficial groin nodes through a posterior treatment port or the need for separate inguinofemoral fields. Posterior portal shown by dotted line.

tion. Providing split course irradiation is employed, subcutaneous fibrosis over the anterior lower abdomen has not been observed despite the relatively higher entrance dose. The smaller posterior port is readily treated through most cutout sections in the therapy couch of isocentric ^{60}Co teletherapy or linear accelerator units, eliminating the need to rotate patients into a prone position.

Irradiation of the pelvic and groin lymphatics inevitably causes a substantial radiation dose to gonadal tissues. It has not been our practice to attempt sparing of ovarian function by the surgical displacement of the ovaries outside the treatment field since staging laparotomy has been considered to have only selective indications. Partial success with surgical fixation of the ovaries in the midline has been reported however.[22] For testicular shielding, the combination of 2 methods has proven relatively effective. Adequate shadow tray shielding affords 96 per cent attenuation of the exposure dose to the testicles. Further shadow tray shielding is relatively less effective because of internal scatter contribution. Conical gonadal cups (Fig. 7-22) constructed from $\frac{1}{4}$ inch lead sheet and lined with disposable plastic bags serve to reduce markedly the scatter contribution. For ^{60}Co teletherapy, direct measurements have shown reduction of the testicular dose from 225 to 275 rads for shadow tray blocking only to 75 to 125 rads using a combination of shadow tray and gonadal cup shielding when a tumor dose of 4,000 rads is delivered to the pelvic-groin lymph nodes.

and inguinofemoral lymph nodes. The anterior treatment portal encompasses the iliac and groin nodes in continuity, the latter receiving a tumor dose roughly 50 per cent higher than that delivered to the midpelvic nodes from an anterior field. Using an abbreviated posterior field as shown, the groin nodes eventually receive an absorbed dose almost identical to that given the midpelvic nodes when treatment is weighted with 2 anterior exposures for each posterior irradia-

Indications for Total Nodal Irradiation

A major restructuring of attitudes toward the biologic behavior of Hodgkin's disease has occurred in the past decade. There is now widespread awareness of the fallacy in relying upon available diagnostic tests, including surgical exploration of the abdomen, for accurately determining the *true* extent of disease. It is not surprising that the most recent

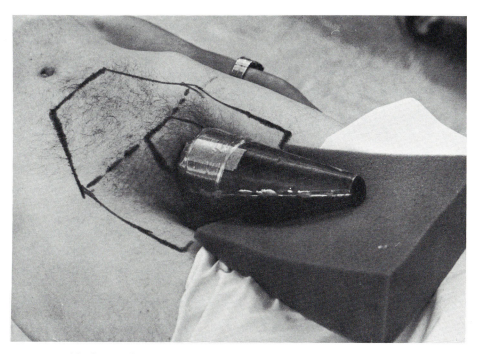

FIG. 7-22. Conical lead cups effectively reduce the scattered radiation dose to testicles.

clinical trials have demonstrated that extensive prophylactic irradiation is imperative for optimal results for this reason.[3] An impression of limited disease far too often is misleading and the concept of *TNI*, with selective modifications, thus deserves rapid acceptance.

Exceptions to the requirement for classical *TNI* of all major lymph node areas exist, the most frequent being the presentation of disease above the diaphragm with a histologic subclassification of nodular sclerosis. Despite normal results of a bipedal lymphogram[9] and the absence of splenomegaly, occult disease is present in the upper abdomen with sufficient frequency to warrant routine prophylactic irradiation of the aortic nodes and the spleen (including the pedicle) for all patients with disease in the lower neck or supraclavicular region. However, we have observed extension of disease below the bifurcation of the aorta in less than 5 per cent of Stages I to II (above the diaphragm) patients having nodular sclerosis histology.

Routine prophylactic irradiation of the pelvis thus offers little prospect if improving the over-all results. Further, the detection of occult disease in the upper abdomen by staging laparotomy should not change this treatment decision as the clinical stage (and experience relating thereto) remains the same. When defined as the irradiation of all high-risk areas, *TNI* for these Stages I to II nodular sclerosis patients will consist of treating all major lymph node areas with the empiric exclusion of the pelvic and groin regions. This approach is particularly desirable for young females in whom reproductive capacity is thereby preserved.

Another recognized manifestation of Hodgkin's disease which deserves a modified treatment approach is the localized unilateral involvement of lymph nodes in the very high cervical region. Whereas initial extension of disease below the diaphragm is extremely uncommon in this situation, recurrence of disease in Waldeyer's ring has been observed in a sufficient number of cases to warrant prophylactic irradiation of Waldeyer's ring when very high cervical nodes are involved. Therefore, while not all patients require classical *TNI,* the decision to use a modified technique should be based not on whim but rather on a complete understanding of the behavior of the disease in its protean clinical manifestation.

Results and Complications

Past years have witnessed uncertainty as to the role of prophylactic irradiation for Hodgkin's disease.[23] This uncertainty resulted, as has often been the case in medicine, from the drawing of conclusions not from prospective study but rather from retrospective examination of clinical experience.[23,21] In the one instance where randomly assigned controls were used for comparison,[18] the type of prophylactic irradiation was too limited to permit identification of improved survival. Not until our recently reported clinical trial[12,13] has scientific data been available to dispel the myth enshrouding the subject of prophylactic irradiation for Hodgkin's disease. It can now be confidently stated that comprehensive treatment is essential at the time of initial therapy for Hodgkin's disease, even for the early clinical stages of disease (Fig. 7-23). The 5-year survival rate for Stages I and II nodular sclerosis patients has been comparable (92 per cent) to that for other cell types of similar stage but did not necessitate irradiation of the pelvic-groin lymph nodes as discussed above. Whereas some oncologists have persistent reservations about the primary management of clinical Stage III patients with radiation therapy, even our initial experience has been reasonably encouraging (Fig. 7-24) and it should be improved with more precise definition of extent of disease.[7]

Normal tissue complications resulting from *TNI* have usually reflected the effect of local irradiation on specific organs rather than being related to *TNI per se.* These local complications are inversely related in fre-

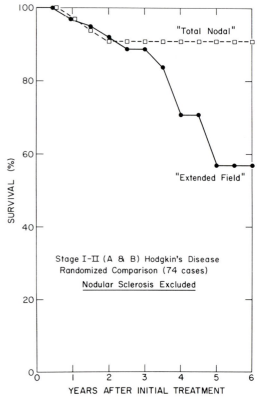

FIG. 7-23. Improved survival for Stages I to II Hodgkin's disease using *TNI* compared to that for limited prophylactic irradiation. Randomized comparison includes patients with and without constitutional symptoms excluding cases with nodular sclerosis histology (see text).

quency to the precision of treatment planning and the protraction of the radiation dose-time schedule. As commented on, it has been determined that virtually all serious local complications have now been eliminated with the adoption of split-course irradiation and that the major considerations with respect to toxicity are systemic in nature, namely hematologic and immunologic.

There is a recognized propensity for Hodgkin's disease to produce or to be associated with immunologic incompetence[1] and intensive chemical or radiation therapy certainly contributes, at least transiently, to suppression of the immune mechanism. Despite this, there has not been an unusual

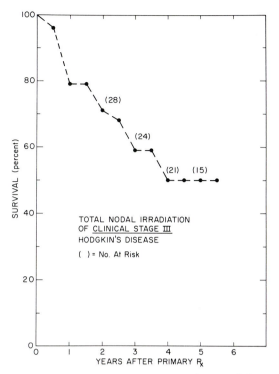

FIG. 7-24. Survival rates for the initial group of clinical Stage III patients treated with *TNI* is shown. Included are all cases ("A" and "B") with generalized lymph node involvement.

number of infections following *TNI* with the exception of a high incidence of herpes zoster.[28] As might be anticipated, however, those patients who have not remained free of Hodgkin's disease have experienced the usual secondary infections which generally complicate the progression of any lymphomatous process.

Hematologic toxicity from *TNI* is widely appreciated and constitutes the most frequent constraint to the completion of treatment. A minimum interruption of therapy for one month is essential at some point during *TNI* if serious bone marrow depression is to be avoided. When suitable (implying flexibility) caution is practiced, almost every patient should complete the planned course of therapy, including those older patients with less hematopoietic resilience. Short-term recovery of the peripheral blood

counts following *TNI* has been described[11] and we recently have summarized the 5-year hematologic values for the initial 56 patients following completion of classical *TNI* to all major lymph node areas. The data shown in Figure 7-25 should prove reassuring to those with any concern that secondary bone marrow failure will prove an obstacle to the adoption of *TNI* as a therapeutically effective *and* tolerated form of treatment.

Discussion

There inevitably will be an increased acceptance of *TNI* as embodied in the concept of primary irradiation of all areas with a significant risk of involvement in contrast to the policy of limited treatment followed by "wait-and-watch." With selective modification, *TNI* offers the prospect of cure to 80 per cent of all Stages I and II patients combined and a 5-year survival rate of at least 90 per cent. It likewise appears reasonable to estimate that future cure rates for Stage III patients should approximate 50 per cent although this figure will obviously be substantially higher in series which include early clinical stage patients considered Stage III on the basis of surgical findings at laparotomy. At the present time, the potential role for *TNI* has not been determined for the non-Hodgkin's lymphomas but certain aspects discussed in this chapter, such as dosimetry and field shaping, are certainly relevant to the treatment of local regional manifestations of non-Hodgkin's lymphomas.

In addition to the need for meticulous treatment planning, there is a compelling requirement for the careful monitoring of patients during *TNI*. The extent of disease, which clinically is appreciated, may change during the therapy of any patient and appropriate studies must be serially made. For example, unexpectedly severe hematologic depression observed during irradiation may clearly dictate the interruption of treatment in some instances. Equally important is the re-evaluation for possible bone marrow in-

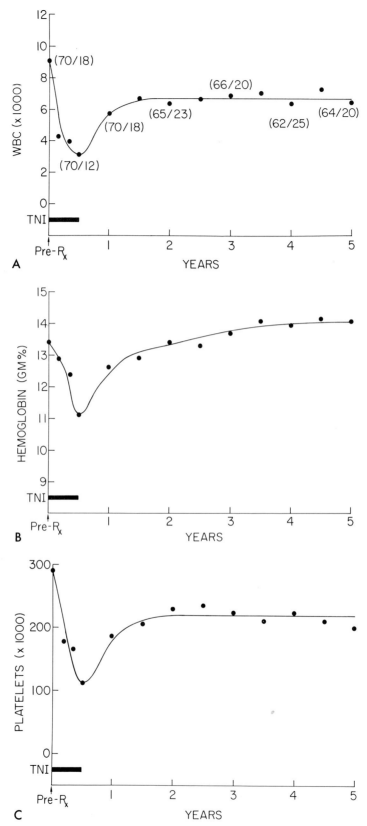

FIG. 7-25. Recovery of peripheral blood counts following treatment with classical *TNI* for initial 56 patients over a 5-year period. **A.** White blood count, **B.** Hemoglobin, **C.** Platelets.

Ratios in parentheses along the leukocyte curve refer to the neutrophil counts: lymphocyte percentages on differential count. All counts represent mean values.

volvement by Hodgkin's disease in this situation. Empiric continuation of radiation therapy once initiated will otherwise serve only to further reduce the bone marrow reserve and hamper, if not negate, the subsequent administration of effective chemotherapy.[3]

In summary, our experience has demonstrated that *TNI* can be completed without excessive morbidity, providing sufficient attention is devoted to treatment planning and the monitoring of patients during therapy. The improvement in survival rates with *TNI* as compared to less aggressive therapy is now a matter of record and radiotherapists are obliged to develop skill in using some carefully planned technique for *TNI*. The only reasonable alternative is the referral of patients to medical centers where adequate therapy *is* available. It is also true that one may "skin-the-cat" in different ways. Quite acceptable alternative techniques for *TNI* are practiced with excellent results in other centers. The methodology described here is presented as one approach which, through trial and quite often error, has evolved to a relatively high degree of reliability.

BIBLIOGRAPHY

1. Aisenberg, A. C.: Hodgkin's disease-prognosis, treatment, and etiologic and immunologic considerations, *New Eng. J. Med.*, 270, 617, 1964.
2. Anderson, R. E., D'Angio, G. J., and Khan, F. M.: Dosimetry of irregularly shaped radiation fields, *Radiology*, 92, 1097, 1969.
3. Curran, R. E., and Johnson, R. E.: Tolerance to chemotherapy after prior irradiation for Hodgkin's disease. *Ann. Int. Med.*, 72, 505, 1970.
4. Faw, F. L., and Glenn, D. W.: Further investigations of physical aspects of multiple field radiation therapy, *Amer. J. Roentgen.*, 108, 184, 1970.
5. Faw, F., Johnson, R. E., Glenn, D. W., and Warren, C. A.: A standard set of "individualized" compensating filters for mantle field radiotherapy of Hodgkin's disease, *Amer. J. Roentgen.*, 111, 376, 1971.
6. Friedman, M., Pearlman, A. W., and Turgeon, L.: Hodgkin's disease; tumor lethal dose and iso-effect recovery curves, *Amer. J. Roentgen.*, 99, 843, 1967.
7. Fuller, L. M.: Results of large volume irradiation in the management of Hodgkin's disease and malignant lymphomas originating in the abdomen, *Radiology*, 87, 1058, 1966.
8. Glatstein, E., Trueblood, H. W., Enright, L. P., Rosenberg, S. A., and Kaplan, H. S.: Surgical staging of abdominal involvement in unselected patients with Hodgkin's disease, *Radiology*, 97, 425, 1970.
9. Johnson, R. E., and Cook, P. L.: Hodgkin's disease: the negative lymphogram in guiding radiotherapy, *Amer. J. Roentgen.*, 102, 883, 1968.
10. Johnson, R. E.: Modern approaches to the radiotherapy of lymphoma, *Semin. Hemat.*, 6, 357, 1969.
11. Johnson, R. E., Kagan, A. R., Hafermann, M. D., and Keyes, J. W.: Patient tolerance to extended irradiation in Hodgkin's disease, *Ann. Int. Med.*, 70, 1, 1969.
12. Johnson, R. E., Thomas, L. B., Schneiderman, M., Glenn, D. W., Faw, F., and Hafermann, M. D.: Preliminary experience with total nodal irradiation in Hodgkin's disease, *Radiology*, 96, 603, 1970.
13. Johnson, R. E., Glover, M. K., and Marshall, S. K.: Results of radiation therapy and implications for the clinical staging of Hodgkin's disease, *Cancer Res.*, 31, 1834, 1971.
14. Johnson, R. E.: Is staging laparotomy routinely indicated in Hodgkin's disease? *Ann. Int. Med.*, 75, 459, 1971.
15. Kagan, A. R., Morton, D. L., Hafermann, M. D., and Johnson, R. E.: Evaluation and management of radiation-induced pericardial effusion, *Radiology*, 92, 632, 1969.
16. Kaplan, H. S.: Radical radiotherapy of regionally localized Hodgkin's disease, *Radiology*, 78, 553, 1962.
17. Kaplan, H. S.: Evidence for a tumoricidal dose level in the radiotherapy of Hodgkin's disease, *Cancer Res.*, 26, 1221, 1966.
18. Kaplan, H. S.: Clinical evaluation and radiotherapeutic management of Hodgkin's disease and the malignant lymphomas, *New Eng. J. Med.*, 278, 892, 1968.
19. Landberg, T.: Radiosensitivity of mediastinal lymphomas in Hodgkin's disease treated with split-course radiotherapy. A retrospective study, *Acta Radiol.*, 9, 177, 1970.

20. Meurk, M. L., Green, J. P., Nussbaum, H., and Vaeth, J. M.: Phantom dosimetry study of shaped Cobalt-60 fields in the treatment of Hodgkin's disease, *Radiology,* 91, 554, 1968.

21. Peters, M. V.: Prophylactic treatment of adjacent areas in Hodgkin's disease, *Cancer Res.,* 26, 1232, 1966.

22. Ray, G., Trueblood, H. W., Enright, L. P., Kaplan, H. S., and Nelson, T. S.: Oophoropexy: a means of preserving ovarian function following pelvic megavoltage radiotherapy for Hodgkin's disease, *Radiology,* 96, 175, 1970.

23. Rubin, P., and Kurohara, S. S.: Has prophylactic irradiation proved itself in the treatment of localized Hodgkin's disease, *Radiology,* 87, 240, 1966.

24. Salzman, F. S., Smedal, M. I., Wright, K. A.,

Trump, J. G.: Two MeV wide field irradiation of lymphoma, twelve year experience, *Amer. J. Roentgen.,* 92, 124, 1964.

25. Scott, R. M., and Brizel, H. E.: Time-dose relationships in Hodgkin's disease, *Radiology,* 82, 1043, 1964.

26. Svahn-Tapper, G., and Landberg, T.: Mantle treatment of Hodgkin's disease with cobalt 60: technique and dosimetry, *Acta Radiol.,* 10, 33, 1971.

27. Van Dorssen, J. G., Mellink, J. H., and Thomas, P.: Construction of auxiliary diaphragms for megavoltage irradiation of large, irregularly shaped fields, *Radio. Clin. Biol.,* 39, 47, 1970.

28. Wilson, J. F., Marsa, G. W., and Johnson, R. E.: Herpes zoster in Hodgkin's disease: clinical, histologic, and immunologic correlations, *Cancer,* 29, 189, 1972.

8. Pediatric Tumors

Radiation Therapy of Cancer in Childhood

I. G. WILLIAMS

Introduction

Tumors in children classified on a histogenic basis show that the commonest arise from mesodermal cells, and 60 per cent are embryonic in origin.[32] One-third arise in the central and sympathetic nervous system, one-third in the hemopoietic tissues (including leukemia) and the remainder in the kidney, urogenital tract and connective tissues.

Most childhood tumors are radiosensitive, but this advantage may be lost as far as the therapeutic ratio of tumor-lethal and tissue tolerance dose is concerned by increased normal tissue sensitivity compared with the adult. Apart from some cerebral tumors, small volume radical radiotherapy is rarely possible.

In a child the adequate treatment of a neoplasm may involve wide regional irradiation; with the proximity of essential normal structures it is not possible to lay down rigid rules or specific dose levels.

The lethal dose for embryonal tumors is not known but bearing all facts in mind, the doses to be used lie between 3,000 to 4,000 r (megavoltage) in 4 to 5 weeks depending upon the site, the volume and perhaps the age of the patient. In the palliative treatment of disseminated radiosensitive tumors much lower doses are given in a shorter period of time for the object here is relief of pain, of pressure, or of ugly tumor masses. On the question of tabular estimates of dosage published by various authors, Paterson[24] advises that they should be regarded only as an initial guide. A real knowledge of tolerance and lethality can only be gained by personal clinical experience by an individual using his own apparatus and dosimetry and having regard to the type of patient seen.

Reactions and Tissue Tolerance

The Hemopoietic System

The effects of irradiation on the hemopoietic system are similar to those in adults, *i.e.,* leukopenia affecting the lymphocytes, and then the polymorphonuclear leukocytes, a fall in the platelet count and later a red cell anemia. When large volumes are being irradiated this effect may be sudden and severe and this entails a careful watch. The white cell count differs from the adult count; at birth the total white count is about 18,000 gradually declining up to the 12th year to the adult total. At the 12th day of life, the lymphocytes comprise about 55 per cent. At 4 years the proportion of lymphocytes and polymorphs are equal at 40 per cent, thereafter the polymorphs gradually increase until adult proportions are reached at the 12th year. Radiotherapy should be suspended if the leukocytes fall to a total of 2,000 cells or the platelets 100,000.

Brain and Spinal Cord

The tolerance of the brain or cord of a child is of the same order as that of the adult. It was considered that the radiation injury was due to damage to the vascular supply, but neuroglial tissue is also affected and repair processes are interfered with. Tolerance is related to volume irradiated. For small volume brain irradiation this is of the order of 5,000 r megavoltage in 6 weeks, and for whole brain 4,000 r in 6 weeks. In the cord volume is related to length. Paterson suggests that the critical length is 20 cm. For 20 cm and over we consider 3,000 r in 5 to 6 weeks the limit of tolerance, while shorter lengths may absorb 4,500 r in 5 to 6 weeks without permanent injury.

The Lungs

When the lungs are directly exposed some degree of radiation pneumonitis always occurs, but irreversible changes are related to dose. In thoracic bath treatment of pulmonary metastases (Wilms' tumor), dose is also dictated by the body volume dose and its consequent reactions. Up to the age of 6 years we have delivered 1,200 r to 1,500 r in 2 weeks measured as a central dose. After the age of 10 years full adult doses will be tolerated. In conjunction with Actinomycin-D, D'Angio[8] advises a dose of 1,200 r in 10 treatments over 2 weeks measured in the center of the thorax. These doses cause no clinically evident pulmonary reaction.

The Kidneys

Adult renal tolerance has been studied by Kunkler et al.[17] From a study of their dose levels they state that: 1) 1,700 r in 5 weeks is tolerated, 2) 2,800 r in 5 weeks results in radiation nephritis in a high proportion of cases, and 3) protection of leaving renal tissue outside the beam will minimize this risk. We have accepted these dose levels as applying to children. One patient aged 18 months with bilateral Wilms' tumors survives symptom-free 16 years following nephrectomy (left) and irradiation of the right kidney to a dose of 1,600 r in 4 weeks.

The Ovary and Testicle

There is no permissible dose level. These organs must be totally screened or totally irradiated. Complete ovarian ablation does not seem to have necessarily any ill effect as far as the growth and secondary sexual characteristics of the female are concerned (see nephroblastoma).

Effects on Bone Growth

Deformity of developing bone can result from the irradiation of active bone growth centers. Neuhauser et al.[22] state that doses above 2,000 r result in retardation of bone growth irrespective of the child's age. The most commonly reported is scoliosis due to vertebral irradiation in the treatment of spinal, thoracic, or abdominal tumors. Rubin et al.[28] studied 12 patients with measurable scoliosis. All were under the age of 18 months when treated, and received minimal doses of 3,000 r in the midplane of opposing fields and were followed up for a period of 5 to 25 years. In their experience deformity became apparent 12 months after therapy and was related to dose and age. There was not much deterioration in the degree of curvature with the passage of time, but once established it was permanent. It did not appear to be related to whether the fields were unilateral or included the whole width of the vertebrae, the result being a unilateral wedge effect. Vaeth et al.[31] described the main radiological changes in the growing spine as scoliosis, irregular epiphyseal lines, transverse growth disturbance lines, abnormal contour of the vertebra, and hypodevelopment. These workers advise that meticulous radiotherapy, constant observation in the post-treatment period, and orthopedic care in the early stages may minimize this postural disability.

Apart from the vertebral changes, bone, soft tissue, and skin can also be affected, resulting in maldevelopment, atrophy and interference with function. This is particularly so around the shoulder and hip joints.

Irradiation Sarcoma

Irradiation sarcomas have been reported[4,7,27] and we have three examples in our records.

The Lens

Merriman and Focht[21] on the question of the relative sensitivity of young lenses state that animal work suggests a greater sensitivity of young lenses to radiations compared with adults. In their series it appeared that the lenses of children below the age of 1 year showed a higher incidence of cataracts which develop more rapidly. They classify radiation cataracts according to whether they are progressive until the opacity is complete, or small early ones which progress for a few months and then remain stationary. The time of onset in 8 children below the age of 1 year varied between 1 year and 7 months to 4 years 1 month, average 2 years and 7 months. In these it tended to be progressive. In 9 children aged 1 to 4 years the interval was 1 year 8 months to 6 years 9 months, average 3 years and 8 months. Over the age of 1 year it would appear that lenses of children had the same sensitivity as adults. They state that if a lens receives 750 to 950 r in 3 weeks to 3 months the patient has a 60 per cent chance of developing a cataract, in 50 per cent of whom it would be progressive.

We have treated bilateral retinoblastoma when large and in the remaining eye after removal of the other, by direct irradiation through an anterior field. We have delivered below the age of 1 year 3,000 to 3,500 r and above this age up to 4,000 r in 4 weeks. Reactions in the eye have been slight, when ^{60}Co is the source. With x-rays, reactions and consequence have been more serious. In cases with large tumors or tumors in multiple sites, the aim has been to reduce the size to such dimensions that the residue could be destroyed by a radioactive applicator sutured to the sclera. All these patients develop an irradiation cataract of some degree but only in very few is it complete enough to warrant surgical treatment.

The General Management of Children Undergoing Radiotherapy

The general management of children undergoing radiotherapy is directed towards gaining and keeping their confidence, and in general medical care, corrections of nourishment, fluid intake, electrolyte balance and blood state, are more important than sedation. The general ill effects of radiation are not common in children but when the general reaction occurs, especially nausea, refusal to take food, vomiting and diarrhea, its significance is greater because of the rapid dehydration and loss of weight which may occur. Washing and bathing is allowed in warm water with gentle drying and the use of a bland dusting powder.

In practice the condition of an anemic child in pain with neuroblastoma may improve rapidly during therapy. A child should never be forceably tied or fixed on the treatment couch but adequately supported with blankets and side bags, and the arms may have to be gently restrained by similar means. Oral sedation or light anesthesia with rectal pentothal is essential in almost all babies below the age of 1 year and in most up to the 4th or 5th year. In fractionated therapy the course should start slowly with small doses of 30 r to 50 r and increase in 3 to 4 sessions to the daily dose necessary to deliver the prescribed dose. Skin reactions with megavoltage therapy will only be slight, and it is accepted practice never to proceed to second degree reactions or fibrinous mucosal reactions.

Palliative Therapy

In palliative radiotherapy the guiding principle is to deliver the minimal dose which will achieve the desired effect, relief of pain, relief of pressure, or the shrinkage of a disfiguring mass. In such it is justifiable to deliver the dose as quickly as possible. Such therapy contributes not only to the welfare of the patient but also to the morale of the nursing staff and especially the morale and happiness of the parents. Most treatments are planned as 5 in 7 days or 10 in 14 days and dose levels will depend upon the volume irradiated, the sensitivity of the neoplasm and perhaps the extent of the dissemination. A slower rate is absolutely indicated in all ill, anemic children for it is quite unjustifiable to risk causing radiation sickness.

Reticuloendothelial Tumors Including Leukemia

Leukemia

Leukemia is the commonest malignant disease process in children.

Radiotherapy

CHRONIC MYELOID LEUKEMIA

This is exceedingly rare in children. In 2 patients aged 8 and 12 years (2 per cent of leukemia admissions) there was a long history and considerable splenomegaly. Treatment was by transfusions and splenic irradiation. There are no differences in technique to that in adults and the main indication and value of radiotherapy is reduction in size of the enlarged spleen. One starts with 50 *r* increasing to 150 *r* depending on speed of fall of white count. In one of the above, the spleen was enlarged to the pelvis and interfered with movement. Reduction in size was gradual and maintained with considerable symptomatic benefit.

ACUTE LEUKEMIA

The Meningeal Syndrome. A meningeal syndrome has been described in 25 per cent of patients treated with cortisone or chemotherapy.[30]

This is due to leukemic infiltration of nerve roots, meninges and perivascular cuffing. It can be intracranial or affect the spinal cord and spinal nerve roots. Hemorrhages ranging from petechia to massive bleeding can also occur. In the Boston series[10] in 50 per cent the neurological condition arose during a remission and in 10 per cent as a presenting symptom. Antileukemic drugs may fail to pass the blood brain barrier in sufficient concentration to influence the intracranial infiltrations. There is often evidence of raised intracranial tension with widening of the sutures and raised cerebrospinal fluid pressure. Treatment is given to the whole head through opposing fields with protection of the eyes but if the cerebrospinal fluid pressure is raised lumbar puncture may be necessary and the initial dose is kept low (25 *r*). The dose is gradually increased to deliver between 400 and 600 *r* in 10 treatments over 14 days. If recurrence occurs after an interval of 2 months, retreatment can be given.

Bone and Joint Pain. Apart from gross effects such as fractures and epiphyseal separation, leukemic infiltrations can occur subperiosteally and are often evident radiologically. Single doses of 50 *r* will often relieve this pain but total doses of the order of 400 to 600 *r* fractionated over 2 weeks produces more lasting benefit.

Skin and Mucous Membrane. The most common sites to be affected are the buccal mucosa, the lips, and the fingers and toes. The infiltrations present as nodular masses and these break down to form deep infected ulcerations. In the fingers and toes the appearance simulates a whitlow and will respond in the majority to similar order of dosage (400 to 600 *r* fractionated). Leukemic infiltrations in other sites such as the kidneys, ureters and bladder with hematuria apart from that due to thrombocytopenia are sensitive to similar dose levels in a small proportion of patients.

Malignant Reticuloendothelial Tumors

This group of tumors includes lymphosarcoma, reticulosarcoma, and lymphadenoma as well as a group with different clinical and pathological patterns, the reticuloendotheliosis (syn: xanthomatosis, lipogranulomatosis, histiocytosis X).

Reticuloendotheliosis

These diseases are characterized by proliferation of the reticulum cells which are widely distributed throughout the body. They have a common factor in a disturbance of lipoid metabolism, which appear to be built up and retained within the cell. Only those conditions where radiotherapy may be of assistance in treatment will be considered.

HAND-SCHULLER-CHRISTIAN SYNDROME AND EOSINOPHILIC GRANULOMA

As the ultimate healing is by fibrosis, care has to be exercised in selection of cases for radiotherapy. In the lungs there is proliferation of reticuloendothelial cells containing lipoid and if healing occurs these cells are gradually replaced by a diffuse interstitial fibrosis which in some results in cyst formation and a honeycomb appearance. Similarly the granulomatous hepatic infiltration heals, if the patient survives, by fibrosis. Irradiation in such may lead to a greater or more rapid fibrosis, progressive invalidism and death. These patients with visceral or widely disseminated disease are better treated by chemotherapy, which can also produce a response in bony defects.[11] The bone lesions offer radiotherapy the greatest scope in control management, although soft tissue and cerebral deposits can also be considered for this treatment in particular instances. Radiotherapy as a method of treatment is rational because of the sensitivity of its parent tissue, the cells of the reticuloendothelial system, while the mixture of eosinophils, mononuclear cells, lymphocytes, polymorphonuclear cells and phagocytic giant cells are all radiosensitive. 250 Kv x-rays *HVL* 2.0 mm. Cu is used but megavoltage can be employed should site warrant this. Single fields are adequate in most sites. Fractionated therapy of the order of 50 to 200 *r* daily dose, 5 days per week to a total of 1,000 to 1,500 *r* throughout the lesion in Hand-Schuller-Christian disease and 2,000 *r* in eosinophilic granuloma. Large soft tissue masses may regress quickly at a lower dose level and in such clinical judgment is exercised when to stop.

In eosinophilic granuloma the lesion is radiosensitive, pain being rapidly relieved, and function or mobility inasmuch as this is limited by muscle spasm, is restored. Soft tissue masses regress rapidly but healing of bony defects is slow and may take up to 12 months to fill in completely. These defects leave a healed area which is indistinguishable from the surrounding bone, without any line of demarcation.

GAUCHER'S DISEASE

The bone lesion is often in the metaphysis and distortion of joints occurs. Severe hip joint pain, or spinal pain, responds dramatically to radiotherapy. One patient aged 7 who had been bedridden for 4 months because of bilateral hip joint disease with severe pain responded to 600 *r* delivered in 1 week. This relief of pain may persist in spite of increased deformity in the joint with the passage of time.

Lymphosarcoma and Reticulosarcoma

These names are applied to tumors of the lymph nodes; lymphosarcoma, denoting the well differentiated lymphocytic form, and reticulosarcoma, a poorly differentiated tumor of the same class. Very occasionally a follicular lymphosarcoma occurs in children in the older age groups. Males are more often affected than females.

Lymphosarcoma

The tumors arise from lymphoid tissue in lymph nodes or mucous membranes.

CLINICAL FEATURES

The features are the same as in adults, important similarities and differences being as follows. The initial complaint is often enlargement of cervical nodes but sometimes the origin is in special sites.

Mediastinum. This can vary from a small mass to massive involvement of mediastinal nodes. In some instances, these form a bulky tumor and some can be confused with thymic tumors which, being also lymphocytic, renders interpretation difficult.

Intestine. Although most often involved as part of a generalized disease, the small intestine especially can be a site of primary lymphosarcoma. In very rare instances this can be a single circumscribed tumor amenable to surgical removal.[12] Very rarely, a child can present with intussusception.

Nasopharynx. The tumor can originate in the nasopharynx and be visible behind the palate, in the nose, or involve the middle ear. Occasionally, the onset is with the symptoms due to general disturbance, with fever and pruritis. In children lymphosarcoma is closely related to acute lymphatic leukemia, the blood and marrow changes occurring after the appearance of the enlarged nodes.

TREATMENT AND PROGNOSIS

The principles of radiotherapy are similar to those in adults.

Hodgkin's Disease

The clinical features of Hodgkin's disease in children are the same as in adults. By far the commonest site of origin is the cervical lymph glands. Boys are affected more than girls and while there is no record of a case below the age of 2 years, it rarely occurs below the age of 4 years. The disease is treated aggressively. Between 4 and 10 years of age involved sites are treated to a dose of 3,000 *r* in 3 weeks. Peter's technique may be used where neighboring gland sites without clinical evidence of disease are treated

to a level of 1,000 *r*. After the age of 12 years full adult doses will probably be tolerated.

Neuroblastoma and Ganglioneuroma

These tumors arise from the adrenal medulla or the ganglia of the sympathetic chain at any level from the neck to the presacral region. Neuroblastoma infiltrates and invades adjacent tissues making complete surgical excision impossible. In the abdomen the large vessels are imbedded in growth and the viscera are involved. In the thorax the spine and spinal cord are involved either by direct extension or the growth extends through an intervertebral foramina into the vertebral canal, forming the "dumbbell" tumor. Metastases occur widely by blood stream embolism to liver, lungs, bone, meninges, and other sites, and lymph nodes are also often grossly involved. Bone metastases stimulate the formation of new subperiosteal bone in spicules or "onionskin" layers. Most often affecting many bones, when single deposits occur with no evidence of a primary, especially in older children, the appearance is that of an "Ewing's Tumor." Willis[32] maintains that mistaken diagnosis of Ewing's is made in cases of unsuspected neuroblastoma with skeletal mestastases. The bone marrow may be extensively involved with a consequent secondary anemia.

Treatment and Prognosis

The ganglioneuroma is a radioresistant tumor and as it is often compact, is amenable to surgical removal. The neuroblastoma is invasive and radiosensitive but in spite of this it is worthwhile exploring and removing tumor masses in the thorax and pelvis and adrenal also, in order to relieve pressure symptoms and to establish the diagnosis. Sensitive tumors can readily be destroyed by irradiation but the widespread metastases nearly always results in death. Depending upon the tumor volume, its site, and the age of the patient, doses of the order of 1,500 to 3,500 *r* in 3 to 4 weeks to a primary compact mass will cause complete resolution, and these doses are also used in postoperative treatment following incomplete surgical removal. With megavoltage (^{60}Co) simple field arrangements, opposing and parallel, with the employment of penumbra trimmers give optimum dose distribution. In palliative therapy for painful or ugly deposits fractions of the order of 150 *r* single field can be applied and the treatment terminated at 1,000 or 1,500 *r* when the desired effect is obtained. Simultaneous administration of vitamin B$_{12}$ has been advocated.[2]

Nephroblastoma (Wilms' Tumor)

Nephroblastoma is a malignant embryonic tumor of the kidney arising from the mesodermal tissues which take part in the formation of the kidney, and which presents in early infancy.

The tumor consists of two main parts: 1) The embryonal blastoma consisting of formed or abortive renal elements, and 2) a supporting connective tissue of spindle cells, which are also malignant.

Spread occurs by direct infiltration, the lymphatics, and the blood stream.

Direct Infiltration

As the tumor grows it compresses the renal substance around it. Eventually, this capsule of renal tissue is infiltrated and through this, adjacent structures, the peritoneum, the suprarenal gland, the bowel and the liver. Very rarely is the renal pelvis and ureter involved. The tumor may, however, grow to a very large size before it commences to infiltrate. It grows forward and across the midline, as a lobulated heavy mass, but if growth is rapid it may be partly cystic.

Lymphatic Spread

The lymphatics drain into para-aortic nodes lying between the inferior mesenteric artery and the crura of the diaphragm. Lymphatic involvement is not common, even in the presence of other spread, and large fleshy nodes found at operation are often histologically found not to contain tumor.

Blood Stream Spread

A tumor thrombus grows into the capsular veins and eventually into the renal vein. Here it progressively grows to reach the inferior vena cava, where it can then extend across to the opposite renal vein or upwards into the right atrium. Tumor emboli are detached and metastases occur in lungs, liver, or indeed, any organ may be involved. Tumor emboli may spread down to the testicular veins to form nodules on the epididymus in the scrotum. Pulmonary and other metastases can occur without evidence of gross venous involvement.

Treatment

SURGERY

Nephrectomy is advised in all cases in order to remove the tumor and to tie off the veins by which the tumor spreads. This is done within 48 hours of admission and prior to operation; examination and palpation of the tumor is allowed only in so far as the establishing of the clinical condition and confirmation of the diagnosis.

RADIOTHERAPY

While it is universally recognized that radiotherapy is required in the treatment of most patients, controversy exists as to whether this should be given preoperatively, postoperatively, or both pre- and postoperatively. The tumor cells are radiosensitive, in some instances highly radiosensitive, both the embryonic renal tissue and the supporting but malignant connective tissue, evidence for this being the rapid shrinking in size of large tumors under treatment, and histological examination of tumors removed after preoperative irradiation. In view of the morbidity associated with radiation, the question arises today, that while in the majority of cases both methods of treatment may have to be used, are there types and conditions where surgery alone can be relied upon? Each patient is an individual problem and the necessity for radiotherapy or its sequence in relationship to the surgery must be carefully assessed.

SURGERY WITHOUT RADIOTHERAPY

In our experience in the Hospital for Sick Children, 1925 to 1944 series, the examination of conditions at operation, and the gross specimen, are more valuable, than the pathology, for we could find no correlation between histology and survival.[16] Fixation of the tumor indicating a tissue reaction to neoplastic infiltration and enlarged lymphatic nodes are definite indications for radiotherapy, as are the presence of tumor thrombi in capsular veins or the main renal veins. The indications for radiotherapy are clear cut in undifferentiated tumors with evidence of spread within or outside the tumor. In the case of a child below the age of 1 year with a well-differentiated tumor confined in its capsule and without evidence of venous lymphatic or tissue invasion, there is probably no indication for radiotherapy.

PREOPERATIVE IRRADIATION

It is our practice to restrict this to the management of very large tumors which, because of their size and fixity, the surgeon considers irremovable. The argument for routine preoperative irradiation in all cases is based on the known radiosensitivity of the tumor cells and the lysis of these cells, which can be demonstrated histologically. The hope is that it will sterilize the tumor zone and diminish the viability of the cells, so that if at operation, they escape into the circulation they will not survive or graft and develop secondary tumors. Such a contention pre-

supposes affecting cells which have not already escaped and it would appear more rational to close the pathways by surgery as soon as possible. Gross and his colleagues[15] found that routine preoperative radiotherapy gave worse results than postoperative and this has been our experience. We thus irradiate large tumors considered inoperable to such a level that when the surgeon considers the operation technically possible the tumor is removed. Postoperative irradiation is then given in the usual way.

POSTOPERATIVE IRRADIATION

Currently we use megavoltage ^{60}Co in all cases. In older children full cooperation is usual, but in babies and infants some form of sedation may be necessary. The position of the remaining kidney must be accurately known so that it may be accurately screened during therapy. Through anterior and posterior fields the renal bed and the lymph drainage area from the level of the inferior mesenteric artery to the crura of the diaphragm is treated in one block to a central dose of 3,000 r in 4 weeks. The size of the fields and total dose will vary from 2,500 r to 3,500 r depending upon the age and the size of the child. In special circumstances of widespread tumor the method in use at the Christie Hospital may be employed. This is based on the high sensitivity of the tumor cells and their tendency to spread within the abdomen. The fields extend from the nipple line to the pelvic floor. With megavoltage this is done with opposing fields with protection of the femoral heads and at a dose level of 2,000 r the normal kidney is shielded. This whole volume is treated to a dose of 2,500 r in 5 to 6 weeks.[24]

IRRADIATION OF THE LUNGS

This is not advocated as a routine measure for the over-all cure rate today is high and the consequences of radiation pneumonitis are serious. A guide to its routine use is gleaned by study of prognosis. In the first year of life it is about 80 per cent, diminishing steadily each year until after the 5th year it is almost nil. This fact, together with a study of histological differentiation and morbid anatomy, may give clues to the wisdom or otherwise of routine irradiation of the lungs. In the presence of pulmonary metastases the whole chest is irradiated.

The whole of both lungs and the entire extent of the pleural surface is irradiated through anteroposterior fields to 2,500 r uniform dose in 4 to 5 weeks, with protection of the larynx and humeral heads. Treatment is started slowly with 50 r, increasing gradually to the daily dose necessary to give the prescribed dose. The treatment is controlled by regular blood counts. The dose of 2,500 r in 4 weeks may be considered low, but the limit is set by the tolerance of the pulmonary tissues. From the theoretical aspect cells are more sensitive than tumor masses and this dose could be sufficient. At the Children's Medical Center,[9] Boston, Farber and his colleagues advise a dose of 1,200 r in 10 treatments over 2 weeks, in combination with Actinomycin D. We use Actinomycin D in the presence of definite metastases in the last 2 weeks of our irradiation as a potentiator of radiation effect. The hope is to try to affect the most resistant cells remaining at the end of therapy. Currently we give 1,500 r in 2 weeks, measured in the mid point of two opposed fields.

None of the patients we have treated by radiation alone or radiotherapy and Actinomycin D have survived for 4 and 2 years. Pearson *et al.*[25] report from the Christie Hospital, Manchester, that of 25 patients (14 per cent) survived 3 years and over. Two are alive over 10 years and 1 died 18 years after therapy from cor pulmonale due to radiation fibrosis.

Two in the Hospital for Sick Children series survive 8 and 9 years following surgical removal (lobectomy) for a single metastasis which appeared 2 years after nephrectomy. In one recent case a solitary metastasis disappeared after irradiation. Detailed radiology failed to demonstrate any abnormality but it recurred in the same site and so was excised. This patient also survives 4 years.

COMPLICATIONS OF TREATMENT

In the Christie Hospital series Pearson *et al.*[25] reports the above boy with cor pulmonale. Two patients treated before the risk of radiation nephritis was appreciated died from acute renal damage 4 and 7 months post-treatment. All the surviving children have long legs in relation to body height, but this growth disturbance is symmetrical and there are no instances of lateral spinal deformities. In girls who survive 1 has amenorrhea and lack of sex development and 2 have normal development but complete amenorrhea, and 2 have normal development and normal menstruation.

Embryonic Sarcomas

These sarcomas, without or only very rare counterparts in adult life, form a classical group of childhood embryonic tumors. They are sarcomas which arise from embryonic tissue before it attains its adult mature differentiation. Histologically, they consist of a cellular mesenchyme in which is found myxomatous tissue with or without anomalous differentiation, especially rhabdomyoblastic.[32] They fall into one of three entities: 1) Rhabdomyosarcoma, 2) embryonic sarcoma, and 3) botryoid sarcoma. The distinction between rhabdomyosarcoma and embryonic sarcoma is based on the presence or absence of striped muscle fibers for otherwise they are identical in their clinical appearance, sites, and behavior. When related to a mucous membrane they present as a grape-like polypoid tumor, covered with epithelium, the sarcoma botryoides.

Head

The primary site is most often in the nasopharynx, but palate, middle ear, mastoid and orbit are also involved. It is often impossible to define the exact origin. In a recent case the tumor presented in botryoid form in the nasopharynx, the external nares and the external ear. In another there was complete nasal obstruction with visible tumor, which could also be seen in the mouth.

Female Urogenital Tract (Sarcoma Botryoides)

It arises in the vaginal walls, and as the most common origin is deeply on the anterior wall, treatment is rendered difficult because of its proximity to the urethra. This structure and the bladder can be the primary site but most often they are secondarily involved as is the body of the uterus. The uterus itself is probably never the primary site.

Embryonic Sarcoma of the Male Urogenital Sinus

Rhabdomyosarcoma which mimics the vaginal tumor occurs in the bladder in either sex as a sarcoma botryoides and in boys in the prostate as a diffuse bulky enlargement of the organ. The clinical and pathological features are similar in both sexes, but these tumors tend to give rise to symptoms of urinary obstruction and earlier death from uremia or infection.

Treatment and Results

Treatment of this group involves surgery, radiotherapy as a primary or postoperative or palliative measure, and chemotherapy.

SURGERY

In nasopharyngeal tumors this often amounts only to incomplete removal in order to restore the airway. In the urogenital sinus tumors, radical surgical excision of the whole potential field of involvement is a practical procedure. It is questionable whether these formidable operations are however justified, not only because of the mutilation, but also because recurrence occurs even after such a wide excision.

Radiotherapy. The tumor cells are radiosensitive, but in spite of the primary regression, recurrence within the irradiated field is common, while the onset of distant metastases is not affected. In recent cases, we have used megavoltage (^{60}Co) and planned the therapy on a regional basis. As most of the children are under the age of 5 years, the maximum modal dose has been 3,500 *r* in the planned volume in a period of 4 to 5 weeks. The combination of Actinomycin D and irradiation has been used by Pinkel and Picknen.[26]

Teratoma

Willis defines an embryonic tumor as one which arises from particular viscera in their immature stages and thus contains tissue representing that of the embryonic visceral parenchyma. While nephroblastoma and hepatoblastoma are thus recognized, Willis gives reasons for including adenocarcinoma of the infant's testis as orchioblastoma. Teratomas are embryonic tumors but differ from the above in being devoid of any organ specificity and produce tissues foreign to the organ in which they grow.

Sacrococcygeal. This tumor is often manifest at birth and all occur below the age of 2 years. Females exceed males in the ratio 4 to 1. It forms a bulky tumor presacral and precoccygeal most often, projecting externally but sometimes intrapelvic. It is attached to the coccyx but the bones are normally developed. Seventy per cent are benign and circumscribed, but 30 per cent contain a carcinomatous malignant growth. The primary treatment in all cases is surgical and in spite of their bulk this is highly successful. Gross *et al.*[14] reported 26 cures out of 29 operated on in infancy and in 3 out of 8 in a later age group. The cancerous type is highly malignant and rapidly fatal, disseminating to the abdominal and inguinal lymph nodes and via the blood stream to the lungs and liver. The discovery of malignancy is an indication for urgent postoperative radical radiotherapy to the pelvis and lymph drainage areas.

Testicular Teratoma. These tumors are all present at birth and the majority are detected before the age of 2 years. In this series the ages at treatment varied from 5 months to 14 years. Clinically the testicle is replaced by a tumor which is cystic but some contain more solid areas. In infancy the tumor is benign, but in later childhood (and adult life) they are invariably malignant. In 2 patients in this series the growth was malignant and disseminated widely. Treatment is by orchidectomy and the discovery of malignancy is an indication for radiotherapy to the lymph drainage areas on conventional lines as for such tumors in adults.

Teratomas in other sites are invariably benign tumors and radiotherapy is not indicated.

Orchioblastoma. This is a term applied by Willis[32] to an undifferentiated embryonal carcinoma. Clinically it presents between birth and the second year of life with enlargement of a testicle. The growth is an adenocarcinoma of low grade of malignancy. The importance of the recognition of this tumor is that it has a good prognosis following treatment.[1,19] While the prognosis following orchidectomy is good, the fact that it is a malignant metastasizing tumor is indication for postoperative radiotherapy applied to the lymphatic drainage areas. That this can be successful in the presence of metastatic disease is illustrated by the following record.

H. G., aged 6 months. In the first 3 months right hydrocele aspirated many times. At 6 months left testis replaced by hard tumor. At operation testis and fundiculus replaced by whitish tumor extending through inguinal canal to a large retroperitoneal mass. Scrotal tumor removed. X-ray therapy to abdominal tumor. Using 10 × 8 cm anterior, lateral and posterior fields 1,500 r applied to each in 48 days. He remained well for 20 years when he died suddenly of coronary occlusion, without recurrence of his neoplasm.

Tumors of Bone

Willis[32] classifies tumors of the skeleton which affect children as follows:
  Benign osteoma and chondroma
  Osteosarcoma and chondrosarcoma
  Osteoclastoma, benign and malignant
  Ewing's tumor and reticulum-celled sarcoma
  Sundry benign or false tumors (osteoid osteoma, benign osteoblastoma, chondroblastoma (Codman's tumor), chondromyxoid fibroma, nonosteogenic fibroma)
  Fibromas and ossifying fibromas of jaws
  Extraskeletal bony or cartilaginous tumors
  Hemangioma and adamantinoma may be added.

Osteosarcoma and Chondrosarcoma

The mainstay of treatment has been radical surgery (amputation). In tumors remote from the trunk this is so, but in tumors near the trunk in infants and children, results do not justify the mutilation of a hindquarter or forequarter amputation. Chemotherapy has not proved of value, but Actinomycin D is advocated to enhance radiation effects. Experience is not sufficiently large to comment on this at this time.

In view of the above, radiotherapy could be the mainstay of treatment, serving one of three purposes: 1) Palliative therapy; to relieve pain and to avoid fungation. The tumor cells vary in their radiosensitivity, and these objectives can be achieved while the more merciful death from metastases ensues. 2) As a preamputation measure. 3) As definitive radical therapy with the aim to cure. In the latter two, practice has been influenced by the teaching of Cade.[3] From a critical appraisal of the results of other workers and his own extensive experience, Cade[3] advocates radiotherapy as the primary approach to treatment. His reasons are as follows: 1) The overall results of amputation alone are so poor that another approach is justifiable. 2) The delay of preamputation radiotherapy is not detrimental to the patient, indeed it may be beneficial. 3) While most osteogenic sarcomata are radioresistant, some are sensitive and as the degree of response cannot be predicted clinically, it is legitimate to offer radiotherapy as a preliminary to amputation, in view of the extremely bad results from surgery. 4) Response to radiation can be assessed in 4 to 8 weeks. If this is favorable, amputation can be delayed. Complete, although temporary arrest, and restoration of the bone to normal has been achieved in a few by radiation. In very few selected cases, amputation can be avoided, but on the whole it is considered safer to amputate than to await reactivation of the tumor cells. Even if response to treatment is negligible, amputation has the same safety and uncertainty as if no radiotherapy had been given. 5) The results are improved at 3 and 5 years.

THE RATIONALE FOR RADIOTHERAPY IN OSTEOGENIC SARCOMA

The rationale for radiotherapy in osteogenic sarcoma can be considered from the clinical and radiobiological aspects.

Clinical. The malignancy of osteogenic sarcoma is very variable. Some are rapidly fatal, others are slower, the average duration of life from diagnosis being 12 to 18 months. In the highly malignant type, surgery imposes needless mutilation and mental discomfort to the patient who will die in any case. In the slower growing type, time is on our side and operation may be avoided.

Radiobiological. Changes due to irradiation are brought about by direct destruction of the malignant cell, enhanced by the vascular effect, and the promotion of healing. Radiation properly applied arrests the mitosis of the neoplastic spindle cells, the stromal cells then invading and destroying them. Calcification and even ossification then occur in the tumor and the bone from which it arises.

TECHNIQUE AND DOSAGE

Cade advised slow irradiation to high dosage. With megavoltage, doses of 7,000 *r* to 8,000 *r* were delivered uniformly throughout the tumor and to the normal bone immediately beyond and around the actual tumor in a period of 8 weeks. Relief of pain occurs early within 1 week in some cases. Decrease in size of a tumor is seen in 3 to 4 weeks, while radiological changes become apparent after 4 to 6 weeks. In a recent review of Cade's and his own patients Lee[18] now advocates a dose in the 6,000 to 7,000 *r* range. In the very young these doses may have to be adjusted but over the age of 10 years they probably will be tolerated.

Osteoclastoma, Benign and Malignant

This tumor shows no difference in its clinical features, prognosis or treatment to its counterpart in adults. A benign tumor, in some cases in recent years the high proportion of malignant metastasizing types has been recognized.

TREATMENT

Cook *et al.*[6] state that all cystic lesions in children (apart from giant-celled tumors) respond to small fractionated doses of radiation to a tumor dose of 1,200 *r*. If after several weeks the desired result is not obtained, surgery can still be carried out, but biopsy may be initially indicated to exclude a malignant growth, if the diagnosis is not clear cut. In true giant-celled tumors the recognition of the malignant types is important and for these doses of the order of 6,000 to 7,000 r megavoltage in 6 to 8 weeks are necessary. For the benign types 4,000 to 5,000 r in 4 to 5 weeks are essential for recurrence and failure to control the tumor is high with doses of a lower order. Four to 5 weeks after the completion of treatment there may be a great increase of osteolysis, the trabeculae and capsule disappearing. During this phase the bone will have to be supported while calcification and ossification is proceeding. In small children the dose will be varied by considerations of age and site and here clinical and therapeutic judgment must be the guides. In Thomson's[13] series from the Middlesex Hospital, out of 34 cases of true giant-celled tumors, 10 died, 2 from fatal local extension and 8 from metastases. Twenty recurred after the initial radiotherapy (to lower dose levels than the above) and 16 had to suffer amputation. These facts outweigh considerations of affecting bone growth or potential carcinogenic effects of irradiation.

"Ewing's Tumor" and Reticulum-celled Sarcoma of the Bone

Since 1921 when Ewing described a tumor of bone marrow in children and adolescents which he called a diffuse endothelioma, and 1939 when Parker and Jackson described a primary reticulum-celled sarcoma of bone marrow, world authorities have expressed controversial opinions on the identity of a distinct tumor, "Ewing's Tumor." Willis[32] maintains that it is not a pathological entity but a clinical syndrome caused by several different kinds of metastatic tumor, the commonest being neuroblastoma. It produces a syndrome of an osteogenic round-celled radiosensitive tumor usually in the long bone of a young subject and promotes osteogenic activity in the periosteum. Magnus and Wood[20] believe that reticulum-celled sarcoma is identical with Ewing's tumor and that both should be regarded as a definite

clinical and pathological entity, an opinion which is shared by Stout[29] and others.

Features of Ewing's Tumor and Reticulum-Celled Sarcoma

In spite of the opinion of authorities based on the histogenesis and histological studies of these tumors, there is no doubt that clinically they are different tumors. Ewing's tumor is classically identified as a tumor of early life (4 to 25 years) affecting the femur or tibia in 50 per cent of cases, and most commonly in the shaft of a long bone. It produces a very painful, elongated swelling, often with a fever and a relatively short history, and sometimes it is associated with lymph node enlargement. The tumor lies in the medulla and subperiosteally with the cortical bone in between. New bone is laid down in "onion peel" layers along the shaft but radiologically osteolysis and sun-ray spicules may also be seen. The gross specimen shows the tumor tissue to be an amorphous grey-like substance. The tumor is exceedingly radiosensitive with rapid relief of swelling and pain. Ultimately the bone may return to a normal appearance. The prognosis is grave, death being due to deposits in other bones, especially the skull, the lungs and lymph nodes, the 5-year survival being 10 to 15 per cent. Reticulum-celled sarcoma occurs in a later age group (20 to 40 years) and affects the metaphysis of long bones or the flat bones. The pain and swelling are not so severe and of longer duration, 6 months to 6 years, the average being about 1 year. The first sign may be a fracture produced by a trivial injury. Fever is uncommon. Radiologically there is a patchy, spongy osteolysis, not necessarily diagnostic. The tumor is radiosensitive to higher doses, but after treatment the bone becomes more dense. The prognosis is fair, about 40 per cent survive 5 years, death being due to generalized disease or pulmonary metastases.

Treatment

EWING'S TUMOR

It is doubtful whether surgery plays any part in the treatment of this tumor, for the local bone manifestation appears to be part of a general process. Radiotherapy can invariably control the bony focus, and this being so, if Willis is correct in his interpretation, there is no purpose in amputation. Using megavoltage radiation (^{60}Co), the entire bone shaft and surrounding soft tissue is irradiated to a dose of 4,000 to 6,000 *r* in 4 to 6 weeks depending on the age and site. Lymph node and other metastases will also respond, but in these cases lower doses are given.

After separation of other groups no patient with this diagnosis treated by amputation and/or radiotherapy before 1959 has survived. The majority died within 2 years. One patient lived 7 years, untimately dying from mediastinal pulmonary and pleural metastases. One, a girl aged 10 years, with a tumor in the femur was alive and well at her 5th anniversary. This patient had a mediastinal metastasis treated $4\frac{1}{2}$ years ago. She then developed pulmonary metastases and died.

RETICULUM-CELLED SARCOMA

This tumor being radiosensitive and radiocurable should also be treated primarily by irradiation to doses of 4,000 to 6,000 *r* in 4 to 6 weeks megavoltage. As the disease tends to extend down the shaft from the metaphysis, a long margin of normal bone should be included.

Soft Tissue Tumors

This term is applied to a group of tumors which arise in mesenchyme, but excluding embryonic sarcoma, tumors of the skeleton and of the hemopoietic system. They arise in connection with the connective tissue of muscle, tendon sheaths, joints, fascia, and nerves.

Fibrosarcoma

It is by far the commonest tumor type. The youngest in our experience was an infant 6 months old with a fibrosarcoma of the scapular region. Treated by wide excision and radiotherapy he remained well for 3 years when a recurrence was excised. A further recurrence outside the treated area was again excised later, but he is now well, 18 years since the first diagnosis. While the majority occur in the limbs, in children they seem more prone to occur in odd sites such as around the jaws and sinuses. It is important to recognize this because bold treatment can be curative even in infants. Where wide excision means complete removal, this is curative, but where there is any doubt about the completeness of excision, postoperative irradiation is indicated and our policy is to proceed to high dosage with prolonged fractionation.

Synovial Tumors

Although uncommon, malignant synovioma is more common than benign tumors of synovium in children. In a limited experience of these tumors in adults, the tumor has proved moderately radiosensitive and control of both primary and metastatic disease has been achieved by irradiation.

Juvenile Angiofibroma of the Nasopharynx

This is an uncommon tumor which occurs at puberty and is entirely confined to the male sex. It is not a childhood tumor, most cases occur between 16 and 20 years of age.

It is not malignant; indeed many doubt whether it is a true tumor, but it is included here for the radiotherapist may be consulted concerning treatment. Eighteen cases are available for study, 4 from St. Bartholomew's Hospital and 14 from Middlesex Hospital by courtesy of Windeyer.

Treatment Policy

Osborn[23] states that the natural history of the disease is obscure but that the observation of Gosselin (1873) on the tendency to regress after reaching sexual maturity dominated opinion for many years. This opinion has not been fully substantiated and it is not felt that this justifies withholding therapy. Capps[5] treated 4 cases by surgical removal, but in 1 case this was incomplete and a very vascular residue had to be implanted with radon seeds. Windeyer[33] in his early cases based on the absence of knowledge of radiosensitivity states that the first approach was orientated to the idea that they should be removed surgically. As a non-malignant tumor, supposed to regress in adult life, this seemed the ideal procedure, provided the problem of its extreme vascularity could be overcome technically. The first 6 cases were treated thus, but because of an unsatisfactory surgical approach, the vascularity, the broad base, and the many adhesions, adequate surgical removal was not achieved and the incomplete surgery was followed by radium needle implantation and teleradium in 1, and external deep x-ray therapy in 5. The first remains well 20 years later; in the others there was marked tumor regression, but 2 needed diathermy coagulation of the base for residual disease. It was obvious that high dosage was necessary for complete resolution. As a result of this experience, Windeyer employed megavoltage therapy as the initial therapy in the next 8 cases. In every case there has been marked regression of tumor but in 4 it has been necessary to employ further treatment by irradiation and/or surgery for residual tumor recurrence. The surgical approach to the nasopharynx has been by a transpalatal fenestration as devised by C. P. Wilson, leaving a permanent opening into the nasopharynx. Windeyer advocates the use of megavoltage, giving between 6,000 and 6,800 r at the rate of 900 r per week, followed by surgery, in order to treat residual disease,

to control hemorrhage, and for adequate inspection at follow-up examination.

Results

Of these 18 cases, 10 remain well and free of disease 5 to 20 years following treatment. In the management of these patients, Windeyer emphasizes that radiotherapy is of value, and that the treatment complicated by the vascularity of tumor may entail a prolonged overall treatment time and call for surgical measures such as diathermy coagulation of tumor remnants or to control hemorrhage. One of his patients was under treatment for 31 months with an 8 months respite, while 2 others were 5 and 6 years from the time of their first operation until their last treatment. Even the most straightforward have taken 3 to 4 months.

BIBLIOGRAPHY

1. Abell, M. R., and Holtz, F.: Testicular neoplasms in infants and children, *Cancer*, 16, 965, 1963.
2. Bodian, M.: Neuroblastoma, *Arch. Dis. Child.*, 38, 606, 1963.
3. Cade, S.: Soft tissue tumors: Their natural history and treatment; president's address, *Proc. Roy. Soc. Med.*, 44, 19, 1951.
4. Cahan, W. G., Woodard, H. Q., Higinbotham, N. L., Steward, F. W., and Coley, B. L.: Sarcoma arising in irradiated bone; report of 11 cases, *Cancer*, 1, 3, 1948.
5. Capps, F. C. W., Irvine, Q. N., and Timmis, P.: Four recent cases of juvenile fibroangioma of the post nasal space, *J. Laryng.*, 75, 924, 1961.
6. Cook, J. D., Krabbenhoft, K. L., and Songe, R.: Radiation therapy of solitary benign cystic-appearing lesions involving the long bones of children, *Amer. J. Roentgen.*, 80, 505, 1958.
7. Cruz, M., Coley, B. L., and Stewart, F. W.: Postradiation bone sarcoma; report of eleven cases, *Cancer*, 10, 72, 1957.
8. D'Angio, G. J.: Clinical and biological studies of Actinomycin D and roentgen irradiation, *Amer. J. Roentgen.*, 87, 106, 1962.

9. D'Angio, G. J., Farber, S., and Maddock, C. L.: Potentiation of x-ray effects by Actinomycin D, *Radiology*, 73, 175, 1959.

10. D'Angio, G. J., Evans, A. E., and Mitus, A.: Roentgen therapy of certain complications of acute leukemia in children, *Amer. J. Roentgen.*, 82, 541, 1959.

11. Dargeon, H. W.: *Tumors of Childhood: A Clinical Treatise*, London, Henry Kimpton, p. 433, 1960.

12. Eisenhoff, H. M., Klinger, L. H., and Sherwin, B.: Lymphosarcoma of the intestine; report of a case in a 10-year-old child, with 7-year cure, *Amer. J. Dis. Child.*, 89, 54, 1955.

13. Eyre-Brook, A. L., Thomson, A. D., and Sissons, H. A.: Discussion giant-celled tumors of bone and related conditions, *Proc. Roy. Soc. Med.*, 49, 409, 1956.

14. Gross, R. E., Clatworthy, H. W., Jr., and Meeker, I. A., Jr.: Sacrococcygeal teratomas in infants and children; report of 40 cases, *Surg. Gynec. Obst.*, 92, 341, 1951.

15. Gross, R. E.: *The Surgery of Infancy and Childhood*, Philadelphia, W. B. Saunders Company, 1953.

16. Innes-Williams, D., Rigby, C., Williams, I. G.: "Tumors of the Kidney and Ureter", *Neoplastic Diseases in Various Sites*, Riches, E., Ed., Edinburgh, E. & S. Livingstone, Vol. 5, 1964.

17. Kunkler, P. B., Farr, R. F., and Luxton, R. W.: The limit of renal tolerance to x-rays; investigation into the renal damage occurring following treatment of tumors of testis by abdominal baths, *Brit. J. Radiol.*, 25, 190, 1952.

18. Lee, E. S., and Mackenzie, D. H.: Osteosarcoma: A study of the value of preoperative megavoltage radiotherapy, *Brit. J. Surg.*, 51, 252, 1964.

19. Magner, D., Campbell, J. S., and Wiglesworth, F. W.: Testicular adenocarcinoma with clear cells, occurring in infancy, *Canad. Med. Ass. J.*, 86, 485, 1962. Also: *Cancer*, 9, 165, 1956.

20. Magnus, H. A., and Wood, H. L. C.: Primary reticulo-sarcoma of bone, *J. Bone Joint Surg.*, 38B, 258, 1956.

21. Merriman, G. R., Jr., and Focht, E. F.: A clinical study of radiation cataracts and the relationship to dose, *Amer. J. Roentgen.* 77, 759, 1957.

22. Neuhauser, E. B. D., Wittenborg, M. H., Berman, C. Z., and Cohen, J.: Irradiation effects of roentgen therapy on growing spine, *Radiology*, 59, 637, 1952.

23. Osborn, D. A.: The so-called juvenile angiofibroma of the nasopharynx, *J. Laryng.* 73, 295, 1959.

24. Paterson, R.: *The Treatment of Malignant Disease by Radiotherapy*, 2nd ed., London, Edward Arnold & Company, 1963.

25. Pearson, D., Duncan, W. B., and Pointon, R. C. S.: Wilm's tumors—A review of 96 consecutive cases, *Brit. J. Radiol.*, 37, 154, 1964.

26. Pinkel, D., and Picknen, J.: Rhabdomyosarcoma in children, *J.A.M.A.*, 175, 292, 1961.

27. Reese, A. B.: *Tumors of the Eye*, 2nd ed., New York, Hoeber Medical Division, Harper & Row, 1963.

28. Rubin, P., Duthie, R. B., and Young, L. W.: Significance of scoliosis and postirradiated Wilm's tumor and neuroblastoma, *Radiology*, 79, 539, 1962.

29. Stout, A. P.: A discussion of the pathology and histogenesis of Ewing's tumor of bone marrow, *Amer. J. Roentgen.*, 50, 334, 1943.

30. Sullivan, M. P.: Intracranial complications of leukemia in children, *Pediatrics*, 20, 757, 1957.

31. Vaeth, J. M., Levitt, S. H., Jones, M. D., and Freter, C. H.: Effects of radiation therapy in survivors of Wilm's tumor, *Radiology*, 79, 560, 1962.

32. Willis, R. A.: *Pathology of Tumors of Children*, London, Oliver & Boyd, 1962.

33. Windeyer, B. W.: Personal communication, 1964.

Irradiation and Chemotherapy in Pediatric Tumors

CARLOS H. FERNANDEZ, and WATARU W. SUTOW

CHEMOTHERAPY IN PEDIATRIC CANCER

Chemotherapy is particularly important in the management of children with cancer.[20] Childhood cancers have the propensity to metastasize early and distantly via the bloodstream instead of spreading locally and regionally. Unlike surgery and irradiation, which are target-limited treatment modalities, the chemotherapeutic agents are systemically active and affect all susceptible malignant cells if sufficient drug concentration can be attained. The clinical areas in which drug treatment has definitely established its effectiveness include the following:

1) for treatment of systemic involvement (acute leukemia).

2) for curative therapy for susceptible tumors (Burkitt's lymphoma, choriocarcinoma).

3) for treatment of widely disseminated disease (metastatic neuroblastoma, Stage III-IV Hodgkin's disease).

4) as adjuvant chemotherapy with surgery and irradiation in primary treatment for Wilms' tumor. It is presumed that chemotherapy effectively eradicates distant, occult metastatic foci.

5) for preoperative use in Wilms' tumor to produce tumor shrinkage and to convert an inoperable to an operable situation.

6) for reduction of tumor mass prior to planned radiation therapy so that a smaller field may be used (Hodgkin's disease, rhabdomyosarcoma).

7) to take advantage of possible synergism with radiation therapy (it has been suggested that actinomycin D potentiates radiotherapy effect).

8) to provide additive antitumor effect in multimodal therapy regimens. The better results now being obtained in children with rhabdomyosarcoma (and possibly in children with Ewing's sarcoma), probably represent at least the summation of the separate effects of each treatment modality. Chemotherapy also appears to be contributing to more long-term control of disease in brain tumors, embryonal carcinomas, and ovarian cancers.

9) for curative therapy with irradiation and/or surgery in Wilms' tumor metastatic to lungs and/or liver.

Improved results have followed the use of drugs in combination. Such a combination consists of a drug, each when administered alone shows definite antineoplastic activity, has a different biochemical site of action and manifests different types of major toxicity. Thus, tumor cell populations resistant to one drug may still be vulnerable to another drug in the combination. Differences in toxicity pattern permit the concomitant use of more than one drug in full therapeutic dosages.

The side effects of chemotherapy must be fully appreciated in the multimodal management of childhood cancer. The skin reaction, for example, within the irradiation treatment field, may be considerably greater in patients receiving actinomycin D than in patients being treated by irradiation alone. The mucositis in children during irradiation and drug therapy for head and neck lesions may be extremely severe and require massive degrees of supportive care. Cyclophosphamide (obtained in the United States under trade name "Cytoxan"), can cause severe and protracted chemical cystitis. When the bladder mucosa is included in the irradiation field, the selection of the dosage and schedule of the cyclophosphamide regimen may present problems. Many chemotherapeutic agents, particularly when used in combinations and intensive courses produce marked suppression of bone marrow activity. The chemotherapist and the radiotherapist, therefore, must anticipate these potential hazards and must plan each multimodal treatment program jointly to minimize and/or circumvent any interruption of scheduled treatment.

RADIOTHERAPY FOR CHILDHOOD CANCER

Radiotherapy. The radiotherapy techniques for pediatric patients require modification, both in dose and in the extent of the irradiated volume, from those employed for the treatment for adult patients. Most pediatric patients receive chemotherapy as a part of the management of their tumors. This also necessitates modification of the radiotherapy.

The age of the host at the time of irradiation influences the tolerance of the tissues and their potential for further growth, development, and function. The younger the host, the more extensive will be the radiation injury for any given amount of irradiation. The chronological age at which development to mature size and function occur differs among the organ systems. The central nervous system anatomically is nearly fully developed at the age of 2 years. The spine, which houses the spinal cord, reaches approximately the same stage of development at 10 years of age. Therefore, one would not expect to see spinal cord damage when treating a Wilms' tumor postoperatively in a 4-year-old, but instead must anticipate growth and development problems related to the spine.

If the patient has had surgery, time is allowed for healing and resolution of any possible infection. If the patient has been receiving chemotherapy, it is preferable to wait for bone marrow recovery before attempting curative radiotherapy. This is especially applicable when large volumes are to be treated.

When patients are receiving chemotherapy concomitantly with radiotherapy, careful monitoring of the patient's status must be employed to avoid the possibility of sudden or severe combined toxicity. Usually, therapy can be continued as long as the absolute neutrophil count is above 1,000 cells per mm^3 and the platelet count is above 50,000. Continued radiotherapy below these minimums is risky and should be used only when the necessary supportive care is available and the seriousness of the circumstances warrants such risks.

Treatment is given 5 days a week at the rate of 1,000 rads tumor dose per week, for limited volumes. In the patients in whom there is major life-threatening, impaired function, such as airway impairment or elevation of the cerebrospinal fluid pressure, it is necessary to lessen the daily dose of radiation. Also, it is necessary to reduce the weekly tumor dose in patients receiving irradiation to large volumes (*e.g.*, total abdomen with pelvis) and in patients receiving intensive chemotherapy.

Ewing's Sarcoma

For the past several decades the published survival rates for patients with Ewing's sarcoma have been uniformly poor, ranging around 10 per cent although an occasional report gave a survival rate as high as 24 per cent.[3] The initial assessment of the impact of adjuvant chemotherapy on the survival rates suggests that some improvement may be occurring. Studies still in progress indicate that the median time to development of metastases is lengthening and that the percentage of patients remaining free of disease 2 to 5 years after diagnosis is increasing.

A more optimistic attitude regarding patients with Ewing's sarcoma has appeared since a report in 1968 by Hustu *et al.*[7] that 5 of 5 patients treated by radiation therapy and prolonged chemotherapy with cytoxan and vincristine were alive and well at 12 to 38 months after the start of treatment. There are now other papers which lend support to that early experience.[13]

OVER-ALL PLAN OF
TREATMENT-PRIMARY LESION

Chemotherapy and radiotherapy are started simultaneously.

RADIATION THERAPY TECHNIQUES
AND DOSE LEVELS

The basic treatment plan is the administration, with ^{60}Co, of 5,000 rads in 25 fractions over a 5-week period (5 fractions per week) to the entirety of the affected bone (Fig. 8-1A). At the 5,000 rad dose level, the fields are reduced so that the clinically and radiographically evident tumor is included with a rather small margin of apparently unaffected normal tissue for the next 1,000 rads (Fig. 8-1B). Therefore, according to this treatment plan, the area clinically affected by disease receives a final dose of 6,000 rads in 6 weeks. An important detail of treatment planning is that even for the first 4 to 5 weeks of treatment, fields are drawn to spare as much normal tissue as possible. For example, if the disease is affecting the upper portion of the femur, then the field would be drawn relatively generously around the primary lesion and soft tissue swelling. But for coverage of the distal shaft and condyles of the femus, the fields are drawn only wide enough to cover the bone structure.

Shaped fields are employed throughout the entire treatment; other appropriate techniques are utilized to minimize irradiation of

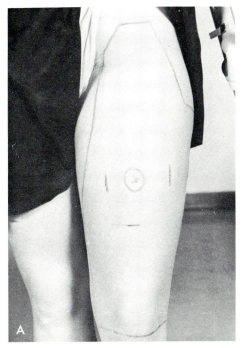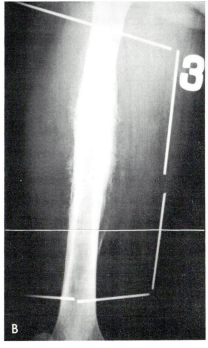

FIG. 8-1. **A.** Fourteen-year-old girl. Diagnosis of Ewing's sarcoma of the left femur. Figure A demonstrates the anterior field; entire bone, fall-off externally, sparing of soft tissues at inner aspect of thigh. The dose given was 5,000 rads in 5 weeks, from August 1971 to October 1971. Vincristine and cyclophosphamide were given concomitantly. In July 1972, local control was still maintained.

    B. Portal film of the reduced field to deliver the last 1,000 rads in 1 week. Total tumor dose, 6,000 rads in 6 weeks.

tissue unintentionally. Irradiation of the full circumference of the limb, even for the first portion of the treatment, is avoided if possible. If "fall-off" is required on one side of the limb, some normal tissues are shielded, if possible, on the other side. These special efforts to protect normal tissues permit tolerance of high doses and retain good function in a painless and nonedematous limb.

There is a definite increase in reaction of normal tissue in patients receiving concomitant cytoxan and vincristine. If reaction is severe, a dose lower than 6,000 rads may be indicated.

CHEMOTHERAPY

Intensive multidrug chemotherapy is now being given along with radiotherapy in the effort to eradicate subclinical metastases. The regimen used at *MDAH* consists of the administration of cylophosphamide and vincristine with radiotherapy in a schedule shown in Figure 8-2.[12]

Cyclophosphamide is given orally or intravenously. Older children and adolescents do not tolerate the high dose very well; severe abdominal pain, nausea and vomiting may occur.

The addition of drug-induced myelosupression to the radiation effect when a large volume of bone marrow is in the treatment field may produce severe leukopenia and thrombocytopenia. These problems are anticipated and vigorous supportive measures are instituted as necessary. The inclusion of the bladder in the treatment field when the tumor involves the pelvic bones may potentiate the development of hemorrhagic cystitis as a side effect of cyclophosphamide.

In this regimen, all chemotherapy is discontinued after the 33rd week of chemotherapeutic treatment.

METASTATIC LESIONS

Although we have not instituted the prophylactic treatment to the lungs, it now is under study.

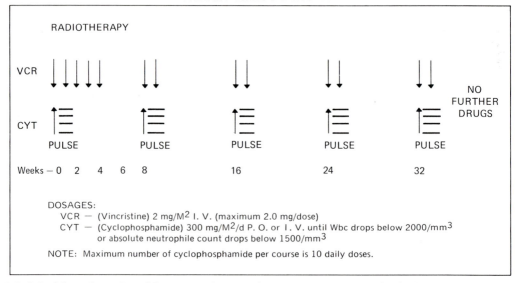

CHEMOTHERAPY SCHEDULE
PRIMARY EWING'S SARCOMA

DOSAGES:
VCR — (Vincristine) 2 mg/M^2 I. V. (maximum 2.0 mg/dose)
CYT — (Cyclophosphamide) 300 mg/M^2/d P. O. or I. V. until Wbc drops below 2000/mm^3 or absolute neutrophile count drops below 1500/mm^3
NOTE: Maximum number of cyclophosphamide per course is 10 daily doses.

FIG. 8-2. Schema for multimodal regimen utilizing combination chemotherapy and radiotherapy in the management of patients with Ewing's sarcoma. Cyclophosphamide is available in the United States under the trade name of Cytoxan. (Courtesy: Suit, Martin, and Sutow, *Clinical Pediatric Oncology*, Sutow, Vietti, and Fernbach, Eds., C. V. Mosby Co., St. Louis, Mo., In press.)

For existing metastases in the lungs, both lungs are treated with 1,500 rads *TD* in 2 weeks, with no lung correction factor. If lesions are still present at that time, an additional 1,500 rads *TD* in 2 weeks are delivered to small areas. Metastases to other organs are treated with a curative aim and doses are adopted according to the supportive structures.

FOLLOW-UP EXAMINATIONS

The patient is under almost constant medical supervision during the first 6 months. After the chemotherapy has been completed, follow-up examinations are performed at 2 monthly intervals for the next 12 months. Then the patients are seen at 3-month intervals until the 36th month after start of treatment. At these follow-up visits, special attention is paid to the status of the primary lesion and the lungs. Any vague symptoms of bone or joint discomfort is investigated promptly because of the frequency of metastasis to bone.

Leukemias

The leukemias, both acute and chronic, are generalized neoplastic diseases that require systemic chemotherapy for control. The clinical circumstances under which radiotherapy may be indicated are:

a) the acute requirement for amelioration of symptoms resulting from infiltration of extramedullary sites by leukemic cells, and

b) treatment program to eradicate leukemic cells in pharmacologic sanctuaries to achieve "total leukemic cell kill" or "cure."

CENTRAL NERVOUS SYSTEM LEUKEMIA

Prior to the use of prophylactic craniospinal irradiation, the frequency with which leukemic involvement of the central nervous system (*CNS* leukemia or meningeal leukemia) complicated the clinical course has been as high as 50 per cent to 83 per cent.[1]

Pathologically, there is leukemic infiltration of the dura, leptomeninges, and perivascular spaces. Infiltrations of the brain are rare. Involvement of the pituitary gland and choroid plexus has been noted occasionally. *CNS* leukemia commonly occurs in the presence of a bone marrow remission.

CHEMOTHERAPY FOR CNS LEUKEMIA

In the treatment of the child with the initial episode of *CNS* leukemia or in the treatment of the child with recurrent *CNS* leukemia in the presence of a bone marrow relapse, it has been the general procedure at *MDAH* to institute multidrug intrathecal chemotherapy.[14]

RADIOTHERAPY OF CNS LEUKEMIA

The pathogenesis of this manifestation of the disease has been attributed to the harboring of leukemic cells in the central nervous system where diffusion of cytocidal concentrations of drugs is prevented by the "blood-brain barrier." Radiation has been an accepted treatment modality for meningeal leukemia from the time this complication of the disease was recognized clinically. Currently, the indications for radiation therapy in *CNS* leukemia include the following:

a) there is involvement of the dura or of the deep structures of the brain, such as the hypothalamus or cerebellum.

b) there is infiltration of the facial nerve.

c) there is infiltration of the spinal nerves and nerve roots.

d) intrathecal chemotherapy fails to control the *CNS* disease.

e) intrathecal chemotherapy is not tolerated.

f) the initial episode of *CNS* leukemia occurs in a child who is maintaining a bone marrow remission of long standing. In such patients, the 3-drug combination is given intrathecally 2 times weekly for 4 doses. Chemotherapy is then followed by craniospinal radiation treatment.

At *MDAH*, the entire neural axis receives

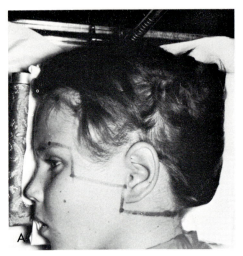 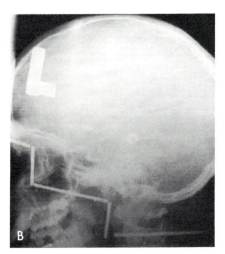

FIG. 8-3. **A**. Thirteen-year-old boy with a diagnosis of acute lymphocytic leukemia in bone marrow remission, but with positive leukemic cells in cerebral spinal fluid. He did not tolerate intrathecal drugs. Figure of parallel-opposed cranial fields. A tumor dose of 3,000 rads in 4 weeks was given at midline. **B**. Portal film.

3,000 rads in 4 weeks. The cranial fields are parallel opposed (Fig. 8-3). Each field is treated every other day with the aim of giving 150 rads midline dose per day. The structures included are: retroorbital space, peripheral portion of the 7th nerve, outlets of the base of the skull and fall-off at contour of the scalp. The lower margins of the head fields are at the level of C2. The posterior spinal fields start at 1.5 cm below the head fields (Fig. 8-4). The spinal canal receives 3,000 rads in 4 weeks (the average depth is usually 4 cm as determined by cross-table lateral films). The lower limit of the spinal fields is at S2, *i.e.* ending of epidural sac. The junction of the fields is moved every week to avoid areas of under- or over-dosage.

When an isolated affected area corresponds to the 7th cranial nerve, unilateral or bilateral facial paralysis occurs. In this situation it is preferable to treat as soon as possible, even immediately after the diagnosis is made. The fields used include the central and peripheral portions of this nerve (Fig. 8-5). The dose calculated at midline is 2,500 rads in 2½ weeks. In approximately half of the cases, the result is dramatic and motion of face is recovered.

PROPHYLACTIC CNS IRRADIATION

There is mounting evidence that "prophylactic" radiotherapy directed to the craniospinal axis results in better control of the leukemic state in children[1,11] because this anatomic site may serve as a reservoir from which the bone marrow may be reseeded by leukemic cells.

In one comparative study, prophylactic 2,400 rads craniospinal irradiation early in remission delayed the onset of *CNS* leukemia and prolonged the duration of complete remission. Two of 45 children who received prophylactic craniospinal irradiation eventually relapsed with *CNS* involvement whereas there were 27 *CNS* relapses among 49 children who did not receive such irradiation. The data also showed that the dose of 2,400 rads produced better results than lower doses and that intrathecal methotrexate used prophylactically was not as effective as prophylactic craniospinal irradiation.[11]

OTHER EXTRAMEDULLARY LEUKEMIC INFILTRATES

Kidneys. Postmortem examinations of the kidneys of 158 leukemic children at *MDAH*

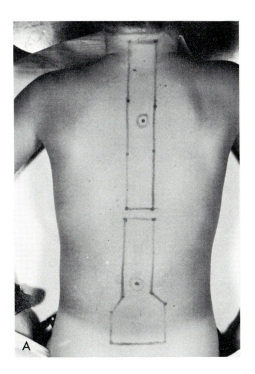

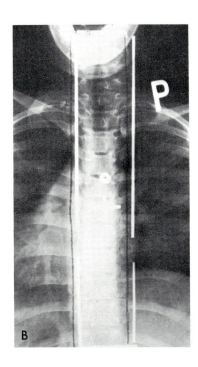

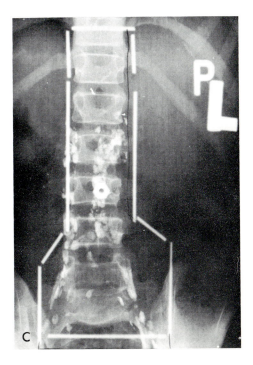

FIG. 8-4. **A.** Spinal fields in same patient as Figure 8-3. Separation between fields is 1.5 cm and this is moved every week. A tumor dose of 3,000 rads in 4 weeks; the depth is calculated at the level of spinal canal as determined by cross-table lateral film.

B & C. Portal of the spinal fields, upper level at *C2*, lower level at *L2* (ending of epidural sac), 6 cm wide.

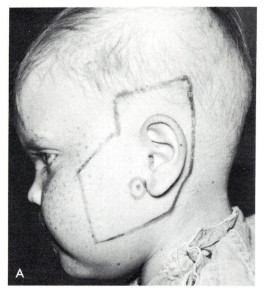

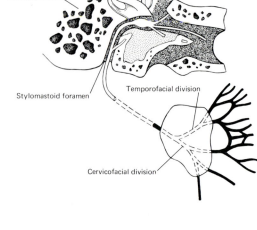

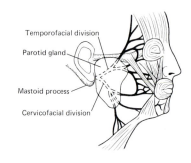

FIG. 8-5. A. Seven-year-old boy with acute lymphocytic leukemia in bone marrow remission but
in central nervous system relapse. He had
radiation therapy to the entire central nervous system in another institution. Later he
presented with bilateral facial paralysis. A
tumor dose of 2,500 rads was given in $2\frac{1}{2}$
weeks. Regression of facial paralysis was
observed after completion of radiation.

  B. Anatomical diagram to stress the distribution of the 7th nerve.

showed in 20 per cent of the patients the
kidneys to be $2\frac{1}{2}$ times or more than normal
weight. Radiotherapy should be considered
when impending renal dysfunction is suspected or documented.[15]

The contribution of this manifestation of
extramedullary disease to bone marrow relapse and subsequent decrease in survival are
not known. In the past, radiotherapy has
been postponed until some evidence of other
renal function had become apparent. The
radiation dosage administered was usually
palliative. At *MDAH*, 10 children have received radiotherapy to the kidneys and the
radiation dosage has exceeded 1,500 rads in
only 3 patients. Significant clinical benefit
resulted in 2 of these children and in 1 additional child who received only 600 rads. Sys-

tematic treatment with radiation to organ
tolerance has not been undertaken and is
now being studied. The pretreatment evaluation consists of plain film of the abdomen
and intravenous pyelogram because renal
masses are not palpable until considerable
size has been obtained. Pyelography is suggested at the time of diagnosis, at the time
of each relapse, and whenever renal masses
are thought to be probable. Increased renal
length, increased cortical thickness and/or
distortion in elongation of the calyceal system should be demonstrated on the pyelogram. Renal biopsy is not considered a requirement for the diagnosis. The initiation
of treatment is to be delayed until stable
bone marrow remission is obtained. The
radiotherapy is done with ^{60}Co or any mega-

voltage equipment. The tumor dose is calculated in rads of the midplane with no corrections for air or bone absorption. The intravenous pyelogram is used for localization. Treatment is delivered through parallel opposed fields anterior and posterior with 1 : 1 loading. The field includes both kidneys with 5 half-value layers midline shield covering the spinal cord. Localization films are obtained and the treatment is begun with the prescribed dose of 2,000 rads in 4 weeks, 5 fractions per day.

Testes. Microscopically, testicular infiltration has been reported in 48 per cent to 92 per cent of leukemic boys. Although regression of enlarged testes frequently may be induced with drugs, either orchiectomy or radiation therapy may be required in persistent or recurrent testicular enlargement which becomes symptomatic.

For the treatment of testicular infiltrations by leukemia, a given dose of 2,500 rads is delivered in 10 fractions with ^{60}Co. Treatment is initiated after the biopsy site is healed completely. Both testicles are included in the treatment field. The testicles are supported posteriorly on a lead block which also shields the perineum (Fig. 8-6). The urethra is excluded from the field by fixing the penis over the symphysis pubis.

Bone. Radiologic evidence of bone involvement ranging from translucent bands to osteolytic lesions to periosteal elevations are common. Frequently the lesions cause severe pain. Radiotherapy produces spectacular responses. Doses in the range of 1,000 to 1,500 rads are delivered with simple techniques. There is no need to include all the bone.

Eye. Infiltration of the optic nerve or the retina may cause visual disturbances. Nonsymptomatic retinal lesions also occur. Radiotherapy through a unilateral field or parallel opposed portals, 2,500 rads *TD* in 2½ weeks is beneficial. If one field is used, the *TD* is

at 3 cm depth; the field is usually 3 × 4 cm starting at the orbital rim (Fig. 8-7).

Other Organs. Almost every organ of the body, not already mentioned, may be infiltrated by the leukemic process. Fortunately, regression of the lesions accompany the achievement of remissions by chemotherapy. When necessary, some degree of palliation can be provided by appropriate radiotherapy in most cases. The spleen is an example. The patient may have great discomfort and pain because of splenomegaly. The techniques of treatment have varied but generally the plan is to start with very low dose, 50 rads *TD*, continue 2 or 3 days, increase to 100 rads *TD* for 3 or 4 days with the aim of a total dose of 1,500 rads. Benefit has been obtained in relieving the pain and in some instances greatly reducing the tumor mass; the patients have splenectomy at a later date.

PROGNOSIS

Utilizing multidrug combinations, more intensive chemotherapy schedules and concomitant radiotherapy of *CNS,* sanctuary sites, treatment for childhood leukemia has become increasingly more successful. Five-year survival rates exceeding 20 per cent have been documented and 5-year survival rates approximating 25 per cent have been projected for children already under therapy.[5,11]

Neuroblastoma

Neuroblastoma is highly invasive locally and up to 70 per cent of the patients already have metastases at the time of diagnosis. Skeletal spread is characteristically common and periorbital ecchymoses and proptosis resulting from skull metastases are almost pathognomonic findings. The bone marrow is frequently invaded. Lymph node spread is common. In about a fourth of the cases, the liver is involved. Pulmonary metastases are less frequent findings.

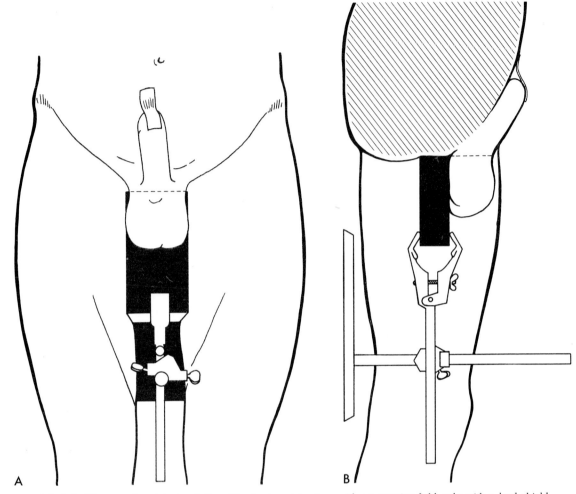

FIG. 8-6. Diagram of testicle irradiation. The treatment is given with an anterior field only with a lead shield
under the testicles to spare the perineum. The penis is taped against the abdomen. A given dose of
2,500 rads is delivered in 10 fractions.
  A. Anterior view.
  B. Lateral view.

CLINICAL STAGING

James,[8] Pinkel *el al.,*[10] and Thurman and Donaldson[21] have suggested classification of patients into prognostic categories. The most recent classification proposed by Evans *et al.*[4] recognizes an unique group (Stage IV-S) consisting of patients, generally under one year of age, with a very good prognosis in spite of liver, skin, and bone marrow (but not bone) metastases. The 2-year survival in this special group of patients under one year of age was 94 per cent[18,19] in one series.[2]

PROPOSED CLINICAL STAGING FOR CHILDREN WITH NEUROBLASTOMA

Stage I—tumor confined to the organ or structure of origin.

Stage II—tumors extending in continuity beyond the organ or structure of origin but not crossing the midline. Regional lymph nodes on the homolateral side may be involved.

Stage III—tumors extending in continuity beyond the midline. Regional lymph nodes may be involved bilaterally.

Stage IV—remote disease involving skeleton organs, soft tissues, or distant lymph node groups.

Stage IV-S—patients who would otherwise be Stages I or II but who have remote disease confined only to one or more of the following sites: liver, skin, or bone marrow (without radiographic evidence of bone metastases on complete skeletal survey).

SURGERY

Surgical extirpation of the tumor remains the best treatment for neuroblastoma. In situations where complete removal of the tumor is not feasible, Koop has advocated a "major surgical insult to the tumor" by removing as much of the tumor as possible.[6]

CHEMOTHERAPY

The value of chemotherapy as an adjuvant measure (so effective in Wilms' tumor) remains unestablished in the treatment of non-metastatic neuroblastoma. The over-all survival pattern following the introduction of a number of drugs appears not to have improved significantly. The disappointing results preclude at this writing the selective consideration of any chemotherapy regimen.[18]

Sporadic responses, occasionally to a spec-

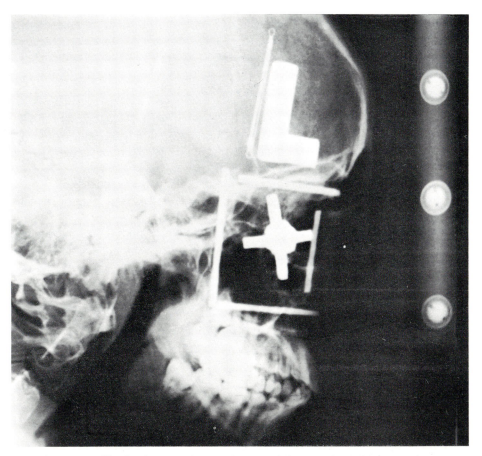

FIG. 8-7. Eighteen-year-old girl with a 3-year history of acute undifferentiated leukemia in bone marrow remission that had had leukemic infiltration of numerous organs (kidneys, central nervous system, etc.). She had received radiation therapy to the calvarium but the retinae were not treated. She developed retinal infiltration. The figure shows the field of treatment. Dose: 2,500 rads tumor dose at 3 cm depth.

tacular degree, have occurred in children with metastatic disease after the administration of a variety of chemical agents including mannitol mustard, cyclophosphamide, vincristine, daunomycin, and adriamycin. These documented responses justify the persistent exposure of the patient with metastatic disease to potentially helpful agents such as cyclophosphamide, vincristine, and daunomycin initially and investigative agents later. The biologic behavior of neuroblastoma in a given patient is notoriously unpredictable and apparent cures under seemingly hopeless conditions are not rarities.

If immunologic considerations (currently under active investigation) become important, the addition or deletion of both radiotherapy and chemotherapy may have to be re-evaluated in terms of the host's (patient) response to the tumor (neuroblastoma).

RADIOTHERAPY

Patients with lesions in the retroperitoneal or posterior mediastinum have been treated postoperatively with parallel-opposed fields. A tumor dose of 3,000 rads in 4 weeks is considered a curative dose. Radiotherapy is beneficial in controlling symptoms produced by metastatic disease. The usual spread includes skull bones, long bones, and liver. Simple field arrangement is used with margins around the metastasis. A dose of 2,000 rads *TD* in 2 weeks produces relief of the symptoms.

PROGNOSIS

In one study, the 2-year survival rates for children with neuroblastoma, all stages combined, were: those under 12 months of age, 51/69 (74 per cent); those 12 through 24 months of age 12/47 (26 per cent); and those over 24 months of age, 16/130 (12 per cent).[2] The data indicated that both age and stage (extent of disease) were factors in determining prognosis, even after statistically ad-

justing for the effects of each.[2] In the presence of skeletal metastases, long term survival is extremely unusual, regardless of age. The currently available clinical experience suggests that the various treatment programs (including vigorous chemotherapy) has not significantly changed the survival figures during the past decade.[18] Other factors that have been related to survival of patients include the site of origin of the primary tumor (mediastinal tumors are considered to have better prognosis) and the degree of histologic differentiation (improved prognosis is correlated with greater degrees of "differentiation").[6]

Rhabdomyosarcoma

Histopathologically, the embryonal rhabdomyosarcomas predominate. Only about 20 per cent of the rhabdomyosarcomas in children are alveolar in type and the pleomorphic rhabdomyosarcomas are very rare. Sarcoma botryoides is a term applied to embryonal rhabdomyosarcoma that originates beneath a mucosal surface (such as the vagina, bladder or larynx) eventually forming polypoid grape-structures.

Rhabdomyosarcoma is locally infiltrative at quite a distance and metastasize early and widely. Metastases are most commonly found in lymph nodes, the lungs, bone, bone marrow, liver, brain, and breast.

TREATMENT

The treatment for rhabdomyosarcoma requires the integration of all effective modalities: surgery, radiotherapy, and intensive chemotherapy. Such a program is outlined in Figure 8-8.

SURGERY

In accessible anatomic sites, surgical excision of the primary lesion is carried out. While the infiltrative behavior of this tumor had previously led the surgeons to recom-

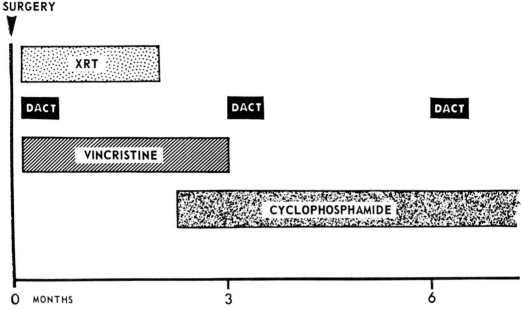

FIG. 8-8. Schema for multimodal therapy for rhabdomyosarcoma. Drugs and irradiation are used postoperatively. Abbreviations: *XRT,* irradiation; *DACT,* dactinomycin (Actinomycin D); cyclophosphamide is the generic name for Cytoxan. (Courtesy: Sutow, In *Neoplasia in Childhood,* Year Book Medical Publishers, Chicago, Ill., p. 201, 1969.)

mend wide and radical excision of the lesion, the good results obtained recently with combined chemotherapy and radiotherapy suggest that a more conservative surgical excision of the tumor may be adequate.

CHEMOTHERAPY

The regimen using the 3-drug combination of vincristine, actinomycin D, and cyclophosphamide *(VAC)* has been outlined in Figure 8-8.[17]

In this *VAC* regimen, vincristine *(VCR)* and actinomycin D *(AMD)* are begun simultaneously with the initiation of radiotherapy. The dose of *VCR* is 2 mg/m^2 (maximum single dose of 2 mgm); IV weekly for a minimum of 8 doses and a maximum of 12 doses. The occurrence of symptomatic neuropathy generally presages limit of tolerance for *VCR.* Each course of AMD consists of the total dose of 75 mcg (micrograms)/kg body weight given intravenously in divided doses over a period of 5 to 7 days.

Many older children do not tolerate more than 500 mcg *AMD* per dose. In such children, 500 mcg is given daily until the cumulative total dose reaches 75 mcg/kg. The side effects of *VCR* and *AMD* have been outlined elsewhere in Table 8-2.

Cyclophosphamide is started after radiotherapy is completed to avoid overlapping suppressive effect on the hematopoietic tissues. The dose of the drug is 2.5 mg/kg body weight daily by mouth.

In more recently treated patients, the cyclophosphamide has been administered in large intermittent "pulses" of 10 mg/kg body weight intravenously or orally daily for 7 to 10 days or until a leukopenia of 1,500/mm^3 or a granulocytopenia of 1,000/mm^3 is achieved. Such pulses are repeated at 3-week intervals initially, then at longer intervals after several pulses have been given.

The side effects of cyclophosphamide include alopecia, bone marrow, depression, and hemorrhagic cystitis (the latter generally after a long period of drug administration).

VCR is not repeated after the initial course. Pulses of *AMD* are given every 3 months for a total of 5 courses. Cyclophosphamide is continued for 2-years elapsed time from initial surgery.

RADIOTHERAPY

For the head and neck, radiotherapy techniques are those of the epithelial tumors for the anatomical sites of involvement. The dose is 5,500 rads *TD* $5\frac{1}{2}$ weeks to 6,000 rads *TD* in 6 weeks.

For other sites of involvement, for example the genitourinary tract, the management of tumor itself and the combination strategy of radiotherapy, chemotherapy, and surgery have to be devised individually. In some cases, when large masses are present, an attempt may be made to shrink the tumor with chemotherapy first, if possible, before attempting radiotherapy. The techniques of the radiotherapy are parallel-opposed fields with the aim of 5,000 rads in 5 weeks with ^{60}Co. Tumors located in the superficial tissues of the lumbar area or abdominal wall are, after surgical excision, given postoperative radiotherapy with electron beam or paired wedged fields with the aim of giving 5,000 rads in 5 weeks. For retroperitoneal tumors, the plan would be partial or complete excision of the mass followed by chemotherapy and radiotherapy, with a dose of 5,000 rads *TD* in 5 weeks.

The combination of drug treatment and radiation therapy is associated with considerable toxicity, including local tissue reactions and severe bone marrow depression. Mucositis becomes particularly distressing when head and neck lesions are being treated. Vigorous and supportive measures are required. When the treatment involves the abdomen, problems with nausea, vomiting, and diarrhea may occur. Severe skin reactions can develop.

In regard to late complications, one must avoid as much as possible the irradiation of unnecessary structures; such damage may be deleterious to the future development of the child. Inclusion of the mandible in the treatment field has produced severe trismus and lack of development of the mandible. Similar growth defects may result from irradiation of the vertebrae.

PROGNOSIS

The reported over-all 5-year survival rate in children with rhabdomyosarcoma has varied from 12 per cent to 35 per cent.[19] The factors that seem to be associated with better survival include aggressive and intensive therapy, younger age (under 7 years), favorable primary site (such as the orbit), and favorable histologic type (embryonal rather than alveolar). Prior to the use of drug combinations and multimodal approach, the survival rate among children with extensive, inoperable, or metastatic disease had been poor. In the *MDAH* experience, none of 24 children survived more than 30 months. With the use of intensive multimodal treatment regimens, the 2- to 4-year survival data indicate improvement among both the nonmetastatic and the metastatic cases.

Wilms' Tumor

Wilms' tumor metastasizes most frequently to the lungs and to the liver. In contrast to neuroblastoma, skeletal metastases develop rarely. Bone marrow infiltration is also uncommon. Lymphatic spread to lymph nodes can occur. Less frequently the extradural spaces, brain, soft tissues, and testicles may be other metastatic sites.

STAGING

One scheme for the staging of the extent of the disease has been formalized by the National Wilms' Tumor Study and is based on clinical, surgical, and pathological considerations[9] (Table 8-1).

Table 8-1. *Assessment of Extent of Disease in Children with Wilms' Tumor per National Wilms' Tumor Study*

Stage or Group	Criteria (clinical, surgical and pathological)
I	Tumor is contained within kidney capsule and is completely resected.
II	Tumor extends locally beyond the kidney (penetration into peri-renal soft tissues; peri-aortic node involvement; tumor thrombus in renal vessels) but is completely resected.
III	Postsurgically, there is residual tumor confined to abdomen (biopsy or rupture of tumor; peritoneal implants; involved lymph nodes beyond the abdominal peri-aortic chains; incomplete resection of tumor).
IV	Distant (Hematogenous) metastases are present.
V	Bilateral renal involvement is present.

TREATMENT

The current treatment for the child with Wilms' tumor is a closely coordinated program utilizing prompt surgical extirpation of the tumor, postoperative radiation therapy, and intensive adjuvant chemotherapy.

SURGERY

The generally accepted principles in the surgical treatment for Wilms' tumor include: a) the transabdominal approach, b) inspection and palpation of the contralateral kidney, c) marking the extent of tumor for guidance of postoperative radiotherapy, d) removal of the primary tumor in its entirety, e) marking with clips any residual tumor, f) thorough inspection of abdominal cavity and viscera, and g) documentation of any rupture or tumor spillage. Routine periaortic node dissection has been recommended by some surgeons. The primary tumor should be removed even when pulmonary metastases are already evident since curative therapy for the metastases is still possible.

Under certain circumstances, surgery is also used as curative therapy for metastatic disease. Surgical excision of a single or even multiple pulmonary nodule has resulted in cures. Hemihepatectomy has been done successfully to control liver metastases. Surgery, further, provides palliation in relieving pressure symptoms such as those resulting from extradural metastases with spinal cord compression.

CHEMOTHERAPY

1) Chemotherapy used in conjunction with surgery and radiotherapy has significantly improved survival rates among children with Wilms' tumor.[18]

2) Two active agents, actinomycin D and vincristine, are equally effective. There is no cross-resistance between them. The possibility that the administration of both drugs may be more effective than either drug used singly is being investigated clinically.[9]

3) In selected situations where the tumor was considered to be inoperable and the diagnostic studies indicated a high probability of Wilms' tumor, the preoperative administration of 2 to 3 weekly doses of vincristine has produced a rapid shrinkage of tumor to permit subsequent nephrectomy. Postoperative radiotherapy was possible without any modification.[16]

4) Actinomycin D and vincristine, either singly or in combination, have been used concomitantly with radiotherapy and/or surgery in the curative approach to patients with metastases to the liver and/or lungs.

5) Studies with actinomycin D suggest that "maintenance" chemotherapy courses for 15 months postsurgery produced better survival rates than short-term adjuvant therapy with the same drug.[22]

6) In patients with widespread metastatic disease, significant palliation has been achieved with the use of actinomycin D and

Table 8-2. *Chemotherapy Regimens for Actinomycin D (AMD) and Vincristine (VCR) in Children with Wilms' Tumor*

Drug	Dose	Regimen	Side Effects
AMD	15 micrograms/kg body weight IV daily 5 per course	Begin initial course on day of surgery. Repeat courses at 6 wk., 3 mos., 6 mos., 9 mos., 12 mos., and 15 mos. discontinue chemotherapy thereafter.	Nausea, vomiting, abdominal pain, depressed blood counts (especially platelets), mucositis, alopecia, skin reaction over previously irradiated sites.
VCR	1.5 to 2.0 mg/m^2 body surface area (maximum dose 2.0 mg) IV	Begin as soon as postoperative status stabilizes. Drug is given weekly for 8 wks. then 2 doses a wk. a part at 3 mos., 6 mos., 9 mos., 12 mos., and 15 mos. Discontinue chemotherapy thereafter.	Abdominal pain, severe obstipation, paresthesia, neuropathy, alopecia.
AMD + VCR	Same doses as above	Both drugs given at same time on same schedules as above	
VCR (preop)	Same dose as above	Administer weekly for 2 or 3 doses. If sufficient regression does not occur, consider preop. irrad.	Be on alert particularly for gastrointestinal side effects of vincristine.

vincristine. Temporary regression of tumor masses has also been produced by pulse doses of cyclophosphamide and by adriamycin.

7) The currently used chemotherapy regimens have been outlined in Table 8-2.

Radiotherapy

Primary Tumor

STAGING

There is increasing clinical experience that postoperative irradiation of the tumor bed may not be necessary if the primary lesion is completely excised (Stage I).[9] In the National Wilms' Tumor Study (Stage I), patients are randomly allocated to a group receiving or to a group not receiving postoperative irradiation.

Patients with disease in Stages II or III and most Stage IV's who have evidence of tumor outside the confines of the kidney should receive postoperative irradiation. The treatment is started as soon after surgery as possible, usually within 48 hours of the surgical procedure.

TECHNIQUES OF TREATMENT FOR STAGE II

Postoperative radiation is given to the tumor bed as determined by the preoperative intravenous pyelogram and the surgical findings. The tumor area and renal fossa on the affected side is considered "contaminated" and all of this volume is included within the treatment field. The field extends across the midline to include all the veretebral bodies at the level concerned to prevent scoliosis, but the contralateral kidney is not included in the field (Fig. 8-9). Opposing anterior and posterior portals are used and the usual tumor dose calculated at midline is:

Birth to 18 months........1,800 to 2,400 rads tumor dose
19 to 30 months ....2,400 to 3,000 rads tumor dose
31 to 40 months ....3,000 to 3,500 rads tumor dose
41 to 50 months ....3,500 to 4,000 rads tumor dose

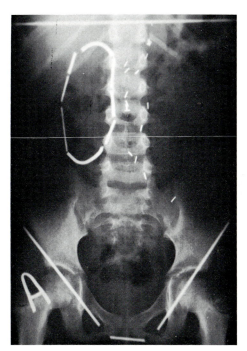

FIG. 8-10. Total abdomen irradiation for a Wilms' tumor on the left in a 10-year-old girl who had received preoperative chemotherapy. The figure demonstrates blocking of remaining kidney front and back with 4 *HVL*. The midline dose was 3,000 rads in 4 weeks.

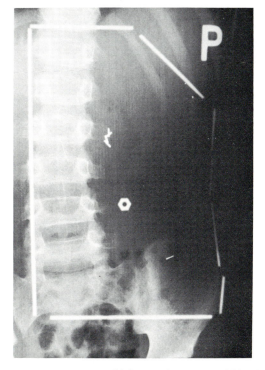

FIG. 8-9. Nine-year-old boy with recurrent Wilms' tumor in right kidney. He received post-operative radiation to tumor bed in combination with chemotherapy. A tumor dose of 3,500 rads calculated to midline were given in 4½ weeks. Figure shows the tumor bed; the whole spine is included to avoid scoliosis.

STAGE III

The entire abdominal cavity (Fig. 8-10) receives a dose of 3,000 rads in 4 weeks adjusted for age. Additional treatment should be given to areas of known residual tumor. The remaining kidney is shielded anteriorly and posteriorly not to exceed 1,500 rads in 4 weeks. The liver is excluded, partially from the beam so the dose to the entire organ does not exceed 2,500 rads in 3 weeks.

STAGE IV

Surgery plays a role in treatment for metastatic disease. Frequently, persistent or recurrent masses are best managed with surgery and one should not be hesitant to advise such treatment. Metastatic disease is generally treated concomitantly with chemotherapy.

Metastases

METASTASES TO THE LIVER

Only metastases that are nonresectable because of location or extent receive radiotherapy. The entire liver is included to receive a tolerable dose of 2,500 rads in 3 weeks or 3,000 rads in 4 weeks. This is done in combination with chemotherapy.

METASTASES TO THE BRAIN, BONE, LYMPH NODES, ETC.

Patients with cerebral metastasis receive whole brain radiation to doses of 3,000 rads

in 3 weeks. An additional 500 or 1,000 rads will be added through a reduced field over the known tumor volume.

The entire bone need not be treated for bony lesions. A dose of 4,000 rads is used routinely if the joint surface and plate can be spared. The fields include the known disease with the margin of not less than 3 cm in any direction. The lymph nodes and soft tissue masses are handled in a similar manner.

METASTASES TO THE LUNGS

Metastases to the lungs are treated using total lung fields for 1,500 rads *TD* in 2 weeks. An additional 1,500 rads *TD* in 2 weeks can be added to localized areas (Fig. 8-11).

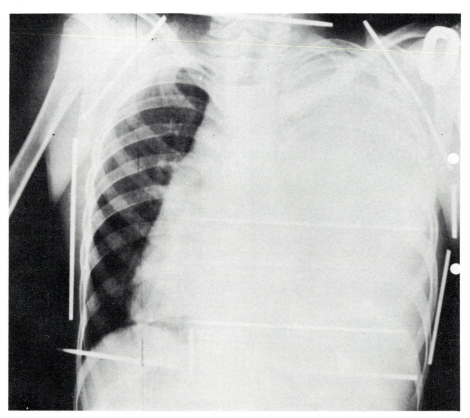

FIG. 8-11. Nine-year-old boy with diagnosis of Wilms' tumor of the right kidney who developed right lung metastases with pleural effusion. The figure shows the portal film of total lung irradiation with planned midline dose of 1,500 rads in 2 weeks.

Treatment of Bilateral Wilms' Tumor

Treatment of the patient with bilateral Wilms' tumor is individualized. The volume and anatomic location of the tumor in each kidney and the mass of functional renal tissue determine the extent of surgery possible. Maximum use of chemotherapy is essential both in terms of intensity and of duration. Radiation therapy is administered only in the dose safely tolerated by the kidney to avoid radiation nephritis, (2,000 rads in 4 weeks).

PROGNOSIS

The pattern of the significant improvement that followed the introduction of adjuvant chemotherapy is indicated in Figure 8-12.[18] The survival curves for 1956 represent the cases that were treated just prior to the wide-spread use of actinomycin D. By 1962, in addition to actinomycin D, vincristine was available for clinical trial. The age of the child at diagnosis emerged as another significant prognostic factor. Best survivals occur in children under the age of 2 years.

The prognosis for long-term survival, even in the children who have metastases at diagnosis or who subsequently develop metastases is not hopeless. Up to one third of these children are being "salvaged" by intensive, persistent multimodal therapy.

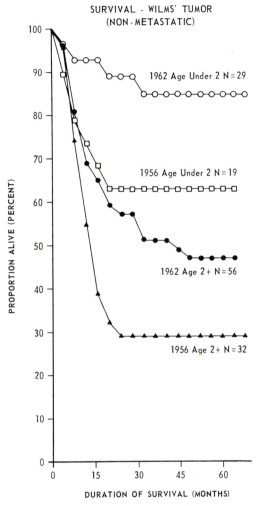

FIG. 8-12. Survival among patients with nonmetastatic Wilms' tumor shown for 2 age groups under and above 2 years for 2 time periods. In 1956, adjuvant chemotherapy was not being used; by 1962, both actinomycin D and vincristine were widely available. N represents the number of cases in each category. (Courtesy: Sutow, Gehan, Heyn, Kung, Miller, Murphy, Traggis, *Pediatrics,* 45, 800, 1970.)

BIBLIOGRAPHY

1. Aur, R. J. A., Simone, J. V., Hustu, H. O., and Verzosa, M. S.: A comparative study of central nervous system irradiation and intensive chemotherapy early in remission of childhood acute lymphocytic leukemia, *Cancer,* 29, 381, 1972.
2. Breslow, N., and McCann, B.: Statistical estimation of prognosis for children with neuroblastoma, *Cancer Res.,* 31, 2098, 1971.
3. Dahlin, D. C.: *Bone Tumors. General Aspects and Data on 3987 Cases,* 2nd Ed., Charles C Thomas, Springfield, Illinois, p. 285, 1967.
4. Evans, A. E., D'Angio, G. J., and Randolph, J.: A proposed staging for children with neuroblastoma, *Cancer,* 27, 374, 1971.
5. Holland, J. F.: Hopes for tomorrow versus realities of today; therapy and prognosis in acute lymphocytic leukemia of childhood, *Pediatrics,* 45, 191, 1970.

6. Horn, R. C., Jr., Koop, C. E., and Kieswetter, W. B.: Neuroblastoma in childhood, *Laboratory Investigation,* 5, 106, 1956.

7. Hustu, H. O., Holton, C., James, D., Jr., Treatment of Ewing's sarcoma with concurrent radiotherapy and chemotherapy, *J. Pediat.,* 73, 249, 1968.

8. James, D. H., Jr.: Proposed classification of neuroblastoma, *J. Pediat.,* 71, 764, 1967.

9. National Wilms' Tumor Study Protocol. G. J. D'Angio, Chairman, Memorial Hospital, N.Y., N.Y.

10. Pinkel, D., Pratt, C., Holton, C., James, D., Jr., and Hustu, H. O.: Survival of children with neuroblastoma treated with combination chemotherapy, *J. Pediat.,* 73, 928, 1968.

11. Pinkel, D., Simone, J., Hustu, H. O., and Aur, R. J. A.: Nine year's experience with "total therapy" of childhood acute lymphocytic leukemia, *Pediatrics,* 50, 246, 1972.

12. Suit, H. D., Martin, R. G., and Sutow, W. W.: Malignant tumors of bone, In *Clinical Pediatric Oncology,* Sutow, W. W., Vietti, T. J., and Fernbach, D. J., Eds., C. V. Mosby Co., St. Louis, Mo., In press.

13. Suit, H. D. Fernandez, C., Sutow, W., Samuels, M., and Wilbur, J.: Radiation therapy and multi-drug chemotherapy in management of patients with Ewing's sarcoma, Presented at Colston Research Society Symposium, Bristol, England, April 1972, In press.

14. Sullivan, M. P.: Current management of acute leukemia in children, *The Cancer Bulletin,* 24, 12, 1972.

15. Sullivan, M. P., and Hrgovcic, M.: Extramedullary leukemia, In *Clinical Pediatric Oncology,* Sutow, W. W., Vietti, T. J., and Fernbach, D. J., Eds., C. V. Mosby Co., St. Louis, Mo., In press.

16. Sullivan, M. P., Sutow, W. W., Cangier, A., and Taylor, G.: Vincristine sulfate in management of Wilms' tumor—replacement of preoperative irradiation by chemotherapy, *JAMA,* 202, 381, 1967.

17. Sutow, W. W.: Chemotherapeutic management of childhood rhabdomyosarcoma, In *Neoplasia in Childhood,* Year Book Medical Publishers, Chicago, Ill., p. 201, 1969.

18. Sutow, W. W., Gehan, E. A., Heyn, R. M., Kung, F. H., Miller, R. W., Murphy, M. L., and Traggis, D. G.: Comparison of survival curves, 1956 versus 1962, in children with Wilms' tumor and neuroblastoma, *Pediatrics,* 45, 800, 1970.

19. Sutow, W. W., Sullivan, M. P., Reid, H. L., Taylor, H. G., and Griffith, K. M.: Prognosis in childhood rhabdomyosarcoma, *Cancer,* 25, 1384, 1970.

20. Sutow, W. W., and Valeriote, F.: General aspects of chemotherapy, In *Clinical Pediatric Oncology,* Sutow, W. W., Vietti, T. J., and Fernbach, D. J., Eds., C. V. Mosby Co., St. Louis, Mo., In press.

21. Thurman, W. G., and Donaldson, M. H.: Current concepts in the management of neuroblastoma, In *Neoplasia in Childhood,* Year Book Medical Publishers, Inc., Chicago, Ill., p. 175, 1969.

22. Wolff, J. A., Krivit, W., Newton, W. A., Jr., and D'Angio, G. J.: Single versus multiple dose dactinomycin therapy of Wilms' tumor, *New Eng. J. Med.,* 279, 290, 1968.

9. Thorax

Radiation Reactions of Normal Tissues

FERNANDO G. BLOEDORN

The thoracic structures which may be included in the irradiated volume are the lungs, the mediastinal organs, and the spinal cord.

LUNG

The tolerance of the lung to irradiation is limited. It is considered that doses in the range of 2,000 rads delivered in 1 to 2 weeks will produce permanent changes in the lung. Irradiation changes in the lung are generally produced in two separate, well-defined periods. First, there is a period of acute reaction with inflammatory changes including congestion, exudate, and infiltration. The acute reaction usually develops during the third week after therapy, especially if the dose has exceeded 4,000 rads, and reaches maximum intensity 4 to 6 weeks after the treatment is finished. This reaction tends to be "subclinical" and asymptomatic. In some patients, because of individual sensitivity or a concomitant infection, a clinical syndrome develops with slight fever, coughing, bronchial secretion, and x-ray manifestations of spotty pneumonitis. The patient then enters a latent period which varies from 6 to 12 months, when a second episode of pneumonitis develops. The radiographic manifestations are more obvious in this second period, which is the beginning of progressive fibrotic changes over the years.

These fibrotic changes constitute the late sequelae, varying from minimal patchy or streaky fibrosis to a complete fibro-thorax with retraction of the mediastinum, chest wall, and diaphragm. The intensity of the changes are related to the total dose and volume of lung irradiated. The radiographic changes are principally in the irradiation field and at the beginning of the process quite often will have a geometric shape corresponding to the irradiated volume (Fig. 9-1). In most patients, even with intense fibrosis, the symptoms are minimal.[1,5] An occasional patient will develop progressive dyspnea, severe cough, and pain. Death may occur because of right heart failure. These late changes may be mistaken for tumor recurrences.

MEDIASTINAL REACTION

The mediastinal structures have been considered quite resistant to irradiation. With megavoltage and larger doses delivered in less time, transient esophagitis occurs. With doses over 4,500 rads given in 4 to 5 weeks and with large volume irradiated, mild exudative asymptomatic pericarditis may occur. With larger doses pericardial effusion may occur and constrictive pericarditis can follow. It is possible that destruction by irradiation of tumor invading the pericardium and myocardium is responsible for the production of ulceration with exudate formation and subsequent fibrosis.

ESOPHAGUS

The esophagus is able to tolerate irradiation doses adequate for tumor control. Epi-

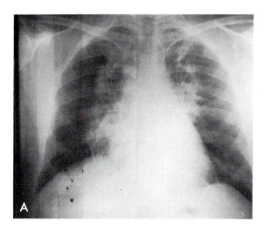

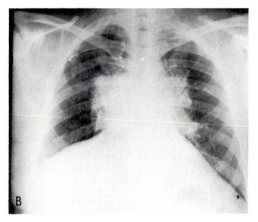

FIG. 9-1. Patient treated for oat-cell carcinoma with bilateral mediastinal nodes. The treatment was finished April 1, 1960.

    A. July 7, 1960, the reaction of the lung outlines the treatment fields.

    B. September 4, 1960, the reaction is more marked in the area of the small volume (higher dose) irradiation.

    During all this period the patient was asymptomatic.

thelitis is produced after 3,000 rads delivered in $2\frac{1}{2}$ to 3 weeks. The dysphagia produced by the reaction subsides within 2 to 3 weeks.[2,3,4]

The production of fistulae or massive hemorrhage due to breakdown of the esophageal wall and rupture into a hollow viscus or a large vessel of the mediastinum occasionally occurs during or immediately after treatment. It results from tumor regression when the tumor had grown into the esophageal wall and destroyed the full thickness of its musculature (Fig. 9-10). These complications should not be considered due to excessive radiation dosage.

With adequate megavoltage techniques, 6,000 rads can be delivered to the whole length of the esophagus in 6 weeks without risk of permanent symptomatic changes. Narrowing of the esophagus at the level of the lesion often follows the treatment for an extensive cancer. In most cases, this narrowing is due to healing by scar tissue in an area of tumor destruction in the wall of the organ rather than from excessive irradiation.

NORMAL TISSUES SURROUNDING THE ESOPHAGUS

Various degrees of fibrosis develop in the structures surrounding the esophagus and, in most cases, are asymptomatic. The tolerance of the organs and tissues that surround the subdiaphragmatic esophagus is considerably less than those in the upper mediastinum.

SPINAL CORD

Myelitis is the most severe complication and results from a poor treatment plan. The tolerance of the spinal cord to irradiation is limited. The level of tolerance is related to dose and time, and the length of spinal cord exposed to irradiation. Maximum doses of 5,000 rads in 5 weeks for small fields and 4,000 to 4,500 rads for large fields have been established for the spinal cord. Myelitis can be avoided by not exceeding this dose.

BIBLIOGRAPHY

1. Bloedorn, F. G., Cowley, R. A., Cuccia, C. A., and Mercado, R., Jr.: Combined therapy: Irradiation and surgery in treatment of bronchogenic carcinoma, *Amer. J. Roentgen.*, 85, 875, 1961.

2. Jennings, F. L. and Arden, A.: Acute radiation effects in the esophagus, *Arch. Path.,* 69, 407, 1960.
3. Moss, W. T.: *Therapeutic Radiology,* St. Louis, C. V. Mosby Company, 1959.

4. Seaman, W. B. and Ackerman, L. V.: The effect of radiation on the esophagus, *Radiology,* 68, 534, 1957.
5. Smart, J.: Can lung cancer be cured by irradiation alone?, *J.A.M.A.,* 195, 8, 1966.

Lung

FERNANDO G. BLOEDORN

The treatment for carcinoma of the lung is a challenging problem for the therapist. It is possible that a more aggressive and optimistic approach in the therapy of lung cancer may improve the results. This section outlines the fundamental basis and reasoning for each modality of treatment.

To control malignant tumors, it is necessary to treat the whole volume of tissues "potentially" involved by the growth. It is recognized that in some anatomical areas the extension of the tumor will not be clinically detectable ("subclinical disease"). A good treatment should be applicable to patients with early as well as advanced disease provided the tumor is still limited to the primary tumor and to the regional lymph node areas.

The curability of any patient with cancer is determined mainly by the natural history of the disease. The cancer which remains localized for a long period of time is highly controllable. Conversely, one which spreads early and widely is seldom brought under control. Cancer of the lung is in the latter group.

Pathology

Malignant epithelial tumors of the lung are generally divided into four groups; 1) squamous cell carcinoma, 2) anaplastic carcinoma (small or oat cell and large-cell carcinoma),

3) adenocarcinoma, and 4) a group of epithelial tumors without definite morphologic characteristics called undifferentiated carcinomas (unclassifiable). Two other groups of tumors can acquire malignant characteristics either locally or by producing metastases: the bronchial adenomas and alveolar cell tumors (also called pulmonary adenomatosis).

Before making a positive diagnosis of adenocarcinoma of the lung, there should be a thorough investigation to rule out a primary tumor elsewhere in the body. A high percentage of the so-called adenocarcinomas of the lung are metastatic tumors from occult primaries located elsewhere in the body, usually the gastrointestinal tract or kidney.

The histology of our series is shown in Table 9-1.

Complex of Potentially Involved Tissues in Bronchogenic Carcinoma

PRIMARY TUMOR AND LOCAL EXTENSIONS

When patients come for diagnosis and therapy, only 15 per cent will have localized disease. Another 30 per cent will have evidence only of regional spread and 55 per cent will have demonstrable distant metastases.[4,14]

By the time the diagnosis is made, most

Table 9-1. *Histology of Lesions from 192 Patients with Bronchogenic Carcinoma Seen at The University of Maryland Hospital*

Histology	Number	Per Cent
Squamous Cell Carcinoma	118	61.3
Undifferentiated Carcinoma	32	16.7
Anaplastic Carcinoma	24	12.6
Adenocarcinoma	16	8.4
No histology (rib erosion)	2	1.0
Total	192	100%

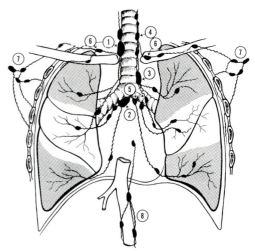

FIG. 9-2. Schematic illustration of the lymphatics of the lung and pleura. 1) azygos node (most commonly involved), 2) intertracheobronchial nodes, 3) paratracheal nodes, 4) supraclavicular nodes, 5) hilar nodes, 6) supraclavicular nodes, 7) axillary nodes, and 8) paraaortic nodes. Modified from: Ackerman, L. V. and Del Regato, J. A., *Cancer: Diagnosis-Treatment-Prognosis,* 3rd ed., St. Louis, The C. V. Mosby Company, p. 463, 1962.

bronchogenic carcinomas have invaded the organs at the site of origin. Not only are there tumor extensions which are visible on x-ray films or by gross examination, but there is microscopic invasion through the intercellular spaces and invasion of capillary lymphatics and blood vessels. In a bronchogenic tumor originating in the hilum (where two thirds of the tumors originate), all these extensions occur in the mediastinal structures which involve vital organs such as the pedicle of the heart, pedicle of the lung, the heart itself, the esophagus, and the trachea.

REGIONAL EXTENSION (LYMPH NODE METASTASES TO THE FIRST AND SECOND ECHELON OF THE TRIBUTARY AREA)

Extension into the lymph nodes of the lung pedicle, the mediastinum, and the supraclavicular area is a frequent occurrence with bronchogenic carcinoma (Fig. 9-2). This type of extension increases in frequency from the squamous cell group to the undifferentiated and anaplastic groups.

Ordinarily over 60 per cent of patients with operable squamous cell carcinoma and adenocarcinoma have metastases to the first or second lymph node echelon. Such metastases occur in close to 100 per cent of patients with anaplastic carcinomas; in patients with undifferentiated carcinoma the incidence of metastases is between 60 to 100 per cent.

In any patient with bronchogenic carcinoma, when the parietal pleura, tissues of the chest wall, or base of the neck are involved, direct spread to axillary and supraclavicular nodes is frequent. When the diaphragm is involved, there may be direct extension into the periaortic nodes of the abdomen.

The incidences given may be lower than the actual incidences because of inability to detect microscopic invasion of the nodes. Obviously, if these extensions are neglected in the treatment, either by resection or irradiation, the treatment will fail.

BLOOD VESSEL INVASION

Bronchogenic carcinoma has a marked tendency to invade blood vessels, usually capillaries and veins. Vascular invasion is present in over 85 per cent of the cases carefully studied. The incidence of vessel invasion varies with the tumor histology. It increases from about 30 per cent for squamous cell carcinoma, to about 60 per cent for undifferentiated carcinoma, to 100 per cent for adenocarcinoma and anaplastic carcinoma. In patients with distant metastases, blood vessel invasion is almost invariably present.

As in any other tumor, veins are the most commonly involved large vessel. Pulmonary veins have been found involved by tumor in 40 per cent of resected specimens. The importance of this finding, from the standpoint of treatment and prognosis, is obvious. For patients with proven blood vessel invasion, the incidence of distant metastases is greater and the prognosis is worse.

SEEDING OF TUMOR

Bronchogenic carcinoma has a high potential for seeding and grafting onto tissues, producing secondary growths. Seeding can be produced spontaneously two ways: 1) via the bronchial tree, producing approximately 10 per cent of secondary pulmonary growths, and 2) with tumor at the surface of the lung, the pleural cavity can be seeded resulting in the production of pleural metastases. It can also be seeded by surgical manipulation into the blood stream or in the operative field.

DISTANT METASTASES

Bronchogenic carcinoma produces distant metastases with high frequency. This tendency is probably caused by a combination of factors: primarily invasion of blood vessels, great motility of the organs involved, and the continuous changes of pressure in the tumor area. The propensity to produce distant metastases is more obvious in some histological forms: anaplastic tumors and adenocarcinomas. The higher incidence of metastases in these groups is probably caused by extensive vascular invasion and decreased cohesion between cells.

CLINICOPATHOLOGIC GROUPS

Bronchogenic carcinoma, from the therapist's viewpoint, can be divided into several groups representing different diseases, each with its own treatment approach.

Squamous Cell Carcinoma. Hilar and Parahilar: This is the most common type of lung carcinoma (about 75 per cent). Originating in the main bronchi, it generally grows around the hilum of the lung obstructing the airways. Growth tends to be slow, producing metastases to the hilar, paratracheal, and subcarinal lymph nodes in about 60 to 70 per cent of the patients when first seen. It is radiographically demonstrable as a mass situated in the hilum or very near it, generally associated with partial, lobular, or complete lung atelectasis.

Because of the primary tumor's central location and proximity to vital nonresectable organs, or the presence of inoperable mediastinal metastases only a low percentage of these tumors is resectable even when the disease appears clinically to be in an early stage. According to autopsy reports, 1 of 4 patients will die with local extension of the tumor without nodal or distant metastases.

Peripheral: These are "coin" lesions which appear commonly as a solitary mass of variable size. The incidence of mediastinal lymph node metastases is between 25 and 50 per cent, depending upon the length of time it has been present and degree of differentiation of the tumor. The primary may be quite small or even radiographically undetectable with the lymph node metastases in the mediastinum being the outstanding feature. In other sites, the tumor is seen radiographically as two masses—the primary mass and the mediastinal mass close to the hilum or trachea. If located in the middle of the lung parenchyma these tumors are highly resectable with a good chance for cure providing mediastinal metastases are not present. If the mediastinal nodes are involved or if the tumor grows to the periphery of the lung and involves the pleural surface and the chest wall, control of disease by surgery alone decreases to a very low percentage.[14]

Apical Tumors. Apical tumors may be centrally placed in the apex of the lung or they originate in the region of the superior sulcus. In general, they are slow growing with less propensity for spread to lymph nodes and distant metastases than are the hilar tumors. Mediastinal node metastases are present in 30 per cent. The relatively low incidence of metastases is probably related to less motility and poor vascularization of the apical area of the lungs. When superior sulcus tumors invade beyond the visceral pleura with involvement of the tissues of the chest wall, spine, ribs, and nerve roots, Pancoast's syndrome is produced. Most of these tumors are unresectable because of early invasion of bone, viscera, or nerves. The pathology includes squamous cell, undifferentiated, anaplastic, and adenocarcinoma; the most common is squamous cell carcinoma.

Anaplastic Carcinoma. Anaplastic carcinomas are generally divided into two groups: 1) oat cell or small-cell carcinoma, and 2) large-cell carcinoma. Oat cell carcinoma is more common and is a very malignant, rapidly growing tumor. Patients with this tumor usually present a poor general condition with sallow color, lack of appetite, and weight loss. The primary tumor is variable in size and location. It may be peripheral or centrally placed, but generally mediastinal metastases are prominent and may be multiple, sometimes bilateral, resembling lymphoma. Supraclavicular, axillary, and distant metastases are common findings in the evolution of oat cell carcinomas. The incidence of lymph node metastases in the mediastinum is 90 to 100 per cent and invasion of blood vessels is usually present. Even if locally resectable, cure by surgery is rare. The histologic diagnosis of anaplastic carcinoma is currently considered a contraindication to surgery.

Undifferentiated Carcinoma. These carcinomas, located either in the central or peripheral areas of the lungs, have mixed characteristics of squamous cell and anaplastic carcinomas, with specific differentiation. The incidence of lymph node and distant metastases is between those of squamous cell and anaplastic carcinomas.

Adenocarcinomas. Adenocarcinomas may be peripheral, central, or apical in location. They are usually highly malignant with mediastinal lymph node metastases in approximately 60 per cent of the patients when first examined. The high incidence of blood vessel involvement is responsible for the early development of multiple distant metastases. Their evolution is capricious and unpredictable.

Mediastinal Syndrome. The mediastinal syndrome can occur with bronchogenic carcinoma of any pathology. It results from tumor compression and/or destruction of the superior vena cava, trachea, and/or the main nerves of the mediastinum, mainly phrenic and recurrent left laryngeal. Two groups of metastatic nodes are frequent causes of the mediastinal syndrome, the aortic window, and the azygous nodes.

Treatment

Place of Radiotherapy in the Treatment of Bronchogenic Carcinoma

Bronchogenic carcinomas had been controlled by irradiation before the first successful pneumonectomy was performed by Graham and Singer in 1933.[6] Radiation therapy, however, has been reserved for patients with inoperable tumors, or who are poor operative risks, or who have refused operation. In patients with resectable tumors, surgical procedures have been the treatment of choice.

The action of irradiation upon bronchogenic carcinomas has been demonstrated—large masses disappear and, in many patients, the tumor is locally controlled. Rissanen[15] found approximately 30 per cent local control of disease when the dose received with megavoltage was 5,000 to 6,000 rads. Kligerman[12] and Bloedorn,[3] with the use of preoperative irradiation, have demonstrated rates of sterilization of the primary which are 30 and 35 per cent respectively. Smart[16] and Hilton[11] treated 40 patients who had biopsy-proven operable lesions with 4,000 rads to 5,500 rads (using orthovoltage and lower doses for anaplastic tumors) given in various total treatment times. The 5-year survival was 22.5 per cent. Davies[5] describes the Christie Hospital experience with small-field megavoltage treatment in 17 patients without evidence of lymph node involvement with a 5-year survival of 41 per cent. These results are comparable with those reported in the best surgical statistics[14] which gives a 42 per cent 5-year survival in a large series of patients. In all radiation series, squamous cell carcinomas have proven to be the most curable.

No major attempt has been made to study the effects of irradiation upon either the primary lung tumor or upon nodal metastases in the mediastinum, scalene, and supraclavicular areas. With megavoltage therapy and better techniques, it may be possible to deliver, in a single volume, a cancerocidal dose to the primary tumor in the lung, the lymph node bearing areas of the mediastinum, scalene, and supraclavicular regions without producing significant damage in the normal tissues. After radical irradiation, surgery is possible without unduly increased morbidity.

Tumor Doses

The response of bronchogenic tumors to irradiation varies with the histology, size of tumor, and site of the growth (tumor bed). There are reports of tumor control with doses of 3,000 rads delivered in 3 to 5 weeks with kilovoltage therapy. Contrary wise, in our experience,[4] there have been adenocarcinomas of small size which did not respond

to 6,000 rads in 6 weeks. In the Maryland series, with irradiation of similarly sized lesions, the order of tumor sensitivity was, from the most sensitive to the least: anaplastic, oat cell, undifferentiated, squamous cell, adenocarcinoma, and alveolar cell carcinoma.

The use of preoperative irradiation has provided a unique opportunity to estimate the sterilization rate of lung tumors and of mediastinal and supraclavicular metastases. Of 98 patients who received preoperative irradiation at the University of Maryland Hospital[3,4] and were subsequently operated upon, the primary tumor was sterilized in 35 per cent. Of the patients who had biopsy-positive mediastinal nodes before radiotherapy, 60 per cent were negative at the second operation. The same study also showed that:

1. Cavitated tumors, if not infected, will respond like solid tumors.

2. Patients with severe infections and/or abscesses tolerated treatment poorly.

3. Contrary to general belief, mediastinal lymph node metastases are more sensitive to radiation, even when larger than the primary, probably due to differences in the tumor beds.

The possibility seems to be lower in controlling nodal metastases in the supraclavicular nodes than in the mediastinum.

Work-Up

Before treatment is selected, complete diagnostic information, the possible disease extensions, a complete history, bronchoscopy findings or other exploration, should be available to the therapist. Details of surgical exploration are also of value.

Chest roentgenograms, *AP* and lateral, must be recent. Tomograms of the mediastinum and, if necessary, of the lung fields in both sagittal and coronal plane, as well as a barium swallow and azygograms, are of great help in studying tumor extension and mediastinal metastases. If there is bone pain, a skeletal x-ray survey is mandatory. Liver function tests and a liver isotope scan assist in detecting liver metastases.

There are some features of the physical examination of special significance for the therapist. Paralysis of vocal cord movement indicates tumor compression of the recurrent laryngeal nerve. A careful search for metastases to the cervical and supraclavicular lymph nodes and to the peripheral lymph node bearing areas is essential. If the liver is palpable, characteristic nodularities produced by metastases should be looked for.

Diagnosis is proved only by histology or cytology. Exploratory thoracotomy should be avoided if possible in those patients who are to receive irradiation only or preoperative irradiation. Such a procedure would risk dissemination of malignant cells within and outside the chest. If cytologic proof is unavailable several efficient diagnostic procedures have been developed recently that can replace open thoracotomy. The procedures which may be attempted in successive order are: 1) Percutaneous needle biopsy under fluoroscopic control, and 2) limited anterior mediastinal exploration through the second intercostal space.[14] These two procedures, plus biopsy through a bronchoscope and sputum cytology should provide histological proof in almost 100 per cent of patients. Mediastinoscopy can be informative if done properly. Patients with overt or suspected active tuberculosis should be placed on appropriate antibiotic treatment for two weeks before irradiation and for the total period of treatment. Only patients with apical tumors and with evidence of bone erosion could be treated without histological diagnosis.

Care Before and During Treatment

Before starting treatment, consideration must be given to the general condition of the patient, including the hematological picture and possible infection. It is of fundamental importance to improve the patient's general condition and the condition of the tumor bed. A high protein diet, vitamins, antibiotics, and blood transfusions should be used when indicated. If the infection is mild, irradiation is continued; if severe, it calls for temporary interruption of treatment while antibiotics are administered.

The patient is examined weekly and attention is given to the movement of the vocal cords and to palpation for lymph nodes in the neck, supraclavicular, axillary, groin, and paraaortic areas, and for liver metastases. Signs and symptoms of bone and brain metastases require special diagnostic procedures. Roentgenograms of the chest are obtained after 4,000 rads tissue dose and again 1 month after the end of treatment.

Types of Irradiation Treatment

Radiation therapy can be classified as: radical irradiation alone, preoperative irradiation, postoperative irradiation, palliative, and symptomatic therapy.

RADICAL IRRADIATION ALONE

Treatment is radical when the whole volume of the complex of potentially involved tissues is irradiated to a dose which is considered necessary to control the gross and "subclinical" tumor.

Indications. In current medical practice, the main indications for radical radiation treatment for bronchogenic carcinoma are inoperable or unresectable tumors, patients who refuse surgery or have medical contraindications for operation, and the anaplastic (oat cell) carcinomas. From the radiotherapist's point of view, radical radiation should be considered in all clinicopathological groups when:

1. The primary tumor is limited to one hemithorax, regardless of its site or extensions; with or without demonstrable lymph node metastases in the mediastinum (uni- or bilateral); with or without lymph node metastases in the scalene and/or supracla-

vicular areas; without malignant pleural effusion (large effusion, hemorrhagic, or with malignant cells); and without distant metastases. With mediastinal syndrome or with disease involving the chest wall, radiation treatment should also be considered.

2. Exploratory thoracotomy has determined the growth to be unresectable but still within the limits described in the previous group.

3. When the lesion is of doubtful operability.

4. When the lesion is clinically operable but the patient is considered a poor risk for surgery or the lesion is an anaplastic (oat cell or large-cell) tumor.

Contraindications. The contraindications to irradiation are with:

1. Peripheral tumors, well differentiated, without evidence of metastases in the mediastinum. Surgery should be the treatment of choice.

2. Patients in very poor general condition, very old or with severe impairment of respiratory function.

3. Patients with severe infections (abscess, empyema).

4. Patients with malignant effusion.

5. Patients with distant metastases.

Techniques of Treatment

Hilar and Parahilar Tumors. Initially, the primary lesion and mediastinum are covered by fields providing at least 2 to 3 cm clearance around the visible tumor (Fig. 9-3). The mediastinal portion of the field should be no less than 10 cm in width and of sufficient length to extend from the sternal notch to at least 8 cm below the carina (14 to 15 cm is the minimum length). If lung atelectasis conceals the tumor, a rather generous field or a portion of it (about 10 × 10 cm) should include the root of the hilum on the affected side. Roentgenograms should be repeated after each 2,000 rads for definition of the

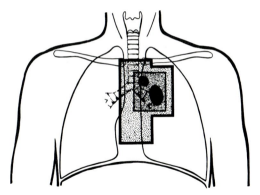

FIG. 9-3. Hilar and parahilar tumors. Well-differentiated squamous cell carcinoma. The larger area is irradiated with two parallel opposing fields. The darker area (small volume) is treated with rotation avoiding the spine.

tumor boundaries when the lung becomes aerated.

Every effort should be made to include the primary tumor and mediastinum in a single irradiation field. In all cases, even without visible mediastinal nodes, the field should encompass the area of the right paratracheal (azygos) node during the large volume portion of the treatment. Parallel opposing portals are recommended to deliver a daily tumor dose of 200 rads, irradiating both fields every day, with a tumor dose of 4,500 rads in 4½ weeks delivered to the midpoint of the thorax at the level of the carina. Anteroposterior and lateral chest x-ray films are obtained after 4,000 rads tissue dose to assess the response to treatment and to plan the final treatment.

The second part of the treatment consists of an additional 1,000 to 1,500 rads tumor dose to a smaller tissue volume, encompassing the primary tumor site and the adjacent mediastinum to 6,000 rads total dose. The field size at this point will be approximately 10 × 12 cm long and 8 × 10 cm wide (Fig. 9-3). To avoid irradiation of the spinal cord beyond tolerance limits, rotational techniques are used. If rotation is not available, a technique of crossfiring with small fields or possibly two parallel or oblique fields which avoid the spine can be substituted.

Peripheral Tumors. This group of tumors includes apical and other tumors located outside the hilar and parahilar regions. More than one field is usually necessary for the first stage of treatment to insure irradiation of the whole disease complex. The placement of fields varies according to the tumor location. The entire treatment is delivered through parallel opposing fields (Figs. 9-4 and 9-5). After 4,500 rads tumor dose, the fields are reduced, if possible, to cover only the detectable tumor and adjacent mediastinum.

When parallel opposing fields are used for small volume, high-dose therapy, the medial limits of the field should not reach the midline, in order to spare the spinal cord. The tissue dose is "boosted" to a total of 6,000 rads in the smaller volume. The daily tumor dose to this small volume is varied from 200 to 250 rads, depending upon the condition of the patient and the size of the irradiated field.

With undifferentiated tumors where upper mediastinal node involvement is detected by x-ray or surgical exploration, both supraclavicular areas are treated (Fig. 9-6). In tumors of the apex with proven or suspected

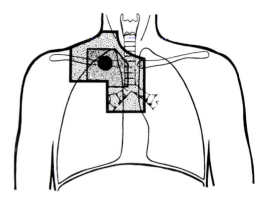

FIG. **9-5**. In apical tumors, the small volume (dark area) is treated with two parallel opposing fields.

parietal pleural involvement (Pancoast's syndrome), the supraclavicular area of the involved side is included in the treatment field (Fig. 9-7). If scalene and/or supraclavicular lymph node biopsies are positive, or if supraclavicular nodes are clinically involved, both supraclavicular areas are treated in addition to the primary and the mediastinum (Fig. 9-6). The given dose (maximum under the skin) delivered to the supraclavicular area is 5,000 rads in 4 to 5 weeks. With proven nodal involvement, the treatment is completed with an additional small field, covering either the palpable mass or the biopsy area plus a 1 to 2 cm margin (field no larger than 5 × 6 cm or 6 × 6 cm). An additional 1,000 rads is delivered to this small field in 3 to 4 days.

Anaplastic Carcinoma. With this histology the aim is to irradiate, in a single volume when possible, the primary, the mediastinum, and the scalene and supraclavicular lymph node bearing areas. The arrangement of the fields is similar to that for well-differentiated carcinomas except that the volume of irradiation should extend more generously beyond the tumor because of probable wider spread of "subclinical" disease.

The supraclavicular areas are treated using an anterior single field extending from the

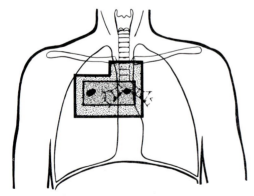

FIG. **9-4**. In these cases the small volume (darker area) is irradiated through two parallel opposing fields, unless it is very close to the mediastinum.

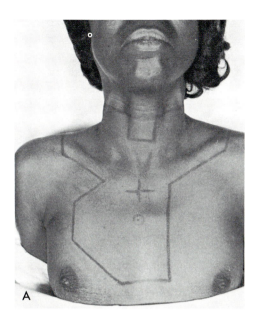

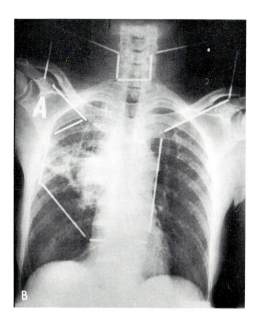

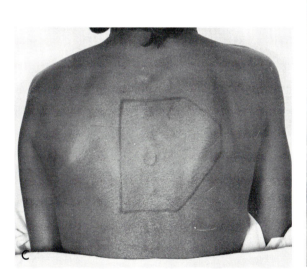

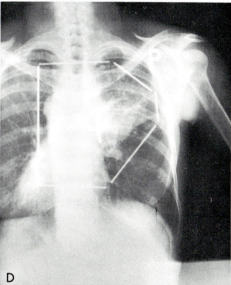

FIG. 9-6. Fifty-two year old Negro woman with a squamous cell carcinoma of the right upper lobe bronchus diagnosed by sputum cytology.

Treatment Plan: The patient received 4,500 rads midplane tumor dose in 4 weeks through portals as illustrated. The anterior portal (*A* and *B*) was treated daily to 5,500 rads given dose in 4 weeks. This is supplemented with a posterior portal encompassing the primary tumor and adjacent mediastinum (*C* and *D*) to bring the midplane tumor dose to 4,500 rads in 4 weeks. The right hilum received an additional 1,500 rads tumor dose in $1\frac{1}{2}$ weeks through a single right posterior oblique portal.

The doses to the tumor at the midplane, the supraclavicular nodes, and the spinal cord at the level of the sternal notch were calculated by the Clarkson method. The supraclavicular fossae received 4,950 rads. Since there was no palpable lymphadenopathy this area received no additional treatment. The maximal spinal cord dose was 4,375 rads.

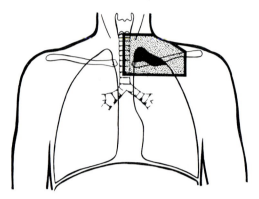

FIG. 9-7. Mallams' technique for apical tumor.

anterior mediastinal field to whatever level of neck is indicated (Fig. 9-6). Four thousand to 4,500 rads tumor dose in 4 weeks is delivered with two parallel opposing fields to the primary and mediastinum. With reduced fields and using rotation whenever possible, an additional 1,500 to 2,000 rads are delivered at the rate of 200 to 250 rads tumor dose daily to cover the detectable residual tumor and adjacent mediastinal area. If no nodes are palpable in the supraclavicular area, the given dose is 5,000 rads delivered in 4 to 5 weeks. If disease is palpable in the supraclavicular area, or the scalene node biopsy is positive, an additional 1,000 rads with a small field is delivered to the node.

Tissue Dose Calculation

The tissue dose is calculated from isodose curves for the two parallel opposing fields. Doses for rotational therapy are calculated using the Johns' central axis procedure. No correction is made for lung transmission because most of the irradiated volume encompasses solid tissue in the mediastinum, tumor, or atelectatic lung. The variation in density between different beam paths, or even within the path of the same beam makes it impossible to use an accurate correction factor. Even though the calculated doses, especially with rotation, are higher than the stated doses, experience shows them

to be well tolerated. Today it is possible to use (for both stationary and rotational fields) dosimetry calculated by computers, which are more accurate and which include tissue inhomogeneity in the dose determination.

Combined Treatment

The techniques described above can be used in treatment for cancer of the lung either by irradiation alone or by preoperative irradiation followed by radical resection.

PREOPERATIVE IRRADIATION

Preoperative irradiation is best undertaken in institutions where there is close cooperation and understanding between thoracic surgeons and radiotherapists, and where specific policies and techniques of treatment have been defined.

The indications for preoperative irradiation in bronchogenic carcinoma are based on the following factors:

1. The high incidence of inoperable and unresectable tumors due to local extension into the mediastinal organs.

2. The high percentage of residual viable tumor at the primary site after radical irradiation (65 per cent in our series).[3,4]

3. The high incidence of lymph node involvement in the hilum and mediastinum, not surgically resectable.

4. The propensity of bronchogenic tumors to invade blood vessels and the possibility of producing metastases during surgical manipulation.

5. The possibility of seeding disease in the operative field.

6. The feasibility of operation after megavoltage irradiation without prohibitive morbidity.[12,14]

7. Lobectomy can replace pneumonectomy in some cases after successful preoperative irradiation.

These features are especially significant for hilar or parahilar tumors. Based on theoretical knowledge as well as on experimental and clinical facts, it seems probable that preoperative irradiation can favorably alter some of the clinical situations described above.

The disadvantages of preoperative irradiation is that the treatment is more difficult, time consuming, and expensive. Several schemes of preoperative irradiation have been developed for the treatment of lung cancer. They can be grouped as listed below.

Low Dose and Short Waiting Period. The dose is generally 500 to 2,000 rads delivered in 1 to 10 treatments completed 1 day to a week before the operation. The aim is to diminish the number of viable cells.

Intermediate Dose and Intermediate Waiting Period. Mallams, Paulson, and Shaw[13] have advocated the use of preoperative irradiation for the treatment of superior sulcus lesions with or without Pancoast's syndrome and without distant metastases.

The treatment technique has been two parallel opposing fields covering the apex of the lung (Fig. 9-7), and delivering 3,000 to 3,500 rads in 10 to 15 treatments. The mediastinum is included in the fields when obvious metastases are present. Four weeks after radiation therapy, en bloc total surgical resection is attempted provided distant metastases or medical contraindications have not developed. Invasion of ribs or vertebrae is not a contraindication to resection.

High Dose with 6 to 8 Weeks Waiting Period. This technique has been developed at the University of Maryland Hospital in a joint study by the Division of Radiotherapy and the Division of Thoracic Surgery.[2,3,4] The maximum dose to the small volume encompassing the detectable tumor is 5,500 rads in $5\frac{1}{2}$ weeks. With this technique resectability was considerably increased. The 5-year survival for initially inoperable patients was increased to 15 per cent in the group that completed treatment. No advantage could be demonstrated for initially operable patients.

The complication rate was high when a) the dose was increased to 6,000 rads in $5\frac{1}{2}$ to 6 weeks, b) the operative procedure was too extensive, with exposure of a large portion of the bronchial tree, or c) the waiting period was longer than 8 weeks.

The main indication for preoperative irradiation is when the tumor is located in the superior sulcus or when the tumor is inoperable. It seems probable that tumors in the hilar region should benefit from this type of therapy but a national cooperative clinical trial with preoperative irradiation failed to show improved results with this treatment.

POSTOPERATIVE IRRADIATION

The rationale for postoperative irradiation is based on the possibility of sterilizing residual tumor or cells seeded during surgery. The main effect of postoperative irradiation perhaps results from irradiation of the areas which surgery has not reached, *i.e.,* direct extension or metastases to the mediastinal, supraclavicular, and scalene lymph nodes.

Postoperative irradiation, if properly indicated, should be considered definitive treatment with a curative aim. Due to the high incidence of lymph node metastases and residual disease after surgery, all bronchogenic carcinomas after resection should be considered for postoperative irradiation with the exception of small, peripheral, well-differentiated tumors or in those patients presenting major postoperative complications.

TECHNIQUES OF TREATMENT

The entire tumor-bearing volume, excluding the area of the primary tumor which was resected, should be treated as described previously (Figs. 9-3, 9-4, 9-5, and 9-6). The larger volume should comprise at least the whole mediastinum and receive 4,500 rads in $4\frac{1}{2}$ weeks. The area of the commonly involved lymph node metastases (small volume) should receive 5,000 to 5,500 rads in 5 to $5\frac{1}{2}$ weeks. If gross residual tumor has been left at operation, it should be included in the small volume receiving 6,000 rads total dose in 5½ to 6 weeks. Parallel opposing fields and rotational therapy should be combined to reduce the dose to the spinal cord.

COMBINED SURGERY AND INTERSTITIAL GAMMA THERAPY

Henschke[7] has developed a technique of interstitial therapy for bronchogenic carcinoma which is performed at thoracotomy. It is indicated for 1) residual tumor after resection, and 2) inoperable tumors localized to the primary and mediastinal areas. Using ^{192}Ir seeds, the dose delivered varied from 15,000 to 25,000 rads to the implanted area.

In some cases, additional external irradiation was added. The complication rate in a series of over 200 cases was negligible. Encouraging results were obtained in these selected patients, especially in those with Pancoast-type lesions (Figs. 9-8 and 9-9).[10] The best results were obtained in patients where higher doses were used and where interstitial therapy was the only therapeutic procedure.

PALLIATIVE TREATMENT

Treatment is palliative when the entire complex of possibly involved tissues is not irradiated or when the dose delivered is less than the dose used for curative therapy. The aim of palliation is to retard the growth of

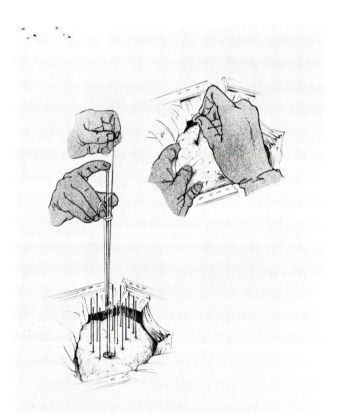

FIG. 9-8. Technique for permanent interstitial implantation of radioactive seeds into unresectable lung cancers. Unloaded hollow needles, each 15 cm long, are first inserted in and around the tumor.
After all needles have been placed, the number of seeds required to deliver the desired dose to the implanted volume is calculated. These seeds are then inserted through the needles by help of a special inserter equipped with a depth gauge. (Courtesy: Henschke, *Amer. J. Roentgen.,* 90, 386, 1963.)

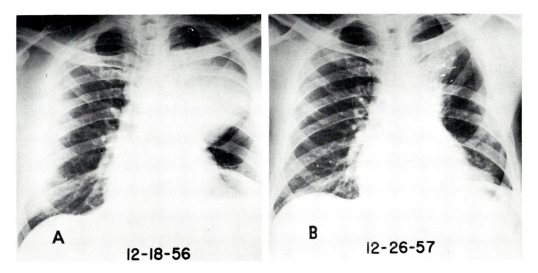

FIG. 9-9. Example of response of an unresectable bronchogenic carcinoma to interstitial implantation.

　A. Biopsy showed epidermoid carcinoma. The tumor was unresectable, due to invasion of the pericardium, mediastinum, and anterior chest wall. Fifty-seven radon seeds of 1.5 mc were inserted through 14 needles during thoracotomy. The calculated Paterson-Parker dose was 7,900 rads. No postoperative x-ray therapy was given (December 1957).

　B. The tumor showed good regression and the patient was free of symptoms and able to work for a full year. Symptoms from brain and liver metastases then appeared, and he died in May 1958, 16 months after implantation. (Courtesy: Henschke, *IXth International Congress of Radiology, Transactions,* Stuttgart, Georg Thieme Verlag, p. 580, 1960.)

disease, to delay the appearance of tumor extension and the symptoms of the invading tumor, or to alleviate existing symptoms.

Indications. The indications for palliative treatment are when the disease is considered beyond control because of the advanced stage, presence of distant metastases, very poor general condition of the patient, or the presence of severe infection. It should also be considered for existing or impending mediastinal syndrome from centrally placed tumors or brachial plexus syndrome in apical tumors even in the presence of metastases.

Techniques. The irradiation field should include the detectable primary disease and the lymph node metastases when clinically evident. It is important to deliver treatment in the shortest possible time compatible with minimal untoward reactions for the patient. If there are distant, supraclavicular, or cervi-

cal node metastases or a positive scalene biopsy, no attempt is made to cover these disease extensions unless it is anticipated that they will become symptomatic. Parallel opposing fields are used to deliver 3,000 rads in 2 weeks or 4,000 rads in 3 weeks.

A split-course of treatment may present advantages for some patients. In the first course 2,000 rads tumor dose in 5 to 7 treatments are given. This dose is repeated after 2 to 3 weeks. If the patient's general condition deteriorates or if distant metastases appear during the waiting period, the second course is omitted.

SYMPTOMATIC TREATMENT

The symptoms to be relieved by irradiation may be produced by either the primary or metastases and are: pain, hemorrhage, superior vena cava syndrome, malignant pleural effusion, and cough. Treatment for symptomatic relief should be given in the shortest possible time compatible with the lowest incidence of adverse reactions. A single field and single treatment should be used when possible, especially for peripheral bony metastases. One thousand to 1,700 rads tumor dose is delivered in one treatment, depending on the site and field size. A maximum of 5- to 10-day treatment, delivering 2,500 to 3,000 rads tumor dose, is used for spinal metastases with a single field or 140-degree posterior arc rotation.

To relieve mediastinal syndrome, it is not necessary, to avoid complications, to start with a low daily irradiation dose. Decompression is most rapidly obtained with a high dose in a short time using the split-dose technique. The same technique is used for the relief of bronchial obstruction. Another indication for palliative treatment of the primary tumor is to stop hemoptysis. The shortest treatment course is indicated (1,000 to 2,000 rads tumor dose in 3 to 5 days) with small fields.

Malignant pleural effusions are usually massive, hemorrhagic, and recurrent. If intrapleural chemotherapy fails to control the effusion, radioactive colloidal gold or chromic phosphate are used intrapleurally. With radioactive colloidal gold, 100 cc to 150 cc are used per treatment. The treatment is repeated 2 or 3 weeks later if partial regression has been obtained, provided the white count is satisfactory.

BIBLIOGRAPHY

1. Ackerman, L. V. and del Regato, J. A.: *Cancer: Diagnosis-Treatment-Prognosis*, 3rd ed., St. Louis, The C. V. Mosby Company, p. 463, 1962.
2. Bloedorn, F. G. and Cowley, R. A.: Irradiation and surgery in treatment of bronchogenic carcinoma, *Surg. Gynec. Obstet.*, 111, 141, 1960.
3. Bloedorn, F. G., Cowley, R. A., Cuccia, C. A. and Mercado, R., Jr.: Combined therapy: Irradiation and surgery in treatment of bronchogenic carcinoma, *Amer. J. Roentgen.*, 85, 875, 1962.
4. Bloedorn, F. G.: In *Progress in Radiation Therapy*, Vol. 2, New York, Grune & Stratton, Inc., p. 114, 1962.
5. Davies, E. S.: Does postoperative irradiation improve survival in lung cancer?, *J.A.M.A.*, 195, 8, 1966.
6. Graham, E. A. and Singer, J. J.: Successful removal of entire lung for carcinoma of bronchus, *J.A.M.A.*, 101, 1371, 1933.
7. Henschke, U. K.: Interstitial implantation in the treatment of primary bronchogenic carcinoma, *Amer. J. Roentgen.*, 79, 981, 1958.
8. Henschke, U. K.: In *IXth International Congress of Radiology, Transactions*, Stuttgart, Georg Thieme Verlag, p. 580, 1960.
9. Henschke, U. K., Hilaris, B. S., and Mahan, G. D.: Afterloading in interstitial and intracavitary radiation therapy, *Amer. J. Roentgen.*, 90, 386, 1963.
10. Hilaris, B. S., Luomanen, R. K., and Beattie, E. J., Jr.: Integrated irradiation and surgery in the treatment of apical lung cancer, *Cancer*, 27, 1369, 1971.
11. Hilton, H.: In *British Practice in Radiotherapy*, London, Butterworths & Company Ltd., p. 258, 1955.
12. Kligerman, M. and Order, S.: Integrated therapy for lung carcinoma, *Cancer Therapy by Integrated Radiation and Operation*, Charles C Thomas, Springfield, Illinois, p. 67, 1968.
13. Paulson, D. L.: The role of preoperative radiation therapy in the surgical management of carcinoma of the superior sulcus, In *Frontiers of Radiation Therapy and Oncology*, University Park Press, Baltimore, p. 177, 1971.
14. Paulson, D. L.: A philosophy of treatment for bronchogenic carcinoma, *Ann. Thorac. Surg.*, 5, 289, 1968.
15. Rissanen, P. M., Tikka, U., Holsti, L. R.: Autopsy findings in lung cancer treated with megavoltage radiotherapy, *Acta Radiologica Therapy*, 7, 433, 1968.
16. Smart, J.: Can lung cancer be cured by irradiation alone?, *J.A.M.A.*, 195, 1966.

Esophagus

FERNANDO G. BLOEDORN

Esophageal cancer constitutes 3 per cent of all carcinomas. The maximum incidence is in males between 60 and 70 years of age. The ratio between males and females varies between 3:1 to 5:1. It frequently occurs with complicating diseases of the cardiovascular system, liver, or other systems. Patients with esophageal carcinoma have an unusually large number of consecutive or concomitant cancers in other locations, often in the head and neck area.

In a significant percentage of cases, esophageal cancer remains localized in the primary site until death occurs. Merendino,[5] in a careful analysis of 100 cases with either postmortem or surgical exploration, showed that about 20 per cent were "potentially curable." The cure rate, however, is disappointingly low.[1] Radical surgery, considered the treatment of choice in most centers, has not yielded better results than modern radiotherapy except for tumors of the infradiaphragmatic portion of the esophagus. In the last 10 years, the results have been slightly improved by more and better use of irradiation alone or combined with surgery.

Histological Classification

The malignant tumors encountered in the esophagus are squamous cell carcinoma, adenocarcinoma, adenoacanthoma, sarcomas (leiomyosarcomas and fibrosarcomas), melanoma, and lymphoma.

Squamous cell carcinoma, which occurs in more than 90 per cent of these cases, is frequently poorly differentiated, spreading locally and metastasizing more widely than when originating in the oral cavity. Adenocarcinomas constitute most of the remaining 10 per cent of malignant tumors, occurring almost exclusively in the supracardiac portion of the esophagus. They should be classified separately from gastric tumors which have invaded the inferior esophagus.

Clinical Features

Site of Origin

The natural history of esophageal carcinoma varies according to the site of origin and the anatomical relations of the organs at different levels of the esophagus. About 20 per cent of the lesions originate in the upper third, about 40 per cent in the middle third, and about 40 per cent in the lower third.

Growth Pattern

The esophagus is a thin-walled organ that is not covered by a serosal lining except for the most distal portion where it is covered by peritoneum. It is in intimate relation to the vital structures of the neck and mediastinum. Grossly, the tumors may be fungating or exophytic, ulcerated, infiltrative, or scirrhous. The principal symptom, dysphagia, results from some degree of obstruction of the gullet either by circular infiltration or by a fungating mass growing into the lumen. Very rarely the tumor grows superficially without much obstruction, producing a shallow ulceration. In most patients, extensive local spread with involvement of vital structures occurs early and is present when the tumor is first diagnosed.

Squamous cell carcinoma of the esophagus spreads both longitudinally and through the esophageal wall. The tumor extends along the mucosal layers, the intermuscular spaces, and the lymphatic vessels of the submucosa. Anaplastic tumors in particular tend to spread extensively along the length of the esophagus. The extent of mucosal involvement can usually be determined by x-ray and esophagoscopic examinations. Submucosal lymphatic extension, which is common, may be in continuity with the tumor but often isolated foci may be found extending cephalad to the main tumor and as much as 20 cm beyond it. These foci may form indurated nodules in the submucosa or may be microscopic. Perineural lymphatic invasion has been observed 8 cm cephalad from the tumor.

Invasion of the various mediastinal structures depends upon tumor location. In the cervical esophagus, tumor spreads to the larynx, thyroid, recurrential nerve, and vascular structures. In the mediastinal portion, tumor spreads to the trachea and bronchi (34 per cent), and to the pleura, pericardium, recurrent and phrenic nerves, and aorta and other vascular structures. The involvement of these structures and ulceration of the tumor are responsible for esophageal perforation into the mediastinal large vessels and/or into hollow organs such as the trachea (Fig. 9-10). Fistulae develop in about 15 per cent of the cases at postmortem examination. In the subdiaphragmatic portion of esophagus, due to the lack of contiguous hollow structures, the tumor less frequently causes fistulae.

Lymph Node Metastases

Lymph node metastases occur in a high percentage of squamous cell carcinomas of the esophagus. In published series of post-

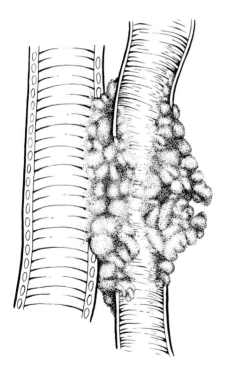

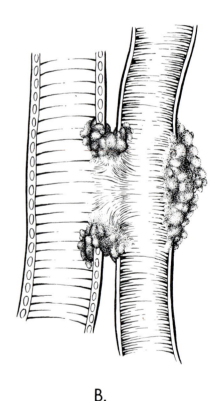

A.

B.

FIG. 9-10. **A.** Illustrates how an advanced tumor destroys the walls of the esophagus, and grows outside of the organ into another hollow viscus whose walls are also destroyed.

    B. Shows the result of the tumor regression by irradiation. Due to the destruction of the continuity of the walls of two neighboring hollow viscera, a wide communication (fistula) between them is produced.

mortem examinations, lymph node metastases are found in approximately 70 per cent. The incidence is highest in anaplastic and extensive tumors. The distribution of positive nodes varies with the site of origin and they are found in the cervical, supraclavicular, mediastinal, and subdiaphragmatic areas. In general, the current of lymph node metastases is from the upper third of the esophagus down to the paratracheal and carinal nodes and from the lower two-thirds toward the abdomen. The right paratracheal nodes are more often involved than those on the left side due to the distribution of the lymphatic vessels.

Left supraclavicular metastases (Virchow's node) are present in less than 10 per cent of tumors of the esophagus. Of 100 patients with squamous cell carcinomas in the lower half of the esophagus with lymph node metastases, 70 had metastases in the abdomen. Tumors in the upper third of the esophagus will produce metastases in the celiac and perigastric lymph nodes in approximately 10 per cent; those in the middle third, 25 per cent; and those in the lower third, about 45 per cent.

Distant Metastases

Three out of 10 patients with squamous cell carcinoma of the esophagus will develop distant metastases at sometime in the evolution of their disease. Widespread metastases may be seen late in the liver, lung, and bones, and less often to other organs.

Merendino[5] in a review of the world literature on postmortem examinations, found that 20 to 48 per cent of patients died with local extension of only the tumor and without lymph node or distant metastases.

Diagnosis of the Tumor and Its Spread (Local, Region and Distant)

Cancer of the esophagus is rarely diagnosed early since dysphagia, usually the first symptom to appear, generally becomes evident only when the tumor has grown beyond the limits of the organ. The principal diagnostic tests are x-ray examination with barium and esophagoscopy. Biopsies of doubtful lesions should be taken and repeated if necessary when symptomatology and barium swallow suggest a tumor.

The following studies will help define the extent of the tumor. Patients with lesions in the middle third of the esophagus should have bronchoscopy and biopsy of the bronchial area or lower trachea and/or carina if there is compression, edema, or suggestion of tumor invasion. Tomograms taken simultaneously with barium swallow will often help to define the tumor mass growing beyond the esophageal wall. The vocal cords should always be examined to detect recurrent nerve paralysis, indicative of direct tumor extension or lymph node metastases and compressing the nerve. Paralysis of one half of the diaphragm is indicative of phrenic nerve involvement. The supraclavicular areas (particularly the left) should be examined carefully for lymph node metastases. Metastases to the liver and epigastric area should be looked for, especially with tumors located in the lower half of the esophagus. A liver scan is indicated in doubtful cases. Because of the high incidence of epigastric (celiac and perigastric) node metastases, some authors recommend laparotomy with exploration of the lymph node bearing areas and biopsy as a necessary diagnostic procedure to determine the actual extension of disease. In tumors of the lower half of the esophagus, laparotomy should be done routinely prior to radical treatment.

Treatment

Localization Technique

With contrast material in the esophagus and markers on the skin or a special bridge (Fig. 12-1), films are taken to determine the treatment fields (Fig. 9-11). On the basis of

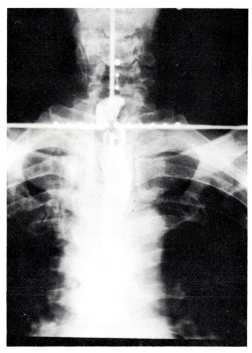

FIG. 9-11. Localization films taken on the bridge in a lesion of the upper third of the esophagus.

the esophagus on the portal films when ^{60}Co is being used, we position a plastic tube in the esophagus. Lead beads (4 mm BB shots) are inserted 1 cm apart for the last 10 cm (Figs. 9-12 and 9-13) in this tube. The tube is passed through the tumor whenever possible; if not, the point at which it is held up shows the tumor level and the position of the esophagus. When the portal fields have been checked and the necessary corrections made, the final treatment fields are marked on the patient.

Preliminary Care before Radiotherapy

At the time of diagnosis, it is probable that most squamous cell carcinomas of the esophagus have been present for over a year. Further limited delay should not greatly increase tumor extent and one should take the time needed to improve the patient's general condition for better treatment tolerance.

these films, fields are drawn tentatively on the patient. Precise measurement of the distance of the esophagus to the table top should be obtained if horizontal rotation is contemplated. As a next step portal films are taken either with the treatment machine or a simulator unit. To visualize the position of

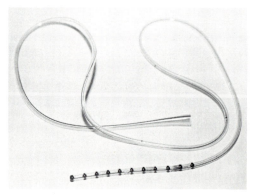

FIG. 9-12. Plastic tubes with lead beads used for the portal films taken with megavoltage radiation.

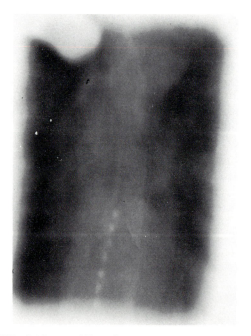

FIG. 9-13. Portal films taken with telecobalt equipment. The lead beads show the position and direction of the esophagus.

Many patients require hospitalization before and during treatment. If the patient can swallow, a diet rich in vitamins, proteins, and calories should be instituted. If the patient can swallow fluids only, a feeding tube should be passed into the stomach. If this is not possible, gastrostomy or bypass procedure (colon transplant) must be considered. At laparotomy, careful examination of the lymph nodes under the diaphragm should be done. With the patient hospitalized, daily observation of vital signs and weight and weekly examinations for possible metastases (liver, epigastrium and supraclavicular area) should be carried out.

Control of the Primary Tumor

With megavoltage irradiation, permanent control of squamous cell carcinoma of the esophagus has been achieved with relatively low doses: 5,000 rads in 6 to 6½ weeks.[2] The best results achieved have been with 5,000 rads in 4 weeks or 5,500 rads in 4½ weeks.[8,9] In our study, 5 of 15 surgical specimens were free of tumor after doses of 6,000 rads in 5 to 6 weeks.

In at least three-fourths of the patients receiving at least 5,000 rads, marked tumor regression can be obtained. With radical doses, approximately 50 per cent of the patients will have local control of disease.[9]

Lymph Node Metastases

There is direct evidence that lymph node metastases from squamous cell carcinoma of the esophagus can be controlled by irradiation:

1) After high dose (5,000 to 6,000 rads) preoperative irradiation, the incidence of nodal metastases in the treated area has been extremely low in our own and other published studies.[3]

2) Histologically proven metastases to the supraclavicular, mediastinal, and abdominal lymph nodes have been controlled by irradiation in our series and others.

Clinical studies have shown that subclinical lymph node metastases can be controlled by considerably smaller doses of irradiation (5,000 rads or less) than gross metastatic nodes. This means that subclinical metastases in the neck, mediastinum, or even in the epigastrium can be controlled with doses of irradiation which are within tolerance of the normal tissues of the area.

Other Types of Tumors

Adenocarcinomas of the lower third of the esophagus can be treated successfully by irradiation, the main limitation in radical treatment being the lower tolerance to irradiation of the abdominal contents. The response to irradiation of other types of tumors, such as sarcomas originating in the muscle or in the connective tissues, is not well known. We have treated a huge leiomyosarcoma of the upper esophagus to a dose of 5,700 rads in 5½ weeks with a remarkably good response.[10]

Radical Irradiation

Megavoltage external beam techniques should be used for irradiation of carcinomas of the esophagus. Other techniques such as intracavitary radium or interstitial therapy should be considered only in special situations, such as "boost" treatment for residual disease after external beam therapy.

SELECTION OF PATIENTS

Certain categories of patients should not be considered for radical irradiation:

1) Patients who are of extreme age, very ill, or cachetic due to advanced disease.

2) Patients in apparently fair general condition who have evidence of lesions which are too advanced locally, *i.e.*, tracheo- or bronchoesophageal fistulae, or biopsy proven tracheobronchial invasion.

3) Patients with retrosternal pain, low grade fever, and rapid pulse rate.

4) Patients with repeated or persistent hemorrhage from an advanced lesion.

5) Patients with distant metastases.

The two groups of patients presenting with signs of advanced disease comprise about 10 per cent of all patients with esophageal cancer. Additionally, radical therapy for some patients is of doubtful value; if the tumor is longer than 10 cm, if a deeply penetrating ulcer is demonstrated by x-ray examination, if there is boring pain radiating toward the back, and if there are left supraclavicular metastases. However, in order to achieve palliation most of these patients must receive radical therapy.

VOLUME

Cervical esophagus. The field size should be between 8 to 12 cm × 8 to 10 cm to cover the lesion with ample margins and the lymph nodes of both carotid and jugular chains. Both supraclavicular areas should be included.

Upper third of thoracic esophagus. The field size should be 15 cm × 8 to 10 cm to include the lesion with a generous superior margin. In all cases, the supraclavicular and lower neck areas and the subcarinal lymph nodes (at least 6 cm below the carina) must be included.

Midthoracic esophagus. Almost the entire esophagus should be included using fields 15 to 20 cm × 9 to 10 cm. The field will include the most commonly involved lymph node bearing areas of the mediastinum.

Lower one third of the esophagus. The field size should be 15 cm × 10 to 12 cm to include the lesion with ample lateral margins and the celiac and perigastric lymph node areas.

The field should *always be reduced to the size of the originally detectable disease with a small margin* (8 to 10 cm × 6 to 8 cm) after completion of the first part of treatment.

TOTAL TIME AND DOSE

Two treatment plans can be used.

1) For large lesions or for lesions of the lower esophagus where part of the abdomen is included in the volume of irradiation, we use a total tumor dose of 6,000 to 6,500 rads in 6 to 6½ weeks. Four thousand five hundred rads in 4½ weeks are given to the larger volume, to be followed by 1,500 to 2,000 rads tumor dose in 1 to 2 weeks after the field has been reduced in size. In some exceptional cases, where the abdominal esophagus is not involved, after further reduction of the field 500 to 700 rads can be added to bring the total tumor dose to the smaller volume to 7,000 to 7,200 rads.

2) For earlier lesions we give a total tumor dose of 5,000 to 5,500 rads in 4 to 4½ weeks with reduction of field size at 4,000 rads. Larger doses greatly increase the incidence of severe complications without improving the control rate.[1,8,9] The best results in treatment for cancer of the esophagus have been published by Pearson[8,9] who used this dosage in a large series of patients in Southeastern Scotland.

TREATMENT GEOMETRY

Cervical and thoracic inlet esophagus. We use two parallel opposing fields plus an additional single field to the supraclavicular areas for upper cervical lesions, and 140-degree arc rotation or two wedge filters for lower cervical and thoracic inlet lesions.

Upper and middle third of thoracic esophagus. Using two parallel opposing fields throughout the whole treatment is not advisable, because a large volume of normal tissues, including the spinal cord, will be exposed to a high radiation dose.

Rotation technique is ideal for small lesions. In large lesions, two parallel opposing fields are indicated for the first portion of the irradiation followed by 360-degree rotation with smaller fields.

Lower third of the esophagus. The oblique direction of the esophagus at this point in both lateral and anteroposterior directions makes the use of rotation with a narrow field inadvisable. The combination of two parallel opposing fields for the first portion of the treatment and cross-firing or rotation for the final portion is a satisfactory technique.

We strongly believe that horizontal rotation presents the double advantage of: a) having a more comfortable patient who can maintain treatment position without effort and b) having the table top as a reference for daily treatment.

Intracavitary and Interstitial Gamma Therapy

A linear source of radium carried in a specially made bougie can be used to give additional irradiation at the completion of external beam therapy when residual tumor is present or suspected. Delivering an additional 1,000 to 1,500 rads to the surface of the applicator could increase local control without compromising normal tissue tolerance in the mediastinum. This technique is hazardous because of the possibility of perforation and should be used with caution and only in carefully selected cases. Dickson[4] has used the technique for retreatment with some success.

The insertion of radioactive seeds (radon, gold, iridium) can be used to give additional treatment for residual tumor after external irradiation for lesions of the abdominal esophagus. About 2,000 rads can be added with a proper implant *limited to the residual tumor and residual metastatic nodes in the area.*

Care During and Immediately After Treatment

In our service, a barium study is done after 4,000 rads in order to assess tumor regression, the development of complications, and to determine the completion of treatment. When a patient is responding well to treatment, swallowing should improve after the second or third week. If there is a sudden worsening in swallowing, it is generally due to blockage by ingested material at the point of tumor narrowing. If barium swallow confirms this diagnosis, suction under esophagoscopy should be done.

Reactions and Complications During Treatment

Most patients who are receiving radical treatment, after the first period of improvement, will again have increased dysphagia after 3,000 to 4,000 rads due to esophagitis; this is sometimes accompanied by retrosternal pain which is never severe unless some complication is present. Persistent boring pain, high pulse rate, fever and persistent hemorrhage all suggest perforation. If x-ray examination with a barium swallow confirms the threat of perforation, treatment should be discontinued.

Results

Improvement in swallowing is obtained in at least 80 per cent of patients who have been properly selected for therapy. About 50 per cent of the patients will have almost normal swallowing toward the end of the treatment and some will continue to improve up to 6 to 8 weeks thereafter.

Complications After Treatment

Persistent dysphagia with retrosternal pain rarely occurs after treatment. These may occur if the patient was too old or in poor general condition, if the tumor was very extensive, or if the dose of irradiation was too high. Perforation, hemorrhage, and late stenosis of the gullet in the area of the lesion are, in most cases, due to tumor destruction by irradiation. Perforation occurs during or immediately after treatment. The symptoms of obstruction generally start 4 to 6 months after therapy and progress for at least one year, sometimes requiring periodic dilatation. The effect of excessive irradiation is manifested by necrotic ulceration, generally painful, with concomitant stenosis. This should not be mistaken for recurrent or persistent tumor; biopsy will provide the real diagnosis. Extensive lung fibrosis is not seen when proper megavoltage techniques are used. Radiation myelitis also can be avoided with proper techniques and dosimetry.

Postoperative Irradiation

Postoperative irradiation is indicated when there is disease left after radical surgery. The residual disease can be peripheral extension of the primary tumor or metastases in the lymph nodes or may be subclinical disease. It is doubtful if postoperative irradiation is ever indicated for abdominal spread of disease. Treatment should include either the whole mediastinum or the neck and upper mediastinum, depending upon the location of the tumor and the type of operation performed. The technique most commonly used is two parallel opposing fields. Smaller fields or rotation may be used toward the end of treatment to give a total dose of 5,000 rads in 5 weeks for subclinical disease and 6,000 rads in 5½ to 6 weeks when known gross disease remains after the operation.

Preoperative Irradiation

Even with well-executed irradiation the disease may not be controlled locally and/or vertical spreading of disease may be missed. Postirradiation resection of an extensive segment of the esophagus, or, if possible, total esophagectomy, could be curative in both eventualities. Severe complications may be eliminated by surgical resection of the treated segment of the esophagus; patients may die as a result of esophageal narrowing or other local complications without having active tumor.

Preoperative irradiation should be used only in selected patients in good general condition and who

are relatively young, otherwise, the operative mortality could counteract the advantages of the procedures.

Preoperative irradiation can make operable originally inoperable tumors,[1,3] simplify the surgical procedure because of regression of the total tumor; reduce the possibility of tumor seeding through surgical manipulation and control lymph node metastases. Several preliminary studies[1,3] have demonstrated the feasibility of combined therapy for carcinoma of the esophagus without increasing the surgical morbidity.

INDICATIONS

We use preoperative irradiation in all extensive tumors (operable or not) and in all tumors of the upper two thirds of the thoracic esophagus.

TECHNIQUES

Several techniques are presently in use.

1) Nakayama[6] uses 2,000 rads delivered in 3 days (48-hour interval between first and last treatment) with rather small fields (10 to 12 × 6 to 7 cm) and a waiting period between 4 and 7 days.

2) Parker[7] uses 4,500 rads in 3 weeks with a waiting period of 2 months. No field size is stated.

3) Cliffton[3] uses doses in the range of 5,500 to 6,000 rads in 5 to 6 weeks with a waiting period between 6 to 8 weeks. Large fields, 15 to 20 cm × 8 to 10 cm, are used for at least two thirds of the treatment. We use a similar technique.

It is important, no matter which technique is used, to make sure that the suture line in the esophagus lies outside the irradiated area.

Palliative Irradiation

The main indications for palliation of the primary tumor are to improve swallowing and to prolong the useful life of the patient. Palliative irradiation is not indicated with extremely advanced disease even if limited to the mediastinum, in patients with mediastinal abscesses, huge ulcerations, constant hemorrhage, or with tracheobronchial fistula (present or imminent).

In advanced cases, with the presence of symptomatic distant metastases, when the complicating factors mentioned above are lacking, palliative treatment directed to the esophageal lesion itself is justified. In cases where only the local obstruction is to be relieved, short treatment with the simplest technique available is indicated: rotation with a field that will cover the detectable disease with a small margin, delivering 4,000 rads in 3 weeks or 2,500 to 3,000 rads in 2 weeks. Two parallel opposing fields can also be used. Split-course therapy may be used (2,000 rads in 5 treatments, 2 to 4 weeks waiting period, and then repeat the same treatment).

BIBLIOGRAPHY

1. Bloedorn, F. G. and Kasdorf, H.: Radiotherapy in squamous cell carcinoma of the esophagus, to be published in the *Proceeding of the Tenth Interamerican Congress of Radiology.*

2. Buschke, F.: Surgical and radiological results in the treatment of esophageal cancer, *Amer. J. Roentgen.,* 71, 9, 1954.

3. Cliffton, E. E., Goodner, J. T., and Bronstein, E.: Preoperative irradiation for cancer of the esophagus, *Cancer,* 13, 37, 1960.

4. Dickson, R. J.: Radiation therapy in carcinoma of the esophagus, A review, *Amer. J. Med. Sci.,* 241, 662, 1961.

5. Merendino, K. A. and Mark, V. H.: An analysis of one hundred cases of squamous cell carcinoma of the esophagus. II. With special reference to its theoretical curability, *Surg. Gynec. Obstet.,* 94, 110, 1952.

6. Nakayama, K.: Preoperative irradiation for cancer—Its theory and practice with reference to esophageal cancer, *Surg. Ther.,* 18, 327, 1968.

7. Parker, E. F. and Gregorie, H. B., Jr: Combined radiation and surgical treatment of carcinoma of the esophagus, *Ann. Surg.,* 161, 710, 1965.

8. Pearson, J. G.: The radiotherapy of carcinoma of the esophagus and post cricoid region in southeast Scotland, *Clin. Rad.,* 17, 242, 1966.

9. Pearson, J. G.: The value of radiotherapy in the management of esophageal cancer, *Amer. J. Roentgen.,* 105, 500, 1969.

10. Wolfel, D. A.: Leiomyosarcoma of the esophagus, *Amer. J. Roentgen,* 89, 127, 1963.

10. Gastrointestinal Tract

Pancreas

LOWELL S. MILLER

Observing that carcinoma of the pancreas is seldom cured by any form of treatment, Miller and Fuller[1] reported in 1958 an average survival of 6.1 months for 118 unirradiated patients, 6.6 months for 91 irradiated patients, with subjective improvement in 29 per cent of the latter ("excellent palliative results" in 10 per cent). Smith et al.[3] noted subjective or objective improvement following irradiation in 20 of a series of 33 inoperable patients. In both studies, doses of the order of 5,000 to 6,000 rads in 4 to 6 weeks are advocated. Henschke[2] has implanted ^{222}Rn, ^{192}Ir, or ^{198}Au in pancreatic cancers in 15 patients in the past 10 years. Two of 9 patients have survived 5 years; 1 patient has survived 10 years.

From 1944 through 1963, only 11 patients with pancreatic cancer were treated with external irradiation at The University of Texas M. D. Anderson Hospital and Tumor Institute, most of them with 22 Mev x-rays through 15 × 15 cm anterior and posterior fields. Aside from one islet cell carcinoma, the tumors were adenocarcinomas, and most were located in the head of the pancreas. The majority received tumor doses of 3,850 to 5,050 rads, usually at a rate approximating 1,000 rads per week.

Survivals have ranged from 1.8 months to 42.5 months, median 4.8 months. There was benefit from irradiation in only 5 cases: reduction in size of mass in 3, decrease in pain in 2 more, duration of benefit varying from 2 weeks to 11 months. The only complications encountered were mild but chronic diarrhea and indigestion in 1 patient—the longest survivor—necessitating treatment with Pancreatin.

The available information indicates that, for nonresectable carcinoma of the pancreas, permanent afterloading implantation with radioactive gold grains should be tried, aiming for a dose of 7,000 to 10,000 rads. Except perhaps to supplement a low-dose implant, external irradiation has little to recommend it, but in doses approximating 6,000 rads in 6 weeks offers the patient for whom interstitial irradiation is not feasible the possibility of short-term palliation.

BIBLIOGRAPHY

1. Miller, T. R., and Fuller, L. M.: Radiation therapy of carcinoma of the pancreas, *Amer. J. Roentgen.*, 80, 787, 1958.
2. Henschke, U. K.: Personal communication, 1965.
3. Smith, I. H., Fetterly, J. C. M., Lott, J. S., MacDonald, J. C. F., Myer, L. M., Pfalzner, P. M., and Thomson, D. H.: In *Cobalt 60 Teletherapy*, New York, Paul B. Hoeber, Inc., p. 269, 1964.

Rectum and Rectosigmoid

LOWELL S. MILLER

Cancer of the rectum and rectosigmoid is almost always adenocarcinoma, and abdominoperineal resection is an effective treatment. When, for any reason, surgical removal of the primary tumor is impossible, 1 Mev x-irradiation in tumor doses of the order of 6,000 r in 6 weeks has been shown by Williams and Horwitz[6] to be of some value, provided the patient is in reasonably good condition and there is no evidence of distant metastases.

That pelvic irradiation before or after resection may be a useful adjuvant is suggested by experience of others[2,3] and by isolated cases of our own, but further investigation is needed.

Bacon and Berkley[1] estimate that over 40 per cent of recurrent carcinomas of the rectum and colon can be resected again, and that one third of these will be alive 5 years later. Williams, Schuleman, and Todd,[7] however, contend that recurrent lesions are "rarely, if ever, amenable to excision," and hence advocate 1 Mev x-irradiation to a tumor dose of 6,000 roentgens in 6 weeks. They have treated 82 patients, with benefit in 87 per cent, 4 patients surviving over 3 years, 2 for over 5 years. Almost identical results have been obtained by Wang and Schulz[5] with 2 Mev x-irradiation to somewhat lower doses ("optimum" 3,500 to 5,000 roentgens in 4 to 5 weeks). Murdock and Kramer[4] have reported results of ^{60}Co irradiation, largely through direct perineal fields to doses of 4,500 to 5,500 roentgens in 4 to $5\frac{1}{2}$ weeks, for perineal recurrences. There was worthwhile palliation in 9 of 10 patients receiving full treatment.

Most radiotherapists agree that high doses are mandatory in even palliative treatment for rectal cancer. Although an occasional lesion is small enough to justify the use of interstitial techniques, the usual tumor, whether an inoperable primary lesion or a pelvic recurrence, is large and requires external irradiation. Approximately the posterior two-thirds of the pelvic cavity must ordinarily be raised to a high dose, and for this megavoltage equipment is essential.

The inoperable primary tumor, in most instances, will already have had its margins defined at laparotomy. (In this regard, personal observation of operative findings is apt to be more informative than the surgeon's description, even when augmented by roentgenograms showing silver clips around the margins of the tumor.) If the tumor is large or obstructing, a preliminary colostomy (placing the stoma well above the intended treatment fields) will lessen the patient's discomfort during the radiation proctitis to follow. A lead-tipped Lucite probe usually can be placed in the rectal lumen to mark the position of the lower end of the tumor in field verification films made with the treatment beam. Localization of other margins of the lesion will sometimes necessitate additional (kilovoltage) radiography, viz., a cross-table lateral film with the patient prone, a small amount of barium in the rectum, and a metal ruler (notched or perforated at 1 cm intervals) marking the position of the skin of the sacral midline and providing at the same time a scale for demagnification of skin-tumor and/or other sagittal distances. If a 22 Mev betatron is available, a four-field box technique similar to that used in treatment for carcinoma of the cervix is suitable, with the single difference that the lateral fields are sufficiently posterior to include the sacral concavity (Fig. 10-1) and are therefore more conveniently irradiated with the patient prone rather than supine. If the only available beam is either ^{60}Co or 2 Mev, rotational techniques are probably to be preferred, basing the choice of field size and placement

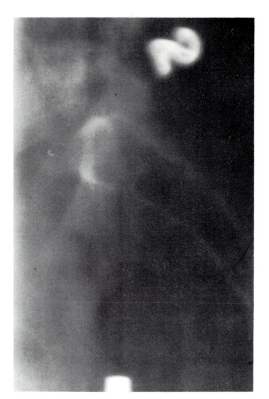

of the axis of rotation upon localization procedures similar to those just mentioned. Minimum tumor dose for radical treatment should approximate 7,000 rads in 7 weeks, reducing field size if appropriate after the initial 5,000 rads of this figure.

In the absence of distant metastases, postoperative patients with pelvic or perineal recurrence should have the benefit of surgical re-exploration to determine extent of disease, with resection if feasible, clip-marking (for subsequent radiotherapy) if not. If a colostomy has not already been created, it should be considered as a preliminary to radiation

FIG. 10-1. Verification film for lateral treatment field showing lead-tipped Lucite probe placed in rectum to mark lower pole of presacral recurrence. Approximately 23 months earlier the patient had undergone anterior resection for adenocarcinoma of the upper rectum. The recurrent mass was discovered on rectal examination and laparotomy gave no evidence of other disease. Rather than risk peritoneal dissemination by biopsy from above, a silver clip was placed on the upper pole of the tumor, the incision was closed, the patient was turned over, and the tumor biopsied through the bed of the resected coccyx.

The film shows only part of the sacral concavity and only a scant margin at the lower pole of the mass. The field was accordingly moved 1 cm farther posteriorly and shifted 1 cm toward the feet.

A four-field 22 Mev x-ray technique was used to deliver a tumor dose of 7,175 rads in 50 days. Rectovaginal fistula required colostomy $2\frac{1}{2}$ years later, but otherwise patient has remained well and active for more than 14 years.

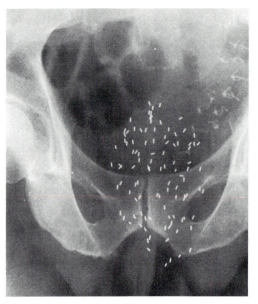

FIG. 10-2. Radioactive gold grains implanted 10-14, 1964 into a 4.5 cm perineal mass of recurrent adenocarcinoma 13 months after abdominoperineal resection for cancer of the rectum. Following laparotomy for access, the patient was placed in dorsal lithotomy position, one hand was inserted into the pelvic cavity from above in order to control the depth of insertion of after-loading transperineal guide needles with the other. Calculated dose was 11,630 rads. Prompt and complete relief of pain; however, patient died in November 1965 with generalized disease.

therapy. Thorough irradiation along the lines just described for inoperable primary tumors will effectively palliate most patients with localized pelvic recurrence, and in a few instances will be curative. Recurrent tumor in the perineum usually is bulky, requiring palliative ^{60}Co or equivalent irradiation through a direct perineal field 10 to 12 cm in diameter (patient in either dorsal lithotomy or knee-chest position) to a given dose of approximately 6,000 rads in 4 weeks. An occasional perineal mass proves less extensive, however, in which case interstitial irradiation (Fig. 10-2) may be considered.

BIBLIOGRAPHY

1. Bacon, H. E., Berkley, J. L.: The rationale of re-resection for recurrent cancer of the colon and rectum, *Dis. Colon Rectum,* 2, 549, 1959.

2. Henschke, U. K.: Radiation therapy of cancer of the colon and rectum, *Dis. Colon Rectum,* 2, 84, 1959.
3. Leaming, R. H., Stearns, M. W., Deddish, M. R.: Preoperative irradiation in rectal carcinoma, *Radiology,* 77, 257, 1961.
4. Murdock, M. G., Kramer, S.: Cobalt 60 therapy in the management of perineal recurrence from carcinoma of rectum and colon, *Amer. J. Roentgen.,* 91, 149, 1964.
5. Wang, C. C., Schulz, M. D.: The role of radiation therapy in the management of carcinoma of the sigmoid, rectosigmoid, and rectum, *Radiology,* 79, 1, 1962.
6. Williams, I. G., and Horwitz, H.: The primary treatment of adenocarcinoma of the rectum by high voltage roentgen rays, *Amer. J. Roentgen.,* 76, 919, 1956.
7. Williams, I. G., Schuleman, I. M., Todd, I. P.: The treatment of recurrent carcinoma of the rectum by supervoltage x-ray therapy, *Brit. J. Surg.,* 44, 506, 1956.

Anal Carcinoma

LOWELL S. MILLER

The most instructive account of radiotherapy for squamous cell carcinomas of the anus is from the Christie Hospital and Holt Radium Institute.[1] Of a total of 171 cases, 106 were treated by irradiation. Interstitial irradiation was considered the method of choice for limited lesions because of the notorious intolerance of perineal tissues for high doses of external irradiation. Of 85 patients followed 5 years or longer, 29 per cent survived 5 years as a result of unassisted irradiation,[2] 43.5 per cent when 12 patients salvaged by subsequent surgery are added. Local necroses occurred in 23 per cent of the histologically proved treated cases. Similar results were reported in 1948 from the Curie Foundation.[4]

Experience with radiotherapy for this disease at the University of Texas M. D. Anderson Hospital and Tumor Institute has been sparse, but most of the successes have been with limited tumors low enough to permit the use of radium needles. The more extensive lesions have usually required external irradiation, either alone or in combination with radium needling; one of the two 5-year survivors in this group was treated with external kilovoltage irradiation alone, the other with a combination of 22 Mev x-irradiation and radium needling.

Interstitial technique ordinarily consists of a single- or double-plane radium needling (rarely volume). Indian club needles are useful for top-crossing, but their active length usually does not exceed 4.5 cm. An afterloading ^{192}Ir technique is useful for implanting higher or more extensive lesions (Fig. 1-35). One of the most common faults in double-plane needlings is cranial divergence of the planes, with consequent higher dose rate at the more vulnerable caudal end of the implant (Fig. 10-3). Convergence at the lower end at times can be prevented by a roll of gauze or an Ivalon sponge cutout sutured into the anal cleft between the two planes of needles. As recommended by Dalby and Pointon,[1] the dose for single-plane implants probably should be limited to 6,000 rγ in 7 days, for two-plane implants to not more than 5,500 rγ in the same period of time.

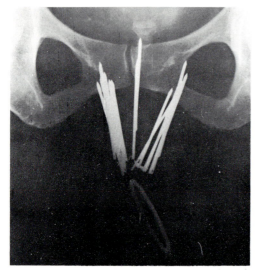

FIG. 10-3. On 11-29, 1952, this 49-year-old white female had partial excision of a papillary 3 × 3 × 2 cm Grade III squamous carcinoma invading the muscularis of the left wall of the anal canal. On 12-29-52, a double-plane radium needling was done. Needles were left in place for 117 hours, providing a dose at the narrowly separated lower ends of the planes of approximately 6,400 rads. During the latter part of the ensuing year, shallow ulceration of the left lateral anal mucosa was noted for several months, but was replaced in 1954 by moderate anal stricture. In 1958, superficial necrosis of anal skin appeared and persisted. In 1966 an abdominoperineal resection was done with no evidence of local recurrence. Patient was last seen in March 1972. Colostomy was functioning well and there was no evidence of disease.

Even with these doses, local necroses are not uncommon and may require major care.

Although with careful nursing, it is possible to get by without preliminary colostomy, we believe that interstitial irradiation should be preceded in every case by diversion of the fecal stream, regardless of tumor size or degree of obstruction, for local reactions are brisk and infection can be fatal.[4]

Techniques for external irradiation are, in general, the same as for adenocarcinoma of the rectum and rectosigmoid—with perhaps greater emphasis on perineal fields because of the relatively lower position of the lesion—and call for minimum tumor doses of the order of 7,000 rads in 7 weeks when used alone, correspondingly less when combined with interstitial irradiation or with surgery.

In the present limited state of our knowledge, it seems reasonable to suggest that low anal cancers, if small and superficial, and if preliminary laparotomy yields no evidence of regional node metastasis, be managed with a temporary colostomy and interstitial irradiation. For higher lesions, for low tumors of moderate extent, and for those found at laparotomy to be associated with regional node metastases, surgical treatment (abdominoperineal resection with dissection of iliac and obturator nodes[3]) is probably more reliable, though experience with isolated cases suggests the combination of surgery with preoperative external irradiation deserves consideration. For irresectable carcinomas, external irradiation either alone or supplemented by interstitial techniques, is the treatment of choice and will occasionally be curative. However, any attempt to control inguinal node metastases should be surgical.

BIBLIOGRAPHY

1. Dalby, J. E., and Pointon, R. S.: The treatment of anal carcinoma by interstitial irradiation, *Amer. J. Roentgen.*, 85, 515, 1961.
2. Dalby, J. E.: Personal communication, 1963.
3. Martin, R. G.: Personal communication, 1965.
4. Roux-Berger, J. L., and Ennuyer, A.: Carcinoma of the anal canal, *Amer. J. Roentgen.*, 60, 807, 1948.

Carcinoma of the Rectum and Colon

CHARLES VOTAVA

Introduction

Adenocarcinoma of the rectum and colon represents the most common internal malignant lesion in population of the United States. Despite stress on early detection, advances in the methods of diagnosis, and surgical techniques, the relative incidence of various stages as well as mortality rates have remained essentially unchanged during the past 30 years. In most series, 50 to 60 per cent of patients have regional node involvement (Dukes' C lesions) at the time of operation.

Until recently relatively little attention has been given to the role of radiotherapy as an adjuvant to improve the results of surgical management. The exact sites of failure are not well described in the literature. This knowledge is important to determine the place of any adjuvant therapy.

Anatomic Considerations

Since the majority of colorectal tumors occur in the rectum and sigmoid colon, a brief anatomic description will be limited to this area.

The rectum is the terminal portion of the large intestine, caudal to the midsacral region. It follows the concavity of the sacrum and coccyx and ends by passing through the levator muscles to become the anal canal which terminates at the anal orifice. The upper one-half to two-thirds of the rectum usually has some peritoneal covering of variable extent. The lower portion of the rectum has no peritoneal covering. The rectum is in direct contact anteriorly with the seminal vesicles, bladder, prostate, ureter, vagina, and uterus. Posteriorly it is in contiguity with the superior hemorrhoidal vessels, sacral nerve plexus, sacrum, and coccyx. There is also contact with coils of ileum in the peritonealized portion. Below the peritoneal reflection the rectum is surrounded by space filled with fibrofatty tissue. The tumor's penetration is perhaps more easily accomplished in this region than in the area covered by a relative barrier of serosa. Patients with rectal cancer are anatomically at risk for recurrence in the many organs, bones, and surrounding fibrofatty tissue which may be involved by direct extension.

The sigmoid colon is not fixed but has a tendency for localization in the left half of the pelvis. It has a complete peritoneal covering and joins the rectum in front of the lower portion of the sacrum. It has an anatomic relationship to loops of small bowel, bladder, uterus, and adnexa.

The blood supply to the upper rectum and left colon is from the branches of the inferior mesenteric artery. The lower rectum receives blood from the branches of the internal iliac (hypogastric) artery. Venous drainage of the rectum is primarily through the superior hemorrhoidal vein and the left colon through the inferior mesenteric veins, both draining to the portal system. The hemorrhoidal plexus has an anastomotic communication with middle and inferior hemorrhoidal veins which drain into the hypogastric vein and the systemic circulation.

The lymphatic drainage of the upper rectum, sigmoid and left colon follow the inferior mesenteric artery to its origin at approximately the midportion of the third lumbar vertebra and then to the paraaortic chain. The mid- and low rectum drain primarily by the internal and occasionally external iliac nodes to the common iliac and then to the paraaortic nodes.

Clinical Pathologic Considerations

Histologically, about 95 per cent of the tumors encountered are adenocarcinomas. The staging system most commonly used has been the Dukes' classification[6] which is a pathologic staging (Table 10-1). There are several modifications of the original staging plan and one must be certain of the definitions when comparing data. The potential for spread is by direct extension, either intramural or to contiguous structures, and via the lymphatic and vascular system. Numerous pathologic studies have correlated the extent of local disease, grade of tumor, the incidence of regional node involvement and blood vessel invasion with ultimate prognosis. It should be pointed out that the data collected with regard to pathologic prognostic factors are based on examination of operative specimens and is applicable, therefore, to only surgically treated patients.

All these factors correlate well with each other to reflect the biologic aggressiveness of a given tumor (Tables 10-2, 10-3 and 10-4). The magnitude of any one observation also reflects prognosis since invasion into the muscle but not through the muscle carries a better prognosis than penetration through the muscle or invasion of adjacent organs. Lymph node involvement is significant since an increased number of involved nodes is associated with decreased survival rates. Metastases to the lymph node chains progress in an orderly systematic basis and rarely do skip areas occur.[8] Blood vessel invasion would appear to be an ominous prognostic sign. However, the data in Table 10-4, similar to that reported by Dukes,[6] show the blood

Table 10-1. *Dukes' Classification*

Class	Description
A	Growth limited to rectum; no extra rectal spread; no lymphatic metastasis
B	Spread by direct continuity into extra rectal tissues; no lymphatic metastasis
C	Lymphatic metastasis present
	MODIFIED DUKES' CLASSIFICATION*
A	Lesion limited to the mucosa
B_1	Lesion extending into but not through the muscular coat without positive nodes
B_2	Lesion extending through the muscular coat without positive nodes
C_1	Lesion limited to the wall with positive nodes
C_2	Lesion extending through all layers with positive nodes

* Astler and Coller, *Ann. Surg.*, 139, 846, 1954.

Table 10-2. *Bowel Wall Involvement With and Without Nodal Metastasis*

Bowel Wall	Nodal Metastasis	No. Patients	Status at 5 years					
			Alive NED*	Dead with Cancer	Alive No Details	Alive with Cancer	Dead No Details	Dead NED
Involvement of mucosa	—	66	71%	6%	0	3%	0	20%
	+	3	67%	0	0	0	0	33%
Involvement into but not through muscle	—	150	61%	18%	1%	3%	0	16%
	+	58	48%	47%	0	5%	0	0
Involvement through muscle	—	379	39%	40%	1%	3%	1%	16%
	+	329	13%	80%	0	2%	2%	3%

* No evidence of disease.
(Adapted from: Copeland, Miller, and Jones, *Amer. J. Surg.*, 116, 875, 1968.)

Table 10-3. *Correlation of Nodal Involvement*

No. Nodes Involved	No. Patients	Status at 5 years			
		Alive NED	Alive With Cancer	Dead NED	Dead With Cancer
None	584	48.5%	3.0%	17.6%	31.9%
1	112	16.8%	3.5%	6.2%	63.5%
2	68	25.0%	2.9%	5.9%	66.2%
3	40	15.0%	2.5%	2.5%	80.0%
4	24	29.1%	4.2%	4.2%	62.5%
5 or more	110	9.1%	0.9%	4.5%	85.5%

Adapted from: Copeland, Miller, and Jones, *Amer. J. Surg.*, 116, 875, 1968.

vessel invasion alone does not indicate a poor prognosis but the combination of lymph node involvement and blood vessel invasion causes a very poor prognosis.

Surgical Considerations

Approximately 10 to 15 per cent of the lesions are within the reach of the examining finger and 65 to 70 per cent are within reach of the sigmoidoscope. Since a number of surgeons use the distance from the anal verge as a factor in determining the type of surgical procedure to be done, it is of interest to see the distribution of these lesions within this 25 cm range (Table 10-5). Considerable stress has been placed on the choice of operation with respect to the distal margin of normal tissue to be removed with the tumor. Various clinical and pathologic studies indicate that distal spread by lymphatics does not occur except when there is gross lymphatic disease with blockage and in those cases prognosis and survival is poor regardless of the margin.[12]

Abdominoperineal resection (Miles' operation) is a major procedure associated with long postoperative convalescence as compared to anterior resection. Healing time for the former is about 2 to 3 months while only 1 month for the latter procedure. A number of surgical reports show no significant difference in local recurrence rates between the two procedures.[3] It would seem that the majority of lesions in the rectum and sigmoid area could be candidates for anterior resection rather than the classical abdominoperineal approach if less than a 5 cm margin were required. More limited margins have not been associated with an increase in recurrence or decrease in survival.[16] Gilbertsen[10] has questioned the indication for the

Table 10-4. *Cancer of Colon and Rectum (1956–1961 Inclusive)*

Involvement		Total Series		Five-year survival
Lymph Node	Blood Vessel	No.	%	
−	−	280	45.9	67.1%
−	+	88	14.4	60.2%
+	−	128	20.9	36.0%
+	+	114	18.7	13.1%

Adapted from: Swinton, Nahra, Khazei, and Scherer, *Dis. Col. Rec.*, 11, 413, 1968.

Table 10-5. *Distance of Lesion to the Anal Verge*

Distance from Anal Verge	Percent of Total Colorectal Cancers
Within 8 cm	13%
8–15 cm	43%
15–20 cm	10%
20–25 cm	5%
Total	71%

(Adapted from: American Cancer Society: Proctosigmoidoscopy for the detection of asymptomatic cancer. 1962.)

Miles' operation on the basis of local extent of disease in the rectum, saying "If the lesion is confined to the wall, the operation is unnecessarily extensive and if it has spread beyond the intestinal wall, it is in fact inadequate." Clinical determination of recurrence is difficult after abdominoperineal resection, especially in the male, since digital examination is impossible. The clinical presentation of recurrence generally is shifted from the anastomotic site (which is often extra-anastomotic as well) following anterior resection to the perineal area after abdominoperineal resection. Perineal or sacral pain, either alone or associated with walking or sitting, should alert one to suspect pelvic recurrence following either procedure.

Site and Magnitude of Recurrence

The incidence of local recurrences seems to be greater than generally presumed. Morson and Bussey[17] report 16 per cent local recurrence with Dukes' C lesions of the rectum. The majority of the recurrences were after abdominoperineal resection.

Taylor[20] analyzing autopsy material of 125 patients dying after palliative and curative resection for cancer of the colon and rectum, demonstrated that 79 and 72 per cent of patients respectively had "local continuance or recurrence" as a principal cause of death by cancer.

Gilbertsen analyzed 125 patients who died

following curative resection for carcinoma of the rectum (operative deaths excluded) and found evidence of recurrence in 93 of 125 patients or 74 per cent.[10] Half of these recurrences were known to be local, in the pelvic area within a few centimeters of the boundaries of the scope of the operative procedure (Fig. 10-4). In an earlier publication, he presented data on a series of 89 patients who had an abdominoperineal operation for rectal carcinoma.[9] Thirty-two of these patients had a local component of recurrence with the distribution shown in Table 10-6.

Cohn[4] states that most series report 1 to 12 per cent recurrence at the suture line with colonic cancers. In a select group of patients subjected to re-exploration or autopsy, recurrence was found in 36 per cent of the patients at the anastomosis.

A most revealing study is that of the so-called second look operation. The University of Minnesota group under the direction of Dr. Wangensteen began using this procedure in 1948 with the idea of attempting surgical salvage of recurrent disease. Asymptomatic patients having had previous visceral cancer with spread to lymph nodes at the time of the primary extirpation performed for cure were subjected to a planned reoperation of the abdomen. These operations were carried out at 6- to 8-month intervals as long as residual cancer was found or until the tumor had obviously spread beyond surgical control. Twenty of 44 asymptomatic patients with Stage C carcinoma of the rectum[11] having had curative resection had recurrent disease at the first reoperation. Thirty-six of 98 patients with cancer of the colon had recurrent cancer at the second look. Although specific sites of active disease were not tabulated it had been noted, as in earlier reports, that these were mainly in the vicinity of the original cancer. In comparatively favorable cases, the most frequent sites of residual disease were in lymph node chains beyond the reach of the original dissection, *i.e.* para-aortic lymph nodes in left-sided lesions and paravenacaval nodes in right colonic lesions.

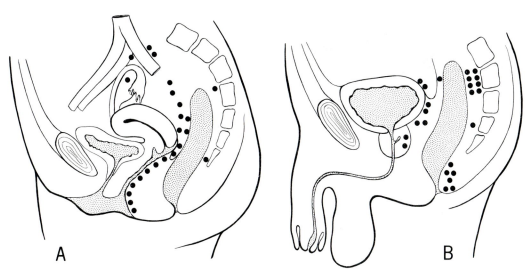

FIG. 10-4. The location of local recurrences in (A) female and (B) male patients having had previous resection for carcinoma of the rectum. (Adapted from: Gilbertsen, V. A., *Surg. Gyn. & Obstet.* 124, 1253, 1967.)

In rectal carcinoma almost all recurrences in the failure group were pelvic and abdominal with a poor salvage rate by re-excision.

The above data would indicate that recurrence within the operative site and the regional nodes accounts for a considerable number of patients having uncontrolled disease.

Table 10-6. *Local Recurrence Following Abdominoperineal Excision-Adenocarcinoma of Rectum*

Location	Number	
	Men	Women
Vaginal wall, cul-de-sac	0	7
Urinary bladder	3	1
Periureteral area	3	0
Prostate gland	1	0
Posterior pelvic, presacral-coccygeal, sacral plexus, sciatic area	13	1
Aortic bifurcation, iliac artery area	1	1
Obturator area	1	1
Perineum	5	0
Left pelvic area	1	0

(Courtesy: Gilbertsen, *Ann. of Surg.*, 151, 340, 1960.)

Radiation Therapy

A good over-all view of the role of radiation therapy in carcinoma of the rectum has been presented by Horwitz.[14] Primary radiotherapy for locally advanced rectal cancer, treatment for recurrent tumor in the pelvis following surgical resection and treatment for distant metastases are essentially palliative with a low rate of cure. An important role of radiation could be its use combined with the surgical procedure in order to reduce the incidence of local recurrences and increase survival rates in those patients with pathologic findings carrying a poorer prognosis (Dukes' *B* and *C* lesions). When residual disease remains or there has been transection of the neoplasm at the time of operation, improvement of local control rate should be expected.[13] For tumors of the rectum and sigmoid, radiation portals can adequately cover the primary sites including the known lymphatic metastatic pathways and relatively high doses can be delivered.

Preoperative Irradiation

The often-quoted and well-publicized data of Stearns[18] concerning a retrospective study of patients with carcinoma of the rectum having received preoperative low dose radiation showed in patients with Dukes' C lesions a 5-year survival rate of 37 per cent versus 23 per cent in those patients having had no irradiation. The 10-year survivals were 23 and 10 per cent respectively.

As a result of this report, a large-scale cooperative VA study was done utilizing 2,000 rads tumor dose to the midplane of the pelvis in 2 weeks followed by surgical resection. Although initially there seemed to be little difference in results between the two groups, a recent analysis[7] suggests improvement in those patients having received irradiation.

Since May 1960, Allen and Fletcher[1] have given 5,000 rads preoperatively to patients with rectosigmoid carcinoma, either with resectable or unresectable lesions. The portals were 10 × 10 cm and did not include the regional node bearing areas. The preoperative dose of 5,000 rads to this region was well tolerated and caused no significant difficulty with subsequent surgical procedures. Fifty-two patients had the preoperative irradiation and surgical resection. Eight of 16 originally unresectable lesions were converted to a resectable situation. No gross tumor was found in 10 of 52 cases completing the combined therapy; 5 had no carcinoma histologically and 5 had only carcinoma *in situ*.

Kligerman[15] conducted a randomized preoperative radiation study in patients with rectal cancer delivering 4,500 rads in $4\frac{1}{2}$ weeks to the pelvis with a narrow extension superiorly to the level of the body of the fourth lumbar vertebra. The field is now extended superiorly to the body of the second lumbar vertebra so that the lymph nodes which accompany the inferior mesenteric vessels are included. More Dukes' A lesions than would be anticipated were found in the pathologic specimen supporting the value of preoperative irradiation. Of significance is the fact that 6 of 16 patients in the control group and 1 of 13 in the irradiation group had metastatic lesions to the liver found at

the time of surgery. This points out one of the difficulties in using preoperative irradiation in this disease as well as other abdominal and pelvic malignancies as one is unable to demonstrate regional and occasionally metastatic disease prior to exploration.

Postoperative Irradiation

Substantial clinical evidence has accumulated to show that postoperative irradiation is effective. The advantage of postoperative treatment in this region may overbalance the theoretical advantages of preoperative therapy. The early lesions (Dukes' A) can be adequately treated with surgical resection alone, and delivering irradiation to large volumes in patients with liver metastases is less than desirable.

Principles and Technique of Postoperative Irradiation

The patients who are candidates for postoperative irradiation are those who have had a curative resection but in whom there are high risk factors such as penetration of the bowel wall, involvement of regional lymph nodes, blood vessel and lymphatic invasion and those having known residual disease left at surgery but no distant metastases.

Radiotherapy is started 1 to 3 months following surgery depending upon the surgical procedure and the degree of healing obtained. The earlier time is preferable and is usually possible in those patients having had an anterior resection. Before starting irradiation, a base-line barium enema is advisable in those patients not having had the rectum removed in order to observe the contour of the rectum and the position of the anastomosis. Silver clips should be placed at surgery to outline the margins of resection, as well as any area of known or suspected residual. A plain film of the abdomen will then indicate whether adjustment to the basic portal arrangement is necessary and to define the residual volume requiring additional dosage.

The radiation portals cover the pelvis and lymphatic drainage to the top of the third lumbar vertebra, incorporating the operative site (Fig. 10-5). The width of the pelvic portion of the field should extend 1 to 2 cm beyond the bony margin at its widest point. The inferior border is placed at the bottom of the obturator foramina. The portals average a 15 to 16 cm width at the level of the pelvis and a 22 to 24 cm length. A metallic seed is placed in the perineum in patients having had abdominoperineal resection. A perineal portal is used to supplement dosage to this area if opposed portals cannot be extended to deliver adequate dosage (Fig. 10-6). The perineum is more difficult to cover in the male since the lower margin may include too great an extent of the base of the penis and scrotum, producing moderate acute reactions and undesirable chronic sequelae. Occasionally slight caudal angulation of the anterior portal may adequately cover the perineum and avoid this problem. Various sized templates cut from clear x-ray film are used to trace out the portals on the patient's skin and alterations are made after localization films are obtained.

Through parallel opposed anteroposterior portals, treating each field daily 5 days per week, 5,000 rads tumor dose is delivered to

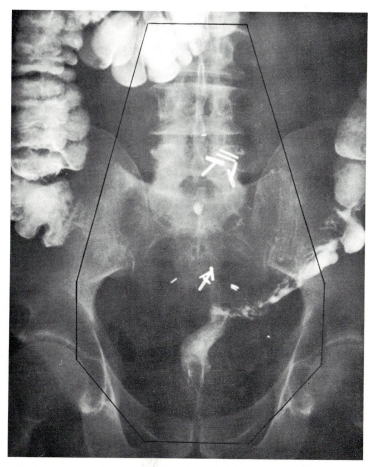

FIG. 10-5. This patient had an anterior resection for a Dukes' C lesion of the sigmoid. Metallic vascular clips placed at the edges of the unresected mesentery were then opposed by closure bringing them to near the midline. In 5 weeks, 5,000 rads were delivered to the midplane.

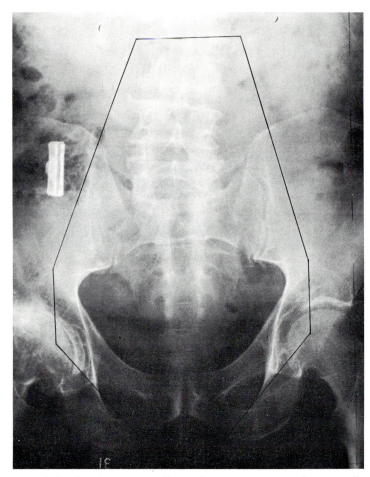

FIG. 10-6. Metallic seed placed in the perineum. Opposed anteroposterior portals can usually adequately cover the region. If this is not possible, a perineal portal is used. With 300 Kv an adequate surface dose is delivered through an 8 to 10 cm round perineal cone which compresses the tissues producing a more uniform surface.

the midplane in $5\frac{1}{2}$ to 6 weeks. A weekly dose rate of 850 to 900 rads is better tolerated and is generally preferred for these large portals. Patients with known residual at surgery but without distant metastases receive 6,000 to 6,500 rads using reduced field, which incorporates only the region of known residual, after 5,000 rads.

The dosage levels in the range recommended here have been used following surgery for gynecologic neoplasms with no significant long term problems. Experience is still being accumulated with respect to delayed effects in those treated following colorectal surgery, especially following abdominal perineal resection, since frequently a larger volume of small bowel is located within the irradiation portals.

BIBLIOGRAPHY

1. Allen, C. V. and Fletcher, W. S.: Observations on preoperative irradiation of rectosigmoid carcinoma, *Amer. J. Roentgen.,* 108, 136, 1970.
2. Astler, V. B. and Coller, F. A.: The prognostic significance of direct extension of carcinoma of the colon and rectum, *Ann. Surg.,* 139, 846, 1954.

3. Butcher, H. R.: Carcinoma of the rectum: Choice between anterior resection and abdominal perineal resection of the rectum, *Cancer,* 28, 104, 1971.

4. Cohn, I., Jr.: Cause and prevention of recurrence following surgery for colon cancer, *Cancer,* 28, 183, 1971.

5. Copeland, E. M., Miller, L. D., and Jones, R. S.: Prognostic factors in carcinoma of the colon and rectum, *Amer. J. Surg.,* 116, 875, 1968.

6. Dukes, C. E.: The pathology of rectal cancer, In *Cancer of the Rectum,* C. Dukes, Editor, Edinburgh, G. & S. Livingston Ltd., 1960.

7. Dwight, R. W., Higgins, G. A., Roswit, B., LeVeen, H. H. and Keehn, R. J.: Preoperative radiation and surgery for cancer of the sigmoid colon and rectum, *Amer. J. Surg.,* 123, 93, 1972.

8. Gabriel, W. B., Dukes, C., and Bussey, H. J. R.: Lymphatic spread in cancer of the rectum, *Brit. J. Surg.,* 23, 395, 1935.

9. Gilbertsen, V. A.: Adenocarcinoma of the rectum: Incidence of locations of recurrent tumor following present-day operations performed for cure, *Ann. Surg.,* 151, 340, 1960.

10. Gilbertsen, V. A.: Improving the prognosis for patients with intestinal cancer, *Surg. Gynec. & Obstet.,* 124, 1253, 1967.

11. Griffen, W. O., Jr., Humphreys, L., and Sosin, H.: The prognosis and management of recurrent abdominal malignancies. In *Current Problems in Surgery,* Chicago, Year Book Medical Publishers, Inc., 1969.

12. Grinnel, R. S.: Lymphatic block with atypical and retrograde lymphatic metastases and spread in carcinoma of the colon and rectum, *Ann. Surg.,* 163, 272, 1966.

13. Guttmann, R.: Significance of postoperative irradiation in carcinoma of the cervix: A ten year survey, *Amer. J. Roentgen.,* 108, 102, 1970.

14. Horwitz, H.: Radiotherapy in carcinoma of the rectum and anal canal, In *Disease of the Colon and Anorectum,* R. C. Turrell, Editor, Philadelphia, W. B. Saunders Company, 1969.

15. Kligerman, M. M., Urdaneta, N., Knowlton, A., Vidone, R., Hartman, P. V., and Vera, R.: Preoperative irradiation of rectosigmoid carcinoma including regional lymph nodes, *Amer. J. Roentgen.,* 114, 498, 1972.

16. Loffgren, E. P., Waugh, J. M. and Dockerty, M. B.: Local recurrence of carcinoma after anterior resection of the rectum and the sigmoid, *A.M.A. Arch. of Surg.,* 74, 825, 1957.

17. Morson, B. C., and Bussey, H. J. R.: Surgical pathology of rectal cancer in relation to adjuvant radiotherapy, *Brit. J. Radiol.,* 40, 161, 1967.

18. Stearns, M. W., Jr., Deddish, M. R., and Quan, S. H. Q.: Preoperative roentgen therapy for cancer of the rectum, *Surg. Gynec. & Obstet.,* 109, 225, 1959.

19. Swinton, N. W., Nahra, K. S., Khazei, A. M. and Scherer, W. P.: The evolution of colorectal cancer, *Dis. Col. Rec.,* 11, 413, 1968.

20. Taylor, F. W.: Cancer of the colon and rectum: A study of routes of metastases and death, *Surgery,* 52, 305, 1962.

11. Female Pelvis

Squamous Cell Carcinomas of the Uterine Cervix

Spread

The squamous cell carcinomas of the uterine cervix are generally fairly anaplastic and could be classified as Grade III.

The main routes of extension are:

1) Into the vaginal mucosa, for a considerable distance beyond palpable or visible disease.

2) Into the myometrium of the lower uterine segment. This type of extension is more likely to occur in carcinomas originating in the endocervix.

3) Into the network of paracervical lymphatics surrounding the ureters lateral to the internal *os* and the lower uterine segment. These lymphatics are often involved even in small lesions.[19] The next spread is to the regional lymphatics through the lymphatics of the broad ligaments. The incidence and location of involved lymph nodes, and their relationship to the bony structures are now well established[18,36] (Fig. 11-1). The obturator node (principal node) lies on the wall of the true pelvis, superimposed on the obturator nerve as it courses along the pelvic wall. The hypogastric nodes cluster around the hypogastric artery from the bifurcation of the common iliac as it enters inferomedially into the pelvis. The other regional nodes are located outside the true pelvis along the external iliac and common iliac arteries.

4) Directly into the parametria.

5) Uncommonly to the uterosacral ligaments.

Clinical Varieties

The three main clinical varieties—exophytic, infiltrative, and ulcerative—exhibit varying anatomical shapes, depending on the origin either on the portio vaginalis or in the endocervix.

Some lesions produce a concentric enlargement of the cervix and may reach huge dimensions, extending from one pelvic wall to the other. They either protrude downward into the vagina, or when they originate in the endocervix, they are palpated on rectopelvic examination as a "barrel-shaped" mass at the level of the isthmus.

Large tumor masses are, in patients with Stages I and II disease, a definite cause of central failure associated with a high incidence of metastasis.[7]

Correlation of Staging with Bulk of Disease

The following substaging is related to bulk of disease:

Stage I_B: Invasive squamous cell carcinoma up to 1 cm in diameter.

Stage I_C: Lesion larger than 1 cm in diameter or two or more positive quadrant biopsies.

Stage II_A (early): Involvement of vagina or medial parametria.

Stage II_B (late): Lesion occupying more than half of the pelvis.

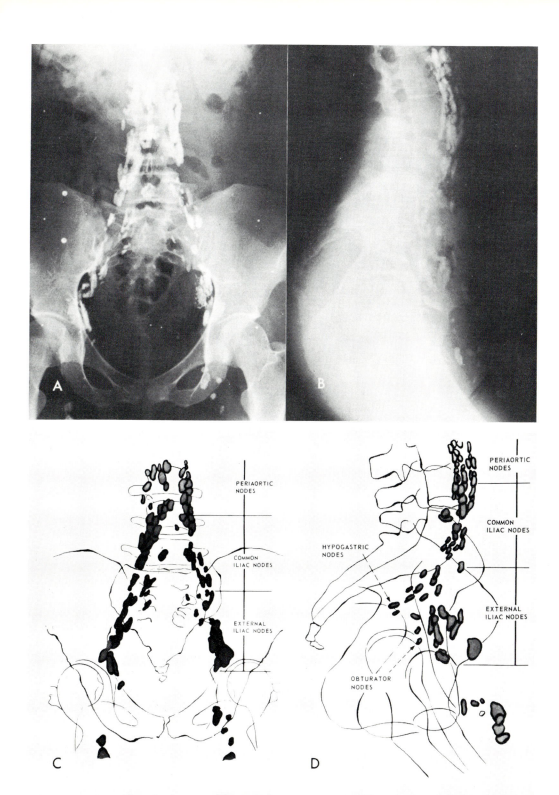

FIG. 11-1. Anteroposterior (A) and cross-table lateral (B) orthogonal radiographs of a patient with a normal lower extremity lymphangiogram. The adjacent line drawings (C and D) illustrate the regional lymphatics of the pelvis and lower lumbar area and the terminology that is used in this chapter. With the exception of the obturator nodes located inside of the acetabula, some of the hypogastric and uterosacral nodes, the nodes are not on the pelvic walls. (Courtesy: Durrance and Fletcher, *Radiology, 91,* 140, 1968.)

Stage III$_A$: Involvement of one pelvic wall or lower third of the vagina.

Stage III$_B$: Both pelvic walls or one pelvic wall and lower third of the vagina.[16]

Stage IV$_A$: Biopsy-proven rectal or bladder involvement.

Stage IV$_B$: Distant metastases.

This substaging is a yardstick in planning treatment to gauge the radicalism of therapy required against the extent of the disease and its potential spread to the regional lymphatics and the paraaortic nodes.

So-Called Radioresistance and Dose Response Curve

Biological radioresistance must not be confused with inadequate irradiation. Because of the steep fall-off of dose with intracavitary radiation therapy, underdosage can easily occur. Sherman[28] studied the distribution of radiation around radium sources and found that the main causes of failure were: 1) a gap between the intrauterine radium and vaginal radium, and 2) downward displacement of the radium.

An accurate correlation of tumor dose with control of cancers of the uterine cervix is not possible because the usual method of treatment has been intracavitary radium therapy which delivers extremely high doses to the cervix and vaginal mucosa, with a steep gradient toward the pelvic walls. Therefore, an average tumor dose is not delivered throughout the involved area. Only small series of patients have been treated by external irradiation alone and information therefore is fragmentary. In patients with Stages I, II, and III$_A$ disease who could not be given local therapy, 5,000 rads in 5 weeks produced no control, 6,000 rads in 6 weeks produce a significant percentage of control and 7,000 rads in 7 weeks excellent local control.[2]

Slow Regression

Retrospective analysis of cancers in human beings have shown that tumors regressing rapidly are just as likely to recur as those which have regressed slowly.[33] In several patients with Stage III disease treated with only 6,000 or 7,000 rads of external irradiation, permanent control was obtained although the clinical impression at the end of treatment was that there was residual disease.[2]

Therefore, the clinical evaluation at the end of treatment of "no evidence of disease" versus "probable residual disease" because of palpable induration should not lead to the decision to perform a hysterectomy.

Traditionally, the viability of tumor cells in the operative specimen has been based on their normal morphological appearance. When a hysterectomy has been performed a few weeks after irradiation, one cannot conclude that the added surgical procedure salvaged the patients even if morphologically normal looking tumor cells are found in the specimen.[32] The value of adding a hysterectomy after irradiation can only be evaluated by a randomized clinical trial.

Spread to the Endometrium

Endometrial curettings in the presence of a primary growth on the cervix contain at times squamous cell carcinoma. A few of these patients had a hysterectomy after irradiation but too few of the uteri findings were positive for disease to justify this surgical practice. Negative findings in the surgical specimen suggest that either the endometrial sample was contaminated as the curette was withdrawn through the cervical canal, or if the fundus contained metastatic cancer, that the amount was small and destroyed by irradiation so that the hysterectomy was unnecessary.

Intracavitary Radium Therapy

History of Intracavitary Radium Therapy

Innumerable techniques have been devised utilizing intracavitary or interstitial radium therapy, transvaginal therapy, external irradiation, or combinations thereof. The design of the applicators, the number and fractionation of the applications, and the dose rate (hourly intensity) have been the main sources of variations in intracavitary radium therapy techniques.

The Stockholm technique (Radiumhemmet) and the Paris technique (Curie Foundation) have evolved as the most successful radium techniques. Many institutions throughout the world use them, either in their original form or with modifications. They represent two distinctly different techniques, both in the physical properties of the applicators and in the duration and intensity of irradiation. The Radiumhemmet technique utilizes short applications of high intensity radium irradiation repeated two or three times in three weeks. The original Stockholm technique has been considerably modified since 1948 by greater individualization, radicalization of radium therapy, and by more elaborate external irradiation.[20,22,37]

The Paris technique delivers low intensity radium irradiation over one week. The Manchester technique is an evolution of the Paris technique.

Excessive Hemorrhaging and Initiation of Tumor Regression

TRANSVAGINAL THERAPY

Transvaginal irradiation is largely used before the start of external radiotherapy for large lesions to produce hemostasis and accelerate shrinkage produced by subsequent whole pelvis irradiation. A dose of 1,000 or 1,500 rads given in two or three daily treatments of 500 rads each usually controls even severe bleeding. There is a fast fall-off of the depth doses even with 300 Kv unit so that almost all of the energy is absorbed in the large central tumor mass. Therefore, the dosage from the initial transvaginal therapy is usually disregarded in planning the subsequent external beam and intracavitary radium therapy.

INTRACAVITARY RADIUM

If a kilovoltage unit is not available and a patient is bleeding from an expanding endocervical lesion, the 24-hour application of a tandem loaded essentially at the level of the isthmus and endocervix to give 1,000 to 1,500 mg-hr in 24 hours will stop bleeding. This amount of radium therapy is not counted in the total treatment plan.

Treatment Planning

External irradiation and intracavitary radium therapy are used in various combinations. When the patient is first seen, gynecologist and radiotherapist together must form a plan of treatment. Initial evaluation of the patient's general condition must be made in order to correct associated diseases, nutritional deficiencies, anemia, etc.[17] Each phase of the treatment must be reviewed and changes made as needed.

Intracavitary radium therapy, with its rapid fall-off is ideally suited for the treatment of early lesions. A minimum radium system of a three-source tandem and two small colpostats adequately irradiates the mucosa of the upper third of the vagina and the lymphatics in the paracervical areas and is equivalent to a hysterectomy with a wide vaginal cuff and dissection of the paracervical tissues (Schauta-type hysterectomy). External irradiation with midline shielding is added for irradiation of parametrial spread and regional lymph node metastases (Fig. 11-2A). Whole pelvis irradiation, producing a uniform dose distribution throughout the pelvis, becomes a major part of the therapy in the advanced stages of disease (Fig. 11-2B).

Because of a T-shaped or linear arrangement of radioactive sources there is a precipitous fall-off of dose from the surface of the radium applicators to the periphery of the pelvis and, therefore, there is no "dose" at "a point" or "a surface" which is representative of the volume distribution in the pelvis. The rules of combination of intracavitary radium and external irradiation can

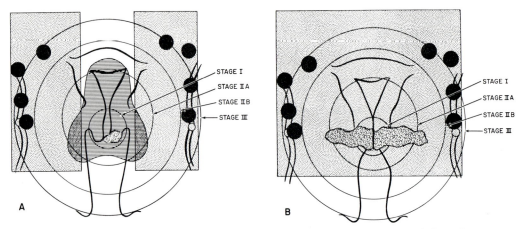

FIG. 11-2. A. Pear-shaped volume distribution resulting from T-shaped arrangement of the radium sources superimposed on the pelvic anatomy to demonstrate that in Stages I and II$_A$ the entirety of the palpable and visible disease is encompassed by a zone of adequate irradiation from the radium (Schauta-type hysterectomy). Parametrial and regional node irradiation supplements the dose to more lateral disease.

B. En bloc irradiation of the whole pelvis is indicated in Stages II$_B$, III, and IV because the wide spread of disease throughout the pelvis and regional lymphatics is largely outside the reach of radium therapy.

only be obtained through trial and error and cannot be reduced to a statement of dose at a point or surface. Furthermore, as various types of vaginal applicators have substantially different volume distributions and are used with different dose rates and fractionation schedules, a set of rules cannot be extrapolated from one system to another.

Tables 11-1 and 11-2 summarize the basic treatment techniques used at M. D. Anderson Hospital.

Initial intracavitary radium is only effective, even in Stages I and II cases, in "nonbulky lesions," with a good local anatomy. It is most important to shrink by external irradiation the bulky ($\geq$ 3 cm) asymmetrical or endocervical cancers to make the subsequent radium applications effective. Radium insertions must be spaced at least two weeks apart or even further apart when more shrinkage is needed. Whole pelvis irradiation is used to make up for diminished effectiveness of the radium therapy when the vault is narrow.

When only external irradiation is used in a patient with early disease because of inadequate anatomy for an effective radium

application, the portal need not necessarily be 15 × 15 cm. *AP* and *PA* portals 10 × 10 cm which cover adequately a small uterus, vagina, and paracervical area, are used to allow delivery of 7,000 rads with good tolerance and low risk of complications.

External irradiation may be omitted in patients with early invasive squamous cell carcinoma ($\leq$ 1 cm) if the radium system is good because the insignificant incidence of regional node metastases ($\leq$ 5 per cent) does not warrant the routine radical treatment.

Patient Care During Intracavitary Radium Therapy

The night before therapy a vaginal douche is given with Betidine 1:1,000 and an *S.S.* enema is ordered. General anesthesia is used unless only colpostats are placed. Packing is used with gauze soaked in 1:2,000 Zephiran solution or in Furacin-impregnated roller gauze.

Films are reviewed with dummy inserters and then the radium placed in the patient's room.

The patient remains in the recumbent po-

Table 11-1. *Policies of Treatment for Squamous Cell Carcinoma of the Cervix on Intact Uterus*†

Stage		
I_B	≤ 1 cm diameter	Radium only[1] maximum 10,000 mg-hrs
I_C	≥ 1 cm diameter or 2 or more positive quadrant biopsies	9,000 to 10,000 mg-hrs radium; parametrial irradiation—3,000 to 4,000 rads[2]
II_A	Medial parametrial involvement and/or spread to upper two-thirds of vagina	Treatment same as Stage I
	Exceptions: (I_C and II_A)	
	Bulky exophytic lesions, or unfavorable anatomy for radium system (narrow vault—short uterine canal, asymmetrical fornices)	2,000 rads whole pelvis irradiation 1st; 8,000–9,000 mg-hrs radium;[3] then 1,000–2,000 rads[2] additional to parametria (4 cm central shielding)
		or
		4,000 rads whole pelvis irradiation; 5,500–6,500 mg-hrs radium[3]
II_B	Lateral parametrial involvement (with or without upper vaginal extension); or massive involvement of corpus (barrel shape)[4]	4,000 rads whole pelvis irradiation; 5,000–6,500 mg-hrs radium[3]
III_A	One pelvic wall or lower one third of vagina	
	Favorable: One wall involved—not massively—and primary not too massive	4,000 rads whole pelvis irradiation; 5,500–6,500 mg-hrs radium,[3] 1,000–1,500 rads[2] added on side involved (15 × 6 cm portal)
	Unfavorable: More disease than above—still confined to this stage	5,000 rads whole pelvis irradiation; 4,000–5,000 mg-hrs radium[3] possibly added 1,000 rads (15 × 6 cm portal) on side involved
III_B	Both pelvic walls *or* one wall plus lower one third of vagina	6,000 rads[5] whole pelvis irradiation; 3,000–4,000 mg-hrs radium[3]
		7,000 rads whole pelvis irradiation
IV		7,000 rads[5] whole pelvis irradiation

Special Clinical Situations	
Pregnancy	
Up to 6 months gestation (all stages)	4,000 rads whole pelvis, then individualize
Postcesarean section and up to 1 year postpartum	Stages I and II, 4,000 rads whole pelvis followed by 5,500–6,500 mg-hrs
PID* or recent surgery	No more than 5,000 rads whole pelvis
Perforation or conization	Always whole pelvis first; usually 2,000 rads
No room for radium or TV cone†	5,000 rads whole pelvis (15 × 15 cm fields to 10 × 10 cm depending on amount of disease). The last 2,000 rads are given surely with fields reduced to 10 × 10 cm.

[1] Provided there is optimal geometry, otherwise external irradiation with or without shielding of the midline is used to build up the dose to the paracervical areas. The portals may be smaller than 15 × 15 cm. The low incidence of nodal metastases (<5%) in these early lesions does not warrant routine parametrial irradiation.

[2] The dose for parametrial irradiation depends upon: 1) extent of disease 2) amount and distribution of the radium sources, 3) location of the radium system within the pelvis.

[3] The larger figures for radium dose are used for lesions which are more infiltrative, endocervical, or have not clinically disappeared at the time of the second radium insertion.

[4] When a hysterectomy is performed after radiation therapy either for adenocarcinomas or large endocervical squamous cell carcinomas, a maximum of 5,000 mg-hrs radium is used.

[5] After 5,000 rads whole pelvis, the pelvic fields should be reduced to 12 × 12 cm parallel opposing portals and to 10 × 10 cm above 6,000 rads.

* *PID*-Pelvic inflammatory disease.

† With 3–6 Mev beams 850 rads are given weekly, *AP* and *PA* fields treated every day. The total dose is increased by 500 rads. For extended fields, even with 20–25 Mev, the weekly dose is 850 rads, the total dose being increased by 10 per cent.

(Courtesy: Fletcher and Rutledge, In *Modern Radiotherapy*, T. J. Deeley, Ed., London, England, Butterworths, 1971.)

Table 11-2. *Squamous Cell Carcinoma of the Cervix on Intact Uterus Maxima for Combining Whole Pelvis Irradiation and Intracavitary Radium Therapy*

Stage	Whole Pelvis	Maximum Hours[1]	Maximum Mg-hr[1,2]	Parametrial
I ≤ 1 cm		72—2 wks—72	10,000	
I ≥ 1 cm		72—2 wks—72	10,000	3,000–4,000 rads
and	2,000	48—2 wks—72[3]	9,000	1,000–2,000 rads
II$_A$	4,000	48—2 wks—48	6,500	
II$_B$*	4,000	48—2 wks—48	6,500	
	4,000	48—2 wks—48	6,500	1,000–1,500 rads on side involved
III$_A$	5,000	72[4] or 48— 2 wks—24-48[3]	5,000	Possibly 1,000 rads on side involved
III$_B$	6,000	72[4]	4,000	
and				
IV	7,000			

[1] Use whichever maximum occurs first, either the time or the mg-hrs.
[2] May be exceeded for unusual tumor size, then use 3 insertions, each 2 weeks apart.
[3] May use the longer time first if the vault size may not permit 2 colpostats for the second application.
[4] If the status of central disease indicates it, the time may be increased beyond 72 hours or above 5,000 mg-hrs. Then split into 48 hrs—2 weeks—24 to 48 hours.
Note: A tandem with a protruding source and a 3 cm diameter vaginal cylinder should have a 20 mg source in the cylinder with one and a half sources protruding. The loading is 15-10-20; 15-10-10-20, etc.
* Whole pelvis irradiation may be carried to 5,000 rads if regression is slow.
(Courtesy: Fletcher and Rutledge, In *Modern Radiotherapy*, T. J. Deeley, Ed., London, England, Butterworths, 1971.)

sition and absolute bed rest is required only when vaginal cylinders are in place since it is difficult to maintain a cylinder in position. With low vaginal cylinders, the patient lays on the back with legs straight. Otherwise, the patient may have a 15-degree head elevation and may move her legs freely. She may turn the upper part of her trunk to eat.

Antibiotics are given only if there is a pyometra or adnexal infection. All patients get Azogantrisin because of the irritation of the Foley catheter.

If the patient's temperature rises to 102 degrees, the radium is removed and antibiotics are given to control the infection during the time before the radium is reinserted.

Physics of Brachyradium Therapy

Figure 11-3 illustrates the influence of the inverse square law on the depth dose from the colpostats and the uterine tandem; Figure 11-4 depicts its influence on the combined contribution of the uterine and vaginal radium to the paracervical areas. Several conditions have to be met for successful radium therapy:

a) The geometry of the radium sources must prevent underdosed regions on and around the cervix.

b) Adequate dose has to be delivered to the paracervical areas.

c) Mucosal tolerance has to be respected.

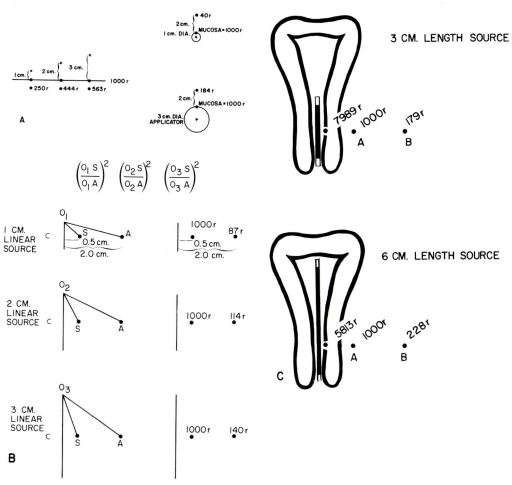

FIG. 11-3. A. The depth dose from a point source increases as treatment distance increases. In this instance, two points are 1 cm apart and the dose at the near point is limited to 1,000 *r*. The dose to the far point increases as the distance to the near point increases from 1 to 3 cm.

The principle of the inverse square law is applied to the design of radium applicators; an applicator of larger diameter produces a greater depth dose in surrounding tissues.

B. Dose contribution from the center of the source (C) to point A is $\left(\dfrac{0.5}{2}\right)^2$ or $\frac{1}{16}$ of that to point S.

As source length increases, $\left(\dfrac{OS}{OA}\right)$ approaches unity.

When this occurs, dose contribution from point O, the end of the source, to points A and S approaches equality $\left(\dfrac{OS}{OA}\right)^2 \rightarrow 1$.

The addition of nearly equal doses to points A and S, already connected by the very steep dose gradient from point C, produces a decrease of that gradient; i.e., an increase in the depth dose.

C. The dose at point A is kept constant at 1,000 *r*. As the length of the source increases, the dose to the mucosa decreases and dose at point B increases.

In view of this, the linear source used in a uterine tandem should be as long as the anatomy will permit. (Courtesy: Fletcher, Stovall, and Sampiere, In *Carcinoma of the Uterine Cervix, Endometrium, and Ovary,* Chicago, Year Book Medical Publishers, Inc., p. 69, 1962.)

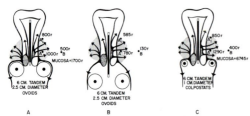

FIG. 11-4. Variations in dose to the vaginal mucosa, to the paracervical area, and at a point 5 cm lateral to the internal *os* with three different radium systems using a total of 1,000 mg-hrs. A tumor originating on the portio is illustrated on the right lip of the cervix; on the left side of each diagram, a tumor originating in the endocervix. The likelihood of involvement of the myometrium of the lower uterine segment is greater with an endocervical lesion. The paracervical areas lateral to the internal *os*, the endocervix and the lower uterine segment, thus, are not a point. They are represented by the stippled areas. Calculations have been made for two points, A and A₁.

   A. 2.5 cm colpostats are used with the tandem reaching the top of the fundus. The relationship between the dose to the vaginal mucosa and the dose to the paracervical areas is good. The dose at point B, 5 cm lateral to the midline, is still favorable.

   B. The same two medium ovoids are used, but because of a cone-shaped vault, they have been displaced downward, the tandem keeping the same position in relation to the colpostats as in a one-piece applicator. There is a sharp drop in the dose to the paracervical areas, the parametria (point B), and the myometrium.

   C. With small diameter colpostats, the doses to the paracervical areas and point B are not as favorable as with large colpostats. If 7,000 or 8,000 mg-hrs are given, or if 7,000 *r* are delivered at point A, the mucosal dose is in the neighborhood of 35,000 *r*. (Courtesy: Fletcher, Stovall, and Sampiere. In *Carcinoma of the Uterine Cervix, Endometrium, and Ovary*. Chicago, Year Book Medical Publishers, Inc., p. 69, 1962.)

In the delivery of adequate dose to the periphery of a tumor, the magnitude of the dose to the mucosa of the vaginal vault could be so great that necrosis would often ensue in spite of the high tolerance to radiation of this area. The dose gradient can be reduced

by the use of large colpostats (Figs. 11-3, 11-4).

Radium Stock, Applicators, and Loading Facilities

The radium stock should consist of 25, 20, 15, and 10 mg tubes with 1 mm *Pt* filtrations. The quantity of radium available depends upon the number of insertions probable at any one time.

A common source length being 2.2 cm (active source length 1.5 cm), small plastic spacers, whenever necessary, are added between sources to produce a physical length of one inch. This does not produce a significant fall-off between sources.

Applicators must be flexible to meet various situations (Fig. 11–5). There is no reason for ovoid-shaped colpostats. Dummy plastic colpostats should be available for fitting in the clinic.

FIG. 11-5. A. From left to right: Afterloading colpostats (2 cm in diameter), and plastic jackets used to increase the size to medium (2.5 cm diameter) and large (3 cm in diameter).

   Half cylinders (0.8 cm in radius for narrow vaults (maximum diameter with the afterloading tandem in between equals 3 cm), designed to have the vaginal sources perpendicular to the vaginal axis in order to minimize the dose to the bladder and rectum as compared to protruding sources with the axis parallel to the vaginal axis. The depth dose is not as good as with one 3 cm colpostat. Uterine afterloading tandems (the three most useful curvatures) with metal flange with "keel" (to stabilize the tandem by means of proper packing around it) and without (to be used with vaginal cylinders).

   Inserters for the colpostats and Teflon tubing to insert radium in the tandems.

   B. Sample of vaginal cylinders of different diameters and length to be used for the irradiation of a selected part or the whole of the vagina.

   C. Form used to record the radium applications. (A—Courtesy: Fletcher and Rutledge, *In Modern Radiotherapy*, T. J. Deeley, Ed., London, Butterworths, 1971.)

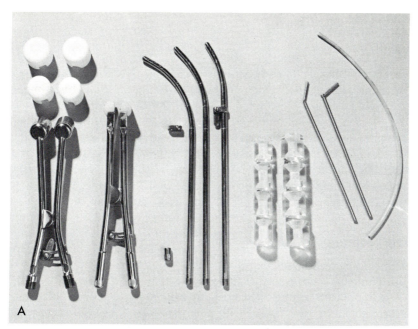

A

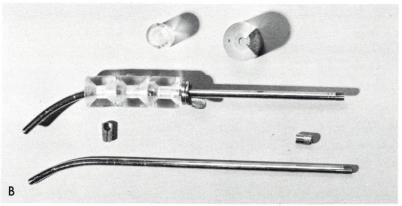

B

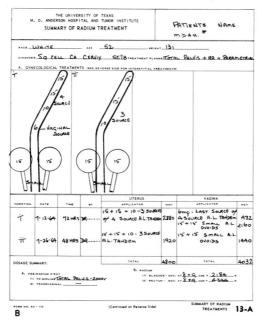

THE UNIVERSITY OF TEXAS
M. D. ANDERSON HOSPITAL AND TUMOR INSTITUTE
SUMMARY OF RADIUM TREATMENT

PATIENTS NAME
M.D.A.H. #

RACE __WHITE__   AGE __52__   WEIGHT __131__

DIAGNOSIS __SQ CELL CA CERVIX ST.ŤB__ TREATMENT PLANNED __TOTAL PELVIS + RR + PARAMETRIAL__

A. GYNECOLOGICAL TREATMENTS (SEE REVERSE SIDE FOR INTERSTITIAL TREATMENTS)

INSERTION	DATE	TIME	BY	UTERUS		VAGINA	
				APPLICATOR	MGH	APPLICATOR	MGH
T	7-12-64	72 HRS	DR------	15 + 15 + 10 - 3 SOURCE of 4 SOURCE A.L. TANDEM	2880	6mg - LAST SOURCE OF 4 SOURCE A.L. TANDEM	432
						15 + 15 SMALL A.L. OVOIDS	2160
TT	7-26-64	48 HRS	DR------	15 + 15 + 10 - 3 SOURCE A.L. TANDEM	1920	15 + 15 SMALL A.L. OVOIDS	1440
				TOTAL	4800	TOTAL	4032

DOSAGE SUMMARY:

A. PRE-RADIUM X-RAY
  (1) TO MIDLINE __TOTAL PELVIS -2000r__
  (2) TRANSVAGINAL _____

B. RADIUM
  (1) BLADDER - MAX. AT __8 + 9__ CMS = __2184__ r
  (2) RECTUM - MAX. AT __8 + 9__ CMS = __2388__ r

FORM NO. AH - 110   (Continued on Reverse Side)   SUMMARY OF RADIUM
                                                            TREATMENTS   13-A

B

C

All gamma-ray emitting isotopes produce essentially the same volume distribution and have the same biologic action. However, tolerance and regression rates obtained with specific treatment times cannot be extrapolated to other treatment times. ^{137}Cs, which has a long half life, can be used for a relatively long period without recalculation of treatment times.

Afterloading Techniques

By using afterloading techniques, exposure to all but ward nursing personnel has become nil.[31] The applicators are inserted unloaded. Verification films are taken with dummy metal sources. Depending on the geometry of the system, any necessary adjustment in loading can be made. The active sources are inserted later on the ward in less than thirty seconds.

TANDEM

The afterloading tandem has the advantage of always having adequate length and of producing almost automatic reduction of anteflexion or retroflexion. The tandem that is to be chosen should be as straight as possible, locating the uterine radium high and back which results in a better contribution to the regional lymphatics.[5]

It is important that the radium sources in the uterus reach the fundus. This is necessary to produce adequate irradiation of the lower uterine segment and paracervical tissues (Figs. 11-3, 11-4) and to decrease the dose gradient in these areas, preventing gross overdosage of the mucosa (Fig. 11-4C). Exception is made when the uterine canal measures more than 4 inches in length (*i.e.*, able to accommodate at least four intrauterine sources) and if the lesion is located on the portio, a plastic spacer may be used instead of a highest source. The contribution to the paracervical areas from sources at so great a distance is relatively small and dose to the small bowel is unnecessarily increased.

The basic loading in the tandem is 15-10, 15-10-10 mg or 15-10-10-10 mg, depending upon the length of the uterine canal. This may be altered to fit any existing situation. With endocervical carcinoma, the distribution might be 15-10-15 mg or 15-10-15-10 mg; with positive endometrial biopsy, it could be 15-15-10 mg, 20-15-10 mg, depending upon the size of the uterus.

In order to avoid an area of underdosage at the midarea, a protruding source is placed between the vaginal colpostats when the lateral sources are separated by a distance of more than 5 cm. The protruding source is usually 10 mg and each colpostat loading is lightened by 5 mg. Conversely, if the endocervical source partially protrudes between two small colpostats close together, a 15-15 mg-dummy is used instead of 15-10-10 mg.

COLPOSTATS

The small colpostats measure 2 cm in diameter, the medium 2.5 cm, the large 3 cm; their basic loading is 15, 20, and 25 mg respectively. In most cases, only a transient fibrinous mucositis occurs on the cervix.

The colpostats should be as large as vault size will permit in order to minimize the mucosal dose but the colpostats should lie in the lateral fornices, to each side of the cervix; one may choose a smaller size colpostat to achieve this location. When one fornix is obliterated, the colpostats can be of different sizes, if necessary staggered, and the handles being fastened with adhesive tape.

While maximum separation of the colpostats is desirable for irradiation of the paracervical and parametrial areas, only gentle pressure should be applied to the handles. In roomy vaults, optimal separation often conforms with the anatomy of the fornices. In the advanced stages of cervical cancer, and with increasing frequency from middle age on, the vaginal canal is often narrow. The vault then forms the truncated apex of a narrow cone. When small colpostats can still be fitted side by side at this apex, any at-

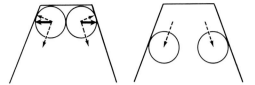

FIG. 11-6. In cone-shaped vaginal canals, lateral separation can only be obtained at the expense of downward displacement of the colpostats.

tandem and one colpostat (Fig. 11-7). Separate insertions are necessary. When a protruding source is used, its strength is less than the strength used in a crossed colpostat (15 and 20 mg for 2.5 and 3 cm diameter cylinder) to avoid overdosage to the anterior rectal wall. When the vault is so narrow that there is no room for a single colpostat, a plastic cylinder of appropriate diameter, is fastened around the level of the protruding source (Fig. 11-8). Gauze packing is used if a small size cylinder cannot be fitted. One and one-half sources should protrude.

Significant shrinkage of the vaginal vault occurs during radium therapy. Colpostat size will therefore be reduced with each application. When only two closely approximated colpostats can be snugly inserted at the time of the first application, the diameter of the vault at the time of the second insertion will be such that either one protruding source in

tempt at lateral separation will automatically result in their direct downward displacement away from the tumor. This can be demonstrated by a vector diagram (Fig. 11-6). Efforts to resist this downward displacement would result only in tearing the vaginal walls.

Not infrequently, the diameter of the vault is such that only a single colpostat can be inserted. A protruding source in the tandem does not provide the same distribution as

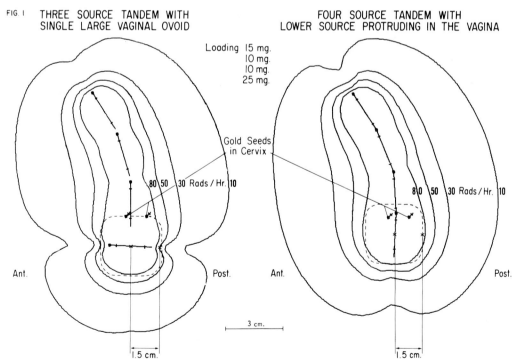

FIG. 11-7. The dose to the anterior rectal wall at the level of the posterior fornix is significantly greater with the linear source arrangement but the dose 2 cm lateral to the internal *os* (point A) is not altered. (Courtesy: Stockbine, et al, *Amer. J. Roentgen.*, 108, 293, 1970.)

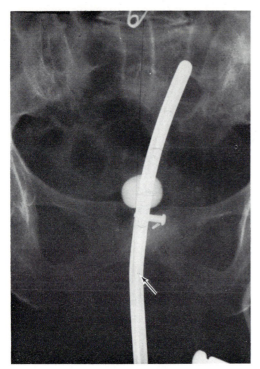

FIG. 11-8. Patient, age 65, with a Stage II$_A$ squamous cell carcinoma of the cervix with involvement of the upper third of the vagina. The vault was narrow, and because of poor geometry 4,000 rads were given first to the whole pelvis.

Although the uterine cavity was 2.5 inches long, five sources (15-10-10-10-20 mg) were used on the first insertion and four sources (15-10-10-20 mg) on the second insertion; the total dose was 5,580 mg-hrs.

One can see the silver clip which identifies the lowest palpable vaginal disease below the screw of the plastic sleeve.

The arrow points to the end of the fifth source in the first insertion.

a cylinder or separate insertions with a large colpostat are used.

Position and Loading of the Radium System

Silver clips are inserted in the anterior and posterior lips (Fig. 11-9) with a radon seed inserter to help visualize the relationship of the colpostats to the lips of the cervix.

The axis of the tandem should be equidistant from the colpostats and bisect their height (Fig. 11-9). The distal end of the endocervical source should slightly overlap the cephalad rim of the colpostats if there is separation. With close small colpostats it is best to use 15-15 mg-dummy to avoid an excessive dose to the vault which results from the crowding of the radioactive sources.

To maintain the position of the tandem, packing surrounds the tandem laterally to prevent deviation toward either colpostat. After the tandem has been positioned at midheight of the colpostats it is kept in this plane by posterior packing. This is important because the colpostats have a tendency to lie somewhat anteriorly even in normal vaults.

Since the colpostats are relatively long, packing in front and back of them is not necessary to spare rectum and bladder. Packing in front or back is used only for those lesions located on the anterior or posterior lips to produce a location of the colpostats circumscribing the lesion (Fig. 11-10).

Thus, a lesion on the anterior lip may be circumscribed by approximating the vaginal sources to its inferior aspect and the intrauterine sources to its posterior surface at the canal. The plane of the tandem will then lie behind the plane of the colpostats. The colpostats are applied in a reverse fashion for a lesion of the posterior lip.

Additional packing is added around the tandem and the handles of the colpostats to produce the frictional resistance on the vaginal walls necessary to prevent downward slipping of the system.

Packing fixes the radium system tautly in the vagina so that no motion of the system is possible. Packing the whole vagina also moves the entire radium system upward with increased contribution of radiation to the parametria and regional lymphatics. It lessens the doses delivered to the bladder and

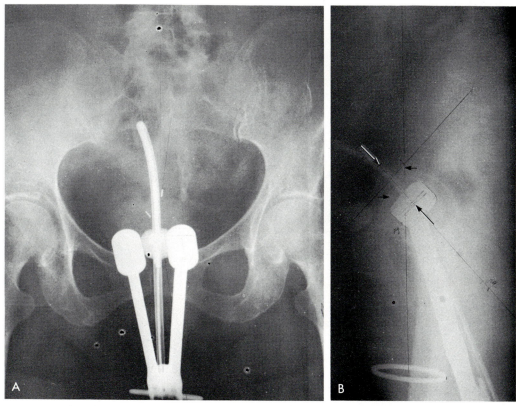

FIG. 11-9. Silver clips (small arrows on Fig. B) are inserted with a radon seed inserter in the anterior and posterior lips of the cervix to determine the position of the colpostats to the cervix.

A plane perpendicular to the radium system passing through the center of the colpostats and the cephalad end of the endocervical source (large arrows) is taken for lateral throw-off calculations. (Courtesy: Fletcher and Rutledge, *Modern Radiotherapy*, T. J. Deeley, Ed., London, Butterworths, 1971.)

rectum since the radium system is partially removed from a location between these two organs. However, in young patients with very distensible vaults, this upward displacement can be excessive as the radium could be moved almost out of the true pelvis.

By favoring the uterine canal with a slightly larger radium load than the vaginal vault, one maximizes the dose contribution to the regional lymphatics without impairing adequate irradiation of the portio.

ADAPTATION TO DISTORTED ANATOMY

Carcinoma of the cervix is often an asymmetrical lesion producing pronounced distortion of the local and pelvic anatomy. Common patterns of distortion may be briefly summarized (Fig. 11-11).

1) Lesions restricted mainly to one lip.

2) Invasion of one fornix.

3) Parametrial shortening. This usually produces deviation of the uterus with angulation of the tandem.

4) Growth along vaginal wall(s).

5) Massive central lesion expanding the cervix and/or the isthmus.

Initial whole pelvis irradiation minimizes the consequences of marked distortion by shrinkage of the tumor and/or making up for poor anatomy.

In a bulky lesion of a lateral lip, the ipsi-

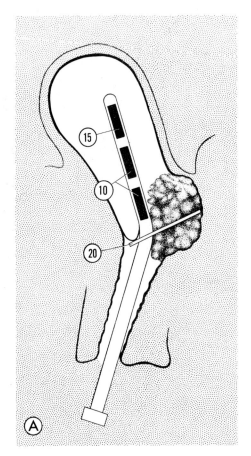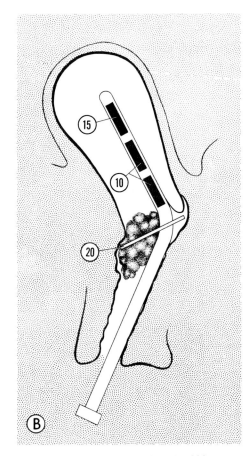

FIG. 11-10. A. Disease on the cervix can originate primarily on the posterior lip. The tandem should be anterior to the colpostats so that the radium sources circumscribe the lesion.

    B. The lesion is on the anterior lip. The tandem should be posterior for the vaginal sources to circumscribe the disease.

lateral colpostat will be displaced away from the tandem; to prevent underdosage of this lip, loading of the displaced colpostat is increased. When the uterine canal is pulled toward one wall by parametrial shortening, a high dose will develop in the acute angle encompassed by the tandem and the colpostat. Loading of the ipsilateral colpostat may be lightened by 5 mg; if the displacement is significant, an equal amount may be added contralaterally to avoid underdosage of the opposite lip. For tumor extension along the vaginal wall(s), a composite applicator (colpostats and vaginal cylinder, referred to at M. D. Anderson as Bloedorn applicator) may

best be suited after whole pelvis irradiation has flattened out the vaginal disease.

Number of Radium Insertions and Treatment Time

Radium therapy must be protracted, both in the number of applications and dosage rate. Total insertion time varies from 120 to 144 hours, and is divided into two applications not less than two weeks apart. Should one insertion be less than optimally placed, it is then shortened and the next application proportionally lengthened, or three applications are used.

If tandem and colpostats are used separately, or for not longer than 48 hours together, the insertions may be spaced only one week apart if shrinkage of the lesion is not a problem. However, if, even after 4,000 rads to the whole pelvis, a large tumor is still present, the insertions should be fractionated over two or even three weeks using tandem and colpostats separately.

The uterine radium is usually increased in loading (15-10-10) and time. A common treatment schedule is tandem 48 hours–2 weeks colpostats 72 hours–2 weeks tandem 48 hours. This widens the dose distribution for the expanding lesions without increased risk of complications as the uterine radium is surrounded by the expanded lesion, so diminishing the dose to the bladder and bowels.

If the os cannot be found, external irradiation and vaginal radium are used followed by an extrafascial conservative hysterectomy. If there is contraindication for the surgical procedure external irradiation only is used.

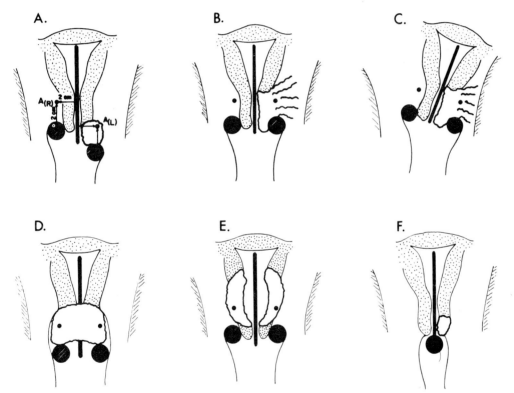

FIG. 11-11. **A.** Point A is displaced downward on the left and lies in midst of tumor growing into the fornix. Dose rate at Point A on the left is lower than on the right.

  B. The significance of dose rate at Point A on the left side, in the middle of tumor in the parametrium, bears little relation to its counterpart on the right.

  C. Parametrial shortening secondary to parametrial invasion, can produce anatomical asymmetry.

  D. A large exophytic mass does not allow insertion of the vaginal applicators into the fornices, thus placing Point A in the middle of bulky neoplasm.

  E. In a barrel-shaped cervix enlarged by massive tumor, both Points A are buried within the depth of the lesion.

  F. A narrow vault with or without encircling disease is often encountered in elderly patients. In the absence of fornices, the position of Point A cannot be determined. (Courtesy: Schwarz, *Amer. J. Roentgen.,* 105, 579, 1969.)

Dosimetric Procedures in Intracavitary Radium Therapy

The structures involved in the dosimetric procedures for intracavitary radium therapy are:

1) Portio, endocervix, endometrium, and myometrium.

2) Paracervical areas and medial parametria.

3) Bladder and rectum.

4) Sigmoid colon and small intestine.

UTERUS

The radiation tolerance of the cervix, endocervix, endometrium, and myometrium is practically limitless. These structures receive extremely high doses in the zones immediately adjacent to the tandem and colpostats. Atrophy of the uterus and cervix follows intracavitary radium therapy, but no complications develop provided the dose to the vault and immediate underlying tissues is not excessive. Extra care must be exercised after conization.

VAGINAL MUCOSA

With colpostats of 2, 2.5, and 3 cm in diameter, doses of 13,000 to 11,000 rads are delivered to the mucosa in 144 hours total time. Larger fractions of this dose are delivered to the submucosal tissues with the larger diameter colpostats. Furthermore, when large colpostats are used a longer length of vaginal sheath is adequately irradiated because of the mucosa of the fornices and of the upper third of the vagina being stretched over them.

PARACERVICAL AREAS AND MEDIAL PARAMETRIA

Only three-dimensional isodose surfaces give complete information of the dose distribution in the corpus, paracervical areas, and parametria. These isodose surfaces for each patient can be made with computer programs.

Points of reference have been used in the Manchester system.[35] Theoretically, point A lies in the paracervical area at the crossing of the uterine artery and the ureter. It is not, as a rule, superimposed on any definite pelvic structure, as has been demonstrated by extensive studies.[24] The anatomic location of point A is even more fallacious if it is determined in relation to a rigid one-piece applicator because bulky lesions, cone-shaped vaults, or obliterated fornices displace the radium system downward. Point A determined by coordinates 2 cm from the cervical end of the tandem and 2 cm laterally may then come to lie in the paracolpos. Furthermore, tumor size or location are distorting. Figure 11-11 illustrates several situations.

A plane passing through the internal *os* and the center of the colpostats bisects the lower uterine segment and the paracervical areas (Fig. 11-9). This plane has been chosen for isodose curve calculation. Calculations are made for each radium insertion and then compounded. The isodose curve of 3,500 rads has been arbitrarily chosen for each insertion. Dose calculation techniques are briefly described in Figs. 1-23, 1-24, and 1-25.

The following information is obtained from these curves in the frontal plane:

1) The presence of cold spots on and around the cervix. Separation between the tandem and the colpostats, or asymmetrical location of the external os, are common causes of cold spots.

2) The amount of lateral displacement of the 7,000 rads curve (compounded curve adjusted for two routine insertions) when the uterus is drawn to one side of the pelvis. This is taken into account for external irradiation with central shielding.

The data must be used semiquantitatively because of the steep gradient of dose rate, but they help in evaluating the adequacy of the radium insertion and in making adjustments for unfavorable anatomic situations.

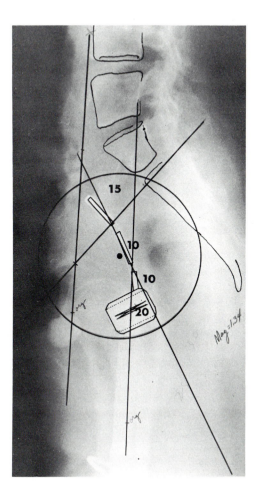

FIG. 11-12. Pelvic fibrosis and sigmoiditis should be related to the total dose from external irradiation and the dose from intracavitary radium in the hollow of the sacrum obtained with computer dosimetry. The dose calculated on a sphere 10 cm in diameter centered over the weighted geometric center of the radium system would be an adequate approximation.

For the same number of rads on that sphere, the doses to the tissues in the immediate vicinity of the cervical canal and fornices is much greater with a small radium system than with a large radium system.

For instance:

   20 1 cm from midcervix 100 rads/hr.

with 15-10-10   or 5-fold

   20 5 cm from midcervix 21 rads/hr.

   1 cm from midcervix 120 rads/hr.

BLADDER, RECTUM, AND SIGMOID

With afterloading tandems, anteflexion, retroflexion, and retroposition are automatically reduced and direct measurements have been discontinued.

As an adequate approximation for tolerance of the sigmoid, the dose to the sigmoid from external irradiation and intracavitary radium therapy, can be obtained by adding the dose from whole pelvis irradiation to the contribution by the radium on a 10 cm diameter sphere centered on the weighted geometric center of the radium system (Fig. 11-12). The dose on that sphere is the number of mg-hrs. multiplied by 8.25 and divided by 25. Therefore, the only variable is the number of mg-hrs. For the same dose on that sphere, a small radium system delivers a much higher local dose than a large radium system; an occasional catastrophic local necrosis has happened with small radium systems.[30]

It is mainly the radium in the tandem which irradiates the small intestine because loops are wrapped around the uterus. In the absence of adhesions, the loops of small intestine change positions, so that excessive doses are not given to any one segment and only mild diarrhea occurs. Adhesions resulting from pelvic surgical procedures or inflammatory disease bind down the loops of bowel.

REGIONAL NODES

The dose contribution of the radium system to the regional nodes depends upon several factors:

1) Total number of milligram hours.

2) The relative radium distribution in the tandem and colpostats.

3) The location of the system, primarily the tandem, within the pelvis.

with 15-15-25   or 10-fold

   5 cm from midcervix 12.5 rads/hr.

(Courtesy: Fletcher, *J. Radiol. Electr.*, **49**, 629, 1968.)

The location of the radium system within the pelvis varies considerably (Fig. 11-13). In young patients with roomy and distensible vaults, the location is high; in old patients and also in patients in whom the vagina is extensively involved by disease, the vagina is short and the radium system therefore lies low.

Direct measurements while the radium is still *in situ* have shown that uterine radium contributes more than vaginal radium to the regional nodes because it is more centrally located and, therefore, closer to the nodes.[10,20] The tandem is best located back, closer to the common iliac nodes. Minimal or no curvature tandem is used unless a curvature is needed to insert the tandem in an anteflexed uterus.

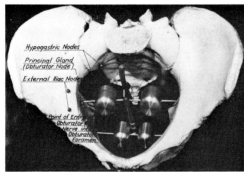

FIG. 11-13. Variations in location of the radium system within the pelvis. Markers have been pinned on a bony pelvis to identify node groups according to lymphadenectomy findings. Two actual radium systems have been reconstructed in space, showing the difference in their relationship to the pelvis and nodes. The lower radium system was used in the treatment of an elderly patient with a short, narrow vagina. The upper radium system was used in the treatment of a young patient with a roomy, distensible vagina and produces a more significant contribution to the pelvic walls because of its central position. (Courtesy: Fletcher, Wall, Bloedorn, Shalek and Wootton, *Radiology,* 61, 885, 1953.)

The dose at Point B is not representative of the dose to the regional lymphatics. Even when the radium system is high it only represents the dose to the obturator nodes (Fig. 11-14).[27]

A plane can be constructed extending upward to the region of the bifurcation of the aorta and points can be chosen at which computer calculations can give estimates of dose rates to the external iliac, common iliac, and low paraaortic lymph node chains (Figs. 11-15 and 11-16).

Direct measurements at laparotomy showed a good correlation[5] with the calculated data at the location of silver clips marking the lymph node areas. Study of representative patients with high radium systems, widely separated vaginal colpostats, colpostats with little separation, and of patients with intrauterine tandem and a protruding source in the upper vagina in a plastic cylinder have established the following points:

1) Most of the dose to the lymph nodes comes from the uterine tandem, best located back close to the common iliac nodes.

2) Highly located vaginal radium contributes a significant dose to the obturator and external iliac lymph nodes, with a smaller dose to the common iliac nodes.

3) In medium and low radium systems, the tandem may deliver a significant dose to the external iliac lymph nodes but contributes relatively little to the low common iliac ones.

With roomy, distensible vaults, 14 to 18 rads per hour are given to the obturator nodes and 10 to 13 rads per hour to the external iliac nodes; whereas with a low radium system, only 8 to 13 rads and 6 to 10 rads are given respectively to the obturator and external iliac nodes.[5]

Computer calculated isodose curves (Fig. 11-17) are obtained in all intracavitary radium insertions. The doses delivered to the low common iliac and the external iliac nodes are averaged for the right and left sides.

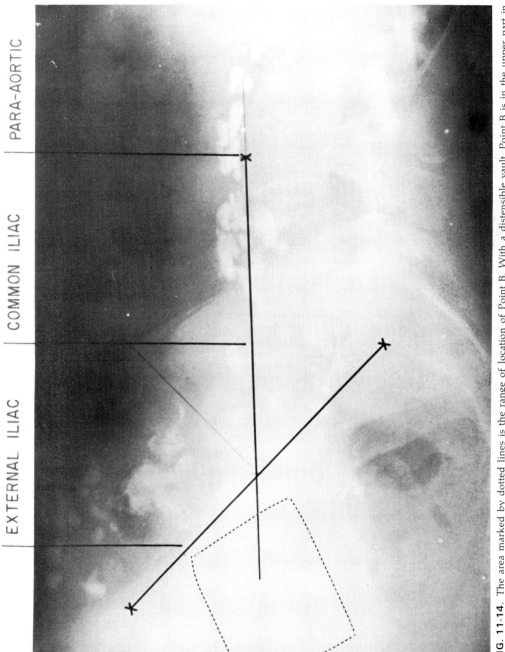

EXTERNAL ILIAC | COMMON ILIAC | PARA-AORTIC

FIG. 11-14. The area marked by dotted lines is the range of location of Point B. With a distensible vault, Point B is in the upper part in the vicinity of the obturator nodes which are located inside the acetabula; with a short vagina, caused by either age or disease, it is in the lower part a great distance from any node area. It therefore cannot be used for the dosimetry of regional lymphatics irradiation. (Courtesy: Schwarz, *Amer. J. Roentgen.,* 105, 579, 1969.)

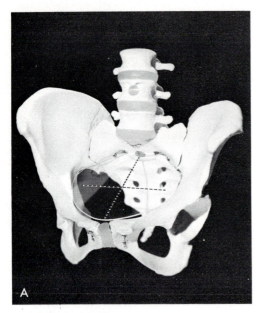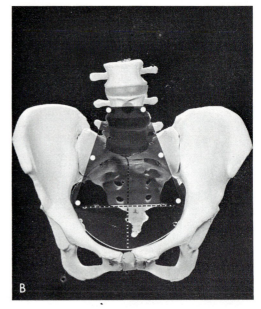

FIG. 11-15. A. The model of the pelvis illustrates the basic reference line extending from the upper aspect of the pubis to the anterior aspect of the S1, S2 junction. The transverse line is shown bisecting the basic reference line at its midpoint.

B. The trapezoid constructed out of dark plastic is shown extending from the transverse line to the anterior aspect of L4. The white dots at the lower end of this figure are 6 cm from the midline and are representative of the midexternal iliac lymph nodes. The white dots at the top of the figure are 2 cm from the midline and represent the low paraaortic lymph nodes. The center dots are halfway between these two points and represent the location of the low common iliac lymph nodes. (Courtesy: Durrance and Fletcher, *Radiology,* 91, 140, 1968.)

Interstitial Radium Therapy

Interstitial gamma-ray therapy, using low intensity radium needles or ^{192}Ir with afterloading technique, is used in the following special situations:

1) When the os cannot be located and the vagina is too narrow to accommodate a transvaginal cone, a cluster of needles is placed in the vault. In recent years, external irradiation only to a tumor dose of 7,000 rads is preferred.

2) When the os is asymmetrical, a cluster of 0.66 mg/cm needles is inserted into the endocervix and corpus through the adjacent vault (Fig. 11-18). The needles are left in place as long as the tandem.

3) When a bladder mass is felt anterior to the tandem, insertion of 0.66 mg/cm needles through the mass and into the base of the bladder is performed with an open bladder.

4) When there is extensive disease in the vagina, a cylindrical volume implant is best suited for disease in the upper two thirds of the vagina; a tandem is also inserted if the os is located (Fig. 11-19). For lower vaginal disease, a double-plane implant is used (Fig. 11-20).

Volume implants for carcinoma of the stump, or recurrent carcinoma, or invasion of the anterior vaginal wall and base of the bladder have been performed with a suprapubic cystotomy (Fig. 11-21). The anterior needles are inserted through the vagina with one hand, with the other hand in the bladder to guide their direction under the base of the bladder and upper parametria. When the anterior half of the implant is completed, the posterior needles are inserted with a finger in the rectum to guide them in the direction of the lateral parametria, uterosacral ligaments, and into the rectovaginal septum.

External Irradiation

The geometrical and anatomical planning varies with the purpose of external irradiation. The structures to be covered are checked by verification films with the patient in the exact treatment position either on the therapy machine or a simulator. Type "M" industrial film by Kodak or equivalent show adequately the body landmarks.

For external iliac nodes coverage, the width of the portals is 15 or 16 cm depending on the beam definition.

Regional Lymphatics Irradiation Only

If therapy begins with a radium application, lymphatics irradiation starts immediately thereafter, to be interrupted 10 days later by the second radium insertion. *AP* and *PA* portals 15 × 15 cm are used.

The central structures irradiated by the intracavitary radium are protected by a lead shield 10 cm placed high in the midline or shifted laterally to follow the position of the radium (Fig. 11-22). The width of shielding at midpelvis is 3 or 4 cm, depending on the radium isodose pattern. With a narrow pattern, a 3 cm shield might be used for the first

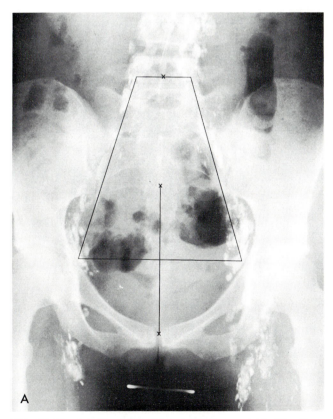
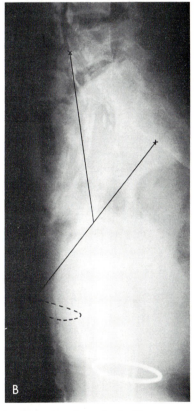

FIG. 11-16. Anteroposterior (A) and lateral cross-table (B) orthogonal radiographs of a patient with a normal lower extremity lymphangiogram. The basic reference line is from the top of the symphysis to the junction of S1-S2 (Fig. B). A line is drawn from the midpoint of the basic reference line to the middle of the anterior aspect of L4. Figure A shows a trapezoid defined by points 6 cm from midline and 2 cm from midline at L4. (Courtesy: Durrance and Fletcher, *Radiology,* 91, 140, 1968.)

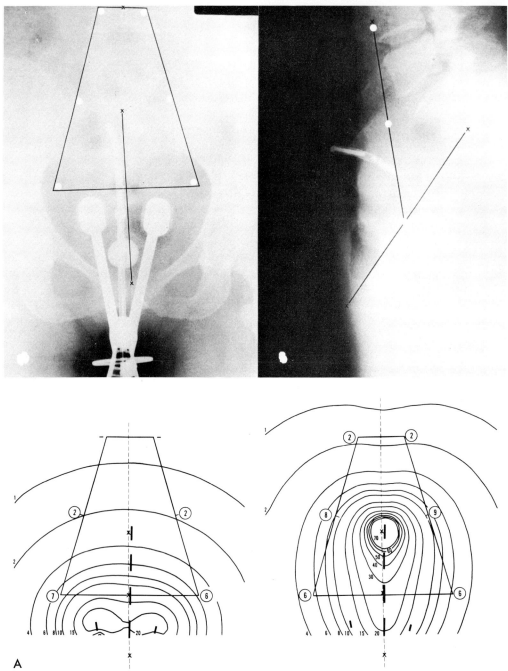

A

FIG. 11-17. A. *AP* and lateral orthogonal radiographs of a high radium system (the tandem should have less curvature to give an even more favorable lymph node dose) with drawing of the trapezoid used for dose calculation. The isodose curves with contributions from the ovoids only and the tandem only are shown.

About half of the dose to the external iliac lymph nodes comes from the ovoids and about half from the tandem. Most of the dose to the low common iliac lymph nodes is contributed by the tandem.

A line is drawn from the junction of *S*1-*S*2 to the top of the symphysis. Then a line is drawn from the middle of that line to the middle of the anterior aspect of *L*4. A trapezoid is constructed in a plane passing through the transverse line in the pelvic brim plane and the midpoint of the anterior aspect of the body of *L*4. A point 6 cm lateral to the midline at the inferior end of this figure is used to give an estimate of the dose rate to the midexternal iliac lymph nodes. At the top of the trapezoid, points 2 cm lateral to the midline at the level of *L*4 are used to estimate the dose to the low paraaortic area. The midpoint of a line connecting these two points is used to estimate the dose to the low common iliac lymph nodes. C and D show respectively the isodose curves from the radium in the colpostats and the radium in the tandem.

NAME _____ No. _____

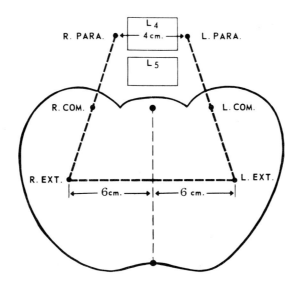

RIGHT

POINTS		R. EXT.		R. COM.		R. PARA.	
No.	Hrs.	DOSE RATE	TOTAL RADS	DOSE RATE	TOTAL RADS	DOSE RATE	TOTAL RADS
TOTAL							

LEFT

POINTS		L. EXT.		L. COM.		L. PARA.	
No.	Hrs.	DOSE RATE	TOTAL RADS	DOSE RATE	TOTAL RADS	DOSE RATE	TOTAL RADS
TOTAL							

B

FIG. 11-17. B. Routine lymph node dosimetry form.

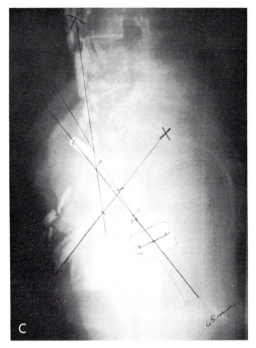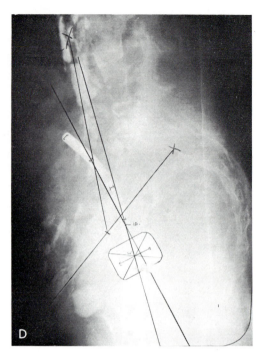

FIG. 11-17. C, D. Contrast 2 insertions in the same patient within D (repositioned insertion) the tandem being higher and more posterior than in C.

    The doses to the common iliac node is increased from 835 rads to 1,365 rads for a 65 hour insertion. (Courtesy: Durrance and Fletcher, *Radiology,* 91, 140, 1968.)

2,000 rads, and widened to 4 cm for the remaining 1,500 to 2,000 rads. The entire treatment can be given through parallel opposing fields with a 22 Mev beam or a ^{60}Cobalt unit. The weekly dose is 1,000 rads with the 22 Mev beam. With a 3 to 6 Mev beam, *AP* and *PA* portals should be treated every day to diminish late fibrosis.

The dose given to the parametria at mid-distance of the anteroposterior diameter varies from 3,000 to 4,000 rads, depending upon the following three factors:

1) Extent of disease.

2) Adequacy of the individual radium system.

3) Location of the radium within the pelvic cavity, correlated with computer calculated doses to the regional nodes.

If 2,000 rads have been given to the whole pelvis, the added parametrial irradiation follows the same anatomical and dosimetric guidelines. The external parametrial therapy is adjusted so that right and left external iliac nodes receive a total tumor dose of about 5,500 rads.

Whole Pelvis Irradiation

Its purpose is to treat the disease in its entirety. Whole pelvis irradiation is given entirely prior to radium therapy. Additional parametrial irradiation may be given after intracavitary radium.

A 22 Mev betatron has been used for whole pelvis irradiation with either parallel opposing or four-field techniques (Fig. 11-23A and B). When the field size does not exceed 15 × 15 cm, 1,000 rads per week are given with the 22 Mev beam. With a 3 to 6 Mev beam, the midline dose is delivered at the rate of 850 rads a week with parallel opposing portals (*AP* and *PA* portals treated every day) and should not exceed 5,500 rads in order to avoid late subcutaneous, fat, and muscle fibrosis resulting from higher doses to the lateral tissues (Fig. 11-23C).

The tilt of the pelvis in the prone and supine positions varies with individuals and the length of the vagina changes with age and disease; therefore, the central mobile struc-

tures show no consistent relationship to the surface landmarks and the bony pelvis. Hence, if the cervix, the paracervical areas, and the involved part of the vagina are to be included, a method of projecting these structures on the anterior and posterior surface of the body must be used[11] (Fig. 11-24).

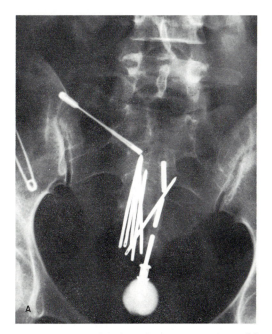 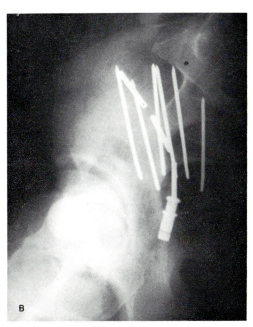

FIG. 11-18. A and B show the anteroposterior and lateral films of a tandem insertion combined with a cluster of radium needles.

This 35-year-old white patient was seen on 4-26-60 with a huge squamous cell carcinoma of the cervix which bled profusely and extended almost from one pelvic wall to the other.

Because of the profuse bleeding, four treatments of 400 rads each were given on consecutive days with transvaginal therapy. The bleeding stopped, and a detailed, thorough pelvic and rectal examination was possible. The cervical mass was estimated to be 8 cm in diameter and the parametria were involved almost to the pelvic walls: the lesion was staged II$_B$. After 5,500 rads to the whole pelvis, the *os* was located eccentrically in the vault.

A tandem with 15-10-10-mg sources was placed in the uterus (one source protruding) and six 4.5 cm active length needles, 0.66 mg per cm were inserted to the left of the *os*. The tandem and the needles were left in place for 72 hours and no attempt was made to calculate the implant. The total number of mg-hrs from the needles and the tandem was 3,096 in the uterus and 720 mg-hrs in the vagina.

Two weeks later, two small ovoids, 15 mg each, were left in place for 48 hours. The total dose in mg-hrs for both insertions was 5,256 mg-hrs.

The patient was discharged on 6-26-60 with almost complete regression, not only of the exophytic mass, but also of the infiltrative part of the tumor.

In November, 1970 the patient was without evidence of disease. (Courtesy: Fletcher, Stovall, and Sampiere, In *Carcinoma of the Uterine Cervix, Endometrium, and Ovary*, Chicago, Year Book Medical Publishers, Inc., p. 69, 1962.)

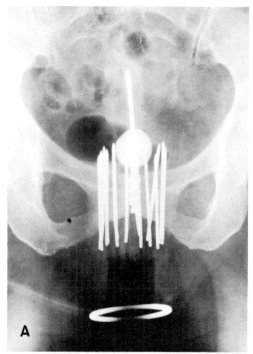
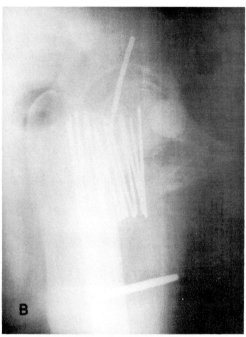

FIG. 11-19. *AP* (A) and lateral (B) films of a combination of uterine tandem and volume implant for disease involving the upper and middle thirds of the vagina. This 52-year-old patient had a squamous cell carcinoma extending to both pelvic walls (Stage III$_B$). There was also a nodule at 3 o'clock and a 2 cm plaque at 12 o'clock in the middle third of the vagina. Biopsy specimens of both the nodule and the plaque were reported to be positive for squamous cell carcinoma. The patient was treated with 6,000 *r* (5,600 rads) in 6 weeks to the whole pelvis with fields covering the entire vagina. Following external irradiation, both the nodule and the plaque were no longer palpable. There also was marked regression of the parametrial infiltration. The vagina was narrow and short; the uterine canal measured 2.5 inches in length. Radium therapy was planned to consist of a tandem, with a source protruding into the vault, combined with a volume implant of the vagina. It was performed immediately after external irradiation; 16 radium needles were used in the implant.

    Type implant: Cylinder
    Radium:

    16 × 1.94 mg (dumbbell, 4.5 cm active length) = 31.04 mg.

    The needles were equally spaced around the surface of a plastic cylinder that was 4.0 cm in diameter and implanted in the vaginal wall. The dose rate at a point 0.5 cm outside the cylinder was calculated by considering the needles as linear sources.

    Dose rate: 48.5 *r*/hr.
    Aim: 4,500 *r*
    Time: 93 hours

    A tumor dose of 4,600 rads was delivered in 96 hours, and the tandem was left in place for the same time. Three months later, a mass in the right groin was excised. At the same time a pelvic lymphadenectomy was performed; six nodes were positive for squamous cell carcinoma. The patient died six months later from generalized peritoneal carcinomatosis. (Courtesy: Fletcher, Stovall, and Sampiere, in *Carcinoma of the Uterine Cervix, Endometrium and Ovary,* Chicago, Year Book Medical Publishers, Inc., p. 69, 1962.)

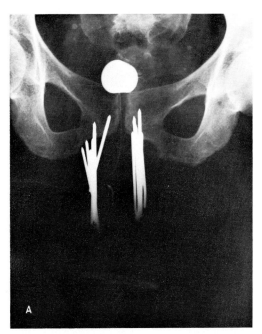
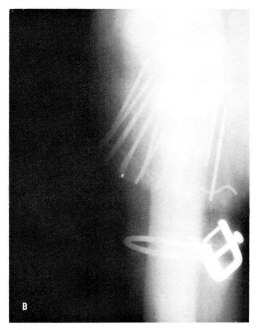

FIG. 11-20. *AP* (A) and lateral (B) films of a double-plane implant for low vaginal disease. This 55-year-old patient was seen on 11-30-58 with poorly differentiated adenocarcinoma. The cervix was replaced by an ulcer measuring approximately 2.5 cm in diameter and 1 cm in depth, covered by a gray necrotic film. The endocervix was barrel-shaped and hard. There was marked limitation of the mobility of the uterus. The right parametrium was infiltrated with disease to the pelvic wall and the left was also involved, but not to the pelvic wall. The left uterosacral ligament was indurated. A 5 mm nodule was palpated on the right side of the introitus at the hymenal ring. A biopsy specimen was reported as metastatic adenocarcinoma in vaginal mucosa. The case was staged III$_B$ because of fixation to the right pelvic wall and disease at the introitus. The whole pelvis was irradiated with 6,000 rads, including the whole length of the vagina. During treatment, another nodule, approximately 1 cm in diameter was felt in the lower vagina. At the completion of the 6,000 rads, a tandem, 15-15-10 mg and two small ovoids, each 12 mg, were left 72 hours for a total of 4,600 mg-hrs. A week later, a double-plane implant was performed for the lower vaginal disease.

Type implant: Double plane.
Radium:

12 × 1.70 mg (Indian club, 4.5 cm active length) = 20.40 mg
4 × 2.91 mg (Indian club, 4.5 cm active length) = 11.64 mg

Total: 32.04 mg

The separation of the planes was measured directly on the anteroposterior radiograph as 3.0 cm. Area of right plane was 25.0 sq cm. Area of left plane was 21.0 sq cm. The dose rates at 0.5 cm medial to each plane were calculated: Right plane, 47.2 *r*/hour; left plane, 51.4 *r*/hour. The average dose rate was used to determine the duration of the implant.

Dose rate: 49.3 *r*/hour
Aim: 4,000 *r*
Time: 81 hours

Three weeks after the completion of treatment, there was marked reaction of the vaginal mucosa and marked parametrial induration. The patient did not return for follow-up and died on 4-2-59. (Courtesy: Fletcher, Stovall, and Sampiere, In *Carcinoma of the Uterine Cervix, Endometrium and Ovary*, Chicago, Year Book Medical Publishers, Inc., p. 69, 1962.)

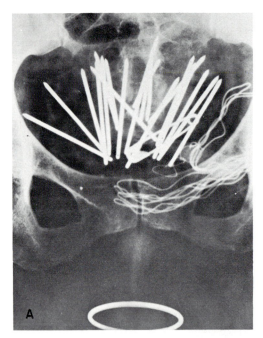
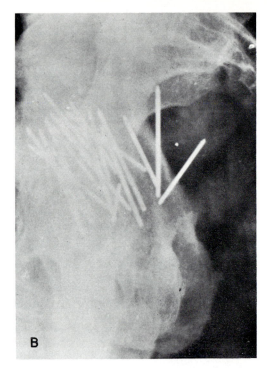

FIG. 11-21. *AP* and lateral films of a volume implant inserted with an open bladder. This 39-year-old woman had a hysterectomy for squamous cell carcinoma of the cervix in 1952, followed by external irradiation to a tumor dose of approximately 2,000 *r*. The patient was first seen at M. D. Anderson Hospital in January 1954. There was a granular recurrence on the vault of the vagina as well as extensive involvement of the base of the bladder, which was detected by cystoscopy. Both the vaginal recurrence and the bladder recurrence were proved by positive biopsy. An implant of the vault and base of the bladder through the vagina with an open bladder (suprapubic cystotomy) was done on 2-12-54. Because of invasion of the left parametrium, an extra plane of needles was placed there.

> Type implant: Volume implant
> Volume: 78.8 cm^3
> Total radium:

14 dumbbells—4.5 cm active length (0.65 mm Pt)
7 dumbbells—3.0 cm active length (0.6 mm Pt)

One posterior and two lateral needles were considered outside the volume and were not included in the calculations.

> Effective radium:

$$12 \times 1.94 \ (4.5 \text{ cm DB}) = 23.28 \text{ mg}$$
$$6 \times 1.47 \ (3.0 \text{ cm DB}) = \underline{\ 8.82 \text{ mg}}$$
$$32.10 \text{ mg} \ (0.5 \text{ mm Pt})$$

Paterson-Parker dose rate

$$= \frac{32.10 \times 1,000}{627} - 51.2 \ r/hr \ (46.1 \text{ rads/hr})$$

Total dose = 51.2 × 134 hrs − 6,861 *r* (6,177 rads)

Following this implant, a tumor dose of 4,000 rads was given in 26 days to the lateral aspects of the parametria and the pelvic walls with a kilocurie ^{60}Co unit. Central shielding and wedge filters were used. The patient had an uneventful therapeutic course. The vault healed rapidly. During the first two or three years, there were a shallow ulceration and small calculi on the base of the bladder. The patient was last seen in April 1964, and in the last 4 years cystoscopies were negative except for telangiectasia. The vault is soft and there is little pelvic fibrosis. (Courtesy: Fletcher, Stovall, and Sampiere, In *Carcinoma of the Uterine Cervix, Endometrium and Ovary,* Chicago, Year Book Medical Publishers, Inc., p. 69, 1962.)

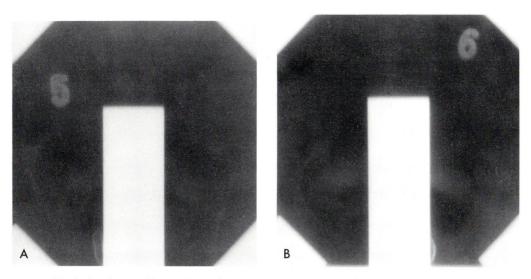

FIG. 11-22. **A.** Localization film (22 Mev) of a 15 × 15 cm anterior portal with a center block, 4 cm in width, 10 cm high, used for peripheral lymphatics "U" shaped field.

    The lower margin should glance the upper aspect of the obturator foramina as the nodes at the entrance of the obturator foramina are rarely involved. The obturator nodes project over the posterior iliac spine and therefore are well within the fields. The sacroiliac joints and part of *L5* are seen.

    B. The same lower margin is used for the posterior portal. (Courtesy: Fletcher and Rutledge, In *Modern Radiotherapy*, T. J. Deeley, Ed., London, Butterworths, 1971.)

Lateral Portals in Whole Pelvic Irradiation

The promontory must be included by a substantial margin to assure coverage of the hypogastric and low common iliac nodes (Figs. 11-1B, 11-24D). The acetabula must also be seen.

The center of the portal is first determined with the caliper on the stand between the patient's legs. A verification film is taken and adjustments are then made both along the cephalocaudad and anteroposterior planes. Day-to-day treatment reduplication is assured by use of a Lucite bridge (Fig. 11-24B).

Regional Lymphatics Irradiation with Extended Fields

In our lymphadenectomy studies,[26] a high percentage of control was obtained in external iliac and obturator nodes with doses ranging from 5,000 to 6,000 rads given in 5 to 7 weeks, compared to the data in the literature.[18] The percentage of patients with positive nodes in the common iliac nodes was high (21 of 28 patients with positive nodes).[9]

Kottmeier[21] reported that in 19 patients with positive node biopsy prior to treatment, six patients were alive with no evidence of disease (*NED*) three and one-half to 12 years with doses of no more than 4,000 rads adding the contribution from intracavitary radium to the dose from external irradiation.

Patients with bulky disease, even if Stages I and II$_A$ or with Stages II$_B$, III, and IV lesions have an initial lymphangiogram. Patients with a negative lymphangiogram are treated with 15 cm high fields. Patients with only positive external iliac nodes are treated with extended fields to include the body of *L4* (Fig. 11-25A). If the common iliac or paraaortic nodes are involved, the extended field includes the entire paraaortic lymph node chain (Fig. 11-25B). The dose in both instances is 5,500 rads *TD* in 6½ weeks deliv-

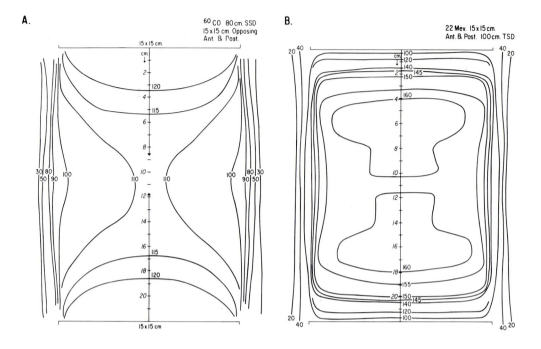

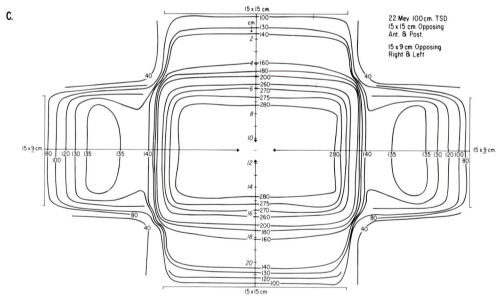

FIG. 11-23. Comparative volume distributions for 22 cm *AP* diameter between a ^{60}Co and 22 Mev beam. The ratio of central dose to the dose in the lateral tissues is in favor of the 22 Mev beam.

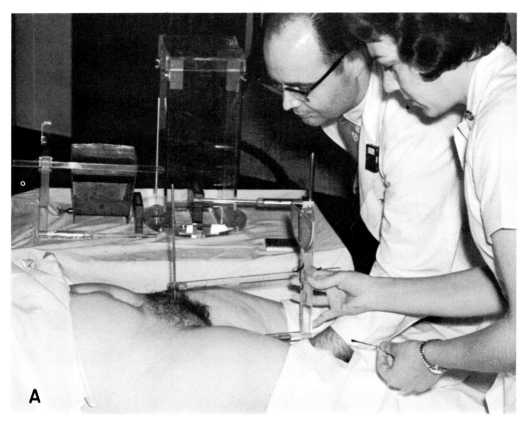

FIG. 11-24. A. Projection of vaginal disease onto the surface of the body. The cervical localizer, seen on the left side of the tray, consists of a plastic rod with a lead plug at its tip and a fluid level to assure its horizontal position. The plastic rod is introduced into the vagina, guided by the examining finger until contact is made with the lowest palpable vaginal disease. As the rod is then attached to the stand at exactly this level, the vertical pointer which is in line with the tip of the rod, will project the location of the lowest palpable vaginal disease onto the surface of the body. The lower margin of the portal is drawn 2 cm below that projection. A verification film is taken immediately and adjustments are made until the field includes approximately 1 cm of tissue below the lead plug, which means that there will be at least 2 cm of normal vaginal tissues in the irradiated field.

Also seen on the tray are the compression cone for the 22 Mev betatron with the lead blocks to shield respectively 2 and 4 cm of tissue at 10 cm depth. The end of compression cone for the ⁶⁰Co unit is made of copper mesh to minimize secondary electron emission. The lead blocks can slide sideways to fit the isodose curves of the individual radium system.

ered at the rate of 850 rads a week. *AP* and *PA* portals must be irradiated every day with 3 to 6 Mev beam.

External Irradiation Alone

External irradiation alone is used when:

1) Vault is too narrow for colpostats or the uterine cavity is short (<2 inches).

2) The os cannot be found.

3) Stump carcinoma with poor geometry for intracavitary radium and too narrow for at least a 3.5 cm diameter cone.

4) Disease too massive for effective intracavitary radium therapy.

5) Posthysterectomy recurrent disease.

It has been shown[5] that 6,000 rads in six weeks is a minimum dose to assure permanency of control. Extended fields are used for positive regional lymphatics.

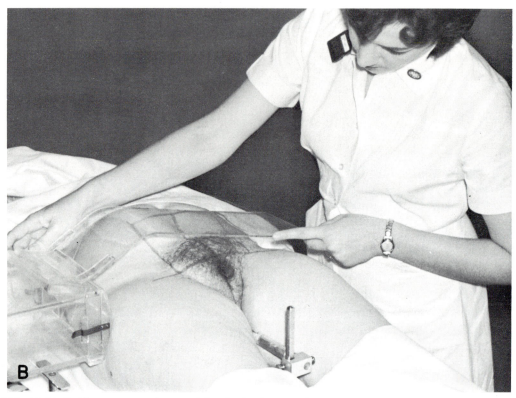

FIG. 11-24. B. The same procedure used for the localization of the lowest palpable disease is also used to determine the center of the lateral portals. A Lucite bridge used for daily treatment duplication is also shown.

For Stages I and II cases, after 5,000 rads are given with large fields, one can use 10 × 10 cm or even 8 × 8 cm portals centered over the apex of the vagina to give extra 2,000 rads. For Stage I or II cases with a small central lesion (≤1 cm) and therefore a low risk of lymph node metastases, 10 × 10 cm or even 8 × 8 cm portals are used to irradiate the vault and proximal parametria.

For Stages III$_B$ and IV cases, the portals are reduced to 12 × 12 cm from 5,000 to 6,000 rads, then 10 × 10 cm for 6,000 to 7,000 rads; for Stage III$_B$, occasionally 15 × 15 cm portals are used to deliver up to 6,000 rads.

Carcinoma of the Cervical Stump

The absence of the uterine cavity makes intracavitary radium therapy less effective than when the uterus is present because the zone of effective irradiation does not reach the end of the stump (Fig. 11-26) and radiation sources inserted up to the fundus are necessary to achieve adequate irradiation of the paracervical areas. Whole pelvis external irradiation is used to compensate for the absence of uterine radium. Since 1954, when megavoltage became available, all patients but those with very early Stage I lesions have been treated with initial whole pelvis irradiation using a 22 Mev beam.

If the disease is early and apparently limited to the lips of the cervix and the cervical canal is deep enough to accommodate at least one radium source and the vault is adequate for two colpostats, two intracavitary radium applications may be performed two weeks apart, as for carcinomas of the intact uterus. As a rule, a 25 mg source is placed in the canal.

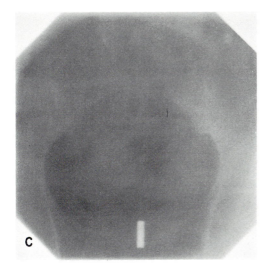

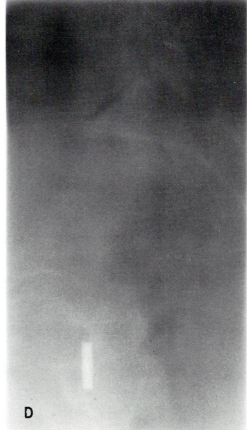

FIG. 11-24. **C.** Verification film of an *AP* portal. The four corners are shielded by triangular lead plugs.

D. Verification film of a lateral portal. The portal was moved 1 cm cephalad.

When there is no room for any type of radium source in the cervical canal, combined transvaginal therapy, with 150 Kv, and vaginal radium is used. Vaginal radium alone does not give an appreciable depth dose to the end of the stump. Transvaginal therapy adequately irradiates to a depth of 3 to 4 cm but does not give a sufficient dose to the vaginal mucosa outside the aperture of the cone. Vaginal radium supplements the dose to the vaginal mucosa.

Table 11-3 outlines the treatment schemes used to combine whole pelvis irradiation, transvaginal therapy, and intracavitary radium, depending upon the stage of the disease and the availability of residual cervical canal as a container for radium. The sequence of treatment may vary depending on the local anatomy and the extent of the local disease. For example, although the lesion calls for 4,000 rads whole pelvis first, one may use first 25 mg in the remaining canal because after 4,000 rads the canal may be too short.

Clinical Situations
Post-simple Hysterectomy

Patients seen after a simple hysterectomy for cervical cancer fall into several radiotherapeutic groups (Table 11-4 and 11-5).[6]

1) Early localized disease with apparent surgical clearance around the specimen; colpostats are applied twice for 48 hours each with two-weeks interval. If the vault is narrow 10 × 10 cm or even 8 × 8 cm parallel opposing portals are used to deliver 6,000 rads in six weeks.

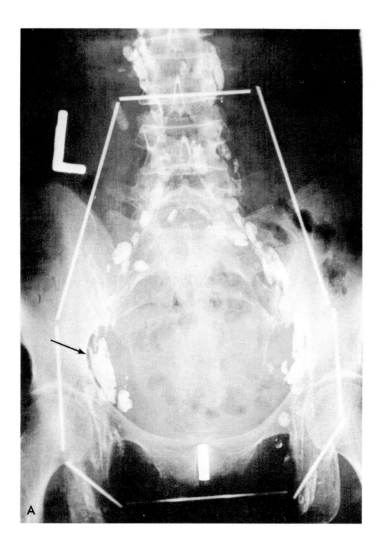

FIG. 11-25. Verification films taken with simulator. **A.** Extended fields to *L*4 (17-20 cm high) to include common iliac nodes in a patient with Stage III$_A$ disease. Oblique films of the lymphangiogram had shown involved external iliac node where the arrow points to.

2) If gross tumor is shown to have been transected at the surgical margin, 5,000 to 6,000 rads are given to the whole pelvis since tumor cells have been spread at time of surgery. This is followed by vaginal radium therapy (2,000 to 3,000 mg-hrs) or 2,000 rads transvaginal irradiation.

3) Recurrences following hysterectomy are handled by using principles similar to those guiding therapy of untreated lesions. If disease is widespread in the pelvis, 6,000 rads is given to the entire pelvis. If a recurrence is localized at the vault, 5,000 rads to the pelvis may be followed by intracavitary or interstitial irradiation, or up to 7,000 rads

with reduced *AP* and *PA* portals. A volume implant with an open bladder technique may be most effective (Fig. 11-21).

The risk of injury to the small bowel is increased since fixed loops of bowel, bound by postoperative adhesions may be re-irradiated daily. Therefore, even in cases of clear-cut surgical transection or definite pelvic recurrence where the additional risk is justified, doses of 5,000 rads are not exceeded with 15 × 15 cm portals. Depending on the extent of disease, portals from 12 × 12 cm to 8 × 8 cm are used to give a total dose of 7,000 rads. In case of a resection with no margin, the dose should be 6,000 rads.

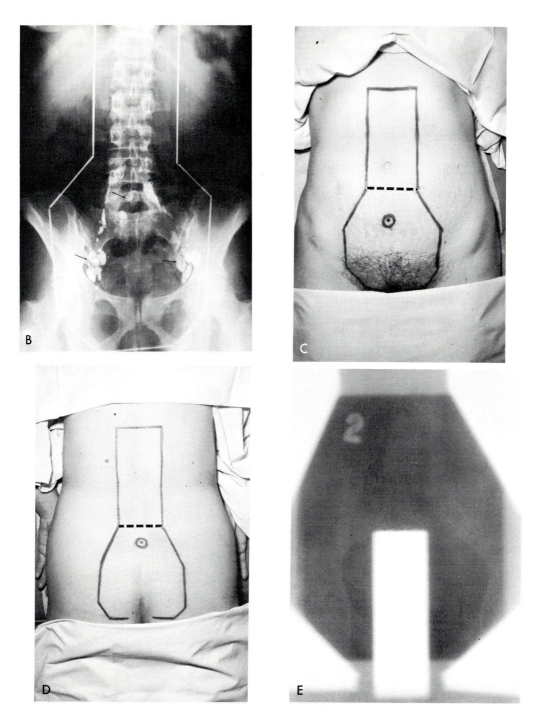

FIG. 11-25. B. Extended fields to level of diaphragm (8 cm wide over paraaortic nodes; 28–30 cm high) to include paraaortic nodes in a patient with Stage I disease. Arrows point to involved nodes.

 C and **D.** Photograph of portals. Dotted line shows the difference in the two types of extended fields.

 With extended fields, 850 rads a week are given to improve small bowel tolerance. The total dose is 5,500 rads in $6\frac{1}{2}$ weeks.

 E. Initial verification film of an extended field to L4 with central shielding. Corrections were made for size and asymmetry. This illustrates the necessity of verification films for pelvic portal. (A and B—Courtesy: Fletcher and Rutledge, In *Modern Radiotherapy*, T. J. Deeley, Ed., London, Butterworths, 1971.)

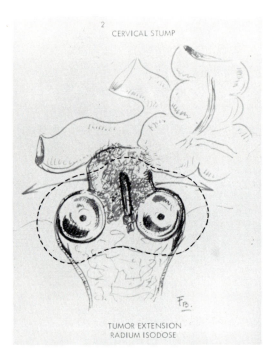

FIG. 11-26. Inadequate volume distribution with radium in the remaining cervical canal. The bowels are not pushed away by the body of uterus. (Courtesy: Wimbush and Fletcher, *Radiology,* 93, 655, 1969.)

In Situ and Microinvasive Carcinoma

Although conization or hysterectomy is the treatment of choice for these lesions, there are patients who for various reasons may be treated with irradiation. The risk of spread to the regional lymphatics is for all practical purposes nonexistent. The irradiation should be the equivalent of an extrafascial conservative hysterectomy.

Intracavitary radium alone is used, if feasible, for *in situ* lesions, one insertion of 72 hours is adequate. For microinvasive carcinoma, one may increase the dose to 2 × 48 hours which gives a dose to the paracervical areas adequate to eradicate potential small deposits of cancer cells in this proximal relay of lymphatics.

Irradiation Combined with Hysterectomy

For central bulky lesion with no fornices or parametrial involvement, 4,000 rads (4,500 rads, 850 rads per week with 4 to 6 Mev) followed by one 72 hours radium insertion are given prior to Class I hysterectomy.

If nodes are involved, 5,500 rads (850 rads per week) with central shielding after 4,500 rads followed by one 72 hour radium insertion are given prior to Class I hysterectomy.

In selected patients with a massive central lesion and some parametrial involvement, 5,000 rads at a weekly rate of 850 rads (central shielding after 4,500 rads) followed by one 72 hour radium insertion are given prior to a Class II hysterectomy.

An exenteration (anterior usually) can be performed safely after 4,000 rads (1,000 rads per week) or 4,500 rads (850 rads per week).

Modified Treatments

Modified treatment is in order for:

1) Patients with associated conditions, such as: a) Psychosis: Those patients who can benefit by intracavitary radium therapy only, have occasionally been thus treated while being kept under narcosis for periods of three to five days.

b) Coexistence of another cancer: A diagnosis of squamous cell carcinoma of the uterine cervix is occasionally made in patients with another cancer. Control of the cervical cancer may or may not be attempted, depending on the status of the other primary. For instance, even in the presence of generalized bone metastases from a breast cancer, an almost radical treatment of a uterine cancer may be worthwhile since the patient may still have a significant period of life expectancy. Conversely, if there is a diffuse carcinomatosis, the symptoms from the cervical disease may be insignificant in the over-all picture.

For lesions which are locally curable, a single 96 hour application of the radium sys-

Table 11-3. *Carcinoma of the Cervical Stump*

Stages	Whole Pelvis Irradiation††	Cervical Canal 1½″ or more†		Shallow Cervical Canal*†		Additional Parametrial Irradiation
		TV**	RADIUMΨ (at least 1 cervical source + ovoids)	TV**	RADIUMΨ (ovoids)	
≤ 1 cm		3,500 rads and	1 × 72 hrs	6,000–7,000 rads or 5,000 rads and	1 × 48 hrs	
≥ 1 cm II$_A$§	2,000 rads	3,500 rads and	1 × 48 hrs	5,000–6,000 rads or 3,500 rads and	1 × 48 hrs	2,000 rads
II$_B$	4,000 rads	2,500 rads and	1 × 48 hrs	4,000–5,000 rads or 2,500 rads and	1 × 48 hrs	
	5,000–6,000 rads∇		1 × 72 hrs	3,000–3,500 rads		
III$_A$	5,000–6,000 rads∇		1 × 72 hrs	3,000–3,500 rads		1,000 rads to 1 side?
III$_B$ IV	7,000 rads 7,000 rads					

*When no room for either radium or transvaginal cone, the whole pelvis is irradiated to 5,000 rads in 5 wks (15 × 15 cm fields), then fields are reduced to 10 × 10 cm or even 8 × 10 cm and additional 2,000 rads TD are given in 2 weeks.
†Each case is judged individually to determine whether transvaginal therapy alone or combined with radium is best. Transvaginal therapy may precede or follow radium depending upon bulk of primary and diameter of vault, etc.
Ψ25 mgm source is placed in canal; if canal is longer the treatment is like with intact uterus. If canal is not of adequate depth, transvaginal therapy is increased to compensate. If vagina is too stenosed for ovoids or transvaginal cone, a volume radium implant may be used (3,000–5,000 rads depending on dose to whole pelvis and size of volume implant).
§If the vault is narrow, the treatment is like for a Stage II$_B$ case.
∇Within each stage whole pelvis irradiation is increased as extent of disease increases (last 1,000 rads, above 5,000 rads 12 × 12 cm AP and PA portals are used and 10 × 10 cm above 6,000 rads).
**150 Kv should be used.
††With 3–6 Mev beam 850 rads per week. The total dose is increased by 10 per cent.

tem, normally used twice for 72 hours, is quite effective. This will usually produce good control of the local lesion for a sufficient period of time.

c) Other medical conditions. Marked hypertension, diabetes, and tuberculosis are rarely contraindications unless they are very severe. Changes in treatment planning may be necessary.

2) Aged patients. Patients over the age of 80, even with Stage III$_A$ lesions, are treated; but when the lesion is Stage III$_B$ or Stage IV, even if limited to the pelvis, treatment has been found to be most unrewarding.

3) Early or moderately advanced pelvic disease with distant metastases. These cases are treated by radium to control the primary lesion. If there is a solitary pulmonary metastasis, full treatment is carried out and a resection of metastasis is performed.

Palliative Techniques

For advanced lesions, no benefit is derived from even 5,000 rads.[2] At least 6,000 rads must be given to achieve even temporary control.

Pain caused by sciatic nerve involvement

Table 11-4. *Treatment Plan after Conservative Hysterectomy for Invasive Cancer of the Cervix*

Groups	Treatment Plan
Patients with microscopic evidence of invasive cancer found incidentally in hysterectomy specimen.	Local irradiation to the vaginal apex with vaginal radium in colpostats.
Gross tumor in the surgical specimen with apparent surgical clearance.	Whole pelvis irradiation to 3,500–4,000 rads followed by one 72 hour vaginal radium application or two 48 hour applications, two weeks apart.
Tumor cut through at the margins of surgical resection but no known gross residual disease.	Whole pelvis irradiation to 5,000 rads followed by one 72 hour vaginal radium application.
Patients with one or any combinations of: 1) known gross residual tumor following surgery 2) positive biopsy at the time of admission 3) clinical evidence of residual or recurrent pelvis disease referred for radiotherapy less than six months after surgery.	1) Whole pelvis alone. 2) Whole pelvis followed by transvaginal therapy or vaginal radium.
Patients with one or any combination of the above referred for radiotherapy more than six months after surgery.	1) Whole pelvis alone. 2) Whole pelvis followed by transvaginal therapy or vaginal radium.

Table 11-5. *Dosage Combinations of Whole Pelvis Irradiation with Intracavitary or Transvaginal Therapy after Conservative Hysterectomy for Invasive Cancer of the Cervix*

Whole Pelvis* (Tumor Dose** in Rads)	None	3,500–4,000	5,000	6,000†	7,000†
Vaginal Radium†† (Surface Dose in Rads)	48 hrs–48 hrs (8,000–9,000)	72 hrs (5,000–6,000) or§ 48 hrs–48 hrs (7,000–8,000)	72 hrs (5,000–6,000)	48 hrs (4,000)	None
Transvaginal Therapy (Given Dose in Rads)	6,000	4,000	3,000–3,500	2,500 3,000	None

*If small amount of cancer in surgical specimen and therefore low risk of metastases, 10 × 10 cm portals are used, the purpose of external irradiation being only to enlarge the zone of adequate irradiation around the vault.

**1,000 rads per week with 20–25 Mev; 850 rads per week with 3–6 Mev beam.

†12 × 12 cm or 10 × 10 cm portals after 5,000 rads whole pelvis.

††Times refer to time of colpostat application required to give the specified surface dose at the vaginal apex using the standard loadings of 15 mg–15 mg in 2 cm in diameter; 20 mg–20 mg in 2.5 cm in diameter; 25 mg–25 mg in 3 cm in diameter colpostats.

§Depending on extent of disease and therefore probability of microscopic cut-through and also on irregularity of apical scar which determine the depth dose from the surface of the applicators.

is rarely relieved unless considerably high doses are given. Neurosurgical procedures or alcohol blocks are preferable. In selected patients, gold grain implantation to a dose of 7,000 to 10,000 rads may produce pain relief.

Low Vaginal Metastases

Low vaginal metastases are best handled with double plane or volume implant, delivering approximately 5,000 rads in 4 to 5 days.

Metastases at the introitus may at times be satisfactorily managed with cone therapy, using 140 Kv unit, with air doses of 5,000 to 6,000 rads given in three weeks. Most of the patients die from disseminated cancer but a few do survive even if inguinal nodes are involved.[4]

Care During and After Radiation Therapy

Douches with a solution of one full tablespoon of white vinegar to a quart of warm water are prescribed twice a day during and after radiotherapy.

After treatment is completed, intercourse is advised. Patients are instructed to insert daily plastic candles up to the apex to prevent adhesions. This practice is to be maintained forever.

Approximately 5 per cent of all patients develop a superficial vault necrosis in the months following treatment. An antibiotic cream is prescribed and occasionally a power spray or a tampon saturated in Zephiran concentrate diluted 1:1,000 in glycerin. If pain is present, buccal Varidase may be helpful. These superficial vault necroses usually heal within three to six months.

Infection

Infection is now rare. If a tubo-ovarian abscess is diagnosed, it should be surgically removed prior to initiating treatment. External irradiation is then given first, irrespective of the stage of the disease. During the period of external irradiation, the cervical os should be gently dilated at least three times weekly to facilitate pyometrial drainage. Antibiotics are always given during radium application as prophylaxis against recrudescence.

Anemia

Garcia[17] has shown that cure rates are significantly lower in patients with hemoglobin levels of less than 11 grams. This clinical observation conforms with the known role of oxygen tension in radiation response.

Hemorrhage, if profuse, must be stopped as soon as possible by either transvaginal therapy or intracervical canal radium application.

Simultaneously, transfusions are given until the hemoglobin level is restored to 12 grams.

Diarrhea and Dysuria

Diarrhea during external irradiation is caused by irritation of the small bowel, and if mild, can be stopped by giving a mixture of Kaopectate, 5 ounces, and Paregoric, 3 ounces, one tablespoon, after each bowel movement and thirty minutes before meals. Also Lomotil (diphenoxylate with atropine), 2.5-5.0 mg *t.i.d.* can be prescribed. If diarrhea continues or becomes more severe, straight Paregoric is given.

Patients take Pyridium (phenazopyridine hydrochloride), 100 mg *t.i.d.-q.i.d.* for dysuria and frequency of urination.

Coexisting pyelonephritis or cystitis should be actively treated.

Nutritional Status

Patients with good nutritional status have a better prognosis. A diet adequate in proteins and vitamins should be prescribed, and occasionally high protein formulae should be used.

Iron compounds may be given if the hemoglobin is low, but if diarrhea occurs, the medication should be stopped.

Results and Complications

Results in Squamous Cell Carcinoma

The 5- and 10-year survival rates are shown in Table 11-6. In addition, data must be obtained on the three main sites of failure:

1) Central (or local) disease in the vault of the vagina or the remaining uterus or the immediate parametria.

2) Pelvic and regional lymphatic disease is disease anywhere in the pelvic structures and/or in the regional lymphatics. The diagnosis of active disease in the bladder or rectum can be confirmed by endoscopy and

biopsy. Following irradiation there is always a certain amount of fibrosis of the pelvic structures, usually bilateral. Our experience indicates that the triad of sciatic pain, hydronephrosis, and leg edema is never produced by fibrosis alone, but by active disease.

3) Distant metastases detected by usual means of palpation of the superficial lymphatics, x-ray examination, etc.

4) Intercurrent disease.

Table 11-7 shows the sites of failures in patients treated with modern technique of metavoltage therapy from September 1, 1954, through December 1963 by stages and substages.[25] Although all patients at the time of the analysis did not have 5-year follow-up, the percentage will not be changed significantly as various studies have shown that most deaths and recurrences do appear within 24 months.[34]

Table 11-6. *Survival Rates for Squamous Cell Carcinoma on Intact Uterus, Sept. 1954–Dec. 1963, 1,705 Patients**

Stage	Five-Year Survival Rate† Per Cent Megavoltage	Ten-Year Survival Rate† Per Cent Megavoltage
I	91.5	90.0
II$_A$	83.5	79.0
II$_B$	66.5	57.0
III$_A$	45.0	39.5
III$_B$	36.0	30.0
IV	14.0	14.0

Carcinoma of Cervical Stump 189 Patients		
I	97.0	97.0
II$_A$	93.0	89.0
II$_B$	67.0	67.0
III$_A$	61.0	61.0
III$_B$	32.0	32.0
IV	0	0

* Includes patients treated incompletely or for palliation.
† Modified life table.
Patients dying from intercurrent disease are excluded.
(Courtesy: Fletcher and Rutledge, In *Modern Radiotherapy*, T. J. Deeley, Ed., London, England, Butterworths, p. 11, 1971.)

Table 11-7. *Status of Disease in Patients Dead up to 5 Years—1,705* Patients with Megavoltage External Irradiation, Sept. 1954–Dec. 1963, Analysis March 1966*

Stage	No. Pts.	Pts. with Central Active Disease Alone or at Other Sites	Disease Within Irradiated Area or Complications**	DM + ID only	No Data
I	407 ⎫	1.5% (12)	4.2% (17)	24	2
II$_A$	327 ⎭		8.0% (29)	28	6
II$_B$	291	5.0% (15)	18.9% (55)	34	9
III$_A$	324	7.5% (24)	33.6% (109)	44	8
III$_B$	275	17.0% (49)	48.0% (132)	21	12
IV	81	39.0% (32)	72.8% (59)	5	—
Total	1,705†	132	401	156	37

*Includes patients treated incompletely or for palliation.
**Includes disease in the pelvis and in the regional lymphatics.
†Three cardiac patients in Stages II$_B$, III$_A$, and III$_B$ died during treatment.
DM—Distant Metastasis.
ID—Intercurrent Disease.
(Modified from: Paunier, et al., *Radiology*, 88, 555, 1967.)

Central Recurrences in Stages I and II

The incidence of central recurrences in patients with Stages I and II squamous cell carcinoma of the cervix on intact uterus treated at the M. D. Anderson Hospital from 1954 through 1963 is 1.5 and 4.5 per cent respectively, low compared with other figures cited in the literature.[1,22,23] Some of these central recurrences were late (over 5 years) having the clinical appearance of a new primary lesion.[7] This reflects the individualization of treatment for each patient with carcinoma of the cervix[8] with the sequential use of whole pelvis irradiation prior to radium for patients with bulky lesions, or with poor radium geometry.[14]

The barrel-shaped lesions, *i.e.*, the endocervical lesion with myometrial involvement account for a high proportion of the central recurrences in Stage II carcinoma of the cervix. The patients with bulky endocervical lesions who had a planned conservative hysterectomy as a part of their treatment have had a few failures.[7]

Complications in Patients Treated by Irradiation Only

URETERAL STRICTURE

Ureteral strictures which can be attributed solely to radiation fibrosis are rare. In our material, there are five partial and/or unilateral ureteral strictures which can be attributed solely to fibrosis in 1,749 patients treated from September 1954 through June 1966 by irradiation only.[29]

Troublesome Cystitis and Bladder Ulcers

These high dose effects in the bladder are generally caused by unusual proximity of the radium sources to the bladder floor, and generally seen in the very anteflexed uterus.[12] With 4,000 rads to the whole pelvis cystitis and bladder ulcers are uncommon because of the diminished radium.[3] Several severe cystitis or bladder ulcers developed in patients who had received extra interstitial gamma-ray therapy or vaginal radium in cylinders for anterior vaginal wall disease.

RECTAL ULCERS

Rectal ulcers arise from over-dosage to the anterior rectal wall at the level of the posterior fornix. They had been almost unknown until 1961 when it became a practice to use protruding sources in the vagina in the afterloading tandem instead of inserting separately tandem and colpostat.[30] A few ulcers also appeared when additional vaginal radium was used in a cylinder because of extensive vaginal disease.

FISTULAE

At least 90 per cent of the vesico- or rectovaginal fistulae have developed when there was massive central disease or extensive vaginal involvement.[30] In both instances, therapy had to be extraradical, at times with additional interstitial gamma-ray treatment in the form of sources in the vagina or interstitial implant. In a few patients, a fistula developed when a compact radium system consisting only of an afterloading tandem with a protruding source was used with heavy radium loading.

SIGMOIDITIS

The location is always in the loops of sigmoid (Fig. 11-27).[3,30] The changes range from temporary spasms of the sigmoid with some bleeding and intermittent periods of diarrhea (sigmoiditis, Stage I), to permanent narrowing (sigmoiditis, Stage II) to complete obstruction or necrosis necessitating surgical intervention (sigmoiditis, Stage III). The severity and incidence increase with amount of whole pelvis irradiation. In addition to dose, old age, previous pelvic inflammatory disease, or surgical procedures creating adhesions binding the loops of sigmoid to the uterus are significant contributing factors.[9,30] After 4,000 rads to the whole pelvis, location

of the radium system in a retroposed fashion in the hollow of the sacrum is also a factor (Fig. 11-27).

OTHER BOWEL COMPLICATIONS

With whole pelvis irradiation of 4,000 rads or more, a few patients with severe rectal bleedings have been seen without concomitant rectal ulcer or sigmoiditis. There also have been a handful of small bowel necroses, as a rule with the history of previous surgical procedures or perforation at the time of the radium insertions. Loops of small bowel bound to the uterus receive high doses which, with the already partially disturbed blood supply by the adhesions, is a contributing factor to ischemic necrosis.

MISCELLANEOUS COMPLICATIONS

There is only one instance of necrosis of the femoral head which can be attributed to irradiation. In less than 10 per cent of the patients, pelvic fibrosis has been noted repeatedly at follow-up examinations, more in the patients treated since 1959 when there was an increase of 7 per cent dose determination. This pelvic fibrosis is asymptomatic.

Vault necrosis, self-healing in a few months with conservative care, appears in a small percentage of the patients. There have been three vault necroses which were complicated with severe hemorrhage, two being fatal. In these two fatalities, the treatment had been extraradical because of massive central lesions with a higher loading than average of the radium system.

COMPLICATIONS IN STAGES I AND II

Between September 1, 1954 through June 1966, 1,030 patients with Stages I and II lesions have been treated by irradiation only.[8] In that group there are 83 patients with some type of problem, 22 of which are severe complications (fistulae, sigmoiditis, ileitis, fatal vault necrosis, ureteral stricture requir-

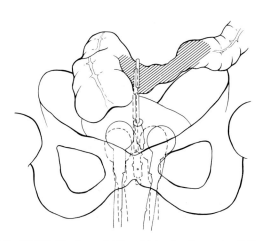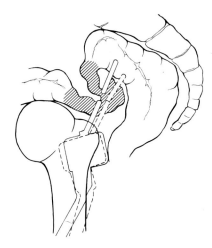

FIG. 11-27. Tracings of *AP* and lateral radiographs. Patient, age 58, with squamous cell carcinoma of the endocervix producing a barrel-shaped mass more than 6 cm in diameter. There was also positive endometrial biopsy and shortening of the right parametrium.

   The patient first received 4,000 rads in 4 weeks through 2 parallel opposing portals, 15 × 15 cm
with the 22 Mev beam. The patient then had two radium applications, the first one with a tandem
15-15-6 mg and 2 small ovoids 15 and 15 left for 30 hours. The second application 1 week later
with a tandem 15-15 and small ovoids 10-10 left for 72 hours. The total of mg-hrs was 5,580. The
treatment was completed on 11-17-61. On 9-11-62 the patient was admitted with possible bowel
obstruction with bloody discharge from the rectum. Barium enema showed a lesion in the loops of
sigmoid. On 12-4-62 there was improvement of symptoms; on 3-5-63 there was evidence of a rectal
ulcer 6 cm inside the anal opening.

   The patient had until 1964 some inconvenience with some episodes of diarrhea and constipation
and occasional bleeding. From 1965 until 4-30-68 the patient was completely asymptomatic. Diffuse
intense fibrosis in both parametria is the only finding on palpation. (Courtesy: Stockbine, et al., *Am.
J. Roentgenol.*, 108, 293, 1970.)

ing an ileoconduit). Seventeen of the 22 patients had received 4,000 rads or more whole
pelvis irradiation because of extensive central
or late Stage II disease. Some patients had
additional vaginal therapy or interstitial radium implant because of extensive vaginal
wall disease.

COMPLICATIONS IN PATIENTS HAVING HAD 4,000 RADS OR MORE WHOLE PELVIS IRRADIATION

   Eight hundred and thirty-one patients
treated between September 1, 1954 through
June 1966 received 4,000 rads or more to the
whole pelvis.[30]

   There are 46 severe bowel complications
(fistulae or sigmoiditis). If one keeps in mind

that failure to control disease locally, in the
pelvis and the regional lymphatics in those
patients having had a complete treatment
with the 22 Mev beam followed by intracavitary radium is respectively 16, 26, and 37
per cent for Stages II_B, III_A, and III_B, this
incidence of complications is not prohibitive.

AVOIDANCE OF COMPLICATIONS

   Several analyses done have indicated some
factors producing complications which can
be corrected. The use of an afterloading tandem which reduces anteflexion and retroflexion diminishes the incidence of bladder
ulcers, bothersome cystitis, and sigmoiditis
appearing at the 4,000 rad level. When the
vault is narrow and can accept only one

colpostat, it is best to use separate insertions rather than one single insertion with a linear arrangement of protruding sources. In the presence of a small radium system, one must not use a heavier loading, for instance 20-15-20, to avoid prolonged treatment times, but one should use two insertions with 15-10-10 mg sources. If, after 5,000 rads whole pelvis irradiation with 15 × 15 cm or extended fields, intracavitary radium therapy is not indicated, the treatment is carried with portals 12 × 12 cm and eventually 10 × 10 cm to 7,000 rads.

BIBLIOGRAPHY

1. Bourne, G. R., and Mead, K. W.: A proposed method of selecting patients with carcinoma of the cervix for radiotherapy or surgery, *Radiology*, 90, 139, 1968.
2. Castro, J. R., Issa, P., and Fletcher, G. H.: Carcinoma of the cervix treated by external irradiation alone, *Radiology*, 95, 163, 1970.
3. Chau, P. M., Fletcher, G. H., Rutledge, F. N., and Dodd, G. D., Jr.: Complications in high dose whole pelvis irradiation in female pelvic cancer, *Amer. J. Roentgen.*, 87, 22, 1962.
4. Delclos, L.: Analysis of 19 cases of low vaginal metastases in previously treated patients with carcinoma of the cervix or cervical stump, In *Cancer of the Uterus and Ovary*, Chicago, Year Book Medical Publishers, Inc., p. 331, 1969.
5. Durrance, F. Y., and Fletcher, G. H.: Computer calculation of dose contribution to regional lymphatics from gynecological radium insertions, *Radiology*, 91, 140, 1968.
6. Durrance, F. Y., and Fletcher, G. H.: Treatment of carcinoma of the cervix following inadequate surgery, In *Cancer of the Uterus and Ovary*, Chicago, Year Book Medical Publishers, Inc., p. 229, 1969.
7. Durrance, F. Y., Fletcher, G. H., and Rutledge, F. N.: Analysis of central recurrent disease in Stage I and II squamous cell carcinoma of the cervix on intact uterus, *Amer. J. Roentgen.*, 106, 831, 1969.
8. Easley, J. D., and Fletcher, G. H.: Analysis of the treatment of Stage I and II carcinoma of the uterine cervix, *Amer. J. Roentgen.*, 111, 243, 1971.
9. Fletcher, G. H.: Cancer du col uterin, stade III, *J. Radiol. Electr.*, (Paris), 49, 629, 1968.
10. Fletcher, G. H., Wall, J. A., Bloedorn, F. G., Shalek, R. J., and Wootton, P.: Direct measurements and isodose calculations in radium therapy of carcinoma of the cervix, *Radiology*, 61, 885, 1953.
11. Fletcher, G. H., and Calderon, R.: Positioning of pelvic portals for external irradiation in carcinoma of the uterine cervix, *Radiology*, 67, 359, 1956.
12. Fletcher, G. H., Brown, T. C., and Rutledge, F. N.: Clinical significance of rectal and bladder dose measurements in radium therapy of cancer of the uterine cervix, *Amer. J. Roentgen.*, 79, 421, 1958.
13. Fletcher, G. H., Stovall, M., and Sampiere, V.: In *Carcinoma of the Uterine Cervix, Endometrium and Ovary*, Chicago, Year Book Medical Publishers, Inc., p. 69, 1962.
14. Fletcher, G. H., Watanavit, T., and Rutledge, F. N.: Whole pelvis irradiation with 4,000 rads in Stage I and II cancers of the uterine cervix, *Radiology*, 86, 436, 1966.
15. Fletcher, G. H., and Rutledge, F. N.: Carcinomas of the uterine cervix, In *Modern Radiotherapy*, Thomas J. Deeley, Editor, London, England, Butterworth & Co. Publishers, p. 11, 1971.
16. Garcia, M.: Further observations on tissue dosage in cancer of the cervix uteri, *Amer. J. Roentgen.*, 73, 35, 1955.
17. Garcia, M.: The effect of anemia and uropathy on the curability of carcinoma of the cervix, Read before 58th Annual Meeting, American Roentgen Ray Society, 1957.
18. Graham, J. B., and Graham, R. M.: The curability of regional lymph node metastases in cancer of the uterine cervix, *Surg. Gynec. Obstet.*, 100, 149, 1955.
19. Henriksen, E.: The lymphatic spread of carcinoma of the cervix and the body of the uterus; study of 420 necropsies, *Amer. J. Obstet. Gynec.*, 58, 924, 1949.
20. Kottmeier, H. L.: Studies of the dosage distribution in the pelvis in radium treatment of carcinoma of the uterine cervix according to the Stockholm method, *J. Fac. Radiol.*, 2, 321, 1951.
21. Kottmeier, H. L., and Forssner, E.: Die Entwicklung der Therapie des Kollumkarzinoms am Radiumhemmet, *Muenchener Medizinische Wochenschrift*, 32, 1028, 1955.

22. Kottmeier, H. L.: Current treatment of carcinoma of the cervix, *Amer. J. Roentgen.*, 76, 243, 1958.

23. Kottmeier, H. L.: Surgical and radiation treatment of carcinoma of the uterine cervix, *Gynaecol. Clinic Radiumhemmet*, 43, 1, 1964.

24. Lewis, G. C., Jr., Raventos, A., and Hale, J.: Space dose relationships for points A and B in the radium therapy of cancer of the uterine cervix, *Amer. J. Roentgen.*, 83, 432, 1960.

25. Paunier, J., Delclos, L., and Fletcher, G. H.: Causes, time of death, and site of failure in squamous cell carcinoma of the uterine cervix on intact uterus, *Radiology*, 88, 555, 1967.

26. Rutledge, F. N., and Fletcher, G. H.: Transperitoneal pelvic lymphadenectomy following supervoltage irradiation for squamous cell carcinoma of the cervix, *Amer. J. Obstet. Gynec.*, 76, 321, 1958.

27. Schwarz, G.: An evaluation of the Manchester system of treatment of carcinoma of the cervix, *Amer. J. Roentgen.*, 105, 579, 1969.

28. Sherman, A. I.: A study of radiation failures and the role of radioresistance in the treatment of cancer of the cervix, *Amer. J. Roentgen.*, 85, 466, 1961.

29. Slater, J. M., and Fletcher, G. H.: Ureteral strictures after radiotherapy for carcinoma of the uterine cervix, *Amer. J. Roentgen.*, 111, 269, 1971.

30. Strockbine, M. F., Hancock, J. E., and Fletcher, G. H.: Complications in 831 patients with squamous cell carcinoma of the intact uterine cervix treated with 3,000 rads or more whole pelvis irradiation, *Amer. J. Roentgen.*, 108, 293, 1970.

31. Suit, H. E., Moore, E. B., Fletcher, G. H., and Worsnop, R.: Modification of Fletcher ovoid system for afterloading, using standard-sized radium tubes (milligram and microgram), *Radiology*, 81, 126, 1963.

32. Suit, H. D., and Gallager, H. S.: Intact tumor cells in irradiated tissue, *Arch. Path.*, 78, 648, 1964.

33. Suit, H. D., Lindberg, R. D., and Fletcher, G. H.: Prognostic significance of extent of tumor regression at completion of radiation therapy, *Radiology*, 84, 1100, 1965.

34. Suit, H. D., Wette, R., and Lindberg, R. D.: Analysis of tumor recurrence times, *Radiology*, 88, 311, 1967.

35. Tod, M. D., and Meredith, W. J.: Treatment of cancer of the cervix uteria—a revised "Manchester method", *Brit. J. Radiol.*, 26, 252, 1953.

36. Twombly, G. H.: Female pelvis in relation to cancer of the cervix, *Amer. J. Roentgen.*, 77, 796, 1957.

37. Walstam, R.: The dosage distribution in the pelvis in radium treatment of carcinoma of the cervix, *Acta. Radiol.*, 42, 237, 1954.

38. Wimbush, P. R., and Fletcher, G. H.: Radiation therapy of carcinoma of the cervical stump, *Radiology*, 93, 655, 1969.

Adenocarcinoma of the Uterus

In Collaboration with

FELIX N. RUTLEDGE, and LUIS DELCLOS

Introduction

Traditionally, adenocarcinoma of the cervix has been distinguished separately from adenocarcinoma of the endometrium. Most clinicians associate adenocarcinoma of the cervix more closely with squamous cell carcinoma of the cervix than with adenocarcinoma of the endometrium.

The late stages of adenocarcinoma of the cervix spreads upward to involve the corpus. Endometrial cancer grows downward into the cervix; when both sites are positive, the lesion is designated corpus et collum. Sometimes the site of origin cannot be established. The fractional curettage, so helpful in distinguishing cervical from endometrial cancer, yields indefinite information. A large factor of inaccuracy is introduced when the gross clinical features are the basis for determining whether the cancer should be classified as adenocarcinoma corpus et collum developing from the cervix or from the endometrium.[15,16,18] The three types of involvement are discussed together because of some common factors, best illustrated by the operative findings as shown on Table 11-8.

Disease has been found in the pelvic structures (*i.e.*, ovaries, tubes, and peritoneal surface of the pelvic cavity) in 7 per cent of the patients with endometrial cancer. In only one of 66 lymphadenectomies were nodes found to contain cancer (this patient also had tumor in the pelvic structures). This low incidence of involved regional nodes is not caused by previous irradiation, since intracavitary radium alone, as used in most patients, contributes little radiation to the regional lymphatics.

Of the patients with corpus et collum cancer, 6 per cent had pelvic structures involved, primarily resulting from implants on the serosal surface of the uterus or pelvic organs, with local lesions apparently of small size. The incidence of positive involvement of regional and paraaortic nodes is 7 per cent which is higher than for the endometrial group. This low incidence partially may result from external irradiation which was given either in the form of parametrial or whole pelvis irradiation.

The incidence of positive nodes in adenocarcinoma of the cervix only is low (2 of 57 patients had positive regional nodes; one also had positive paraaortic nodes). Here again, external irradiation, often having been given in many instances, may be partially responsible for the low incidence of positive nodes; however, it seems that adenocarcinoma of the cervix does not spread as often to the regional lymphatics as does squamous cell carcinoma. Pelvic structures were rarely found to be involved.

The relatively high incidence of involvement of the paraaortic nodes without involvement of the regional lymphatics can be

Table 11-8. *Operative Findings (Radiation and Surgery) Adenocarcinoma of the Uterus Jan. 1948 through Dec. 1964*

	Endometrium		Corpus et collum		Cervix, Stages I & II	
	Number of Patients	Dead of Tumor	Number of Patients	Dead of Tumor	Number of Patients	Dead of Tumor
Negative Uterus	145	6	35	2	28	1
Positive Uterus Only	69	7	33	5	26	5
Positive Regional Lymphatics Only	0	0	5	3	1	1
Positive Pelvic Structures*	13**	6	4	3	0	0
Positive Para-aortic Nodes	6†	5	5††	5	2	2§
Totals	233	24	82	18	57	9

*Tubes, ovaries, peritoneal surface of pelvic walls, bladder, rectum, and sigmoid.
**One also had regional nodes.
†3 also had pelvic disease.
††One had pelvic disease and one also had regional nodes.
§One also had regional nodes.
(Courtesy: Delclos, et al., *Amer. J. Roent.*, 105, 603, 1969.)

explained on the basis that the primary lymphatics of the corpus drain upward via the infundibulopelvic ligament. Thus, the first group of nodes encountered are the common iliac, lumbar, and paraaortic clusters.

Involvement of pelvic structures can perhaps be explained by tumor invading the myometrium and spreading through the serosa and/or through the fallopian tubes to the abdominal cavity.

Adenocarcinoma of the Cervix

As a rule, adenocarcinomas of the cervix are of endocervical origin. They commonly invade the myometrium and may grow to large lesions at the level of the endocervix and isthmus. This pattern of local growth allows them to remain longer in Stages I and II than do the squamous cell carcinomas. The tissues of the bladder, rectum, and ureters are more apt to be pushed aside by the expanding growth, rather than being incorporated into the cancer as with squamous cell carcinoma.

Only patients with very small lesions of adenocarcinoma of the cervix should be selected for treatment by extended hysterectomy alone. For the younger patients the ovaries may be conserved. There should be little need for a small dose of preoperative irradiation. Although the total disease, adenocarcinoma of the cervix, may be managed quite effectively by intracavitary radium and external roentgen therapy, some patients are candidates for additional conservative hysterectomy. The survival rates for Stages I and II are respectively 94.5 and 65.5 per cent as good as those for squamous cell carcinomas.[21]

The primary radiotherapeutic management of adenocarcinomas limited to the cervix is that of the squamous cell carcinomas. Because of a lesser probability of lymphatic spread, there is a tendency to accentuate local radium therapy and de-emphasize external irradiation. For example, in a Stage IIB lesion, only 2,000 rads may be delivered to the whole pelvis while the dose from radium

is correspondingly increased. There is no need for extended fields when whole pelvis irradiation is used to shrink lesions prior to intracavitary radium.

The hysterectomy is conservative; the uterus is removed without an additional vaginal cuff, with minimum dissection of the bladder, ureters, and rectosigmoid colon. As much tissue as possible is removed with the cervix, without dissecting the ureters from their paracervical position. The conservative procedure has few complications and is adequate to remove any residual cancer remaining within the myometrium. The procedure supplements the irradiation which gives an adequate dose to the vaginal mucosa and the paracervical areas, but which may be somewhat inadequate in reaching cancer cells deep in the myometrium. This type of hysterectomy would not be applicable to patients with advanced disease or would not be necessary for those very small lesions. These patients would be treated by irradiation alone.

Stages I and II adenocarcinoma on the cervical stump can be treated satisfactorily by radiotherapy only.[23] It seems that the absence of the corpus gives no opportunity for spread of disease to the myometrium.

Control of disease in the irradiated area for the Stage III adenocarcinomas on intact uterus is poor.[11] There is also a difference in the sites of failure. Whereas 90 per cent of the failures are due to regional lymphatics involvement in the squamous cell carcinomas, there is more often invasion by the adenocarcinomas of pelvic structures such as corpus, uterosacral ligaments, low vagina or diffuse spread in the pelvis.[11]

Table 11-9 summarizes the treatment planning.

Corpus et Collum

Although we customarily think of the cervix and the corpus as opposite poles of the uterus, cancer may develop at the juncture of these sites. Adenocarcinoma of the cervix regularly arises in the endocervix higher in

Table 11-9. *Adenocarcinoma of the Cervix*

Clinical Situations	Treatment
	TREAT LIKE SQUAMOUS CELL CARCINOMA
Stages I & II	Tandem and Colpostats 72 hrs × 2, 2 wks apart
SMALL LESION	?Parametrial irradiation
Stages I & II	4,000 rads whole pelvis MEDICALLY INOPERABLE
LARGE CENTRAL	Tandem and Colpostats, 72 hrs 4,000 rads whole pelvis
LESION	hysterectomy 4–6 wks Tandem and Colpostats
	post-radiation 48 hrs × 2, 3 wks apart
Stages II & III	*TREAT LIKE SQUAMOUS CARCINOMA*
PARAMETRIAL	External Irradiation 4,000 rads whole pelvis
INVOLVEMENT	Tandem and Colpostats 48 hrs × 2, 2 or 3 wks apart
OR FIXATION	or
	6,000 rads whole pelvis
	Tandem and Colpostats, 72 hrs

(Modified from: Fletcher, Rutledge, and Delclos, In *Frontiers of Radiation Therapy and Oncology, Vol. V,* Karger-Basal Publishing Co., p. 262, 1970.)

the uterus than squamous cell carcinoma. Endometrial cancer may develop in the lower segment of the corpus. Endometrial cancer spreads downward and adenocarcinoma of the cervix spreads upward, readily causing these two tumors to occupy common tissues. This confuses the diagnosis, but more importantly, the entire uterus is suspected of harboring tumor.

Both adenocarcinomas of the cervix and of the endometrium remain localized in growth process until large tumor bulk is formed before the outward spread becomes clinically evident.

Although the incidence of lymph node metastases according to stage is lower than that for squamous cell carcinoma, adenocarcinomas of the cervix and the endometrium will spread to the regional lymph nodes (Table 11-8).

Adenocarcinoma, irrespective of origin, that involves both the cervix and corpus cannot receive both standard treatments designed for each site. The total dose would be excessive and not uniform. Therefore, the cervix and surrounding structures should receive therapeutic irradiation since denuding the ureters cannot be done without risk. The corpus, in turn, should be treated surgi-

cally since it is more accessible for excision.

Because the spread to the vagina and the parametria is similar to that of adenocarcinoma of the cervix, intracavitary radium therapy is of the same type as for squamous cell carcinoma of the cervix. The Heyman packing technique is not used preoperatively; instead a tandem is used to give maximum paracervical irradiation combined with the same type of vaginal radium therapy that is used for squamous cell carcinomas.

Whole pelvis irradiation is emphasized for large uteri and/or anaplastic tumors because the chances are greater that the tumor will reach the serosal surface of the uterus. It has been shown previously that whole pelvis irradiation for adenocarcinoma of the fundus and corpus et collum is locally effective with doses from 4,000 to 5,000 rads.[7]

If there is doubt that a hysterectomy can be performed because of medical contraindications, or if the disease is so advanced as to produce a large bulky corpus, the uterus is packed by Heyman's technique (2,500 mg-hrs each packing), while vaginal ovoids irradiate the vault to the same doses as in cervical cancer. Longer fractionation is used, with as many as 3 packings at 2 week intervals. If the disease is clinically unresectable and the uterine cavity is enlarged, the Heyman packing technique may be used after whole pelvis irradiation.

Table 11-10 summarizes treatment planning for the corpus et collum cases.

Endometrium

MICROSCOPIC PATTERN OF CANCER OF THE ENDOMETRIUM

In some endometrial carcinomas, the reproduction of the endometrial glands is so complete that the tissue is quite similar to benign endometrium and is described as a well-differentiated tumor. At the other extreme, only single cells or fragments of glands suggestive of the mother structure are present; this is described as a poorly differentiated tumor. In even more severe degrees of undifferentiation, the microscopic appearance is so amorphous that the tumor cannot be distinguished from sarcoma. When the cell type is one which apparently stems from the stroma of the endometrium, the diagnosis of sarcoma can be accurately made. In approximately 15 per cent of the very poorly differentiated tumors, the pathologist has difficulty distinguishing adenocarcinoma from sarcoma.

SPREAD INTO THE MYOMETRIUM

Gusberg has observed that in tumors with a high degree of differentiation, myometrial invasion was only present in 20 per cent, whereas in Grade III tumors, it was present in more than half of the cases.[13]

SPREAD TO THE VAGINA

Vaginal metastases present when the patient is first seen, as a rule, indicate widespread disease.[20] A 10 to 15 per cent incidence of later spread to the vagina, mostly in the upper third, is reported in many series.[3,13,14] The mechanism of this spread is unknown.

SPREAD TO PELVIC STRUCTURES

Spread to the broad ligaments, the fallopian tubes, and the ovaries is common. Excision of these tissues is a necessary part of

Table 11-10. *Adenocarcinoma of the Corpus and Cervix*

Clinical Situations	Treatment	
SMALL OR NORMAL UTERINE CAVITY	Tandem and Colpostats 72 hrs and 48 hrs (Like SCC of cervix) 2 wks apart ?Parametrial Irradiation Hysterectomy, 4–6 wks	
ENLARGED UTERINE CAVITY No extension beyond uterus or cervix	4,000 rads whole pelvis Tandem and Colpostats 72 hrs (Like SCC of cervix) Hysterectomy, 4–6 wks.	MEDICALLY INOPERABLE 4,000 rads whole pelvic Tandem and Colpostats 48 hrs × 2, 3 wks apart
Extension beyond uterus and cervix	4,000–6,000 rads whole pelvis Heyman packing or Tandem & Colpostats 3,500–4,000 mg-hrs to uterus 4,000 rads surface dose to vagina	

(Modified from Fletcher, Rutledge, and Delclos, In *Frontiers of Radiation Therapy and Oncology, Vol. V,* Karger-Basel Publishing Co., p. 262, 1970.)

the surgical procedure. The frequency of occurrence of these metastases is too great to allow preservation of the ovaries even when the patient is not of menopausal age.

DISTANT METASTASES

The distribution of distant metastases is not similar to the patterns of spread from cancer of the cervix. Generalized implantation metastases on the abdominal serosa is more prevalent than in cervical cancers because the cancer penetrates the wall of the uterus and seeds the abdominal cavity. Cul-de-sac implants, masses in the omentum and ascites may signal such spread. When lymphatic spread occurs, there is a greater incidence of bypass, or skipping the pelvic nodes. The cancer may travel via the ovarian vascular drainage pathway and metastasize to the paraaortic nodes near the level of the renal vascular pedicle.

PREOPERATIVE IRRADIATION

When the uterus is of normal size and the tumor well differentiated, preoperative irradiation is probably of no value.[14]

Intracavitary radium in the uterus and the vagina,[1,3,4,16] external irradiation alone,[19,22] and a combination of both[7] have seemingly achieved equal survival rates and prevented recurrent disease in the vagina.

With the more anaplastic tumors and/or an enlarged uterus, one should emphasize whole pelvis irradiation. In the poorly differentiated carcinomas resembling sarcoma and the mixed mesodermal tumor, whole pelvis irradiation of at least 4,000 rads is given first.

Table 11-11A. *Adenocarcinoma of the Endometrium Technically and Medically Operable*

Clinical Situations	Treatment to Uterus	Treatment to Vagina
SMALL uterine cavity well-differentiated tumor	Hysterectomy only	Wide vaginal cuff
SLIGHTLY ENLARGED uterine cavity, well-differentiated tumor	Radium 1–72 hr tandem or 3,000 3,500 mg-hrs with packing Hysterectomy	Colpostats 7,000 rads surface dose in one application
MODERATELY ENLARGED uterine cavity (6–8 wks size) well-differentiated tumor	Radium 2,000 mg-hrs × 2–3 wks apart or 4,000 rads whole pelvis and radium 1 Heyman packing 2,500 mg-hrs or tandem 72 hrs with 15 and 10 mg sources Hysterectomy	Colpostats 4,000 rads surface dose × 2 3 weeks apart 4,000 rads surface dose 1 application
LARGE uterine cavity or anaplastic tumor	4,000 rads whole pelvis and radium 1 Heyman packing 2,500 mg-hrs or tandem 72 hrs with 15 and 10 mg sources Hysterectomy	Colpostats 4,000 rads surface dose 1 application

(Courtesy: Fletcher, Rutledge, and Delclos, In *Frontiers of Radiation Therapy and Oncology, Vol. V,* Karger-Basel Publishing Co., p. 262, 1970.)

Table 11-11A summarizes the policies of treatment and details of technique.

Two thousand five hundred (2,500) mg-hrs of radium are given twice in the uterine cavity, 3 weeks apart. If there is a question about performing a hysterectomy because of the patient's poor general condition, the dose is increased to 3,000 mg-hrs twice given 3 weeks apart.

Vaginal radium is an important part of preoperative irradiation. Most vaginal recurrences develop on the vault and seldom develop in the lower third of the vagina.[3,9,20] Only colpostats are used or, in case of a narrow vagina, a small vaginal cylinder. If possible, the colpostat applications are carried out at the time of the Heyman's packings with a total surface dose of approximately 8,000 rads. If the vagina is narrow, the application is done at one time between the 2 Heyman packings with 6,000 to 7,000

rads surface dose given in 72 to 96 hours. Twenty per cent lesser dose can be used for the well differentiated lesion.

RADIATION ONLY

For advanced disease, 4,000 rads to the whole pelvis followed by 2,500 to 3,000 mg-hrs to the uterus and 4,000 rads surface dose to the upper vagina, is used. If disease is very advanced, one may give 6,000 rads (reduce portal size of 12 × 12 cm at 5,000 rads) to the whole pelvis and no radium.

Table 11-11B outlines treatment planning.

Because spread to the regional lymph nodes is uncommon, 12 × 12 cm anterior and posterior portals may be used to cover the uterus and upper half of the vagina or even the whole vagina in more extensive or anaplastic lesions. Portals 15 × 15 cm are used if the uterus is too large to be included in 12 × 12 cm portals or if the tumor is very

Table 11-11B. *Adenocarcinoma of the Endometrium Technically Operable but Medically Inoperable Or Technically Inoperable*

Clinical Situation	Treatment to Uterus	Treatment to Vagina
SMALL uterus, well-differentiated tumor	TANDEM (20-15-10) 2 × 72 hrs (6,000 mg-hrs)	COLPOSTATS 4,000 rads surface dose × 2
SLIGHTLY ENLARGED uterus, well-differentiated tumor	Heyman Packing 3,000 mg-hrs × 2 or 2,500 mg-hrs × 3	COLPOSTATS 4,000 rads surface dose × 2
MODERATELY ENLARGED uterus or Anaplastic tumor	External Irradiation 4,000 rads whole pelvis Heyman packing or tandem applications—3,500-4,000 mg-hrs	COLPOSTATS 4,000 rads surface dose
LARGE UTERUS	External Irradiation 4,000–6,000 rads whole pelvis ?May add 1 or 2 radium applications depending on response	COLPOSTATS 4,000 rads surface dose if whole pelvis stopped at 5,000 rads
TECHNICALLY INOPERABLE	External Irradiation 4,000 rads/4 wks to 6,000 rads/6 wks May add 1 packing if response to external therapy is satisfactory	COLPOSTATS Surface dose 2,500–4,000 rads dose depending upon external irradiation

anaplastic because the spread to lymph nodes may be more frequent.

POSTOPERATIVE IRRADIATION

Following hysterectomy, radiation therapy may be requested. Table 11-12 outlines various situations.

Intracavitary Radium Therapy

Intrauterine gamma-ray therapy can be applied with a tandem, if the uterine cavity shows no gross irregularity and the uterus is of normal size, in one insertion of 72 hours (Fig. 11-28). In recent years, we have improved the packing method by adding an afterloading tandem, instead of the larger capsule used in the past, which allows us to choose the necessary radium to irradiate the lower segment more adequately. Furthermore, the addition of the tandem, used as a lever, decreases severe anteflexions, reducing unnecessary high doses to the base of the bladder (Fig. 11-29), or retroflexions. Figure 11-30 shows the form used for recording the intracavitary radium treatment.

The uterine cavity size is estimated by bimanual palpation. However, patients are often obese and associated uterine myomata hamper accurate evaluation. Both the shape and size of the cavity are best judged by rotating a curved probe and measuring the depth from the cervix. One then selects the most suitable size of capsules to allow insertion of 10 to 15 capsules. The use of external irradiation has been recently emphasized when the uterus is larger or the tumor is undifferentiated, therefore we used almost exclusively the No. 1 capsule, with 5 mg tubes; the exposure to the personnel involved in the procedure is reduced to half and it is easier to match the time the tubes will be left in place to deliver the vaginal surface dose from the ovoids which is aimed at 4,000 rads for each insertion.

TANDEM

If the uterine cavity shows no gross irregularity and the uterus is of normal size, Heyman's packing technique offers little advantage over a tandem either for preoperative irradiation or, in a case of medically unsuited patients, for radiation only, as the number of sources will not be significantly different. Loading of the tandem for instance, for a 3-source tandem, is 20-15-10 mg.

As a preoperative procedure in a uterus of normal size, only one insertion of 72 to 96 hours is performed. If hysterectomy is not contemplated, a 72-hour insertion followed 3 weeks later by 48-hour insertion would constitute a good treatment.

Table 11-12. *Adenocarcinoma of the Endometrium Postoperative Irradiation*

Clinical Situation	Whole Pelvis Irradiation	Vagina
Normal size uterus with well-differentiated, superficial tumor		
Normal size uterus with well-differentiated tumor, limited myometrial invasion		COLPOSTATS 7,000 rads surface dose 1 application
Enlarged uterus, Deep myometrial invasion, Anaplastic tumor, Residual disease	5,000 rads/5 weeks up to 7,000 rads*/7 weeks	COLPOSTATS 4,000 rads surface dose if external stopped at 5,000

*Reduced fields after 5,000 rads.

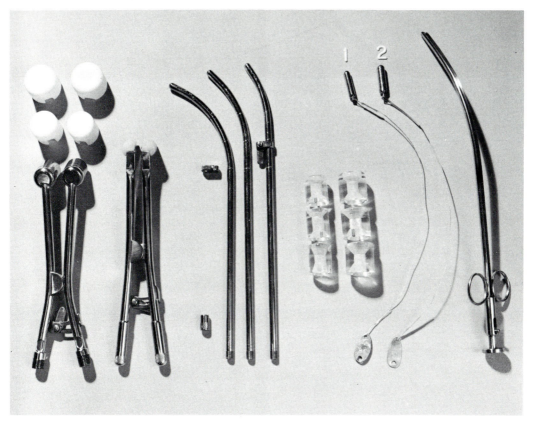

FIG. 11-28. Two sizes of Heyman's capsules (No. 1 and 2) shown with the inserter. The capsules are numbered so that the proper sequence is followed at removal. No. 1 capsules are loaded with 5 mg radium tubes. No. 2 capsules are loaded with 10 mg. The use, in recent years, of more external irradiation for the larger uterus and more undifferentiated tumors makes the No. 2 capsules almost unnecessary. In addition there is less exposure to the personnel involved in the procedure, the time is protracted and easier to match with the surface dose of the vaginal radium. An intrauterine tandem is added for a better coverage of the endocervix.

For routine preoperative vaginal radium therapy, the ovoids shown are used.

Cylinders of various diameter and size, or a combination of vaginal cylinder linked with ovoids (Bloedorn applicators) are only used in cases of already existing low vaginal spread, vagina too narrow for ovoids, or for the treatment of recurrences.

HEYMAN'S PACKING TECHNIQUE

Cancer of the endometrium often grows into the uterine cavity in an everting manner. This gross tumor will hold a tandem at an excessive distance from the tumor base (Fig. 11-31). Small irradiators can be better adapted to the distorted uterine cavity and can be arranged so that the sides and the base of the tumor mass receives more effective irradiation.

The uterus with cancer remains a distensible organ. With care it can be stretched and will then accommodate more radium containers (Fig. 11-32). Three advantages of stretching are gained:

1) A more homogeneous distribution of irradiation is delivered to the tumor mass and to the uterine wall which is apt to contain nests of cancer cells.

2) Stretching of the uterus thins the wall, thereby shortening the distance for intra-

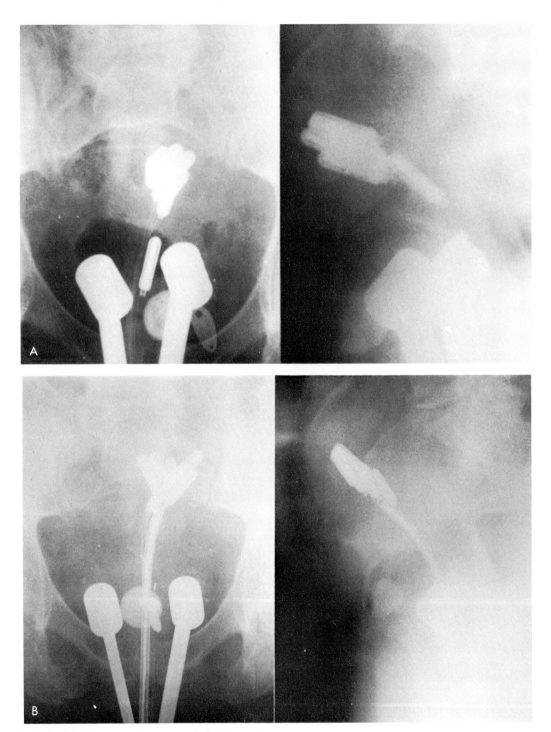

FIG. 11-29. Heyman packing with afterloading tandem.

The use of an afterloading tandem in addition to the Heyman capsules allows a better irradiation of the endocervical canal. In addition, by using the rigid tandem as a lever one decreases severe anteflexion or retroflexion, and so reduces unnecessary high doses to the base of the bladder or rectum. The tandem is loaded as required for a better irradiation of the endocervix and paracervical area (for instance 5-5-15 when No. 1 capsules with 5 mg each are used, or 10-10-15 when No. 2 capsules with 10 mg each are used).

The use of the afterloading colpostats or vaginal afterloading cylinders as indicated allows one to determine appropriate radium sources for a desired surface dose. (Courtesy: Delclos, and Fletcher, In *Cancer of the Uterus and Ovary,* Chicago, Year Book Medical Publishers, Inc., p. 62, 1969.)

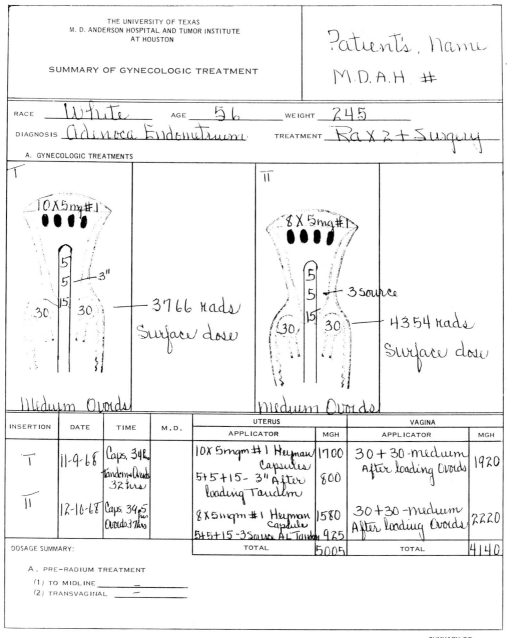

THE UNIVERSITY OF TEXAS
M. D. ANDERSON HOSPITAL AND TUMOR INSTITUTE
AT HOUSTON

SUMMARY OF GYNECOLOGIC TREATMENT

Patient's Name

M.D.A.H. #

RACE *White*   AGE *56*   WEIGHT *245*

DIAGNOSIS *Adenoca Endometrium*   TREATMENT *Ra X 2 + Surgery*

A. GYNECOLOGIC TREATMENTS

I — 10 X 5 mg # 1 — 3″ — 30 15 30 — 3766 rads Surface dose — Medium Ovoids

II — 8 X 5 mg # 1 — 3 source — 30 15 30 — 4354 rads Surface dose — Medium Ovoids

INSERTION	DATE	TIME	M.D.	UTERUS		VAGINA	
				APPLICATOR	MGH	APPLICATOR	MGH
I	11-9-68	Caps. 34 hrs Tandem+Ovoids 32 hrs		10 X 5 mgm # 1 Heyman Capsules	1700	30 + 30 - medium After loading Ovoids	1920
				5+5+15 - 3″ After loading Tandem	800		
II	12-10-68	Caps. 34.5 Ovoids 37 hrs		8 X 5 mgm # 1 Heyman Capsule	1580	30 + 30 - medium After loading Ovoids	2220
				5+5+15 - 3 Source AL Tandem	925		
				TOTAL	5005	TOTAL	4140

DOSAGE SUMMARY:

A. PRE-RADIUM TREATMENT
   (1) TO MIDLINE _____
   (2) TRANSVAGINAL _____

SUMMARY OF
GYNECOLOGIC TREATMENTS

FIG. 11-30. Form used for recording the intracavitary radium treatment.

uterine irradiation to reach the outermost layers.

3) Folds and ridges of cancer resulting from growth, may be stretched out to make the tumor flatter and shallower. The flattened tumor is then more effectively irradiated.

The two major risks in packing the cancerous uterus are perforation of the wall and rupture (split) of the cervix. The latter is unnecessary since the cervical canal does not need to be dilated to cause a tear; if proper diameters of the capsules are selected, the

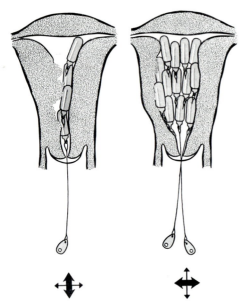

FIG. 11-31. Graphic illustration of the advantage of stretching the uterine cavity.

cervix will accommodate them with moderate dilation. With large uterus, the large endometrial cavity, where larger diameter capsules are needed, almost certainly the cervical segment can be dilated safely. Tears of the cervix occur when a capsule of excess size is forced into a small uterus.

Perforation of the uterus occurs easily. The top capsule may be forced through the fundus wall when pushed by another capsule (Fig. 11-32). If a perforation has happened external irradiation is often substituted for radium.

As the capsules are inserted, thought must be given to their removal. To make certain that capsules are removed in the reverse order of insertion, the retention wires are tagged and numbered. As they are placed, the number is recorded. Jamming of the capsules which prevents extraction rarely occurs if orderly removal is practiced.

Dosage

UTERINE RADIUM

If a hysterectomy is contemplated, 2,500 mg-hrs are given in the uterine cavity twice, 3 weeks apart. If there is a question that the hysterectomy may not be performed, the dose is increased to 3,000 mg-hrs twice, also 3 weeks apart. In cases where hysterectomy is not contemplated and the uterus is large, one uses 2,500 mg-hrs 3 times, each insertion being 2 weeks apart. Alternately 4,000 rads whole pelvis are given followed by 2,500 to 3,000 mg-hrs to uterus and 4,000 rads to vaginal mucosa.

VAGINAL RADIUM

Vaginal radium is an important part of preoperative irradiation. Most vaginal recurrences develop on the vault and rather infrequently in the lower third of the vagina.[3,9,20] Only ovoids are used; in case of narrow vagina, a small vaginal cylinder is used. If possible, the ovoid application is carried out at the time of the Heyman's packing with a total surface dose of approximately 8,000 rads. If the vagina is narrow, the application is done at one time between the two Heyman's packings with 7,000 rads surface dose in 72 to 96 hours. Table 11-13 and 11-14 are useful for quick calculation of surface doses.

Management of Vaginal Recurrences after Hysterectomy

A common site for a single recurrence is the vagina. Usually these patients' vaginas were not irradiated, otherwise, the vaginal recurrence would have been prevented. Therefore this region can now be irradiated effectively.

Individualization is made according to site. The suburethral location was not the rule in the patients referred with a vaginal recurrence.[7] Several patients had also clinically pelvic disease. A recurrence at the vault is likely to be isolated whereas in the lower third of the vagina it is usually one manifestation of disease noted.

As vaginal recurrences generally are associated with pelvic disease, the treatment

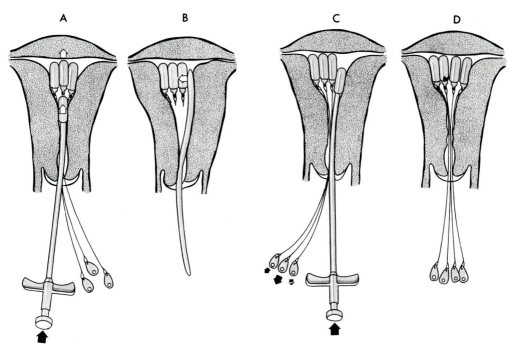

FIG. 11-32. The force exerted to find a place for another capsule must be spread broadly against the uterine wall and not through any one capsule placed before. This is prevented by holding the retention wires of all capsules in the uterus at the same level, causing them to resist being pushed forward by additional sources inserted from below.

Holding the wires firmly tends to align the capsules parallel unless the uterine cavity and its tumor masses direct them otherwise. A uterine dilator of a diameter near the size of the capsules used serves as a suitable instrument to arrange the capsules that lie obliquely and perpendicular to others so that a maximum number will be accommodated.

should be comprehensive, *i.e.,* irradiation of the whole pelvis to a minimum of 4,000 rads plus additional local treatment with the most suitable modality of radium procedure for each case. This will prevent discomfort from tumor growing in the vagina.

Vaginal recurrences in the lower third of the vagina can be treated by double plane or volume implant; often preferably with afterloading ^{192}Ir technique. Superficial recurrences located higher on the lateral wall can be treated with a vaginal cylinder. Superficial vault recurrences can be treated by transvaginal therapy (5,000 to 6,000 rads in 3 weeks), or by using a Bloedorn applicator or vaginal ovoids. Unless lesions are very superficial most of the treatment should be given with megavoltage external irradi-

ation. Portals 15 × 15 cm, 12 × 12 cm, or 10 × 8 cm, are used depending upon how widespread the disease is throughout the pelvis. The vault is identified with the cervical localizer (Fig. 11-33). With small fields, doses of 7,000 rads given in 7 weeks are well tolerated and are not fraught with late complications, because the volume of irradiated bowel and sigmoid is small.

Moderately infiltrative lesions about the lower third of the vagina may have 4,000 to 5,000 rads given with external irradiation plus a surface dose of 4,000 to 5,000 rads given by carefully individualized intracavitary applicator. At the mid- and upper levels a radium applicator suits superficial lesions. The vaginal cylinder, the Bloedorn applicator or vaginal ovoids serve well. The surface

Table of surface dose in rads per hour for three sizes of vaginal ovoids.

When the vaginal ovoids are used concomitantly with Heyman's packing, one estimates the number of 5 mg (or 10 mg) sources to deliver 2,500 to 3,000 mg-hrs in the uterus. The loading of the ovoids is determined to give a surface dose of approximately 4,000 rads to each of the two insertions. Adjustments of loading can be made up at the second insertion to approximate a total surface dose of 8,000 rads.

When the vaginal radium insertion is done separately, one can determine exactly the loading of the vaginal ovoids to give 7,000 rads in one treatment usually of 72 to 96 hours.

Table 11-13. *Metal Ovoids: Surface Vault Dose*

Small Ovoid—2.0 cm diameter								
	6 mg	10 mg	12 mg	15 mg	20 mg	25 mg	30 mg	35 mg
rads/hr	34.9	58.2	69.9	87.3	116.5	145.6	174.7	203.8
rads 24 hours	840	1400	1680	2100	2800	3490	4190	4900
rads 48 hours	1680	2790	3360	4190	5590	6990	8390	9780
rads 72 hours	2510	4190	5030	6290	8390	10,490	12,580	14,680
rads 96 hours	3450	5590	6710	8380	11,180	14,000	16,770	19,560

Medium Ovoid—2.5 cm diameter								
	6 mg	10 mg	12 mg	15 mg	20 mg	25 mg	30 mg	35 mg
rads/hr	23.5	39.2	47.1	58.8	78.5	98.1	117.7	137.3
rads 24 hours	560	940	1130	1410	1880	2350	2820	3290
rads 48 hours	1130	1880	2260	2820	3770	4710	5650	6590
rads 72 hours	1690	2820	3390	4230	5650	7060	8470	9880
rads 96 hours	2260	3760	4520	5640	7540	9420	11,300	13,180

Large Ovoid—3.0 cm diameter								
	6 mg	10 mg	12 mg	15 mg	20 mg	25 mg	30 mg	35 mg
rads/hr	16.8	28.1	33.7	42.1	56.1	70.2	84.2	98.2
rads 24 hours	400	670	810	1010	1350	1680	2020	2360
rads 48 hours	810	1350	1620	2020	2690	3370	4040	4710
rads 72 hours	1210	2020	2430	3030	4040	5050	6060	7070
rads 96 hours	1610	2700	3240	4040	5390	6740	8080	9430

dose should be 7,000 rads for a single application or 8,000 rads in 2 applications. Superficial vault recurrences can be treated by transvaginal therapy (5,000 to 6,000 rads in 3 weeks).

The long-term results of recurrences after treatment are poor because single site recurrences are rare. Vaginal recurrences generally are associated with pelvic disease. A recurrence at the vault is likely to be isolated whereas in the lower third of the vagina it is usually one manifestation of disease elsewhere.

Retreatment of the Corpus

Patients with a recurrence in the corpus following intracavitary radium therapy can be retreated safely. We have done so in several instances, using two Heyman's packings

Table for 3 cm diameter cylinders. Similar tables are available for cylinders with diameters of 2 to 5 cm.

Table 11-14. *Vaginal Cylinders—3 cm diameter Dose at 0.25 cm beyond surface*

Without Spacers			With Spacers			Name _____
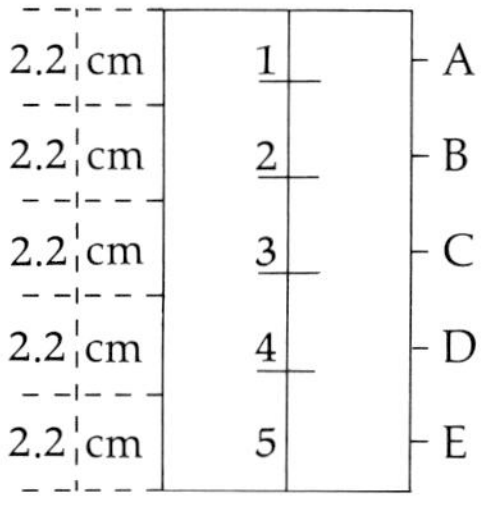 2.2 cm	1	A	2.5 cm	1	A	Hosp. # _____
2.2 cm	2	B	2.5 cm	2	B	Date of Insertion _____
2.2 cm	3	C	2.5 cm	3	C	Number of Hours _____
2.2 cm	4	D	2.5 cm	4	D	Calculated by _____ Date __
2.2 cm	5	E	2.5 cm	5	E	Checked by _____

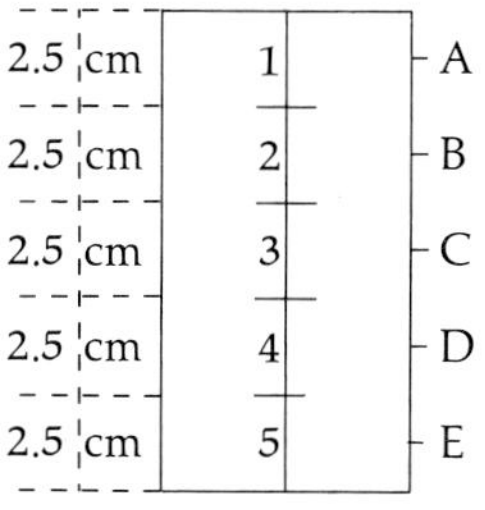

Sources without spacers

	A	B	C	D	E
Mg	rads/mgh	rads/mgh	rads/mgh	rads/mgh	rads/mgh
1	2.23	0.86	0.26	0.10	0.05
2	0.86	2.23	0.86	0.26	0.10
3	0.26	0.86	2.23	0.86	0.26
4	0.10	0.26	0.86	2.23	0.86
5	0.05	0.10	0.26	0.86	2.23

Total Dose Rate

Hrs ×
Total Dose Rate

Sources with 0.3 cm spacers (inch)

	A	B	C	D	E
Mg	rads/mgh	rads/mgh	rads/mgh	rads/mgh	rads/mgh
1	2.23	0.72	0.20	0.08	0.04
2	0.72	2.23	0.72	0.20	0.08
3	0.20	0.72	2.23	0.72	0.20
4	0.08	0.20	0.72	2.23	0.72
5	0.04	0.04	0.20	0.72	2.23

Total Dose Rate

Hrs ×
Total Dose Rate

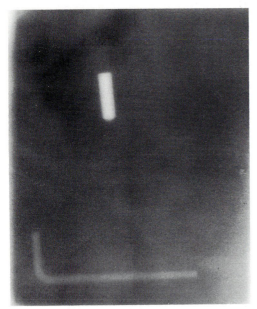

FIG. 11-33. In October 1963, patient, aged 71, had a total abdominal hysterectomy and bilateral salpingo-oophorectomy for adenocarcinoma of the endometrium. In July 1964, the patient was seen because of vaginal bleeding. Pelvic and rectal examination showed three areas of recurrence; one located at the right vaginal apex, another on the anterior vaginal wall, and a third on the posterior vaginal wall slightly above the introitus.

A tumor dose of 7,000 rads in 7 weeks was given through 2 parallel opposing portals on the 22 Mev betatron. For the first 5,000 rads the portals were 10 × 8 cm and for the last 2,000 rads they were reduced to 8 × 6 cm.

Verification films were taken with vaginal caliper placed at the apex and projection of the introitus on the surface of the body identified with lead wire. Film shows that both apex and introitus are adequately covered.

with the usual dose of 2,500 mg-hrs. No vaginal radium has been used. Worthwhile control has been obtained.

Survival Rates and Sites of Failure

The patients with adenoacanthoma have the same survival rate as those with adeno-

carcinoma exhibiting a similar clinical behavior.[2]

For the lesions limited to the cervix, the survival rates are equally as good as for squamous cell carcinoma.[21] There is no evidence in Stage I cases that the addition of hysterectomy is of benefit; however, despite the small numbers there is the suggestion that additional hysterectomy is worthwhile in Stage II cases. If no lymphadenectomy is performed, the complications of conservative hysterectomy are minimal. Therefore, when one deals with an endocervical and somewhat bulky lesion, the uncertainty of how much of the myometrium is involved justifies adding conservative hysterectomy to the plan of treatment to increase its effectiveness.

The results in corpus et collum cases are not as good as are those in patients with disease limited to the endometrium or the cervix.[8]

Concerning the endometrial cancers, review of the undifferentiated tumors for the separate group of mixed mesodermal sarcomas survival rates were superior when preoperative irradiation was used.[10] It is of interest that there were instances of tumor sterilization of mixed mesodermal sarcomas in the operative specimen.

A review of the sites of failures for the technically operable cases shows that pelvic failures were about the same in the three groups. Distant metastases are the main cause of death of patients with tumors of the corpus et collum. Vaginal metastases are rare after preoperative irradiation[5,6,9,13,17,19,20] which is also confirmed in our material. To prevent vaginal recurrences, it is not necessary to treat the whole vagina, since in the M. D. Anderson Hospital material, as in other series[9] the observed recurrences primarily are on the vault. Recurrences are rarely solitary but are but one manifestation of diffuse spread.

BIBLIOGRAPHY

1. Arneson, A. N.: Long term follow-up observations in corporeal cancer, *Amer. J. Roentgen.*, 91, 3, 1964.

2. Boronow, R. C.: Carcinoma of the corpus, In *Cancer of the Uterus and Ovary*, A Collection of Papers Presented at the Eleventh Annual Clinical Conference on Cancer, 1966, at The University of Texas M. D. Anderson Hospital and Tumor Institute at Houston, Texas, Chicago, Illinois, Year Book Medical Publishers, Inc., p. 35, 1969.

3. Chau, P. M.: in *Carcinoma of the Uterine Cervix, Endometrium and Ovary*, Chicago, Year Book Medical Publishers, Inc., p. 235, 1962.

4. Costolow, W. E., Nolan, J. F., Budenz, G. C., and DuSault, L.: Radiation treatment of carcinoma of the corpus uteri, *Amer. J. Roentgen.*, 71, 669, 1954.

5. Dobbie, M. D.: Vaginal recurrences in carcinoma of the body of the uterus and their prevention by radium therapy, *J. Obstet. Gynec. Brit. Emp.*, 60, 702, 1953.

6. Davis, E. W., Jr.: Carcinoma of the corpus uteri, *Amer. J. Obstet. Gynec.*, 88, 163, 1964.

7. Delclos, L., and Fletcher, G. H.: Malignant tumors of the endometrium: Evaluation of some aspects of radiotherapy, In *Cancer of the Uterus and Ovary*, A Collection of Papers Presented at the Eleventh Annual Clinical Conference on Cancer, 1966 at the University of Texas M. D. Anderson Hospital and Tumor Institute at Houston, Texas, Chicago, Year Book Medical Publishers, Inc., p. 62, 1969.

8. Delclos, L., Fletcher, G. H., Gutierrez, A. G., and Rutledge, F. N.: Adenocarcinoma of the uterus, *Amer. J. Roentgen.*, 105, 603, 1969.

9. Douglas, R. G.: Personal communication, 1964.

10. Edwards, C. L.: Undifferentiated tumors, In *Cancer of the Uterus and Ovary*, A Collection of Papers Presented at the Eleventh Annual Clinical Conference on Cancer, 1966 at the University of Texas M. D. Anderson Hospital and Tumor Institute at Houston, Texas, Chicago, Year Book Medical Publishers, Inc., p. 84, 1969.

11. Fletcher, G. H.: Cancer du col uterin, Stade III, *J. Radiol. Electr.*, 49, 629, 1968.

12. Fletcher, G. H., Rutledge, F. N., and Delclos, L.: Adenocarcinoma of the uterus, in *Frontiers of Radiation Therapy and Oncology, Vol. V*, A Collection of Papers Presented at the Fifth Annual San Francisco Cancer Symposium, 1969, San Francisco, California, Karger-Basel Publishing Co., White Plains, New York, p. 262, 1970.

13. Gusberg, S. B., Jones, H. C., Jr., and Tovell, H. M. M.: Selection of treatment for corpus cancer, *Amer. J. Obstet. Gynec.*, 80, 374, 1960.

14. Gusberg, S. B., and Yannopoulos, D.: Therapeutic decisions in corpus cancer, *Amer. J. Obstet. Gynec.*, 88, 157, 1964.

15. Heyman, J., Reuterwall, O., and Benner, S.: The Radiumhemmet experience with radiotherapy in cancer of the corpus of the uterus, *Acta Radiol.*, 22, 14, 1941.

16. Hunt, H. B.: Comparative radiotherapeutic results in carcinoma of the endometrium as modified by prior surgery and postirradiation hysterosalpingo-oophorectomy, *Radiology*, 66, 653, 1956.

17. Ingersoll, F. M., and Meigs, J. V.: *Proc. Sec. Nat. Cancer Conf.*, 1952, p. 747, New York, American Cancer Society, 1954.

18. Kottmeier, H. L.: Carcinoma of the corpus. Its classification and treatment, *Gynaecologia*, 138, 287, 1954.

19. Lampe, I.: Endometrial carcinoma, *Amer. J. Roentgen.*, 90, 1011, 1963.

20. Rutledge, F. N., Tan, S. K., and Fletcher, G. H.: Vaginal metastases from adenocarcinoma of the corpus uteri, *Amer. J. Obstet. Gynec.*, 75, 167, 1958.

21. Rutledge, F. N., Gutierrez, A., and Fletcher, G. H.: Management of stage I and II adenocarcinomas of the uterine cervix on intact uterus, *Amer. J. Roentgen.*, 102, 161, 1968.

22. Sala, J. M., and del Regato, J. A.: Treatment of carcinoma of the endometrium, *Radiology*, 79, 12, 1962.

23. Wimbush, P. R., and Fletcher, G. H.: Radiation therapy of carcinoma of the cervical stump, *Radiology*, 93, 655, 1969.

Tumors of the Vagina and Female Urethra

In Collaboration with

JOSEPH R. CASTRO, GEORGE R. BROWN

and FELIX N. RUTLEDGE

The treatment of the primary and metastatic tumors of the vagina and female urethra will be dealt with together in this chapter because of the similarities in treatment techniques. The management of these tumors is determined both by the extent of disease and the location.

Primary Tumors of the Vagina

Primary tumors of the vagina are usually squamous cell carcinoma, generally Grade II or Grade III lesions.[2,6,7] According to the International Classification Committee,[5] the tumor should not be allocated to the vagina unless the cervix is free of tumor or the tumor is an obvious vaginal primary extending to minimally involve the cervix but not the external os. Primary adenocarcinoma of the vagina should not be diagnosed unless adenocarcinoma of the endometrium has been excluded. Occasional rare sarcomas or tumors of embryonal origin are encountered.

The following staging classification is useful in carcinoma of the vagina:

Stage 0: Carcinoma in situ, intraepithelial carcinoma.

Stage I: The carcinoma is limited to the vaginal wall.

Stage II: The carcinoma has involved the subvaginal tissues but has not extended to the pelvic wall.

Stage III: The carcinoma has extended to the pelvic side wall or to the pubic symphysis.

Stage IV: The carcinoma has extended beyond the true pelvis, or has involved the mucosa of the bladder or rectum, or there is fixation to the pubic symphysis. Bullous edema alone of the bladder does not permit allotment of a case to Stage IV.

In Situ Carcinoma

Carcinoma in situ of the vagina may be multicentric, and often is part of a sequential involvement of different sites in the female genital tract. Nearly half of the patients seen with in situ carcinoma of the vagina at Anderson Hospital had a previous history of carcinoma in situ of the cervix. Some patients treated for in situ lesions of the vaginal vault later develop lesions in the distal vagina or vulva. Care must be taken to obtain adequate biopsies to exclude invasive cancer.

A limited lesion anywhere in the vagina may be treated locally by irradiation or excision or observed carefully. Previously, treatment policy excessively emphasized prophylactic treatment of the whole vagina, because some patients demonstrated a trait for eventually developing other carcinomata along the entire genital tract. This total prophylactic treatment by vaginectomy or whole vaginal radiation may not be required for localized lesions. A more flexible management plan is now advocated according to the size of the lesion, its location, and the patient's age[1] in order to preserve sexual function.

If the lesion is localized to the vault and the cervix is still present, irradiation can be given with an intrauterine tandem and colpostats; the vault dose is 6,000 to 7,000 rads in 72 hours or 8,000 to 9,000 rads in 2 insertions of 48 hours each separated by 1 week.

If previous hysterectomy has been done, colpostats or a specially designed vaginal applicator (colpostat(s) plus vaginal cylinder(s)—so-called "Bloedorn" applicator) are utilized to deliver 6,000 to 7,000 rads surface dose in 72 hours.

Care must be taken to avoid overdosage

which can lead to severe mucosal reaction and/or vaginal stenosis. The length of vagina irradiated is the most significant factor in later vaginal stenosis.

Only 4 of the 34 patients with in situ carcinoma of the vagina had recurrent disease in the irradiated area. Two of these 4 patients have no evidence of disease 5 and 7 years after biopsy only of the recurrent in situ carcinoma. One patient died 3 years after biopsy with intercurrent disease and 1 patient subsequently had carcinoma of the vulva and urethra following vaginectomy for the in situ vaginal recurrence. An additional 2 of the 34 patients developed in situ carcinoma below the radiation field, one on the vulva and the other on the introitus. Both were treated by surgery and have no evidence of disease at $1\frac{1}{2}$ and 8 years posttreatment.

Invasive Carcinoma of the Vagina

Stage I or Stage II lesions of the upper vagina are treated with techniques similar to that for carcinoma of the cervix. External irradiation is utilized first to flatten the lesion and render intracavitary irradiation effective since the radiation dose from cylindrical vaginal applicators falls off sharply. The usual dose is 4,000 rads in 4 weeks with the 22 Mev photon beam. Providing the vault is adequate, vaginal ovoids (plus intrauterine tandem if the cervix is present) can then be utilized to deliver vaginal surface doses in the range of 8,000 rads in 2 applications of 48 hours each separated by 2 weeks.

Stage I or Stage II carcinomas of the vaginal walls or introitus are best treated by interstitial irradiation, (Fig. 11-34), either ra-

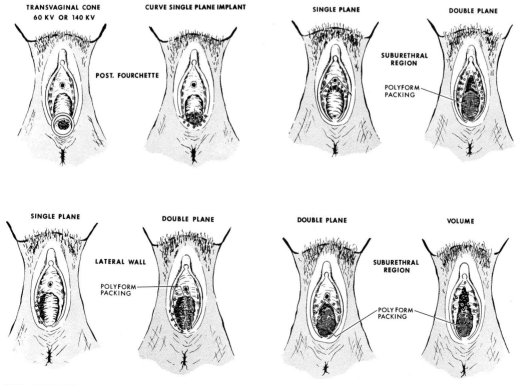

FIG. 11-34. Tumors on the introitus. (Courtesy: Chau, *Amer. J. Roentgen.,* 89, 502, 1963.)

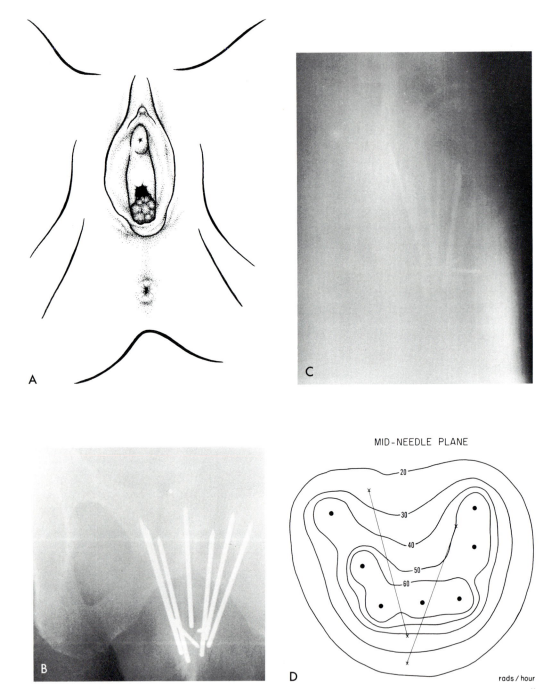

FIG. 11-35. A. Fifty-one year old white female with invasive squamous carcinoma, arising in the posterior wall of the vagina. The lesion was approximately 1 to 1.5 cm in thickness. **B.** *AP* radiograph of radium needle implant using 4.5 cm active length needles of 0.5 mg/cm intensity; 2.0 cm needles (0.66 mg/cm) were used to cross the distal end of the implant. **C.** Lateral radiograph of the same implant. **D.** The volume enclosed within the 45 rad/hr isodose received 6,500 rads in 145 hours. The patient had a persistent posterior rectal ulcer for several years with eventual biopsy proven recurrence at 5½ years posttreatment, excised with surgically clear margins.

dium needle or [192]Iridium wire implant. Planning must be individualized depending on the extent and thickness of the lesion. Single (Fig. 11-35) or double plane implants or, in some instances, volume implants may be used. Preneedling external irradiation is given in the amount of 2,000 to 4,000 rads in 2 to 4 weeks to thick lesions to flatten the tumor allowing an implant to be more effective. Often the lesion is too long for radium needles of 4.5 cm active length. Stainless steel hollow needles of greater length (4.5–8 cm) after-loaded with [192]Iridium wire (Fig. 11-36) provide more effective coverage. An Ivalon sponge packing placed in the vagina allows volume implants to be performed more effectively since some needles are placed in the vaginal packing to complete the volume distribution. If the lesion reaches the vault near the base of the bladder, a suprapubic cystotomy allows one finger to be placed in the bladder to provide accurate guidance for implantation of the needles through the vagina and near the base of the bladder without puncturing it.

Doses in the range of 6,000 to 7,000 rads in 5 to 7 days are given if the treatment is entirely by interstitial irradiation. When preneedling external irradiation is given first, 2,000 to 4,000 rads in 2 to 4 weeks preferably with the 22 Mev betatron (photon beam) are given through anterior and posterior fields

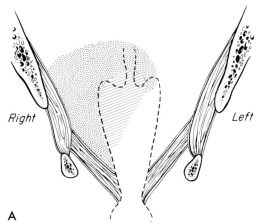

FIG. 11-36. A. This 47-year-old white female had a previous hysterectomy for carcinoma *in situ* of the cervix, followed by partial vaginectomy for carcinoma *in-situ* of the vaginal vault. An invasive squamous carcinoma of the vagina then developed and infiltrated the right parametrium and was fixed to the right pelvic wall.

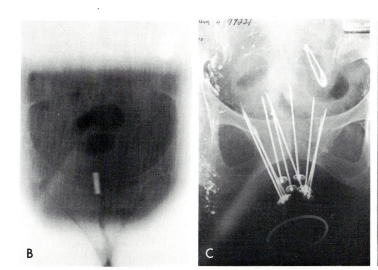
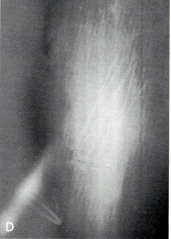

FIG. 11-36. B. Five thousand rads in 5 weeks were given through *AP-PA* portals with the 22 Mev betatron (photon beam).

C, D. Anterior and posterior radiographs of an ^{192}Ir implant which delivered 3,000 rads in 94 hours. Seven and 8 cm length needles were required because of the extent of the lesion.

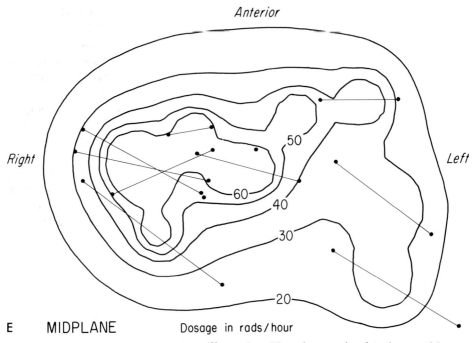

FIG. 11-36. E. Isodose distribution around the ^{192}Ir implant. The volume enclosed in the 32 rad/hour isodose received 3,000 rads.

followed by an additional 4,000 to 5,000 rads in 3 to 5 days from the interstitial needling. External radiation portals are localized using a lead-tipped Lucite probe to mark the inferior limit of the tumor (Fig. 11-37).

Stage III and Stage IV lesions may require treatment entirely with external irradiation. As much of the pelvic lymphatics as is possible should be covered by the radiation portals since larger tumors have a greater chance of lymphatic metastases. AP-PA 15 × 15 cm fields are used for the initial 5,000 rads, followed by reduction to 10 × 10 cm or 10 × 12 cm fields over the residual tumor for an additional 1,000 to 2,000 rads. When feasible, external irradiation is stopped at 5,000 rads and an interstitial implant is performed to deliver an additional 2,500 to 3,000 rads in 3 to 4 days. An extra plane of needles may be required in the paracolpos if the lesion extends to the pelvic wall. The results of treatment for invasive carcinoma of the vagina are shown in Table 11-15 and Table 11-16.

Table 11-15. *Sites of Failure in Vaginal Tumors*

Clinical Stage	Number of Patients	Recurrence in Treated Area	New Disease Below Treated Areas
0	34	4	2
I	21	2	
II	26	3	
III	16	4	
IV	13	7	

Mesonephric Adenocarcinoma

Occasionally primary adenocarcinoma of the vagina is found to arise from mesonephric duct remnants. Six such patients have been treated with techniques ranging from interstitial radium implants for lesions of 0.5 to 1.5 cm thickness to combinations of external irradiation and radium needling for bulky and infiltrating lesions. The interstitial radiation dose is 6,000 to 7,000 rads in 4 to

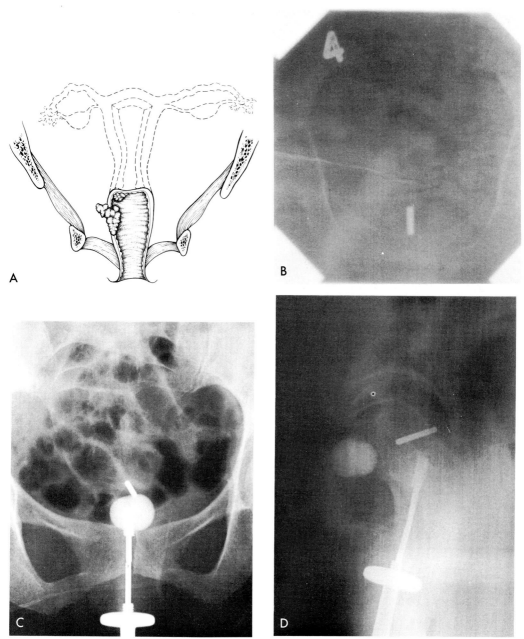

FIG. 11-37. **A.** Fifty-two year old white female with previous hysterectomy for endometrial hyperplasia. She presented with an exophytic squamous carcinoma of the right vaginal wall with right paravaginal infiltration. (Stage II)

    B. Four thousand rads in 4 weeks were given with *AP-PA* 15 × 15 cm 22 Mev betatron portals (photon beam). A lead-tipped Lucite rod was used to localize the lesion. Almost the entire remaining vagina was irradiated. An additional 2,000 rads dose in 2 weeks was given with reduced (12.5 × 9 cm) fields over the vagina and right paracolpos.

    C, D. *AP* and lateral films of the intracavitary radium application with a specially designed vaginal applicator (colpostat(s) and vaginal cylinder(s)) which delivered 2,000 rads surface dose in 27 hours. Patient was alive with no evidence of tumor 4 years posttreatment.

Table 11-16. *5-Year Survival of Patients with Invasive Squamous Cell Carcinoma of Vagina*

Clinical Stage	Absolute Survival	Intercurrent Disease	Lost to Follow-up	Determinate Survival
I	11/16 (69%)	2	1	11/13 (85%)
II	13/19 (68%)	1	1	13/17 (76%)
III	4/15 (27%)	5		4/10
IV	0/11	2		0/9

5 days. Four thousand rads in 4 weeks with the 22 Mev photon beam through opposed anterior and posterior portals have been utilized in larger tumors followed by an additional 3,000 to 4,000 rads in 3 to 4 days with radium needling.

These 6 patients have no evidence of tumor from 37 to 84 months posttreatment. Four patients were treated entirely with irradiation; 1 patient had vaginectomy following 5,000 rads tumor dose in 5 weeks with the 22 Mev betatron and 1 patient was treated by anterior exenteration. Although this group of patients with primary vaginal mesonephric adenocarcinoma is small, the results suggest that irradiation is to be preferred over mutilating surgery.

Metastatic Carcinoma of the Vagina

Metastases from adenocarcinoma of the endometrium occur in the following order of frequency:

1) Vaginal vault.
2) Distant third of the vagina near introitus and/or urethra.
3) Vaginal walls.

Metastases appearing in the distal third of the vagina or at the introitus are usually a sign of disseminated disease. However, local control of the lesion is useful in preventing distressing, painful tumor growth with bleeding. Interstitial irradiation techniques are utilized for introital lesions delivering doses of 6,000 to 7,000 rads in 4 to 5 days.

Metastases in the upper vaginal walls or vaginal vault are best treated by external irradiation using limited *AP-PA* portals of 8 × 8 or 10 × 10 cm to deliver doses of 4,000 to 5,000 rads in 4 to 5 weeks. Supplemental interstitial radium may be added at times with a suprapubic cystotomy to deliver an additional 3,000 to 4,000 rads mucosal dose.

Although local control of vaginal metastases is usually obtained, the ultimate outlook is poor because of the frequency of other metastases.[3]

Squamous carcinoma of the cervix rarely shows metastases to the distal one third of the vagina.[4] These patients are treated with interstitial techniques since the upper vagina has previously usually been irradiated. Most of these patients may be significantly palliated but almost all die from other distant metastases and/or pelvis disease.

Carcinoma of the Female Urethra

Tumors of the female urethra are usually squamous or transitional cell carcinomas. Classification by treatment technique and location is shown in Table 11-17. Thirty-seven such patients were treated during the period from 1948 through 1967[8] with local control in 18 of these patients (Table 11-18).

Table 11-17. *Treatment and Location of Carcinoma of the Urethra*

	Limited to Anterior Urethra	Entire Urethra Periurethral Extension	Urethra + Vulva	Urethra + Bladder Neck	Urethra Vulva Bladder Neck
Interstitial	8	—	2	1	—
External only	2	4	2	2	1
External, interstitial and/or intracavitary	2	3	—	6	—
Surgery only for primary	1	1	—	1	1

Treatment techniques included: 1) Surgical excision for small lesions at the external meatus. 2) Interstitial implants for small- or moderate-sized lesions of the distal urethra. 3) Combinations of external irradiation and interstitial implants for extensive tumors or if the tumor invaded the bladder neck, treatment entirely by external irradiation. The tumor doses range from 5,000 to 7,000 rads in 4 to 7 days if treated entirely by interstitial irradiation. Four thousand to 5,000 rads in 4 to 5 weeks were given with opposed *AP-PA* 22 Mev photon beam portals, or [60]Cobalt perineal field, followed by 3,000 to 4,000 rads from radium needling. A few patients received 5,000 to 7,000 rads in 5 to 7 weeks entirely by external irradiation.

Techniques of implantation were similar to those of carcinoma of the vagina. An open bladder implant is necessary for lesions occupying the proximal aspect or entire length of the urethra. This affords direct visualization of extension into the bladder, in which case, external radiotherapy may be preferred to interstitial therapy. If the tumor is suitable for implantation, a finger placed

Table 11-18. *Local Control vs. Primary Site and Extent in Patients at Two Years in Carcinoma of the Urethra February 1948–December 1967*

Location of Primary Tumor	Number of Patients	Control in Treated Area	Sites of Failure				Unknown
			Urethra	Vagina	Bladder Neck	Urethra + Bladder Neck	
Limited to distal urethra	11	7	3				1§
Entire urethra + periurethral extension	9	1	6	1†			1
Urethra + vulva	4	2	2				
Urethra + bladder neck	11	6*				5	
Urethra, vulva + bladder neck	2	1†				1	
Totals	37	17	11	1		6	2

*Two patients treated only by surgery (local excision).
†Anterior exenteration.
§Controlled to death at 5 months.

in the bladder guides the radium needles which are inserted through the vagina.

Urethral function following radiotherapy is good providing local control is achieved. The best local control occurs in small-to-moderate-sized lesions of the anterior urethra. Extension to bladder, vulva or extensive paraurethral infiltration worsens the outlook.

BIBLIOGRAPHY

1. Brown, G. R., Fletcher, G. H., Rutledge, F. N.: Irradiation of *"in situ"* and invasive squamous cell carcinomas of the vagina, *Cancer*, 28, 1278, 1971.
2. Chau, P. M.: Radiotherapeutic management of malignant tumors of the vagina, *Amer. J. Roentgen.*, 89, 502, 1963.
3. Delclos, L., Fletcher, G. H.: Malignant tumors of the endometrium: evaluation of some aspects of radiotherapy, *Cancer of the Uterus and Ovary*, Year Book Medical Publishers Inc., p. 62, 1969.
4. Delclos, L.: Analysis of nineteen cases of low vaginal metastases and previously treated patients with carcinoma of the cervix or cervical stump, *Cancer of the Uterus and Ovary*, Year Book Medical Publishers, Inc., p. 331, 1969.
5. Kottmeier, H. L.: Problems relating to classification and stage grouping of malignant tumors in the female pelvis, *Cancer of the Uterus and Ovary*, Year Book Medical Publishers Inc., p. 25, 1966.
6. Livingstone, R. G.: *Primary Carcinoma of the Vagina*, Springfield, Illinois, Charles C Thomas, 1950.
7. Rutledge, F.: Cancer of the vagina, *Am. J. Obstet. & Gynec.*, 97, 635, 1967.
8. Taggart, C. E., Castro, J. R., and Rutledge, F. N.: Carcinoma of the female urethra, *Amer. J. Roentgen.*, 114, 145, 1972.

Tumors of the Ovary

LUIS DELCLOS, and JULIAN P. SMITH

Most of the reports in the medical literature have grouped all ovarian cancers together and/or have frequently utilized one of several different staging schemes in reporting the results of treatment.[11,9,17] This means that the treatment results of the epithelial cancers of the ovary, the most common ovarian malignancies, have been confused by the treatment results of the uncommon malignancies, and the results of treatment often cannot be compared due to the different staging schemes. Because of the wide variation in 1) malignancy, 2) sensitivity to ionizing radiation, 3) sensitivity to chemotherapy, and 4) pathways of metastases, the several groups of ovarian cancers such as the epithelial cancers, the stromal cancers, and the germ cell cancers should be considered separately. The Cancer Committee of the International Federation of Gynecology and Obstetrics have recognized this problem and have proposed a staging (Table 11-19) and histologic classification (Table 11-20) that should lead to more uniformity in our evaluation of results of the treatment of ovarian cancer.[1]

Since the ovaries are confined within the bony pelvis, most patients are unaware of their tumors until the neoplasm enlarges enough to extend into the abdomen, causes ascites or produces some hormonal abnormality. This period of silent intrapelvic growth allows ovarian cancers to spread beyond the ovary to adjacent pelvic or abdomi-

Table 11-19. *Stage-Grouping for Primary Carcinoma of the Ovary**

(To be used from January 1, 1971)

Stage I: Growth limited to the ovaries.

Stage I_A: Growth limited to one ovary; no ascites; (1) capsule ruptured, (2) capsule not ruptured.

Stage I_B: Growth limited to both ovaries; no ascites; (1) capsule ruptured, (2) capsule not ruptured.

Stage I_C: Growth limited to one or both ovaries; ascites present with malignant cells in the fluid; (1) capsule ruptured, (2) capsule not ruptured.

Stage II: Growth involving one or both ovaries with pelvic extension.

Stage II_A: Extension and/or metastases to the uterus and/or tubes and/or other ovary.

Stage II_B: Extension to other pelvic tissues.

Stage III: Growth involving one or both ovaries with widespread intraperitoneal metastases.

Stage IV: Growth involving one or both ovaries with distant metastases.

Special Category:

      Unexplored cases which are thought to be ovarian carcinoma.

*From: The Cancer Committee of the International Federation of Gynecology and Obstetrics (January 1971).

nal viscera before they are discovered. Eighty per cent of the patients with ovarian cancer when first seen at this institution have cancer spread beyond the ovary (Stage II) and 69 per cent have cancer spread into the abdomen (Stage III).

Most of the patients referred to The University of Texas M. D. Anderson Hospital and Tumor Institute at Houston with ovarian cancer have had surgery by the referring physician with removal of as much of the ovarian tumor as possible. An occasional patient has had only a unilateral oophorectomy before her referral because the referring physician was unaware of the diagnosis or was not acquainted with the frequency of

bilateral ovarian involvement in most patients with ovarian cancers. Patients with one of the common epithelial cancers who only have had an oophorectomy before referral and who have cancer limited to the ovary will have removal of the opposite ovary and the uterus before receiving radiotherapy or chemotherapy.

Table 11-20. *Histologic Classification of the Common Primary Epithelial Tumors of the Ovary**

I. *Serous cystomas.*
   a) Serous benign cystadenomas.
   b) Serous cystadenomas with proliferating activity of the epithelial cells and nuclear abnormalities but with no infiltrative destructive growth (low potential malignancy).
   c) Serous cystadenocarcinomas.

II. *Mucinous cystomas.*
   a) Mucinous benign cystadenomas.
   b) Mucinous cystadenomas with proliferating activity of the epithelial cells and nuclear abnormalities but with no infiltrative destructive growth (low potential malignancy).
   c) Mucinous cystadenocarcinomas.

III. *Endometrioid tumors* (similar to adenocarcinomas in the endometrium).
   a) Endometrioid benign cysts.
   b) Endometrioid tumors with proliferating activity of the epithelial cells and nuclear abnormalities but with no infiltrative destructive growth (low potential malignancy).
   c) Endometrioid adenocarcinomas.

IV. *Mesonephric tumors.*
   a) Benign mesonephric tumors.
   b) Mesonephric tumors with proliferating activity of the epithelial cells and nuclear abnormalities but with no infiltrative destructive growth (low potential malignancy).
   c) Mesonephric cystadenocarcinomas.

V. *Concomitant carcinoma, unclassified carcinoma* (tumors which cannot be allotted to one of the groups I, II, III or IV).

*From: The Cancer Committee of the International Federation of Gynecology and Obstetrics (January 1971).

Epithelial Tumors

Except for the pure dysgerminomas, the other malignant ovarian tumors have a limited sensitivity to ionizing radiation and require relatively high doses of radiation to kill the tumor cells.

The müllerian or epithelial cancers of the ovary (serous, mucinous, undifferentiated adenocarcinoma, endometrioid, and mesonephric) account for 86.3 per cent of the ovarian cancers seen at this institution and 85.4 per cent (Table 11-21) of the tumors treated with irradiation. Since these cancers comprise the majority of the malignant tumors of the ovary, probably arise from the same stem cells, respond similarly to irradiation and chemotherapy, and spread by similar mechanism, they should be considered separately from the other ovarian cancers of stromal or germ cell origin. Although the epithelial cancers behave similarly, they exhibit a different degree of malignancy, the mucinous cancers having the best prognosis and the undifferentiated adenocarcinomas having the poorest prognosis.

At this institution, the diagnosis of mesonephric or endometrioid cancers[2,3,4,8,10,12,13,14,15] of the ovary is seldom made, as these two cancers are considered variants of serous carcinomas.

Treatment Policy and Techniques

The primary treatment for all ovarian carcinomas is surgical excision. All patients with suspected ovarian tumor should have an exploratory laparotomy to establish the diagnosis. Borderline malignancies are treated with surgery only, unless they have spread beyond the ovaries. Although, in most patients it will not be possible to completely remove all the tumor, it is beneficial to remove as much tumor as possible without removing the adjacent viscera such as the colon or bladder, leaving only small aggregates of malignant cells, which are more radiosensitive than larger masses. Larger

Table 11-21. *M. D. Anderson Hospital and Tumor Institute Distribution of Ovarian Cancers by Histology Treated by Surgery and Postoperative Irradiation July 1947–Dec. 1967*

Histology	Per Cent
Serous*	62.7
Mucinous	10
Undifferentiated adenocarcinoma	12.7
Others	14.6

*Endometrioid and mesonephric are included in this group.

unresectable tumor masses are better treated with chemotherapy[16] as will be discussed later. The location of the tumor remaining after surgery is also important in planning postoperative treatment. Tumor masses in front or behind the liver or overlying the kidneys cannot be irradiated effectively because of the limited tolerance of these structures to irradiation.

Patients with small amounts of residual tumor following surgery should receive irradiation to the entire abdomen plus additional irradiation to the pelvis, because the abdomen and the pelvis are a continuous cavity and once tumor cells are free in this cavity, they do not remain in the pelvis. Twelve of 20 patients with cancer originally confined to the ovary (Stage I) and 35 of 87 patients with cancer outside of the ovary but confined to the pelvis (Stage II) developed metastatic cancer in the abdomen (Table 11-22) above the pelvis.

The [60]Co Moving Strip Technique

When irradiation is delivered through large portals (Fig. 11-38), marked systemic reactions can be avoided only by protraction of treatment. Often treatment has to be interrupted because of nausea, diarrhea, malaise, or depression of the blood count; a tumor dose of 3,000 rads calls for 5 to 6 weeks of

Table 11-22. *Site of Recurrence of Ovarian Cancer by Stage (260 Patients with Recurrent Cancer after Irradiation)*
July 1947–Dec. 1967

Site of Recurrence	Stage I	Stage II	Stage III	Stage IV	Unknown	Total
Abdomen only	4	6	13	0	1	24
Abdomen and pelvis	8	29	91	6	1	135
Pelvis only	4	30	16	2	0	52
Distant metastases alone or with abdominal disease.	1	16	10	4	0	31
Site Unknown	3	6	9	0	0	18
Total	20	87	139	12	2	260

treatment. It is unlikely that this dose of irradiation will be lethal to the epithelial cancers. The "moving strip" technique (5) allows the delivery of a tumor dose of 2,600 to 2,800 rads in 12 doses. This technique can be used with any megavoltage unit by proper correction of the depth dose and penumbra effect provided the beam is wide enough to cover the abdomen from side to side.

The abdomen, or the volume to be irradi-ated, is divided into contiguous segments, or "strip" of 2.5 cm (Fig. 11-39). To avoid the edge effect and therefore improve the toler-ance, our present practice is to treat front and back daily (Fig. 11-40). The treatment field is increased by 1 strip every 2 days until 4 strips (10 cm) have been treated. Then the 10 cm segment (Fig. 11-41) is moved up every 2 days (2.5 cm), until the last strip is reached. The field is then reduced progres-

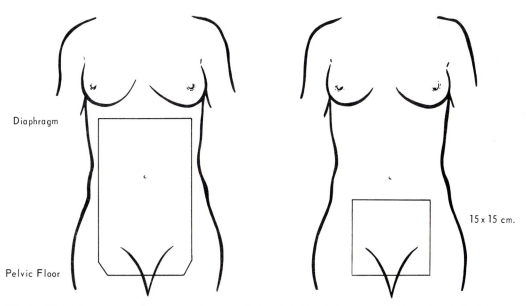

Diaphragm

Pelvic Floor

15 x 15 cm.

FIG. 11-38. Volume covered with megavoltage irradiation. Left: Parallel opposing fields to the whole abdomen with open fields. A dose of 3,000 rads in 5 to 6 weeks can be given with proper shielding of the kidneys and liver. Right: Pelvic irradiation (15 × 15 cm fields). Lower border at midpubis for adequate coverage of pelvis floor.

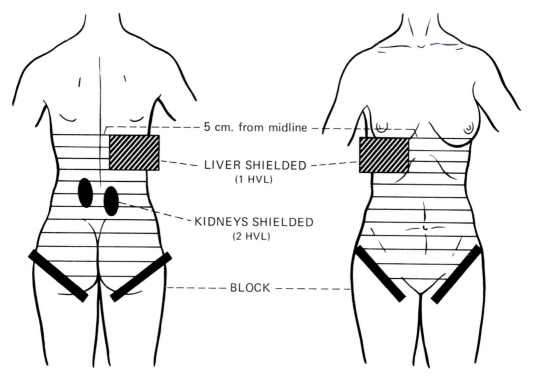

5 cm. from midline

LIVER SHIELDED
(1 HVL)

KIDNEYS SHIELDED
(2 HVL)

BLOCK

FIG. 11-39. Volume covered with the megavoltage moving strip technique.

    The kidneys are shielded from the posterior beam by 2 *HVL* of lead placed on a satellite platform (this will reduce the dose to the kidneys to about 50 per cent of the tumor dose). The right side of the liver (3 strips) is shielded both front and back with 1 *HVL* of lead.

    To compensate for the lower dose at both ends of the irradiated volume, we start one strip below the lower margin of the pelvic field (which is placed at midpubis) and complete the treatment one strip above the diaphragm.

sively by 1 strip (2.5 cm). On the last 2 days of treatment a single 2.5 cm strip is irradiated.

    With this technique, each strip of the abdomen is irradiated 8 days from the front and back by the main beam and 4 days by the penumbra, a total of 12 days of irradiation. It requires 30 to 40 days to treat the entire abdomen from the pelvic floor to the diaphragm. A tumor dose of 2,600 to 2,800 rads, measured at the midline along a saggital plane, can be delivered safely. This dose to the tumor has a greater biological effect because it is given in a shorter time than with the static field technique.

    Since only a small portion of the abdominal cavity is irradiated at any one time the

treatment is well tolerated.[6] It has been found that the patient's weight remains unchanged during the treatment despite the nausea and diarrhea. The hemoglobin and hematocrit remains also unchanged but on the first 2 weeks of treatment the lymphocytes and platelets drop to about 60 per cent of their initial values. After the second week there is a slow decrease in values, both returning to normal after completion of treatment (Fig. 11-42). Diarrhea usually begins during the second week of treatment and then decreases as the treatment field moves up the abdomen. Nausea is most common in the fifth or sixth week while irradiating the upper abdomen.

    The kidneys are shielded from the back

with 2 half value layers of lead (Fig. 11-39 and 11-41B), which reduces the dose to the kidneys by 50 per cent.

In the majority of patients, the liver has been either partially excluded or it was in the area of fall-off in the upper edge of the irradiated area. Because cancer developed under the diaphragm in one patient, the whole liver was included in the treatment fields in 1965. Several cases of radiation hepatitis, some fatal, occurred in these patients.[7,18] Since July 1967, the right side of the liver both front and back is partially shielded (Fig. 11-39). Since 1970, one half value layer of lead is used.

An additional 2,000 rads in 2 weeks is given to the pelvis with the 22 Mev betatron (photon beam) through parallel opposing 15 × 15 cm portals before the abdominal irradiation (Fig. 11-38).

Results

Thirteen patients with Grade I cancer of the ovary had tumors that were confined to one ovary (Stage I_A). All of these patients survived 2 years regardless of the irradiation treatment they received. Eleven of these patients were treated more than 5 years ago and all have survived 5 years without evidence of recurrence. The results of treatment in these patients with Grade I lesions suggest that these tumors of low grade malignancy are not truly malignant and do not require additional treatment after removal of both ovaries. Eighty-four per cent of patients with Grade II or Grade III, Stage I_A cancers survived 2 years after receiving postoperative irradiation, and 81 per cent survived over 5 years.

Our data provide a unique opportunity to

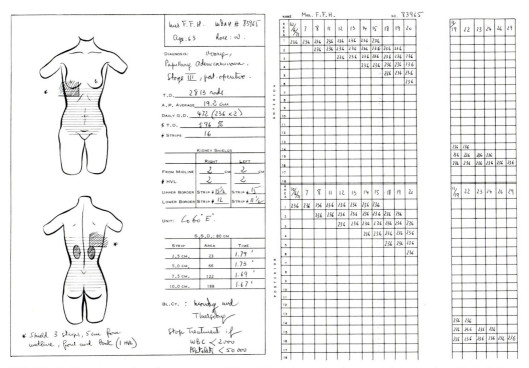

FIG. 11-40. Prescription sheet for treatment of the whole abdomen by the megavoltage moving strip technique. Note that both front and back are treated daily to avoid the edge effect and therefore to increase the tolerance.

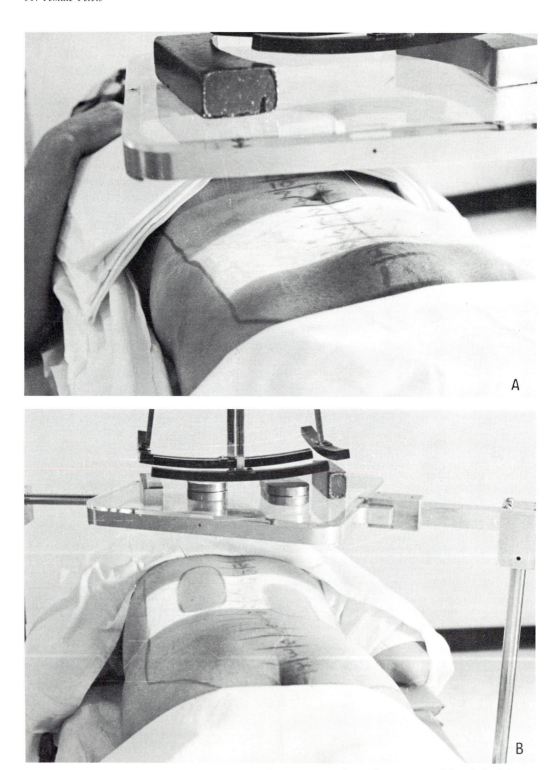

FIG. 11-41. Photographs of patient showing skin marks 2.5 cm apart during the treatment of the whole abdomen by the ^{60}Co moving strip. Note the kidneys are shielded (2 *HVL* lead) when treating the back (B).

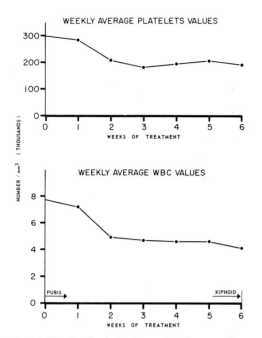

FIG. 11-42. Graph of platelets and leukocytes during treatment of the whole abdomen by the megavoltage moving strip technique. There is a rapid fall during the first two weeks of treatment with stabilization thereafter. (Courtesy: Delclos, *Amer. J. Roentgen.*, 96, 75, 1966.)

radiotherapists, and diagnosed by the same pathologists.

Table 11-23 shows the number of patients treated by each irradiation technique.

The results of treatment at 2 and 5 years are shown in Tables 11-24 and 11-25. It can be seen that the results in all stages are better when treatment is given to the whole abdomen with additional irradiation of the pelvis, except for treatment of Stage I where [198]Au instilled into the abdomen is as effective as external irradiation. Since only a minimal number of cells should be free in the abdomen or the pelvis when the primary cancer was confined to the ovaries, treatment with radioactive colloidal gold which circulates freely throughout the abdominal cavity should be effective in eradicating these cells.

When the different methods of irradiation are compared for all stages combined, whole abdominal irradiation with the [60]Co "moving strip" plus additional pelvic irradiation is superior to the other methods (Fig. 11-43).

In Table 11-26 the results of treatment are tallied according to the size of the residual cancer remaining after surgery. As might be expected, the results are better when all or almost all the tumor was removed. Because of the poor results obtained with irradiation when treating patients with residual masses larger than 2 cm, it is our present policy to treat patients with chemotherapy when

compare the results of several treatment methods for the epithelial cancers of the ovary, in patients who have been evaluated by the same observers, treated by the same

Table 11-23. *M. D. Anderson Hospital and Tumor Institute Irradiation Techniques in Ovarian Cancer July 1947–Dec. 1967*

Histology	Whole Abdomen Plus Pelvis	Whole Abdomen Only	Pelvis Only	[198]Au	Other	Total
Serous	137	55	33	50	6	281
Mucinous	14	7	4	17	3	45
Undifferentiated adenocarcinoma	15	12	10	20	0	57
Dysgerminoma	8	11	3	0	1	23
Others	12	13	11	6	0	42
Total	186	98	61	93	10	448

Table 11-24. *Results of Treatment by Stage NED—2 Years*
July 1947–Dec. 1967

| Treatment | Stage I | | | Stage II | | | Stage III | | | Stage IV | |
	No. Pts.	NED No.	%	No. Pts.	NED No.	%	No. Pts.	NED No.	%	No. Pts.	NED No.
Abdomen and pelvis	28	23	82	71	35	49	64	17	27	3	1
Abdomen only	20	13	65	23	8	35	28	4	14	2	0
Pelvis only	5	5	100	18	3	17	22	1	4	1	0
[198]Au	19	16	84	16	5	31	48	6	12	2	0
Other	2	2	100	4	1	25	0	0	0	3	0

Table 11-25. *Results of Treatment by Stage NED—5 Years*
July 1947–Dec. 1967

| Treatment | Stage I | | | Stage II | | | Stage III | | | Stage IV | | |
	No. Pts.	NED No.	%	No. Pts.	NED No.	%	No. Pts.	NED No.	%	No. Pts.	NED No.	%
Abdomen and pelvis	21	16	76	38	13	35	49	11	22	1	0	0
Abdomen only	14	7	50	17	4	24	24	1	4	2	0	0
Pelvis only	5	4	80	17	3	18	20	1	5	1	0	0
[198]Au	18	14	78	16	3	19	47	4	8	4	0	0
Other	2	2	100	4	1	25	0	0	0	3	0	0

known or palpable residual masses are larger than 2 cm.

Chemotherapy

In addition to the patients with residual tumor masses larger than 2 cm, patients with ascites, intestinal obstruction, or general debility are treated with chemotherapy, since intensive irradiation is poorly tolerated by these patients.

Several of the alkylating agents, Thiotepa, cyclophosphamide, chlorambucil and Melphalan are probably equally effective in patients with ovarian epithelial malignancies. Melphalan is the drug of choice at this institution. It is well tolerated, is effective by both intravenous and oral administration and does not require careful monitoring of the blood counts for proper control of therapy.

Melphalan is given orally in a dose of 1 mg/kg of body weight in 3 or 4 divided doses daily for 5 days. These 5 courses of chemotherapy are repeated every 4 weeks if the white blood count returns to 3,000 per

Table 11-26. *Results of Treatment Epithelial Cancers of the Ovary by Size of Residual Tumor after Surgery (All Irradiation Techniques)*
July 1947–Dec. 1967

Size of Largest Mass	NED—2 Years Per Cent	NED—5 Years Per Cent
None	66.2	57.1
<2 cm	31.5	27.5
2–4 cm	25.7	17.2
4–6 cm	14.3	10.5
6–10 cm	3.0	0
>10 cm	3.4	3.5

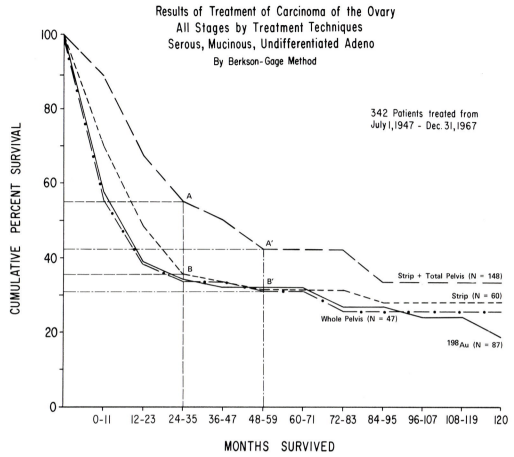

FIG. 11-43. Graph of results of treatment of all stages of the epithelial cancers of the ovary by different treatment technique. At 3 years, 55 per cent of patients treated with irradiation to the entire abdomen by the moving strip technique plus additional irradiation to the pelvis are alive as compared to 35 per cent of patients treated with the other techniques. At 5 years, 42 per cent of patients treated with "strip plus total pelvis" are alive as compared to 31 per cent of patients treated with the other techniques.

cubic millimeter and the platelet count returns to 150,000 per cubic millimeter. If the blood count does not return to these levels in 4 weeks, Melphalan is withheld until the levels are satisfactory.

Forty-five per cent of the patients with the common ovarian cancers treated with Melphalan had a partial or complete response for 3 months or longer. An additional 10 to 20 per cent had tumors which did not progress for at least 3 months after this treatment[16] (Table 11-27).

A combination of Actinomycin D, 5-

fluorouracil and cyclophosphamide is equally effective in treating patients with the common ovarian cancers and is also effective in patients with cancers that do not respond to Melphalan (Table 11-28).

Several patients who had residual cancers that were too large for treatment with irradiation when first seen have had a "second look" operation after several courses of chemotherapy in an attempt to integrate the several methods of treating ovarian cancer, utilizing each modality when it was most effective.

Table 11-27. *Response of Epithelial Cancers of the Ovary to Melphalan**

	Complete Response		Partial Response		No Change		Increasing Cancer	
	No.	%	No.	%	No.	%	No.	%
Serous	74	22	88	27	51	16	116	35
Mucinous	10	22	10	22	9	20	16	36
Undifferentiated adenocarcinoma	16	13	35	29	12	10	57	48
Total	100	20	133	27	72	14	189	38

*(p-di (2-chloroethyl) amino-L-phenylalanine) also called L-Sarcolysin, *PAM* and Alkeran.

Table 11-28. *Response of Epithelial Cancers of the Ovary to ActFuCy* After Treatment with Melphalan*

	Complete Response		Partial Response		No Change		Increasing Cancer	
	No.	%	No.	%	No.	%	No.	%
Serous	3	9	11	32	6	18	14	41
Mucinous	0		0		0		5	
Undifferentiated adenocarcinoma	1	12	3	38	1	12	3	38
Total	4	9	14	30	7	15	22	47

*Actinomycin-D, 5-Fluorouracil and Cyclophosphamide (cytoxan).

Dysgerminoma

Patients with pure dysgerminoma are given 2,000 rads to the entire abdomen by the "moving strip" technique with the ^{60}Co unit. An additional 2,000 rads are given to the pelvis. The paraaortic nodes receive additional treatment if indicated by the findings at surgery and/or lymphangiography. Prophylactic irradiation is given to the mediastinum and the left supraclavicular area after 3 to 6 weeks of rest if metastatic tumor is found in the paraaortic lymph nodes at surgery or by lymphangiogram. These areas receive 2,500 rads in 3 weeks.

Patients with dysgerminomas mixed with other malignant germ cell elements, being less sensitive, are given 2,600 to 2,800 rads to the entire abdomen by the ^{60}Co "moving strip" technique, plus 2,000 rads in 2 weeks to the pelvis. The paraaortic nodes are given additional treatment if indicated.

Twenty-three patients with dysgerminomas have received postoperative irradiation. Three of these patients had received irradiation in another hospital and had recurrent disease or new distant metastases. Two of the patients had mixed tumors with other germ cell elements present, and both of these patients were dead less than 2 years after treatment.

Three of 7 patients with Stage IV, 3 of 6 with Stage III, and 3 of 5 with Stage II dysgerminomas were alive and well without evidence of disease more than 2 years after treatment. Most of the patients with Stage I dysgerminoma did not receive postoperative irradiation. Since most patients are young, prophylactic irradiation is usually withheld unless they have evidence of spill at surgery, lymph node metastases by lymphangiogram, bloody ascites, other germ cell elements, or very large primary tumors.

Granulosa Cell Cancers

Twenty-five patients with granulosal cell cancers of the ovary were given postoperative irradiation. These patients were treated the same way as patients with epithelial cancers.

Although the granulosa cell cancers frequently recur late, the 2-year and 5-year survivals were similar. Thirty-six per cent of the patients treated with irradiation were alive and well at 5 years and 3 of 12 patients (25 per cent) with Stage III and IV disease were among these survivors.

Other Ovarian Cancers

Irradiation is of very limited value in treating the teratomas, embryonal carcinomas, and rare sarcomas of the ovary. One patient with an extremely rare and very malignant embryoma of the ovary which was confined to one ovary is living and well more than 5 years after being treated with irradiation to the entire abdomen by the moving strip technique plus additional irradiation to the pelvis with the 22 Mev betatron.

BIBLIOGRAPHY

1. The Cancer Committee of the International Federation of Gynecology and Obstetrics. *Acta obstet. gynec. scan.*, Vol. 50, No. 1, p. 1, 1971.

2. Charles, D.: Endometrial adenoacanthoma. A clinicopathological study of 55 cases, *Cancer,* 18, 737, 1965.

3. Czernobilsky, B., Silverman, B. B., and Mikuta, J. J.: Endometrioid carcinoma of the ovary. A clinicopathologic study of 75 cases, *Cancer,* 26, 1141, 1970.

4. Czernobilsky, B., Silverman, B. B. and Enterline, H. T.: Clear cell carcinoma of the ovary. A clinicopathologic analysis of pure and mixed forms and comparison with endometrioid carcinoma, *Cancer,* 25, 762, 1970.

5. Delclos, L., Braun, E. J., Herrera, J. R., Jr., Sampiere, V. A., and Van Roosenbeek, E.: Whole abdominal irradiation by ^{60}Cobalt moving strip technique, *Radiology,* 81, 632, 1963.

6. Delclos, L., and Murphy, M.: Evaluation of tolerance during treatment, late tolerance, and better evaluation of clinical effectiveness of the ^{60}Cobalt moving strip technique, *Amer. J. Roentgen.*, 96, 75, 1966.

7. Delclos, L., and Quinlan, E. J.: Malignant tumors of the ovary treated with megavoltage postoperative irradiation, *Radiology,* 93, 659, 1969.

8. Gray, L. A., and Barnes, M. L.: Endometrioid carcinoma of the ovary, *Obstet. & Gynec.*, 29, 694, 1967.

9. Hanks, G. E., and Bagshaw, M. A.: Megavoltage radiation therapy and lymphangiography in ovarian cancer, *Radiology,* 93, 649, 1969.

10. Long, M. D., and Taylor, H. C., Jr.: Endometrioid carcinoma of the ovary, *Amer. J. Obstet. & Gynec.*, 58, 943, 1949.

11. Munnell, E. W., and Taylor, H. C., Jr.: Ovarian carcinoma. A review of 200 primary cases and 51 secondary cases, *Amer. J. Obstet. & Gynec.*, 58, 943, 1949.

12. Sampson, J. A.: Endometrial carcinoma of the ovary, arising in endometrial tissue in that organ, *Arch. Surg.*, 10, 1, 1925.

13. Santessen, M. D., and Kottmeier, H. L.: General classification of ovarian tumors, In *Ovarian Cancer,* UICC Monograph Series, Vol. II, New York, Springer-Verlag, p. 1, 1968.

14. Schueller, E. F., and Kirol, P. M.: Prognosis in endometrioid carcinoma of the ovary, *Obstet. & Gynec.*, 27, 850, 1966.

15. Scully, R. E., and Barlow, J. F.: "Mesonephroma" of ovary. Tumors of müllerian nature related to the endometrioid carcinoma, *Cancer,* 20, 1405, 1967.

16. Smith, J. P., and Rutledge, F. N.: Chemotherapy in the treatment of cancer of the ovary, *Amer. J. Obstet. & Gynec.*, 107, 691, 1970.
17. Taylor, H. C., Jr., and Munnell, E. W.: In *Treatment of Cancer and Allied Diseases,* 2nd ed.,

Pack and Ariel, (eds.), New York, Paul B. Hoeber, Inc., 1962.
18. Whaton, J. T.: Radiation hepatitis in ovarian carcinomas treated by whole abdominal irradiation, *Amer. J. Roentgen.*, 67, 73, 1972.

Management of Bowel and Bladder Complications from Irradiation to Pelvis and Abdomen

JULIAN P. SMITH

Acute Problems During Treatment

Intestinal Reactions

Pelvic irradiation frequently causes loose stools and lower abdominal cramps. These complaints frequently can be controlled with a low residue bland diet. If the symptoms persist, drugs such as diphenoxylate hydrochloride with atropine sulfate (Lomotil, G. D. Searle and Co., Chicago, Ill.), 2 tablets 3 or 4 times each day are often helpful. If the patient develops diarrhea, paregoric (4 ml) or tincture of opium (.4 ml) after each loose stool is usually more effective than the diphenoxylate with atropine combination. If the diarrhea persists or becomes more severe, the radiation should be stopped temporarily and the patient should be given only clear liquids such as tea and boullion. If this is not effective, the patient should be hospitalized, treated with intravenous fluids, placing the intestinal tract at complete rest with feeding nothing by mouth.

When the mid- or upper abdomen is radiated, symptoms such as anorexia, nausea, vomiting, and abdominal cramping are more common. A low residue bland diet may be helpful; but if these symptoms persist or become severe, a liquid diet should be ordered and antiemetics such as prochlorperazine (Compazine, Smith Kline and French Laboratories, Philadelphia, Pa.) 5 mg every 4 to 6 hours or prochlorperazine with isopropamide capsules (Combid, Smith Kline and French Laboratories, Philadelphia, Pa.) every 12 hours may be helpful.

If nausea and vomiting persist or increase in severity after treatment with a liquid diet and antiemetics, radiation should be stopped, the patient hospitalized, treated with intravenous fluids, and given nothing by mouth. Occasionally the vomiting will continue and nasogastric suction, or intubation of the small intestine with a long intestinal tube and continuous suction will be necessary. All patients requiring hospitalization should have the serum electrolytes measured and any abnormality should be corrected.

Rarely, despite these measures, a patient will have severe abdominal pain with guarding of the abdomen and symptoms of peritonitis. These patients should be managed conservatively despite the indications of peritonitis unless the attending physician is convinced that an intra-abdominal catastrophe has occurred. None of the patients at the M. D. Anderson Hospital taken to surgery with these symptoms have been found to have had peritonitis or any correctable surgical condition and all treated conservatively have recovered although an occasional patient has required as much as 10 to 14 days of careful observation.

The new low-residue products for oral alimentation may prove helpful to patients with severe diarrhea or severe nausea and vomiting. These supplements are mixtures of amino acids, triglycerides, and dextrose and are absorbed in the upper gastrointestinal tract. They reportedly reduce the secretion of digestive enzymes produced in the stomach, pancreas, gallbladder, and duodenum. These enzymes contribute to the injury of the intestine after radiation by digesting the surface epithelium producing mucosal ulcers and hence should be prescribed with great caution.

Bladder Reactions

Urinary frequency, urgency, dysuria, and pain with urination are quite common during irradiation of the pelvis. These symptoms are frequently associated with bacterial cystitis and are usually controlled by appropriate antibacterial therapy. Urinary antispasmodics such as a mixture of potassium citrate and tincture of hyoscyamus are frequently effective in controlling bladder symptoms in the absence of bacterial cystitis.

Posttreatment Complications

Vaginal Vault Necrosis

Radiation necrosis of the upper vagina requires vigorous and immediate treatment. If this necrotizing process cannot be controlled quickly it often progresses to rectovaginal, vesicovaginal, and occasionally enterovaginal fistulae. To successfully treat vault necrosis it is necessary to eliminate the anaerobic infection that is responsible for this complication. Vaginal douches two or three times each day with either a solution of $3/4$ per cent hydrogen peroxide (3 per cent hydrogen peroxide diluted 3:1 with water) or half strength Dakin's solution (.25 per cent sodium hypochlorite solution) are frequently beneficial.

It is very important that the patient is instructed in douching properly. She should lie in the bathtub to douch and intermittently occlude the vagina by squeezing the labia majora together with her hand. This intermittently irrigates the entire vagina with the douche solution. Douching over the toilet irrigates only the lower vagina and the vault is seldom irrigated properly.

Bowel

The acute symptoms of irradiation enteritis may persist for several weeks after treatment. After 4 to 8 weeks more serious changes in the intestinal tract, however, must be suspected. The histological findings in the intestine during treatment consist of inflammatory changes in the mucosa with occasional loss of epithelium and edema of the intestinal wall. These changes are usually self-limited and regress completely. Of patients treated at M. D. Anderson Hospital it is uncommon for the patients who develop severe symptoms during their treatment to develop a bowel injury which requires surgery following treatment. The patients who developed injuries requiring surgery, as a group, tolerated their irradiation very well and had nothing during their treatment to suggest that they would have difficulty at a later date.

The majority of large intestine injuries occur in the first 2 years after treatment, however, an occasional injury will occur after 2 years. The large bowel injuries that are seen following irradiation include rectal ulcers, proctosigmoiditis, rectosigmoid obstruction, rectovaginal fistula, sigmoid perforation and rarely enterocolonic or vesico-colonic fistulae.

Proctosigmoiditis which is the most common large bowel injury seen should be treated expectantly and conservatively. Symptoms such as rectal bleeding, excess mucous formation and rectal tenesmus can often be controlled with a low residue bland diet, psyllium hydrophilic mucilloid (Metamucil, G. D. Searle and Co., Chicago, Ill.) 2 or 3 times daily and a sedative anticholinergic drug combination before each meal and at bedtime. We have found that the use of hydrocortisone enemas, hydrocortisone rectal foam or systemic steroids are completely ineffective in controlling rectal symptoms.

Occasionally a patient will require a diverting colostomy because of proctosigmoiditis. Although the colostomy frequently can be closed at a later date this severe treatment should be reserved for patients who require repeated transfusions because of rectal bleeding and the occasional patient whose rectal pain and tenesmus is severe and not relieved by medical management.

Excision of the injured proctosigmoid has no place in the treatment of this complication. Because of the poor healing of tissues injured by radiation, the surgical procedures are associated with a high mortality, a high incidence of complications, and a low rate of success. The other large bowel complications secondary to irradiation such as rectovaginal fistula and rectosigmoid obstruction should be treated with a diverting colostomy.

Patients with small intestine injuries secondary to irradiation should have surgery as soon as the diagnosis is made. Perforation of the small bowel with peritonitis or intestinal necrosis with local peritonitis carries a high mortality. If these patients are to be helped they should have surgery before these complications develop. Surgical by-pass of the injured area of intestine in the absence of perforation or necrosis is the procedure of choice and is the least radical procedure to alleviate the intestinal obstruction that almost always is present.

Bladder

Vesicovaginal fistulae and hemorrhagic cystitis are the two most common bladder complications seen following pelvic irradiation. Most of the vesicovaginal fistulae seen at M. D. Anderson Hospital are secondary to vaginal necrosis and are best managed by urinary diversion with an ileoconduit. An occasional small fistula in a patient who has not received high-dose external irradiation can be treated by colpocleisis or a simple closure of the fistula with the closure covered by the gracilis muscle from the medial thigh or the bulbocavernosis fat pad.

Hemorrhagic cystitis can be a very difficult problem. If the hematuria is not severe the patient should be treated with a diet which eliminates all known bladder irritants such as coffee, tea, alcohol, pepper, chili powders, and other spicy foods. The urine should be acidified with mandelic acid, ascorbic acid, or cranberry juice. Substances such as fruit juice and milk products which cause the urine to be alkaline should be eliminated from the diet. If an infection is present, appropriate antibiotic or antimicrobials should be given.

If the bleeding is severe and eliminating bladder irritants and acidifying urine is not effective the patient should be hospitalized and a large Foley cathether placed in the bladder. If the hematuria does not stop after several days of catheter drainage, a large 3-way catheter should be placed in the bladder and the bladder irrigated continuously with .5 per cent acetic acid or 1 to 10,000 potassium permanganate solution. It is extremely important to remove all the clots in the bladder before attempting continuous irrigations. This can be done through vigorous irrigation of the bladder with saline or through the cystoscope.

Occasionally an isolated bleeding spot can be found by cystoscopy and the area fulgurized. Unfortunately the bleeding usually occurs from multiple sites. Installation of hydrocortisone into the bladder has been disappointing. If continuous irrigation with the 3-way catheter is not effective, a suprapubic cystotomy should be performed and the bladder irrigated from above with the irrigation solution running into the bladder from the cystotomy tube and out through the urethra.

Several patients have had ileal urinary conduits constructed with diversion of the urine through the abdominal wall. A few have continued to have severe hematuria despite the urinary diversion. Cystectomies done because of the persistent bleeding have been associated with severe complications and even death.

Summary

1) Intestinal complaints during irradiation treatment should be managed symptomatically. If symptomatic treatment is not effective and the symptoms are severe, irradiation should be stopped and the intestine allowed to recover.

2) Large bowel injuries following irradiation can usually be managed conservatively with a low residue bland diet, antispasmodics, and psyllium hydrophilic mucilloid.

3) Large bowel complications such as rectovaginal fistulae and obstruction should be managed by diverting colostomies.

4) Radiation injuries of the small intestine following radiation should be treated surgically as soon as the diagnosis is made. The surgical procedure should be as conservative as is possible, consistent with eliminating the problem.

5) Irradiation cystitis should be treated by eliminating the known bladder irritants from the diet and acidifying the urine. Severe bladder bleeding should be treated by constant irrigation of the bladder.

BIBLIOGRAPHY

1. Smith, J. P., Golden, P. E., and Rutledge, F.: The surgical management of intestinal injuries following irradiation for carcinoma of the cervix. *Cancer of the Uterus and Ovary*, A Collection of papers presented at the Eleventh Annual Clinical Conference on Cancer, 1966 at The University of Texas at Houston M. D. Anderson Hospital and Tumor Institute, Houston, Texas, Year Book Medical Publishers, Inc., p. 241, 1969.

Surgical Procedures Associated with Radiation Therapy for Cervical Cancer

FELIX N. RUTLEDGE, and J. TAYLOR WHARTON

Variations in Radicality of Hysterectomy for Cancer of the Cervix

The following types of hysterectomy have been defined in our service to allow ease and precision in documenting the radicality of the operation.

Class I (Extrafascial Hysterectomy)

The procedure which separates the cervix and upper vagina in a plane outside the pubocervical fascia may be described as an extrafascial hysterectomy. There are two variations of this operation and in both instances there is minimal disturbance of the ureters and bladder base which lessens the risk of urinary complications.

The following description explains the rationale and technique:

PRIMARY TREATMENT

This operation may be used as primary therapy for carcinoma in situ and micro-invasive cancer of the cervix. The procedure assures complete removal of the cervix and when desired 1 to 2 cm of vaginal cuff. The inclusion of additional paracervical tissue with the operative specimen reduces the risk of dissection into the side of the cervix should there be deep endocervical gland extension or subclinical foci of cancer contiguous to the cervix. The additional vaginal cuff should be included when the neoplastic changes in the mucosa is noted by colposcopy, iodine staining, or biopsy to extend onto the vagina. The added paracervical tissue also allows a safer margin should invasion be found in the specimen.

METHOD

1) Deflection and retraction of the ureters laterally without dissecting the ureteral bed.

2) Transection of the uterine vessels wider than usual but medial to the ureters, made possible by more complete exposure of the uterine artery and vein.

3) Mobilization of the vagina prior to section for added cuff.

FOLLOWING IRRADIATION

The type of extrafascial hysterectomy (also referred to as a conservative hysterectomy) is a valuable adjunct to irradiation therapy in the treatment of selected patients with bulky tumors confined to the uterus. The operation is designed to simply remove the uterus with minimal inclusion of additional paracervical tissue and vaginal cuff.

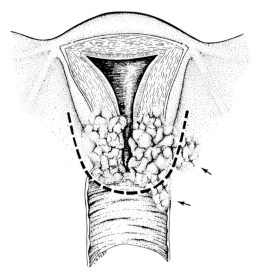

FIG. 11-44. The dotted line represents the extent of the Class I postirradiation hysterectomy. The operation is intended as an adjunct to nearly full-intensity irradiation therapy. The procedure is contraindicated when the disease invades the paracervical tissue or vagina as shown in the drawing (arrows).

Careful selection of the patient for operation is of the upmost importance in that paracervical and parametrial infiltration (Fig. 11-44) and/or vaginal involvement are contraindications since cutting through areas of known involvement with cancer is unsafe. The operation is also discontinued at the time of laparotomy if it is unduly difficult to separate the bladder from the cervix due to fibrosis. Adherence to these guidelines has resulted in few complications.

METHOD

1) Minimal reflection of the rectum, utero-sacral ligaments and broad ligament.

2) Sharp dissection of the bladder to the level to allow excision of the entire cervix.

3) Retraction of the ureters laterally without dissection.

4) Transection of the uterine vessels adjacent to the cervix.

Class II (Extended Hysterectomy)

This operation is classed as a radical hysterectomy because extra tissue is excised with the uterus. The pelvic surgeon may employ the Class II extended hysterectomy as primary treatment for microinvasive cancer when occult invasion cannot be ruled out or for selected patients with invasive cancer after near full intensity irradiation.

The moderately radical operation may be performed safely following 4,000 rads whole pelvis irradiation by preservation of more blood vessels to local segments of the ureters and base of the bladder. These patients usually have "barrel-shaped" lesions with bulging of the cancer into the parametrium but still confined to the cervix or very large tumors that fail to regress with whole pelvis irradiation. This procedure is also used in certain patients where uterine radium cannot be inserted because of inability to find the endocervical canal or in pregnant patients who do not abort following whole pelvis irradiation. A higher incidence of postoperative complications will be encountered when this extended hysterectomy is done following whole pelvis irradiation.

METHOD

1) Mobilization of the ureters but maintenance of their attachment to the uterine and superior vesicle vessels.

2) The uterosacrals ligaments and surrounding peritoneum, medial two-third parametrium and paravaginal tissue and upper one-third vagina are excised.

Class III (Conventional Radical Hysterectomy)

The Class III radical hysterectomy may be used as primary treatment when the cancer is confined so that a tumor-free margin can be obtained. The patient should have youthful strength for recovery and a healthy physical reserve.

METHOD

1) The uterine vessels are transected at their origin but the superior vesicle artery is conserved.

2) The uterosacral ligaments extending down into the pillars of the rectum are transected near the pelvic wall.

3) The parametrium is divided at the pelvic wall attachment.

This wide resection can be achieved only after detachment of the ureter and bladder from the cervix and the upper vagina. Since the important blood supply from the uterine artery is sacrificed, collateral circulation through the superior vesicle artery is preserved. Bladder atony becomes evident after operation since there is significant resection of the neural supply to the bladder and lower ureters that courses via the uterosacral ligaments, periureteral tissues and parametrium. This loss of nerve supply is manifest by urinary retention, a condition favorable for infection. The surgeon who is alert to the postoperative urinary changes protects and avoids most of the infections that may follow incomplete voiding. To escape the more serious complications of the urinary fistulae the surgeon must be able in proper selection of patients and skilled during the operation.

Class IV (Extended Radical Hysterectomy)

A more radical hysterectomy is performed representing an expansion of the scope of a Class III operation. Such a procedure should be reserved for patients unfavorable for an alternate treatment (irradiation) or a condition discovered first at laparotomy. Patients who develop recurrent cancer of the cervix after irradiation treatment may qualify.

Resection of the advanced cancer requires sacrifice of additional blood supply to the ureters, bladder, and rectum. This increases the risk for necrosis and development of fistula. These patients require extra care to offset the increased complications.

METHOD

1) The superior vesicle artery and bladder pillars (pubovesicle ligaments) are excised.

2) Three-fourths of the vagina is often included in the specimen.

3) The extent of the disease may force additional dissection in selected patients in whom division and excision of the internal iliac system and/or total resection of the vagina will be necessary to remove the cancer.

Class V (Ultraradical Hysterectomy)

The purpose of this procedure is to expand the Class III and IV operation for the more advanced or recurrent cancers. The necessity to deviate from a planned conventional radical hysterectomy may become evident at laparotomy. Such operations as the Class *V* hysterectomy are not advised for primary treatment and may be discontinued to favor irradiation since the hazards of this procedure are obvious. Successful treatment of patients with recurrent carcinoma after irradiation is dependent upon surgical management since there is no alternative. Certain patients may be suited for the Class *V* modifications and an exenteration may be avoided.

METHOD

In addition to wide resection of the uterus and pelvic wall lymph nodes, a portion of the bladder or bowel or a segment of ureter is removed to encompass the cancer. Reconstruction of the defect will differ among patients. Various techniques include primary closure, ureteral reimplantation, or the use of a portion of small bowel to bridge the ureter (ileoneocystotomy) to the bladder.

Pelvic Exenteration

If cancer recurs after full dose irradiation, surgery is the preferred treatment because a second course of radical irradiation has prohibitive hazards. Surgery after radical irradiation also has some unavoidable and serious complications. The radical hysterectomy may be suitable for a recurrent, centrally localized lesion, however, more advanced cancer demands a more aggressive approach.

When the bladder and rectum are involved by recurrent cancer, the only recourse is pelvic exenteration. Extensive involvement is best treated by a total exenteration. Recurrent disease involving only the bladder may be treated with an anterior exenteration whereas posterior vaginal wall and rectal disease may require only a posterior exenteration.

These more radical procedures are controversial because of the serious operative mortality and postoperative complications. The mortality rates and complications can probably be reduced with improved techniques. Our own series, in recent years, show a definite reduction of the operative mortality and postoperative complications. Some patients have benefitted by pelvic exenteration in terms of life prolongation and increased comfort, but evaluation of the exenterative procedures in cancer control is not possible at this time.

Microinvasive Carcinoma of the Cervix

Microinvasive carcinoma is an established pathological entity. The International Federation assigns a substage (Stage 1A) to this disease. However, the management is still unresolved. Among those who have acquired some experience in treatment for this cancer there is a tendency to treat the patient conservatively. We think this is justified at the present time and agree with the consensus that microinvasive lesions are more nearly related to carcinoma in situ than to invasive cancer.

Microinvasive carcinoma apparently originates from carcinoma in situ involving the epithelial surface of the cervix or extends outward of carcinoma in situ that has replaced endocervical glandular epithelium. The projections are of limited depth and penetrate the basement membrane 3 to 5 mm. These areas may be singular but are often multicentric. The diagnosis may be difficult or impossible to make when histologic sections of the cervix are cut tangentially.

Occasionally small islands of neoplastic cells are isolated some distance from the surface. If these islands are contained in an endothelial-lined space then lymphatic invasion is a possibility and this provides an opportunity for spread within the cervix or to the regional lymphatics.

Treatment

Microinvasive carcinoma usually remains confined near the developing site of carcinoma in situ. The risk of local recurrence or metastasis is small and the Class I hysterectomy has proven adequate therapy and is presently our preference. When there is inconclusive evidence of occult invasion due to tangential sectioning or cancer cells within a space suggesting a lymphatic vessel the Class II hysterectomy may be a solution for treatment because the range of resection is increased with a minimal risk.

Intracavitary radium may also be used if hysterectomy would be difficult or unsafe for the patient. For those patients to whom irradiation is advised we prefer two 48-hour tandem and ovoids insertions at two-week intervals since less intense treatment is necessary than for invasive cancer. There is simply no need for radical irradiation therapy in the treatment of this lesion.

Preirradiation Surgery

Treatment of Pelvic Inflammatory Disease

Acute or subacute pelvic infection may be aggravated by irradiation. Irradiation destroys the inflammatory cells which have entrapped the inflammatory process. This causes an exacerbation of the infection resulting in a pelvic cellulitis which is frequently resistant to antibiotic therapy. This leads to interruption of therapy which is detrimental or even fatal to the patient. All patients with suspected or diagnosed pelvic inflammatory disease should have an exploratory laparotomy with removal of the adnexae, before starting irradiation therapy.

Urinary or Fecal Diversion

Severe obstruction of the ureters caused by cancerous tissues is first aggravated by irradiation because edema is induced in these tissues. Obstruction increases before the cancer can be controlled by irradiation and uremia develops. An ileal conduit should be established before irradiation is begun in patients with bilateral ureteral obstruction especially when there is a concomitant elevation of the blood urinary nitrogen and creatinine.

Intestinal obstruction is rarely caused by cancer of the cervix, yet some patients will need operation to relieve it.

Selective Lymphadenectomy

Analysis of treatment failures and previous experience with postirradiation lymphadenectomies have clearly shown that with treatment policies used at the M. D. Anderson Hospital progressive disease is frequently related to:

1) Cancer involving the common iliac and paraaortic nodes and, therefore, beyond the treatment area of the standard 15 × 15 cm fields (Table 11-29).

Table 11-29. *Incidence of Positive Nodes up to the Bifurcation of the Aorta in Specimens of Lymphadenectomy Performed Three Months After Completion of Radical Irradiation in 148 Unselected Stage IIIA and IIIB Cases*
April 1955–February 1960

Positive Nodes	Number
Only within irradiated area (obturator, external iliac, hypogastric)	7
Only outside irradiated area (common iliac)	10
Both within and outside irradiated area	11
Total	28 or 20%

(Courtesy: Fletcher and Rutledge, *Amer. J. Roentgen.* 114, 116, 1972.)

2) Failure of irradiation to sterilize large matted nodes (excessive tumor volume) within the irradiated area.

Both of these causes of failure may be studied and corrected more efficiently if an exploratory laparotomy is done. The laparotomy will allow determination of the extent of the disease (number and location of lymph node groups involved) and removal of enlarged nodes. The removal of clinically apparent disease, especially cancerous nodes greater than 2 cm in diameter is invaluable in reference to enhancing the efficiency of irradiation therapy. The reduction of the volume of tumor to subclinical aggregates of cancer cells should result in a greater control rate within the irradiated area.

Extended field irradiation is required when cancer has spread to the proximal external iliac, common iliac, or paraaortic nodes. The regional node groups are irradiated one level beyond the group proven to contain metastatic cancer. Patients with positive principal (obturator) and/or adjacent external iliac nodes are irradiated to the level of fifth lumbar (*L5*) vertebrae. Patients with positive proximal external iliac and/or lower common iliac and hypogastric nodes have the

fields extended to the level of the middle of *L4* vertebrae (Fig. 11-25). Proximal common iliac or paraaortic involvement requires treatment to the *T12* level (Fig. 11-25).[4]

With the increase in volume of tissue irradiated, the risk of injury to vital organs (especially the small bowel) is increased. The risk is justified if the patient is known to have disease within the area irradiated.

PATIENT SELECTION

Patients with bulky Stage I or II lesions and all patients with Stage III squamous cell carcinomas who are in good medical condition have lymph nodes removed from the following groups of nodes (Fig. 11-45).

1) Precaval
2) Paraaortic
3) Common iliac
4) External iliac
5) Internal iliac (hypogastric)
6) Principal node (obturator)

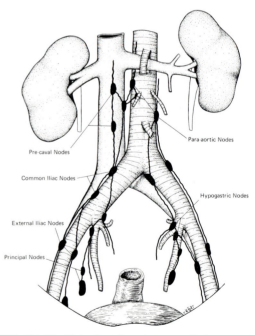

FIG. 11-45. Major lymph node groups that are sampled in patients having a preirradiation therapy selective lymphadenectomy.

The type and number of nodes removed are determined by preoperative lymphangiography, palpation of the node at the time of exploration, and extent of disease (matted, enlarged nodes are removed en bloc).

TECHNIQUE

A midline lower abdominal incision extending from the umbilicus to the symphysis is preferred. Adequate exposure for the paraaortic phase is essential and the surgeon should not hesitate to extend the incision. The peritoneum at the base of the small bowel mesentery is opened from the ileocecal area to the third portion of the duodenum. This will expose the inferior vena cava and abdominal aorta. The lymph nodes anterior and lateral to these vessels extending from the bifurcation of the aorta to the level of the 3rd lumbar vertebrae are removed en bloc. These nodes are in a critical area in reference to therapy planning and the thorough dissection is justified.

The peritoneum over the common iliac and external iliac vessels is opened and selected nodes are removed. Major lymphatic channels must be preserved in this region. The hypogastric and principle node (obturator) groups are then sampled. These nodes frequently are involved with cancer and become enlarged and matted. The iliac vessels may be exposed without opening the round ligament and nodes may be removed without separating the external iliac artery and vein or disturbing their attachment to the psoas muscle.

An attempt is made to tie or clip the major lymphatic vessels related to the nodes since this may possibly prevent the accumulation of lymph and lymphocyst formation. Although it is desirable to maintain lymphatic channels, the dissection is quite radical if matted or enlarged nodes are found. Nodes that are normal to palpation and in appearance are not disturbed other than by the random sampling of the representative group. Each individual node or node group that is removed during the procedure is placed on a plastic template for proper identification (Fig. 11-46).

In order to diminish bleeding and limit growth of the disease, 1,000 rads (500 rads daily for two consecutive days) are given with a transvaginal cone or a tandem is loaded with two 20 mg sources and inserted in the lower segment and endocervix for 24 hours. With a large central lesion this amount of radium is not taken into consideration in the final dose.

RESULTS

Fifty consecutive patients with bulky squamous cell carcinomas of the cervix have had a preirradiation therapy exploratory laparotomy and selective lymphadenectomy (Table 11-30). Twenty-seven of the patients had positive nodes. Preliminary analysis of the data reveals the procedure is safe and that large matted nodes can be removed without undue risk. Six patients have developed lymphocyst during the immediate postoperative period, however, irradiation therapy was not interrupted. The study has been expanded and all patients who are surgical candidates with bulky or advanced cancer of the cervix are included.

As all palpable nodes have been removed, the dose to the lymphatics is only 4,500 rads (850 rads per week). This diminished dosage is because of the adhesions resulting from the surgical procedure.

Adjunctive Hysterectomy

Combined intracavitary radium and external beam therapy are eminently successful for treating patients with carcinoma of the uterine cervix, with the exception of voluminous cancers that concentrically enlarge the cervix. Radical surgery does not provide a solution because an en bloc dissection would very likely necessitate interference with the urinary tract.

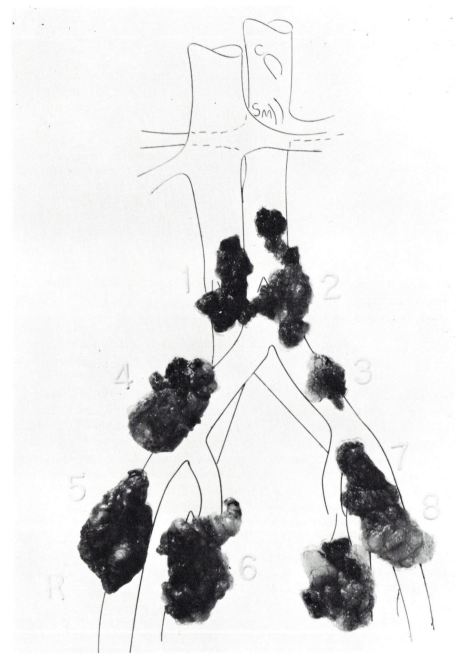

FIG. 11-46. Lymph nodes removed at the time of selective lymphadenectomy are placed on this plastic plate. The device is autoclaved and the surgeon accurately places each node or node group in the exact anatomical position in the operating room. This patient had a bulky Stage II-B squamous cell carcinoma of the cervix and groups 4,5,6, and 8 contained metastatic cancer. Group 5 was matted and adherent to the vessels and measured 3 × 4 cm.

Table 11-30. *Operative Findings by Selective Lymphadenectomy in 50 Consecutive Patients with Bulky Squamous Cell Carcinomas—Cervix July 1971–July 1972*

| †Stage | Number Patients Studied | Number Patients Positive Nodes | Bilateral Lymph Node Group Involvement | *Node Groups Involved | | | | Postoperative Lymphocyst |
				Obturator-hypogastric Complex	External Iliac	Common Iliac	Para-aortic	
I	18	6	2	5	1			3
II$_A$	6	1	1	1				
II$_B$	16	11	3	8	4	2	1	1
III	10	9	4	7	1	2	4	2
Total	50	27	10					6

† *FIGO* Classification—January 1, 1971.
Multiple groups involved in some patients.

Growth Patterns Requiring Special Therapy

Cancer, either squamous cell carcinoma or adenocarcinoma, originating in the endocervix can extend to the lower uterine segment enlarging the endocervix to the same diameter as the fundus producing a barrel-shaped uterus (Fig. 11-47).

This growth pattern produces lesions so large that the distances are too great from the intracavity radioactive source, and furthermore a significant portion of the cells are anoxic with increased radioresistance. Foci of cancer cells escape irradiation destruction and hence produce later local recurrence. Therefore, patients who are candidates for combined therapy are those with bulky Stage I and Stage II cancers. The purpose of the combined treatment is primarily to prevent central recurrences and perhaps increase survival rates.

Result of Combined Therapy

Two hundred and forty-seven patients have had a hysterectomy after irradiation therapy during the years 1952 to 1971. The amount of irradiation, the scope of the surgery, and the clinical indications have been modified as experience was gained.

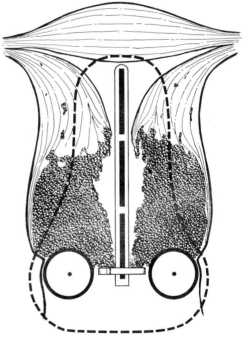

FIG. 11-47. In the bulky, expansile lesions of the endocervix, tumor cells deep in the myometrium are beyond the zone of adequate dosage because of the pear-shaped isodose distribution of the radium system.

Of the 247 patients, 207 had squamous cell carcinoma of the cervix and 40 had adenocarcinoma of the cervix. The amount of irradiation preceding the hysterectomy varied

Table 11-31. *Postirradiation Hysterectomy Type and Amount of Irradiation Received by 247 Patients 1952–1971*

Whole Pelvis Irradiation	Patients
4,000–8,000 rads	34
3,500–4,000 rads	149
2,000–3,500 rads	23
Parametrial irradiation	31
Radium only	10
	247

Table 11-33. *Urinary Tract Fistulae Following Whole Pelvis Irradiation and Class I Hysterectomy 1952–1971*

3,500–4,000 rads	
Vesicovaginal	4
Rectovaginal	3
	7/149
4,000–8,000 rads	
Vesicovaginal	4
Rectovaginal	3
	7/27

(Table 11-31). Class I hysterectomy was done on 220 of these patients and the remaining 27 patients had a more radical procedure (Table 11-32).

The incidence of vesico and rectovaginal fistulae following surgery was influenced by the amount of external irradiation (Table 11-33) and class of hysterectomy performed (Table 11-34). It is evident that patients who have above 4,500 rads whole pelvis irradiation or those in whom a radical hysterectomy is performed, the incidence of fistula is excessive.

The use of an extrafascial hysterectomy as an adjunct to near full intensity irradiation is effective in reducing central recurrences. From 1948 to 1963, 133 patients with endocervical barrel-shaped cancers or positive endometrial biopsy were treated with radiation therapy alone (94 patients) or radiation therapy plus an extrafascial hysterectomy (39 patients). Fourteen patients treated with radiation alone had recurrences in the vault and/or pelvis. Local control was excellent in the radiation plus surgery group in that only

one patient experienced a vault and pelvic recurrence (Table 11-35).

CLINICAL SITUATIONS (INDICATIONS FOR SURGERY) NO LYMPH NODE INVOLVEMENT OR ONLY OBTURATOR OR CAUDAL EXTERNAL ILIAC NODES

These patients receive 4,000 rads whole pelvis irradiation (15 × 15 cm portals), and a uterine tandem and vaginal ovoids for 72 hours insertion (maximum of 5,000 mg hours insertion (maximum of 5,000 mg-hrs). This is followed in 6 weeks with a Class I hysterectomy.

INABILITY TO FIND THE INTERNAL OS

Combination therapy is indicated in treatment for Stage I and II carcinomas of the cervix when the internal os cannot be probed following 4,000 rads whole pelvis irradiation. An additional 5,000 rads surface dose is given to the mucosa of the vaginal apex with ovoids and the Class II hysterectomy is per-

Table 11-32. *Postirradiation Hysterectomy Class of Hysterectomy Received by 247 Patients 1952–1971*

Class I	220
Class II	6
Class III	20
Class V	1
	247

Table 11-34. *Postirradiation Hysterectomy Postoperative Complications—Radical Hysterectomy Following Whole Pelvis Irradiation 1952–1971*

Vesicovaginal fistula	2
Uterovaginal fistula	1
	3/27 (10%)

Table 11-35. *Patients with Endocervical Barrel-Shaped Lesions or Positive Endometrial Biopsy 1943–December 1963*

	NED 3-yr.	Dead	Site of Recurrence & Status of Disease at Time of Death					
			Vault Alone	Vault ± Pelvic Disease ± Distant Metastases	Pelvic Disease Distant Metas.	Inter-current Disease with Negative Vault	Complications	Unk
Radiation Therapy Alone (94)	60 (64%)	34	2	12	17	4	0	0
Radiation Therapy + Conservative Hysterectomy (39)	29 (75%)	10	0	1	6	1	1	1

Note: (1) The patients in the table represent a retrospective selection of Stage II patients with bulky central endocervical lesions or lesions with positive endometrial biopsy.

(2) The table shows low incidence of central recurrence in radiation therapy + hysterectomy group (about 3 per cent) versus about 15 per cent in radiation therapy alone group. There is about the same incidence of distant metastases in both groups. (Courtesy: Durrance, Fletcher and Rutledge, *Amer. J. Roentgen.*, 106, 831, 1969.)

formed 6 weeks later. The lack of the tandem necessitates the Class II procedure since the paracervical areas would be undertreated with the Class I operation.

With the larger lesions, a lymphadenectomy is indicated since the incidence of regional node involvement is significant and in the absence of uterine radiation a dose to most of the lymphatics is only 4,000 rads which is inadequate.

INVOLVEMENT OF PROXIMAL EXTERNAL ILIAC, AND/OR COMMON ILIAC AND/OR PARAAORTIC NODES

Lymph node involvement is determined by lymphangiogram or preferably by selective lymphadenectomy and when present, 5,500 rads are given (850 rads per week) with extended fields. In patients with bulky lesions and no fornices or parametrial involvement, one 72-hour radium insertion is performed followed by a Class I hysterectomy 6 weeks later.

Postirradiation Lymphadenectomy

In the early 1900's, the importance of the spread of the disease was recognized by Wertheim, who, in practicing the extended hysterectomy, removed enlarged and hard lymph nodes.[11] The early experiences were followed by a more extensive dissection, and the proponents of surgical excision were exemplified by Victor Bonney, who obtained a 20 per cent *NED* rate when lymph nodes were positive. This figure is essentially unchanged in all surgical series.[1]

Taussig[10] and Morton[8] in the 1940's showed that the incidence of positive lymph nodes was less in patients who had a lymphadenectomy following irradiation as compared to surgery only. Gorton[6] from Sweden and Gray et al.[7] also confirmed that positive nodes were found less frequently after irradiation than after primary surgical treatment. Despite this information, gynecologists long have had the belief that irradiation cannot be depended upon to sterilize cancer in the regional lymph nodes because of the frequency of recurrences to first appear in these nodes when the primary lesion is healed.

The belief that surgical excision held advantages over external irradiation prompted a program of clinical investigation at The University of Texas M. D. Anderson Hospital and Tumor Institute. A double treatment of the pelvic wall nodes, first by irradiation and then lymphadenectomy seemed logical to improve cure rates.

In order to obtain quantitative information of positive lymph nodes response to irradiation, a systematic study was done. A transperitoneal lymphadenectomy was performed three months after completion of irradiation in 100 consecutive Stage III patients who were medically suitable for operation. The incidence of positive nodes in the regional lymphatics up to the bifurcation of the aorta was found to be 19 per cent. Continued use of lymphadenectomy in this sequence required some statistical proof of benefit of irradiation. Therefore, a randomized study was begun.

This study included 142 patients in the lymphadenectomy group and 169 in the control group treated by irradiation therapy alone.[9] Distribution in Stages I through III was approximately equal. The incidence of positive nodes was low in all stages and particularly in Stage III when compared with the published data. At operation, few patients were found with a single positive node; nodes were usually large, matted and frequently adherent to adjacent structures suggesting extensive pre-irradiation involvement. These nodes could not be resected with adequate margins to totally remove the neoplastic disease.

The patients tolerated the operation well and no unusual technical problems were caused by the irradiation. However, serious problems were encountered in the early postoperative phase. The disrupted lymphatic drainage system of the pelvis and lower extremity did not re-establish collaterals following high-dose irradiation. The

lymph pooled in the pelvis, became encapsulated, producing a lymphocyst. This pseudocyst became a source of discomfort and caused obstructing pressure upon the surrounding blood vessels and ureter. As was often necessary, relief of this pressure by drainage was attempted, infection was induced, and a persistant abscess prolonged the patient's recovery. Approximately 20 per cent of those patients who had lymphadenectomy after radiation therapy had delayed recovery.

Based on this experience with lymphadenectomy, the following conclusions can be drawn:

1. Pelvic node metastasis can be sterilized by external irradiation. Table 11-36 shows the results of a randomized study. When the incidence of positive nodes recovered after irradiation is compared with the incidence in nonirradiated patients, it is evident that half of the nodes with metastasis were sterilized by irradiation.

2. Survival rates were not appreciably improved by lymphadenectomy. In the first series of 100 consecutive patients with Stage III squamous cell carcinoma of the cervix, no patient with positive nodes was cured by lymphadenectomy. In the second series (randomized Stages I through III), the survival time of the lymphadenectomy group and

Table 11-36. *Patients Randomly Selected to have Lymphadenectomy Three Months after Full-Dose Irradiation Therapy for Carcinoma of the Cervix*
Stage I–III
February 1957–February 1960

Stage	No. Pts.	No. Pos. Lymph Nodes	Per Cent
I	30	1	3.3
II$_A$	39	4	10.3
II$_B$	25	5	20.0
III$_A$	23	4	17.4
III$_B$	23	2	8.0

(Courtesy: Fletcher and Rutledge, *Amer. J. Roentgen.*, 114, 116, 1972.)

irradiation only group patients for all stages was almost identical.

3. Lymphadenectomy after high-dose irradiation caused serious complications. Lymphocyst developed in one fourth of the patients producing hydronephrosis and leg edema.

4. Failure of the lymphadenectomy to improve survival rates can be partly attributed to bulky metastatic disease surviving irradiation and the frequent involvement of the periaortic nodes.

Carcinoma of the Cervix Complicated by Pregnancy

The extent of the cancer and the duration of the pregnancy are the important considerations in the management of cancer of the cervix complicated by pregnancy.

Pregnancy induces anatomical alterations of the uterus by expansion of the cervix and lower uterine segment making intracavitary radium less effective. Thus, whole pelvis external irradiation is used initially in all stages. Lymphatic metastasis may occur at an earlier stage, and the en bloc coverage of the pelvis produced by the whole pelvis irradiation is beneficial. A hysterectomy may follow nearly full intensity irradiation and aid in eradicating residual disease remaining in the outer margin of the expanded cervix. The type of hysterectomy performed is governed by the radium system utilized (Table 11-37).

At the present time we are considering the use of the preirradiation selective lymphadenectomy for patients with advanced or bulky disease. A hysterotomy also could be done if the pregnancy is far enough advanced since further delay in starting irradiation therapy would probably not be encountered. This initial evacuation of the uterus would seem highly desirable in patients with advanced cancers and advanced gestation. External irradiation portal size would be determined by the lymph node group involved.

Treatment Policy

Treatment is begun as soon as possible after the diagnostic studies are completed. Prior to 24-weeks gestation the pregnancy is disregarded, and whole pelvis irradiation is given. This will cause fetal death and usually induces abortion by the fourth week of treatment. If abortion is not induced, surgical evacuation of the uterus is required before further radiation therapy can be given.

Therapy is usually delayed after the twenty-fourth week of gestation until viability is reached. A cesarean section is done when the fetus weighs approximately 1,500 gm. Whole pelvis irradiation begins immediately after the surgical wound is healed.

The same basic treatment plans (Tables 11-1 and 11-2) used for carcinoma of the cervix in the nonpregnant patient are applicable. The only difference is the use of 4,000 rads whole pelvic irradiation in patients with Stage I and early Stage II cancers and 5,000 rads in late Stage II and Stage III cases. Standard 15 × 15 cm parallel opposed portals are adequate to encompass the tumor and regional lymph node areas if the preirradiation selective lymphadenectomy is negative or positive only in the obturator or the most caudal external iliac node groups.

Irradiation with Abortion

NONBULKY LESIONS

Stage I and Stage II-A cancers that do not expand the endocervix are best treated entirely with irradiation. The abortion will usually occur during the external therapy, which is continued immediately after evacuation of the uterus. The cervix usually dilates without difficulty to accommodate expulsion of the products of conception, and cervical lacerations or severe bleeding are rarely encountered. The uterus involutes rapidly following evacuation, and intracavitary radium therapy is given according to Tables 11-1 and 11-2.

Table 11-37. *Carcinoma of the Cervix and Pregnancy*

	Up to 24 weeks—disregard pregnancy		
Stage	Whole Pelvis*	Radium**	Surgery

I and II$_A$ — 4,000 rads

- abortion → tandem and colpostats → Endocervical barrel-shaped or bulky disease may require +Class I hysterectomy
- no abortion
  - colpostats only for 72 hours → Class II hysterectomy and pelvic lymphadenectomy
  - surgical evacuation† → tandem and colpostats → Irradiation alone or with +Class I hysterectomy

II$_B$

bulky local—4,000 rads disease barrel-shaped

- abortion → tandem and colpostats → Irradiation alone or with +Class I hysterectomy
- no abortion
  - colpostats only for 72 hours → Class II hysterectomy and pelvic lymphadenectomy
  - surgical evacuation† → tandem and colpostats → Irradiation alone or with +Class I hysterectomy

extensive para-metrial infiltration—5,000 rads

- abortion → tandem and colpostats
- no abortion → surgical evacuation† → tandem and colpostats

III — 5,000 rads

- abortion → tandem and colpostats
- no abortion → surgical evacuation† → tandem and colpostats

From 24 Weeks		

24 to 28 weeks ⟶ await viability of fetus ⟶ cesarean section

after 28 weeks ⟶ cesarean section when fetal weight greater than 1,500 gm

I–II ⟶ 4,000 rads ⟶ See tables 11-1 and 11-2

III ⟶ See tables 11-1 and 11-2

---

* 15 x 15 cm parallel opposing fields—unless extended fields required based on selective lymphadenectomy.
** See tables 11-1 and 11-2.
+Class I hysterectomy is performed 6 weeks following 4,000 rads (or equivalent) whole pelvis irradiation and one 72-hr insertion tandem and ovoids (maximum 5,000 mg/hrs).
† Surgical evacuation is performed by hysterotomy or dilatation and curettage depending on gestational age—If a hysterotomy is done then selective lymphadenectomy is recommended. For patients with advanced disease and advanced gestation, a hysterotomy and selective lymphadenectomy may be done prior to irradiation therapy.

BULKY LESIONS

Stages I, II-A, and II-B cancers that expand the endocervix are very likely to have nests of cancer cells in the outer margin of the expanded cervix or lower uterine segment that survive irradiation therapy. This anatomic pattern is difficult to treat adequately with intracavitary radium which may have an occasional central failure. Therefore, one 72-hour tandem and ovoid insertion is followed in 4 to 6 weeks by Class I hysterectomy.

Irradiation without Abortion

Patients with Stages I and II-A cancers who do not abort following 4,000 rads whole pelvis irradiation may be treated with a 72-hour ovoid insertion followed by a Class II hysterectomy and pelvic lymphadenectomy. Careful selection is important in that only barrel-shaped lesions are treated with an extended hysterectomy.

Patients with extensive parametrial infiltration or Stage III lesions are best treated with evacuation of the uterus followed by intracavitary radium. A dilatation and curettage will suffice for patients with early gestations. If a hysterotomy is required for evacuation of the uterus, the regional nodes should be sampled if a preirradiation lymphadenectomy has not been done. The paraaortic and common iliac nodes are particularly important since irradiation therapy for disease in these nodes would require a supplemental 12 × 8 cm field (5,000 rads in 5 weeks). Suspicious or clinically positive nodes in the pelvis should be removed even though 4,000 rads whole pelvis irradiation has been given.

Results

The over-all results of treatment in Stage I show little difference between the pregnant and nonpregnant patient. In the Stage II category results in the nonpregnant group are slightly superior.[2]

BIBLIOGRAPHY

1. Bonney, V.: Results of 500 cases of Wertheim's for carcinoma of cervix, *J. Obst. & Gynec. Brit. Emp.*, 48, 421, 1941.
2. Creasman, W. T., Rutledge, F. N., and Fletcher, G. H.: Carcinoma of the cervix associated with pregnancy, *Obst & Gyn.*, 36, 495, 1970.
3. Durrance, F. Y., Fletcher, G. H., and Rutledge, F. N.: Analysis of central recurrent disease in Stages I and II squamous cell carcinomas of the cervix on intact uterus, *Amer. J. Roentgen.*, 106, 831, 1969.
4. Fletcher, G. H., and Rutledge, F. N.: Carcinomas of uterine cervix, In: *Modern Radiotherapy—Gynecological Cancer*, Editor, T. J. Deeley, Butterworth and Co., London, England, 1971.
5. Fletcher, G. H. and Rutledge, F. N.: Extended field technique in the management of cancers of the uterine cervix, *Amer. J. Roentgen.*, 114, 116, 1972.
6. Gorton, G.: Radiation therapy and excision of the lymph nodes in cervical cancer, In: *Progress in Gynecology*, Volume 3, Editors, J. V. Meigs, and S. H. Sturgis, Grune & Stratton, Inc., New York, p. 594, 1957.
7. Gray, M. J., Gusberg, S. B., and Guttmann, R.: Pelvic lymph node dissection following radiotherapy, *Amer. J. Obst. & Gynec.*, 76, 629, 1958.
8. Morton, D. G.: Pelvic lymphadenectomy in treatment of cervical cancer, *Amer. J. Obst. & Gynec.*, 45, 19, 1945.
9. Rutledge, F. N., and Fletcher, G. H.: Transperitoneal pelvic lymphadenectomy following supervoltage irradiation for squamous cell carcinoma of cervix, *Amer. J. Obst. & Gynec.*, 76, 321, 1958.
10. Taussig, F. J.: Iliac lymphadenectomy for Group II cancer of cervix, *Amer. J. Obst. & Gynec.*, 45, 733, 1943.
11. Wertheim, E.: Radical abdominal operation in carcinoma of the cervix uteri, *Surg., Gyn. & Obst.*, 4, 1, 1907.

12. Genitourinary

Carcinoma of the Bladder

FERNANDO G. BLOEDORN

Introduction

The role of radiotherapy being the most useful treatment for cancer of the bladder began when megavoltage became readily available and surgeons were convinced that cystectomy proved inadequate for controlling most infiltrating tumors. In many institutions today, irradiation is the treatment of choice for most carcinomas of the bladder. However, even if the results have improved, the cure rate is still low for a disease which, in most patients, remains localized to the pelvis for a long period of time. According to Jewett and Cooling,[4,10] 40 to 50 per cent of the patients failed to show at autopsy extrapelvic extension of their tumor. In spite of the fact that "radical doses" of radiation can be delivered to the pelvis, the rate of local control of disease is disappointingly low; this is probably due to an unfavorable tumor bed produced by altered urologic physiology. It is possible that the results of radiation therapy may improve by better management of the complicating factors, by greater consideration being given to the radiobiological principles, and by development of adequate combinations of radiation and surgery. The diagnosis, treatment, and follow-up of patients with carcinoma of the bladder pose complex and interesting problems that can be mastered only by a team of specialists—urologist, radiotherapist, and pathologist—closely collaborating.

Site of Origin and Multiplicity within the Bladder

According to the Armed Forces Institute of Pathology,[10] of 1,400 cases of bladder tumors, 84 per cent of the tumors were located in the lateral and posterior walls, 40 per cent in the trigone, 10 per cent in the vertex, and 11 per cent in the anterior wall. These percentages include individual count of multiple tumors that originate in different areas of the bladder in the same patient.

Multiplicity is a common fact or in any histological group of bladder cancers. In the carcinoma registry of the American Urological Society, of 643 patients, 250 (28 per cent) had more than one tumor.[12] The multiplicity of tumors, mainly the papillary type, affects not only the bladder mucosa but the mucosa of the whole urinary tract.

Several tumors can be present in the bladder at the same examination or develop consecutively; in either case they result from:

1) Submucosal circumferential lymphatic spread[2,10] which could extend far from the original focus.

2) Some cancerogenic factor acting on all of the bladder epithelium.

3) Tumor cells carried by urine and transplanted from place to place in the bladder mucosa spontaneously or because of instrumentation.

Histological Classification

The most commonly accepted histological classification involves classifying by type, noninfiltrative or infiltrative, and by grade.

Noninfiltrative Type

BENIGN PAPILLOMAS

Benign papillomas do not infiltrate beyond the bladder mucosa, are often multiple (Jewett, 25 per cent),[10] and their history extends over the years. Invasion and metastases in benign papillomas are so rare that they need not be discussed.

MALIGNANT PAPILLOMAS

Malignant papillomas are multiple in a high percentage of cases and are prone to develop into infiltrative carcinoma.

Evidence of true carcinomas has been found 5 years after treatment in about 20 per cent of the patients with histologically benign papillomas and in 50 per cent of those with malignant cells.

Infiltrative Type

There are 4 types of infiltrative carcinomas. They are papillary, squamous cell, transitional cell, and adenocarcinoma.

PAPILLARY CARCINOMA

This carcinoma is papillary in its histological architecture but it infiltrates beyond the basal membrane into the submucosa, muscle, or beyond the bladder wall if left untreated. It originates from a noninfiltrating papillary tumor. It grows slowly and has little tendency to invade lymph or blood vessels.

SQUAMOUS CELL CARCINOMA

Squamous cell carcinoma is a tumor originating in metaplastic cells and has the characteristics of other squamous cell carcinomas, *i.e.*, a local invasion and a marked affinity to produce regional lymph node metastases. There is little tendency for it to invade blood vessels or to produce distant metastases. In most autopsy cases, the extensions of squamous cell carcinoma are limited to the perivesical tissues and pelvic lymph nodes.[10]

TRANSITIONAL CELL CARCINOMA

This is the most common type of infiltrative tumor of the bladder. It originates from the transitional cell epithelium of the urinary tract. When anaplastic, it is the most aggressive bladder tumor and is the highest producer of extravesical extensions and has a high tendency for lymph and blood vessel invasion.

ADENOCARCINOMA

Adenocarcinoma can be divided into 2 groups:

1) Simple or nonmucous forming which is rare.

2) Mucous forming as a result of long-standing cystitis glandularis or because it originates in the urachus. Characteristic of tumors of the urachus is their site of origin in the bladder dome, extension into the urachus remnant as nodular lymphatic seeding, and metastasis to the umbilicus.

Grade of Malignancy

The grade of malignancy from the least to the most malignant tumors is as follows: papillary, well differentiated; papillary anaplastic, well differentiated; transitional cell; squamous cell carcinoma; adenocarcinoma; and transitional cell anaplastic.

Prognostic Factors

Local Extensions and Metastases

The factors which determine the prognosis in a bladder cancer are:

1) Degree of penetration into the bladder wall. Jewett[10] has shown that the production

of metastases and microscopic extravesical extensions in each case are directly related to the depth of infiltration of the tumor. Tumors which do not infiltrate beyond the basal membrane of the mucosa do not produce metastases or microscopic extension beyond the local tumor. Once the basal membrane is penetrated, local spread, lymph node involvement, and distant metastases increase with depth of infiltration. The critical point is half way into the muscle layer thickness. For tumors which do not infiltrate beyond the muscularis, the incidence of regional lymph node metastases is about 20 per cent, whereas when they invade deep into the bladder wall, the incidence is about 50 per cent.[10] Jewett (Rubin's Symposium) also has demonstrated the importance of lymph channel's permeation by tumor cells. Over one third of infiltrative tumors will show lymph channel involvement. Around 90 per cent of patients showing this type of involvement will develop lymph node metastases. The obturator, external iliac, and hypogastric nodes are most commonly involved.[1]

2) Histological type and grade of anaplasticity. The more anaplastic a tumor is, the more aggressive it is with a greater potential for local extensions, and regional and distant metastases for a tumor of the same stage with less anaplasticity. However, when transitional cell carcinomas produce lymph node metastases they generally have islands of squamous cell metaplasia responsible for the metastases.

3) Site of origin. The incidence of lymph node involvement and distant metastases is exceptionally high in the tumors of the dome of the bladder and in the tumors originating at the base of the bladder that have invaded the prostatic gland.

Clinical Staging of the Tumor

Staging: (International Union Against Cancer)

T_1S: Carcinoma in situ

T_1: Tumor with infiltration into subepithelial tissues

T_2: Tumor with infiltration into superficial muscle

T_3: Tumor with infiltration into deep muscle

T_4: Tumor with infiltration into adjacent organs

$N +$ (regional) Tumor with lymph node metastases below bifurcation of iliac arteries

$M +$ (distant) Tumor with distant metastases of lymph node metastases in periaortic region

Clinical staging should be based on clinical, radiographic, endoscopic, and biopsy findings. The important point in staging is the assessment of the degree of infiltration of the tumor through the different layers of the bladder wall or beyond it, degree of fixation to the pelvic wall, detection of nodes either by abdominal or bimanual examination, or by lymphangiography.

Obstruction of one ureter with hydronephrosis indicates that the tumor is in an advanced stage; they should always be staged as infiltrative tumors, even if not palpable by bimanual examination or if there is no evidence of histological invasion of the submucosal muscularis.[11] A dual classification making use of the staging as described and the grade of anaplasticity of the tumor will help in deciding the policy of treatment.

It is to be emphasized that there is a great deal of divergence between clinical and surgical staging by the study of the specimen; usually the surgical specimen shows deeper penetration than the clinical work-up. This difference is to be considered when comparing results between radiotherapy and surgical excision alone or preceded by preoperative irradiation.

Examination and Clinical Evaluation of Tumors of the Bladder

History and Physical Examination

A careful history is necessary to evaluate the natural history of the tumor. The examination should provide information of the extension of the growth, condition of the tumor bed, urinary function, and general condition of the patient. Rectal examination for men is the first step. Basic information about the direct extensions of the tumor can be obtained by palpation of the prostate and tissues immediately above the lateral to the prostate and by rectovaginal examination in women of the tissue anterior and lateral to the uterine isthmus.

Lymph node bearing areas of the groin, iliac fossae, and supraclavicular area should be examined and the liver carefully palpated. If indicated, liver scanning and liver function tests are carried out.

Cystoscopic and bimanual examination under general anesthesia is of utmost importance and the radiotherapist should participate at this particular examination. A pedunculated tumor (large polyp) is seldom palpable and if it is, it is felt as a soft, mobile intravesical mass. A thickening of the bladder wall is generally felt above and/or lateral to the prostate or just above and lateral to the uterine isthmus and represents, as a rule, infiltration of the muscle without extension beyond the vesical wall. A mass with some fixation which can be felt in the previously described areas, usually represents infiltrating carcinoma throughout the bladder wall. If the mass is fixed to the pelvic wall, it is clear that there is extravesical extension easily palpable. Sometimes metastatic lymph nodes are felt as a mass against the pelvic wall or the iliac fossa. Other times an abdominal mass is palpable, mostly in tumors originating in the bladder dome. If the patient has had previous suprapubic cystotomy, the scar on the abdominal wall should be carefully examined for nodularities which represent tumor seeding.

Biopsy

It is useful to take several biopsies from representative areas which will give the histological type of the tumor and its grade. Gradually, deeper biopsy with separate specimens could give information of the degree of infiltration.

X-ray Examination

An *IVP* gives information about possible obstruction, dilation, and also possible presence of tumor in the renal pelvis, calyces, or ureters. If there is an indication, retrograde urograms and separate cytologies from the ureters should be requested.

A cystogram helps define the extension of the tumor into the bladder and/or extravesical spread. In treatment planning, it is an indispensible film for the localization of the bladder and its tumor. Today, all infiltrating carcinomas of the bladder should have lymphangiogram study. It will give information in regard to lymph node metastases in the pelvis and the common iliac and periaortic areas. The technique of treatment should be modified only in cases where the diagnosis of metastatic nodes from the lymphangiogram is unquestionable. Angiograms, with and without air contrast can be of help in better defining the true extension of the tumor. X-ray films of the chest and bones are indicated if there is suggestion of osseous pain.

Action of Radiation on Normal Structures

Bladder

With megavoltage, mucosal reactions start with a mild congestion and edema at 3,000 rads delivered in 3 to 4 weeks increasing sometimes to very severe cystitis when the dose is in the order of 6,000 rads or more delivered in 5 to 7 weeks. In general, the cystitis subsides 2 to 3 weeks after the treatment. The late changes appear generally between 1 and 4 years after treatment and consist of fibrosis of the muscularis, atrophy of the mucosa, and telangiectasis. In some patients, the bladder capacity is reduced and in rare cases periodic hematuria is produced which is seldom profuse. When the bladder has been irradiated beyond the tolerance, necrotic ulcers may result which can be infected and encrusted with calcium deposits. A deep ulcer can lead to the production of rectal and/or vaginal fistulae. Slow-healing ulceration, encrusted with calcium, results after proper treatment of large ulcerated tumors. In these cases symptoms are scarce and spontaneous healing follows several months after therapy. A very uncomfortable late effect of radiation upon the bladder is the so-called retracted bladder which is due to a replacement of the muscle and mucosa by fibrotic tissue so that the bladder is no longer distensible and capacity is reduced to 40 to 80 cc.

With megavoltage and proper technique it is possible to conduct radical treatment with only mild cystitis in most patients and a minimum of complications.[3] In our experience, severe cystitis or a retracted bladder is produced usually in the patient exhibiting factors which enhance the reaction of irradiation. These factors are:

1) Surgical procedures such as transurethral resection, multiple biopsies (with extensive cauterization), suprapubic cystotomy, or segmental resection performed within 3 weeks prior to the beginning of radiation therapy.

2) Obstruction of the bladder neck, prostatic hypertrophy, and urethral obstruction.

3) Gross infection.

4) Repeated multiple cauterizations in years prior to therapy.

5) In extensive ulcerating tumors, there is usually a combination of several of the previous factors. In patients with tumors invading the bladder neck, there are almost always marked reactions (frequency and burning) to the treatment.

Ureter and Urethra

When these organs are in normal condition, they tolerate well radical doses of irradiation. Obstruction can be the result of scarring following tissue destruction pro-

duced by a tumor which was sterilized by irradiation. Late obstruction is usually a sign of residual or recurrent cancer.

Small Intestine

When a large volume of the pelvis is irradiated, often a small intestine enteritis is produced which is manifested by watery diarrhea without tenesmus. It is usually transient and responds well to the usual treatment. Late effects on the small intestine and sigmoid colon can be fibrosis and necrosis with the production of intestinal obstruction and/or fistulae.

Rectum

With radical techniques avoiding irradiation of the whole rectum, rectal reactions are rare. Mild rectitis with tenesmus and production of mucous can appear in some patients. Late complications from irradiation can be narrowing of the rectum, necrotic rectal ulcer, and fistulae formation.

Radiosensitivity of Bladder Tumors

Primary Tumor

There is some gradient of radiosensitivity ranging from that for the anaplastic transitional cell carcinoma to that for the more differentiated squamous cell carcinoma. At the moment, the differences in radiosensitivity between different histological types do not justify changes in dosage. Histology is only one factor in the determination of the response to irradiation of a particular tumor. Other factors are: Size of the tumor, volume of tissue irradiated, condition of the tumor bed, and the general condition of the patient.

A study of the literature shows a wide range in the dose used in treatment for bladder carcinoma. Using 3,000 to 4,000 rads in 3 to 4 weeks preoperatively, Guttmann *et al*[8] have reported a high percentage of sterilization of bladder tumors, whereas local failures of controlling tumor have been reported with a maximum tumor dose of 13,000 rads in 90 days.[6] With megavoltage irradiation the doses commonly used in the treatment of bladder tumors are between 6,000 rads in 5 weeks to 7,000 rads in 7 weeks. With interstitial gamma-ray therapy, 6,000 rads in 5 days to 6,500 rads in 7 days have been commonly used. For intracavitary therapy with a central source, surface doses of 6,000 to 10,000 rads in 15 days have been used. With radioactive colloidal gold, 8,000 rads are generally delivered with 2 to 6 weeks interval between the two applications.

With those doses, local control of the tumor has been only around 50 per cent. Although some failures may be due to geographic misses or not treating in the best optimal physiologic conditions, for the vast majority there is no obvious explanation except that tolerable doses for the whole bladder are still below a high point on the sigmoid response curve of tumor control.

It is possible that after whole bladder irradiation additional procedures such as local implants or central sources of irradiation delivering an extra dose to an area of residual tumor could help improve local results without considerable increase of complications. However, there are several factors that militate against control of the bladder tumor in most cases. These factors are: lack of proper oxygenation, poor tumor bed in most tumors, and, in grave cases, massive size. We have to wait for new laboratory developments in order to dramatically improve the results.

Irradiation does not seem to prevent new tumors. Recurrent tumors after irradiation are often at sites different than the original primary and frequently have different clinical and histological characteristics, mostly better differentiated. In our experience, benign or malignant papillary tumors have developed after irradiation of infiltrating squamous cell or transitional cell carcinomas.

Radiosensitivity of Lymph Node Metastases

By analogy with squamous cell carcinoma of the uterine cervix, where it has been proven that lymph node metastases can be sterilized, one can infer that a certain percentage of metastases from tumors of the urinary bladder can be sterilized. There is some clinical evidence to that effect.

It is to be remembered that subclinical, microscopic metastases can be controlled with much lower doses (around 4,000 rads in 4 weeks) than the doses necessary for the control of the primary.

Radiation Treatment of Bladder Cancer

Factors To Be Considered in Setting a Policy of Treatment

Besides the considerations common to the treatment for any other groups of carcinoma, there are some features peculiar to carcinoma of the bladder which pose special therapeutic problems; they are:

1) The frequent multiplicity of tumors could be responsible for failures when the whole bladder is not included in the treatment.

2) Bladder tumors often originate and grow near the orifices of the ureters and urethra. Obstruction, with resulting urinary retention and infection, is usually produced by the tumor bulk or infiltration. Two thirds of the deaths from bladder cancer are due to renal damage produced by these obstructions.

3) The continuous contact of the tumor with urine is responsible for maceration, necrosis in the tumor, common infection, and other alterations in the tumor bed which modify radiation effect. Transplant of tumor cells might be responsible for some treatment failures.

4) Some bladder tumors are histologically benign, however, they run a clinically malig-

nant course; other benign tumors will degenerate into histologically malignant ones during their evolution.

5) The examination of a patient for diagnosis, treatment, and follow-up of bladder cancer requires special procedures (cystoscopy and bimanual examination under anesthesia) out of the dominion of the radiotherapy department; however, the radiotherapist must familiarize himself with these procedures to evaluate the findings in each case.

6) Bladder tumors are most frequent in patients of extreme age who have other complicating diseases.

All these factors should be considered in planning the treatment of a patient with bladder cancer.

Preparation of the Patient for Optimal Physiologic Conditions

Obstructions should be eliminated by the necessary surgical procedures, *i.e.,* TUR in prostatic adenomas or bladder neck hypertrophy or tumor invasion; sometimes an indwelling catheter or even urinary diversion is required. By correcting the obstruction, treatment of infection is greatly facilitated. Administration of antibiotics during the first 2 weeks of therapy will improve the tolerance in those patients.

The urinary diverting procedures diminish tumor maceration produced by the contact of urine and therefore diminishes necrosis, infection, and the late changes in the bladder. The possibility of transplant of desquamated tumor cells by urine is diminished. Possibly it could also diminish the incidence of new tumors at a later date because the cancerogenic agent responsible for the production of bladder cancers is eliminated.

A minimum waiting period of 4 weeks after any one of the surgical procedures, *i.e.,* transurethral resection, multiple biopsies (with extensive cauterizations), suprapubic cystotomy, or segmental resection will diminish the severity of reactions and the incidence of contracted bladders.

External Radical Irradiation

QUALITY OF RADIATION

Through the years a great variety of treatments have been used in dealing with carcinoma of the bladder. Since the advent of megavoltage, external beam irradiation has established itself as the main modality of treatment. Today, whenever radical treatment is indicated, the use of megavoltage external irradiation is mandatory and all the other modalities of irradiation should be considered as complementary techniques to be used in exceptional cases. The energies of radiation most used are: 1 to 6 Mev and 22 Mev, telecobalt with an *SSD* of 70 cm or over.

LOCALIZATION PROCEDURES

The position and shape of the bladder varies considerably from patient to patient. A cystogram with reference markers on the

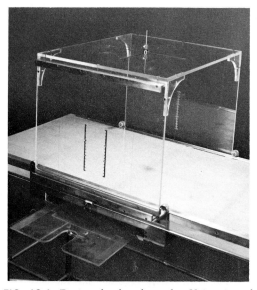

FIG. 12-1. Device developed at the University of Maryland for the localization of tumors in relation to the table top. It carries cassette holders, lateral and vertical markers, and a pointer to relate the position of the bridge with the patient.

patient's skin and/or in reference to the table top (Figs. 12-1, 12-2A and B) is an indispensable first step in any treatment planning; it will give topographic information about the area to be treated and also be helpful in defining the site and extension of the tumor.

Once the cystogram is available, the number, position, and size of the fields are decided and marked on the patient; the bladder is emptied; the 5cc balloon of the already inserted Foley catheter is filled with mercury and 30 cc of air is injected freely in the bladder. Portal films (Fig. 12-3) are taken with the megavoltage machine in the treatment position for each field (90-degree angle; *AP* and lateral at the desired height if rotation

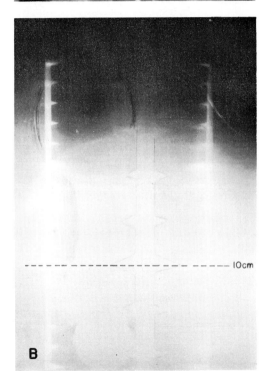

FIG. 12-2. A. Cystogram taken with the localization bridge. The lead bead markers are 1 cm apart, giving references for dimensions and displacement of the fields.

   B. A lateral cystogram taken with the localization bridge. The markers show centimeters from the top of the table.

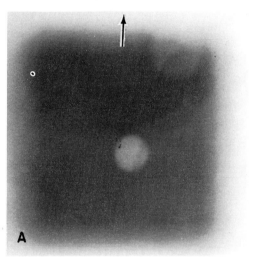

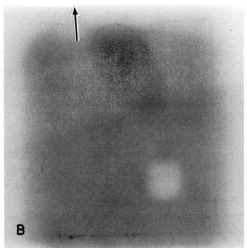

FIG. 12-3. *AP* and lateral localization films taken with telecobalt unit. The air bubble and the mercury bag show the position of the dome and base of the bladder respectively. Adjustments were made in the direction of the arrows.

is planned). If the mercury-filled balloon is kept snugly against the bladder neck, it will outline the position of the trigone; the air will define the dome area. In institutions where simulator equipment is available, the whole cystogram and field localization procedure can be performed outside the treatment room with the same contrast medium.

We prefer to have the bladder emptied immediately before each treatment in order to assure the inclusion of the whole organ within the smallest volume of high-dose irradiation.

TOTAL PELVIS IRRADIATION
(Fig. 12-4A)

The indications for this technique are based on the need to irradiate the whole complex of clinically and potentially in-

volved areas. An effort should be made to irradiate uniformly the whole pelvis sparing the rectum as much as possible without jeopardizing the success of the treatment by missing tumor extensions. The correctness of the irradiation coverage is corroborated when the portal films taken under treatment conditions show the whole bladder, the paravesical tissues, and the lateral walls of the pelvis including the lower half of the sacroiliac joint and the upper half of the obturator foramen. If there is any potential or evident prostatic and/or proximal urethral involvement, the caudal limit of the fields should be extended to cover these organs. With total pelvis irradiation, a daily dose of 200 rads tissue dose is well tolerated by most patients. The main early reaction noticed has been indolent, watery small intestinal diarrhea. Severe cystitis seldom develops during the first 3 weeks of treatment. If either of these reactions are unusually intense, the daily

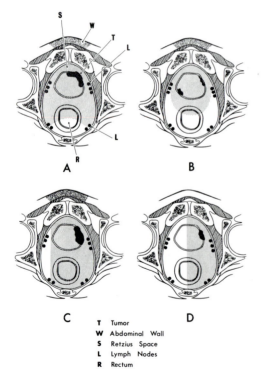

T	Tumor
W	Abdominal Wall
S	Retzius Space
L	Lymph Nodes
R	Rectum

FIG. 12-4. The cross-section of the volume to be irradiated is stippled.

    A. Total Pelvis Irradiation. The area of high dose irradiation should cover the

whole true pelvis, trying to save at least the posterior portion of the rectum whenever possible. The abdominal wall (*W*) and Retzius's space (*S*) should also be included in cases where suprapubic operations have been performed.

    B. Total Bladder Irradiation. The volume of high dose irradiation should include the whole bladder with a margin around it. Most of the rectum should be spared from high irradiation. In cases of suprapubic surgery, the abdominal wall (*W*) and the Retzius's space (*S*) should be included in the high-dose volume.

    C. Whole Bladder to One Pelvic Wall. The volume of high-dose irradiation should include, besides the bladder, the paravesical tissues and lymph node bearing areas of one side of the pelvis (*L*). In cases of suprapubic surgery, the abdominal wall (*W*) and the Retzius's space (*S*) should be included in the high-dose volume.

    D. Irradiation of Residual Tumor, Paravesical Tissues, and Lymph Node Bearing Areas of the Pelvis. The volume of high-dose irradiation should cover only the tumor-bearing areas of the bladder, the paravesical tissues, and the lymph node bearing areas of the pelvis (*L*).

dose should be reduced or even the treatment should be discontinued for a few days. By using higher daily doses, the proportion of early reactions increases sharply as well as the late morbid effects in the bladder, small intestine, sigmoid, and rectum. Total pelvis irradiation is usually indicated as the first phase of the therapy up to a total tumor dose (enough to control subclinical disease outside of the primary tumor) of 4,000 to 4,500 rads in 4 to $4\frac{1}{2}$ weeks to be complemented by one of the techniques described later. Higher doses are possible in some cases without overtaxing the tolerance of the pelvic organs (5,000 to 5,500 rads with 2 Mev or ^{60}Cobalt; 7,000 rads in 7 weeks with 20 Mev). These extremely high doses sharply increase the complication risks, seldom adding to the cure rate.

The most used field arrangement to cover the pelvis is that of 2 parallel opposing fields, cross-fire of 3, 4, or more fields and large-field rotation. The sizes of the fields are between 12 to 14 cm in height and width. The oblique fields on the cross-fire techniques are generally narrower (10 to 12 cm). The 2 parallel opposing fields technique has the disadvantage of irradiating the subcutaneous tissues to levels higher than the pelvic structures. The large-field rotation has little advantage over cross-fire technique in sparing normal tissues and has an added inconvenience in that the cylinder of heavy radiation is not always the best orientation for all variants of pelvic position. The 3-fields technique is especially useful when the patient has had previous suprapubic surgery or tumor extension into the prevesical space requiring higher irradiation in the front.

We use 2 parallel opposing fields in thin patients up to 20 cm in diameter in the rest of the patients, the 4-fields technique is used, except for the very fat patient where we use rotation. We rarely use the 3-fields technique; it is used only when the abdominal wall is to be irradiated. The highest voltage available is always indicated.

TOTAL BLADDER IRRADIATION

This plan of treatment is used when the volume of high irradiation is to encompass the whole bladder with a margin of at least 2 cm around it. The geometry preferred is the one which irradiates the least normal tissues around the bladder with day-to-day accurate reproducibility. The techniques most used are: rotation of either 360 degrees or arc (120 to 220 degrees) or a combination of anterior and posterior arcs or cross-fire of 3, 4 or more fields. Two anterior oblique wedge fields have been used in institutions where 20 Mev or more is available.[13] The whole bladder should show in each of the portal films. The field size required is between 8 to 10 cm per side. Beyond these dimensions the volume irradiated is practically the whole pelvis in a male. The daily dose which is tolerated by most patients is from 200 to 250 rads tumor dose with telecobalt and 2 to 6 Mev. It could be slightly higher with higher energies and better beam collimation. The total dose of 6,000 to 6,500 rads in 5 to 6 weeks for telecobalt and 2 to 4 Mev, 6,500 to 7,000 rads in 6 to 7 weeks with 20 or more Mev. The daily dose and the total dose are to be matched with the field size, the local condition of the bladder, tumor and tumor bed, and the general condition of the patient.

All the techniques described here are useful and the choice should be made according to the position and shape of the bladder and the equipment available. A 360-degree or arc pendular rotation should be the techniques of choice when available. They are easily reproduced and except for larger fields they yield the best distribution of radiation. Using rotation with the patient lying on a flat-top table presents distinct advantages; comfort for the patient with less chances of moving during therapy and the possibility of using the table top as reference, giving more accuracy and easy reproducibility in daily treatments.

OTHER TECHNIQUES

In some cases, there are indications to irradiate the whole bladder along with paravesical tissue and lymph node bearing areas of one pelvic wall (Fig. 12-4C). Rotational techniques, cross-fire 4-field or 2 parallel opposing fields are used in these cases. The size of the fields in these cases should be 12 to 14 cm in height and from 10 to 12 cm in width. We prefer the 4-fields "box" or rotation as the technique which most spares the normal tissues from unnecessary irradiation. In advanced tumors, it may be necessary to increase the irradiation to the lymph node region at the pelvic wall and paravesical tissues at the end of the treatment period with 2 narrow parallel opposing fields of 12 to 14 by 6 to 7 cm (Fig. 12-4D).

Internal Irradiation

IRRADIATION OF THE MUCOSA ONLY

These techniques of treatment have been developed with the idea of delivering radiation only to the whole of the mucosa and submucosal layers and the small papillary tumors originated in it. Most of the procedures devised make use of predominantly beta-emitting isotopes. Due to the slight penetration of these types of radiation only small papillary tumors, about 0.5 cm, can be treated properly. The isotope can be in a thin rubber balloon which fills the bladder or it can be injected freely as a colloidal solution.

Free Colloidal Solution Method. The rationale for the use of this technique is that the beta-emitter in a colloidal solution injected freely will irradiate evenly the bladder surface (mucosa and submucosa), disregarding the shape of the bladder, and will penetrate the multiple spaces among the digitations of the tumor. The absorption of a colloidal solution is negligible.

The most common procedure in use today is instillation of radioactive colloidal gold[5] in 2 applications of 300 mc, mixed with 50 to 60 ml of isotonic saline solution. The solution is retained in the bladder for the time necessary to deliver 3,000 to 4,000 rads (90 per cent beta) in approximately 3 hours. The procedure is repeated 1 month after cystoscopy to check the reaction and tumor regression. The second dose is regulated according to cystoscopic findings.

We inject the solution through a French catheter, which is removed as soon as the gold is injected, to assure proper irradiation of the trigone and bladder neck. Recurrences in these areas have been seen when a retention catheter was used which prevents proper contact between the fluid and the mucosa of the area. The patient should restrain from intaking fluid 12 hours before the treatment and sedation and muscle relaxants are administered. Continuous change of position of the patient assures uniformity of the suspension and contact of the colloidal gold with the mucosa. After the solution is removed through a catheter, the bladder is washed generously with saline solution until the suprapubic count shows radiation level below tolerance. From the 2nd to the 4th weeks after treatment the patient develops reaction cystitis which is generally mild. Late effects of mucosal atrophy and telangiectasia of different degrees are frequent. Severe hemorrhage produced by rupture of dilated vessels seldom occurs.

The use of intracavitary chemotherapy is diminishing the use of radioactive colloids.

Partial Irradiation of the Bladder Mucosa and Muscle

This group of techniques has been developed for the irradiation at different depths of only a segment of the bladder depending upon the procedure required for a primary treatment. The indication for use of these techniques of irradiation are limited. They can be useful, however, for cases where total bladder irradiation is contraindicated (*i.e.* retreatment, palliation) or as a complementary treatment for residual tumors after external irradiation.

Central Intracavitary Source (Walter Reed Technique). This method, developed by Friedman[7] consists of the use of a small but strong intracavitary source of radiation which is maintained in place by a Foley balloon which also maintains constant treatment distance. The aim of the central source technique is the irradiation of the tumor-bearing area of the bladder with a minimum irradiation of the surrounding structures. The treatment distance is about 2 cm. A suprapubic cystotomy assures a better evaluation of the tumor extension and the proper placement of the balloon. Suprapubic drainage of the urine during the application avoids urine accumulating between the balloon surface and the tumor. Roentgenographic control of the application during the treatment is indispens-

able to correct any displacement of the balloon.

Interstitial Methods. The aim of interstitial therapy is to irradiate the tumor and tumor-bearing area of the bladder. This procedure has been developed by the Manchester group.[16,17] It consists of implantation of interstitial sources of gamma radiation into the tumor-bearing area in a single-plane fashion through a suprapubic cystotomy. It will irradiate satisfactorily a slab of tissue 1 cm thick. In exophytic lesions, the surface of the tumor is saucerized by a diathermy loop. The sources of irradiation used have been permanent implants—such as radon seeds (Fig. 12-5), and radioactive gold grains[9] and temporary implants—such as radium needles,[15] radioactive tantalum wire[20] and nylon-threaded radioactive iridium of cobalt seeds.[19] The distribution of the radiation

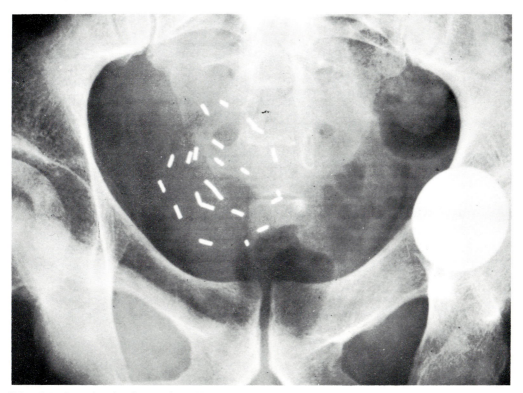

FIG. 12-5. Example of radon implant. (Courtesy: Eric Easson, Christie Hospital and Holt Radium Institute, Manchester, England.)

sources follows the Paterson-Parker system. In the techniques where permanent implants are used, the bladder is closed after the procedure. In the temporary ones, the threads or tubes are brought out through the cystotomy wound and pulled out when the treatment is finished. In all procedures, the dosimetry is based on calculation performed from postoperative films. The dose aimed for is 7,000 rads in 7 days.

These techniques have yielded some satisfactory results in selected cases: well-differentiated tumors producing flat lesions less than 4 cm in diameter "which have not penetrated the muscle coat"[18] and in single lesions or multiple clusters in small areas without obvious changes of the bladder mucosa outside of the tumor. The limitations of these methods are the limited volume of irradiation in area and depth and the possibilities of wound seeding.

Clinicopathological Groups and Therapeutic Indications

Patients with bladder cancer come to the therapist with different types of tumors at varied stages of their disease. These clinicopathological features are grouped in rather constant patterns of clinicotherapeutic significance. These groups and their therapeutic indications are described below.

SINGLE OR MULTIPLE PAPILLOMAS (NONINFILTRATIVE)

Patients in this group come to the therapist with different stages of disease, seldom without previous cauterizations, and commonly after a few or multiple transurethral cauterizations. In general, they have a long history. The tumors are not palpable. A careful study of the whole urinary tract (*IVP*, retrograde studies, and separate cytologies from both ureters) is indispensable to make sure that the disease is limited to the bladder.

In general, this type of disease can be kept under control for many years by surgical procedures, mostly *TUR*. Irradiation is to be

considered only in cases where the recurrences become more frequent and numerous, when the histology of some of the tumors shows malignant changes or when there is infiltration on the base of some of the papillomas. If there is not an infiltrating tumor and the diameter of each of the papillomas is not larger than a half centimeter, intracavitary radioactive gold should be the treatment of choice. If the diameter of one or more of the papillomas is larger, it should be cauterized first and after a resting period of one month the gold can be applied. In all other cases, total bladder external irradiation (if possible with rotation) is the treatment of choice. Permanent control of the disease with this kind of treatment is not very good. In about 30 to 50 per cent of the cases, post-irradiation recurrent papillomas will appear, generally occurring at time periods spaced further and further apart and at slow growing rates. These can be controlled with further cauterization. In other cases, a total cystectomy is required to control the relentless progression of the disease.

EARLY INFILTRATING CARCINOMA (ONE OR MORE TUMORS, BUT GROUPED TOGETHER IN THE SAME SITE OF THE BLADDER)

These patients should have cystoscopic and/or histological proof of muscle infiltration. They are either not palpable or palpable only as thickening of the bladder wall in the area involved by the tumor. In general, they are tumors with infiltration not going beyond the muscular layer.

The minimum treatment should consist of total bladder irradiation with external beam (megavoltage). These types of tumors can be divided into 2 groups:

Well-Differentiated Tumors (Transitional Cell, Squamous Cell, and Adenocarcinoma). These are treated by total bladder technique all the way (Fig. 12-4B). The dose aimed at will be 6,000 to 6,500 rads in 5 to 6½ weeks depending upon the field size, local and general conditions, and reactions produced during the treatment.

Anaplastic. The whole pelvis (3 or 4 fields) (Fig. 12-4A) received up to 4,000 to 4,500 rads tumor dose and then the entire bladder up to a total tumor dose of 5,500 to 6,000 rads by rotation. The total dose will depend upon the field size, the general condition of the patient, and the amount of reaction developed during the treatment. Cross-fire technique or two anterior oblique wedge fields are possible alternatives when rotation is not available. The indication for whole pelvis irradiation is based on the percentage of subclinical spread of the tumor outside the bladder in this group of tumors even in its early stages.

INFILTRATING TUMOR WITH
PALPABLE MASS

In general, these represent tumors which spread beyond the bladder wall. They can be: 1) without obstruction, or 2) with obstruction of the bladder neck and/or unilateral or bilateral obstruction of the ureters.

Without Obstruction. In this group of patients, the minimum volume to be considered for treatment comprises the whole bladder and the paravesical tissue to the pelvic wall of the affected side (Fig. 12-4C), going as low as demanded by the extension to the bladder neck and potential of actual extension to the prostate. In most cases, due to location of the tumor or its extensions not crossing the midline or to the anaplasticity shown by histology, whole pelvis (Fig. 12-4A) irradiation is indicated for the first 4,000 to 4,500 rads; this is followed by rotation or cross-fire technique including the bladder and pelvic wall of the affected side for the remainder of the treatment (up to 6,000 rads). In cases where the tumor presents as a large mass outside of the bladder, it is necessary to add an extra 500 to 700 rads in 2 to 3 treatments with narrow parallel opposing fields (10 to 12 × 6 to 7 cm) (Fig. 12-4D) covering the affected half of the bladder and the paravesical tissues to the pelvic wall.

With Obstruction. Patients with bladder neck obstruction should have the obstruction corrected by *TUR* with a rest period of one month before starting irradiation. The technique of irradiation is the one indicated by the characteristics of the tumor and its extensions; the same policy of treatment applies whether the obstruction is due to prostatic invasion by the bladder tumor or to benign prostatic adenoma. Patients with bladder neck tumor, even without obstruction, tolerate treatment poorly due to painful urination, frequency, and intense burning sensation. We have found it useful to use an indwelling catheter during the treatment and 2 to 4 weeks thereafter. In cases where there is obstruction of one ureter and no previous surgery was indicated, the obstruction often will improve and disappear with the treatment. If there exists an involvement with obstruction of both ureters (even if mild on one side), the patient must have a urinary diversion, preferably ileal pouch, one month before starting irradiation. The technique of irradiation in cases after diversion invariably should be total pelvis first (Fig. 12-4A); 4,500 to 5,000 rads are given in 4½ to 5 weeks. Thereafter, the bladder alone or bladder to pelvic wall receive up to 6,000 to 6,500 rads in 6½ weeks (reducing field size after 5,500 to 6,000) according to the gross extension of the tumor, general and local condition of the patient and the reaction produced during the treatment. After diversion, the irradiation of the bladder is generally better tolerated.

LATE TUMORS WITH EXTENSION OUTSIDE
OF THE BLADDER OR WITH TUMORS
INVOLVING A VERY LARGE SEGMENT
OF BLADDER WALL

These tumors are generally fixed to the pelvic wall, pelvic organs, or to the abdominal wall. It is unusual to have these types of tumors without some kind of obstruction. Most cases will show obstruction as in the previous groups and/or fixation to the pelvic wall. Generally these tumors are present in patients who are very old, in poor general condition, with tumors ulcerated, infected, macerated, and with abnormal urinary physiology.

The first effort in this group of tumors should be concentrated on improving the general condition, local condition, and physiologic flow of urine. Antibiotics are indicated when infection is present. The indications for *TUR* of the bladder neck and/or diversion are as outlined for the previous group. If the patient cannot be put in better physiologic condition, radical treatment is not indicated. In all cases, the first stage of therapy is total pelvis (Fig. 12-4A) irradiation up to 4,500 to 5,000 rads in 4 to 5 weeks. The second portion of the treatment should involve the bladder and paravesical tissues to the pelvic wall of the involved side (Fig. 12-4C) up to 6,000 to 6,500 rads in $6\frac{1}{2}$ weeks. If the amount of residual tumor, general and local condition of the patient, and the reaction developed during the treatment allows, an additional 500 rads in 2 treatments is indicated in the area of remaining tumor (Fig. 12-4C). Two parallel opposing fields or rotation can be used.

In a few cases where the residual tumor mass is of considerable extension, a more localized therapy such as central source or interstitial therapy after 6,000 to 6,500 rads tumor dose has been delivered could be indicated (1,000 to 2,000 rads to the tumor only). We have done it only in a few instances, but it seems probable that higher local doses are necessary to control most of these extensive tumors when they are not resectable after irradiation. This is possible only if the last phase of the treatment is strictly limited to the residual tumor.

SIMULTANEOUS MULTIPLE VARIABLE TYPES (TUMORS OVER A LARGE PORTION OF THE WHOLE BLADDER)

Some of them are of the infiltrating type. Others are noninfiltrating and papillary. At least one or more tumors will be in advanced stages.

In this group of patients, the indication for the technique of treatment to use is indicated by the most advanced and/or anaplastic lesion.

POSTSURGERY

Some patients are referred for therapy after some type of surgical act has been performed. Depending upon the extension of the surgery and the time period since it was performed the patients could be grouped as follows:

1) After exploration and biopsy: Operation performed through a suprapubic approach.

2) After surgical procedures with intent to cure. This could be extensive or repeated transurethral resections, segmental resection or total cystectomy. According to the time elapsed between the surgery and irradiation, these patients can be divided into 2 groups: 1) up to 3 months after the surgical procedure (postoperative therapy); and 2) over 3 months after the surgical procedure has been performed (retreatment).

In all cases a resting period of one month is allowed between the surgical act and the beginning of the irradiation.

Group 1. Due to the possibilities of wound seeding in these patients, the use of a technique which will give a high dose to the anterior abdominal wall and the Retzius's space is indicated. We prefer three-field arrangement for total pelvis (Fig. 12-4A) and anterior arc rotation (140 to 180 degrees) for total bladder irradiation. Otherwise, the indications, techniques, and dosage are given as demanded by the tumor and its extensions.

Group 2. Postoperative therapy: after extensive *TUR* of the tumor and the resting period of 1 month, the therapy is carried out according to the original site, histology, and extension of the tumor as described in previous groups. After segmental resection, all patients should be considered as having residual disease in the bladder and possible seeding in the pelvis and abdominal wall (operative field). Therefore, the technique of irradiation will consist of total pelvis irradiation (Fig. 12-4A) for 4,000 to 4,500 rads in 4 to 4½ weeks, preferably with a three-field arrangement for the first stage of the treatment that should include the bladder, the anterior abdominal wall, and the Retzius's space. For the last portion of the treatment, up to a total of 5,500 to 6,500 rads in 5½ to 6 weeks only the bladder (Fig. 12-4B) is irradiated. The highest dose is used in cases with clinically detectable residual tumor. The patient should be cautiously checked during the treatment, trying to assess his tolerance because these are the patients who develop the most severe early and late reactions to irradiation.

In these cases, the treatment must be guided by the local situation of the tumor and its extension and the other considerations of the patient's general condition and urinary function as in any patient with previous open surgery with cystostomy. Due to the previous surgical manipulation, irradiation of the total pelvis (Fig. 12-4A) and the anterior abdomen is required in all cases where the time elapsed between the operation and irradiation is within a year. It is not unusual to find in this group of patients tumor nodules in the abdominal wall along the surgical scar. In such cases, we add interstitial irradiation (radium needles or nylon-threaded iridium) to the area involved in the abdominal wall at the end of the external irradiation (1,000 to 2,000 rads). It is sometimes necessary to perform a higher transverse laparotomy to place the implant properly with minimum irradiation of the abdominal organs (Fig. 12-6).

After Total Cystectomy Immediately After Surgery (Up to Three Months). In cases with residual disease or seeding, radiotherapy is indicated. A resting period between procedures of at least 3 weeks is necessary. The

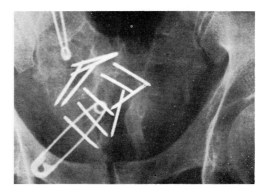

FIG. 12-6 Example of radium implant. The patient had a residual tumor 3 months after external irradiation which delivered, 4,200 r in 5 weeks (200 Kv, 1 ml Cu *HVL*). A single plane implant was performed delivering 6,500 r in 95 hours. The patient is alive with no evidence of disease 6 years later.

total pelvis technique with high irradiation of the abdominal wall (Fig. 12-4A) is indicated in these cases up to 4,500 rads in 4½ to 5 weeks. Thereafter, in accordance with the site and extension of the residual disease, extra treatment (*i.e.* 1,000 to 2,000 rads, small-field 360 degrees rotation) is indicated for prostatic involvement or narrow fields against the pelvic wall for lymph node involvement.

If the patient is to be treated 3 months after surgery for recurrent disease, the treatment is guided by the site, type, and extension of the recurrent tumor. In general, total pelvis and additional treatment by rotation, small-field or interstitial therapy is indicated.

RECURRENT, POSTIRRADIATION

The previous therapy could have been delivered by means of conventional external irradiation, megavoltage, intracavitary, or interstitial irradiation.

Complete radical external irradiation is not advisable after any kind of irradiation (localized or not) has failed in controlling the tumor. In some exceptional cases, when surgery is contraindicated and the location of the recurrence is favorable, an interstitial implant or central source technique could be indicated. In general, the tolerance for retreatment is very limited and the risk of complication is great with a very slim chance for tumor control.

Preoperative Irradiation

In spite of the progress made in the treatment of bladder cancer by irradiation, the analysis of series of patients treated reveals that the results are still unsatisfactory. The local control of the disease is low (less than 50 per cent) and the production of new tumors is frequent. With the present knowledge it is impossible to predict which particular tumor will respond favorably to irradiation; even after treatment, it is impossible to determine when permanent control has been obtained. The results of surgical therapy by itself are even more disappointing in regard to tumor control and complication rates. Based on theoretical reasoning and on the results obtained in a few clinical studies it seems that preoperative irradiation may have a place in treatment for bladder cancer. Preliminary studies have shown that the method is feasible without appreciably increasing the morbidity.[21,22] Preoperative irradiation in treatment for carcinoma of the bladder should only be undertaken where the association between radiotherapist and urologist is very close and the techniques of both modalities of treatment very careful and accurate.

INDICATIONS

Preoperative irradiation may be indicated in the group of tumors where the control of the disease is low with both modalities of therapy: large infiltrating tumors (with palpable mass), tumors with extension outside of the bladder (prostate, perivesical tissue, lymph nodes at pelvic wall), all infiltrating, squamous and adenocarcinomas as well as multiple infiltrative tumors with frequent recurrences or consecutive primaries.

Most cases should have total pelvis irradiation since the rationale is to irradiate the whole of the complex of potentially involved tissue. The surgery indicated is total cystectomy. Two techniques have been developed which proved feasible and safe.

1) Four thousand rads total pelvis in 4 weeks and 8 weeks resting period before surgery.[21]

2) Five thousand to 5,500 rads in $5\frac{1}{2}$ weeks with a minimum of 4,500 rads delivered to the total pelvis[22] with surgery 6 to 8 weeks later.

With the latter technique we have 54 per cent of 37 patients alive and free of disease 3 years or more and 39 per cent of 27 patients with advanced disease free of disease 5 years or over.[22] With either of these techniques, the surgical complications were not higher than without previous irradiation. A well-controlled study is needed to determine the real place of preoperative irradiation in bladder cancer.

PALLIATIVE TREATMENT

In our experience, there are very few indications for palliative irradiation in cancer of the bladder except to stop bleeding. In very advanced tumors with obstruction and infection, the treatment will precipitate or worsen lethal complications, *i.e.* urinary retention with uremia and ascending infection. If a patient with advanced cancer of the bladder has disease beyond the limits of the pelvis (periaortic lymph nodes or distant metastases), the simplest urinary diversion procedure is indicated if there is an obstruction and irradiation is used only to relieve bleeding or pain due to bony metastases.

BIBLIOGRAPHY

1. Ackerman, L. V., and del Regato, J. A.: *Cancer,* 3rd ed., St. Louis, C. V. Mosby Company, 1962.
2. Baker, R.: Lymphatic spread of bladder cancer and surgery, *M. Ann. District of Columbia,* 23, 475, 1954.

3. Bloedorn, F. G., Young, J. D., Cuccia, C. A., Mercado, R., Jr., and Wizenberg, M. J.: Radiotherapy in carcinoma of the bladder: Possible complications and their prevention, *Radiology*, 79, 576, 1962.

4. Cooling, C. I.: In *Tumours of the Bladder*, David M. Wallace, ed., Edinburgh, E. & S. Livingston, Ltd., 1959, vol. 2, pp. 171.

5. Ellis, F., and Oliver, R.: Treatment of papilloma of bladder with radioactive colloidal gold [198]Au, *Brit. Med. J.*, 1, 136, 1955.

6. Friedman, M.: Supervoltage (2-Mvp) rotation irradiation of cancer of the bladder, *Radiology*, 73, 191, 1959.

7. Friedman, M., and Lewis, L. G.: A new technic for the radium treatment of carcinoma of the bladder, *Radiology*, 53, 342, 1949.

8. Guttmann, R., and Bauza, A.: The treatment of advanced carcinoma of the bladder, *Radiology*, 77, 465, 1961.

9. Hodt, H. J., Sinclair, W. K., and Smithers, D. W.: A gun for interstitial implantation of radioactive gold grains, *Brit. J. Radiol.*, 25, 419, 1952.

10. Jewett, H. J.: In *Urology*, 2nd ed., Meredith F. Campbell, ed., Philadelphia, W. B. Saunders & Company, vol. II, p. 1031, 1963.

11. Marshall, V. F., and Whitmore, W. F., Jr.: In *Symposium on Bladder Tumors*, Philadelphia, J. P. Lippincott & Company, p. 67, 1956.

12. Mostofi, F. K.: Pathology of cancer of bladder, *Acta Un. Int. Cancr.*, 18, 611, 1962.

13. Miller, L. S.: Supervoltage irradiation for carcinoma of the urinary bladder, *Radiology*, 82, 778, 1964.

14. Muller, J. H.: Radiotherapy of bladder cancer by means of rubber balloons filled *in situ* with solution of radioactive isotope (^{60}Co), *Cancer*, 8, 1035, 1955.

15. Murphy, W. T.: In *Urology*, 2nd ed. Meredith F. Campbell, ed., Philadelphia, W. B. Saunders & Company, vol. II, p. 1361, 1963.

16. Paterson, R.: *The Treatment of Malignant Disease by Radium and X-rays*, Baltimore, The Williams & Wilkins Company, 1956.

17. Poole-Wilson, D. S.: Surgery and irradiation in treatment of bladder cancer, *Brit. J. Urol.*, 29, 244, 1957.

18. Poole-Wilson, D. S. and Pointon, R. C. S.: In *British Surgical Practice*, London, Butterworth & Company Ltd., p. 62, 1961.

19. Vermooten, V., and Maxfield, J. G. S.: Use of radioactive cobalt in nylon sutures in treatment of bladder tumors; technic and case reports, *J. Urol.*, 74, 767, 1955.

20. Wallace, D. M., Walton, R. J., and Sinclair, W. K.: Preliminary communication on intracavitary irradiation of bladder mucosa by radioactive isotope solution, *Brit. J. Radiol.*, 21, 357, 1949.

21. Whitmore, W. F., Jr., Phillips, R. F., Grabstald, H., Bronstein, E. L., Mackensie, A. R., and Hustu, O.: Experience with preoperative irradiation followed by radical cystectomy for the treatment of bladder cancer, *Amer. J. Roentgen.*, 90, 1016, 1963.

22. Wizenberg, M. J., Bloedorn, F. G., Young, J. D. Jr., et al: Radiation Therapy in the treatment of carcinoma of the bladder; University of Maryland experience, *Amer. J. Roentgen.*, 96, 113, 1966.

Tumors of the Testis

JOSEPH R. CASTRO

The primary tumor in the testis is effectively managed by radical orchiectomy through an inguinal incision with high ligation of the spermatic cord. If the patient has been referred after an incisional biopsy or scrotal orchiectomy, either a radical orchiectomy or resection of the spermatic cord, as needed, is done before proceeding to further therapy.

The exception is the case of pure seminoma where irradiation of the spermatic cord and scrotum may be substituted for further surgery.

The first site of spread from testicular tumors is commonly the regional lymphatics, that is, the periaortic and paracaval nodes in the lumbar region just at or below the level of the renal veins. Other sites of lymphatic metastases include: 1) nodes at the junction of the left spermatic vein and left renal vein which fill directly from the left testicle lymphatics which are along the internal spermatic vessels, 2) the low periaortic nodes and occasionally in cases of massive disease, external or common iliac nodes. The determining factor in survival rate is the proper management of lymphatic metastases by either surgery or radiation or a combination of the two modalities.

The presence of extranodal metastases such as pulmonary nodules heralds a rapidly progressive situation which may be palliated by aggressive chemotherapy and/or radiotherapy, but cure is rarely possible in this clinical setting.

HISTOPATHOLOGICAL CLASSIFICATION

Over 95 per cent of testicular tumors arise from the germinal cells and may be conveniently subdivided according to the classification of Dixon and Moore:[3]

Group I: Seminoma, pure.

Group II: Embryonal carcinoma, pure or with seminoma.

Group III: Teratoma, pure or with seminoma.

Group IV: Teratoma with either embryonal carcinoma, choriocarcinoma, or both, and with or without seminoma.

Group V: Choriocarcinoma, pure or with either seminoma or embryonal carcinoma, or both.

For treatment purposes, pure seminoma is considered as one clinical entity. All of the remaining histologic groups (I through V), hereinafter referred to as "mixed tumors" are considered as another clinical entity for purposes of treatment planning.

Rare miscellaneous tumors noted are interstitial cell tumors, lymphosarcoma, reticulum cell sarcoma, or rhabdomyosarcoma (intrascrotal but probably not of testicular origin).

Table 12-1 shows the incidence and survival as a function of histology in nearly 300 cases treated at M. D. Anderson Hospital and Tumor Institute, Houston, Texas, during the period February 1944 through December 1967.

Clinical Stage

A convenient clinical staging system, modified from Boden and Gibb[1] is as follows:

Stage I—Tumor limited to the testicle with no evidence of spread through the capsule or to the spermatic cord.

Stage II—Clinical or radiographic evidence of tumor beyond the testicle such as regional lymphatics but not beyond the diaphragm. Included are cases with tumor in the spermatic cord, scrotum, inguinal, iliac or periaortic lymph node regions.

Stage III_A—Extension beyond the diaphragm but still confined to the mediastinal or supraclavicular lymphatics; or massive retroperitoneal lymphatic disease.

Stage III_B—Extranodal metastases.

Clinical examination, radiographic studies including intravenous pyelography and lymphangiography, and findings noted as orchiectomy are utilized in the clinical staging. The surgical findings, if a lymphadenectomy is done, do not alter the clinical stage.

Clinical Work-Up

A complete history and physical examination with appropriate laboratory work-up is done including *CBC*, urinalysis, liver function tests and *BUN*. Radiographic studies are obtained including chest x-ray film, intravenous pyelogram, lymphangiogram and inferior vena cavagram if needed.

Table 12-1. *Distribution of Patients and Influence of Histology on Survival Rates March 1944–December 1967*

	Number Patients Treated	3-yr. *NED* Rate (All Stages)
Seminoma, Pure	113 (39%)	85/113 (75%)
Embryonal Carcinoma, pure or with seminoma	78 (26%)	28/78 (36%)
Teratoma, pure or with seminoma	24 (8%)	16/24 (66%)
Teratoma with embryonal carcinoma, or choriocarcinoma, or seminoma	56 (18%)	28/56 (50%)
Choriocarcinoma, pure or with seminoma and/or embryonal carcinoma	13 (5%)	1/13
Miscellaneous	11 (4%)	6/11
Total	295	

The lymphangiogram has proven to be the most accurate test for the evaluation of lymphatic metastases, although it is only useful in the presence of gross deposits in the lymph nodes. Some nodes lying lateral to the upper lumbar nodes just below the level of the renal veins (*L*-1, *L*-2) are not filled by pedal lymphangiography. This fact must be taken into account when planning treatment portals. Inguinal nodes are not ordinarily involved unless there is spread of the primary tumor to the scrotum.

Occasionally, bulky lymphatic metastases may be palpated in the abdomen, left supraclavicular area or rarely in the inguinal area.

Persistent high titers of chorionic gonadotrophin suggests the presence of choriocarcinoma, a bad prognostic sign. Gynecomastia conversely is not a significant prognostic sign; the mechanism for its cause is poorly understood.

Pure Seminoma

This tumor has a tendency for lymphatic spread and is very radiosensitive. Orchiectomy plus radiotherapy results in high survival rates (Table 12-2).

The 3-year *NED* rate is valid for analysis of treatment techniques since almost all recurrences or metastases appear prior to 36 months. Survival without evidence of disease at 3 years or more is excellent in patients with both Stage I (92 per cent) and Stage II (77 per cent) disease. Control within the irradiated area is the rule and the few failures occur because of distant metastases. Once seminoma has extended beyond the lymphatics, either with abdominal visceral or disseminated metastases (Stage III_B) the likelihood of salvage is diminished.

Lymphadenectomy is not indicated since seminoma is radiocurable with moderate doses. Although an anaplastic type of seminoma has been described by some, the treatment is not altered by this finding providing the tumor is pure seminoma.[6] Friedman et al.[4] believes, however, that the prognosis is diminished somewhat with this histologic finding.

The incidence of retroperitoneal node metastases in clinical Stage I seminoma of the testis is thought to lie between 10 to 19 per cent.[7,8,9] Elective irradiation of the iliac and periaortic lymphatics is justified, and the tumor dose is 2,500 rads delivered in 3 weeks. If there is a scrotal incision, it is included in the treatment field together with the in-

Table 12-2. *Patients with Pure Seminoma NED at 36 Months Posttreatment*
March 1944–December 1967

Stage	No. Pts.	Area Treated		Limited field Pal. *XRT*	*NED*
		Iliac and Periaortic only	Iliac, Periaortic, Mediastinum, Lt. *SC**		
I	63	52/56	6/7		
		1-*ENM*†			
		2-2nd primary	1-acute leukemia		58/63
		(opp. testis)			(92%)
		1-uncertain			
II	26	7/10	13/16		
		1-*LFU*Ψ			
		1-rec. medias	2-*ENM* + nodes		20/26
		+ *SC* + *ENM*	1-rad. nephritis		(77%)
		1-met. as embryonal *Ca*			
III$_A$	10		6/10		
			1-uncertain		
			2-*ENM* + nodes		6/10
			1-*ID* (7 mos.)		
III$_B$	14			1/14	1/14

*SC—Supraclavicular area.
†ENM—Extranodal metastases (lung, bone, brain, liver).
ΨLFU—Lost to follow-up.

guinal lymph nodes. The remaining testicle is shielded since the incidence of bilateral tumors is low.[8]

The merit of elective irradiation of the mediastinum and the supraclavicular areas in Stage I seminoma is not proved. The 3-year *NED* rate with irradiation only of the iliac and periaortic areas is better than 90 per cent.

In patients with Stage II seminoma, irradiation of the iliac and periaortic lymphatics is carried to a basic dose of 2,500 rads in 3 weeks. An additional 500 to 1,000 rads may be given through reduced fields to grossly involved nodes. If the nodal disease is very bulky, whole abdomen irradiation with open fields is employed to deliver 2,500 rads in 3 weeks, or 2,000 rads is given with ^{60}Co moving strip technique, after which the fields are reduced for an additional 1,000 to 1,500 rads over the initial nodal mass. Care should be taken to limit the renal dose to no more than 1,500 rads. Since the possibility of oc-

cult metastases to the mediastinum and left supraclavicular area is high and the required dose is low, elective irradiation of these areas is carried out.

Aggressive treatment will salvage many patients with Stage III$_A$ disease (confined to the lymphatics) which is either massive retroperitoneal nodes or more commonly mediastinal and/or left supraclavicular lymphatics. A basic dose of 2,000 to 2,500 rads is given to the whole abdomen in 2½ to 3 weeks followed by an additional 1,000 to 1,500 rads to the areas of bulky nodal disease. Mediastinal and left supraclavicular areas receive similar doses depending on the extent of disease in these areas.

Some patients develop evidence of radiation enteritis such as diarrhea and bowel cramps toward the end of a course of treatment together with mild to moderate hematological depression. For this reason if mediastinal and left supraclavicular irradiation is to be used, a rest period of 3 to 6 weeks is

Table 12-3. *Advocated Treatment Plan for Pure Seminoma*

Primary	Clinical Stage	Iliac-Periaortic Lymphatics		Mediastinum-Left Supraclavicular Area	
Radical Orchiectomy with high Cord Ligation	I	2500 rads/3 wks (Megavoltage)	⎰ Elective ⎱ Irradiation ⎰ Basic ⎱ dose		
	II	2500 rads/3 wks Add			
		1000–1500 rads/1–1½ wks reduced fields over area of initial nodes.	⎰ Bulky ⎱ nodes	2500 rads/3 wks	Elective Irradiation
	III$_A$	2500 rads/3 wks +			
		1000–1500 rads to involved nodes with reduced fields		2500 rads/3 wks +	
		or		500–1000 rads	
		2000 rads whole abd. moving strip + 1500 rads through reduced fields	⎰ Massive ⎰ retro- ⎱ peritoneal ⎱ disease	through reduced fields as needed	
	III$_B$	*XRT* and/or chemotherapy on individualized basis			

often given following the abdominal irradiation.

Extranodal disease (Stage III$_B$), such as pulmonary or bony metastases, is treated locally with similar doses of radiation and/or chemotherapy since even in these instances, long-term palliation or even cures can occasionally be obtained.

Table 12-3 summarizes the advocated plan of treatment for pure seminoma.

Mixed Tumors

The results of treatment for mixed tumors are shown in Table 12-4. Choriocarcinoma has been excluded because of virtually complete failure (only 1 of 13 *NED* at 3 years). Patients with the other mixed tumors have an excellent chance of control in Stage I (81 per cent) whether treated by radiotherapy alone or lymphadenectomy (plus irradiation

Table 12-4. *Patients with Mixed Tumors NED at 36 Months Posttreatment Excluding Choriocarcinoma March 1944–December 1967*

Clinical Stage	Orch. Alone	Orch. + XRT	Orch. + Node Dissection		Orch. + Node Dissec. + XRT		Total
			− Nodes	+ Nodes	− Nodes	+ Nodes	
I	1/1	7/11	39/43*	2/3	5/7	4/6	58/71 (82%)
II		0/5		1/3	5/6†	7/14	13/28 (47%)
III			1—Chemotherapy				1/59

* 1-LFU.
† 1-dead, intercurrent disease (18 months).

if there are positive nodes), but over-all results are considerably reduced in Stage II (48
per cent).

An analysis of sites of failure in patients
with Stages I and II disease is shown in Table
12-5. Of 26 patients with recurrent or metastatic disease, only 3 patients had mediastinal
and/or left supraclavicular lymphatic disease
as the next manifestation of disease and two
of these concurrently had pulmonary metastases. This high frequency of pulmonary or
visceral metastases precludes benefits from
elective irradiation of mediastinum and left
supraclavicular area in patients with Stage I
or II disease.

Treatment for mixed tumors is the same
irrespective of the histologic pattern. Tumor
doses of 5,000 rads in 5 weeks are required.
In some instances, the weekly dose rate is
reduced to 850 rads per week to improve
tolerance. Occasionally a tumor diagnosed as
pure seminoma in the orchiectomy specimen
shows other histologic elements in the lymphatic metastases. The presence of these elements requires doses of 5,000 rads in 5

weeks since the more malignant cells determine the radiosensitivity.

Although a small group of patients with
clinical Stage I tumors have done well with
only irradiation of the periaortic nodes after
orchiectomy (7 of 11 *NED* at 3 years), a
bilateral transperitoneal lymphadenectomy is
advocated in patients with clinical Stage I
mixed tumors. If no tumor is found in the
specimen, no further treatment is needed as
only a rare patient (3 of 43, Table 12-5) will
succumb to distant metastases.

When positive periaortic nodes are found
at lymphadenectomy, local control is improved when irradiation is combined with
the lymphadenectomy (Table 12-6).[2]

In patients with Stage II disease, lymphadenectomy is utilized to remove bulky disease. Then the patient receives 5,000 rads
tumor dose to the iliac and periaortic lymphatics. Fixed nonresectable nodes treated
with irradiation alone are likely to persist
despite doses of 5,000 rads. Resection of as
much disease as possible may improve
results by leaving only microscopic or mini-

Table 12-5. *Sites of Failure in Mixed Tumors
March 1944–December 1967*

Clinical Stage	Orchiectomy + XRT	Orchiectomy + Node Dissection		Orch. + Node Dissection + XRT	
		(−) Nodes	(+) Nodes	(−) Nodes	(+) Nodes
I	4/11 ENM* only—2 ENM + Nodes—1 ID—1	4/43 ENM—3 LFUѰ—1	1/4 Periaortic Nodes + ENM—1	2/7 ENM only—2	3/7 ENM only—1 Periaortic Nodes + ENM—1 Mediast. + ENM—1
II	5/5 Periaortic Nodes + ENM—4 Uncertain—1		3/4 Periaortic Nodes + ENM—3	1/6 ID—1	7/14 Periaortic Nodes—3 ENM only—2† Mediast. + ENM—1 Mediast. + S—C—1

*ENM—extranodal disease.
†One patient alive at 60 months (chemotherapy).
ѰLFU—lost to follow-up.

Table 12-6. *Mixed Tumors Failure in Positive Periaortic Nodes Found at Nodal Dissection With or Without Irradiation March 1944–December 1967*

	Orchiectomy + Node Dissection	Orchiectomy + Node Dissection + Radiation Therapy
No. Positive Periaortic nodes	8	21
No. Failures in Periaortic Area	4	4

mal disease to be controlled by irradiation.

An attempt to facilitate resection of involved nodes by giving preoperative irradiation has been made in a small group of patients. Surgical morbidity has not been increased when 2,500 rads given in 3 weeks with ^{60}Co was delivered to the iliac and periaortic areas. Following lymphadenectomy, an additional 2,500 rads in $2\frac{1}{2}$ weeks are given to areas of involved nodes marked by silver clips. Preliminary results show 10 patients have no evidence of disease at 3 years with negative lymphadenectomy after preoperative irradiation. Three of 4 patients with positive nodes at surgery after preoperative irradiation have no evidence of disease 3 years or more posttreatment.

Patients with minimal changes on the intravenous pyelogram or lymphangiogram probably should not have preoperative ir-

radiation since so many are found to have negative nodes at surgery.

The presence of mediastinal or supraclavicular lymphatic disease in patients with mixed tumors usually means extranodal metastases which quickly become evident. The use of radiotherapy in these cases must be on an individualized basis and often chemotherapy forms the basis of treatment.

The advocated plan of treatment for mixed tumors is summarized in Table 12-7.

Radiation Techniques

Portals

The treatment fields (Fig. 12-7) employed are similar for pure seminoma and mixed tumors. The inguinal nodes are included in the inguinal-iliac fields if the scrotum was

Table 12-7. *Advocated Treatment Plan For Mixed Tumors*

Stage	Primary	Lymphatics	
I	Radical Orchiectomy	Bilateral Lymphadenectomy	Negative nodes: no further treatment
			Positive nodes: postoperative *XRT* 5000 rads to iliac and periaortic areas
II	Radical Orchiectomy	Small or questionably involved nodes on x-ray studies: Lymphadenectomy + Postoperative *XRT*	
		Large nodes on x-ray studies	
		Preoperative *XRT* (2500 rads/3 weeks)	
		Lymphadenectomy 2500 rads/3 weeks to areas of involved nodes	
III A & B	Radical Orchiectomy	Chemotherapy and/or *XRT* on individualized basis	

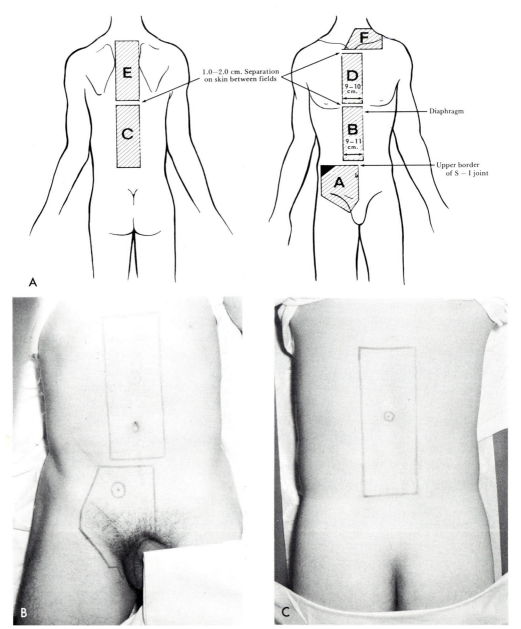

FIG. 12-7. A. Field arrangement for seminoma treated with ^{60}Co. Tumor dose for field A is assessed at 3 to 4 cm anterior to midplane. For fields B and C, tumor dose is assessed at midplane. The usual height of field A is 15 to 18 cm, the width is approximately 10 cm, its medial border being 1 cm past the midline. Fields B and C are 9 to 11 cm wide depending on the lymphangiogram and vary from 18 to 24 cm in length. One to 2.0 cm separation on the skin is ordinarily used between fields depending on the length of the portals. Because of the location of the nodes under the skin, the dose to the supraclavicular field is assessed as given dose.

For tumors other than pure seminoma only fields A, B and C are utilized. (A-Courtesy: Castro and Gonzalez, *Amer. J. Roentgen.*, 111, 355, 1971.)

B. Photographs of inguinal iliac field A and anterior periaortic field B.

C. Photograph of posterior periaortic field C.

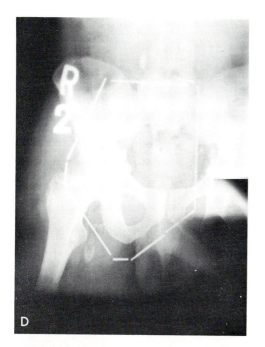

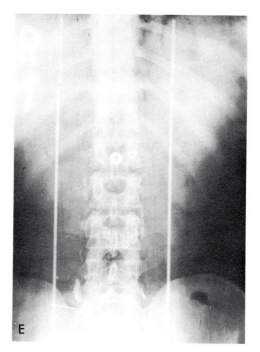

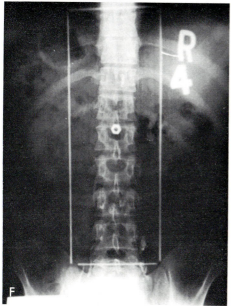

FIG. 12-7. D, E, and F. Portal films of same fields (A,B,C) with lead wire markers outlining treated areas.

involved with tumor. A portion of the scrotum may be included if the orchiectomy incision reaches the scrotum; the opposite testicle is shielded (Fig. 12-8). Because of their anterior location, the inguinal and iliac nodes ordinarily are irradiated through a single anterior field of approximately 15 × 10 cm. The dose is assessed at 3 or 4 cm anterior to midplane depending on patient thickness.

For the periaortic nodes, the tumor dose

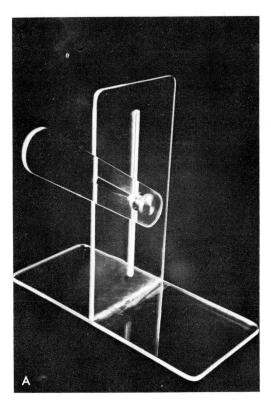

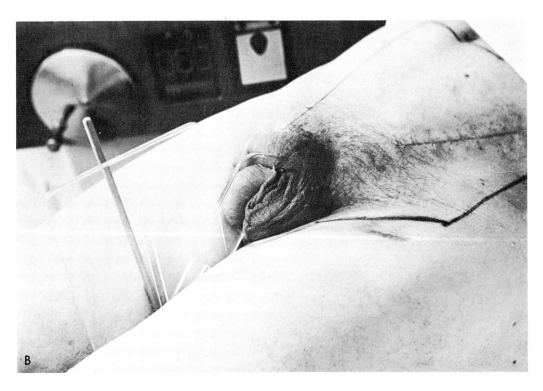

FIG. 12-8. A. Lucite device for isolating remaining testicle from radiation beam. B. Lucite holder in use to exclude remaining testicle from direct radiation beam while irradiating portion of scrotum. (Courtesy: Dr. Luis Delclos, Hospital General De Asturias, Oviedo, Spain).

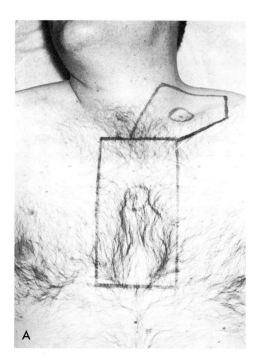

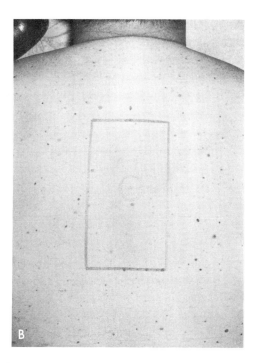

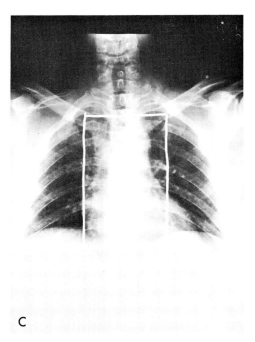

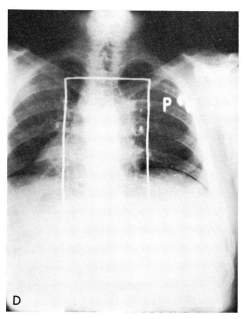

FIG. 12-9. **A** and **B.** Photographs of mediastinal and left supraclavicular fields. **C** and **D.** Portal films of mediastinal and left supraclavicular fields.

is assessed at midplane through opposing anterior and posterior portals. These fields are usually 25 to 30 cm long by 9 to 11 cm wide, utilizing the lymphangiogram to insure proper coverage of the nodes. Care must be taken to include the nodes at the renal hila especially on the left where the spermatic vein enters the left renal vein. Some nodes lying laterally to the lumbar nodes at the level of the renal veins may not be filled by pedal lymphangiography but have been filled by testicular lymphangiography. The bulk of the kidneys is excluded after localization by intravenous pyelograms or renal isotope scans.

Mediastinal and left supraclavicular fields used in pure seminoma are shown in Figure 12-9. The mediastinal fields are 9 to 10 cm wide and the tumor dose is assessed at midplane. Since the supraclavicular nodes lie just under the skin, only an anterior field is used for these and the given dose is assessed to be the tumor dose.

Bulky involvement of periaortic nodes with obstructed lymphatics and collateral lymphatic flow may be better treated by wide fields (12 cm or more) or whole abdomen techniques for the initial 2,000 to 2,500 rads.

^{60}Co moving strip therapy to the entire abdomen (Fig. 12-10) may be employed in patients with massive lymphatic disease which is not suitable for lymphadenectomy, either pure seminoma or mixed tumors. Tumor doses on the order of 2,600 rads (2,000 rads for pure seminoma) are given to each segment of irradiated volume in a period of 9 to 11 days. Following this, an additional boost of 1,000 to 1,500 rads, depending on histology, is given through reduced fields directly over residual lymphatic disease. In mixed tumors, this technique has occasionally salvaged some patients whose disease was nonresectable. Lymphadenectomy following such doses is not advocated because of the morbidity and difficulties with wound healing.

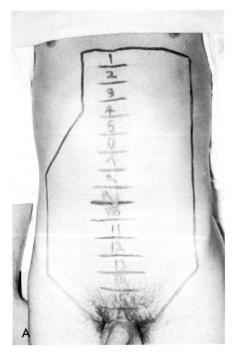 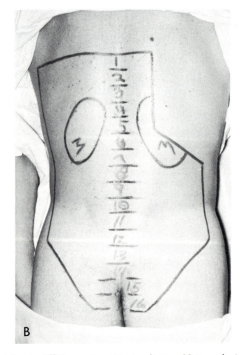

FIG. 12-10. Photograph of typical field arrangements for abdominal ^{60}Co moving strip irradiation. Note exclusion of most of the right lobe of the liver. Kidneys are blocked from posteriorly with two *HVLs* of lead.

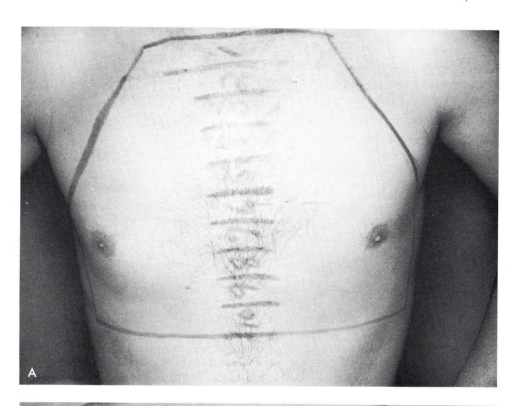

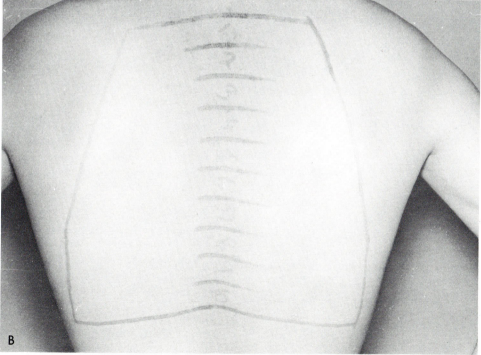

FIG. 12-11. Photograph of pulmonary fields treated by 2,000 rads moving strip ^{60}Co irradiation. No lung correction
is used.

Pulmonary metastases may be effectively treated by utilizing ^{60}Co moving strip technique to deliver 2,000 rads (Fig. 12-11). Alternately, a 2,000 rads midplane tumor dose in 3 weeks to both lung fields may be given with ^{60}Co. Irradiation may be combined with chemotherapy.

Tolerance and Complications

With the doses customarily employed there are few complications in treatment for pure seminoma, providing renal shielding is employed to limit the renal dose of 1,500 rads.

In the mixed histologic groups which require doses in the range of 5,000 rads in 5 weeks, the risk of complications is greater. Doses of this level have been known to cause neurologic and bowel complications and should not be exceeded.

To avoid excess irradiation to the anterior abdominal wall in the ilio-inguinal field, a posterior portal may be required in patients with mixed tumors. Given doses of 6,000 rads to the ilio-inguinal field should not be exceeded. Of 285 patients with germinal tumors, there have been 4 who have had bilateral tumors, 3 with pure seminoma (1 NED at 56 months), and 1 with mixed histology. This low incidence of bilaterality (1.4 per cent) has indicated that the remaining testicle may be shielded rather than irradiated as suggested by some.[5] Nevertheless, some scatter radiation to the remaining testicle unavoidably occurs. By utilizing lithium fluoride dosimetry, it appears that the opposite testis received from 25 to 30 rads per 1,000 rads given to the ilio-inguinal field. A much smaller scatter dose occurs from the periaortic field. This would indicate that the dose to the remaining testicle in the seminoma group is about 75 to 120 rads and in the carcinoma-teratoma group, about 150 to 200 rads. These doses may be reduced by use of hemispherical lead shields about the remaining testis.[8,9] Instances of healthy off-spring born of treated patients have been reported.[8,9]

Pediatric Testicular Tumors

Fourteen patients in the pediatric age group have been treated. None had seminoma; 5 had embryonal rhabdomyosarcoma, and the remainder had mixed tumors.

The treatment has generally consisted of radical orchiectomy and lymph node dissection for the mixed tumor group. Three patients had short courses of cytoxan in addition to surgery. The results have been surprisingly good. In patients with Stage I tumors, 7 of 7 show no evidence of disease at 3 years posttreatment or longer.

The rhabdomyosarcoma group has generally been treated by orchiectomy, lymphadenectomy, and postoperative irradiation (3,000 rads in 4 weeks plus 500 to 1,000 rads to reduced fields over involved nodes in 1 to 2 weeks). Three of these patients have also received chemotherapy consisting of vincristine and/or cytoxan. Four of 5 patients have no evidence of disease for periods of 32 to 66 months.

BIBLIOGRAPHY

1. Boden, G. and Gibb, R.: Radiotherapy and testicular neoplasms, *Lancet*, 2, 1195, 1951.
2. Castro, J. R.: Lymphadenectomy and radiation therapy in malignant tumors of the testicle other than pure seminoma, *Cancer*, 24, 87, 1969.
3. Castro, J. R. and Gonzalez, M.: Results in treatment of pure seminoma of the testis, *Amer. J. Roentgen.*, 2, 355, 1971.
4. Dixon, F. J. and Moore, R. A.: Tumors of male sex organs, *Atlas of Tumor Pathology, Armed Forces Institute of Pathology, Sect. VIII, fasc. 31B and 32.*
5. Friedman, M. and Pearlman, A. W.: Seminoma with trophocarcinoma. A clinical variant of seminoma, *Cancer*, 26, 46, 1970.
6. Gibb, R.: Personal communication.
7. Maier, J. G., Nuttemeyer, B. T. and Sulak,

M. H.: Treatment and prognosis in seminoma of the testis, *J. of Urol.,* 99, 72, 1968.

8. Maier, J. G., Von Buskirk, K. E., Sulak, M. H., Perry, R. H. and Schamber, D. T.: Evaluation of lymphadenectomy in the treatment of malignant testicular germ cell neoplasms, tion of lymphadenectomy in the treatment of malignant testicular germ cell neoplasms,

Trans. Amer. Assoc. GU Surgeons, 60, 71, 1968.

9. Notter, G. and Ranudd, N. E.: Treatment of malignant testicular tumors, *Acta Radiologica,* 2, 273, 1964.

10. Smithers, D. W. and Wallace, E. N. K.: Radiotherapy in the treatment of patients with seminomas and teratomas of the testicle, *Brit. J. Urol.,* 34, 422, 1962.

Chemotherapy of Testicular Tumors

MELVIN L. SAMUELS

Significant results with chemotherapeutic agents were first reported with the use of the alkylating agent, L-sarcolysin (phenylaline mustard) in patients with seminoma.[1] Other alkylating agents, such as chlorambucil in a dose of 10 mg daily for 1 to 2 months, have been found effective in seminoma that has escaped radiotherapy.[2] Nonseminomatous germinal tumors do not generally respond to alkylating agents, and the first objective regressions with these tumors were observed in 50 per cent of tumors, including all histological types, when actinomycin-D, methotrexate and chlorambucil were used concurrently.[2] MacKenzie[3] subsequently reviewed 72 patients who had been treated with this triple drug regime and, again, confirmed objective responses in about half of the patients. However, complete clinical responses of at least one-year duration were noted in only 10 per cent. Like others, we have found actinomycin-D used alone, or in combination, an impressive drug, but it is difficult to use for repetitive courses because of toxicity. The latter includes severe stomatitis, acneiform skin eruption, and myelosuppression. We have had one fatality as a result of acute toxic hepatitis.

At M. D. Anderson Hospital, we have been impressed with vinblastine sulfate.[4]

The dosage employed in testicular cancer has been higher than that administered in Hodgkin's disease. In previously untreated patients, we usually give 0.45 to 0.55 mg/kg total dose over a 2- to 3-day period in 2 or 3 equal fractions. This is repeated every 3 to 4 weeks, as the toxicity is not cumulative. The primary toxic manifestation is myelosuppression. Of 40 patients who have been adequately treated, significant objective and subjective responses have been obtained in 20. Seven of these responses were complete. The median survival of the partial responders was 48+ weeks and 98+ weeks for the complete responders. The nonresponders showed a median survival of only 18 weeks.

Our most recent studies have been with a new agent, Bleomycin, an antibiotic isolated from a strain of *Streptomyces Verticulus* by Umezawa.[5] Although tumor responses have been reported with many tumor types, including squamous cell carcinoma, they are, for the most part, partial responses of brief duration. Complete responses have been reported in a small group of germinal tumors of the testis[6] including choriocarcinoma which has proved the most resistant to conventional agents. These results have been confirmed by our experience at M. D. Anderson Hospital but the responses are short lived. Since the toxicity of Bleomycin is qualitatively different from vinblastine, we have combined the two drugs in full dosage. Bleomycin is given in a dose of 30 mg intramuscularly twice weekly, usually for 5 weeks and vinblastine is given on the first and second treatment days in the previously stated dosage. The dose of Bleomycin is reduced 50 per cent in subsequent courses because of the risk of pulmonary fibrosis when the total dose exceeds 500 to 600 mg. Of 28 evaluable patients, very impressive responses were observed in 21. Four of these responses have been complete. This program has been in effect for only one year so that survival time cannot be appropriately evaluated at this time but it is our impression that survival time will be significantly improved in Stage III disease.

An attempt to improve salvage of patients with pulmonary metastases by chemotherapy is a program which combined whole lung irradiation with hydroxyurea. A tumor dose of 2,000 rads is administered over a 3-week period and hydroxyurea is given in a dosage of 30 mg/kg per day on each treatment day. It has been found necessary to carefully monitor the blood counts as one will generally see significant leukopenia developing about the tenth day of treatment.

Eight patients have completed this program and are evaluable and significant objective remissions were seen in all. However, the median duration of response was only 4 months with the longest extending to 10 months so that this program appears to have only limited usefulness.

BIBLIOGRAPHY

1. Boldkhin, N., Larionov, L., Perenodchikova, L., Chebotareva, L. and Merkulova, N.: Clinical experiences with sarcolysin in neoplastic disease, *Ann. N.Y. Acad. Sc.*, 68, 1128, 1958.
2. Li, M. D., Whitmore, S. F., Jr., Golbey, R., and Grabstalt, H.: Effects of combined drug therapy on metastatic cancer of the testis, *JAMA*, 174, 145, 1960.
3. MacKenzie, A. R.: Chemotherapy of metastatic testis cancer, *Cancer*, 19, 1369, 1966.
4. Samuels, M. L. and Howe, C. D.: Vinblastine in the management of testicular cancer, *Cancer*, 25, 1009, 1970.
5. Umezawa, H., Maeda, K., Takeuchi, T., and Okami, Y.: New antibiotics, Bleomycin A and B., *J. Antibiotics*, 19, 200, 1966.
6. Clinical screening Co-operation Group of the European Organization for Research on the Treatment of Cancer (G. Mathe, H. Redong, M. Hyat) Study of the Clinical Efficiency of Bleomycin in Human Cancer, *Brit. Med. J.*, 2, 643, 1970.

Definitive Megavoltage Radiation Therapy in Carcinoma of the Prostate

MALCOLM A. BAGSHAW

Excluding skin cancer, carcinoma of the prostate is the third most prevalent neoplasm in the male, the incidence being substantially exceeded by carcinoma of the lung but only slightly by colorectal cancer. In 1971, it was estimated that there would be 35,000 new cases of cancer of the prostate in the United States and that this neoplasm would cause 17,200 deaths.[1]

Soon after Young introduced perineal

prostatectomy in 1904, Pasteau in 1911 employed radium as a treatment for prostatic cancer.[27,31] This method was elaborated upon by Barringer[5] and also by Young[32] in 1917. The latter series was described in detail in 1922 by Deming who reported excellent palliation in 75 of 100 patients treated by a variety of radium applications.[13] In the same year, Bumpus reported the results in treatment of 197 cases with several different radium techniques.[9] Barringer pursued the treatment of prostatic cancer vigorously using interstitial implantation and in 1942 reported convincing evidence of sterilization of the neoplasm proven by post-mortem examination in 2 patients 7 and 6 years after treatment.[6] In 1932, Widman reported the palliative value of external irradiation for advanced localized prostatic cancer.[30] His observations were overshadowed by Huggins and Hodges in 1941 who demonstrated the depression of prostatic cancer by deprivation of male hormone.[24] Flocks and coworkers, in 1952, revitalized radiation therapy by infiltrating a radioactive gold suspension directly into the neoplasm or the neoplastic bed after subtotal resection.[16,17] Recently, Hilaris and Whitmore developed an elegant technique for the homogeneous implantation of the prostate with ^{125}I seeds.[23]

In spite of the variety of therapeutic approaches, radical perineal prostatectomy has remained the therapeutic standard with a number of authors reporting 5-year survival rates of between 50 and 91 per cent in carefully selected patients.[22,25,26,29] Among others, Flocks and Franks have stressed, however, that only 2 to 10 per cent of all patients are candidates for radical prostatectomy.[18,19] About 55 per cent of all patients already have metastases when the diagnosis is established. The remaining have either moderately extensive, but still local, neoplasms or local neoplasm plus regional lymph node involvement to which radiotherapists have devoted increasing attention since the mid 1950's. The recent interest in the application of external radiation to treatment for prostatic cancer is the product of the development of megavoltage units which permit the delivery of large doses of ionizing radiation homogeneously to the prostate, the periprostatic region, and the regional lymph nodes without undue injury to other structures.[3,4,7,8,12,21]

In this section, a method of external megavoltage radiation therapy is described which appears to be effective in controlling the local neoplasm. In addition, a method of extended field radiation therapy is discussed which can be used in the treatment of the primary tumor plus the regional adenopathy.

Methods

Selection of Patients

In this series, 360 consecutive patients were considered for definitive radiation therapy for primary carcinoma of the prostate. Among those, 50 were eliminated from the analysis for such reasons as: lack of definitive pathologic diagnosis, the discovery of metastases or concomitant neoplasms during initial evaluation, or previous radical surgery. The age distribution of the 310 patients not eliminated is presented in Figure 12-12. Patients were selected for treatment according to the following criteria: 1) No metastases demonstrable by survey roentgenograms, physical examination or in some patients by scintiscans, 2) primary tumor localized to the prostate, its capsule, or the immediately adjacent periprostatic tissue, including the seminal vesicles, or 3) primary tumor considered by urological consultation to be too extensive for radical prostatectomy; this criterion was not always followed since a few patients were treated who might have been candidates for radical prostatectomy but who had refused the operation.

In order to establish the above criteria, additional pretreatment evaluation has gradually evolved so that now chest roentgenograms, intravenous pyelograms, bone x-ray surveys for metastases, and total serum acid

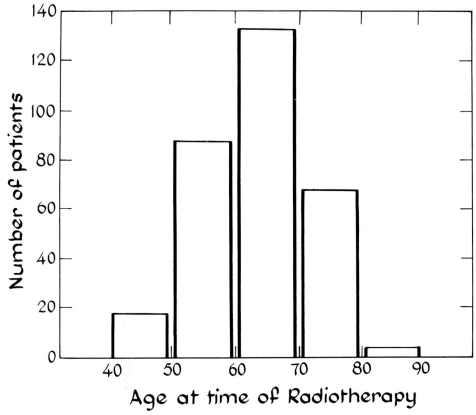

FIG. 12-12. Frequency distribution of age in 310 patients with carcinoma of the prostate. The mean was 62.5 years with a range of 39 to 89 years. There is a significant number of young patients.

and alkaline phosphatase determinations are included. It has not been useful to employ the serum acid phosphatase level as a definitive indicator of metastatic disease.

Recently, several additional tests including fractionated serum acid phosphatase determinations, lower extremity lymphangiography, inferior vena cavography, Strontium-85 bone scintiscans, and Westerman-Jensen posterior iliac crest bone marrow needle biopsy have become routine.[15] These studies have been coupled recently with diagnostic pelvic laparotomy in order to be more precise in the pretherapeutic evaluation of the extent of neoplasm especially with reference to lymph node involvement.

Presenting Symptoms, Pathologic Confirmation, and Extent of Disease

The presenting symptoms are detailed in Table 12-8. Two hundred and fifty patients were symptomatic. On routine digital examination of the prostate, 60 patients were discovered to have signs suggestive of malignancy. Transrectal needle biopsy was the most common and least traumatic diagnostic method, although transurethral resection was also employed frequently.

In asymptomatic patients with a single nodule, the primary tumor occupied less than 25 per cent of either lobe in only 4

Table 12-8. *Carcinoma of the Prostate List of the Frequency of First Symptoms or Multiple Symptoms*

Group			Number of Patients	
Asymptomatic			60	
Symptomatic			250	
			1st. Sx*	Sx* Complex
			223	245
1. Prostatism				

Nocturia	60	Dysuria	16	
Diminished Stream	52	Urgency	13	
Frequency	48	Hematuria	11	
Hesitancy	34	Dribbling	10	
Frank Obstruct.	30	Hematospermia	4	

Group	1st. Sx*	Sx* Complex
2. Anal pain	0	3
3. Perineal pain	5	19
4. Sensation of mass	0	7
5. Bone pain	2	25
Totals	230**	299

*Sx = symptoms.
**20 patients—information unavailable.

patients. Thus, only a small percentage would have been candidates for radical prostatectomy according to the strict criteria for radical prostatectomy set forth by Jewett.[26]

In view of the lack of general agreement on a staging system for prostatic cancer, the 310 patients in this series were divided simply into 2 groups, 160 with the disease limited to the prostate (*DLP*) and 150 with extracapsular extension (*ECE*) as determined by digital examination and when possible by the evaluation of biopsy specimens. Among the patients with extracapsular extension, 44 had tumors so extensive that they were either fixed to the pelvic sidewalls, invaded the bladder, or caused partial occlusion of the rectal lumen. Extension to only the seminal vesicles was noted in 49 patients, to only the lateral sulcus in 14 patients, and to various combinations of lateral sulcus and seminal vesicle involvement in 43.

Technique

An isocentric treatment planning technique with the patient in the standing position was used for all patients in this series. Whether employed with the patient positioned vertically or horizontally this method includes: 1) Physical examination, 2) localization of the position of the tumor with orthogonal diagnostic films after instillation of appropriate contrast media and information derived from lymphangiography and/or diagnostic pelvic laparotomy, 3) isodose contours on a cross-sectional diagram, 4) calculations of dosage, and 5) verification of the position of the therapeutic beam.[20] Because patient morbidity is directly proportional to irradiated volume and the amount of bladder and rectum included in the irradiated volume, care during the localization procedure cannot be overstressed.

With most modern therapeutic equipment tumor localization and treatment planning is best performed with the patient lying supine and by using a simulator which includes as a minimum the following elements:

1) A patient support assembly identical, or at least similar to the actual treatment couch which employs a floating table top capable of either longitudinal or lateral translation and vertical adjustment so that any point within the patient may be moved in three planes without moving the patient relative to the table top.[20]

2) An isocentrically mounted diagnostic x-ray source capable of achieving the same source to axis distance, *SAD*, as that employed with the therapy equipment. This is usually 100 or 80 cm. A film cassette holder which is a constant distance from the radiation source with a sufficient source film distance, *SFD*, to allow the interposition of a patient between the source and the film while maintaining the source axis distance. For radiotherapy equipment having a 100 cm *SAD*, 135 cm is convenient for the *SFD*. A radiation field light localizer in which the center of the field is identified by the projected shadow of cross wires. In addition to this a radiopaque film marker is projected to coincide with the central axis of the treatment beam for the anterior-posterior localization film and a radiopaque lateral film marker is projected to coincide with the lateral localization film. This is conveniently fixed to the table top and is coincident with the central axis crosswire. As an alternate, a lead marker could simply be taped to the skin at the point of entrance of the central axis of the *AP* and lateral beams.

The patient is placed in a comfortable supine position in the middle of the simulator couch. A small foley catheter is passed into the urinary bladder and the balloon is distended with 5 ml of mercury. It is important to use mercury because it is necessary to identify the prostatic urethra especially in the lateral view (Fig. 12-13A & B). Superimposed bone frequently obliterates a less

dense contrast media. Next, 25 ml of renographin are instilled into the bladder in order to establish the superior boundary of the prostate and 100 ml of thin barium are instilled into the rectum in order to delimit the posterior boundary. An anterior localization film is exposed by adjusting the patient's position relative to the table top so that the central axis is centered at the midline either at the level of the pubis for localization of the prostate only, or 3 or 4 cm superior to the pubis for localization of the entire pelvis. The central axis will automatically be projected on the localization film by the *AP* film marker. The entrance point at the central axis is marked on the patient's skin for further reference. Without moving either the patient or the table top the simulator is rotated 90 degrees taking care to assure that the patient is lying perfectly supine. Side lights are an asset in making this determination. A similar lateral localization film is exposed with the central axis at about the mid frontal plane. This is accomplished by simply adjusting the vertical position of the table. The entrance point of the central axis is marked on the skin for future reference. A cross-sectional contour of the patient is made at the level of the central axis skin marks. Molding heavy solder wire to the body surface at the level of the projected index marks is a simple and convenient method for obtaining the contour. The point within the patient which represents the intersection of the central axis of the anterior-posterior localization film and the central axis of the lateral localization film is designated point *R*. This point can be identified on the localization film as indicated in Figure 12-13A and B and also can be identified on the cross-sectional diagram. The isodose distribution is calculated for the appropriate tumor volume, that is either through the midpelvis or through the midprostate. The best isodose pattern usually dictates a change in the central axis of the treatment beam to a new isocenter point. In the case illustrated in Figure 12-13A, the new isocenter point T_1 for the midpelvic treat-

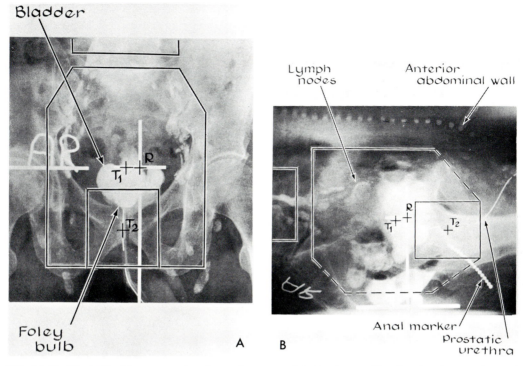

FIG. 12-13. The bold white cross projected near the center of the localization film identifies the central axis of the localization x-ray beam. The reference point, R, represents the provisional isocenter point. After establishing the desired field sizes and dose distributions a new isocenter point is deduced. These are represented as T_1 for the general pelvic volume and T_2 for the prostatic volume. These new points are shifted to the isocenter of the therapy machine by simple adjustment of the patient support assembly. See text for details.

ment plane was established within the midsaggital plane simply by translating the patient support assembly about 1.5 cm from right to left. In the lateral projection, Figure 12-13B, the support assembly was translated 1 cm caudad effectively moving the central ray 1 cm superiorly and lastly, the treatment couch was elevated 0.5 cm, establishing the anterior-posterior position of the isocenter point within the midsaggital plane. The position of T_1 is marked on the skin of the patient by reference to the field-light crosswire shadow, or by side lights if these are available. T_1 is indicated on both the right and left sides of the patient in order to control malpositioning which might occur if the patient were not lying perfectly supine. The corners of the respective fields may be

blocked as illustrated in Figures 12-13A and B and 12-14 in order to avoid unnecessary irradiation of tissue not at risk. Portal films of sufficient quality for verification may be obtained with megavoltage beams but they are of unsatisfactory contrast for illustrations here.

If the therapeutic decision requires a boost of 1,500 to 2,000 rads to the prostatic volume a new treatment isocenter, T_2, may be established from the reference point R by translating the table top and thus the patient from right to left 1.5 cm and by moving the support assembly craniad 4 cm. The new tumor point T_2 is marked on the anterior skin surface as described above for T_1. A similar procedure is followed for establishing the isocenter point for patients treated solely to the prostatic volume except the provisional localization point R, is projected in the midline at the superior margin of the pubis and by convention 11 cm above the table top in the lateral projection. The tumor volume is calculated and the isocenter is adjusted to the new isocenter point T_1 as described above. Thus, it is possible and convenient to establish the isocenter points for a whole pelvic treatment, prostatic boost, or localized prostatic therapy with a single localization procedure.

If the paraaortic lymph nodes are to be treated (Fig. 12-14), it is also convenient to establish the treatment position for the upper abdominal fields at the time of the initial setup. The procedure outlined above is repeated for the upper abdomen and a tumor point is established for the paraaortic lymph nodes. Once this has been established it is easy to deliver a portion of the dose by anterior and posterior opposed fields, by multiple oblique fields, or by a combination of anterior and posterior fields and rotational therapy.

Isodose distributions for small treatment volumes are shown in Figure 12-15. For convenience, the contour receiving the maximum dose is considered 100 per cent. Figure 12-16 shows the distribution obtained by utilizing 2 120-degree lateral sector rotations instead of full 360-degree rotation. This technique has been useful in the patients whose primary tumor extends laterally or in patients in whom it is desirable to reduce the radiation dose to the rectum as much as possible. A 10 per cent reduction in the radiation dose to the rectum results in a notice-

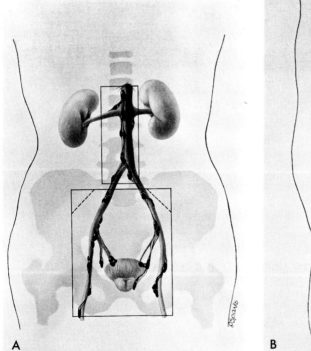
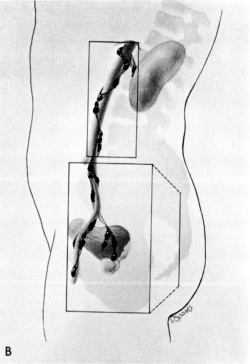

A   B

FIG. 12-14. Representation of large pelvic and paraaortic fields. The posterior margin of the lateral pelvic fields vary with the degree of posterior extension of the primary. Even at the risk of a reduced dose to rarely involved presacral nodes it is desirable to protect the posterior wall of the rectum whenever reasonable. The field arrangement for the prostatic boost is identical to that illustrated in Figure 12-13.

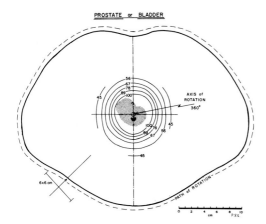

FIG. 12-15. A typical isodose distribution plotted on a cross section of the patient obtained at the level of the superior margin of the pubis and utilizing a 6 × 6 cm field as determined at the axis of rotation. (Courtesy: Bagshaw, *Radiology*, 85, 121, 1965.)

able decrease in rectal morbidity. For these reasons the lateral arc technique has gradually replaced the full 360-degree rotation as the treatment of choice for patients with localized neoplasm. While a ^{60}Co beam has not been utilized in this series, the dosimetry

with a well-collimated isocentric ^{60}Co unit shows a dose distribution nearly identical to a 6 Mev linear accelerator. A rotational volume distribution calculated for ^{60}Co is shown in Figure 12-17. Figure 12-18 shows a volume distribution with parallel opposed anterior, posterior, and lateral fields.

In the rotational treatment of localized carcinoma of the prostate with megavoltage radiation obtained from a well-collimated ^{60}Co unit or linear accelerator, the diameter of the homogeneous high dose volume will be essentially equal to the transverse diameter of the geometrical field measured at the axis of rotation. The caudad-cephalad dimension of the field should be increased about 1 cm over the transverse diameter in order to insure that the axial dimension of the cylindrical treatment volume for rotational therapy will be equal to the transverse diameter at the isocenter. This is necessary

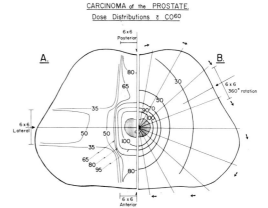

FIG. 12-17. Isodose distribution which may be achieved with a ^{60}Co teletherapy device. The 6 × 6 cm field was determined at a source distance of 95 cm.

A. Distribution obtained from parallel opposing anterior, posterior and right and left lateral fields.

B. Distribution obtained by a full 360° rotation and calculated by the tumor-air ratio method.

If 4 fields are to be employed rather than rotation therapy, all 4 fields should be treated each day in order to assure homogeneity within the treatment volume.

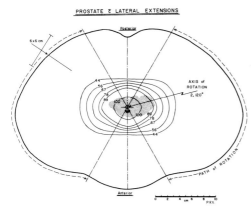

FIG. 12-16. Dosimetric pattern for a patient with carcinoma of the prostate with lateral extension. The elliptical isodose pattern may be achieved by using two lateral arcs of rotation of 120 degrees centered on the same axis. The method slightly reduces the total dose to the rectum. (Courtesy: Bagshaw, *Radiology*, 85, 121, 1965.)

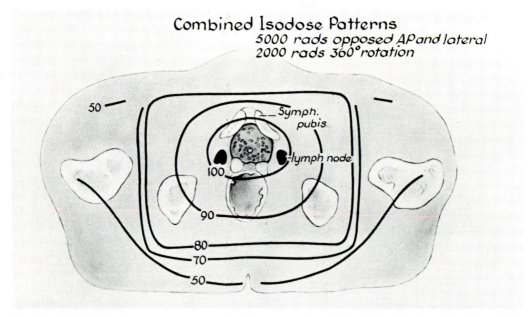

FIG. 12-18. Combined isodose pattern through midprostate, when 5,000 rads is administered by 4 large fields and the prostatic region is boosted an additional 2,000 rads by rotational therapy with 6 × 6 or 7 × 7 cm fields centered on prostate.

in rotational therapy because the dose is slightly lower at the margins of the treatment volume which are parallel to the beam axis because of the penumbra. Therefore, given a table of tumor-air ratios, *i.e.* the ratios of the absorbed dose in tissue to the exposure dose in air as a function of overlying tissue and field cross section, one may easily calculate the dose by simply determining the mean radius of the patient and employing the conventional equation for the determination of tumor dose.

Irrespective of the megavoltage unit if the maximum dose of radiation is limited to the base of the bladder, taking care to include the seminal vesicles, minimum morbidity results and most patients are able to tolerate 7,500 rads absorbed at the 100 per cent contour in $7\frac{1}{2}$ weeks with little more than transient dysuria or diarrhea. Our standard dose in patients with disease limited to the prostate is 7,500 rads calculated at the isocenter and delivered at the rate of 1,000 rads per week. Patients are treated 5 days a week. In

the event that more serious symptoms occur, a split course may be used with treatment discontinued for 2 weeks after a dose of about 4,000 rads has been given. In practice, the patient is asked to report for the daily treatment with a full bladder in order to elevate the dome out of the treatment volume. It is prudent to avoid making the patient wait too long for his therapy.

In patients with proven lymph node metastases or in those with primary neoplasms extending to the pelvic sidewalls, or invading the urinary bladder, or with otherwise massive extraprostatic involvement, a 4-field pelvic technique employing anterior, posterior, left, and right lateral fields is used (Fig. 12-17). Although other therapists might have different methods to achieve the same dose distributions the following method has been used successfully for several years with a minimum of morbidity. The treatment volume extends from the ischial tuberosities to about the superior margin of *L*-5 and laterally approximately 1.5 cm lateral to the pelvic sidewalls in order to include the internal and external iliac lymph nodes (Fig. 12-14A and B). It is best to localize the position of the prostate at the same time the larger pelvic fields are localized so that before the termination of therapy the fields may be reduced to include only the prostatic region. It is important to perform the localization procedure and catheterization well before a pelvic dose of 5,000 rads has been achieved since catheterization of tissues irradiated to this level is more likely to be associated with patient discomfort and an increased probability of secondary bacterial infection. The lateral cutaneous marks, which designate the position of the isocenter for the rotational boost are identified at the time of the initial localization and permanently tatooed on the skin of the lateral thigh.

Five thousand rads are delivered to the treatment volume with the 4-fields and then the fields are reduced and relocated to deliver a boost of 2,000 rads to the more restricted prostatic volume usually with rotational techniques as described above. The pelvic volume is matched at about the level of *L-5* with anterior and posterior fields which cross-fire the paraaortic lymph nodes (Fig. 12-14). The gap between the 2 adjacent fields is calculated carefully in order to avoid either overlap or an anatomic miss and the superior margin of the paraaortic volume extends to about *L-1*. About 3,000 rads are given to the paraaortic nodes with anterior and posterior fields and then up to 5,000 to 5,500 rads with either rotational therapy or isocentrically placed multiple oblique fields. A compromise is achieved between renal and subcutaneous irradiation which assures prevention of later symptomatic subcutaneous fibrosis or radiation nephritis (Fig. 12-19). In the 2 to 10 Mev energy range, large tissue volumes should not receive doses approaching 7,000 rads delivered at 1,000 rads per week

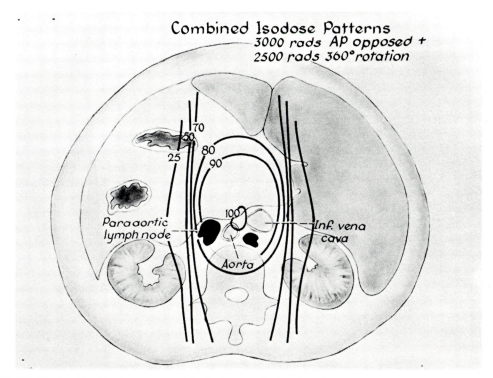

FIG. 12-19. Combined isodose pattern at level of paraaortic lymph nodes.

Table 12-9. *Entire Population—310 Patients*
137 Patients at Risk for 5 Years or More

Group	Total	No. Alive without *Ca*	No. Alive with *Ca*	No. Dead without *Ca*	No. Dead with *Ca*
Disease Limited to Prostate	68	41 (61%)	7 (11%)	9 (12%)	11 (16%)
Extraprostatic Extension	69	25 (36%)	10 (14%)	8 (12%)	26 (38%)

through opposed anterior and posterior radiation portals only. In so doing, one may be erroneously tempted to treat only 1 field per day; this results in unacceptably high increments every other day to the subcutaneous tissues. In patients treated at other institutions by this technique but followed in our clinic, severe late symptomatic subcutaneous fibrosis has been observed in the pubic, sacral, perineal, and gluteal regions. Either the rotational or multiple field method assures the delivery of a homogeneous dose to the entire target volume at each treatment session.

Results

The status of all patients at the time of this analysis who had been at risk for at least 5 years is detailed in Table 12-9. In this tabulation patients examined within 6 months of death, dying prior to the closing date of the study from an obviously unrelated cause, were considered to have died without cancer. Table 12-10 details a similar analysis of the

current status of all patients who have been at risk for 10 years.

The survival data presented in Figure 12-20 is calculated strictly by the actuarial method outlined by Cutler and Ederer and recommended by the American Joint Committee for Cancer Staging and End Results Reporting.[2,11] For each curve, unless otherwise stated, the calculation of actuarial survival is based on data in which all patients who died were scored as having died of cancer and were considered treatment failures. This method presents a conservative estimate of the actual success of the treatment as reflected by survival data since, as noted in Tables 12-9 and 12-10 some patients classified as treatment failures for calculation by the method had died of intercurrent disease without clinical evidence of tumor. Thus patients with limited disease (*DLP*) had actuarial survival rates of 72 and 44 per cent at 5 and 10 years respectively; those with more extensive neoplasm had the 5- and 10-year rates drop to 48 and 27 per cent. These differences were statistically significant

Table 12-10. *Entire Population—310 Patients*
43 Patients at Risk for 10 Years or More

Group	Total	No. Alive without *Ca*	No. Alive with *Ca*	No. Dead without *Ca*	No. Dead with *Ca*
Disease Limited to Prostate	23	9 (39%)	1 (4%)	8 (35%)	5 (22%)
Extraprostatic Extension	20	6 (30%)	1 (5%)	3 (15%)	10 (50%)

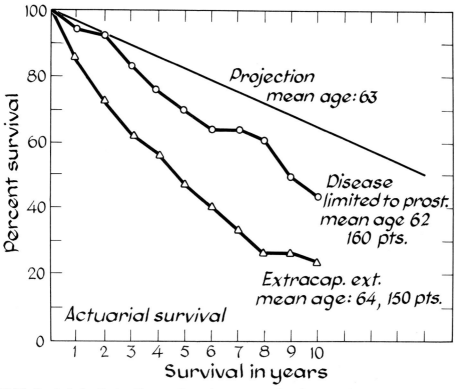

FIG. 12-20. Survival of patients with prostatic carcinoma, comparison by anatomic extent.

(p < 0.05). Bladder invasion was the most significant adverse finding with 9 of 13 patients dead with tumor, 3 alive with tumor and only 1 living without disease at 3 years following therapy. The survival data are not age corrected, although the predicted survival for the male population for the same mean age is presented on the over-all survival curves for the reader's convenience.

A prolonged interval between the diagnosis and treatment also appeared to adversely affect survival. Table 12-11 demonstrates that 62 per cent of the 247 patients who were diagnosed within 1 year prior to treatment were living without evidence of disease as opposed to only 44 per cent of 57 patients whose diagnosis had been established prior to 1 year before beginning radiotherapy.

In addition to the 310 patients presented above, 13 patients who had had prior radical prostatic resections were treated by the techniques described above except that the fields

Table 12-11. *Effect of Interval Between DX and RX Upon Survival*

Group	Aver. Age	Total	Alive NED	Alive with Ca	Dead NED	Dead with Ca	% Survival 5 yrs*
DX <1 yr.	63	247	156 (63%)	33 (13%)	24 (10%)	34 (14%)	61
DX >1 yr.	66	57	25 (44%)	3 (5%)	5 (9%)	24 (42%)	39

* Actuarial.

were somewhat larger.[10] While this is a small group, it is important to record this experience since referral for such treatment is occurring with increasing frequency and only 1 previous series of 4 patients has been reported.[14] Of these 13 patients, 4 were referred during convalescence from surgery because of gross residual tumor; 9 were referred 6 months to $6\frac{1}{2}$ years after surgery because of frank recurrence. Ten of the 13 patients are living, 7 without evidence of carcinoma. The longest follow-up is 4 years. Although the follow-up period is short, aggressive postoperative irradiation in patients in whom the resected specimen demonstrates marginal transection of tumor appears worthy of careful consideration.

Concomitant Hormone Therapy

One hundred and sixty of the 310 patients had neither received estrogen nor been castrated prior to radiation therapy. In general, the survival in this cohort appeared better than in the other, however, statistical significance could not be determined because of differences in staging between the two groups. A more detailed analysis of the influence of concomitant hormone therapy on survival is presented elsewhere.[28]

Morbidity

Symptoms attributed to the treatment were classified as either of major or minor significance and each of these subdivided into acute and chronic. Of major significance were those which interfered with the patient's daily activities or prompted an interruption of the treatment sequence. They were regarded as acute if they were of less than 3 months duration from the date of the last treatment and chronic if they persisted longer than 3 months.

A change in bowel habits was the most common acute symptom and was observed in about 60 per cent of all patients. This was manifested as either nonbloody diarrhea or formed stools with mucus or blood and it occurred during the fourth or fifth week of treatment. Although bloody diarrhea was observed in 9 per cent of the patients, the blood loss was never significant. Proctitis usually responded to treatment with a combination of a low residue diet, a suppository which contained hydrocortisone, and the use of bulk stool softeners such as Colace. If such medication was required during treatment it was usually continued for a month or two after the completion of therapy. The most common chronic rectal sequelae present in 12 patients (4 per cent) was intermittent streaking of the stools with blood which on sigmoidoscopy appeared secondary to an increase in friability of the rectal mucosa and telangiectasia. Seven patients noted persistent tenesmus and in several of these this was severe. This situation usually occurred among patients who had a history of chronic constipation, hemorrhoids, fistulae-in-ano, or previous anal or rectal surgery. Treatment of constipation by bulk stool softeners usually led to gradual improvement.

The most common acute genitourinary symptom was dysuria and/or frequency in about 25 per cent of the patients. Deep perineal pain was noted in 10 per cent and occasionally was severe. Analgesics, especially suppositories containing belladona and opium derivatives usually relieved this difficulty. The symptoms usually disappeared within 2 months of the completion of treatment when there was a satisfactory tumor response. Acute dysuria and frequency was usually alleviated by the administration of topical genitourinary analgesics such as phenazopyridine HCL (Pyridium). When these symptoms occurred, the patient was investigated for urinary infection and when documented, it was treated vigorously throughout the remaining course of therapy and for about one month thereafter with the appropriate antibiotics.

Chronic urethral stricture occurred in 14 patients. In 2 of these patients, the local neoplasm persisted and the stricture was attributed to this cause. Eleven other patients had had more than one transurethral resection prior to irradiation. In 3, there was severe obstruction requiring a urethral catheter for a prolonged period either before or during irradiation. In 9 of these patients who were treated during the early years of this program, the tumor dose at the 100 per cent isodose contour exceeded 7,700 rads.

If the patient developed symptoms of radiation sequelae, the symptoms were usually multiple and involved both the lower gastrointestinal and urinary systems. The most frequent combination included a change in bowel habits, urinary frequency, and dysuria. Therefore, 7,500 rads delivered in $7\frac{1}{2}$ weeks is rarely exceeded at the present time. If a relatively large volume (such as that encompassed by an 8×8 cm field) must be irradiated, or if the patient presents a past history which includes one or more of the factors known to predispose to an increase of radiation sequelae, then the dose may be reduced to 7,000 rads in 7 weeks or a 2 week split may be allowed after 3,500 to 4,000 rads are given. Although no significant difference in the incidence of sequelae was observed in comparing patients who had been treated with the 120-degree lateral arc rotation versus those treated with full 360-degree rotation, bowel sequelae following the 120-degree arc technique occurred later and were less severe.

Since all of these patients have been treated with rotational therapy there has been no incidence of either acute cutaneous reactions or late subcutaneous fibrosis. Similarly, in the patients treated more recently with an extended treatment plan, using combinations of fixed field and rotational therapy, there has been no evidence of either early or late cutaneous reactions.

Potency

Sexual histories were considered sufficiently complete for analysis in 164 patients. Fifty-two (32 per cent) of these were impo-

tent prior to therapy. The remaining 112 indicated that they were capable of maintaining erections and performing sexual intercourse prior to either treatment or diagnosis. Of the potent group, 70 per cent maintained essentially the same degree of potency after therapy, while 30 per cent either reported no return of potency after the pretherapeutic diagnostic procedure or a gradual decline in the ability to maintain erections; the decline commenced from several months to several years following therapy.

Discussion

Three conclusions can be drawn from the group of patients presented here:

1) The survival among those patients with disease limited to the prostate is significantly better than those with extraprostatic extension.

2) Prior or concomitant hormone therapy does not alter the over-all survival in patients irradiated in the prostatic region.

3) Sexual potency is preserved in a high proportion of patients who are potent at the start of radiation therapy in marked contrast to the nearly 100 per cent incidence of impotency which accompanies radical prostatectomy.

Thus, for patients with disease limited to the prostate, the survival approaches that achieved with radical prostatectomy. For those with more extensive disease, a higher survival might be achieved by the employment of extended radiation which would include the pelvic and/or paraaortic lymph nodes. In order to better evaluate the degree of extension, recently lymphangiography has been employed as a staging aid (Fig. 12-21). Among some 70 lymphangiograms which have been performed on patients with prostatic carcinoma, 20 patients were selected for laparotomy in order to confirm the lymphangiogram. In 16 patients the lymphangiogram findings were confirmed—10 having had unequivocally positive studies. A larger

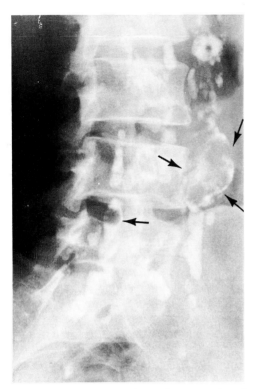

FIG. 12-21. Two common iliac nodes, one on the right and one on the left are clearly partially and nearly totally replaced by filling defects. Both of these nodes were pathologically positive. The patient had a single 2 × 2 × 2 cm nodule in the superior pole of the right lobe of the prostate with modest extension to the region of the right seminal vesicle.

number of patients were not subjected to pelvic and paraaortic exploration because in some the lymph nodes clearly appeared positive and the need for pathological confirmation evolved during the study of the lymphangiograms in this initial group of patients. Although it is far from established at this time that lymphangiography can be relied upon for definitive staging unless it is clearly positive, this remains a subject for intensive further study.

Radiotherapy of Metastases From Prostatic Carcinoma

External irradiation of either osseous metastases or soft tissue metastases, such as

hilar lymph nodes may offer considerable palliation to the patient. Often a patient with extensive skeletal metastases will complain of pain in a specific site even though the general progress of the disease is suppressed by endocrine therapy. External irradiation in doses of 2,000 to 4,000 rads, fractionated at the rate of 200 to 300 rads per day will almost always produce significant and prolonged relief of pain.

Similarly, symptoms of bronchial obstruction may be relieved and the progression of mediastinal metastases arrested by doses in the range of 4,000 rads fractionated at the rate of 1,000 to 1,500 rads per week.

BIBLIOGRAPHY

1. American Cancer Society: 1971 Cancer Facts and Figures, 1970 copyright.
2. American Joint Committee for Cancer Staging and End Results Reporting: Reporting of cancer survival and end results, 55 East Erie Street, Chicago, Ill., 1963.
3. Bagshaw, M. A., and Kaplan, H. S.: Radical external radiotherapy of localized prostatic carcinoma, Tenth International Congress of Radiology, Montreal, Canada, Abstract, 1962.
4. Bagshaw, M. A., Kaplan, H. S., and Sagerman, R. H.: Linear accelerator supervoltage radiotherapy. VII. Carcinoma of the prostate, *Radiology,* 85, 121, 1965.
5. Barringer, B. S.: Radium in the treatment of carcinoma of the bladder and prostate; review of one year's work, *JAMA,* XVIII, 1227, 1917.
6. Barringer, B. S.: Prostatic carcinoma, *J. Urol.,* 47, 306, 1942.
7. Bennett, J. E.: Treatment of carcinoma of the prostate by cobalt-beam therapy, *Radiology,* 90, 532, 1968.
8. Budhraja, S. N., and Anderson, J. C.: An assessment of the value of radiotherapy in the management of carcinoma of the prostate, *Brit. J. Urol.,* 36, 535, 1964.
9. Bumpus, H. D.: Roentgen rays and radium in the diagnosis and treatment of carcinoma of the prostate, *Amer. J. Roentgen.,* 9, 269, 1922.
10. Cassady, J. R., Bagshaw, M. A., and Ray, G. R.: Radiation salvage following radical prostatectomy for prostatic carcinoma, Submitted to *J. Urol.*

11. Cutler, S. J., and Ederer, F.: Maximum utilization of the life table method in analyzing survival, *J. Chron. Dis.*, 6, 699, 1958.

12. Del Regato, J. A.: Radiotherapy in the conservative treatment of operable and locally inoperable carcinoma of the prostate, *Radiology*, 88, 761, 1967.

13. Deming, C. L.: Cancer of the prostate and seminal vesicles. Results in one hundred cases of cancer of prostate and seminal vesicles, treated with radium, *Surg. Gynec. and Obst.*, 34, 99, 1922.

14. Dykhuizen, R. F., Sargent, C. R., George, F. W., III, and Kurahara, S. S.: The use of cobalt 60 teletherapy in the treatment of prostatic carcinoma, *J. Urol.*, 100, 33, 1968.

15. Ellis, L. D., Jensen, W., and Westerman, M. P.: Needle biopsy of bone and marrow, *Arch. Internal. Med.*, 14, 213, 1964.

16. Flocks, R. H., Kerr, H. D., Elkins, H. B., and Culp, D.: Treatment of carcinoma of the prostate by interstitial radiation with radioactive gold (^{198}Au): A preliminary report, *J. Urol.*, 68, 510, 1952.

17. Flocks, R. H.: Combination therapy for localized prostatic cancer, *J. Urol.*, 89, 889, 1963.

18. Flocks, R. H.: Current Cancer Concepts. Present status of interstitial irradiation in managing prostatic cancer, *JAMA*, 210, 328, 1969.

19. Franks, L. M.: Some comments on the long-term results of endocrine treatment of prostatic cancer, *Brit. J. Urol.*, 30, 383, 1958.

20. Gardner, A., Bagshaw, M. A., Page, V., and Karzmark, C. J.: Tumor localization, dosimetry, simulation and treatment procedures in radiotherapy: The isocentric technique, *Amer. J. Roentgen.* (In Press).

21. George, F. W., III, Carter, E. C., Jr., and Dykhuizen, R. F.: Cobalt-60 teletherapy in the definitive treatment of carcinoma of the prostate: A preliminary report, *J. Urol.*, 93, 102, 1965.

22. Gilbertsen, V. A.: Cancer of the prostate gland. Results of early diagnosis and therapy undertaken for cure of the disease, *JAMA*, 215, 81, 1971.

23. Hilaris, B. S., Whitmore, W. F., Grabstald, H., and O'Kelly, P. J.: A new approach to radical radiation therapy of cancer of the prostate using interstitial and external sources, *Clinical Bulletin of Memorial Hospital* (In Press).

24. Huggins, C., and Hodges, C. V.: Studies on prostatic cancer, effect of castration of estrogen and of androgen injections on serum phosphatase in metastatic carcinoma of the prostate, *Cancer Res.*, 2, 293, 1941.

25. Jewett, H. J., Bridge, R. W., Gray, G. F., Jr., and Shelley, W. M.: The palpable nodule of prostatic cancer. Results 15 years after radical excision, *JAMA*, 203, 403, 1968.

26. Jewett, H. J.: The case for radical perineal prostatectomy, *J. Urol.*, 103, 195, 1970.

27. Pasteau, O.: Traitement du cancer de la prostate par le radium, *Rev. des mal. de la Nutrition*, 363, 1911.

28. Ray, G. R., Bagshaw, M. A., and Cassady, J. R.: Definitive radiation therapy of carcinoma of the prostate. A report of 14 year's experience, Submitted to *Radiology*.

29. Turner, R. D., and Belt, E.: A study of 229 consecutive cases of total perineal prostatectomy for cancer of the prostate, *J. Urol.*, 77, 62, 1957.

30. Widmann, B.: Cancer of the prostate. The results of radium and roentgenray treatment, *Radiology*, 22, 153, 1934.

31. Young, H. H.: The early diagnosis and radical cure of carcinoma of the prostate: Being a study of 40 cases and presentation of a radical operation which was carried out in four cases, *Bull. Johns Hopkins Hosp.*, 16, 315, 1905.

32. Young, H. H., and Frontz, W. A.: Some new methods in the treatment of carcinoma of the lower genitourinary tract with radium, *J. Urol.*, 1, 505, 1917.

Irradiation of Prostatic Cancer Combined with Abdominal Exploration

PHILIP T. HUDGINS

Small field radiation therapy for cancer of limited extent offers the distinct advantage of improved tissue tolerance and thus less risk of complication. However, the difficulty of evaluation of the extent of disease and the inaccuracy of beam directioning from uncertainties in precise positioning of the volume to be treated negate any beneficial effect of small field therapy if there is a geographic miss of the prescribed treatment.

Clinical staging of carcinoma of the prostate has been described by Willet Whitmore, Jr.[1] and generally accepted as:

Stage A: Clinically latent cancer which is identified only by histologic examination of prostatic tissue removed by surgery.

Stage B: Clinically early cancer characterized by the presence of a palpable nodule confined to the prostatic capsule and no evidence of metastases.

Stage C: Locally invasive, extending through the capsule and still no evidence of metastatic disease.

Stage D: Clinically evident metastases characterized by radiographic bone disease or pulmonary metastases or occult metastases evidenced by an increase in the serum acid phosphatase.

A Stage B lesion may be fairly large, that is 4 cm or more in diameter, without extension beyond the capsule. Some Stage C lesions extending into the seminal vesicles may be small. There is a great range of size in Stage C as these may extend all the way to the pelvic side walls. In our experience and the experience reported by others[2] in which there has been surgical exploration of the patients following clinical staging, clinical staging is found to be highly inaccurate.

Clinical Stage B's have been found to be Stage C upon exploration in 50 per cent of the cases. With these facts in mind, the following policy has been outlined.

While patients with Stage A and B lesions classically have been considered as candidates for radical prostatectomy, we have had an increasing number of these patients who have come to primary radiation therapy. Some of these patients are poor surgical risks and others refused surgery because of the complication of virtually 100 per cent impotency. Furthermore, there is an appreciable incidence of incontinence and fistula formation following a radical prostatectomy. Patients with Stage A, B and limited C lesions (that is no larger than an estimated 6 cm in diameter) have retropubic surgical exploration for the purpose of surgical staging and implantation of the primary tumor with radioactive gold grains. The surgical procedure consists of mobilization of the prostate gland so that it can be visualized and palpated in its entirety and evaluation of the pelvic lymph nodes. Palpable nodes are removed. If none are palpated, random biopsy samples are obtained. Approximately 85 per cent of those patients surgically explored meet the criteria of having no more than limited Stage C disease surgically, and radioactive gold grains are implanted for the purpose of getting a boost dose of radiation in the primary tumor and to provide radiopaque markers for beam directioning (Figs. 12-22 and 12-23). Interstitial radiation dosages generally are planned not to exceed 3,000 rads to total decay to the volume of interest. Detailed computer calculations of interstitial isodose curves are seldom used since they

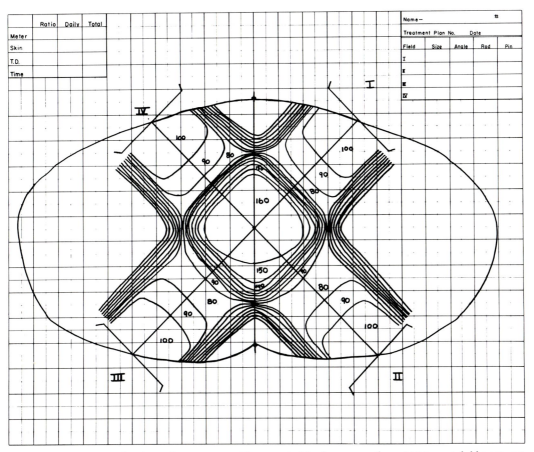

FIG. 12-22. An example of a patient contour with summated isodose curves for a 6 × 6 cm 4-field treatment plan on a ^{60}Co unit.

have not caused us to alter our external beam therapy. It is recognized and accepted that there will be inhomogeneity of dose. Dose is estimated on the basis of a central placement of sources and considered as one point source in a sphere of prostatic tissue, even though the actual placement is attempted in as near homogeneous dose distribution as is practical. The radioactivity of the gold grains at the time of an implant is in the range of 2 to 9 mc per grain. The following table is used to estimate radiation dose from the implant.

Dose in R/mc ^{198}Au at the periphery of a sphere for a central point source:

Diameter in cm	Dose
1	1000
2	250
3	110
4	65
5	40
6	30

External beam therapy is initiated in 2 weeks allowing time for the patient to recover from surgery. A 4-field cross-firing technique (Fig. 12-24) as well as rotational therapy techniques with a ^{60}Co unit or a 8 Mev linear accelerator have been used to complement the interstitial dosages of radia-

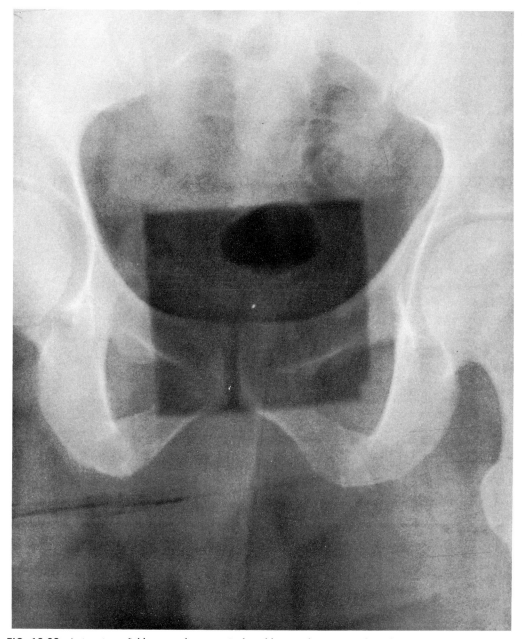

FIG. 12-23. A 6 × 6 cm field centered over a single gold grain that was implanted in a 1 cm nodule of prostatic carcinoma at the time of surgical exploration. Activity of gold grain 3.7 mc estimated dose to 1 cm volume 3,700 rads.

tion. The cross-fire field size or rotational techniques have not exceeded 8 × 8 cm. If large volumes are treated, opposed fields are used. External beam is planned for a total of 5,000 rads in 4 weeks given on a 4 day per week schedule.

Transient mild symptoms of proctitis and cystitis are frequent side effects during therapy. These symptoms are generally easily controlled symptomatically and abate within 2 to 3 weeks of completion of treatment. In over 100 patients treated during the past 6

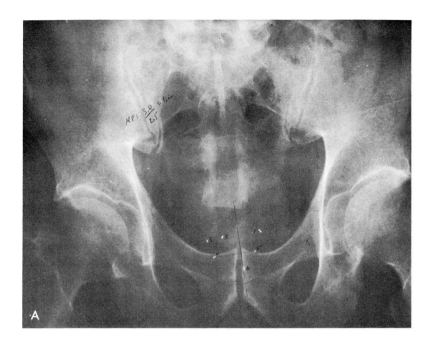

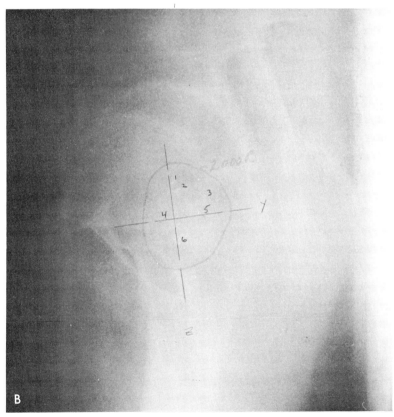

FIG. 12-24. **A.** *AP* radiograph of gold grain implant on a patient with limited Stage C disease. At the time of surgical exploration, iliac node biopsies were negative and a 5 cm prostatic cancerous mass was implanted with 6 gold grains of 8.3 mc activity each, estimated dose is 2,000 rads to total decay for a 5 cm sphere. A 2,000 rad isodose curve based on multiple point sources as determined computer calculations from the multiple point sources is superimposed, and correlates closely with the estimated dose. External beam therapy of 5,000 rads in 4 weeks supplemented the interstitial therapy. **B.** Lateral radiograph depicting implant and dose distribution in the sagittal plane.

years with this approach, there have been only two serious complications, one a hemorrhage from the prostate requiring multiple transfusions and the other a necrotic fistula leading to septicemia and death.

In those patients treated who have Stage *A, B* or limited *C* disease, the aim of treatment is cure. Such patients should not be placed on hormone therapy or have orchiectomy. Routine prophylactic hormone therapy does not increase longevity and should be reserved for management of the patient when there is evidence of persistent or recurrent disease.

BIBLIOGRAPHY

1. Whitmore, W. F., Jr.: The rationale and results of ablative surgery in prostatic cancer, *Cancer,* 16, 1119, 1963.
2. *Ibid.*

Penis and Male Urethra

FERNANDO G. BLOEDORN

Penis

Squamous cell carcinoma of the penis is rare, never seen in the male who was circumcized at birth. It occurs most often in patients with phimosis.[2] It is encountered primarily between the age of 50 to 70, but in 30 per cent of the patients it develops between the age of 30 and 50. This tumor develops almost exclusively in patients with low hygienic standards. Treatment by irradiation should be tried when proper clinical indications are present in order to save the organ.

With the exception of rare histological patterns squamous cell carcinomas, as a rule well differentiated, constitute the large majority of the cases. In addition to the cancerous lesions there are precancerous ones, leukoplakia ordinarily of the verrucous type or the intraepithelial tumor known as Queyrat's erythroplasia. The various degrees from precancerous states to infiltrative squamous carcinoma may be seen in the same patient.

The clinical varieties of ulcerative, infiltrative, and exophytic tumors are seen. The exophytic type is less aggressive and responds better to irradiation.

The tumors are usually diagnosed late often showing signs of maceration and infection especially if phimosis is present.

Routes of Spread

LOCAL EXTENSION

Squamous cell carcinoma of the penis remains localized in the primary site for a long period of time in most patients. The infiltration in depth is impaired by Buck's fascia that acts as a temporary barrier but when perforated the corpus cavernosum will be invaded (20 per cent of the cases). The corpus spongiosum is the last to be involved. Once the erectile organs are invaded the progression of the disease is accelerated not only locally but also by the involvement of the lymph vessels and nodes. The urethra is seldom involved even in the advanced cases.

LYMPH NODES

Metastases are seen more commonly in younger patients with undifferentiated carcinomas and when the tumor originates on the glans or has infiltrated the erectile organs.

The group of nodes commonly involved are the superficial and deep inguinal nodes if the cancer is limited to the prepuce and glans. The deep iliac nodes may be involved when tumor has invaded the cavernous bodies or originated in the urethra.

Because of the commonly superimposed infection, enlargement of nodes in the groins are not always metastatic in origin, around 50 per cent being inflammatory. Conversely, a certain percentage of groin nodes are involved with cancer without being palpable. When a node is larger than 3 cm in diameter or is fixed or ulcerated, it is more likely to be metastatic.

Aspiration biopsy of palpable nodes is indicated but is of value only if positive.

Distant metastases are uncommon and only seen in the late stages of the disease and can be anywhere in the body.

PATIENT CARE

A dorsal slit of the foreskin or a total circumcision is necessary to determine the diagnosis of the tumor and its extension in patients with induration palpable through a phimotic prepuce. Circumcision is preferred except in patients whose prepuce is involved by tumor.

Infection has to be dealt with actively, therapy is not started until it is under control and the incision wound well healed (2 to 4 weeks).

Reaction to Radiation

PENIS

The tolerance and reactions of the mucosa of the glans and urethra are similar to those of the mucosa of the oral cavity. Dysuria and burning sensation on urination are common during treatment because of epithelitis. The tolerance of the erectile tissues, especially those of the corpora cavernosa is diminished by tumor infiltration and concomitant infection; however, the tolerance is better with the use of megavoltage irradiation.

Cancerocidal doses result in some atrophy and fibrosis of the treated areas. Meatal atrophy, and coronal sulcus obliteration due to adhesions are produced by scarring in areas of tumor destruction or excessive radiation reaction. Erectile function is changed but not abolished and with proper protection of the testicles libido can be preserved. Excessive doses can lead to painful necrosis requiring amputation.

GROIN

Because of moisture and friction the skin of the groins has worse tolerance than in any other part of the body. Megavoltage and/or interstitial gamma-ray therapy are imperative for any treatment in this area.

Tumor Response

PRIMARY TUMOR

According to Murphy[3] the radiation response of the squamous cell carcinoma of the penis is similar to squamous cell carcinoma of the lip. The only difference is difference in tumor bed.

LYMPH NODES

Little information is available; however, probably one can control disease with megavoltage irradiation and, if necessary, with additional interstitial gamma-ray therapy to residual tumor. The use of elective irradiation of lymph node bearing areas when only microscopic seedings are present could also be of value in increasing cure rates.

Type of Irradiation: Indications and Techniques

RADICAL IRRADIATION

All modalities of irradiation have been used in treatment for cancer of the penis. We shall refer only to those of practical present use.

Low Energy Irradiation (60 to 140 Kv). Low energy irradiation can be used with 5 to 20 cm *FSD* providing the lesion is small, its extensions in depth are not beyond a few millimeters from the surface, and only small areas of normal tissue of the penis are irradiated. A margin over half a centimeter should be allowed beyond the visible and palpable disease. The dose-time schedule indicated for this type of therapy is of 5,000 to 6,000 rads in 3 to 5 weeks. The highest filtration should be used. Single direct fields are used in these cases.

Megavoltage Irradiation. This type of irradiation is mandatory in the treatment of all other infiltrating lesions and in advanced carcinomas of the penis and for treatment of lymph node bearing areas. In order to avoid the low surface dose due to the electronic build-up, when using high energy irradiation, bolus should be added in all cases; therefore, irradiation through a special device becomes indispensible (Fig. 12-25). Two parallel opposing fields produces homogeneous irradiation throughout the gadget. The dose-time will vary between 5,000 rads in 3 to 4 weeks to 6,000 rads in 5 to 6 weeks depending upon the volume; the highest dose and the shortest protraction are used for the smaller volume irradiation.

Interstitial Therapy: Radium Implants or Other Gamma Emitters. Exceptional cases, where a circumscribed lesion, limited to the surface of the organ and of a well-differentiated type, can be treated by a single planar implant covering the lesion with adequate margins of normal tissue. The Paterson-Parker rules of source distribution are followed, delivering 5,000 to 6,000 rads in 5 to 6 days. An implant, however, is better indicated as complementary treatment to residual tumor after external irradiation has been delivered. In these cases the implant should be limited to the tumor itself with minimal irradiation to the normal neighboring tissues. No crossing needles are needed. In this way 1,000 to 1,500 rads can be added to the external irradiation.

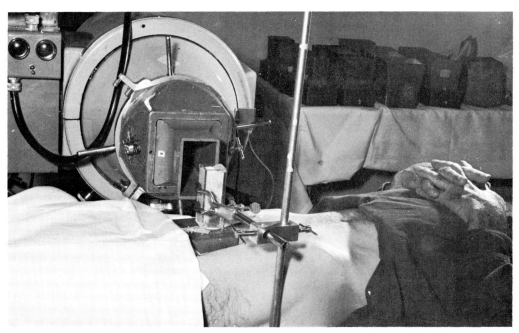

FIG. 12-25. Jig used at M. D. Anderson Hospital and actual set-up for the treatment of penile cancer with telecobalt therapy.

Molds. Radium, or other artificial gamma emitters as radium sources, can be used. The indications are based on the special anatomy of the organ and the advantages of high energy irradiation. Today, this technique is still an excellent treatment in well-selected cases; the late changes produced by this modality of treatment are minimum. Care should be taken for the distance between the radioactive sources and the abdominal wall and the scrotum to be longer than the treatment distance.[4] The distal radium sources should go far enough beyond the tip of the penis to make sure that the tip will be included in the volume of high irradiation. The use of an indwelling catheter during each treatment will avoid treatment interruption because of

difficulty of urination and help to maintain the organ in proper position. This modality of therapy is best suited for the irradiation of the distal half of the organ; it should not be used for obese patients with a short penis. Most molds used for this purpose have been of cylindrical shape with several rows of short needles following the Manchester rules.[4] This source arrangement, in general, gives a higher dose of irradiation to the surface of the organ than in the axis.[4] I have developed a simpler mold which by compressing the organ will adapt it to the inside of the mold delivering very uniform irradiation throughout the desired area of the distal half of the organ (Fig. 12-26).

A dose in the order of 5,500 rads in 8 days

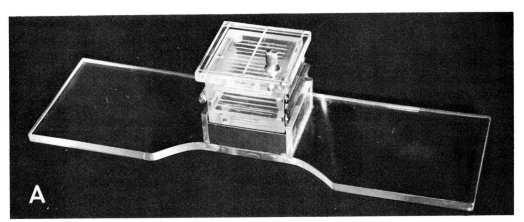

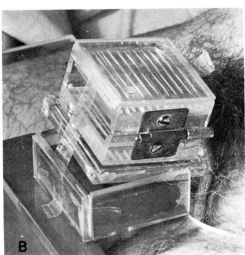

FIG. 12-26. A. Box mold. The inner surface of the mold is grooved to avoid motion of the organ. The plate on top of the box is the radium carrier. It is perforated in the periphery and in the middle to allow the introduction of needles (their loading follows Paterson-Parker rules). It is used in each side of the box on alternate days, 6 to 8 hours per day.

B. Actual application of the mold.

is indicated with the box-mold. With a cylindrical mold a maximum of 6,000 to the skin and 4,000 to 5,000 rads to the central axis in 8 days should not be exceeded.

Treatment of the Lymph Node Bearing Areas

For this portion of the treatment the volume of irradiation should include the groin, external iliac and hypogastric lymph node bearing areas. The use of megavoltage therapy is mandatory to take advantage of its skin sparing effect since high tumor doses are to be delivered through areas of poor skin tolerance. In most cases, bilateral irradiation is indicated through narrow rectangular fields with protection of the midline, as in parametrial irradiation. We have used a longer anterior field covering the lymph node bearing areas of the pelvic wall and groin and a posterior field that will oppose only the pelvic portion of the anterior field. The dose to be delivered will vary according if one is irradiating potentially microscopic seeding or metastases of several centimeters in diameter. For elective treatment of cases without detectable metastases, tumor doses of the order of 5,000 to 5,500 rads in 5 to 5½ weeks are indicated. In cases with proven metastases, the minimum tumor dose should be 6,000 rads in 6 weeks with the addition of 1,000 to 2,000 rads by interstitial gamma therapy to any residual tumor. The needles are so inserted to give a minimum irradiation to the skin of the area (Fig. 12-27). With the treatment indicated here a sharp epithelitis develops in the groin folds especially in obese patients where the incidence of the beam is tangential to the skin surface.

Clinicopathological Groups

NONPALPABLE LYMPH NODES

In Situ Carcinoma (Queyrat's Erythroplasia). The lesion appears shallow, generally with multicentric patches of exulcerations of the

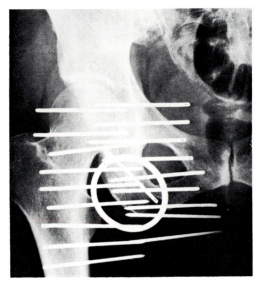

FIG. 12-27. Groin implant consisting of an angulated single plane with an extra needle placed where the residual tumor was thicker. The patient had extensive, inoperable groin metastases treated with external irradiation (5,000 rads in 5 weeks) prior to this implant that irradiates only the residual disease.

mucosa of the glans and/or prepuce and/or sulcus (bright red); patches of leukoplakia are sometimes present. The treatment consists of irradiation of the whole glans to cancerocidal level. Radium mold is the treatment of choice. In exceptional cases where the lesion is limited, superficial irradiation could be used.

Squamous Cell Carcinoma. **A.** Well-differentiated squamous cell carcinoma limited to the prepuce without invasion of the balanopreputial sulcus should be treated by total circumcision. If the lesion is near or just invading the balanopreputial sulcus, circumcision is indicated even if the incision could be close or through the margin of the tumor; postoperative irradiation by megavoltage or mold of the distal third of the organ must follow. Irradiation of the lymph node areas is not indicated.

B. In patients over 40 years of age with

well-differentiated lesions up to 2 cm in diameter, plaque-like exophytic tumor, without deep infiltration or ulceration the tumor bearing area only is to be treated. A radium implant and for the small superficial lesions low energy irradiation (60 to 100 Kv) is indicated.

C. In cases with deeper infiltration and/or larger lesions the distal one-third of the organ is to be treated. Megavoltage with jig and bolus or radium mold is indicated.

D. In younger patients or in anaplastic tumors larger volumes of irradiation are indicated; the minimum being the distal half of the organ. Lymph node bearing areas should be treated electively in these patients.

E. Tumors involving large portions of the glans with or without invasion of the prepuce, deeply ulcerating and infiltrating lesions. These cases should have irradiation of the distal half of the organ as a minimum. The main technique indicated here is megavoltage with jig and bolus. Lymph node bearing areas should be treated electively.

F. All other more extensive tumors with obvious invasion of the erectile tissues should have irradiation of the whole shaft. Megavoltage irradiation as described is indicated in all cases. Lymph node bearing areas should be treated electively.

G. Recurrent tumor after irradiation. Surgery is indicated.

PATIENTS WITH PROVEN LYMPH NODE METASTASES

If the nodes are mobile and operable, node dissection should be the treatment of choice. If they are inoperable or surgery is not possible for other reasons (refusal or poor risk), they should have megavoltage irradiation plus radium implant as described.

Postoperative Irradiation. When indicated, postoperative irradiation should be started after complete healing of the operative wound has taken place. If the surgical excision is localized, the technique of irradiation and the volume to be included should be the same as if the surgery has not been performed. In most cases, however, the patient is referred for therapy after amputation when tumor has been found at the edges of the specimen. In these cases only external irradiation with megavoltage is indicated. The technique to be used should be adapted to the case.

Palliative Treatment

Palliative treatment is indicated only in hopelessly advanced cases with complete destruction of the penis and invasion of the scrotum and abdominal wall and/or large ulcerated fixed necrotic nodes in the groin or when there are distant metastases. In most of these cases the use of a direct field covering obvious disease only, primary and/or lymph node metastases, is indicated. With megavoltage irradiation, the shortest possible treatment is preferable: 3,000 to 4,000 rads in 2 to 3 weeks is given to reduce or heal the ulceration, to reduce tumor size, and to lessen the probability of profuse bleeding.

The symptomatic treatment of distant metastases is similar to any other metastatic squamous cell carcinoma.

Care During Treatment

Scrupulous hygiene of the organ is important throughout the treatment. Bathing the penis and cortisone ointment dressing help diminish the symptoms produced by radiation reactions that are oftentimes severe, especially where the whole shaft is irradiated.

Complications

During and immediately after the treatment infection can complicate the reactions produced by irradiation. This should be avoided by proper care and the use of antibiotics when necessary. A necrotic ulcer developing immediately or a few months after treatment has been finished, is always due to over-irradiation or some faulty technique. Conservative treatment is generally indicated. In cases of severe necrosis, amputation has to be carried out. Late effects such as atresia of the meatus, adhesion between prepuce and glans, massive edema in the preutial remains may be corrected by proper conservative therapy.

Results in Carcinoma of the Penis

The expected results following proper treatment are: almost 100 per cent cure in early lesions (less than 2 cm in diameter), about 75 to 80 per cent in larger lesions but still limited to the distal end of the organ and about 65 per cent of all patients treated. It is to be emphasized that the use of irradiation with radical doses does not preclude the use of surgery in the cases where the irradiation has failed to control the disease locally.

Male Urethra

Cancers of the male urethra are rare. The maximum incidence occurs between 50 and 60 years of age without distinction of race or environmental influence. Longstanding strictures, especially the congenital ones, seem to act as predisposing factors.

The male urethra can be divided into the anterior or penile urethra, the most distal portion of which is called the fossa navicularis, bulbomembranous urethra, and posterior prostatic.

There is a group of noninfiltrating papillary tumors which can be either single or multiple and may at times form part of a generalized urinary papillomatosis. These tumors are generally treated by cauterization only. We shall refer here to a different group of tumors which main characteristics consists of their infiltration beyond the mucosa.

Anterior Urethra

The main epithelial lining of the anterior urethra is of a columnar variety except for small islands throughout it and the whole fossa navicularis where the epithelium is of the squamous cell type.[1]

The tumors originating in the anterior urethra are usually well-differentiated squamous cell carcinomas remaining localized for long periods of time, seldom producing metastases.

The lymphatic drainage is to the inguinal, iliac, deep femoral, and eventually pelvic lymph nodes in a fashion similar to that of the penis.

Because of coexistent inflammatory infection, enlarged nodes are often inflammatory and should have a biopsy before making the diagnosis of metastasis.

Bulbomembranous Urethra and Posterior Urethra (or Prostatic Urethra)

The epithelium is columnar with islands of mucoid glands. The tumors of this site are either transitional cell carcinomas or adenocarcinomas. The tumors extend quickly into the bladder, prostate, and into the tissues of the perineum. With adenocarcinoma the differential diagnosis with primary adenocarcinomas of the prostate is often impossible.

The lymphatic drainage is similar to that of the bladder and of the ejaculatory system, that is, drainage of the hypogastric and eventually to the common iliac nodes.

Treatment

The response and tolerance of the normal tissues of the urethra is as discussed for the penis and bladder.

The squamous cell carcinomas or transitional cell carcinomas exhibit response to irradiation similar to those originating in the bladder or penis. As a rule tumor response is diminished by infection, necrosis, and urimaceration, factors which jeopardize treatment. The common presence of abscesses or fistulae makes the management of these tumors less satisfactory.

PRELIMINARY CARE BEFORE RADIOTHERAPY

Except for the rare cases of early tumors and tumors of the navicular fossa, most patients come to the radiotherapist with obstruction and infection and some have a fistula present. The infection should be treated by antibiotics and drainage incision of abscesses. In order to avoid continuous maceration and necrosis and to control better infection, all patients with advanced tumors should have a temporary cystostomy prior to the treatment. This preliminary procedure will ensure a better response to the treatment.

VOLUME TO BE IRRADIATED

Tumors of the Fossa Navicularis. Here, a small margin of 1 cm beyond the tumor is required. No irradiation of the lymph node bearing areas is indicated unless proven positive. Tumors of the rest of the anterior urethra require larger margins of at least 2 cm around the tumor; the lymph node bearing areas should be treated when metastases, proven by biopsy, are present or when the primary is extensive and/or anaplastic. In most patients with tumors of the posterior urethra, the treatment should include the primary site with very wide margins and the lymph node bearing areas of the pelvis. It should start with total pelvis irradiation, including the perineum, up to 4,500 rads in $4\frac{1}{2}$ weeks, followed by local irradiation to the tumor bearing area with small margins up to 6,000 to 6,500 rads in $5\frac{1}{2}$ to 6 weeks.

Techniques of Treatment. In tumors of the anterior urethra the same principles, modalities and techniques of treatment apply as for penile cancers; the tumors of the posterior urethra are treated in a similar way as for bladder and prostatic tumors. For the tumors of the anterior urethra, in the final stage of the treatment, an intracavitary linear source of radium or other similar gamma emitters could be useful to reduce the volume of irradiation to the required area. An interstitial implant, permanent or temporary (seeds or needles), could be useful for the final portion of the treatment for tumors of the membranous urethra that are accessible from the perineum or through a cystotomy.

Treatment of the Lymph Node Metastases. The indications and techniques are the same as for cancer of the penis.

PALLIATIVE IRRADIATION

The same indications and techniques as for cancer of the penis are applied. In most cases of very advanced tumors of the urethra the performance of a cystostomy alone will provide the best relief of symptoms. In such cases irradiation is only indicated if it could add to the patient's comfort.

BIBLIOGRAPHY

1. Dean, A. L.: Carcinoma of the male and female urethra; Pathology and diagnosis, *J. Urol.*, 75, 505, 1956.
2. Marcial, V. A.: Carcinoma of the penis, *Radiology*, 79, 209, 1962.
3. Murphy, W. T.: *Radiation Therapy*, Philadelphia, W. B. Saunders Company, 1959.
4. Paterson, R.: *Treatment of Malignant Disease by Radiotherapy*, Baltimore, The Williams & Wilkins Company, p. 390, 1963.

Renal Parenchyma and Pelvis

LOWELL S. MILLER

The course of carcinoma of the renal parenchyma is usually rapid, but most series of patients, including our own, contain examples of extremely slow progression of the disease. There are, moreover, reports of recurrences and/or metastases discovered as late as 31 years after treatment. This variability of behavior and the relative rarity of the disease (2 per cent of all malignant tumors) help explain the lack of agreement in the urologic and radiologic literature on the worth of irradiation as an adjuvant to surgery.

Cancer of the renal pelvis may be transitional or squamous cell carcinoma; it occurs in a ratio of about 1:8 to parenchymal cancer, and is allegedly radioresistant. Histologically similar tumors often are found in ureter and/or bladder after or even before discovery of the renal lesion.

Irradiation has been used chiefly in one of four clinical situations: 1) alone when surgical resection is not possible, 2) postoperatively, 3) preoperatively, and 4) for postoperative recurrences in the renal fossa. In all four circumstances, the same field geometry is required. The adult kidney lies nearly in the coronal midplane of the abdomen, so that an ordinary opposed anteroposterior pair of treatment fields usually suffices. ^{60}Co gamma- or 2 Mev x-irradiation is adequate for most cases, but in the exceptionally obese patient 22 Mev x-rays are an advantage. Addition of a third field laterally is of doubtful value except under special circumstances (unusually great *AP* diameter, unusual lateral extension of tumor). Fields must of necessity be generous, *viz.*, 15 × 12 cm or more, and if possible these should be reduced medially after 4,500 rads in an effort to prevent cord injury. Lateral fall-off of appositional fields

at lower energies may be useful if there has been contamination of (or recurrence in) the scar in the flank.

Tissue doses of the order of 5,000 rads and more especially 6,000 rads can be expected to produce gastrointestinal complications in a significant percentage of cases (see Testis), for there is no way to deliver a reasonably homogeneous dose of ionizing radiation to the kidney without exposing at least some segment of the gastrointestinal tract to approximately the same dose. The radiotherapist is therefore limited in most cases to doses of about 5,000 rads in 5 weeks.

M. D. Anderson Hospital Experience

1944–1963 Irradiation Alone

Of 5 patients with inoperable parenchymal carcinoma, palliative irradiation in varying dosage yielded reduction in size of palpable masses in 2 patients, cessation of gross hematuria in a third, but no improvement in the 2 remaining patients. Four of the 5 patients were dead within a year, but the fifth patient, with the help of chemotherapy, irradiation of a spine metastasis, and supportive management survived for 42 months.

There were 2 patients with inoperable carcinomas of the renal pelvis. Neither received any clearcut benefit from palliative irradiation.

Postoperative Irradiation

Eleven patients with parenchymal cancer were irradiated postoperatively with doses ranging from 4,500 to 6,000 rads in 5 to 6 weeks. Five had gross residual tumor (transected in stump of renal vein in 3, metastatic in unresected paraaortic nodes in the other 2) and have fared badly—4 have died in 50 months or less (2 with proven local failure); the fifth patient is living at 2 years, but with probable pulmonary metastases. Of the 6 patients without gross residual tumor, 1 died with distant metastases at 17 months, but the others are clinically well at 6 years, 5, 4, 3 years, and 1 year respectively. Because the stomach is more radiovulnerable than the small bowel or colon, the absence of complications in this group is perhaps related to the fact that 8 of the 11 tumors were on the right.

None of the 3 patients irradiated postoperatively for cancer of the (left) renal pelvis had any gross residual tumor. Tumor doses were in the same range as for parenchymal carcinoma. One died of distant metastases at 15 months; another is living but with distant metastases at 47 months; the third patient required subtotal gastrectomy approximately 7 months after irradiation for gastric ulceration, but at 44 months is well and working.

Preoperative Irradiation

Three patients with inoperable parenchymal cancer received preoperative doses of 4,000 to 5,000 rads with only questionable reduction in tumor volume by the time of transperitoneal (right) nephrectomy 5 to 11 weeks later. There were no technical difficulties attributable to radiotherapy, but one patient died a few hours postoperatively of a surgical complication (hemorrhage from a branch of the renal artery). Of the remaining 2 patients, 1 died at 12 months with a hard recurrent mass in the renal fossa; the other remains alive (though with probable distant metastases) at 48 months.

No patients with carcinoma of the renal pelvis have received preoperative radiotherapy.

Irradiation for Postoperative Recurrence

Five patients with parenchymal cancer were irradiated for postoperative recurrences in the renal fossa and/or the surgical scar. Of the 4 whose treatment was palliative, 1 enjoyed restraint of his tumor's growth for approximately 5 months, but the other 3 were not benefited. The lone patient treated definitively (5,650 rads in 44 days) has not been followed in this hospital. His outside physician reports that the mass in the left renal fossa grew for 5 months after the end of radiotherapy; a course of Mustargen was then followed by improvement. At approximately 2½ years a perforating gastric ulcer required subtotal gastrectomy. The patient is still living (though with a palpable calciferous mass) more than 8 years postradiation.

Only one patient with cancer of the renal pelvis has been treated for postoperative recurrence. A tumor dose of 5,975 rads in 37 days was delivered without untoward incident. Cause of his death 4 weeks later has not been determined.

Discussion

Windeyer and Riches[3] no longer advocate routine postoperative irradiation except when there has been extension beyond the renal capsule and/or metastases to regional lymph nodes, especially if extirpation is known to have been subtotal. Flocks' current policy[1] is identical. Noting especially the favorable experience of Flocks and Kadesky's[2] with 25 patients irradiated preoperatively, and adding 11 cases of their own, Windeyer and Riches now hold that "If radiotherapy has any routine place in association with surgery, it is more rational to give it as a preoperative treatment." The dose recommended for preoperative use is 3,000 roentgens in 3 weeks, the optimum interval before nephrectomy about 3 weeks.

In view of the limited nature of our own experience, we are not yet prepared to make a recommendation with respect to preoperative irradiation. We are inclined, however, to agree with Windeyer and Riches and with Flocks that postoperative irradiation be reserved for high-risk cases, and suggest that if all gross tumor is believed to have been removed the dose be 5,000 rads in 5 weeks; if gross tumor is known to be residual, 6,000 rads in 6 weeks probably should be ventured. When gross tumor has recurred after surgery, and in the case of the irresectable or medically inoperable primary tumor, the latter dose is certainly justified. When only short-term palliation is intended, a smaller dose should be considered, but probably not less than 3,000 rads in 2 weeks.

BIBLIOGRAPHY

1. Flocks, R. H., Personal communication, 1965.
2. Flocks, R. H. and Kadesky, M. C.: Malignant neoplasms of the kidney: An analysis of 353 patients followed five years or more, *J. Urol.,* 79, 196, 1958.
3. Windeyer, B. and Riches, E.: In *Monographs on Neoplastic Disease,* D. W. Smithers, ed., Baltimore, The Williams & Wilkins Company, vol. V, p. 291, 1964.

13. Soft Tissue Sarcoma

HERMAN D. SUIT

Soft tissue sarcoma is the conventional designation for malignant tumors which arise from one of these supporting tissues: connective or fibrous, fat, muscle, synovium, vascular, and coverings of peripheral nerves. Usually the tumors of peripheral nerves are put into this category also. Accordingly, these tumors are designated as fibrosarcoma, liposarcoma, rhabdomyosarcoma, leiomyosarcoma, angiosarcoma, neurofibrosarcoma and neurosarcoma. There are many subclassifications within each of these major groups. As would be expected, these tumors do in fact appear at virtually every site within the body. That is, not only in connective tissue and muscles of the extremities, torso, head and neck region, retroperitoneal area, etc., but also in the various organs (breast, lung etc.).

The vast majority of the lesions develop in the extremities and the torso. Age distribution of patients presenting with tumors of this group covers the entire age span with a median age at diagnosis being in the fourth decade. Rhabdomyosarcomas are relatively more common in the pediatric age group than the other sarcomas while liposarcomas tend to appear in older persons. Males and females are afflicted with approximately the same frequency.

Clinical history of these tumors usually is not impressive; a "knot" or "lump" is detected accidently by the patient. Pain is usually not a symptom until the lesion has become quite large. A history of antecedent trauma is not usual, but occasionally there is a history of a significant or unusual injury at the specific site of tumor several months to years before the tumor is noted. The relationship between trauma and tumor remains undefined.

There are a number of benign lesions which can easily be confused histopathologically and clinically with sarcoma. One should request additional pathological opinion in all cases where there is any question of the malignant nature of the tumor or where the malignancy is low grade. Some of the processes which may be confused with sarcoma are nodular fascititis, organizing hematoma, infiltrating lipoma, benign atypical histocytoma, myxoma, myositis ossificans, etc.

After a lesion has been diagnosed as malignant, there is practical value in determining into which histopathologic category it should be placed. This is true because lesions which are high grade should be treated with much more generous fields than lesions which are low grade or well differentiated. A significant pathological fact is that these lesions often exhibit considerable variation in histopathological pattern from one region to another region in the same tumor. Accordingly, a better appreciation of the nature of the tumor is obtained if a generous biopsy specimen has been provided. Needle biopsies suffer from the limited nature of the samples. In a single lesion there may be areas which show relatively acellular myxoid tissue with practically no mitotic figures and in other areas the tumor may be quite cellular with a high mitotic index.

Traditions in Management of Patients with Sarcoma of Soft Tissue

A strong tradition has developed over the past 40 years that the only effective treatment for soft tissue sarcoma is surgical and that this should be radical wide excision for torso lesions and selected lesions of the extremity with ablation of the affected part of the extremity for the remainder.

Usually the patient presents for definitive treatment shortly following an "excisional biopsy," a simple excision, or "shelling out of tumor" at the community hospital. In some instances there has been an attempt to excise adjacent normal tissue after the principal mass was removed. Early surgical experience has amply demonstrated that such procedures are associated with an extremely high local recurrence rate, *viz.* 80–100 per cent.[1,2,3,4,8] Simple procedures are ineffective because these tumors are not truly encapsulated, *i.e.* there are micro-extensions of tumor beyond the apparent limits of the tumor mass. Accordingly, if the primary tumor or the surgical wound following excisional biopsy is to be treated surgically the resection must be radical. For this to be effective there must be a removal of the skin overlying the tumor mass with a generous margin of normal tissue around the lesion or suspected site of lesion. It is essential that the surgical margin be sufficiently great that tumor is not visualized during the procedure and that on gross pathological examination of the resected specimen that there be substantial margin of normal tissue in all directions. If this cannot be achieved because of likely involvement of critical vessels, nerves etc. the procedure must be judged incomplete and the patient subjected to amputation if the treatment is surgical.

Cantin et al.[5] published a detailed analysis of local recurrence frequency in 653 patients who had soft tissue sarcoma of the extremity or trunk and who were treated by a radical surgical procedure at Memorial Hospital of New York. Of this group, 187 patients or 29 per cent developed local recurrence. Results according to histopathological variety of sarcoma are reproduced in Table 13-1. In this series local results were not dependent upon histopathology. They also observed that recurrence frequency increased with size of tumor and with extent of infiltration of adjacent structures. Also, frequency of local fail-

Table 13-1. *Local Recurrence Rate After Primary Treatment at Memorial Cancer Center, New York*

	No. of Pts.	Recurrences
Unclassified sarcoma	163	42 (26%)
Liposarcoma	116	30 (26%)
Rhabdomyosarcoma	109	29 (27%)
Fibrosarcoma	97	35 (36%)
Synovioma	81	24 (30%)
Neurosarcoma	43	15 (35%)
Embryonal rhabdomyosarcoma	23	6 (26%)
Others	21	6 (29%)
Total	653	187 (29%)

Adapted from: Cantin, McNeer, Chu, and Booher, *Ann. of Surg.,* 168, 47, 1968.

ure was higher for treatment of recurrent lesions than for primary lesions. Their results are quite similar to recurrence rate of 28 per cent in 243 patients treated by radical surgical excision or amputation as reported by Martin et al.[9] from the M. D. Anderson Hospital at Houston, Texas. These experiences represent two of the largest reported. As their recurrence rates are among the lowest published, the 28 to 29 per cent recurrence rate is used here as a reference figure. There are many reports of higher recurrence frequencies, however, a literature review will not be included in this presentation.[1,2,6,9,10,12,13]

Past Experience with Radiation Therapy for Sarcoma of Soft Tissue

Radiation therapy has not been considered to be an effective treatment modality for sarcomas of soft tissue. This attitude has had a good basis on clinical experience of the premegavoltage therapy period. In that early period there were numerous clinical testings of x-ray therapy (up to 400 Kv), radium packs, etc. but usually with unsatisfactory results and not competitive with those of surgery. A partial explanation may be that the early work was characterized by: 1) radiation dose was limited by skin reaction to levels which would now be considered modest, 2) massive primary lesions were accepted for treatment, and 3) the clinician expected the rate of regression of sarcoma to be comparable to that observed in the treatment of epithelioma of tonsil (we now know that sarcomas even when successfully treated often regress slowly, *i.e.* regression rate is not a good indication of ultimate response). One of the earliest papers to give an enthusiastic account of the role of radiation therapy for this group of tumors was that by Cade in 1951.[3] He described results of management of 153 patients with malignant tumors of soft tissue treated during the years of 1920–1950. There are several significant points in his presentation: 1) 6 of 16 patients treated by radiation alone survived free of disease for 5 years, 4 of the 6 being fibrosarcoma; 2) in his analysis of results of treatment by wide excision combined with radiation therapy, better results were apparently obtained than if amputation were performed; 3) he concluded that radiation therapy was most effective when combined with surgery. This was a strong encouragement to evaluate the role of radiation therapy in the management of soft tissue.

Introduction of megavoltage equipment into clinical practice provided an additional excellent reason for further study of the effectiveness of radiation therapy for this group of lesions. There have appeared over the past 10 to 15 years a number of papers[1,7,8,11,12,14,15] which continue to attest to the fact that excellent results may often be obtained by radiation therapy either alone or in combination with surgery. For example, Windeyer et al. treated 22 fibrosarcomas (11 primary lesions and 11 postsurgical recurrences) by radical dose radiation therapy; 9 or 41 per cent survived free of disease 28 to 75 months. An interesting finding by McNeer et al.[11] was that a number of patients treated by radiation alone did quite

well following modest doses in the range of 2,500 to 5,000 rads (megavoltage and orthovoltage techniques).

Experience at M. D. Anderson Hospital Using Radiation Therapy in Management of Patients with Soft Tissue Sarcoma

Because of the high incidence of local failure following radical surgical procedures performed by expert and competent surgeons, a clinical study of the role of radical dose radiation therapy in the management of patients with sarcoma of the soft tissue has been performed at the University of Texas at Houston M. D. Anderson Hospital.

Results from this study have shown that simple excision of small to moderately advanced lesions of the extremities followed by radical dose radiation therapy to the operative site and adjacent tissues likely to be involved yields a very high local control rate with preservation of satisfactory functional state of the treated limbs in most patients. A similar approach has been applied in a smaller group of patients in the management of lesions in the torso.

The basic concept is that by removing all gross disease surgically, readily tolerated radiation doses would be effective in destroying the small number of cells not removed in the surgical specimen. An important fact is that radiation treatment fields may be planned on the basis of probable areas of involvement without concern for location of vessels, nerves, or tendons. This combined modality approach is applicable only to the early or moderately advanced lesions on the extremity. Extensive or massive lesions cannot be properly treated by this approach in most instances because a simple excision is not possible. Probably patients with such lesions should be submitted to an amputation without attempted radiation therapy. The decision to employ radiation therapy alone for massive lesions can be justified only for limited palliation and in special circumstances, *e.g.* rhabdomyosarcoma, highly cellular and undifferentiated lesions, etc.

Patient Evaluation

Patients should be examined jointly with a surgical colleague. Assuming that a simple excision has been performed, copies of the surgical and pathological report are reviewed. In addition, the case should be discussed with a pathologist. Points of special interest are: 1) was the tumor visualized during the surgical procedure; 2) was the lesion attached to vessels and/or nerves; 3) was the lesion removed *in toto* or in fragments; 4) was gross tumor left behind; 5) was the lesion invading adjacent structures; and 6) specifications of muscle group or other anatomical structures involved? From the report of the pathological examination determine the following: 1) description of gross appearance of lesion; 2) nature and extent of infiltration of adjacent structures; 3) apparent adequacy of surgical margin; and 4) histopathological diagnosis. On review of the histological material, it is often desirable to request the tissue blocks so that special stains may be prepared. For example, the *PAS* stain may be helpful (if it is positive after diastase treatment) in the diagnosis of rhabdomyosarcoma. Further work-up and treatment are influenced by the findings mentioned above. For example, if the simple excision was not obviously complete for a lesion in the thigh or in the fleshy parts of the torso a re-excision is indicated. In a number of such cases we have often found considerable additional tumor which should be removed before starting therapy.

Treatment Planning

Arteriographic study is often helpful in detecting residual tumor or the presence of satellite tumor nodules. We now perform lymphangiogram on patients with rhabdomyosarcoma or high grade synovial sarcoma.

In this group, approximately 15 per cent of patients will exhibit metastasis to the regional lymph nodes as the first sign of metastatic disease. If re-excision is planned, this must be discussed with the surgeon to ascertain that location and length of scar will be compatible with a proper course of treatment. Also the stab wound for the drain must not be placed at an awkward site for positioning of treatment fields. In all instances the surgical wound must be healed (not almost healed) before irradiation is started.

Field size and arrangement are critically dependent upon the histopathological diagnosis and the gross local character of the lesion. For example, if the tumor were read as an embryonal rhabdomyosarcoma which had been "excised" from hamstrings of the thigh, fields would have to cover the entirety of the muscles involved, or in this example extend from the knee to the origin of these groups on pubis and ischium. In this instance, including the femoral and external iliac nodes would be part of the treatment of the muscle groups. Treatment would probably best be effected through an anterior-posterior pair of parallel opposed fields. Dose in this instance might be 5,000 rads in 5 weeks to such long fields. Following this, fields should be reduced and then again at the 6,000 rad level. This final dose at the immediate region of primary lesion is 7,000 rads in 7 weeks. Because of the frequency of involvement of regional nodes on patients with rhabdomyosarcoma and high grade synovial sarcoma, we now treat the first relay of nodes to 4,500–5,000 rads in $4\frac{1}{2}$–5 weeks. In the example just given, the nodes would be included in the fields covering the origin of the involved muscle.

In contrast, consider the problem presented by a patient who has had a well differentiated neurofibrosarcoma removed by simple excision from the volar surface of the wrist. Assuming that the lesion did not demonstrably invade adjacent tendons, muscles, etc., then relatively small fields should be employed initially. No intent to include all the length of adjacent nerve, tendon, or muscle is warranted. Treatment fields have to be planned in relationship to the clinical problem. Neurofibrosarcomas do not, as a rule, infiltrate along the nerve to which they are attached so that there is no need to cover the peripheral nerve for any particular length.

Synovial sarcomas usually do not arise directly from the synovial membrane of a joint. Accordingly, in most patients there is no need to cover the entirety of the nearest joint. If the tumor invades the joint, then the entirety of the synovial membrane of the affected joint should be covered for the initial 5,000 rads. There are practical limits to the extent of fields. For example, a synovial sarcoma arising in the thenar eminence of the hand could theoretically spread throughout the entirety of the hand, digits, and up into the forearm for some distance because of the interconnection of the synovial spaces around the tendons of the hand. Based on our rather limited experiences, the treatment fields can be drawn on a much more limited basis as these lesions apparently tend to infiltrate only immediate local tissue.

There are several major rules of treatment planning: 1) acceptance for radiation therapy requires that fully adequate coverage be obtained without including the full circumference of the extremities. This is necessary because of the severe constricting fibrosis which results from treatment of the entirety of the extremity, 2) even on the affected side, the skin and subcutaneous tissue should be included only in the immediate area of the surgical field, *i.e.* "fall-off" should be allowed over a minimal area, 3) for radiation therapy at all other sites, treatment plans should make full use of all available techniques to minimize irradiation of normal tissue which are not to be included in the treatment volume by intent. Specifically, wedge filters, compensator filters, complex field arrangements, etc. are to be employed where appropriate.

There are several technical points which may be given here: 1) for lesions in the knee region, arrange fields so that all or at least part of the patella is excluded. This is a region which is especially vulnerable to trauma and also to the constant irritation of the rubbing of the trouser leg, or stocking, 2) for lesions of the upper medial thigh, caution should be exercised so as to treat a minimum amount of skin and subcutaneous tissue because of the chronic damage produced by the rubbing of the inner aspects of the thigh in some people, 3) the anterior tibial chin is frequently bumped or otherwise injured so that in treatment of lesions in the leg special effort should be made to reduce dose in this region, 4) in treatment of lesions on the foot or ankle, employ medial and lateral fields so as to avoid the soles, back of heel and Achilles tendon if at all possible, 5) where quite long regions must be treated and two abutting fields are required to provide adequate coverage, a safe rule is to use 1 cm between the fields and to move this 1 cm zone 1 cm each week, *i.e.* a moving field abutment, and 6) treat all fields each day, 7) use bolus to achieve build up over the scar for the first 5,000 rads (bolus should be only slightly wider than the scar).

Dose Level

Treatment is given at 1,000 rads per week and 200 rads per session. The dose is calculated as a minimum dose in the volume of tissue suspected of being involved by tumor. However, the maximum difference between maximum and minimum should not exceed 10 per cent; if the best dose distribution achieved has a maximum-minimum difference of 15 per cent, the tumor dose should be calculated on a depth dose that was 10 per cent less than maximum. This is necessary to avoid regions of overdose which might result in severe fibrosis at a later date. The initial 5,000 rads is administered to relatively generous fields which encompass tissues likely to be involved by microscopic foci of disease. At the completion of this portion of the treatment, the fields are reduced to cover just the tissues manipulated at the surgical procedure. Then at 6,000 rads, fields are again reduced to include only the scar (or central region of scar if it is very long) and the actual site of the initial lesion. Therefore, the stated dose of 7,000 rads in 7 weeks is actually the dose given to the central region of the involvement. Several illustrative cases are described:

Case I. A twenty-year-old girl first noticed a painful mass in the left anticubital space in October 1967. A simple excision was performed and the diagnosis was fibrosarcoma, Grade III. On examination, there was a well healed scar of 9 cm length and there was no palpable evidence of tumor.

The recommended surgical procedure was disarticulation as the scar came well up onto the upper arm. The patient was accepted for treatment and 7,100 rads in 35 fractions over a total period of 51 days were administered according to the diagram in Figure 13-1. The

initial field was 30 cm long. Because of the high histological grade of the lesion, large fields were selected. Fields were medial-lateral opposed with the olecranon excluded. This treatment was well tolerated. She is now 44 months after treatment without evident local, regional, or distant disease. As evidence of the functional state of the arm this patient has graduated from college as an organ major and now has a position as an organist.

Case 2. For about 4 months this 37-year-old man had a mass on the lateral aspect of his left ankle. This was removed by simple excision at his local hospital. It was 3 cm in diameter and not encapsulated. Histopathologically this tumor was cellular, with many mitotic figures (1-2/HPF), and was interpreted as a synovial sarcoma, Grade II, showing a biphasic pattern. The recommended surgical procedure was amputation. This patient was treated by the tourniquet technique and received 14,000 rads in 14 fractions over a total time of 43 days (Fig.

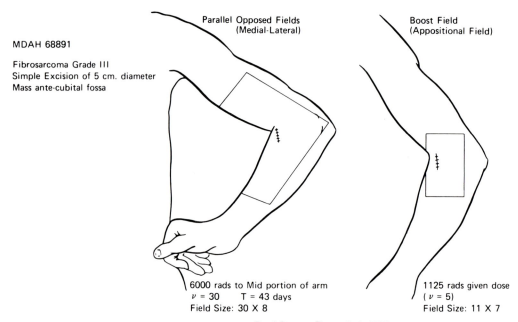

MDAH 68891

Fibrosarcoma Grade III
Simple Excision of 5 cm. diameter
Mass ante-cubital fossa

Parallel Opposed Fields
(Medial-Lateral)

Boost Field
(Appositional Field)

6000 rads to Mid portion of arm
$\nu = 30$ T = 43 days
Field Size: 30 X 8

1125 rads given dose
($\nu = 5$)
Field Size: 11 X 7

Total Dose to Tumor Bed: 7000 rads
$\nu = 35$ T = 51 days

FIG. 13-1. Treatment plan.

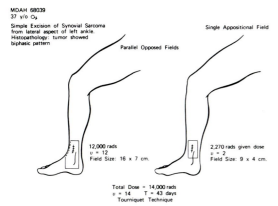

MDAH 68039
37 y/o ♂

Simple Excision of Synovial Sarcoma
from lateral aspect of left ankle.
Histopathology: tumor showed
biphasic pattern

Single Appositional Field

Parallel Opposed Fields

12,000 rads
υ = 12
Field Size: 16 x 7 cm.

2,270 rads given dose
υ = 2
Field Size: 9 x 4 cm.

Total Dose = 14,000 rads
υ = 14   T = 43 days
Tourniquet Technique

FIG. 13-2. Treatment plan.

13-2). Here the Achilles tendon, back of heel, and heel pad were excluded. There was a modest dry desquamation at the completion of treatment, with a few small patches of moist change. This subsided quickly. At present, this patient is without evidence of disease and quite active at 40 months after treatment.

Case 3. This 75-year-old man had a mass on the medial aspect of the left thigh removed by simple excision at his local hospital. Gross pathology showed the mass to be 30 × 29 cm. There was a local recurrence detected at 28 months. At this point he was initially seen at the M. D. Anderson Hospital. Radical resection was attempted but abandoned because of tumor extension to and partly around the shaft of the femur. On

examination by the radiotherapist, there was an ill-defined 8 × 8 cm mass beneath the healed scar. The histopathologic diagnosis was malignant fibrous histiocytoma, Grade I. The plan of treatment is shown in Figure 13-3. This tumor was given 7,000 rads in 35 fractions over a period of 49 days. Some 6–9 months were required for the mass to regress. This patient is alive and well and free of evident disease at 24 months.

Case 4. A 61-year-old woman had a history of a mass in the right buttock for several months. She presented at the M. D. Anderson Hospital with a 20 × 15 cm mass which involved most of the right buttock, as shown in Figure 13-4A. Histopathologically, the tumor was a malignant fibrous histiocytoma. The lesion was to have been treated by radical resection. This was not achieved because of spillage of tumor and gross cut-through. As soon as the wound was healed, radiation therapy was initiated, employing a very large angle wedge pair. Figure 13-4B and 13-4C illustrate the treatment plan. The total dose was 7,000 rads in 46 days. Despite the extent of prior surgery and the size of fields employed, this patient has done well. At more than 2 years she is free of evident disease; there is no pain and no edema of the leg. She carries a normal work load as a secretary. The appearance of treated area at 18 months is shown in Figure 13-4D.

Case 5. This 16-year-old girl noted a pain-

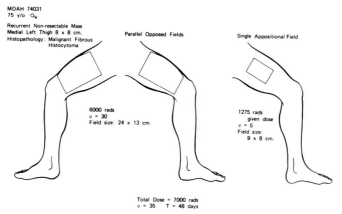

MDAH 74031
75 y/o ♂

Recurrent Non-resectable Mass
Medial Left Thigh 8 x 8 cm.
Histopathology: Malignant Fibrous
Histocytoma

Parallel Opposed Fields

Single Appositional Field

6000 rads
υ = 30
Field size: 24 x 13 cm.

1275 rads
given dose
υ = 5
Field size:
9 x 8 cm.

Total Dose = 7000 rads
υ = 35   T = 48 days

FIG. 13-3. Treatment plan.

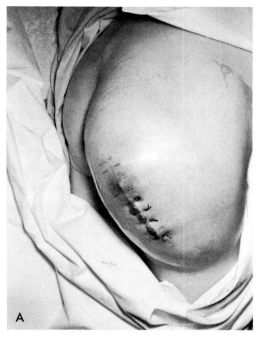

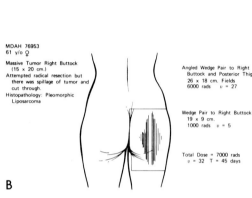

MDAH 76953
61 y/o ♀

Massive Tumor Right Buttock
(15 × 20 cm.)
Attempted radical resection but
there was spillage of tumor and
cut through.
Histopathology: Pleomorphic
Liposarcoma

Angled Wedge Pair to Right
Buttock and Posterior Thigh
26 × 18 cm. Fields
6000 rads   υ = 27

Wedge Pair to Right Buttock
19 × 9 cm.
1000 rads   υ = 5

Total Dose = 7000 rads
υ = 32 T = 45 days

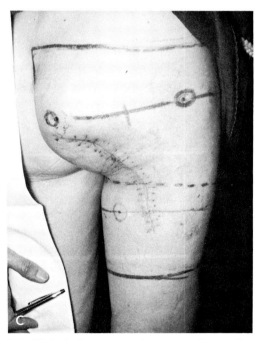

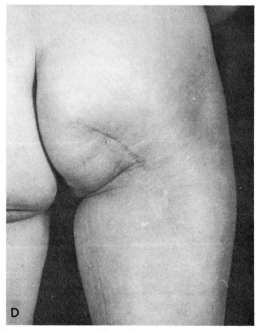

FIG. 13-4. A. Presentation of massive malignant fibrous histiocytoma in right buttock area. Patient seen shortly after incisional biopsy. **B.** Treatment plan. **C.** Treatment fields as applied to patient. Generous margin of fields were employed around the surgical wound. **D.** Appearance of treated area at 18 months after treatment.

less swelling on the ulnar aspect of the left hand and was promptly seen by her local physician. An excision biopsy of the mass showed alveolar rhabdomyosarcoma. On examination an enlarged epitrochlear node was observed, which was proven to contain metastatic sarcoma. Treatment was given according to the plan shown in Figure 13-5. The primary site received 6,500 rads in 32 fractions over 44 days. The doses to the epitrochlear node area and the axillary-supraclavicular area were 5,000 rads in 5 weeks. The intent here was to irradiate one node group past the level of clinical involvement by tumor. Because of the high likelihood of occult metastatic tumor, a course of vincristine and cytoxan therapy had been given (6 cycles over a period of almost one year). At present, the patient is free of evident tumor and enjoys normal function of the affected part.

Results of Treatment

LESIONS OF THE EXTREMITIES

Results achieved in 57 patients treated 2–10 years ago are presented in Table 13-2. Those patients received radical dose radiation therapy, *viz.* 6,300 rads or more in 6 weeks. Further, there was no clinical evi-

Table 13-2. *Results in 57 Patients with Sarcoma of Soft Tissue Treated by Radical Dose Radiation Therapy 2–10 Years Ago*

Site	Local Control
Elbow	8/8
Forearm	10/10
Wrist-Hand	7/7
Knee-Popliteal	9/9
Leg	6/6
Ankle-Foot	6/6
Arm	2/4
Thigh	2/7
Total	50/57 = 87%

dence of distant metastasis at the start of treatment. Local control has been obtained in 50 of the 57 patients, *i.e.* 87 per cent. Eleven of these patients were treated for an unresected primary lesion or for grossly recurrent tumor. In this subgroup of 11 patients, local control has been achieved in 9. Local recurrence has occurred in 5 of the 46 patients who were treated after simple excision. The anatomical site of tumor appears to be important in success rate of radiation therapy. Local control has been obtained in 46 of 46 patients treated 2–10 years ago for lesions of the distal extremities (elbow—hand; knee—foot). In contrast, only 2 of 7

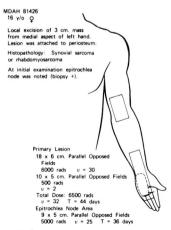

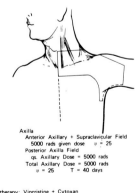

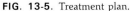

FIG. 13-5. Treatment plan.

lesions of the thigh and 2 of 4 lesions of the upper arm have been controlled locally. However, of 15 patients treated 6 to 22 months ago for lesions in the thigh all have local control and retain good function of the limb.

As there have been only 7 recurrences, no correlation between histopathology and local recurrence can be made. The pathological diagnoses in these 7 tumors were: neurofibrosarcoma-2, malignant fibrous histiocytoma-2, pleomorphic rhabdomyosarcoma-1, and synovial sarcoma-1.

Good function of the treated limb has been retained in 34 of the 57 patients. All of the necroses or instances of severe damage occurred in the first 18 patients in this series when the full width of the limb was included in the treatment field. Accordingly, functional results are very much better in more recently treated cases where precision techniques have been employed.

The metastasis free survival figure of 58 per cent at 2 or more years shown in Table 13-3 is fully comparable to results from the previously mentioned surgical series. As the median time for detection of metastases in this series is 11 months, there is expected to be very few additional losses due to metastasis. Survival rate depends upon the histopathology to some extent. Four of 11 and 0

of 2 patients with a diagnosis of rhabdomyosarcoma and leiomyosarcoma are free of metastatic disease. In the group of 9 patients diagnosed as neurofibrosarcoma, 6 are alive (one patient died of a cerebral vascular accident).

Because of the high frequency of distant metastasis in patients with rhabdomyosarcoma and high grade synovial sarcoma, there is justification for instituting chemotherapy at the time of radiation therapy. This has been the treatment of several patients over the recent years and the results appear promising, but no conclusion regarding the efficacy of this approach is warranted at this time.

An assessment of the results of treatment given under tourniquet induced hypoxia is interesting. Thirty of 30 lesions on the distal extremities treated to 8,100 rads in 23 days to 14,000 rads in 43 days have had local control. Similarly, 16 of 16 lesions on the distal extremities which were treated to 6,300 rads to 7,500 rads by conventional techniques have been controlled. That is, no recurrence in either group. Further, there was no advantage in terms of tolerance of normal tissue in the tourniquet technique treated patients. Accordingly, this experience does not provide an indication that the tourniquet technique is an advance in the treatment of soft tissue sarcoma on the distal extremity.

LESIONS AT OTHER SITES

Eleven patients had lesions located in buttock-hip, abdominal wall, and chest wall regions. These have been treated to doses in the range of 6,500 to 7,000 rads following resection. No recurrence has been observed in this group.

EFFECT OF LOCAL RECURRENCE ON SURVIVAL

Patients whose tumors recur do less well than those who never experience recurrence because of a greater frequency of developing

Table 13-3. *Metastasis Free Survival for Two to Ten Years After Radical Dose Radiation Therapy According to Histopathological Type*

Neurofibrosarcoma	6/9
Fibrosarcoma	3/5
Synovial Sarcoma	8/14
Clear Cell Sarcoma	2/2
Liposarcoma	3/4
Malignant Fibrous Histiocytoma	5/7
Rhabdomyosarcoma	4/11
Leiomyosarcoma	0/2
Unclassified Sarcoma	1/2
Angiosarcoma	1/1
Total	33/57 = 58%

distal metastasis. This has been indicated by the analysis of Cantin et al.,[5] van der Werf-Messing and van Unnik[13] and Brennhovd.[2] Further, each additional recurrence complicates the next attempt at surgery and/or radiation therapy. Accordingly, the first attempt at treatment should be comprehensive and as aggressive as the particular situation permits.

DISTANT METASTATIC DISEASE

Treatment of patients with distant metastatic disease is complex and often disappointing. However, the first metastatic lesions should be subjected to an intensive course of treatment, surgical or radiologic and usually chemotherapeutic. Treatment of patients at this or later stages must be highly individualized and selective.

Summary

The treatment policy which the author favors would be to administer radiation therapy postoperatively for all soft tissue sarcoma, except for low grade lesions which appear to be encapsulated and were removed with good margins of normal tissue in all directions. For lesions of the rhabdomyosarcoma, high grade synovial sarcoma or unclassified sarcoma, the first relay of clinically uninvolved nodes are being treated to 5,000 rads. In addition, these patients are being treated by a multi-drug chemotherapy program.

Further, even in a situation where surgery is not feasible and radiation doses must be limited, the patient should be accepted for moderate dose radiation therapy because some occasional good results have been obtained after modest dose levels.[10]

BIBLIOGRAPHY

1. Atkinson, L., Garvan, J. M., and Newton, N. C.: Behavior and management of soft connective tissue sarcomas, *Cancer,* 16, 1552, 1963.
2. Brennhovd, I. O.: The treatment of soft tissue sarcomas—a plea for a more urgent and aggressive approach, *Acta Chir. Scand.,* 131, 438, 1966.
3. Cade, S.: Soft tissue tumors: Their natural history and treatment, *Proc. Royal Soc. of Med.,* 44, 19, 1951.
4. Cadman, N. L., Soule, E. H., and Kelly, P. J.: Synovial sarcoma, an analysis of 134 tumors, *Cancer,* 18, 613, 1965.
5. Cantin, J., NcNeer, G. P., Chu, F. C., and Booher, R. J.: The problem of local recurrence after treatment of soft tissue sarcoma, *Ann. of Surg.,* 168, 47, 1968.
6. Coran, A. G., Crocker, D. W., and Wilson, R. E.: A twenty-five year experience with soft tissue sarcomas, *Amer. J. Surg.,* 119, 288, 1970.
7. Flatman, G. C.: Some observations on the treatment of certain radioresistant tumors, *J. of the Faculty of Radiologists,* 10, 21, 1959.
8. Hare, H. F., and Cerney, M. J.: Soft tissue sarcoma, *Cancer,* 16, 1332, 1963.
9. Martin, R. G., Butler, J. J., and Albores-Saavedra, J.: Soft tissue tumors: Surgical treatment and results. In *Tumors of Bone and Soft Tissue,* Chicago, Year Book Medical Publishers, Inc., 1963.
10. Mattheiem, W., and Smets, W.: Les sarcomes des tissus mous (Experience de l'Institut Jules bordet), *Bull. Du Cancer,* 54, 349, 1967.
11. McNeer, G. P., Cantin, J., Chu, F., and Nickerson, J. J.: Effectiveness of radiation therapy in the management of sarcoma of the soft somatic tissues, *Cancer,* 22, 391, 1968.
12. Shieber, W., and Graham, P.: An experience with sarcomas of the soft tissue in adults, *Surg.,* 52, 295, 1962.
13. van der Werf-Messing, B., and van Unnik, J. A. M.: Fibrosarcoma of the soft tissues—a clincopathologic study, *Cancer,* 18, 1113, 1965.
14. Windeyer, Sir B., Dische, S., and Mansfield, C. M.: The place of radiotherapy in the management of fibrosarcoma of the soft tissue, *Clin. Radiol.,* 17, 32, 1966.
15. Zuppinger, A.: Radiation therapy of sarcoma of the bone and soft tissue, *Amer. J. Roentgen.,* 99, 435, 1967.

14. Palliative Radiotherapy in The Management of Metastatic Disease Excluding Breast Cancer

ELEANOR D. MONTAGUE

Palliative radiotherapy is given 1) for relief of symptoms such as pain, malodorous discharge, hemorrhage, prevention of symptoms due to increasing pressure of impending paralysis, or 2) for temporary arrest of the tumor.

Various schemes of dose and fractionation have been employed depending on the tolerance of the surrounding tissues. Effective palliation is a balance of dose and time involved for the patient, the facilities, and the available personnel. The specific schedule for palliative irradiation is dependent upon, 1) site and occasionally the histology of tumor, 2) volume, and 3) life expectancy.

Five thousand rads tumor dose given in 5 weeks is effective palliation for almost any troublesome metastatic site, but the time and expense of such treatment are impractical for many palliative situations. If there is evidence of rapid tumor growth or early dissemination of disease after definitive treatment, long protracted palliative courses are impractical. Conversely, massive fractions such as 1,500 rads in 2 consecutive days or 1,000 to 1,500 rads in one fraction have yielded only temporary significant symptomatic improvement. Attempts at retreatment with recurrence of symptoms are fraught with poor control and complications and, therefore, the few high-dose fraction schemes should be used only in patients with a short life expectancy.

There is, of necessity, great individualization depending on specific patient problems. For example, bony metastases from prostatic adenocarcinoma respond well to the same dose level used for metastatic disease from breast cancer. Metastatic adenocarcinoma to bone from the gastrointestinal tract, kidney, and thyroid frequently has produced a large area of destruction which becomes symptomatic only after large volumes of bone have been destroyed. For even modest palliation, 4,000 rads in 4 weeks to 5,000 rads in 5 weeks are necessary. Treatment should encompass the involved area plus generous margins. For the pelvic bone, involved bone should be treated, i.e., the entire ileum, but not the entire hemipelvis. The whole brain is treated even if there is clinical evidence of only one area involved because the probability of multiple metastatic foci is high (Fig. 14-1).

Table 14-1 shows various treatment schemes suggested for specific sites, related to prognosis for life, volume to be irradiated, and vital structures in the field of irradiation.

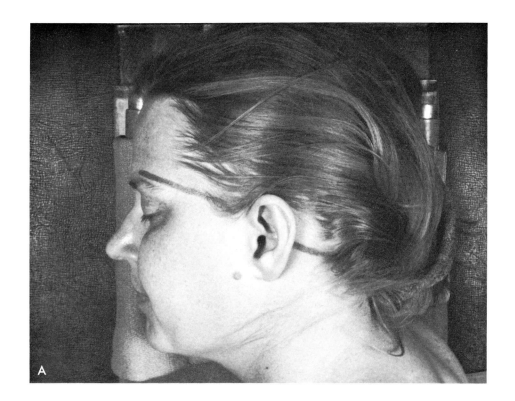

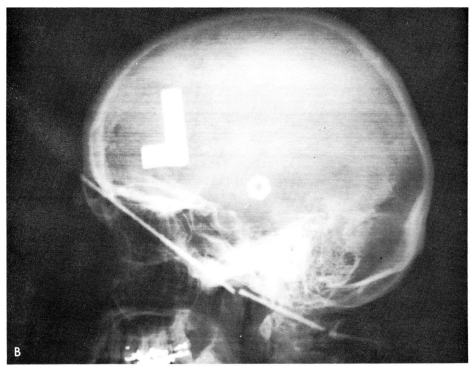

FIG. 14-1. Female, age 40 with a metastasis in the frontal area of the brain from a bronchogenic carcinoma. A midplane dose of 3,950 rads in 19 treatments in 25 days was given.

    A. Treatment portal.

    B. Verification film.

Table 14-1. *Management of Common Metastatic Sites**

Site	Prognosis 3-6 Months or Small Volume and no Vital Structures Involved		Prognosis 6 months or Large Volume or Vital Structures Involved
NODES: Squamous cell Adenocarcinoma	Massive Fractions		
NECK: Supraclavicular	1,000–1,500 GD/1 rx 1,500 GD/2 rx	5,000 GD/ 10 rx	6,000 GD/4 wks
AXILLA			
Appositional field		2,500 GD/5 rx 3,500 GD/7 rx	
Parallel opposed		3,000/2 wks	5,000/5 wks
INGUINAL	2,500 GD/5 rx 3,500 GD/7 rx	4,000 GD/ 3 wks	5,000 GD/5 wks
PARAAORTIC			4,000–5,000/4–5 wks
LUNGS			
Solitary (Surgery preferable)	2,100/3 rx	3,000/2 wks	4,000–5,000/4 wks
MEDIASTINAL		3,000/2 wks	4,000/4 wks
BRAIN			
Whole brain irradiation	1,000/1 rx	3,000/2 wks	4,000/4 + 1,000 (?)
Limited fields: Retro-orbital			
Base of brain involvement		3,000/2 wks	4,000/4 wks
SPINAL CORD INVOLVEMENT			4,000–5,000/4–5 wks
PRE-SACRAL NERVE PLEXUS			5,000/5 wks
BONE	Massive w/ fracture		
squamous cell carcinoma	1,000/1 rx 1,500/1 rx		See Breast Chapter 6
Adenocarcinoma			4,000/3–4 wks
Internal fixation procedures			4,000/3–4 wks entire bone
RECTOSIGMOID CANCER**			
Pelvic recurrence		3,000/2 wks	5,000/5 wks
Perineal recurrence		3,000/2 wks	5,000–6,000/4–5 wks**
PANCREAS		3,000/2 wks	
SOFT TISSUE			4,000–5,000/4–5 wks

*Tumor dose in rads unless specified.
**Significant and long-term pain relief in only 50 per cent of patients. Treatment should be given electively postoperatively.

15. Clinical Experimental Radiotherapy

HERMAN D. SUIT

Clinical experiments in radiation therapy currently are based predominately on one of four approaches for improving the differential killing of cells of normal and malignant tissue. First, elimination of oxygen tension differential between tumor tissue and normal tissue is the best understood and most intensively studied approach. Second, modification of tumor cell radiosensitivity is being attempted by exposing the cells to one of several of the pyrimidine or purine analogs that increase cell radiosensitivity by being incorporated into the cellular *DNA*. Third, enchancement of effectiveness of radiation therapy is being investigated by combining radiation and certain chemotherapeutic agents, *i.e.* cell toxic agents that might have a preferential killing effect against tumor cells. The effects of the latter type of chemotherapeutic agents would be additive to those of the irradiation, whereas the radiation sensitizer would act synergistically with the radiation. Finally, there is a renewed clinical interest in evaluation of the effectiveness of different regimens of dose fractionation or even of different dose rates.

The success of these endeavors to improve the efficacy of radiation therapy should be evaluated in terms of local results as well as patient survival. Specifically, for a new treatment method to represent an advance, the recurrence rate must be demonstrated to be reduced for a specified complication rate, or for a given tumor control frequency the complication rate must be lessened. Furthermore, the most meaningful treatment results will come from a planned clinical trial, *viz.*

the patient assigned to either the new or the conventional treatment group by a random number procedure after having been judged suitable for treatment by either of the two methods.

Tissue Oxygen Tension and Clinical Radiotherapy

Molecular oxygen is one of the most potent radiation sensitizers yet studied. The ratio of radiosensitivities or D_{37} values for anoxic cells to aerobic cells is in the range of 2 to 3. This is of special relevance to clinical radiotherapy because oxygen is normally present in body fluids and tissues, and for most tissues, oxygen is maximally sensitizing at physiological concentrations. There has been intensive interest in oxygen tension of tumor cells as a factor in clinical radiation therapy since the symposium organized by L. H. Gray et al.[15] when it was suggested that in many human tumors there might be anoxic but viable tumor cells at the edge of necrotic regions. These anoxic (radio-resistant) cells could account for some of the failures of radiotherapy. A histological study by Thomlinson and Gray[35] showed that in human bronchogenic carcinomas, areas of necrosis were at distances from capillaries predicted to be anoxic on the basis of 1) oxygen diffusion coefficient, 2) metabolism of oxygen by cells between capillary and necrotic areas, 3) oxygen tension and blood flow rate through the capillary, and 4) capillary length and diameter. No areas of necrosis were found at less than 160μ from a capillary, and all tumor tissue $\geq 200\,\mu$ distant from a capillary was necrotic.

If small foci of anoxic cells cause failures, a major improvement in the efficacy of radiation therapy should result from employment of techniques which eliminate oxygen tension differentials between tumor and normal tissue or by the use of a radiation beam whose biological effectiveness is less dependent on oxygen tension than is the case for standard x-ray beams (high *LET*, reduced oxygen enhancement ratio or *OER*). Three different approaches are currently being attempted, 1) increasing pO_2 in all the cells of the tumor by allowing the patient to respire pure oxygen at normal or increased pressure, 2) decreasing pO_2 of all cells of tumor and the surrounding normal tissue to hypoxic levels and 3) using high *LET* and low *OER* radiations, *e.g.* fast neutrons, negative pions.

High Pressure Oxygen and Clinical Radiotherapy

The most extensively explored technique to reduce the oxygen tension differential between tumor cell and normal cell has been to place patients in special chambers and exposing them to 100 per cent oxygen at 3 or 4 atmospheres pressure absolute. When breathing air at one atmosphere of pressure, the oxygen tension of arterial blood is 100 mm Hg; 19 ml of oxygen per 100 ml of blood (0.25 ml of oxygen is simple solution in plasma) almost all of which is present as oxyhemoglobin. As 95 per cent of the hemoglobin is in the oxyhemoglobin form, any substantial increase in the oxygen content of blood would be as oxygen dissolved in the plasma. During respiration of 100 per cent O_2 at three atmospheres of pressure the pO_2 of arterial blood goes up to $\approx 2,200$ mm Hg; the total oxygen content increases to 26 ml per cent, 6 ml being in solution in the plasma.[7] This represents a highly significant increase because tissue oxygen needs are met by 5 ml per cent in plasma. This is confirmed by the observation that the pO_2 of venous

blood is ≈ 700 mm Hg or substantially higher than for normal arterial blood. The result is that oxygen tension of the various normal tissue is sharply increased.

Even under these special conditions, oxygen tension in all parts of a tumor may not be raised to aerobic levels. If the rate of blood flow through a capillary is slow or the capillary is longer than normal, as is often true for tumor vessels, then oxygen tension at the venous end of the capillary could be quite low and the adjacent tumor tissue hypoxic. This is illustrated in Figure 15-1. Despite these possible limitations, the use of oxygen under high pressure as an adjunct to radiation therapy has been attractive because the hypoxic regions are quire narrow (≤ 3 cells) and pO2 need be increased only up to 10 mm Hg for a near maximum effect.

Churchill-Davidson at St. Thomas Hospital of London[8,9] initiated clinical work with radiation therapy and hyperbaric oxygen. The encouraging results from his experience have stimulated a number of centers to con-

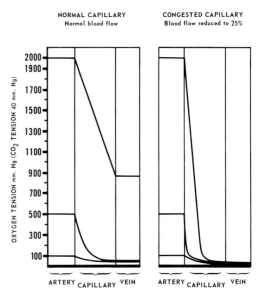

FIG. 15-1. Oxygen tension variation along capillary length as modified by capillary blood flow and pO$_2$ in arterial blood. (Courtesy: Churchill-Davidson, *Brit. J. Radiol.*, 30, 406, 1957.)

duct clinical trials of hyperbaric oxygen as a potentiator of radiation therapy. Data from those trials indicate that better results are obtained by hyperbaric oxygen and radiation therapy than radiation therapy alone, especially for treatment given in 4 to 10 treatments over a period of $\approx$3 weeks. These results come from studies of squamous cell carcinoma of the head and neck region[16,39] and of carcinomas of the urinary bladder.[39] When the radiation dose has been given in 27–40 fractions over 5 to 8 weeks in treatment of carcinoma of uterine cervix and urinary bladder there is only a weak suggestion of an improvement.[10,37] There are data from other centers; in general, they also indicate that local results are improved slightly by treating while the patient respires pure oxygen under increased pressure. A critical point is that although the available results provide evidence for an "oxygen effect" in clinical radiation therapy they, in fact, do not document a better clinical result than is achieved by well applied conventional radiation therapy.

Radiation Therapy Given Under Local Hypoxia

The most straight forward approach to elimination of differentials in oxygen tension between normal and tumor tissues would appear to be the reduction of oxygen tension to very low levels by occlusion of the arterial supply of the affected part. It is relatively simple to achieve severe hypoxia of an entire limb by applying a high pressure tourniquet to the proximal portion of the limb. A tourniquet left in place for a time sufficient for the tissues to metabolize all oxygen already present would result in severely hypoxic tissues. Polarographic studies on human muscle showed that a tourniquet time of 20 to 30 minutes is required to effect the severe reduction of muscle pO_2 required for this application to hypoxia to radiation therapy.[40]

In several institutions, sarcomas of the distal extremities have been irradiated under conditions of local tissue hypoxia produced by tourniquet application.[3,30,31,40] Suit and Lindberg have described 22 patients with osteosarcoma of distal extremities who were treated by ultra high dose radiation therapy under tourniquet induced hypoxia.[31] A central tumor dose of 1,000 rads (^{60}Co) was given on two successive days for each week of treatment. Total doses were 12,000 rads in 12 fractions in 36 days to 16,000 rads in 16 fractions over 50 days. The results are presented in Table 15-1.

As shown, the frequency of long term local control at 14,000 rads was low. Unfortunately, after 16,000 rads, normal tissue changes were so severe that the technique was judged ineffective as a clinical treatment procedure despite the high local control rate. Van den Brenk[38] also observed recurrences at doses which produced some severe local reactions. The failure to obtain a clinically acceptable result in treatment of osteosarcoma argues against the validity of the premise upon which this study was based.

Table 15-1. *Results of Radiation Therapy by Tourniquet Technique Osteosarcoma*

Dose (Rad/da.)	No. Patients Treated	Dead (12 mos. or less*)	Local Control (longer than 12 mos.)
12,000/36	11	8	1/3
14,000/43	5	1	1/4
16,000/50	6	3	3/3

*Distant metastasis but with local control.

Table 15-2. *Local Control Results in Treatment of Soft Tissue Sarcoma on the Distal Extremities*

Tourniquet Technique	Local Control >24 months
(12,000 rads/36 days 14,000 rads/43 days)*	30/30
Conventional Technique	
(6,300 rads/6 weeks 7,000 rads/7 weeks)	16/16

*There was one marginal recurrence in this group.

Another study of tourniquet technique radiation therapy is in progress using sarcomata of the soft tissues of the distal extremities. These lesions include liposarcoma, neurofibrosarcoma, rhabdomyosarcoma, and synovial sarcoma, etc.;[31] they are located in the elbow, forearm, wrist-hand, knee, leg or ankle regions. The patients were seen after local excision or at the time of a small recurrence. Amputation was the recommended surgical procedure in all patients. A total of 30 patients have been treated by the tourniquet technique at 12,000 rads to 14,000 rads. During this time, 16 patients with comparable lesions were assigned to treatment by conventional technique using doses of 6,300 rads to 7,000 rads in 6 to 7 weeks. Results are given in Table 15-2.

Local recurrence has not been observed in any of the tourniquet or in the control patients. The early and late reactions were approximately comparable in the two groups. Thus the clinical effectiveness of the two treatment methods is approximately the same for soft tissue sarcoma of the distal extremities.

High LET Radiation in Clinical Radiation Therapy

FAST NEURON: EXTERNAL BEAM THERAPY

Employment of high *LET* particles in clinical radiation therapy has been limited almost exclusively to neutron beams. A 6 Mev neutron beam has a depth dose distribution intermediate between that for 250 Kv x-rays and ^{60}Co. At 30 Mev, a neutron beam has a depth dose curve which is marginally superior to that of a ^{60}Co beam. For fast neutron therapy the *LET* would be high throughout the irradiated tissue.

In the period 1937 to 1942, a series of 250 patients with advanced malignant disease were treated by Stone[29] employing a fast neutron beam. The neutrons were produced by 8 to 16 Mev deuterons reacting with a beryllium target. Although local control of disease was achieved, late damage to normal tissues was judged excessive. A recent review of the experience of Stone with fast neutron radiotherapy has been published by Sheline et al. in 1971.[27] Apparently, the severe late reactions can be accepted as due to overdose, because of an error in using *RBE* data. Stone et al. estimated the *RBE* for their neutron beam by comparing response of human skin to *single* doses of x-rays or fast neutrons. They used the resultant *RBE* value to calculate the total neutron dose to be given in a number of small doses. However, it is *now* known that the *RBE* increases with dose fractionation. For example, the *RBE* is 2.5 for single dose and 3.3 for 6 dose irradiation of pig skin.[13] Therefore, the total dose effect was higher than intended.

Because of the severity of the late normal tissue reactions described by Stone, there had been no active interest in further clinical trials of high *LET* particles in clinical radiation therapy until the results of the neutron radiobiological studies became available. A clinical trial of radiation therapy utilizing 6 Mev neutrons is in progress at the Hammersmith Hospital, London.[6]

^{252}CALIFORNIUM

There is another source of neutrons of potential interest for radiation therapy: the radionuclide ^{252}Californium, which yields fission spectrum neutrons. At present small quantities of this material are being made available to radiation therapy departments to evaluate the relative efficacy of ^{252}Cf and radium as sources for interstitial and intracavitary therapy. Physical aspects and clinical prospects for this therapy mode have been reviewed.[1]

NEGATIVE PIONS

The negative pions carry a single negative charge and have a mass of 273 times that of an electron.

The special attraction of these particles results from the fact that at the end of the track length the pion is captured by an atomic nucleus which disintegrates producing energetic protons, alpha particles, neutrons, and other nuclear fragments, a recoil, *i.e.* a number of high *LET* reaction products. In this region of the track the *RBE* is high and the *OER* reduced. This contrasts with the superficial part of the track length where energy loss is low *LET* and correspondingly *RBE* and *OER* should be about the same as for standard photon therapy. Nearly pure beams of negative pions can be extracted so that particle or photon contamination is not a problem. By careful planning of the distribution of pion energies within the beam, the high *LET* region of the depth dose curve can be widened so that it is feasible to treat large volumes of tissue with the high *RBE*-low *OER* part of the beam.[4] Dose distribution patterns can be made to approximate so closely any desired distribution that a limitation in utilizing these beams probably will be the lack of precise knowledge of location and configuration of the tumor. The potential value of the pion beam over a good fast neutron beam lies in the better dose distribution patterns; *OER* is approximately the same for the two radiations.

A basic question in radiation therapy is: how much improvement in results can be expected by further refinements in dose distribution patterns? In many anatomical sites, radiation necrosis develops at the site of the primary tumor (*e.g.* bladder, upper respiratory and digestive tracts, breast), and accord-

ingly clinical results are not likely to be improved greatly due to a better dose distribution. For other sites, complications develop because gross radiation damage appears in tissues which were irradiated incidentally, *e.g.* the eye, spinal cord, etc. In those cases, pion therapy should offer a clinically important advantage over fast neutron beams which have approximately the same *OER*. Proton beams have been employed so as to utilize the high *LET* Bragg Peak[22] and also for the low *LET* region because of an improved dose distribution.[24,36]

Radiation Dose Fractionation Schedules

Another area of interest is the optimization of dose fractionation schedule. The radiation therapist can vary 3 parameters in selecting the fractionation schedule: number of fractions (ν), time between fractions (t_i) and dose rate. Four biological processes occur during each intertreatment interval; these determine radiation dose required to elicit a specified response. These are: repair, redistribution, repopulation, and reoxygenation. It is essentially certain that there are quantitative differences between tumor and normal tissues in one or more of these processes. This means that the standard dose fractionation schedule of 180–200 rads per day for 5 treatments per week is not optimal for essentially all tumor-normal tissue situations. Because of the rate of advance in research in tissue biology and radiobiology, a reasonable expectation is that more effective treatment schedules will be developed for selected tumor-normal tissue situations. For example, on the basis of existing knowledge one might expect that a higher fractionation number might be an advantage in treatment of extensive lymphoma in the abdomen (intestinal crypt cells have high N while the lymphoma cells probably have a small N) or the intertreatment interval might be reduced from the standard 24 hours to 4 to 8 hours in therapy of a fast growing rhabdomyosarcoma in the thigh (tumor cells would be rapidly proliferating while cells of most of the normal tissues would be essentially non-proliferating).

Available clinical data indicate that some fractionation is better than single dose treatment. At present, the scientific basis for preferring one fractionation schedule over another has been poorly developed. Pertinent to this is the fact that one multi-institution study found that 3 fractions per week were as effective as 5 fractions per week in treating carcinomas of the larynx and pharynx (appropriate adjustments of total dose were made).[12] This is interesting, but unfortunately there was no gain in therapeutic results. There are also numerous reports available describing the results of split course therapy (daily treatments for 2 to 3 weeks, a 1 to 3 week rest period, and a final 2 to 3 weeks of treatment). Current results do not indicate superiority for the split course.[25]

Radiation Sensitizing Compounds and Chemotherapeutic Agents Combined with Radiation Therapy

HALOGENATED ANALOGS OF THYMIDINE AND CYTODINE

There are several halogenated analogs of thymidine and cytodine which are powerful radiosensitizers of bacterial and mammalian cells.[11,18,20,26] For sensitization these analogs must be incorporated into *DNA* during the *S* period (time that *DNA* of a cell is replicated). Cells which have only been in G_2 to G_1 phases of the cell cycle when the agent was present show no change in radiosensitivity (D_{37} or N). Analogs of thymidine which are effective sensitizers are 5-bromo-, ido-, or chlorodeoxyuridine (BUdR, IUdR, and ClUdR) but not 5-fluorodeoxyuridine. The latter is not incorporated into *DNA* and does not sensitize. Also bromodeoxycytidine is a potent radiation sensitizer. Magnitude of sensitization is related to extent of thymine or replacement by the analog. These analogs

reduce D_{37} by a factor of 1.5 to 1.7 at drug concentration which do not have demonstrable toxic effects on cells.[26] At higher and toxic drug doses the D_{37} may be reduced by a factor $\simeq 2.5$ and the N may be reduced also. The increased sensitivity of these cells is seen for radiation given under aerobic or under hypoxic conditions.[18,21]

Unfortunately these compounds have only limited stability when injected into an animal. BUdR is rapidly degraded as it passes through the liver.[23] Therefore, clinical use of this compound requires intra-arterial infusion over relatively prolonged periods.

Recently there have been reports which describe sensitization of tumor cells *in vivo* by intraperitoneal injection of IUdR and intra-arterial infusion of BUdR of BrCdR.[5,14,32]

Only limited clinical trials of the efficacy of any of this group sensitizing compounds have been reported. Greatest effect would be expected in tumors composed of rapidly dividing cells but growing in normal tissue whose cells were dividing slowly, *e.g.* muscle, connective tissue, brain. This would enable a large differential in sensitization of tumor and normal cells. Correspondingly, a decreased clinical effectiveness of such a treatment would be expected if the tumor cells divided slowly but were surrounded by normal tissue composed of rapidly dividing cells, *e.g.* bone marrow, gut.

Bagshaw et al. have described results of a trial of intra-arterial infusion of BUdR and radiation therapy based upon head and neck lesions.[2] Although there was enhanced response of the tumor, the net clinical results were less than hoped because of increased reaction of mucous membrane. Hoshino et al.[17] selected malignant glioma for their trial; preliminary results indicate that mean survival time is sharply prolonged.

Chemotherapeutic Agents

5-FLUOROURACIL

This agent is not a radiation sensitizer, but it is an effective chemotherapeutic agent.

Biochemically 5-FU acts to block the action of the enzyme thymidilic synthetase and does prevent cells from entering the *S* or *DNA* synthetic period of the cell cycle. It has other metabolic effects and is incorporated to some extent in the *RNA* molecule. Cells at all phases of the cycle are inactivated by 5-FU.

Five-Fluorouracil has been administered intra-arterially as an adjunct to radiation therapy in the treatment of patients with advanced lesions of the head and neck region and of the uterine cervix and apparently resulted in improved local control and survival rates.[19,28]

In the clinical trial by Vermund et al.,[41] there was evidence of prolongation of survival time of patients with squamous cell carcinomas at several anatomical sites within the head and neck region and bronchogenic carcinoma, who were treated by systemic 5-FU and external irradiation instead of radiation therapy alone.

Another role for utilization of a chemotherapeutic agent and radiation therapy is administration of the former with the intent of inactivation in micro metastases, while the radiation therapy is expected to sterilize the primary tumor. The combination of radiation therapy, surgery and chemotherapy (Actinomycin D) has apparently been operating in this manner in the very successful treatment of patients with Wilms' tumor. Similarly, there is evidence that Actinomycin D, vincristine and cytoxan given concomitantly with radiation therapy for rhabdomyosarcoma of head and neck region of children also yields greatly improved results over radiation therapy alone.[34] Also, patients with Ewing's sarcoma treated by cytoxan-vincristine and radiation therapy experience improved survival as compared with similar patients treated only by radiation therapy.[33]

BIBLIOGRAPHY

1. Atkins, H. L.: The medical use of Californium-252. USAEC Report BNL-12919, Brookhaven National Laboratory, Upton, New York, 1968.

2. Bagshaw, M. S., and Doggett, R. L. S.: A clinical study of chemical radiosensitization, in *Frontiers of Radiation Therapy and Oncology,* Vol. 4, Basel/New York, S. Karger, 1969, pp. 164–173.

3. Balmuhanov, S. B., Gordienko, G. P., Pozdnuhov, L. G., Dosaev, A. K., Kauasev, S. K., Eselbaeva, G. O., Ahtjamov, M. D., and Ectjutina, O. A.: *Radiation Therapy of the Extremities Tumors Under Soncitions of Local Anoxia,* Voprosi Onkologll, Vol. 14, No. 8, 1968, pp. 29–36.

4. Bond, V. P.: Negative pions: Their possible use in radiotherapy, *Amer. J. Roentgen.,* 111, 9, 1971.

5. Brown, J. M., Goffinet, D. R., Cleave, J. E., and Kallman, R. F.: Preferential radiosensitization of mouse sarcoma relative to normal skin by chronic intra-arterial infusion of halogenated pyrimidine analogs. In Preparation.

6. Catterall, M.: Clinical experience with fast neutrons from the medical research council's cyclotron at Hammersmith Hospital, *Europ. J. of Cancer,* 7, 227, 1971.

7. Churchill-Davidson, I.: In *Cancer Progress,* R. Raven, editor, London, Butterworths and Co, Ltd., p. 164, 1960.

8. Churchill-Davidson, I., Sanger, C., and Thomlinson, R. H.: Oxygenation in radiotherapy, II. Clinical application, *Brit. J. Radiol.,* 30, 406, 1957.

9. Churchill-Davidson, I., Chir, B., Foster, C. A., Wiernick, G., Collins, C. D., Pizey, N. C. D., Skeggs, D. B. L., and Purser, P. R.: The place of oxygen in radiotherapy, *Brit. J. Radiol.,* 39, 391, 1966.

10. Dische, S.: Report presentation to Medical Research Council of Britain, September 1970.

11. Djordjevic, B., and Szybalski, W.: Genetics of human cell lines, III. Incorporation of 5-bromo- and 5-iodeoxyuridine into deoxyriboneucleic acid of human cells and its effect of radiation sensitivity, *J. Exper. Med.,* 112, 509, 1960.

12. Ellis, F.: Interim progress report (1969) on the British Institute of Radiology fractionation study on 3-fractions/week or 5 fractions/week treatment of larynx and pharynx. In *Time and Dose Relationships in Radiation Biology as Applied to Radiotherapy,* New York,

Brookhaven National Laboratory report BNL 50203 (C-57), 1969.

13. Fowler, J. F., Morgan, R. L., Silversten, J. A., Bewley, D. K., and Turner, B. A.: Experiments with fractionated x-ray treatment of skin of pigs, *Brit. J. Radiol.,* 36, 188, 1963.

14. Goffinet, D. R., Brown, J. M., Bagshaw, M. A., Kaplan, H. S.: Prolonged carotid arterial radiosensitizer infusion and radiation therapy of mouse gliomas, submitted to Amer. Radium Soc. Meeting, Mexico City, March 1971.

15. Gray, L. H., Conger, A. D., Ebert, M., Hornsey, S., and Scott, O. C. A.: The concentration of oxygen dissolved in tissues at the time of irradiation as a factor in radiotherapy, *Brit. J. Radiol.,* 26, 638, 1953.

16. Henk, J. M., Kunkler, P. B., Shah, N. K., Smith, C. W., Sutherland, W. H., Wassif, S. B.: Hyperbaric oxygen in radiotherapy of head and neck carcinoma, *Clin. Radiol.,* 21, 223, 1970.

17. Hoshino, T., and Sano, K.: Radiosensitization of malignant brain tumors with bromouridine (thymidine analogue), *Acta Radiol.,* 8, 15, 1969.

18. Humphrey, R. M., Dewey, W. C., and Cork, A.: Effect of oxygen in mammalian cells sensitized to radiation by incorporation of 5-bromodeoxyuridine into the DNA, *Nature,* 198, 268, 1963.

19. Jesse, R. H., Goepfert, H., Lindberg, R. D., and Johnson, R. H.: Combined intra-arterial infusion and radiotherapy for the treatment of advanced cancer of the head and neck, *Amer. J. Roentgen,* 105, 20, 1969.

20. Kaplan, H. S., Smith, K. C., and Tomlin, P.: Radiosensitization of *E coli* by purine and pyrimidine analogues incorporated in deoxyribonucleic acid, *Nature,* 190, 794, 1961.

21. Kaplan, H. S., Zavarine, R., and Earle, J.: Interaction of the oxygen effect and radiosensitization produced by base analogues incorporated into deoxyribonucleic acid, *Nature,* 194, 662, 1962.

22. Kjellberg, R. N., Shintani, A., and Frantz, A.: Proton-beam therapy in acromegaly, *NEJ Med.,* 278, 689, 1968.

23. Kriss, J. P., and Revesz, L.: The distribution and fate of bromodeoxyuridine and bromodeoxycytodine in the mouse and rat, *Cancer Res.,* 22, 254, 1962.

24. Larson, B., Leksell, L., and Rexed, B.: The use of high energy protons for cerebral surgery in man, *Acta Chir. Scand.,* 125, 1, 1963.

25. Marcial, V. A.: Studies on the relationships between dose-time fractionation, and rest period in radiation therapy, In *Time and Dose Relationships in Radiation Biology as Applied to Radiotherapy,* New York, Brookhaven National Laboratory report BNL 50203 (C-57), 1969.

26. Mohler, W. C., and Elkind, M.: Radiation response to mammalian cell grown in culture, *Exp. Cell Res.,* 30, 481, 1963.

27. Sheline, G. E., Phillips, T. L., Field, S. B., Breenan, J. T., and Raventos, A.: Effects of fast neutrons on human skin, *Amer. J. Roentgen.,* 111, 31, 1971.

28. Smith, J. P., Kandall, G. E., Rutledge, F., Lindberg, R. D., Castro, J. R., and Fletcher, G. H.: Hypogastric artery infusion and radiation therapy for advanced squamous cell carcinoma of the cervix, *Amer. J. Roentgen.,* 114, 110, 1972.

29. Stone, R. S.: Neutron therapy and specific ionization, *Amer. J. Roentgen.,* 59, 771, 1948.

30. Suit, H. D.: In *Tumors of Bone and Soft Tissue,* Chicago, Year Book Medical Pub., Inc., 1965, p. 143.

31. Suit, H. D., and Lindberg, R. D.: Radiation therapy administered under conditions of tourniquet-induced local tissue hypoxia, *Amer. J. Roentgen.,* 102, 27, 1968.

32. Suit, H. D., Hewitt, R., and Urano, M.: Effect of radiation-sensitizing agents in radiation therapy of mouse mammary carcinoma, *Radiology,* 94, 189, 1970.

33. Suit, H. D., Martin, R. G., and Sutow, W. W.: Radiation therapy for primary sarcoma of the bone in children, In *Clinical Pediatric Oncology* (In preparation).

34. Sutow, W. W.: Personal communication, 1970.

35. Thomlinson, R. H., and Gray, L. H.: The histological structure of some human lung cancers and possible implications for radiotherapy, *Brit. J. Cancer,* 9, 539, 1955.

36. Tobias, C. A., Lawrence, J. H., Born, J. L., McCombs, R. K., Roberts, J. E., Anger, H. O., Lowbeer, B. V. A., and Huggens, C. G.: Pituitary irradiation with high energy proton beam, a preliminary report, *Cancer Res.,* 18, 121, 1958.

37. Tobin, D. A., and Vermund, H.: A random-ized study of hyperbaric oxygen as adjunct to regularly fractionated radiation therapy as clinical treatment of advanced neoplastic dis-ease. (In preparation).

38. Van den Brenk, H. A. S.: The tourniquet technique in radiotherapy of limb tumors, *Nuntius Radiologicers*, 34, 207, 1968.

39. Van den Brenk, H. A. S.: Hyperbaric oxygen in radiation therapy. An investigation of dose-effect relationships in tumor response and tissue damage, *Brit. J. Radiol.*, 102, 8, 1968.

40. Van den Brenk, H. A. S., Madigan, J. P., Kerr, R. C., Cass, N. M., and Richter, W.: The treatment of malignant disease of the ex-tremities by megavoltage irradiation under tourniquet anoxia, *J. Coll. Radiol.*, *Aust*, 7, 142, 1963.

41. Vermund, H., Gollin, E. F., Ansfield, F. J.: Clinical studies of 5-Fluorouracil as adjuvant to radiotherapy, In *Frontiers of Radiation Therapy and Oncology*, 4, 132, 1969.

Index